W9-BLM-597

DISORDERS OF THROMBOSIS AND HEMOSTASIS

CLINICAL AND LABORATORY PRACTICE

THIRD EDITION

DISORDERS OF THROMBOSIS AND HEMOSTASIS

CLINICAL AND LABORATORY PRACTICE

THIRD EDITION

Editor

RODGER L. BICK, M.D., PH.D., F.A.C.P.

Clinical Professor of Medicine and Pathology
University of Texas Southwestern Medical School
Director: Dallas Thrombosis/Hemostasis Clinical Center
Director: ThromboCare Laboratories
Dallas, Texas

LIPPINCOTT WILLIAMS & WILKINS
A **Wolters Kluwer** Company
Philadelphia • Baltimore • New York • London
Buenos Aires • Hong Kong • Sydney • Tokyo

Acquisitions Editor: Ruth W. Weinberg
Developmental Editor: Brigitte P. Wilke
Production Editor: Jonathan Geffner
Manufacturing Manager: Colin Warnock
Cover Designer: Patricia Gast
Compositor: Lippincott Williams & Wilkins Desktop Division
Printer: Maple Press

© 2002 by LIPPINCOTT WILLIAMS & WILKINS
530 Walnut Street
Philadelphia, PA 19106 USA
LWW.com

All rights reserved. This book is protected by copyright. No part of this book may be reproduced in any form or by any means, including photocopying, or utilized by any information storage and retrieval system without written permission from the copyright owner, except for brief quotations embodied in critical articles and reviews. Materials appearing in this book prepared by individuals as part of their official duties as U.S. government employees are not covered by the above-mentioned copyright.

Printed in the USA

Library of Congress Cataloging-in-Publication Data
Bick, Rodger L.
Disorders of thrombosis and hemostasis : clinical and laboratory practice / Rodger L. Bick. — 3rd ed.
p. ; cm.
Includes bibliographical references and index.
ISBN 0-397-51690-8
1. Blood coagulation disorders. 2. Hemostasis. 3. Thrombosis. I. Title.
[DNLM: 1. Blood Coagulation Disorders. 2. Hemostasis. 3. Thrombosis. WH 322 B583db 2002]
RC647.C55 B54 2002
616.1'57—dc21

2002016168

Care has been taken to confirm the accuracy of the information presented and to describe generally accepted practices. However, the authors, editor, and publisher are not responsible for errors or omissions or for any consequences from application of the information in this book and make no warranty, expressed or implied, with respect to the currency, completeness, or accuracy of the contents of the publication. Application of this information in a particular situation remains the professional responsibility of the practitioner.

The authors, editor, and publisher have exerted every effort to ensure that drug selection and dosage set forth in this text are in accordance with current recommendations and practice at the time of publication. However, in view of ongoing research, changes in government regulations, and the constant flow of information relating to drug therapy and drug reactions, the reader is urged to check the package insert for each drug for any change in indications and dosage and for added warnings and precautions. This is particularly important when the recommended agent is a new or infrequently employed drug.

Some drugs and medical devices presented in this publication have Food and Drug Administration (FDA) clearance for limited use in restricted research settings. It is the responsibility of the health care provider to ascertain the FDA status of each drug or device planned for use in their clinical practice.

10 9 8 7 6 5 4 3 2 1

To the memory of my wife, Marcy Ann Bick,
and to my two daughters, Shauna Nicole Bick and Michelle Leanne Bick

CONTENTS

Contributing Authors ix

Preface xi

Acknowledgments xiii

1. Physiology of Hemostasis 1
Rodger L. Bick and Genesio Murano

2. Clinical Assessment of Patients with Hemorrhage 31
Rodger L. Bick

3. Hereditary and Acquired Vascular Thrombohemorrhagic Disorders 39
Rodger L. Bick

4. Platelet-Function Defects 59
Rodger L. Bick

5. Thrombocytopenia and Thrombocytosis 91
Eugene P. Frenkel

6. Hereditary Coagulation Protein Defects 117
Frank A. Nizzi, Jr., Suneeti Sapatnekar, and Rodger L. Bick

7. Disseminated Intravascular Coagulation 139
Rodger L. Bick

8. Thrombohemorrhagic Defects in Liver and Renal Diseases 165
Eberhard F. Mammen

9. Thrombotic and Hemorrhagic Problems During Cardiovascular Bypass Surgery and Cardiovascular Procedures 177
Rodger L. Bick

10. Acquired Blood Coagulation Inhibitors 213
Yale S. Arkel and De-Hui W. Ku

11. Clinical Approach to the Patient with Thrombosis, Thromboembolus, and Pulmonary Embolus 251
Rodger L. Bick and William F. Baker, Jr.

12. Thrombohemorrhagic Defects Associated with Malignancy 265
Eugene P. Frenkel and Rodger L. Bick

13. Hereditary Thrombophilic Disorders 283
Rodger L. Bick and William F. Baker, Jr.

14. Acquired Thrombophilia 303
Rodger L. Bick and William F. Baker, Jr.

15. Thromboprophylaxis and Thrombosis in Medical, Surgical, Trauma, and Obstetric/Gynecologic Patients 325
Rodger L. Bick and Sylvia K. Haas

16. Oral Antithrombotic Therapy: Warfarins and Related Compounds 349
Graham F. Pineo and Russell D. Hull

17. Heparin and Low-Molecular-Weight Heparins 359
Rodger L. Bick

18. Antiplatelet Therapy 379
Hans Klaus Breddin

19. Thrombolytic Therapy 397
William F. Baker, Jr.

20. Hemostatic Factors in Atherothrombotic Disease 421
Yale S. Arkel and De-Hui W. Ku

Subject Index 435

CONTRIBUTING AUTHORS

Yale S. Arkel, M.D. Research Professor, Department of Obstetrics/Gynecology, Maternal/Fetal Medicine, New York University School of Medicine, New York, New York

William F. Baker, Jr., M.D. Associate Clinical Professor, Department of Medicine, Center for Health Sciences, University of California–Los Angeles, Los Angeles, California; Director: Thrombosis, Hemostasis, and Special Hematology, Department of Medicine, Kern Medical Center, Bakersfield, California; and California Clinical Thrombosis Center, Bakersfield, California

Rodger L. Bick, M.D., Ph.D. Clinical Professor of Medicine and Pathology, University of Texas Southwestern Medical Center; Director: Dallas Thrombosis/Hemostasis Clinical Center; Director: ThromboCare Laboratories, 10455 North Central Expressway, Suite 109, PMB 320, Dallas, Texas 75231, rbick@thrombosis.com

Hans Klaus Breddin, Prof. Dr. med, Dr. h.c. International Institute of Thrombosis and Vascular Disease, Frankfurt/Main, Germany

Eugene P. Frenkel, M.D. Professor, Departments of Medicine and Radiology, University of Texas Southwestern Medical School; Faculty Attending Physician, Simmons Cancer Center, Zale–Lipshy University Hospital, Dallas, Texas

Sylvia K. Haas, M.D. Professor, Department of Medicine, Insitut fur Experimentelle Onkologie und Therapieforschung, Technische Universität München, Munich, Germany

Russell D. Hull, M.B.B.S., M.Sc. Professor, Department of Medicine, University of Calgary; Active Staff, Department of Medicine–Hemotology, Foothills Hospital, Calgary, Alberta, Canada

De-Hui W. Ku, Ph.D. Research Assistant Professor, Department of Obstetrics/Gynecology, New York University Medical Center, New York, New York

Eberhard F. Mammen, M.D. Professor Emeritus, Department of Obstetrics/Gynecology, Wayne State University School of Medicine, C.S. Mott Center, Detroit, Michigan

Genesio Murano, Ph.D. Genentech, Inc., South San Francisco, California

Frank A. Nizzi, Jr., D.O. Assistant Professor, Department of Pathology, University of Texas Southwestern Medical Center, Dallas, Texas; Medical Director of Clinical Services, Department of Medical Services, Carter BloodCare, Bedford, Texas

Graham F. Pineo, M.D. Professor, Department of Medicine, University of Calgary; Active Staff, Department of Medicine–Hemotology, Foothills Hospital, Calgary, Alberta, Canada

Suneeti Sapatnekar, M.D., Ph.D. Medical Director, American Red Cross Blood Services, Northern Ohio Region, Cleveland, Ohio

PREFACE

Disorders of thrombosis and hemostasis are common to all medical specialties. Thrombosis is the single most common cause of death in adults in the United States, with four times as many deaths resulting from thrombosis as from cancer annually. In addition, almost six times as many cases of thrombosis as of cancer are diagnosed each year. Thus, disorders of thrombosis and hemostasis constitute major health problems from the standpoints of morbidity, mortality, and healthcare costs.

This textbook, unlike other texts on thrombosis and hemostasis, focuses on the practical aspects of diagnosing and managing thrombosis and hemorrhage. In all instances the etiology, pathophysiology, and clinical and laboratory diagnosis and management are discussed. Basic research, basic physiology, and animal data not yet pertinent to clinical practice are kept to a minimum.

This text is written for the clinician and laboratory scientist who face the multidisciplinary problems relating to the straightforward diagnosis and management of the disorders of thrombosis and hemostasis. Thus, in addition to the pathologist and laboratory technologist, it will be of interest as a guide for a wide variety of medical specialists in the areas of internal medicine, hematology, oncology, cardiology, neurology, obstetrics and gynecology, pediatrics, family practice, and general, vascular, orthopedic, and cardiovascular surgery.

The goal of this text is to address the disorders of thrombosis and hemostasis in a logical, sequential, and practical manner so that those using it will find it of benefit in rendering outstanding medical care to patients with these potentially devastating disorders.

Rodger L. Bick, M.D., Ph.D.
Dallas, Texas

ACKNOWLEDGMENTS

The editor thanks the experts for contributing their experience and knowledge to chapters of this text, as well as Brigitte Wilke at Lippincott Williams & Wilkins for her tireless and extraordinary medical editing.

1

PHYSIOLOGY OF HEMOSTASIS

RODGER L. BICK
GENESIO MURANO

An understanding of basic physiology of hemostasis is important for multiple reasons. Understanding physiology allows one an ability to interpret new laboratory testing modalities, to comprehend the enormously complex nature of most thrombohemorrhagic disease processes, and to understand many new novel targeted pharmacologic agents now being used or assessed for the treatment of thrombotic and hemorrhagic disorders.

The hemostasis system comprises three equally important anatomic compartments, the vasculature, the platelets, and the blood-coagulation proteins; these are depicted in Fig. 1.1 (1,2). These three compartments are very elaborately interrelated and indeed interact with many other physiologic elements, including cytokines, adhesion molecules, neutrophils, lymphocytes, monocytes, and others (1,2), all discussed in this chapter. Disturbances of these delicately balanced interrelations may lead to serious clinical thrombotic and or hemorrhagic consequences (1–4).

VASCULAR FUNCTION

Normal vascular morphology comprises three discrete layers: the intima, the media, and the adventitia (5–7). The intima consists of a monolayer of nonthrombogenic endothelial cells and an internal elastic membrane. The media consists of smooth muscle cells; the size of the media will vary depending on the type (arterial/venous) and size of the vasculature. The adventitia comprises an external elastic lamina or membrane and supportive connective tissue.

Permeability, fragility, and vasoconstriction are properties of the vasculature (1) and are summarized in Table 1.1. Vascular permeability, if increased, results in blood leaving the vessel and is apparent as petechiae and purpura or, in some instances, large ecchymoses. If increased vascular fragility occurs, there can be rupture of the vasculature with ensuing petechiae and purpura, especially in the integument and mucous membranes, large ecchymoses, and potential serious deep-tissue hemorrhage. If vasoconstriction is inappropriately intense, there may be partial or complete occlusion of the vessel, ischemia, and eventual thrombus formation (1,2). Vasoconstriction is under local, neural, and humoral control (1,2). Most important of these is humoral control; as noted in Table 1.1, those compounds that mediate humoral control of vasoconstriction are primarily compounds released from platelets including epinephrine, norepinephrine, adenosine diphosphate (ADP), kinins, and thromboxanes (1–4,8–10). Fibrin(ogen) degradation products (FDPs) liberated when the fibrinolytic system acts on a fibrin clot also modulate vasoconstriction (1,2).

Properties of the endothelium are summarized in Table 1.2, as are basic properties of the subendothelium. Platelet attraction and subsequent activation occur when basement membrane or collagen is exposed. The known mechanisms are depicted in this table. It also should be noted that subendothelial collagen may directly activate factor XII to factor XIIa, as well as factor XI to factor XIa (1–4,11,12). Any of these activation processes, if left unmodulated, may give rise to a local or systemic activation of the hemostatic system (1–4,13). Endothelial cells are contractile and contract when stimulated by histamine, serotonin, kinins, thrombin, or thromboxanes (1). The endothelial cell is the major site of synthesis for von Willebrand factor (ristocetin cofactor) (14,15), tissue plasminogen activator (t-PA), plasminogen activator inhibitor type 1 (PAI-1) (1–4,16–19), tissue factor pathway inhibitor (TFPI), tissue factor, prostacyclins, and protein C activator and inhibitor activity (20). Weibel–Palade bodies are unique to endothelial cells and are thought to be derived from Golgi bodies (21). These are the sites of von Willebrand factor and von Willebrand antigen; P-selectin also is found in and released by Weibel–Palade bodies (22,23). Interleukin-1 (IL-1), endotoxin, mechanical injury, and complement components induce release of the contents of Weibel–Palade bodies, whereas release, and possibly synthesis, is inhibited by

R. L. Bick: Departments of Medicine and Pathology, University of Texas Southwestern Medical Center; Dallas Thrombosis/Hemostasis Clinical Center; ThromboCare Laboratories, Dallas, Texas.

G. Murano: Genentech, South San Francisco, California.

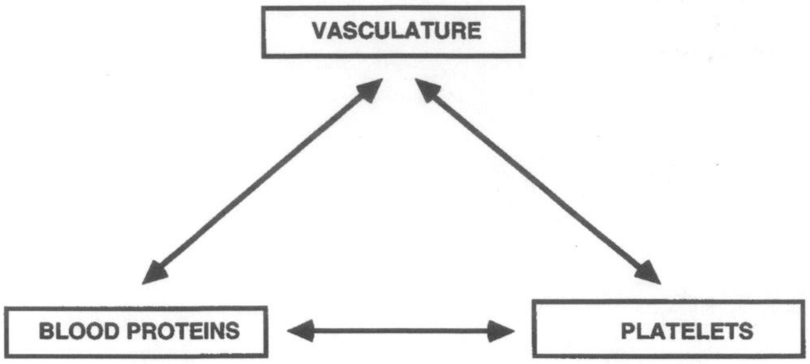

FIGURE 1.1. The three hemostatic compartments.

TABLE 1.2. PROPERTIES OF THE ENDOTHELIUM AND SUBENDOTHELIUM

Endothelium	
	Contraction by histamine, kinins, 5-HT, and thromboxanes
	Synthesis of plasminogen activator activity
	Synthesis of VIII:vW factor
	Synthesis of protein C inhibitor
Subendothelium	
	Platelet activation and attraction
	Factor XII activation
	Factor XI activation

5-HT, serotonin.

tumor necrosis factor (TNF) and interferon-γ (24,25). Endothelial cells constantly secrete nitrous oxide (NO), which relaxes smooth muscle cells and dilates the vessel, thus assuring vascular patency; when the endothelium is damaged, as by thrombin, TNF, and IL-1, or other substances, endothelin-1 and other compounds are secreted (26,27). This induces vasoconstriction; endothelin-1, when released into the circulation by endothelial cells, acts as a chemoattractant and recruits leukocytes and platelets. Endothelin-1, along with thrombin, also induces endothelial expression of various adhesion molecules, including integrins and selectins, which facilitate cellular and platelet adhesion (28). The endothelium also contains numerous vascular proteoglycans, including heparan sulfate, chondroitin sulfate, dermatan sulfate, and thrombomodulin (1). All of these proteoglycans may, to some degree, interact with antithrombin to accelerate inhibition of generated serine proteases. Thrombomodulin is an endothelium-bound proteoglycan with a molecular weight of about 60,000 that acts as a thrombin receptor (29). The role of thrombomodulin is to redirect the procoagulant activity of thrombin such that thrombomodulin-bound thrombin loses ability to convert fibrinogen to fibrin, to activate platelets, and to activate factor XIII; thrombomodulin-bound thrombin activates protein C to activated protein C (protein Ca), thus generating anticoagulant activity (30). Thrombomodulin, like other vascular proteoglycans, also may accelerate the activity of antithrombin for inhibition of generated serine proteases (31). The role of endothelial cell prostaglandin synthesis is discussed in subsequent sections.

TABLE 1.1. VASCULAR FUNCTION

Permeability → Leakage
Fragility → Rupture
Constriction → Occlusion
Neural control (sympathetic system)
Local control (temperature, pH, Pco_2)
Humoral control (Epi, NorEpi, ADP, kinins, FDP)

Epi, epinephrine; NorEpi, norepinephrine; ADP, adenosine diphosphate; FDP, fibrin degradation product.

Figure 1.2 depicts an important pathophysiologic event: endothelial sloughing. This may be induced by a wide variety of insults (triggers) including acidosis, hypoxia, endotoxin, circulating antigen–antibody complexes, and many others (1–4,32,33). Figure 1.3 depicts the first event occurring when endothelial sloughing occurs, with the subsequent exposure of subendothelial collagen and basement membrane. Platelets are immediately recruited to "fill" this endothelial gap (1,34). Subendothelial collagen and/or subendothelial basement membrane recruit platelets with the goal of forming a primary hemostatic plug, thereby stopping blood from leaving the vascular compartment (1). As the primary hemostatic plug is formed, subsequent reparative events ensue as follows: smooth muscle or other cells from the media differentiate, migrate through the internal elastic membrane, and then differentiate into new nonthrombogenic endothelial cells (1,2). If this is a one-time event, then a normal healing process is completed. It

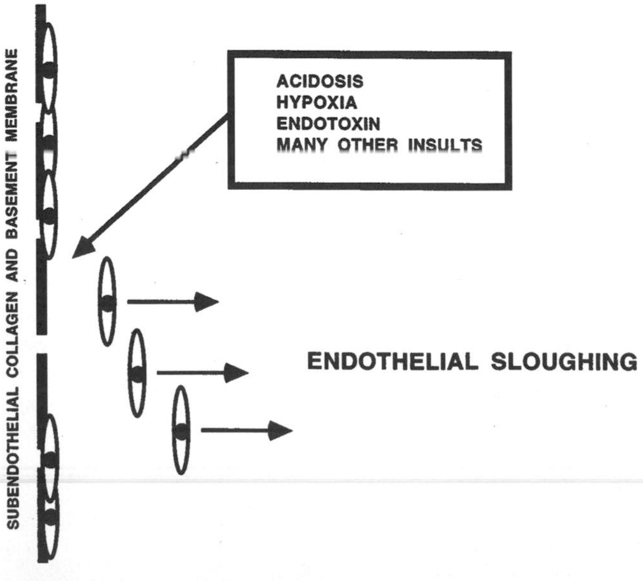

FIGURE 1.2. Endothelial sloughing and exposure of blood to subendothelial collagen/basement membrane.

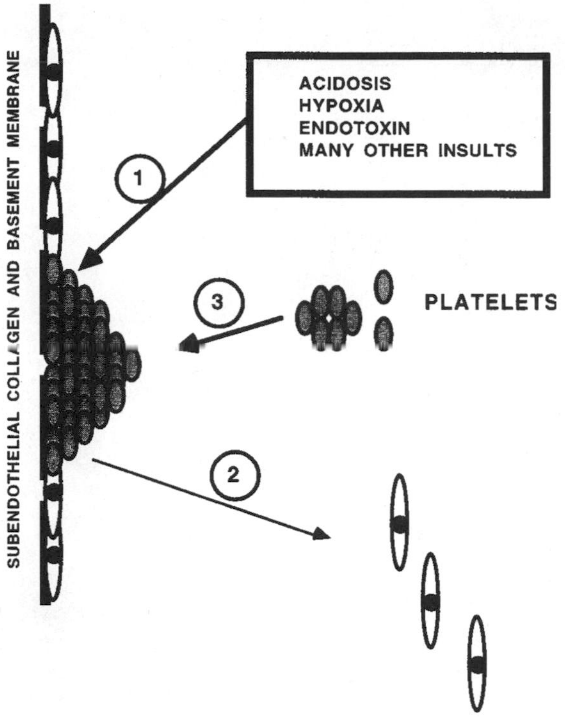

FIGURE 1.3. Platelets filling endothelial gaps.

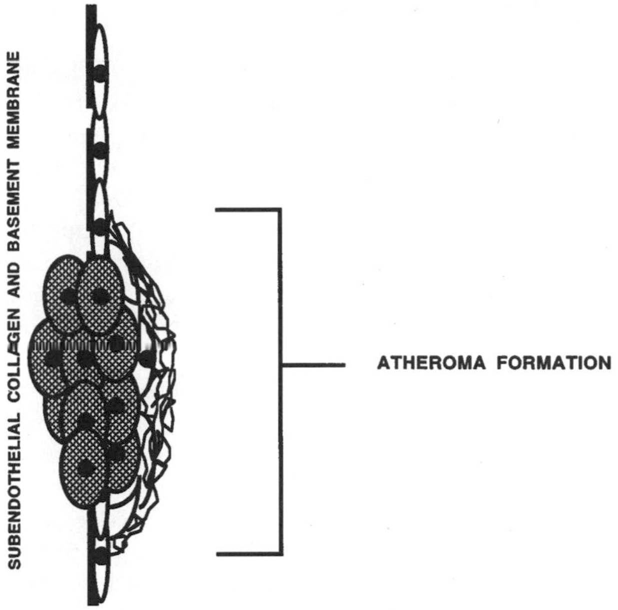

FIGURE 1.4. Endothelial sloughing and atheroma formation.

should be noted, however, that forming the primary hemostatic plug may be an overwhelming event, leading to a large platelet/fibrin thrombus, and impedance of blood flow with resultant end-organ damage through ischemia. Figure 1.4 depicts another event that may occur with endothelial sloughing and damage: atherosclerotic plaque formation (1–4,35–37). If this occurs repeatedly in the same area over a protracted period, then as smooth muscle or other cells differentiate and migrate into the intima, compounds are released that attract macrophages, which then ingest cholesterol and other materials, and an atherosclerotic plaque will eventually develop (1–4). All of these potential events are summarized in Fig. 1.5.

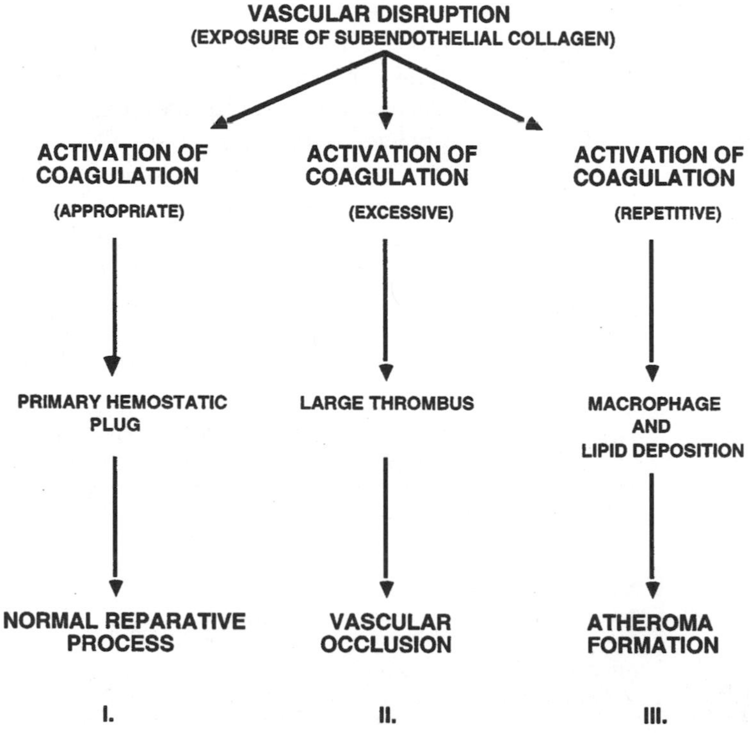

FIGURE 1.5. Vascular damage and consequences (endothelial cell sloughing).

PLATELET FUNCTION

Table 1.3 depicts normal platelet morphology. This morphologic division, although somewhat artificial, facilitates our understanding of relevant biology. In general, the platelet can be envisioned as being composed of three primary zones: (a) a peripheral zone, (b) a sol–gel zone, and (c) an organelle zone (38). The peripheral zone is composed of an extramembranous glycocalyx inside of which is a plasma membrane, similar to any other trilamellar cellular plasma membrane. Under the plasma membrane is an open canalicular system. The sol–gel zone is comprises microtubules and microfilaments, a dense tubular system that contains primarily adenine nucleotides and calcium. In addition, in the sol–gel zone is found the all-important contractile protein, thrombosthenin. Thrombosthenin is similar to actomyosin. The organelle zone comprises dense bodies, α granules, mitochondria, and the usual array of organelles found in other cellular systems, including lysosomes and endoplasmic reticulum. The α granules contain and release fibrinogen, platelet-derived growth factor (PDGF), and lysosomal enzymes, whereas dense bodies contain and release adenine nucleotides, serotonin, catecholamines, and platelet factor 4 (1–4,39–41).

Figure 1.6 depicts a transmission electron micrograph of a platelet, demonstrating many of these constituents and organelles. The open canalicular system, dense bodies, mitochondria, and lysosomes are apparent.

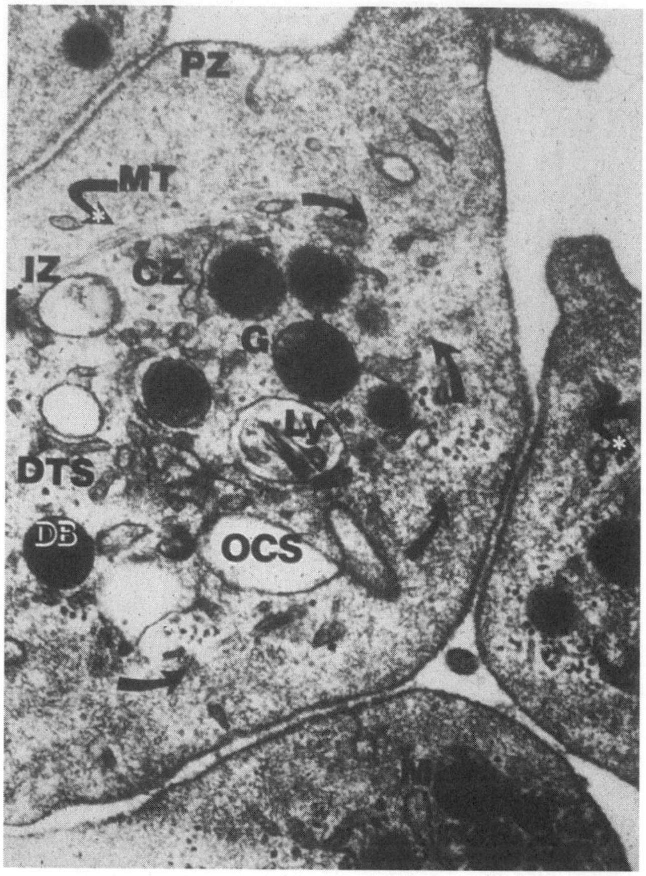

FIGURE 1.6. Transmission electron micrograph of platelet (*OCS,* open canalicular system; *Ly,* lysosome; *PZ,* peripheral zone; *G,* Golgi body; *DB,* dense body; *DTS,* dense tubular system; *MT,* microtubule; *IZ,* inner zone *CZ,* central zone).

Table 1.4 summarizes factors necessary for normal platelet function. An adequate number of platelets must be present for normal platelet function in vivo and in vitro. This is usually defined as approximately 100×10^9/L (1,2). In vitro and ex vivo tests of platelet function, in the face of a platelet count of less than 100×10^9/L, will yield abnormal results; for example, prolonged template bleeding times and abnormal platelet aggregation profiles will usually be noted (1). For normal function, platelets present must have adequate energy metabolism and an adequate number of (and contents of) storage granules capable of releasing their contents when appropriate stimuli are presented. Cationic proteins such as thrombosthenin also must be present. Membrane receptors must be responsive to appropriate stimuli. Platelets require divalent cations, the most important of which is calcium, and, of course, adequate physical conditions such as pH and temperature (1–4).

Table 1.5 summarizes the common platelet proteins. Some are not platelet specific, including numerous plasma proteins that are found in or on the surface of platelets; these include clotting factors II, V, VII, VIII, IX, X, XI, XII, and XIII (42,43). In some instances, these proteins are found in a slightly different molecular form in platelets

TABLE 1.3. PLATELET MORPHOLOGY

Peripheral zone	
	Glycocalyx
	Platelet membrane
	Open canalicular system
Sol–gel zone	
	Microtubules and microfilaments
	Dense tubular system
	Thrombosthenin
Organelle zone	
	Dense granules
	Mitochondria
	α Granules

TABLE 1.4. FACTORS NECESSARY FOR NORMAL PLATELET FUNCTION

Adequate number of platelets (>100×10^9/L)
Adequate energy metabolism
Adequate number and contents of storage granules
Adequate storage granules and release
Adequate cationic proteins
Adequate membrane receptors and responsiveness
Adequate divalent cations (Mg^{2+} and Ca^{2+})
Adequate physical conditions (pH, temperature)

TABLE 1.5. PLATELET PROTEINS

Nonspecific (plasma) proteins
Fibrinogen
Factors II, V, VII, VIII, IX, X, XII, and XIII
Albumin
Plasminogen
Complement components
Specific platelet proteins
Thrombosthenin
Platelet glycoproteins
Platelet factors 2 and 4
Platelet antiplasmin
Cathepsin A
β-Thromboglobulin

when compared with plasma (for example, factor XIII). Platelet-specific proteins also are present, including thrombosthenin, platelet factor 4, β-thromboglobulin, cathepsin A, and others (1–4).

Table 1.6 depicts those platelet factors that have been identified and characterized. Thus far, platelet factors 1 through 7 are recognized. The most important of these are platelet factor 3 (or platelet membrane phospholipoprotein, so-called platelet thromboplastin) and platelet factor 4 (antiheparin factor), which has become one of several important molecular markers of platelet reactivity and activation (44,45).

Table 1.7 summarizes compounds released from platelets. These include the biogenic amines including serotonin, catecholamines, and histamine; the all-important adenine nucleotides: cyclic adenosine monophosphate (AMP), ADP, and adenosine triphosphate (ATP); various enzymes including acid hydrolases; specific ions including calcium, magnesium, and potassium; PDGF and platelet factors, including platelet factor 4, β-thromboglobulin, and platelet factor 3 (1–4). Platelet factor 3 is not actually released but represents a conformational change in the platelet membrane making available activity, referred to as platelet factor 3, on which phospholipid-dependent hemostatic reactions may occur. In addition, other proteins including fibrinogen, other clotting factors, albumin, and other compounds are released from platelets during a release reaction (1).

Many stimuli induce a platelet-release reaction (1). These include subendothelial collagen and basement membrane, as previously mentioned. Additional potent inducers of a platelet-release reaction are thrombin, soluble fibrin monomer (fibrin monomer, which remains solubilized by complexing with FDPs), some FDPs (especially fragment X), endotoxin, circulating antigen–antibody complex, γ-globulin–coated surfaces, various viruses, ADP, catecholamines, and free fatty acids (46–49). Numerous proteolytic enzymes including trypsin, snake venoms, papain, and elastase are used in vitro to study platelet release (1,2). Other in vitro release-reaction techniques include the use of centrifugation, cold fracture, latex particles, carbon particles, kaolin, and celite (1,2).

Figure 1.7 is a scanning electron micrograph of a moderately activated platelet. As platelets become activated, they

TABLE 1.6. PLATELET FACTORS

Platelet factor 1: Coagulation factor V
Platelet factor 2: Thromboplastic material
Platelet factor 3: Platelet thromboplastin (phospholipid)
Platelet factor 4: Antiheparin factor
Platelet factor 5: Fibrinogen coagulant factor
Platelet factor 6: Antifibrinolytic factor
Platelet factor 7: Platelet cothromboplastin

TABLE 1.7. COMPOUNDS RELEASED FROM PLATELETS

Biogenic amines
Serotonin
Epinephrine
Norepinephrine
Histamine
Adenine nucleotides
ADP
ATP
Cyclic AMP
CATIONS
K^+
Ca^{2+}
Platelet factors 3 and 4
Platelet proteins
Albumin
Fibrinogen
Platelet factor 4
Thromboxanes

ADP, adenosine diphosphate; ATP, adenosine triphosphate; AMP, adenosine monophosphate.

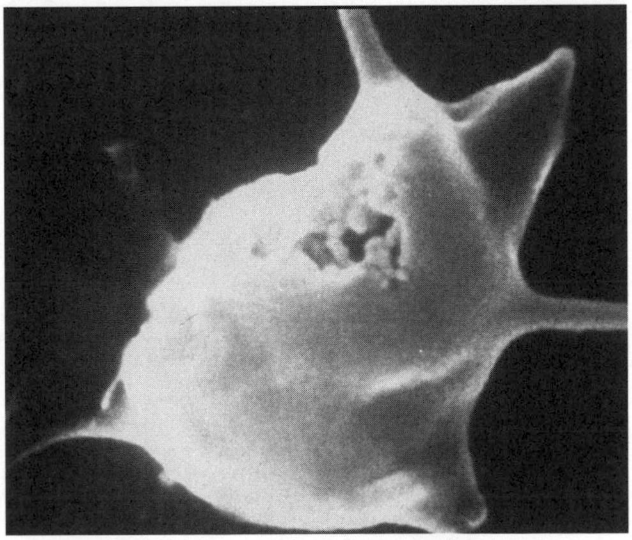

FIGURE 1.7. Moderately activated platelet (original magnification ×5,000).

begin to contract and form pseudopodia. During the process of contraction, the numerous intraplatelet compounds and granules are concentrated at the center of the platelet. As activation progresses, platelets become markedly contracted with pronounced pseudopod formation (1). It is observed that, during this event, the platelet organelles (including α granules and dense bodies) are concentrated at the center of the platelet, where organelle membranes are disrupted, their contents are released and subsequently transported outside the platelet via the open canalicular system. These compounds then interact with platelet membrane receptors of adjacent platelets, causing further platelet activation in a type of amplification process whereby numerous platelets become activated (1,2). In addition, many of these compounds may interact with adjacent endothelium. Pseudopod formation enhances platelet–surface interactions (adhesion) and platelet–platelet interaction (cohesion) (1).

Figure 1.8 shows a scanning electron micrograph of endothelium that has been rendered hypoxic. There are several areas where endothelial cells are missing. Note that these endothelial cell gaps are filled by activated platelets (contracted and with marked pseudopod formation).

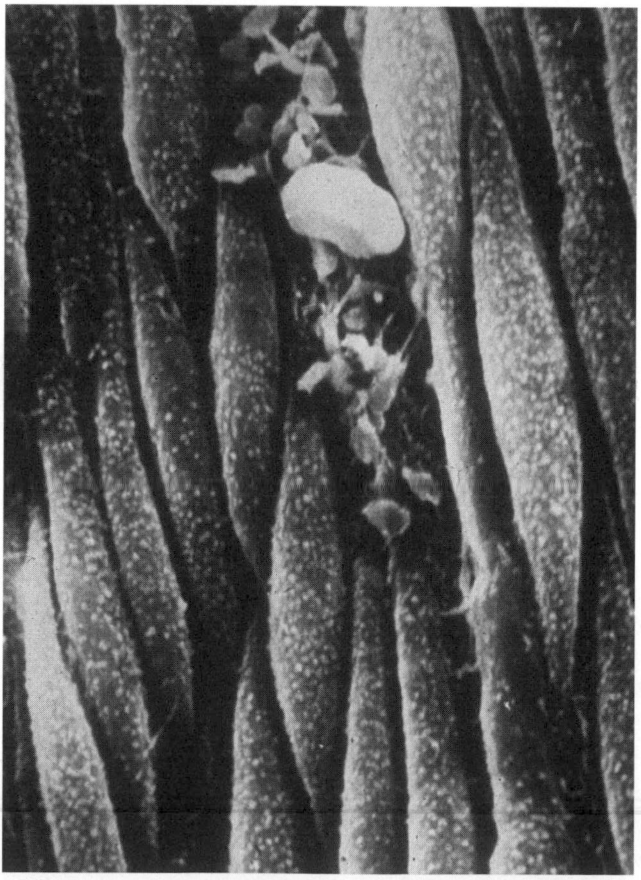

FIGURE 1.8. Endothelium with "gaps." Note: activated platelets fill the gap (original magnification ×10,000).

A summary of platelet function is presented in Fig. 1.9. The first process that occurs during platelet activation is that of platelet adhesion (1,2). The process of platelet adhesion refers to a platelet adhering to something other than another platelet (for example, an artificial surface, or collagen/basement membrane). After platelet adhesion, there is an initial release reaction with the release of intraplatelet ADP. This is a reversible process and accounts for the primary wave on an aggregation pattern. This is referred to as "primary (reversible) aggregation." As the concentration of ADP increases, platelet cohesion occurs. Platelet cohesion refers to platelets adhering to other platelets. As this progresses, more ADP and other compounds (including serotonin) are released. These compounds not only activate adjacent platelets but also induce vascular constriction (to prepare for an effective primary hemostatic plug or primary platelet/fibrin plug). During this increased release reaction, when the ADP concentration reaches a critical point, there ensues an irreversible conformational change in the platelet membrane, making available platelet factor 3 (platelet membrane phospholipid) activity. This material then serves as a primary surface mediating the formation of complexes in the coagulation protein sequence. The sequence of platelet cohesion, increased release reaction, and the conformational changes leading to the availability of platelet factor 3 is an irreversible process and accounts for the secondary wave seen in a platelet-aggregation pattern (1–4). In vivo, the result of all of this is the eventual formation of a platelet/fibrin plug, or "primary hemostatic plug," the function and integrity of which are rendered most efficient by vasoconstriction induced by compounds released from platelets. As α-granule release of procoagulant and platelet activation products occurs, PDGF also is released, and then PDGF binds to receptors, the result of which is inhibition of thrombin-induced aggregation and platelet secretion.

Abbreviated intraplatelet functional and biochemical pathways are outlined in Fig. 1.10. The key modulator of intraplatelet function is cyclic AMP (1,2,50–52). The role of this compound is to combine with a cyclic AMP–dependent protein to generate a kinase activity. The role of this kinase is to phosphorylate a receptor protein, which then binds calcium. When intraplatelet calcium is bound, it is not available to thrombosthenin, rendering the platelet hypoaggregable and hypoadhesible. Epinephrine, thrombin, collagen, and serotonin inhibit the enzyme adenylate cyclase (Fig. 1.10), which is responsible for the conversion of ATP to cyclic AMP. This inhibition results in a decrease in kinase concentration, a decrease in phosphorylated receptor protein, and an increase in ionized calcium concentration, which renders the platelet hyperaggregable (1–4).

The enzyme responsible for converting cyclic AMP into an inactive form is phosphodiesterase (53,54). One popular antiplatelet agent, dipyridamole, inhibits phosphodiesterase (1,2). Caffeine and papaverine also inhibit this enzyme. In

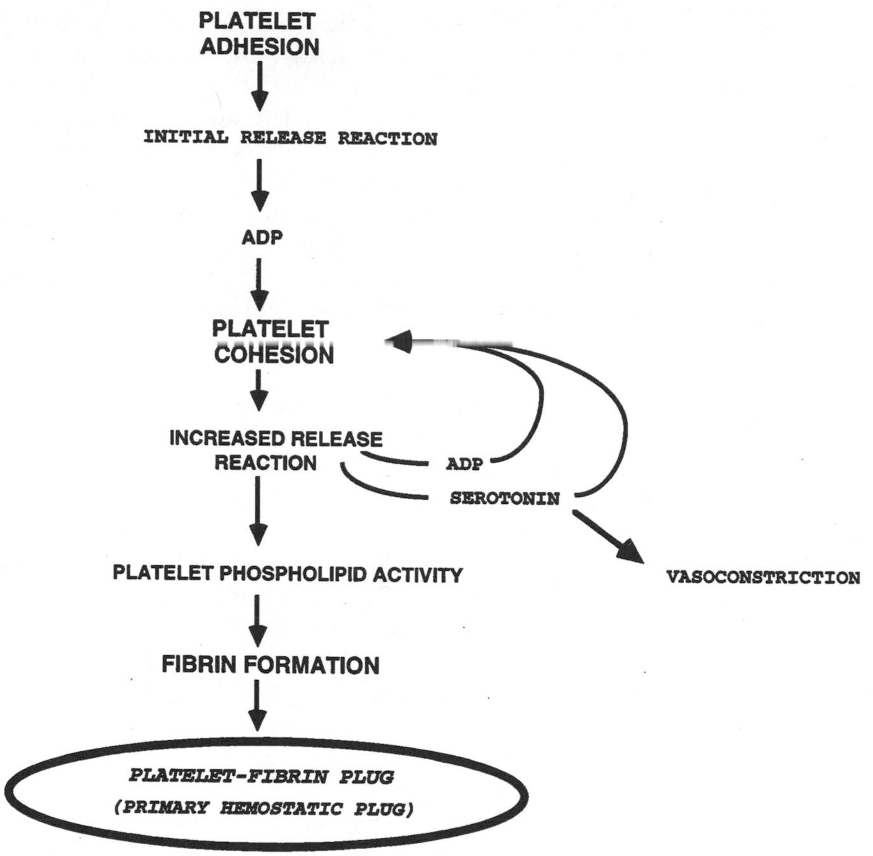

FIGURE 1.9. Simplified platelet function.

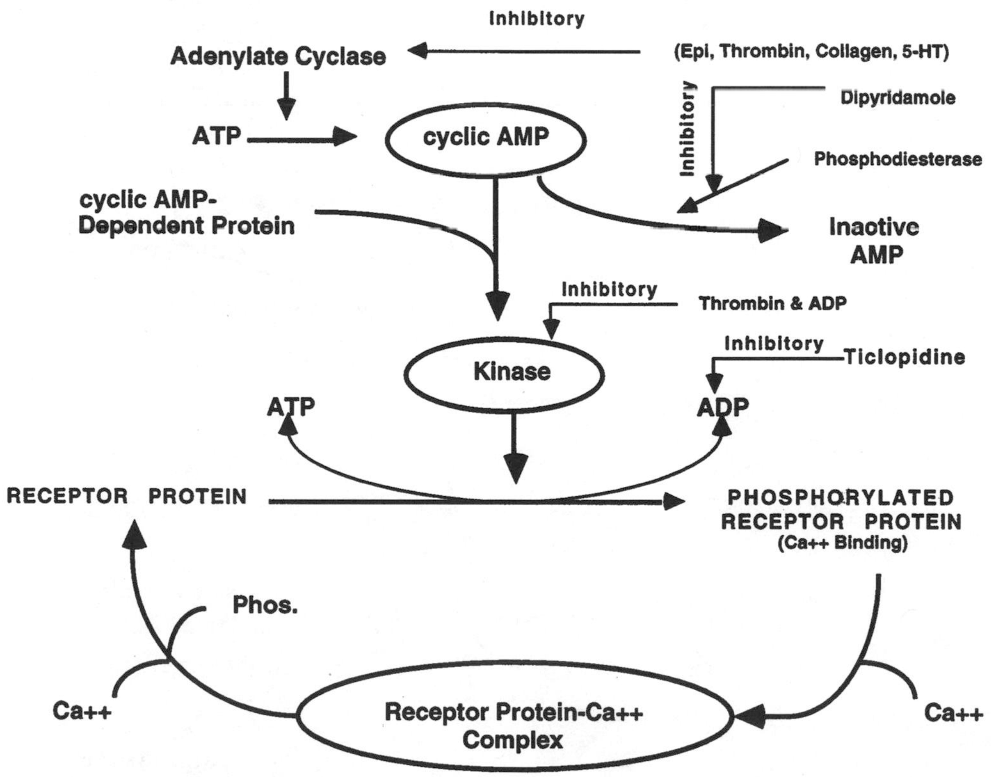

FIGURE 1.10. Intraplatelet biochemistry.

these instances, the concentration of cyclic AMP, kinase, and phosphorylated receptor protein will increase, intraplatelet calcium will become bound, and the platelet will be rendered hypoactive (1–4). Yet another mechanism for regulating the availability of ionized calcium may relate to the activity of membrane-bound alkaline phosphatase, the enzyme responsible for dephosphorylation of the receptor protein–Ca^{2+} complex.

The roles of prostaglandins and derivatives in platelet function are summarized in Fig. 1.11. Platelet and endothelial cell membrane phospholipids are converted into arachidonic acid by the enzyme phospholipase A_2 (PLA_2) (55,56), which is activated by both thrombin and collagen. Arachidonic acid is converted into prostaglandin intermediates, prostaglandin G_2 (PGG_2), and prostaglandin H_2 (PGH_2) by the enzyme cyclooxygenase. In the platelet membrane, thromboxane synthetase converts PGH_2 into thromboxane A_2, one of the most potent aggregating agents described (1,2). Thromboxane A_2 also has very potent vasoconstricting activity (1). In the endothelial cell, as well as in some subendothelial muscle cells, prostacyclin synthetase converts PGH_2 into prostacyclin, which is a very potent aggregation inhibitor and a potent vasodilator (57–59). Cyclooxygenase is inhibited by aspirin and sulfinpyrazone, two popular antiplatelet agents (1,60,61). These two antiplatelet agents' function selectivity is that their activity is directed about 70% toward platelets and only 30% toward the endothelial cell, most likely a manifestation of endothelial cell ability to continue synthesis of prostaglandins, but platelets lack this ability (1–4).

Thromboxane A_2 is a potent inhibitor of adenylate cyclase, and prostacyclin is a potent stimulator of adenylate cyclase. Therefore, the predisposition to bleeding or thrombosis may depend on the relative concentrations of these two compounds. This represents an exquisitely balanced biologic system whereby platelets are synthesizing and releasing into the adjacent milieu, a compound (thromboxane A_2) that promotes platelet function, and the adjacent endothelium is synthesizing and releasing prostacyclin, which inhibits platelet function (1–3).

Platelet interactions with the vasculature (adhesion), with other platelets (cohesion), and with plasma proteins occur at the platelet membrane surface, mediated by various platelet membrane glycoproteins (PMGPs) (62,63). The major PMGPs and their functions, where known, are summarized in Table 1.8. PMGP Ia is complexed to PMGP IIa and adheres platelets to subendothelial collagen independent of von Willebrand factor (64). PMGP Ib has been associated with a number of functions. It has a molecular mass of about 170,000 daltons and comprises an α and a β subunit, one of which fixes it to the platelet membrane. PMGP Ib exists in complex with PMGP IX and V (65). PMGP Ib and IX are absent from platelets in the Bernard–Soulier syndrome (66,67). The PMGP Ib/IX complex serves as a receptor for von Willebrand factor; thus subendothelial von Willebrand factor binding to PMGP Ib/IX is responsible for initial platelet adhesion to the subendothelial surface, the first step in platelet adhesion, usually in response to injury (67). PMGP Ib also is the receptor for quinine and quinidine drug-dependent antibody, which is present in quinine- and quinidine-induced thrombocytopenia (68). PMGP Ib also is part of the thrombin-receptor complex of platelets, and PMGP V is of vital importance in thrombin activation of platelets

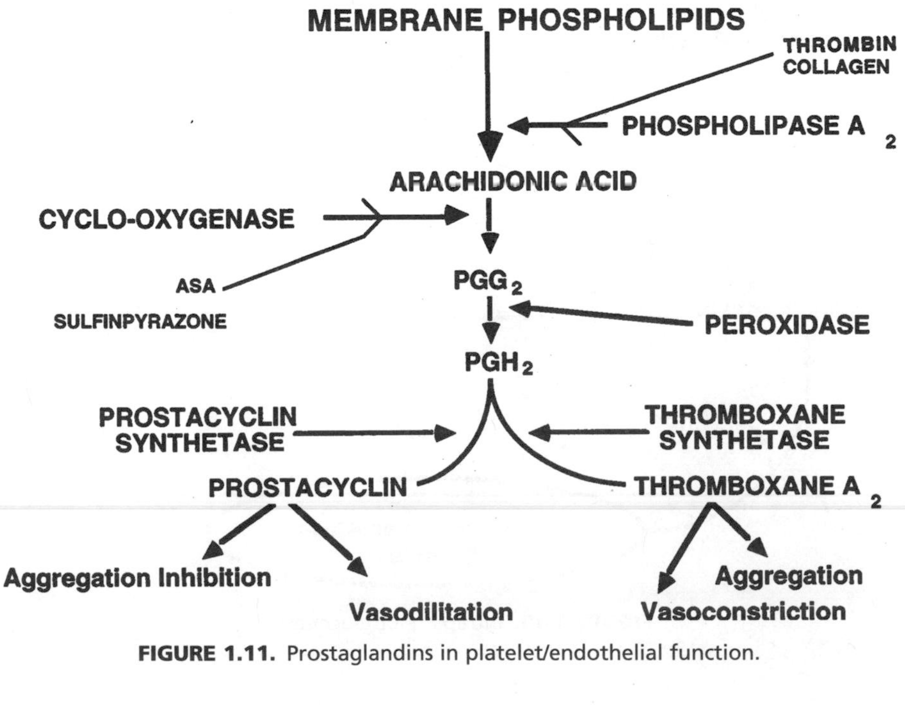

FIGURE 1.11. Prostaglandins in platelet/endothelial function.

TABLE 1.8. PLATELET MEMBRANE GLYCOPROTEINS

Glycoprotein	Function	Characteristic
Ia	von Willebrand–independent receptor for subendothelium	
Ib	von Willebrand receptor	Missing in Bernard–Soulier quinidine-Ab receptor
IIa		
IIb	von Willebrand and fibrinogen receptor	Missing in Glanzmann PLA-1 Ab receptor
IIIa	von Willebrand and fibrinogen receptor	Missing in Glanzmann PLA-1 Ab receptor
V	Thrombin receptor	Missing in Bernard–Soulier
IX	Thrombin receptor ?	Missing in Bernard–Soulier

Ab, antibody.

(69). PMGP IIb/IIIa complex is found in platelet α granules as well as on the membrane (70). PMGP IIb has a molecular weight of about 125,000, and PMGP IIIa, about 93,000. Both are subunits of a single glycoprotein, heavily dependent on calcium for binding of the complex. IIb is a major calcium-binding protein for platelet function (71). PMGP IIa/IIIb is absent or markedly reduced in Glanzmann thrombasthenia, is the binding site for fibrinogen, and serves as the apparent binding site for PLA1 antibody (72,73). The binding of fibrinogen to IIb/IIIa is required for optimal ADP-induced platelet aggregation. GP IIb/IIIa also binds to von Willebrand factor and fibronectin. GP G, also called thrombospondin, has a molecular weight about 180,000 and is partially responsible for thrombin- and collagen-induced aggregation (74,75). PMGPs Ic and IIa have been identified but are, as yet, without clearly defined function in hemostasis. As platelets become activated, catalytic processes remove the GP I, GP V, and P-selectin, and GP IIb/IIIa undergoes change, allowing binding to soluble fibrinogen; the binding to soluble fibrinogen induces altered contractile activity, and clot retraction begins.

Methods to assess platelet activation, based on the previously described physiology, have been developed. As mentioned, several release products, such as platelet factor 4, PDGF, and others, may be indicative of platelet activation. Newer, more specific, methods to assess platelet activation use flow cytometry and monoclonal antibodies to platelet-activation sites. Monoclonal antibodies (mABs) against resting IIb/IIIa complex (CD 41/61) are available (76); however, one mAB (PAC1) is directed against the fibrinogen binding site domain exposed only with platelet activation (77). CD 62P is directed against P-selectin, which mediates adhesion of activated, but not resting, platelets to neutrophils and monocytes (78). Some mABs react with both resting and activated platelets, but with much more avidity to activated platelets. One such mAB is CD 36, directed against PMGP IV (79). The opposite is true of CD 42, directed against GP Ib/IX/V complex; in this instance, there is low avidity for activated platelets and high avidity for resting platelets; thus decreasing avidity is a marker of platelet activation (80).

PLASMA PROTEIN FUNCTIONS

Plasma protein function in hemostasis comprises numerous systems, the five most important of which are depicted in Table 1.9. These systems consist of (a) the coagulation protein system, (b) the fibrino(geno)lytic system, (c) the kinin system, (d) the complement system, and (e) the inhibitors for the first four systems (1–4). Kinin generation and complement activation are often not appreciated as important participants in thrombohemorrhagic disorders. Pathophysiologically, these systems assume extreme importance, especially in disorders such as disseminated intravascular coagulation (81).

The Coagulation Protein System

Coagulation proteins and their synonyms are summarized in Table 1.10. The Roman numeral system is most widely used and is preferred. However, in some instances, no Roman numerals are assigned to factors. Protein C also has been referred to as factor XIV or autoprothrombin II-A. Fletcher factor is synonymous with prekallikrein, and Fitzgerald factor, also called William's factor, Flaujac factor, Reid factor, or Fujiwara factor, is high-molecular-weight

TABLE 1.9. BLOOD PROTEIN FUNCTION: THE FIVE INTERACTIVE SYSTEMS

1. Coagulation protein system
2. Fibrinolytic enzyme system
3. Complement system
4. Kinin system
5. Inhibitors to the first four systems

TABLE 1.10. COAGULATION FACTORS AND SYNONYMS

Factor	Synonym
I	Fibrinogen
II	Prothrombin
V	AC-globulin
VII	Prothrombin conversion accelerator
VIII:C	Antihemophilic factor
IX	Christmas factor (PTC)
X	Stuart–prower factor
XI	Thromboplastin antecedent (PTA)
XII	Hageman (contact) factor
XIII	Profibrinoligase
Fletcher factor	Prekallikrein
Fitzgerald factor	HMW kininogen
Protein C	Xa Inhibitor
Protein S	None

HMW, high molecular weight.

TABLE 1.11. CHROMOSOMAL LOCATION CONTAINING COAGULATION FACTOR INFORMATION

Factor	Inheritance	Chromosome	Region
I	AD	4	q26-31
II	AD	11	p11-q12
V	AR	1	q21-25
VII	AR	13	q34
VII:C	SLR	X	q28
vWF	AD	12	p12-13
IX	SLR	X	q27
X	AR	13	q34
XI	AR	4	q35
XII	AR	5	q33
XIII	AD	6	p24-25
AT III	AD	1	p23
Protein C	AD	2	q13-14
Protein S	AD	3	p21
Plasminogen	AD	6	q26-27
t-PA	AD	8	p12
t-PA-I-1	AD	7	q21-22
t-PA-I-2	AD	18	q21-22
Antiplasmin	AR	18	?
Fletcher	AR	?	?
Fitzgerald	AR	?	?
Heparin Cofactor-II	22	?	

Inheritance, usual mode of inheritance; AD, autosomal dominant; AR, autosomal recessive; SLR, sex-linked recessive; t-PA, tissue plasminogen activator.

TABLE 1.12. THE FOUR KEY PROCOAGULANT REACTIONS

1. Contact activation (generation of IXa)
2. The generation of factor Xa
3. The generation of thrombin (IIa)
4. The generation of fibrin

kininogen (82–84). The chromosome location containing genetic information for synthesis of almost all the coagulation factors is known (1,85,86) and is summarized in Table 1.11.

The formation of a fibrin clot is best thought of as consisting of four key reactions; this concept is helpful to render the procoagulant system easily understandable. The first key reaction is contact activation; the second is the formation of factor Xa; the third is the formation of thrombin; and the fourth is the formation of fibrin. These are depicted in Table 1.12.

Generation of Factor IXa

The contact activation phase of coagulation begins with the activation of Hageman factor (factor XII). There are numerous potential mechanisms by which factor XII can be activated with subsequent activation of factors XIa and IXa; these are depicted in Fig. 1.12. Phospholipids, collagen, subendothelial collagen, and kallikrein (activated Fletcher factor) are capable of converting factor XII to factor XIIa (87–90). Active Hageman factor, a serine protease, then converts factor XI to factor XIa. This reaction occurs quickly in the presence of high-molecular-weight kininogen and occurs more slowly without it, thus accounting for a significantly prolonged activated partial thromboplastin time in its absence (91,92). The role of factor XIa, also a serine protease, is to convert factor IX (in the presence of calcium ions) into factor IXa. Factor IXa is the enzyme responsible for the second key reaction, the generation of factor Xa (1). It also should be noted (Fig. 1.12) that factor XIIa itself is able to convert prekallikrein into kallikrein, which is capable of then converting more factor XII to factor XIIa (2).

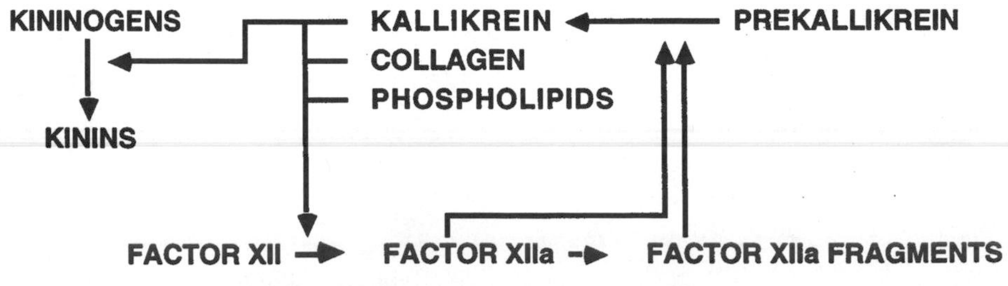

FIGURE 1.12. Mechanisms of factor XII activation.

Generation of Factor Xa

The second key reaction involves two major pathways, "intrinsic" and "extrinsic." Intrinsic activation is depicted in Fig. 1.13. The "extrinsic" pathway of factor Xa formation involves the participation of "thromboplastin" (tissue factor), factor VII, and calcium ions (1). Tissue factor is a membrane-bound protein (lipoprotein) existing in a protected state within the plasma membrane of endothelial cells (93,94). On injury, it is released into the circulation, where it forms a complex with coagulation factor VII (a vitamin K–dependent protein containing γ-carboxyglutamic acid residues) in the presence of calcium ions. The activity of the complex seems to be dependent largely on the concentration of tissue factor. However, the enzymatic activity responsible for the proteolytic activation of factor Xa resides in the factor VII molecule (1).

Factor VII exists in plasma as a single-chain GP, with close structural homology to prothrombin, factor IX, and factor X. Contrary to its analogues, however, factor VII is not a zymogen in the true sense, because it has proteolytic activity, although to a limited extent. In the presence of thrombin or factor Xa and lipids and calcium ions, this activity may be increased as much as 400-fold and is accompanied by the formation of a two-polypeptide-chain molecule. On further incubation, the two-chain form of factor VII becomes inactive, and the rate of inactivation is dependent on the concentration of factor Xa. It has been proposed that in the activation of factor X by factor VII, the continuing generation of factor Xa results in a "pulse of factor X–converting activity that can quickly disappear" (1). The role of and interactions of factor VII, tissue factor, and TFPI are discussed in detail in subsequent sections.

The "intrinsic" formation of factor Xa is a five-component system and requires (a) a substrate (factor X), (b) an enzyme (factor IXa), (c) a determiner or cofactor (factor VIII:C), (d) a surface (platelet factor 3), and (e) calcium ions (1,2). The complex formed is bound together by calcium, depicted by the asterisks in Fig. 1.13. The enzyme factor IXa cleaves a peptide from the substrate (factor X), with resultant exposure of an active serine site. Factor Xa is the product of this reaction. Factor VIII:C is modified and rendered dysfunctional after this reaction.

Tissue Factor and Tissue Factor Pathway Inhibitor

The "extrinsic" pathway of factor Xa formation involves the participation of tissue factor ("thromboplastin"), factor VII, calcium ions, and TFPI (95). Tissue factor (TF) is a membrane-bound lipoprotein existing in a protected state within the plasma membrane of endothelial and other cells (96). TF may be derived from both benign and malignant cells, and cells able to produce this lipoprotein, under appropriate stimulus, include not only endothelial cells, but also the monocyte/macrophage system, and others (97,98). TF is an injury-based lipoprotein of molecular weight 45,000 and functions as a cell-surface receptor for factor VII. TF is activated/released on injury to activate VII to VIIa. On injury, including that induced by endotoxin, interleukin-1 (both α and β), tumor necrosis factor α (TNF-α), complement activation (particularly C5a), lipopolysaccharide, and circulating immune complexes, TF is released into the circulation, forming a complex with coagulation factor VII in the presence of calcium ions (99–103). The activity of this complex is dependent on the concentration of TF (1). However, the enzymatic activity responsible for the proteolytic activation of factor Xa resides in the factor VII mole-

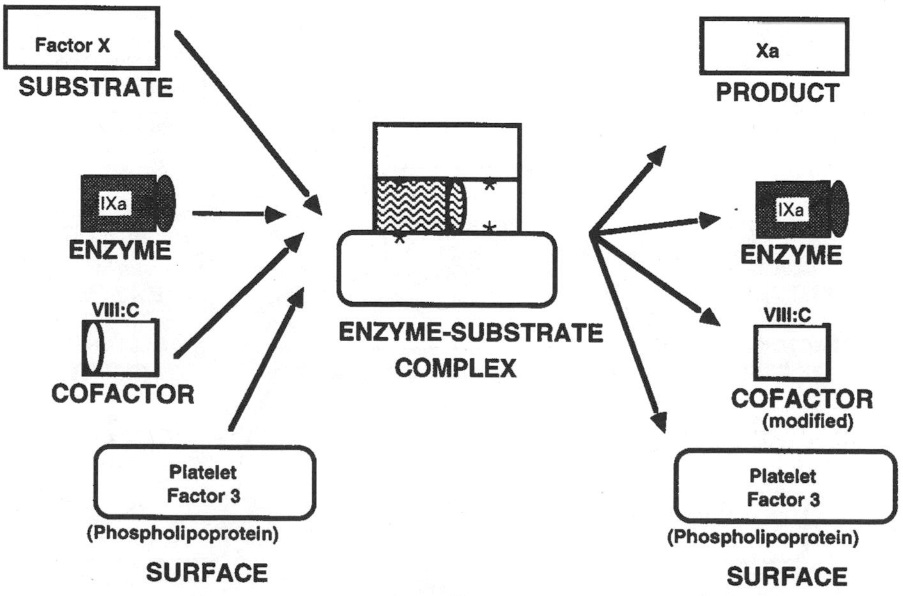

FIGURE 1.13. The formation of factor Xa ("intrinsic activation").

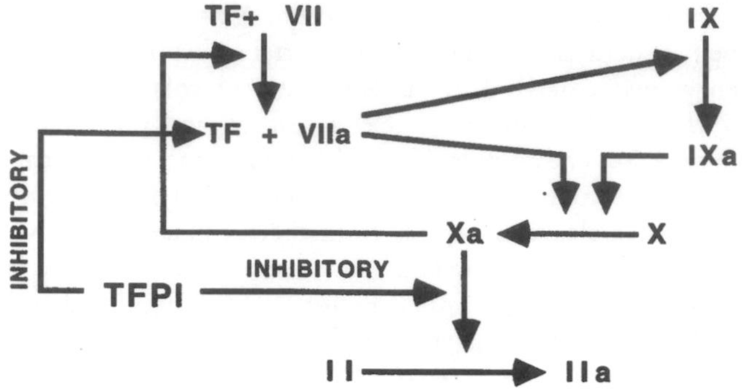

FIGURE 1.14. Tissue factor pathways of activation. *TF,* tissue factor; *TFPI,* TF pathway inhibitor.

cule. Factor VII exists in plasma as a single-chain GP with close structural homology to prothrombin, factor IX, and factor X. Contrary to its analogues, however, factor VII is not a zymogen in the true sense, because it has proteolytic activity, although to a limited extent. In the presence of thrombin or factor Xa and lipids and calcium ions, this activity may be increased as much as 400-fold and is accompanied by the formation of a two-polypeptide-chain molecule (1). On further incubation, the two-chain form of factor VII becomes inactive, and the rate of inactivation is dependent on the concentration of factor Xa. It has been proposed that in the activation of factor X by factor VII, the continuing generation of factor Xa results in a "pulse of factor X–converting activity that can quickly disappear" (1).

The TF/VII complex is able to activate factor X to factor Xa and factor IX to IXa; in addition, factor Xa converts the TF/VII complex to a TF/VIIa complex, which becomes much more potent in activation of factors X and IX (104). The preferential target of the TF/VIIa complex is tissue/cell phospholipid–bound factor Xa (105). This injury-mediated activation process is inhibited by TFPI (106). TFPI is a protease with a molecular weight of 36,000 to 43,000 and contains three Kunitz-type domains (107). The first domain is responsible for inhibition of the TF/VII and TF/VIIa complex. The second domain appears responsible for the mediation/inhibition of factor Xa activity, and the third domain appears to interact with heparin and other proteoglycans (107,108). TFPI binds to endotoxin, thereby inhibiting the cellular effects of endotoxin (109). Sources of TFPI are multiple and include endothelium, hepatocytes, lung tissue, monocytes, renal tissue, and bladder tissue; however, endothelium is the most pronounced source (110). TFPI may inhibit both TF/VIIa and the Xa/TF/VIIa complex. Inhibition of the TF/VII complex is greatly enhanced in the presence of Xa (111). Most TFPI circulates bound to plasma lipoproteins, with the preferential binding being low-density lipoprotein (LDL) greater than high-density lipoprotein (HDL) greater than very low density lipoprotein (VLDL); in addition, about 10% of circulating TFPI is bound to platelets (112). The anticoagulant activity of TFPI resides primarily in the C-terminus portion of the molecule, which is capable of binding TF/VIIa, lipoproteins, and heparin; all of the binding in this region is greatly enhanced by the presence of factor Xa (113). Heparin induces the release of endothelial TFPI, and this is thought to be important in the overall antithrombotic activity of heparin (114). Mechanisms of factor VII, TF, and TFPI are summarized in Fig. 1.14.

Generation of Thrombin

The third key reaction is the formation of thrombin. Figure 1.15 summarizes enzyme–substrate complex formation for this reaction, which also is a five-component system requir-

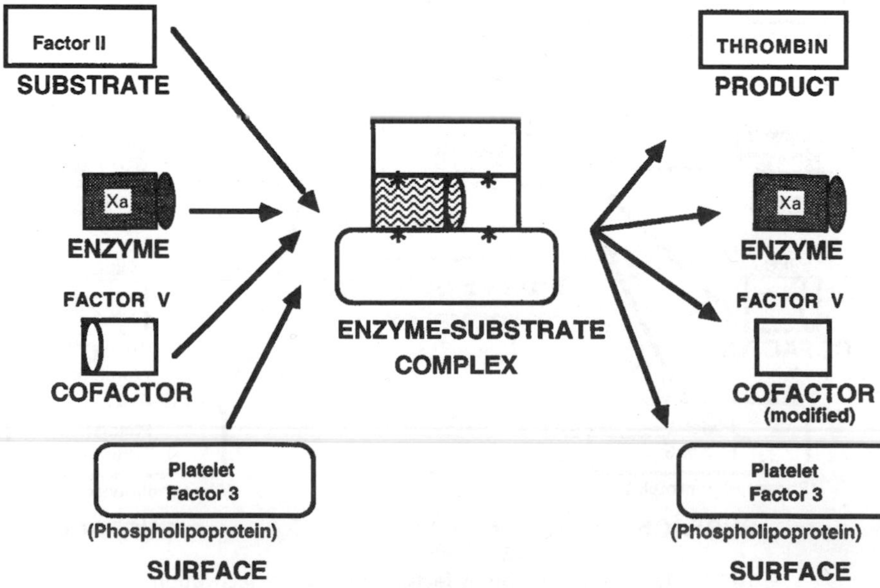

FIGURE 1.15. The formation of thrombin (factor IIa).

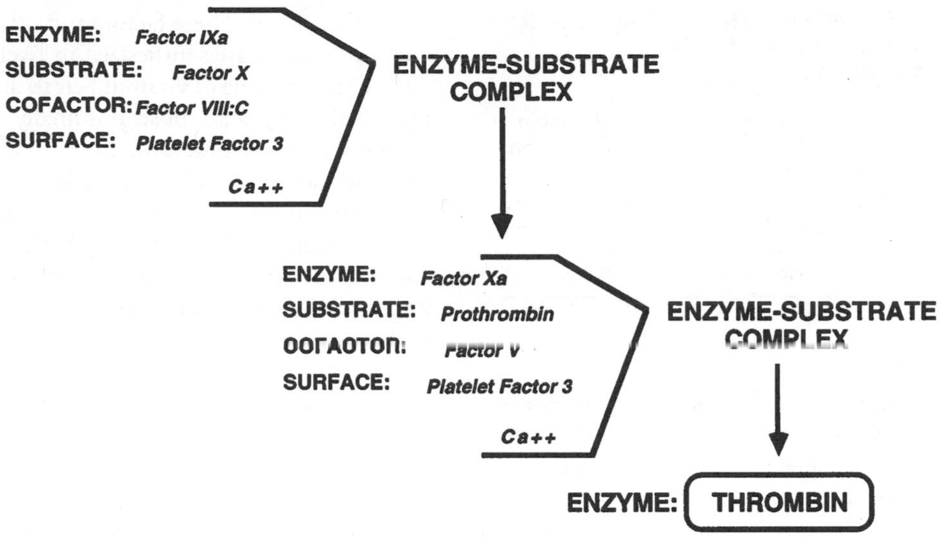

FIGURE 1.16. Summary of the first two key reactions: the formation of Xa and thrombin.

ing (a) a substrate (factor II), (b) an enzyme (factor Xa), (c) a cofactor (factor V), (d) platelet factor 3 or other phospholipid surface, and (e) calcium ions (1,2,115–117). These components form a complex on the phospholipid surface, and a product (thrombin), the new enzyme, is generated. Factor V, like factor VIII:C in the previous reaction, is modified and loses biologic activity. The role of the determiner/cofactor is to ensure that the correct enzyme and substrate enter into complex formation. For example, the presence of factor V enables the enzyme factor Xa to interact with the correct substrate, factor II. Likewise, in the preceding key reaction, factor VIII:C ensures that factor IXa reacts with factor X (1–4).

Figure 1.16 summarizes the similarity of the two five-component system reactions. Figure 1.17 exemplifies the criticality of stoichiometry for these reactions. If any one of

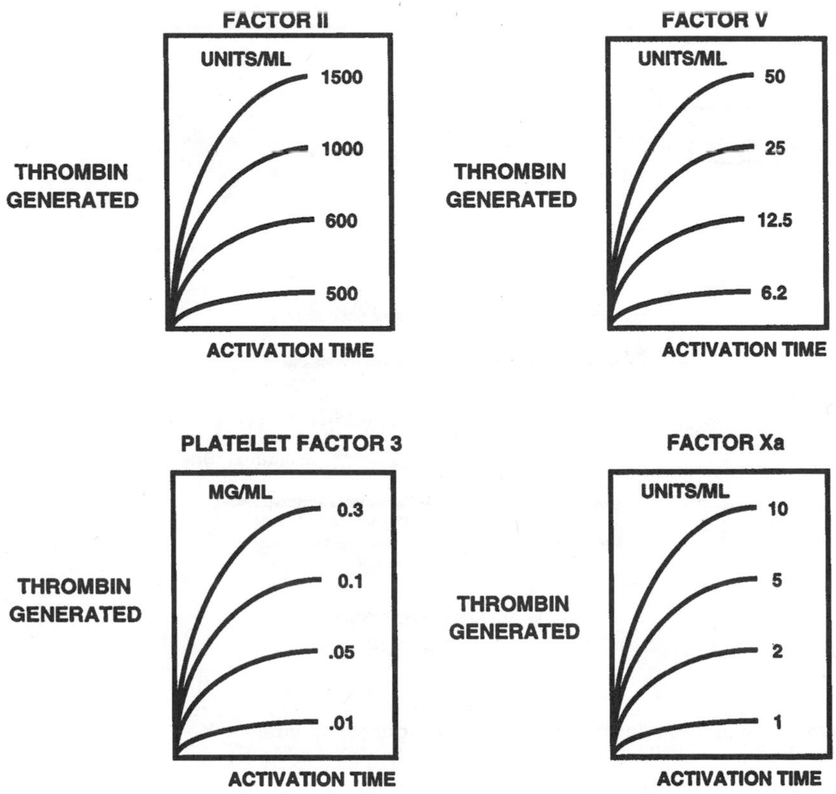

FIGURE 1.17. Necessity of stoichiometry in coagulation reactions.

TABLE 1.13. PLATELET MEMBRANE PHOSPHOLIPID (PLATELET FACTOR 3) SELECTIVITY IN PROCOAGULANT ACTIVITY

Phospholipid Component	Factor Xa Generation	Thrombin Generation
Phosphatidylethanolamine	*Active*	Not active
Phosphatidylcholine	*Active*	Not active
Phosphatidylinositol	Not active	*Active*
Phosphatidylserine	Not active	*Active*

the components is present in less than optimal concentrations, the amount of product generated is reduced. Thus physiologically, all five components must be present in relatively normal concentrations and must be appropriately functional (118).

Platelet membrane phospholipid or platelet factor 3 has many individual constituents. Four of these constituents are selectively active in the second two key reactions; these four constituents and their activities are summarized in Table 1.13. Phosphatidylserine and phosphatidylinositol are active in the third key reaction or thrombin generation. They have no activity in factor Xa formation (1–4). Phosphatidylcholine and phosphatidylethanolamine have no activity in thrombin formation; however, they are active in the formation of factor Xa (1–4).

The generation of factors Xa and IIa (thrombin) are dependent on several vitamin K–dependent factors, factors II, VII, IX, and X. These factors and others, such as protein C and protein S, are synthesized in liver parenchymal cells (119–121). The role of vitamin K is to attach calcium-binding prosthetic groups postribosomally to the N-terminal region of each of these proteins (1). The process involves the introduction of an extra carboxyl group on the side chain (γ position) of several glutamic acid residues, forming γ-carboxyglutamic acid. In the absence of vitamin K, for example, in a patient receiving warfarin therapy, calcium-binding sites are not attached, and although a protein is synthesized, calcium-binding sites are missing, and the protein is dysfunctional. These abnormal vitamin K–dependent factors are referred to as "PIVKAs," or proteins induced by vitamin K absence or antagonists (122). This situation is depicted on the left side of Fig. 1.18. Normal vitamin K–dependent factor synthesis is depicted on the right side of the figure, with the "x" representing the γ-carboxyglutamic acid residues. γ-Carboxyglutamic acid is depicted in Fig. 1.19.

Generation of Fibrin

The fourth key reaction is the formation of fibrin. Figure 1.20 summarizes the conversion of fibrinogen to fibrin. Thrombin removes two small peptides, fibrinopeptide A and fibrinopeptide B, from fibrinogen, leaving fibrin monomer (1–4,123,124). Fibrin monomer polymerizes by aggregating end to end and side to side; these aggregates are stabilized by noncovalent bonds (1,2). This fibrin is referred

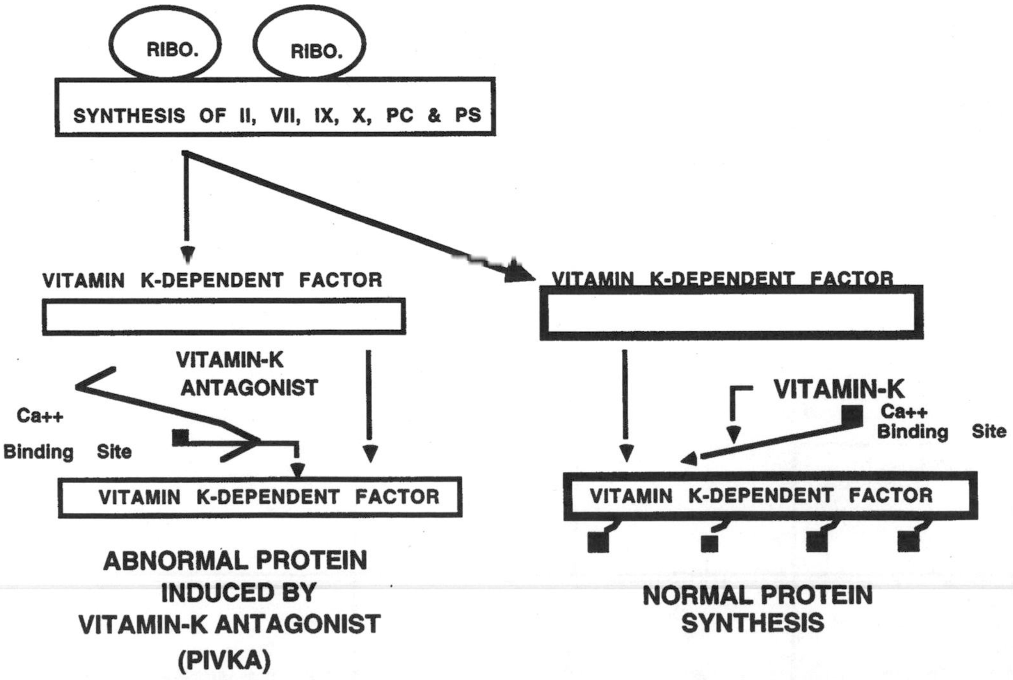

FIGURE 1.18. Vitamin K–dependent coagulation factors and proteins induced by vitamin K absence or antagonists (*PIVKAs*) synthesis.

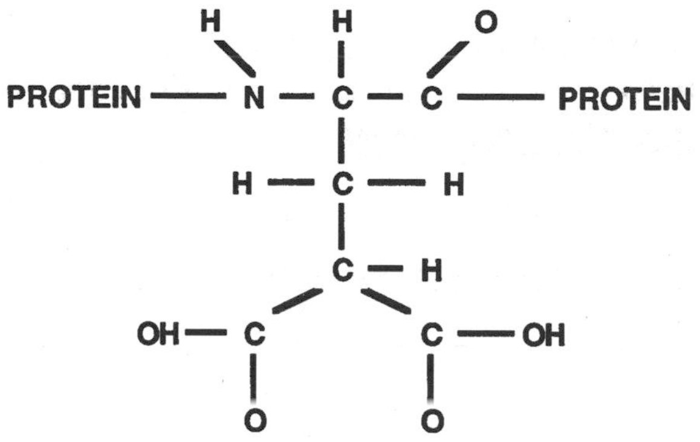

FIGURE 1.19. γ-Carboxyglutamic acid (calcium-binding group).

to as "soluble fibrin" because it dissolves in 5 *M* urea or 1% monochloroacetic acid (1,2). The formation of soluble fibrin monomer aggregates, held together only by hydrophobic bonds, is referred to as polymerization I. Another important role of thrombin is to activate factor XIII (profibrinoligase) to factor XIIIa (fibrinoligase). Factor XIIIa replaces hydrophobic bonds with peptide bonds, rendering insoluble fibrin (125,126). This is referred to as polymerization II. Figure 1.21 depicts fibrinogen. Fibrinogen is a dimer composed of six polypeptide chains, two A-α, two B-β, and two γ chains (127). The role of thrombin is to remove fibrinopeptides A and B proteolytically by cleaving at specific amino acid sites. Fibrinopeptide A is released very rapidly, and fibrinopeptide B, more slowly (1,2). Fibrin monomer aggregation begins as soon as fibrinopeptide A is released, and the B peptide need not necessarily be released for fibrin monomer aggregation to occur (1–4). Fibrinopeptide A consists of 16 amino acids, and fibrinopeptide B consists of 14 amino acids; assays are available for these peptides, and their clinical importance is discussed in other chapters. Figure 1.22 illustrates polymerization I, the α and γ chains held together by hydrophobic bonds before factor XIII (fibrinoligase) activation by thrombin. Figure 1.23 illustrates polymerization II, with factor XIIIa having replaced hydrophobic bonds with peptide bonds.

The Fibrinolytic System

The fibrinolytic system is responsible for the destruction of a fibrin clot. It is generally thought that small amounts of fibrin are constantly being deposited systemically and subsequently lysed (1,4,128,129). The presence or absence of hemorrhage or thrombosis thus may depend on a delicate balance between the procoagulant system and the fibrinolytic system (1,2,130). Figure 1.24 summarizes the biology of the fibrinolytic system, which consists of a proenzyme, plasminogen, which is converted by numerous pathways into the active enzyme, plasmin (131). Unlike the enzyme thrombin, which has very narrow substrate specificity, the serine protease plasmin has a much broader spectrum of activity with a number of substrates. It has similar affinity for both fibrinogen and fibrin, degrading both into FDPs (132). Plasmin also biodegrades factors V, VIII, IX, and XI, adrenocorticotropic hormone (ACTH), growth hormone, insulin, and many other plasma proteins (1,2,130,133–136). There are two primary physiologic activation pathways for the fibrinolytic system. One involves endothelial cell–derived plasminogen activator activity (TPA) (137). The other is Hageman factor (factor XIIa) activation (138). Active Hageman factor converts a proactivator (prekallikrein) into an activator (kallikrein), which then converts plasminogen into plasmin. There also are numerous poorly characterized tissue activators that convert plasminogen to plasmin. Pharmacologic activators are currently used clinically, including streptokinase, urokinase, tissue plasminogen activator (t-PA), and acyl-plasminogen-streptokinase activator complex (APSAC), for therapeutic thrombolysis (139). Urokinase directly activates plasminogen into plasmin; however, streptokinase forms a streptokinase–plasminogen complex; the complex then converts plasminogen into plasmin (1,2,140).

Figure 1.25 summarizes the Hageman factor activation pathway for the fibrinolytic system. Numerous materials are able to convert Hageman factor into active Hageman factor, including collagen and phospholipids. However, endotoxin, antibody–antigen complex, and other pathological materials also may initiate this activation pathway, creating circulating plasmin (1–4,141). Plasmin tends to be a "self-per-

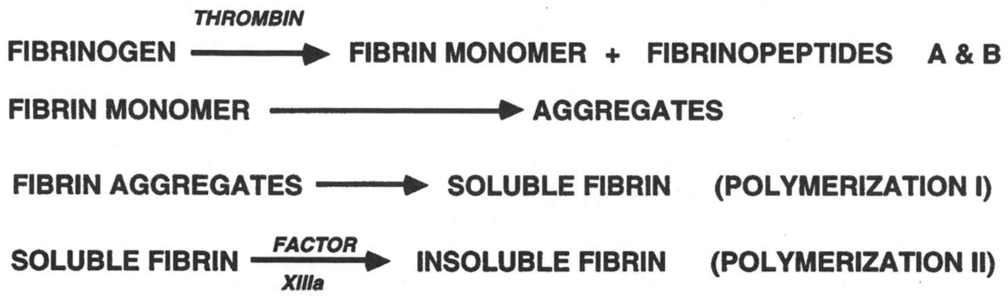

FIGURE 1.20. The conversion of fibrinogen to fibrin.

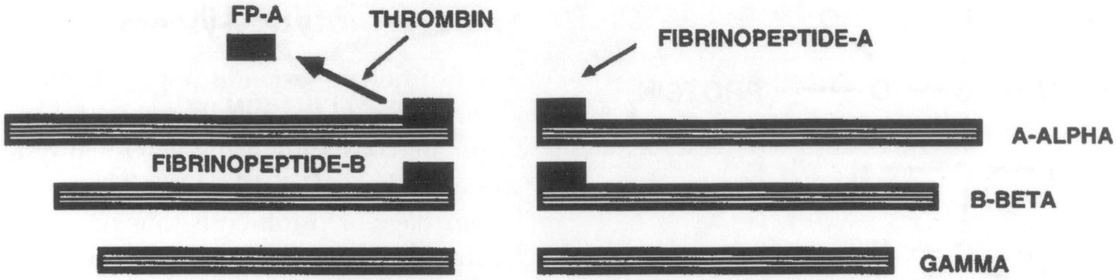

FIGURE 1.21. The structure of fibrinogen.

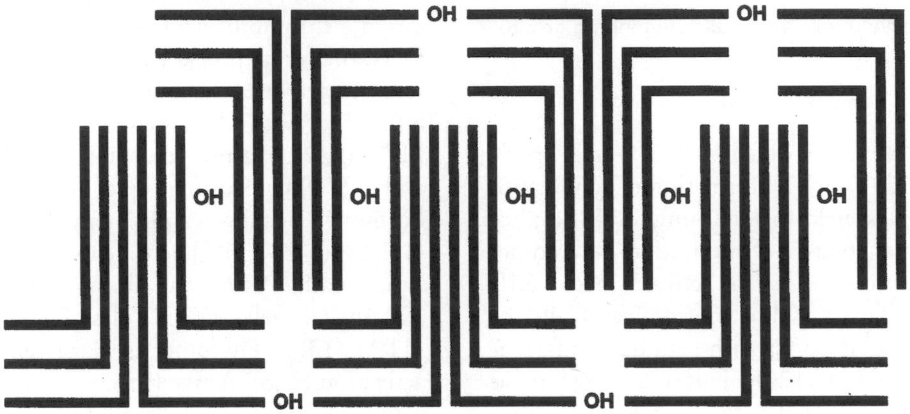

FIGURE 1.22. Polymerization I (soluble fibrin).

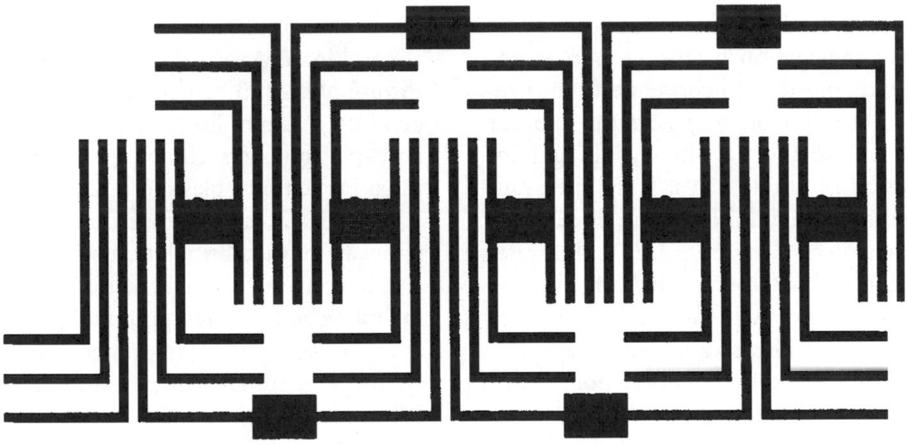

FIGURE 1.23. Polymerization II (insoluble fibrin).

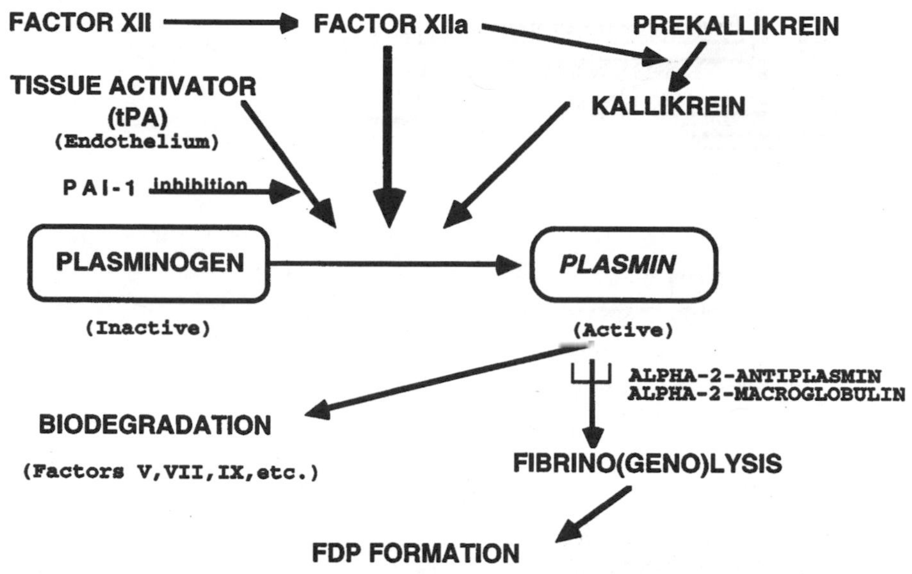

FIGURE 1.24. Physiology of the fibrinolytic system (*PAI-1,* plasminogen activator inhibitor type 1; *FDP,* fibrinogen/fibrin degradation products).

petuating" enzyme, a self-feeding loop generating more plasmin once traces of plasmin are generated through the Hageman factor/prekallikrein activation pathway. The conversion of active Hageman factor into Hageman factor fragments by plasmin will then convert more prekallikrein to more kallikrein and convert more plasminogen to plasmin (1,2,142,143).

The fibrinolytic system is modulated by a number of inhibitors. α_2-Antiplasmin (α_2-AP) is a rapid inhibitor of plasmin activity, and α_2-macroglobulin is an effective although slow inhibitor of plasmin activity (129,144). Although present in very low concentration in plasma, α_2-AP, with an extraordinary affinity for plasmin resulting in an irreversible covalent complex, makes α_2-AP one of the major regulators of fibrinolysis in vivo. There are two known inhibitors of t-PA, t-PA-I-1 [plasminogen activator inhibitor type 1 (PAI-1) and t-PA-I-2 (PAI-2)]; a third (PAI-3) exists but is without clearly defined function at present (1–4,145,146). PAI-1 is the primary modulator. A number of cells produce this protein, including platelets, supporting the hypothesis that at sites of injury, platelet aggregation facilitates the survival of the fibrin and thus the integrity of the hemostatic "plug" (1,147).

In contrast to thrombin, which cleaves fibrinopeptides A and B from the amino-terminal end of fibrinogen, creating fibrin monomer, plasmin begins to degrade fibrin(ogen) at

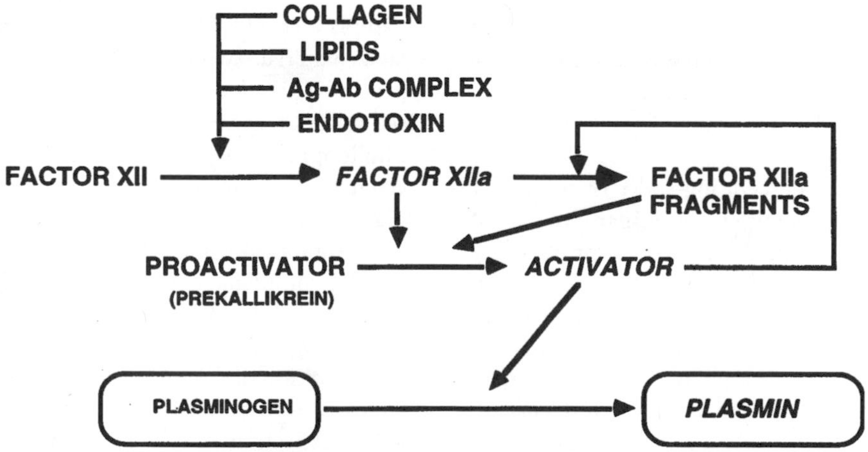

FIGURE 1.25. Factor XII (Hageman factor)–dependent activation of fibrinolysis.

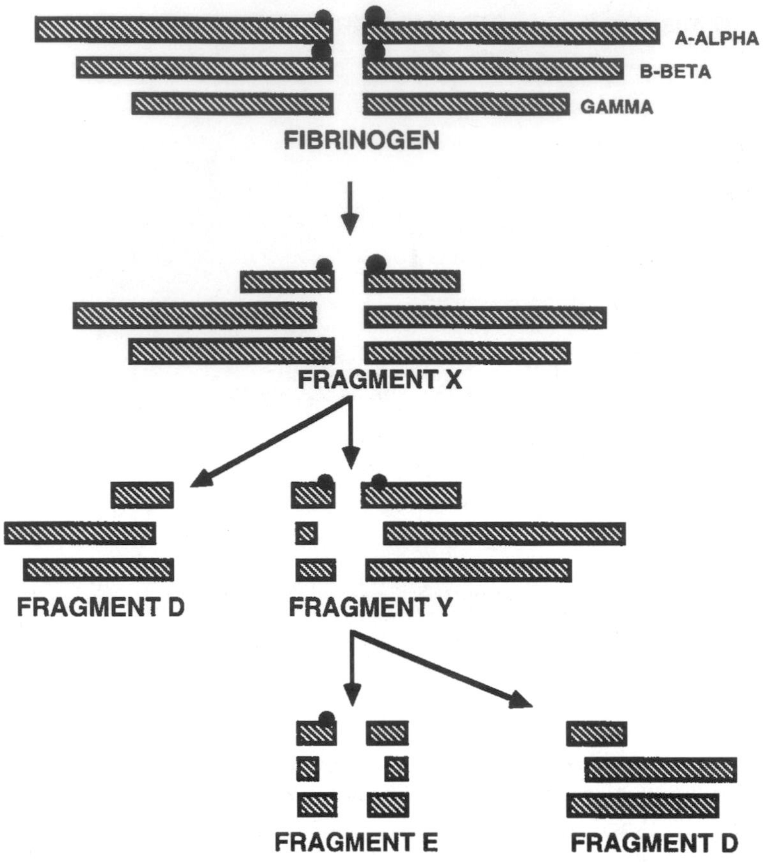

FIGURE 1.26. Formation of fibrin(ogen) degradation products.

the carboxy terminal end of the A-α chain to create degradation products (1–4,130). Figure 1.26 depicts the clinically significant FDPs. At the top of the figure, fibrinogen is depicted as comprising the A-α, B-β, and the γ chains, with the A-peptide and the B-peptide being depicted as small circles. Fibrinogen and fibrin are first degraded into fragment X after plasmin-induced symmetric cleavage of the carboxy-terminal end of the A-α chains. Subsequent digestion of fibrinogen and fibrin by plasmin is then asymmetric and occurs at the amino-terminal end of one portion of the molecule, giving rise to a fragment Y and a fragment D. Further digestion gives rise to another fragment D and a fragment E. The latter constitutes the N-terminal disulfide knot (1–4,130,148,149). Fragments X, Y, D, and E are the clinically significant FDPs measured by commercially available FDP assay kits.

The FDPs are named in descending order of molecular weight, with fibrinogen having a molecular weight of approximately 340,000; fragment X, approximately 265,000; fragment Y, approximately 155,000; fragment D, approximately 95,000; and fragment E, the smallest and last of the fragments, about 50,000 (1,2,130). The presence of FDPs may seriously compromise hemostasis by interference with fibrin monomer polymerization and platelet function (1–4,130,150,151).

Complement Activation and Hemostasis

Although complement activation is generally not considered an integral part of the physiology of hemostasis, its role in the pathophysiology of thrombohemorrhagic disorders is of considerable importance. The complement system is capable of increasing vascular permeability, leading to hypotension and shock, common occurrences in disseminated intravascular coagulation and other thrombohemorrhagic disorders (1,2,152,153). Complement activation to the C8-9 (attack) phase leads to osmotic lysis of red cells and platelets (154,155). This results in release of procoagulant material, which usually accelerates a coagulation process (1,2). For example, if there is complement-induced red cell lysis, there is the release of red cell membrane phospholipoprotein as well as red cell ADP; both serve as procoagulant or coagulation-accelerating materials. Lysis of platelets leads to release of materials, including ADP, which also promote clotting activity (1–4).

The complement system involves a series of sequential reactions similar to the coagulation system and is depicted in Fig. 1.27. A primary "classic" activation pathway involves the activation of C1 by antigen–antibody complexes and an alternate (properdin) activation pathway involving the direct activation of C3 (156,157). The activation of C1

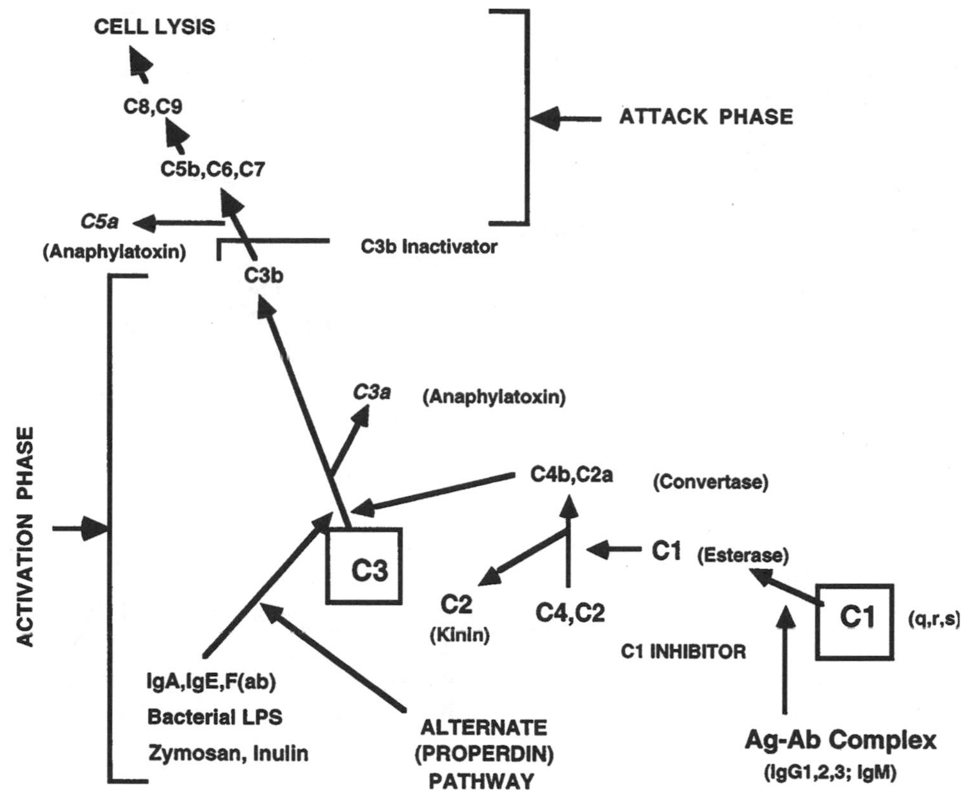

FIGURE 1.27. The complement system.

through C5 is called the "activation phase," and the activation of C5 through C9 is called the "attack phase," leading to osmotic lysis (1). Figure 1.28 summarizes the role of plasmin in complement activation. As previously discussed, factor XIIa converts prekallikrein to kallikrein, which converts plasminogen to plasmin. Plasmin is capable of directly activating C1 or C3, providing two pathways for activation of complement, independent of the presence of antigen—antibody complexes. In many instances of clinically significant thrombohemorrhagic disease, there is plasmin-induced activation of the complement system, leading to serious clinical consequences (1,2,81,134).

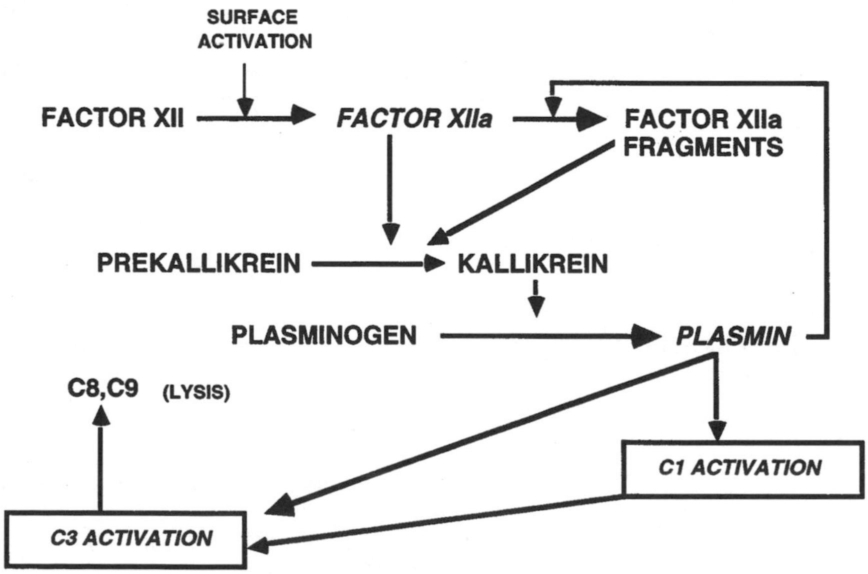

FIGURE 1.28. Complement activation in hemostasis.

Kinins and Coagulation

Only recently has the importance of kinin generation during thrombohemorrhagic disorders been appreciated (1,2). Kinins increase vascular permeability and induce vascular dilatation, leading to hypotension, shock, and other potential end-organ damage (1–4,158–160). Figure 1.29 summarizes pathways of kinin generation. Like complement activation, generation of kinins centers on Hageman factor activation. Factor XIIa converts prekallikrein (Fletcher factor) into kallikrein; kallikrein converts kininogens into kinins. Factor XIIa also is converted into XIIa fragments by plasmin; these fragments also activate prekallikrein to kallikrein, with ensuing generation of kinins. This figure summarizes the interrelations between Hageman factor, the fibrinolytic system, and the kinin system (1,2).

Figure 1.30 illustrates the important interrelations between the coagulation system, the fibrinolytic system, the complement system, and the kinin system. Hageman factor is converted to active Hageman factor by various compounds including collagen and phospholipids; active Hageman factor converts prekallikrein to kallikrein, and this converts plasminogen to plasmin. Plasmin activates C1 and/or C3 of the complement system. Additionally, plasmin-induced Hageman factor fragments convert prekallikrein to kallikrein, which, in addition to generating more plasmin, will convert kininogens to kinins. These activation pathways often lead to catastrophic clinical consequences (1,2).

Inhibitor Systems

Like other biologic processes, the blood-coagulation system is governed by a number of inhibitory devices designed to limit the extent of the various biochemical reactions and possible dissemination of the coagulation process, resulting in pathology. To this extent, the regulation of coagulation is effected by a number of negative-feedback mechanisms, the involvement of many specific inhibitors, and compartmentalization of function, all of which restrict clotting to a localized process. The most important inhibitors of the procoagulant system are antithrombin III, protein S, and protein C (1,2,161–163). These inhibitors, and their deficiencies, are discussed in detail in subsequent chapters. Table 1.14 summarizes inhibitory mechanisms in hemostasis. Most of these inhibitory mechanisms are important physiologically, and some assume major importance in pathophysiology. First, there is inactivation of factors V and VIII:C by thrombin, as well as by activated protein C (protein Ca) and protein S (164,165). In addition, there is inhibition of prothrombin activation and fibrin formation by small fragments generated during the conversion of prothrombin to thrombin (profragments 1 and 2). There is inhibition of factor Xa by modified protein C, and recent evidence suggests that α_1-antitrypsin also may be an inhibitor of factor Xa (166). There is major inhibition of the serine proteases thrombin, factor Xa, factor IXa, factor XIa, factor XIIa, and kallikrein by antithrombin III (AT III) (167–170). The inhibitory activity of AT III is markedly enhanced by heparin (171–173).

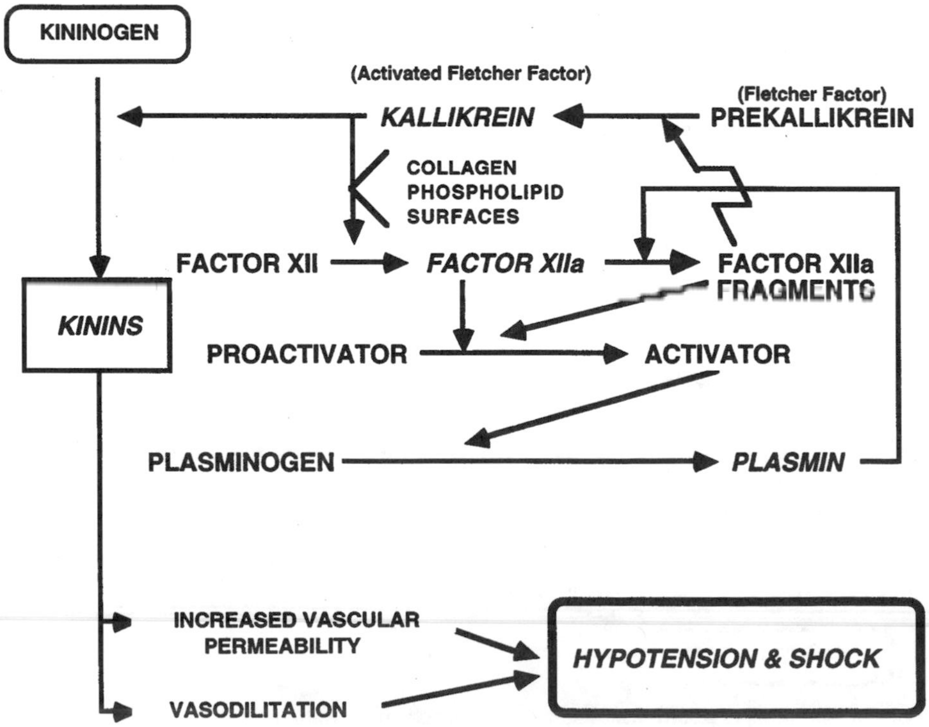

FIGURE 1.29. Kinin generation and hemostasis.

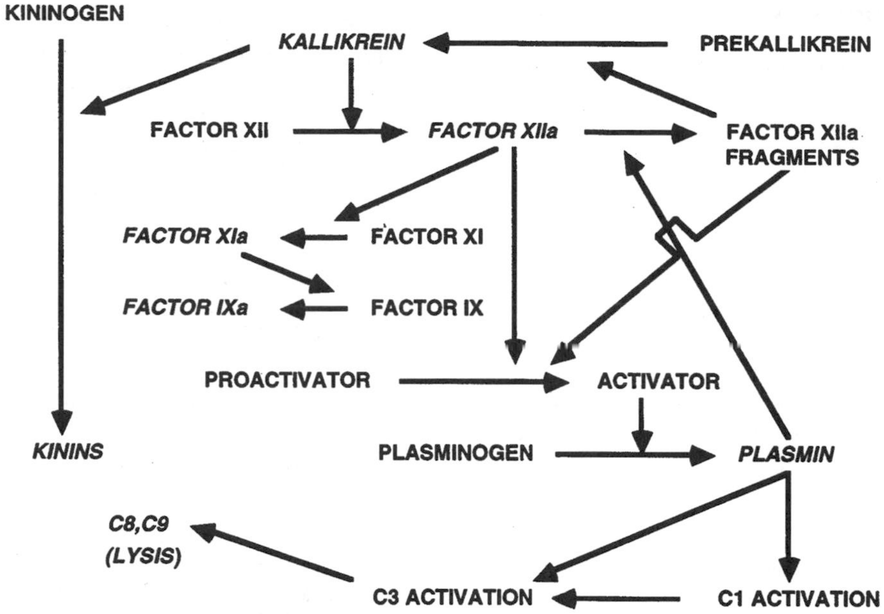

FIGURE 1.30. Interrelations between coagulation, fibrinolysis, kinins, and complement.

Figure 1.31 depicts a model of AT III, illustrating the interaction of AT III with serine proteases. Arginine-rich centers in AT III react irreversibly with the serine center of serine proteases (167,169). In this figure, thrombin is depicted; however, factor Xa, factor IXa, or other serine proteases also could have been illustrated. Serine proteases irreversibly react with arginine of AT III, and the complex is removed from the circulation. Heparin, when used therapeutically, reacts with lysine sites in AT, making the arginine-rich center more available, thereby enhancing AT inhibitory activity. This ternary complex then dissociates to yield an inactive thrombin–AT III complex and free heparin. The elucidation of this mechanism has served as a fundamental premise rationalizing heparin and "miniheparin" therapy.

TABLE 1.14. INHIBITORY MECHANISMS IN HEMOSTASIS

Inactivation of factors V and VIII by thrombin and activated protein C and protein S
Inhibition of prothrombin activation and fibrin formation by prothrombin fragments
Inhibition of factor Xa by activated protein C
Inhibition of thrombin or factor Xa formation by suboptimal "complex" components
Inhibition of thrombin, factor Xa, IXa, XIa, XIIa, and kallikrein by antithrombin
Inhibition of thrombin activity by absorbing to fibrin
Inhibition of fibrin monomer polymerization and platelet function by fibrinolytic degradation products

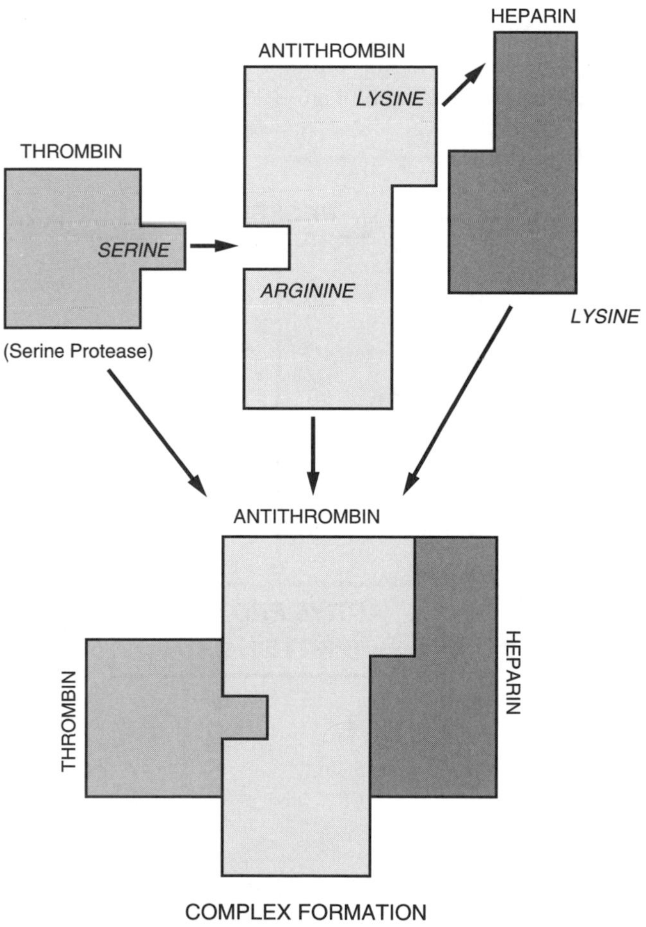

FIGURE 1.31. Antithrombin–heparin inhibitory activity.

TABLE 1.15. FUNCTIONS OF PROTEIN C AND S

Inactivation of factors Va and VIII:Ca (enhanced by protein S)
Enhances fibrino(geno)lysis by depressing inhibitors
Enhances epinephrine-induced platelet aggregation
Related to clot retraction by unclear mechanisms
Competitive inhibition of factor Xa

As fibrin is formed, it absorbs thrombin, thus decreasing thrombin availability. Inhibition of fibrin monomer polymerization and platelet function by FDPs may occur. If FDPs complex with fibrin monomer before polymerization, fibrin monomer becomes solubilized and unavailable for polymerization. Later degradation products, especially D and E fragments, have a high affinity for platelet membranes and render platelets markedly dysfunctional. In some pathological instances, this activity can lead to quite significant clinical hemorrhage through an FDP-induced platelet dysfunction (1,2,130).

Table 1.15 summarizes the functions of proteins C and S. Activated protein C (APC) is capable of the inactivation of factors Va and VIII:Ca; this inhibitory activity is facilitated by protein S, which functions to "bury" APC into the phospholipid moieties of factors V and VIII:C (164,165,174). APC enhances fibrinolysis, perhaps by depressing fibrinolytic inhibitors or enhancing the activity of plasminogen activators. Figure 1.32 depicts the protein C and S system. This system involves the interaction of the enzyme thrombin with an endothelial cell component, thrombomodulin, resulting in an *in situ* complex incapable of converting fibrinogen to fibrin but fully active in converting protein C (a proenzyme) to protein Ca (an enzyme). Protein Ca in turn, and in the presence of protein S, inactivates by proteolysis factors Va and VIII:Ca. This effectively halts further fibrin deposition (1,2).

OTHER INTERACTIVE COMPONENTS

Evidence is mounting that numerous other interactive components of hemostasis, including the vascular proteoglycans, fibronectin, complement derivatives, neutrophils/monocytes, and other as yet unknown components, may have important roles in modulating hemostasis. With time, the interactive activities of these components will become clear; it is anticipated that many other components in the cellular and blood systems will be found to interact with the hemostasis system.

Fibronectin is a high-molecular-weight GP found in its soluble form in plasma (175). An insoluble form is found in connective tissue and basement membranes (176). Fibronectin binds to collagen, fibrin, fibrinogen, and intact cells, especially fibroblasts (176–178). Fibronectin is synthesized by vascular endothelium and also is found in, and is possibly synthesized by, the α granules of platelets (179).

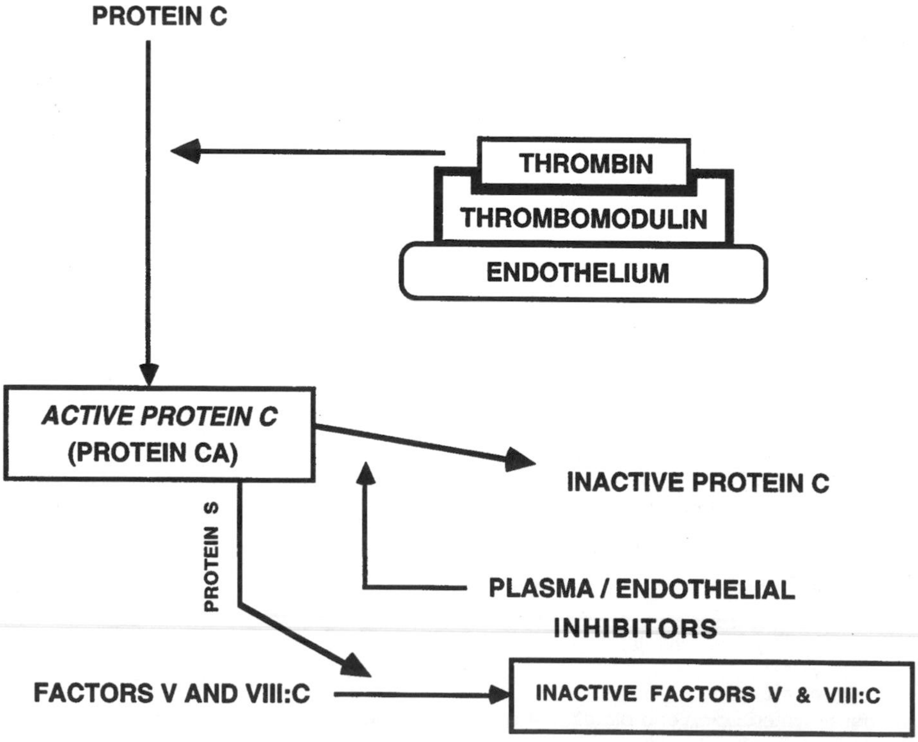

FIGURE 1.32. Protein C and S activity.

Fibronectin is cleaved by thrombin and trypsin and coprecipitates with fibrin (180,181). Fibronectin also is cross-linked by factor XIIIa (180,181). More specifically, fibronectin is covalently cross-linked to a fibrin clot by factor XIIIa. Fibronectin is required to support cell growth, to enhance cellular migration into a fibrin clot, and to provide an extracellular matrix that eventually replaces a fibrin clot. Additional activities are the potentiation of plasminogen activators, thus mediating clot lysis and matrix turnover. Fibronectin mediates activation of platelets by damaged tissue, promotes opsonization of bacteria, and mediates attachment of bacteria to damaged tissues. The fibronectin associated with α granules of platelets is released by collagen or thrombin-induced platelet aggregation; after release, fibronectin binds to the platelet surface. On the platelet surface, fibronectin mediates collagen–platelet adhesion and further stimulates collagen-induced platelet aggregation and release. Other activities of fibronectin include cellular binding, especially to fibroblasts, binding to bacteria, where promotion of opsonization by neutrophils may occur (this requires factor XIIIa), and fibronectin inhibits the endothelial uptake of LDL. Fibronectin interacts intimately with fibrinogen and fibrin. As clot formation occurs, approximately 50% of plasma fibronectin is lost (181). This is enhanced if clot formation occurs at less than 4°C. This loss is due to cross-linking of fibronectin to the α chain of fibrin (by factor XIIIa), thus accounting for approximately 5% of the total protein of a fibrin clot. Fibronectin is necessary for cryoprecipitation of fibrinogen–fibrin complexes and accounts for the laboratory "cryoprecipitation" seen in disseminated intravascular coagulation. The fibrin–fibronectin complex is necessary for the migration and adhesion of cells in an area of thrombus formation. Fibronectin is commonly decreased not only in disseminated intravascular coagulation, but also in postoperative states, in patients sustaining major trauma and especially in burns, and in patients with solid tumor metastases (182). Fibronectin also interacts with collagen and other vascular proteoglycans. Fibronectin binds to collagen; this is mediated by cross-linking of fibronectin to collagen by factor XIIIa. In addition, fibronectin binds to heparin, endogenous heparan sulfate, hyaluronic acid, and chondroitin sulfate. Heparin may accelerate the binding of fibronectin to both fibrinogen and collagen; however, the binding of heparin to fibronectin does not change the "anticoagulant" nature of the bound heparin (182).

Vascular proteoglycans are a heterogeneous group of high-molecular-weight protein polysaccharides consisting of carbohydrate polymers (glycosaminoglycans) covalently linked to a protein core (183). The common vascular proteoglycans are hyaluronic acid, chondroitin-4-sulfate, chondroitin-6-sulfate, dermatan sulfate, keratin sulfate, heparin sulfate, endogenous heparan sulfate, and heparin. Endogenous heparan sulfate differs from USP heparin in that it is a low-sulfated, D-glucuronic acid–rich polysaccharide, whereas USP heparin is a highly sulfated, L-iduronic acid–rich polysaccharide. The amount of each type of vascular proteoglycan depends on the type and portion of the vasculature evaluated. Most of the vascular proteoglycans are concentrated in the intimal layer of the vessel. The concentration of some of the vascular proteoglycans, especially dermatan and heparan sulfate, correlates closely with antithrombotic activity. Selected vascular proteoglycans inhibit collagen and thrombin-induced platelet aggregation and accelerate AT III inhibitory activity directed against thrombin and factor Xa. Vascular proteoglycans induce the release of platelet factor 4. The concentrations of vascular proteoglycans change with the development of atherosclerotic plaques. The physiologic role of vascular proteoglycans is thought to consist of supporting vascular integrity, maintaining the viscoelastic properties of vessels, regulating permeability of macromolecules from the plasma passing through the vessel wall, and regulating arterial lipid deposition. All of these properties encompass modulating functions in the interaction of blood proteins with the vascular wall.

Several complement derivatives, especially C3a and C5a, may play key roles in hemostasis (1–4). These components not only regulate vascular tone but also may induce a neutrophil/monocyte release of enzymes like elastases and collagenases, important in the degradation of fibrinogen, fibrin, and FDPs (184). Additionally, complement derivatives modulate release of granulocyte/monocyte procoagulant activity, may modulate platelet reactivity, and influence the neutrophil/monocyte interaction with fibronectin (185). Granulocytes and monocytes contain procoagulant activity that may be released under pathologic conditions (such as in acute leukemia) and interact with the hemostasis system (186,187).

The hemostasis system also involves interactions between neutrophils (both granulocytes and lymphocytes), monocytes, platelets, and the endothelium (188). These interactions involve cell-to-cell interactions and, after this, intracellular and intercellular biochemical signaling, resulting in cytokine release and other phenomena (1,189). Many of these interactions also are initiated by cytokines. The processes of cell–cell interaction are modulated by a number of compounds, primarily the "adhesion" molecules (190). The adhesion molecules involved in cell–cell interactions pertaining to hemostasis are the integrins, the selectins, and immunoglobulin-like proteins. The selectins are a group of cell receptors composed of three members. E-selectin is synthesized by cytokine-activated endothelial cells; lipopolysaccharide (endotoxin) also may induce E-selectin endothelial expression (191,192). E-selectin also is known as the endothelial leukocyte adhesion molecule (ELAM-1) (193). The adhesion molecules, cells, activity, and alternate names are summarized in Table 1.16. E-selectin binds granulocytes (polymorphonuclear neutrophils) to the endothelium. E-selectin may be useful as a

TABLE 1.16. ADHESION MOLECULES IN HEMOSTASIS AND SYNONYMS

Name	Alternate	Cell(s)	Activity
SELECTINS			
E-Selectin	ELAM-1	Endothelium	Binds granulocytes to endothelium
P-Selectin	GMP-140/PADGEM	Endothelium and platelets	Binds WBCs to activated platelets and activated endothelium
L-Selectin	LAM-1	Lymphocytes	? In hemostasis
Integrins			
LFA-1	CD 11a/CD18	Leukocytes	Receptor for ICAM 1 and ICAM 2
MAC-1	CD 11b/CD18	Leukocytes	Receptor for ICAM 1 and leukocyte binding site for fibrinogen and HMW kininogen
GP 150,95	CD 11c/CD18	Leukocytes	Binds fibrinogen to neutrophils

ICAM, intercellular adhesion molecule; ELAM, endothelial leukocyte adhesion molecule; HMW, high molecular weight.

marker for activated or damaged endothelium (194). P-selectin, also known as granule membrane protein 140 (GMP-140) and PADGEM (platelet-activation-dependent granule to external membrane), or CD-62, is found in platelet α granules and Weibel–Palade bodies of endothelium (195,196). P-selectin is expressed on both activated platelets and activated endothelial cells, and is thus a marker for both activated endothelium and activated platelets (197,198). P-selectin mediates binding of neutrophils, eosinophils, basophils, monocytes, and some T cells to activated platelets and activated endothelium (199,200). L-selectin (LAM-1) is a cytokine-activated lymphocyte adhesion molecule with unclear roles in hemostasis, but demonstrates binding to activated endothelial cells and may modulate binding of neutrophils to the activated endothelium (201). Both P-selectin and L-selectin have been mapped to chromosome 1 bands q23-q25 (202).

The integrin adhesion molecule family comprises three proteins. All are heterodimeric proteins consisting of α and β subunits; varying combinations give rise to unique molecules (203,204). Integrins are primarily leukocyte adhesion molecules. The three leukocyte integrins are LFA-1 (CD11a/CD18), Mac-1 (CD11b/CD18), and glycoprotein 150,95 (GP-150,95) (CD11c/CD18) (205–207). LFA-1 functions as a receptor for intercellular adhesion molecule (ICAM)-1 and -2 (208). The role, if any, of LFA-1 in hemostasis is not yet clear. Mac-1 also binds ICAM-1 and is a leukocyte-binding site for fibrinogen and high-molecular-weight kininogen, thus allowing indirect binding of factor XI and prekallikrein to neutrophils (209,210). This activity may induce release of leukocyte elastase and cathepsins and resultant protease activity, including thrombin and platelet activation and the degradation of fibrinogen, fibrin, and other proteins (211,212). Glycoprotein 150,95 mediates the binding of neutrophils to fibrinogen (213). This complex and rapidly evolving area of hemostasis is summarized in several recent excellent reviews (214–216).

It can be reasonably anticipated that in the future, many other biologic components of the cellular and plasma protein system will be found to interact with and be very important to the physiology and pathophysiology of hemostasis and thrombosis.

SUMMARY

The importance of firmly mastering basic mechanisms and pathways of hemostasis is again emphasized. Subsequent chapters deal with specific disease states, more easily understood by appreciating basic physiology. A working knowledge of basic hemostasis physiology enhances interpretation and understanding of pathophysiology, testing modalities, and thrombohemorrhagic disorders, provides a basis for therapeutic approaches, and implements future development of augmented diagnostic and therapeutic advances.

REFERENCES

1. Bick RL, Murano G. Physiology of hemostasis: clinics lab. *Medicine* 1994;14:677.
2. Bick RL, Murano G. Physiology of hemostasis. In: Bick RL, Bennett JM, Brynes RK, eds. *Hematology: clinical and laboratory practice.* St. Louis: Mosby, 1993:98.
3. Bick RL. Physiology of hemostasis. In: *Disorders of thrombosis and hemostasis: clinical and laboratory practice.* Chicago: ASCP Press, 1992:1.
4. Bick RL. Basic physiology of hemostasis and thrombosis. In: Bick RL, ed. *Disorders of hemostasis and thrombosis: principles of clinical practice.* New York: Thieme, 1985:1.
5. Nawroth PP, Stern DM. Endothelial cell procoagulant properties and the host response. *Semin Thromb Hemost* 1987;13:391.
6. Harker LA, Ross R. Pathogenesis of arterial vascular disease. *Semin Thromb Hemost* 1979;5:274.
7. Schoen FJ. Blood vessels. In: Cotran RS, Kumar V, Robbins SL, eds. *Pathologic basis of disease.* Philadelphia: WB Saunders, 1994:467.
8. Fareed J, Walenga JM, Bick RL, et al. Impact of automation on the quantitation of low molecular weight markers of hemostatic defects. *Semin Thromb Hemost* 1983;9:355.
9. Henry RL. Platelet function in hemostasis. In: Murano G, Bick

RL, eds. *Basic concepts of hemostasis and thrombosis.* Boca Raton, Fla: CRC Press, 1980:17.
10. Bick RL. Platelet function defects. *Semin Thromb Hemost* 1992; 18:167.
11. Walsh P. The effect of collagen and kaolin on the intrinsic coagulation activity of platelets: evidence for an alternative pathway in intrinsic coagulation not requiring factor XII. *Br J Haematol* 1972;22:393.
12. Wilner GD, Nossel HL, LeRoy EL. Activation of Hageman factor by collagen. *J Clin Invest* 1968;47:2608.
13. Muller-Berghaus G. Pathophysiologic and biochemical events in disseminated intravascular coagulation: dysregulation of procoagulant and anticoagulant pathways. *Semin Thromb Hemost* 1989;15:58.
14. Ruggeri ZM Zimmerman TS. von Willebrand factor and von Willebrand disease. *Blood* 1987;70:895.
15. Zimmerman TS, Ruggeri ZM. von Willebrand disease. *Hum Pathol* 1987;18:140.
16. Fareed J, Bick RL, Hoppensteadt D, et al. Molecular markers of hemostasis activation: implications in the diagnosis of thrombosis, vascular and cardiovascular disorders: clinics lab. *Medicine* 1995;15:39.
17. Astrup T. Fibrinolysis: past and present: a reflection of fifty years. *Semin Thromb Hemost* 1991;17:161.
18. Mullertz S. Fibrinolysis: an overview. *Semin Thromb Hemost* 1984;10:1.
19. Lazarus GS, Jensen PJ. Plasminogen activators in epithelial biology. *Semin Thromb Hemost* 1991;17:210.
20. Mammen EF. Inhibitor abnormalities. *Semin Thromb Hemost* 1983;9:42.
21. Weibel ER, Palade GE. New cytoplasmic components in arterial endothelia. *J Cell Biol* 1964;23:101.
22. Ewenstein BM, Warhol MJ, Handin RI, et al. Composition of the von Willebrand factor storage organelle (Weibel-Palade body) isolated form cultured human umbilical vein endothelial cells. *J Cell Biol* 1987;104:1423.
23. McEver RP, Beckstead JH, Moore KL, et al. GMP-140, a platelet-granule membrane protein, is also synthesized by vascular endothelium and is localized in Weibel-Palade bodies. *J Clin Invest* 1989;84:92.
24. Hattori R, Hamilton KK, McEver RP, et al. Complement proteins C5b-9 induce secretion of high molecular weight multimers of endothelial von Willebrand factor and translocation of granule membrane protein GMP-140 to the cell surface. *J Biol Chem* 1989;264:9053.
25. Tannenbaum SH, Gralnick HR. γ-Interferon modulates von Willebrand factor release by cultured human endothelial cells. *Blood* 1990;75:2177.
26. Haller H. Endothelial function: general considerations. *Drugs* 1997;53(suppl 1):1.
27. Dosquet C, Weill D, Wautier JL. Cytokines and thrombosis. *J Cardiovasc Pharmacol* 1995;25(suppl 2):13.
28. Rabiet MJ, Plantier JL, Dejana E. Thrombin-induced endothelial cell dysfunction. *Br Med Bull* 1994;50:936.
29. Ireland H, Kyriakoulis K, Lane DA. Thrombomodulin gene mutations. *Haemostasis* 1996;26(suppl 4):227.
30. Bourin MC, Lunfgren-Akerlund E, Lindhal U. Isolation and characterization of the glycosaminoglycan component of rabbit thrombomodulin proteoglycan. *J Biol Chem* 1990;265: 15424.
31. Esmon CT. The roles of protein C and thrombomodulin in the regulation of blood coagulation. *J Biol Chem* 1989;264:4743.
32. Barnhart MI, Chen ST. Vessel wall models for studying interaction capabilities with blood platelets. *Semin Thromb Hemost* 1978;5:112.
33. Bick RL. Basic mechanisms of hemostasis pertaining to DIC. In: Bick RL, ed. *Disseminated intravascular coagulation and related syndromes.* Boca Raton, Fla: CRC Press, 1983:1.
34. Kehrel B. Platelet-collagen interactions. *Semin Thromb Hemost* 1995;21:123.
35. Ulutin ON. Atherosclerosis and hemostasis. *Semin Thromb Hemost* 1986;12:156.
36. Ruf A, Morgenstern E. Ultrastructural aspects of platelet adhesion on subendothelial structures. *Semin Thromb Hemost* 1995; 21:119.
37. Engelberg H. Endothelium in health and disease. *Semin Thromb Hemost* 1989;15:178.
38. Henry RL. Platelet function. *Semin Thromb Hemost* 1977;4:93.
39. Henry RL. Platelet function in hemostasis. In: Murano G, Bick RL, eds. *Basic concepts of hemostasis and thrombosis.* Boca Raton, FL: CRC Press, 1980:17.
40. Hensby CN, Lewis PJ, Hilgard P, et al. Prostacyclin deficiency in thrombotic thrombocytopenic purpura. *Lancet* 1979;2:748.
41. Hinman JW. Prostaglandins. *Annual Rev Biochem* 1972;41:161.
42. Nachman RL. Platelet proteins. *Semin Hematol* 1968;5:18.
43. Seegers WH. Enzymes in blood clotting. *J Med Enzymol* 1977; 2:68.
46. Davis RB, Mecker WR, Bailey WL. Serotonin release after injection of *E. coli* endotoxin in the rabbit. *Fed Proc* 1961;20: 261.
47. Des Prez RM, Horowitz HI, Hook EW. Effects of bacterial endotoxin on rabbit platelets, I: platelet aggregation and release of platelet factors in vitro. *J Exp Med* 1961;114:857.
48. Mueller-Eckhardt C, Luscher EF. Immune reactions of human blood platelets, I: a comparative study on the effects on platelets of heterologous antiplatelet antiserum, antigen-antibody complexes, aggregation gamma-globulin, and thrombin. *Thromb Diath Haemorrh* 1968;20:155.
49. Pfueller SL, Luscher EF. The effects of immune complexes on blood and their relationship to complement activation. *Immunochemistry* 1972;9:1151.
50. Brodie GN, Bienziger NL, Chase LR. The effects of thrombin on adenylcyclase activity and a membrane protein from platelets. *J Clin Invest* 1972;51:81.
51. Haslam RJ. Interactions of the pharmacological receptors of blood platelets with adenylate cyclase. *Ser Haematol* 1973;6: 333.
52. Salzman EW. Cyclic AMP and platelet function. *N Engl J Med* 1972;286:358.
53. Cole B, Robison GA, Hartman RC. Effects of prostaglandin E and theophylline on aggregation and cyclic AMP levels of human blood platelets. *Fed Proc* 1970;29:316.
54. Horlington M, Watson PA. Inhibition of 3′5′-cyclic-AMP, phosphodiesterase by some platelet aggregation inhibitors. *Biochem Pharmacol* 1970;19:955.
55. Gerrard JM, White JG. Prostaglandins and thromboxanes: "middlemen"modulating platelet function in hemostasis and thrombosis. *Prog Hemost Thromb* 1978;4:87.
56. Nalbandian RM, Henry RL. Platelet-endothelial cell interactions: metabolic maps of structure and actions of prostaglandins, prostacyclin, thromboxane, and cyclic AMP. *Semin Thromb Hemost* 1979;5:87.
57. Day CE. On the newly discovered role of prostaglandins in arteries and its implications for the control of athero-sclerosis, platelets, and thrombosis. *Artery* 1976;2:480.
58. Gryglewski RJ, Bunting S, Moncada S, et al. Arterial walls are protected against deposition of platelet thrombi by a substance (prostaglandin X) which they make from prostaglandin endoperoxides. *Prostaglandins* 1976;12:685.
59. Moncada S, Gryglewski R, Bunting S, et al. A lipid peroxide inhibits the enzyme in blood vessel microsomes that generate from prostaglandin endoperoxides the substance prostaglandin

x) which prevents platelet aggregation. *Prostaglandins* 1976;12: 715.
60. Breddin HK. Antiplatelet agents in cardiovascular and cerebrovascular disease. *Clin Appl Thromb Hemost* 1998;4:87.
61. Gerrard JM, White JG. Prostaglandins and thromboxanes: "middlemen" modulating platelet function in hemostasis and thrombosis. *Prog Hemostas Thromb* 1978;4:87.
62. Berndt MC, Caen JP. Platelet glycoproteins. *Prog Hemost Thromb* 1984;7:111.
63. Nurden AT. Polymorphisms of human platelet membrane glycoproteins: structural and clinical significance. *Thromb Haemost* 1995;4:345.
64. Davies GE, Palek J. Platelet protein organization: analysis by treatment with membrane-permeable cross-linking reagents. *Blood* 1982;59:502.
65. Berndt MC, Gregory C, Chong CH. Additional glycoprotein defects in Bernard-Soulier syndrome: confirmation of genetic basis by parental analysis. *Blood* 1983;62:800.
66. Clemetson KJ, McGregor JL, James E. Characterization of the platelet membrane glycoprotein abnormalities in Bernard-Soulier syndrome and comparison with normal by surface-labeled techniques and high-resolution two-dimensional gel electrophoresis. *J Clin Invest* 1982;70:304.
67. Meyer D, Baumgartner HR. Role of von Willebrand factor in platelet adhesion to the subendothelium. *Br J Haematol* 1983; 54:1.
68. Kunicki TJ, Russell N, Nurden AT. Further studies of the human platelet receptor for quinine and quinidine-dependent antibodies. *J Immunol* 1981;126:398.
69. Berendt MC, Phillips DR. Interaction of thrombin with platelets: purification of the thrombin substrate. *Ann N Y Acad Sci* 1981;370:87.
70. Gogstad GO, Hagen J, Korsmo R. Characterization of the proteins of isolated human platelet alpha granules, evidence for a separate alpha granule pool of the glycoproteins IIb and IIIa. *Biochim Biophys Acta* 1981;670:150.
71. Fujimura K, Phillips DR. Binding of Ca^{++} to glycoprotein IIb from human platelet plasma membranes. *Thromb Haemost* 1983;50:251.
72. White JG. Inherited disorders of the platelet membrane and secretory granules. *Hum Pathol* 1987;18:123.
73. McMillan R, Mason D, Tani P. Evaluation of platelet surface antigens: localization of the pla1 alloantigen. *Br J Haematol* 1981;51:297.
74. Lawler J, Hynes RO. Structural organization of the thrombospondin molecule. *Semin Thromb Hemost* 1987;13:245.
75. Santoro SA. Thrombospondin and the adhesive behavior of platelets. *Semin Thromb Hemost* 1987;13:290.
76. Phillips DR, Charo IF, Parise LV, et al. The platelet membrane glycoprotein IIb/IIIa complex. *Blood* 1988;71:831.
77. Shattil SJ, Hoxie JA, Cunningham M, et al. Changes in the platelet membrane glycoprotein IIb-IIIa complex during platelet activation. *J Biol Chem* 1985;260:11107.
78. Michelson AD. Flow cytometry: a clinical test of platelet function. *Blood* 1996;87:4925.
79. Michelson AD, Wencel-Drake JD, Kestin AS, et al. Platelet activation results in a redistribution of glycoprotein IV (CD 36). *Atheroscler Thromb* 1994;14:1193.
80. Mickelson AD, Benoit SE, Furman MI, et al. The platelet surface expression of glycoprotein V is regulated by two independent mechanisms: proteolysis and a reversible cytoskeletal-mediated redistribution to the surface-connected canalicular system. *Blood* 1996;87:1396.
81. Bick RL. Disseminated intravascular coagulation: pathophysiological mechanisms and manifestations. *Semin Thromb Hemost* 1998;24:3.
82. Colman RW, Bagdasarian A, Talamo RC, et al. Williams trait: human kininogen deficiency with diminished levels of plasminogen proactivator and prekallikrein associated with abnormalities of the Hageman factor dependent pathway. *J Clin Invest* 1975;56:1650.
83. van Iwaarden F, Bouma BN. Role of high molecular weight kininogen in contact activation. *Semin Thromb Hemost* 1987;13:15.
84. Murano G. The "Hageman connection" interrelationships of blood coagulation, fibrino(geno)lysis, kinin generation, and complement activation. *Am J Hematol* 1978;4:303.
85. McKusick VA. Mendelian inheritance. In: *Man: catalogs of autosomal dominant, autosomal recessive and X-linked phenotypes.* 9th ed. Baltimore: Johns Hopkins University Press, 1990.
86. Schriver CR, Beaudet AL, Sly WS. Blood and blood forming tissue (Part 14). In: McKusick VA, ed. *The metabolic basis of inherited disease.* New York: McGraw-Hill, 1989:2107.
87. Kaplan AJ, Meier HL, Mandle R. The Hageman factor dependent pathways of coagulation, fibrinolysis, and kinin-generation. *Semin Thromb Hemost* 1976;3:1.
88. Kaplan AP. Initiation of the intrinsic coagulation and fibrinolytic pathways of man: the role of surfaces, Hageman factor, prekallikrein, high molecular weight kininogen, and factor XI. *Prog Hemost Thromb* 1978;4:127.
89. Meyer KL, Pierce JV, Coleman RW, et al. Activation and function of human Hageman factor. *J Clin Invest* 1977;60:18.
90. Ratnoff OD, Saito H. Coagulation factors and the role of surfaces in their activation. *Ann N Y Acad Sci* 1977;283:88.
91. Griffin JH, Cochrane CG. Recent advances in the understanding of contact activation reactions. *Semin Thromb Hemost* 1979; 5:254.
92. Wiggins RC, Bouma BN, Cochrane CG, et al. Role of high-molecular weight kininogen in surface-binding and activation of coagulation factor XI and prekallikrein. *Proc Natl Acad Sci U S A* 1977;74:4636.
93. Ofosu FA. Anticoagulant actions of tissue factor pathway inhibitor on tissue-factor-dependent plasma coagulation. *Semin Thromb Hemost* 1995;21:240.
94. Jesty J, Wun TC, Lorenz A. Kinetics of the inhibition of factor Xa and the tissue factor- factor VIIa complex by tissue factor pathway inhibitor in the presence and absence of heparin. *Biochemistry* 1994;33:12686.
95. Bach RR. Initiation of coagulation by tissue factor. *CRC Crit Rev Biochem* 1988;23:339.
96. Wada H, Wakita Y, Shiku H. Tissue factor expression in endothelial cells in health and disease. *Blood Coagul Fibrinolysis* 1995;6(suppl 1):26.
97. Osterud B. Cellular interactions in tissue factor expression by blood monocytes. *Blood Coagul Fibrinolysis* 1995;6(suppl 1):20.
98. Osterud B, Berre A, Otnaess B, et al. Activation of the coagulation factor VII by tissue thromboplastin and calcium. *Biochemistry* 1972;11:2853.
99. Broze GJ, Leykam JE, Schwartz BD, et al. Purification of human brain tissue factor. *J Biol Chem* 1981;256:8324.
100. Colluci M, Balconi G, Lorenzet R, et al. Cultured human endothelial cells generate tissue factor in response to endotoxin. *J Clin Invest* 1983;71:1893.
101. Brox JH, Osterud B, Bjorklid E, et al. Production and availability of thromboplastin in endothelial cells: the effects of thrombin, endotoxin, and platelets. *Br J Haematol* 1984;57:239.
102. Ikeda K, Nagasawa K, Horiuchi T, et al. C5a induces tissue factor activity on endothelial cells. *Thromb Haemost* 1997;77:394.
103. Rapaport SI. Regulation of the tissue factor pathway. *Ann N Y Acad Sci* 1991;614:151.
104. Kirshnaswamy S. The interaction of human factor Va with tissue factor. *J Biol Chem* 1992;267:23696.
105. Edgington TE, Mackman N, Brand K, et al. The structural

biology of expression and function of tissue factor. *Thromb Haemost* 1991;66:67.
106. Sanders NL, Bajaj SP, Zivelin A, et al. Inhibition of tissue factor/factor VIIa activity in plasma requires factor X and an additional plasma component. *Blood* 1985;66:204.
107. Girard TJ, Warren LA, Novotny WF, et al. Functional significance of the Kunitz-type inhibitory domains of lipoprotein-associated coagulation inhibitor. *Nature* 1989;338:518.
108. Enjyoji K, Miyata T, Kamikubo Y, et al. Effect of heparin on the inhibition of factor Xa by tissue factor pathway inhibitor: a segment, Gly212-Phe243, of the third Kunitz domain is a heparin-binding site. *Biochemistry* 1995;34:5725.
109. Valentin S, Nordfang O, Bregengard C, et al. Evidence that the C-terminus of tissue factor pathway inhibitor (TFPI) is essential for its in vitro and in vivo interaction with lipoproteins. *Blood Coagul Fibrinolysis* 1993;4:713.
110. Broze G J. The role of tissue factor pathway inhibitor in a revised coagulation cascade. *Semin Hematol* 1992;29:159.
111. Morrison SA, Jesty J. Tissue factor-dependent activation of tritium-labeled factor IX and factor X in human plasma. *Blood* 1984;63:1338.
112. Hubbard AR, Jennings CA. Inhibition of the tissue factor-factor VII complex: involvement of factor Xa and lipoproteins. *Thromb Res* 1987;46:527.
113. Nordfang O, Bjorn SE, Valentin S, et al. The C-terminus of tissue factor pathway inhibitor is essential to its anticoagulant activity. *Biochemistry* 1991;30:10371.
114. Bick RL, Fareed J, Walenga J, et al. Heparin releasable tissue factor pathway inhibitor during interventional cardiovascular procedures. *Blood* 1994;84:81.
115. Seegers WH, Murano G. Blood coagulation: a cybernetic system. *Pol Arch Med Wewn* 1976;55:1.
116. Seegers WH, Hassouna HI, Hewett-Emmett D, et al. Prothrombin and thrombin: selected aspects of thrombin formation, properties, inhibition, and immunology. *Semin Thromb Hemost* 1975;1:211.
117. Seegers WH, Sakuragawa N, McCoy, et al. Prothrombin activation: ac-globulin, lipid, platelet membrane, and autoprothrombin C (Xa) requirements. *Thromb Res* 1972;1:293.
118. Seegers WH. Prothrombin complex. *Semin Thromb Hemost* 1981;7:291.
119. Denson KWE. The levels of factor II, VII, IX, and X by antibody neutralization techniques in the plasma of patients receiving phenindione therapy. *Br J Haematol* 1971;20:643.
120. Pereira M, Couri D. Studies on the site of action of dicoumarol on prothrombin synthesis. *Biochim Biophys Acta* 1971;237:348.
121. Stenflo T. Vitamin K, prothrombin, and gamma-carboxy-glutamic acid. *N Engl J Med* 1977;296:624.
122. Mackie MJ, Douglas AS. Drug-induced disorders of coagulation. In: Ratnoff OD, Forbes CD, eds. *Disorders of hemostasis.* Philadelphia: WB Saunders, 1991:493.
123. Huseby RM. Conformational structure of the fibrinopeptides related during fibrinogen to fibrin conversion. *Physiol Chem Phys* 1973;5:1.
124. Stubbs MT, Bode W. A model for the specificity of fibrinogen cleavage by thrombin. *Semin Thromb Hemost* 1993;19:344.
125. Seitz R, McDonagh J, Egbring R. Factor XIII: state of the art: 1996. *Semin Thromb Hemost* 1996;22:367.
126. Ratnoff OD. The molecular basis of hereditary clotting disorders. *Prog Hemost Thromb* 1972;1:39.
127. Seegers WH. Fibrinogen. *Semin Thromb Hemost* 1981;7:281.
128. Winman B, Hamsten A. The fibrinolytic enzyme system and its role in the etiology of thromboembolic disease. *Semin Thromb Hemost* 1990;16:207.
129. Aoki N, Harpel PC. Inhibitors of the fibrinolytic enzyme system. *Semin Thromb Hemost* 1984;10:24.
130. Bick RL. The clinical significance of fibrinogen degradation products. *Semin Thromb Hemost* 1982;8:302.
131. Castellino FJ. Biochemistry of human plasminogen. *Semin Thromb Hemost* 1984;10:18.
132. Mullertz S. Fibrinolysis: an overview. *Semin Thromb Hemost* 1984;10:1.
133. Bick RL. Disseminated intravascular coagulation. In: Brubaker DB, Simpson MB, eds. *Dynamics of hemostasis and thrombosis.* Bethesda, MD: American Association of Blood Banks, 1995.
134. Bick RL, Arun B, Frenkel EP. Disseminated intravascular coagulation: clinical and pathophysiological mechanisms and manifestations. *Haemostasis* 1999;29:111–134.
135. Ratnoff OD, GB Naff. The conversion of C′1s to C′1 esterase by plasmin and trypsin. *J Exp Med* 1967;125:337.
136. Robbins KM. Present status of the fibrinolytic system. In: Fareed J, Messmore HL, Fenton J, et al., eds. *Perspectives in hemostasis.* New York: Pergamon Press, 1980:53.
137. Bachmann F, Kruithof KO. Tissue plasminogen activator: chemical and physiological aspects. *Semin Thromb Hemost* 1984;10:6.
138. Kaplan AP, Austin F. The fibrinolytic pathway of human plasma: isolation and characterization of the plasminogen proactivator. *J Exp Med* 1972;135:1378.
139. Robbins KC, Barlow GH, Hguyen G. Comparison of plasminogen activators. *Semin Thromb Hemost* 1987;13:131.
140. Bell WR. Thrombolytic therapy: agents, indications, and laboratory monitoring. *Med Clin North Am* 1994;78:745.
141. Stump DC, Taylor FB, Neshein ME. Pathologic fibrinolysis as a cause of clinical bleeding. *Semin Thromb Hemost* 1990;16: 260.
142. Goldsmith GN, Saito H, Ratnoff OD. The activation of plasminogen by Hageman factor (factor XII) and Hageman factor fragments. *J Clin Invest* 1978;21:54.
143. Kaplan AP, Austen KF. A prealbumin activator of pre-kallikrein, II: derivation of activators of prekallikrein from active Hageman factor by digestion with plasmin. *J Exp Med* 1971;133:696.
144. Schreiber AD. Plasma inhibitors of the Hageman factor dependent pathways. *Semin Thromb Hemost* 1976;3:43.
145. Loskutoff DJ, Sawdey M, Mimuro J. Type 1 plasminogen activator inhibitor. *Prog Hemost Thromb* 1989;9:87.
146. Astedt B, Lecander I, Ny T. The placental type plasminogen activator inhibitor: PAI-2 *Fibrinolysis* 1987;1:203.
147. Erickson LA, Ginsberg MH, Loskutoff D. Detection and partial characterization of an inhibitor of plasminogen activator in human platelets. *J Clin Invest* 1984;74:1465.
148. Kudryk B, Collen D, Woods KR, et al. Evidence for localization of polymerization sites in fibrinogen. *J Biol Chem* 1974;249: 3322.
149. Murano G. The molecular structure of fibrinogen. *Semin Thromb Hemost* 1974;1:1.
150. Kowalski E. Fibrinogen derivatives and their biological activity. *Semin Hematol* 1968;5:45.
151. Marder VJ, Shulman NP. High molecular weight derivatives of human fibrinogen produced by plasmin: mechanism of their anticoagulant activity. *J Biol Chem* 1969;244:2120.
152. Rosse WF. Complement. In: Williams WJ, Beutler E, Erslev AJ, et al., eds. *Hematology.* New York: McGraw-Hill, 1977:87.
153. Ruddy S, Gigli I, Austen KF. The complement system in man, I: activation, control, and products of the reaction sequences. *N Engl J Med* 1972;278:489.
154. Coltyen HR. Complement deficiencies. *Annu Rev Immunol* 1992;10:809.
155. Liszewski MK, Faries TC, Lublin DM. Control of the complement system. *Adv Immunol* 1996;61:201.
156. Reid KBM, Porter RR. The proteolytic activation systems of complement. *Annu Rev Biochem* 1981;50:433.

157. Muller-Eberhard HJ, Schreiber RD. Molecular biology and chemistry of the alternative pathway of complement. *Adv Immunol* 1980;29:1.
158. Saito H. Contact factors in health and disease. *Semin Thromb Hemost* 1987;13:36.
159. Ryan JW, Ryan US. Biochemical and morphological aspects of the actions and metabolism of kinins. In: Pisano JJ, Austen KF, eds. *Chemistry and biology of the kallikrein-kinin system in health and disease. DHEW Pub 76-791.* Bethesda, Md: U.S. Department of Health, Education, and Welfare, 1974:315.
160. Van Arman CG, Bohidar HR. Role of the kallikrein-kinin system in inflammation. In: Pisano JJ, Austin KF, eds. *Chemistry and biology of the kallikrein-kinin system in health and disease.* DHEW Publ 76-791. Bethesda, Md: U.S. Department of Health, Education and Welfare, 1974:471.
161. Bick RL, Kaplan H. Syndromes of thrombosis and hypercoagulability: congenital and acquired thrombophilias. *Clin Appl Thromb Hemost* 1998;4:25.
162. Bertina RM. Hypercoagulable states. *Semin Hematol* 1997;34:167.
163. Joist JH. Hypercoagulability: introduction and perspective. *Semin Thromb Hemost* 1990;16:151.
164. Esmon CT. Protein C: biochemistry, physiology, and clinical implications. *Blood* 1983;62:1155.
165. Seegers WH. Protein C and autoprothrombin II-A. *Semin Thromb Hemost* 1981;7:257.
166. Scully MF, Ellis V, Kakkar VV. Studies of anti-Xa activity. *Thromb Res* 1983;29:387.
167. Bick RL. Clinical relevance of antithrombin III. *Semin Thromb Hemost* 1982;8:276.
168. Rosenberg RD. The effect of heparin on factor XIa and plasmin. *Thromb Diath Haemorrh* 1975;33:51.
169. Rosenberg RD, Damus P. The purification and mechanism of action of human antithrombin-heparin cofactor. *J Biol Chem* 1973;248:6490.
170. Seegers WH. Antithrombin III. *Semin Thromb Hemost* 1981;7:263.
171. Jaques LB, McDuffie NM. The chemical and anticoagulant nature of heparin. *Semin Thromb Hemost* 1978;4:277.
172. Rosenberg RD. Biologic actions of heparin. *Semin Hematol* 1977;14:427.
173. Seegers WH. Antithrombin-III: theory and clinical applications. *Am J Clin Pathol* 1978;69:367.
174. Walker FJ. Protein S and the regulation of protein C. *Semin Thromb Hemost* 1984;10:131.
175. Mosseson MW. Cold-insoluble globulin (CIg): a circulating cell surface protein. *Thromb Haemost* 1977;38:742.
176. Pearlstein E, Gold LI, Garcia Pardo A. Fibronectin: a review of its structure and biological activity. *Mol Cell Biochem* 1980;29:103.
177. Couchman JR, Austria MR, Woods A. Fibronectin-cell interactions. *J Invest Dermatol* 1990;94:7.
178. Moser DF. Fibronectin. *Prog Hemost Thromb* 1980;5:111.
179. Zucker MB, Mosesson M, Broekman M, et al. Release of platelet fibronectin (cold-insoluble globulin) from alpha granules induced by thrombin or collagen: lack of requirement for plasma fibronectin in ADP-induced platelet aggregation. *Blood* 1979;54:8.
180. Moser DF, Schad PE, Kleinman HK. Cross-linking of fibronectin to collagen by blood coagulation factor XIIIa. *J Clin Invest* 1979;64:781.
181. Mosseson MW, Umfleet RA. The cold-insoluble globulin of plasma. *J Biol Chem* 1970;254:5728.
182. Mosher DF. Organization of the provisional fibronectin matrix: control by products of blood coagulation. *Thromb Haemost* 1995;74:529.
183. Marcum JA, Rosenberg RD Anticoagulantly active heparan sulfate proteogylcan and the vascular endothelium. *Semin Thromb Hemost* 1987;13:464.
184. Bick RL. Pathophysiology of hemostasis and thrombosis. In: Sodeman WA, Sodeman TA, eds. *Pathologic physiology: mechanisms of disease.* 7th ed. Philadelphia: WB Saunders, 1984:705.
185. Goldstein IM, Perez HD. Biologically active peptides derived from the fifth component of complement. *Prog Hemost Thromb* 1980;5:41.
186. Lisiewicz J. Disseminated intravascular coagulation in acute leukemia. *Semin Thromb Hemost* 1988;14:339.
187. Galloway MJ, Mackie MJ, McVerry BJ. Combinations of increased thrombin, plasmin, and non-specific protease activity in patients with acute leukemia. *Haemostasis* 1983;13:322.
188. Cerletti C, Evangelista V, de Gaetano G. Platelet-polymorphonuclear leukocyte functional interactions: role of adhesion molecules. *Haemostasis* 1996;26(suppl 4):20.
189. Stuhlmeier KM, Tarn C, Czizadia V, et al. Selective suppression of endothelial cell activation by arachidonic acid. *Eur J Immunol* 1996;26:1417.
190. Howiger J. Mechanisms involved in platelet vessel wall interaction. *Thromb Haemost* 1995;74:369.
191. Bevilacqua MP, Nelson RM. Selectins. *J Clin Invest* 1993;91:379.
192. Bevilacqua MP, Stengelin S, Gimbrone MA. Endothelial leukocyte adhesion molecule-1: an inducible receptor for neutrophils related to complement regulatory proteins and lectins. *Science* 1989;243:1160.
193. Phillips ML, Nudelman E, Gaeta FC. ELAM-1 mediates cell adhesion by recognition of a carbohydrate ligand, sialyl-Lex. *Science* 1990;250:1130.
194. Verrier E. The microvascular cell and ischemia-reperfusion injury. *J Cardiovasc Pharmacol* 1996;27(suppl 1):26.
195. Hsu-Lin SC, Berman CL, Furie B. A platelet membrane protein expressed during platelet activation and secretion. *J Biol Chem* 1984;259:9121.
196. Bonfanti R, Furie BC, Furie B. PADGEM (GMP-140) is a component of the Weibel-Palade bodies of human endothelial cells. *Blood* 1989;73:1109.
197. Larsen E, Celi A, Gilbert G. PADGEM protein: a receptor that mediates the interaction of activated platelets with neutrophils and monocytes. *Cell* 1989;59:305.
198. Stenberg PE, McEver RP, Shuman MA. A platelet alpha-granule membrane protein (GMP-140) is expressed on the plasma membrane after activation. *J Cell Biol* 1985;101:880.
199. Gibson RM, Kansan GS, Tedder TM. The lectin and EGF domains of P-selectin at physiological density are the recognition unit for leukocyte binding. *Blood* 1995;85:150.
200. Larsen GR, Sako D, Ahern TJ. P-selectin and E-selectin: distinct but overlapping leukocyte ligand specificity. *J Biol Chem* 1992;267:11104.
201. Bowen BR, Nguyen T, Lasky LA. Characterization of a human homologue of the murine peripheral lymph node homing receptor. *J Cell Biol* 1989;109:421.
202. Tedder TF, Isaacs CM, Ernst TJ. Isolation and chromosomal localization of cDNAs encoding a novel human lymphocyte cell surface molecule LAM-1: homology with the mouse lymphocyte homing receptor and other human adhesion proteins. *J Exp Med* 1989;170:123.
203. Hynes HO. Integrins, versatility, modulation and signaling in cell adhesion. *Cell* 1992;69:11.
204. Williams MJ, Du X, Loftus JC, et al. Platelet adhesion receptors. *Semin Cell Biol* 1995;6:305.
205. Arnaout MA. Structure and function of the leukocytes adhesion molecule CD11/CD18. *Blood* 1990;75:1037.
206. Springer TS. Traffic signals for lymphocyte recirculation and

leukocyte emigration: the multistep paradigm. *Cell* 1994;76: 314.
207. Ruegg C, Postigo AA., Sikorski EE. The role of integrin α4β1 in lymphocyte adherence to fibronectin and VCAM-1 and in homotypic cell clustering. *J Cell Biol* 1992;17:179.
208. Staunton DE, Dustin ML, Springer TA. Functional cloning of ICAM-2, a cell adhesion ligand for LFA-1 homologous to ICAM-1. *Nature* 1989;339:61.
209. Diamond MS, Staunton D, Marlin SD. Binding of the integrin MAC-1 (CD11b/CD18) to the third immunoglobulin domain of ICAM-1 (CD54) and its regulation by glycosylation. *Cell* 1991;65:961.
210. Wachtfogel YT, De La Gardena RA, Kunapuli SP. High molecular weight kininogen binds to MAC-1 on neutrophils by its heavy chain (domain 3) and its light chain (domain 5). *J Biol Chem* 1994;269:19307.
211. Molino M, Blanchard N, Belmonte E. Proteolysis of the human platelet and endothelial cell thrombin receptor by neutrophil derived cathepsin. *J Biol Chem* 1995;270:11168.
212. Kelly SJ, Adams SA, Robson SC. Fibrinogenolysis by a neutrophil membrane protease generates an Aα 1-21 fragment. *Biochem J* 1994;298:689.
213. Loike JD, Sodeik B, Cao L. CD11c/CD18 on neutrophils recognizes a domain at the N-terminus of the Aα chain of fibrinogen. *Proc Natl Acad Sci U S A* 1991;88:1104.
214. Celi A, Lorenzet R, Furie B, et al. Platelet-leukocyte-endothelial cell interaction on the blood vessel wall. *Semin Hematol* 1997; 34:327.
215. Dosquet C, Weill D, Wautier JL. Cytokines and thrombosis. *J Cardiovasc Pharmacol* 1995;25(suppl 2):13.
216. Gillis S, Furie BC, Furie B. Interactions of neutrophils and coagulation proteins. *Semin Hematol* 1997;34:336.

Disorders of Thrombosis and Hemostasis: Clinical and Laboratory Practice, Third Edition, edited by Rodger L. Bick.
Lippincott Williams & Wilkins, Philadelphia © 2002

2

CLINICAL ASSESSMENT OF PATIENTS WITH HEMORRHAGE

RODGER L. BICK

Disorders of hemostasis are common and found in all areas of pathophysiology and clinical medicine. Although many disorders leading to hemorrhage are forthright, many are multifaceted and quite complex with respect to pathophysiology, diagnosis, and management. Disorders of hemostasis associated with bleeding can be divided into hereditary and acquired, with acquired defects being more common than hereditary defects. All hereditary and acquired defects can, moreover, be compartmentalized into defects of the vasculature, defects of platelets, or defects of coagulation proteins. Generally the inherited defects of hemostasis tend to be simple, restricted to one hemostasis compartment, and commonly to one coagulation protein, particularly in most cases of coagulation protein disorders. In contrast, acquired disorders of hemostasis tend to be multifaceted in etiology and in pathophysiology and involve more than one coagulation factor and frequently involve two or all three hemostatic compartments. In assessment of a patient with bleeding or a bleeding history, a methodical and attentive approach to diagnosis is obligatory; my approach is outlined in this chapter.

OBTAINING THE HISTORY

In extracting a current medical history from the patient, we traditionally solicit the chief complaint first by asking the patient to summarize the reason(s) he or she was referred. Precisely who uncovered this disorder and the date the condition was found is important. It also is mandatory to ascertain whether any therapy, including blood or blood products, was administered for the condition; often a patient will be referred for evaluation of a hemostatic problem, and it is found that the patient has recently been transfused with whole blood, fresh-frozen plasma, or other blood components, potentially modifying laboratory results yet to be obtained. The initial encounter with the patient should involve a brief description of the problem(s) in as precise a manner as possible, including a depiction of the primary symptoms and a description of how long the problem has been present. Next, query the patient about all other medical conditions that have been diagnosed and are currently being treated. Regarding this part of the history, a specific drug history is of extreme importance, and all drugs and doses regularly ingested by the patient should be elicited and recorded. Specific attention should be paid to obtaining a history of the ingestion of aspirin, aspirin-containing compounds, antihypertensives, cough medications, digitalis preparations, hormones, cortisone, insulin, diabetes medications, thyroid medications, narcoleptics, analgesics, weight-reducing medications, anticoagulants, dilantin, diuretics, antibiotics, barbiturates, tranquilizers, oral contraceptives, or any type of antidepressant. Particular attention should be paid to drugs interfering with hemostasis, especially platelet function. If the patient is not currently taking any of these medications, a history of former ingestion also should be obtained.

A comprehensive past medical history should be obtained, including a past medical history of childhood illnesses including mumps, measles, chicken pox, rheumatic fever or scarlet fever, and other illnesses including coronary artery disease, heart disease of any type, hypertension, diabetes mellitus, emphysema, recurrent bronchitis, recurrent pneumonia, asthma, tuberculosis, herpes zoster, hepatitis, peptic ulcer disease, liver disease, jaundice, renal disease, hives, venereal disease, anemia, seizures, or mental disease. A rigorous history also should be taken with respect to the type of bleeding the patient has experienced, especially if it has occurred spontaneously. For example, detailed inquiries should be made with respect to the development of petechiae or purpura, to find out whether bruises are spontaneous or accounted for, and to detect if there was a childhood history of epistaxis, umbilical stump bleeding, gingival bleeding with tooth brushing, or easy and spontaneous bruising during earlier years. A thorough past surgical history also should be taken, and the asso-

R. L. Bick: Department of Medicine and Pathology, University of Texas Southwest Medical Center; Dallas Thrombosis/Hemostasis Clinical Center; ThromboCare Laboratories, Dallas, Texas.

ciation of bleeding, or the necessity of blood transfusions should be clarified for each particular surgical procedure. In addition, questions regarding past trauma or dental extraction and associated bleeding and the necessity of transfusions should be asked. The patient also should be specifically asked regarding transfusion reactions or any type of untoward experience occurring with respect to transfusions; it may be expected that the patient, if truly demonstrating a bleeding problem, may require transfusions of one type or another eventually. The patient should be asked about serious injuries or accidents, especially those that have called for hospitalization, and the presence of, and nature of, any particular bleeding associated with injuries or accidents should be noted. The patient should be subjected to a careful allergic history, with particular attention to allergies to any medications.

Next a specific review of systems should be performed, including a meticulous history concerning the type, site, and severity of any bleeding problems, including, as mentioned, the presence or absence of petechiae, purpura, easy or spontaneous bruising, gingival bleeding with tooth brushing, epistaxis, especially bilateral or during childhood, the noting of spontaneous petechiae or purpura, and the development of any mucosal membrane bleeding including gastrointestinal bleeding, genitourinary bleeding, hemoptysis, or blood-tinged sputum. A history of any type of deep tissue bleeding including intracranial hemorrhage, intraarticular bleeding, deep muscle bleeding, or any other similar type of bleeding should be noted when obtaining a comprehensive review of systems. In addition, the patient should be asked about complaints of generalized weakness, chills, drenching night sweats, weight loss, loss of appetite, unexplained fevers, unexplained skin rashes, and an exact description of rashes, poorly healing sores, or enlarging moles. The patient also should be asked about frequent, recurrent, or localized headaches, dizziness, or the loss of consciousness. A history regarding blurred vision, double vision, or persistent scotomata, tinnitus, hearing loss, or sore tongue also is important. The patient also should be asked about oral mucosal bleeding, gingival bleeding with tooth brushing, spontaneous gingival bleeding, epistaxis, the wearing of dentures, frequent upper respiratory infections, difficulty in swallowing, or any unexplained hoarseness. A history of cervical pain or the noting of supraclavicular or cervical adenopathy, chronic cough, hemoptysis, blood-tinged sputum, coughing spells, shortness of breath, paroxysmal nocturnal dyspnea, orthopnea, angina-type chest pain, heart disease of any type, hypertension, the presence of intermittent or persistent tachycardia and palpitations, as well as the presence of or persistence of ankle edema should be noted. A history of preprandial or postprandial epigastric distress, epigastric pain, nausea, emesis, hematemesis, melena, hematochezia, or any changes in bowel habits within the past 6 months should be recorded. A history of hematuria, pyuria, frequency, urgency, renal disease, renal stones, or port wine–colored urine also is obtained. The presence or absence of joint pain, back pain, or bone pain should be documented, and the specific areas noted.

In the female patient, the age of beginning menstruation, the age of first pregnancy, and the presence or absence of continued menses and of menopause, including the year menopause stopped, should be recorded. In addition, a careful history about the degree and length of menstrual periods is of key importance. The prior ingestion of oral contraceptives, the presence or absence of excessive vaginal discharge, recurrent vaginal infections, intramenstrual bleeding, or the noting of nodules, discharge, or irritation of the breasts also should be elicited. The number of children born must be defined, and the female patient should be asked about any potential or real bleeding problems in any of her children, which might have been manifest at childbirth, spontaneously, or in association with surgery. The patient should be asked if she, herself, bled unusually during delivery and whether blood transfusions were required. In the male patient, a history of difficulty in urination, history of prostatic disease, and a history of circumcision, including the presence or absence of unusual bleeding with circumcision, should be noted.

With respect to a personal history, it is of obvious importance to ask the patient about the use of tobacco, and the form in which it is used. An ethanol history also is often difficult to take but must be precisely defined in the patient with a potential or real bleeding/bruising disorder. This should include the type of alcohol used and the amount ingested daily. Questions regarding special diets or food faddism also should be carefully recorded, as the patient may be potentially nutritionally deficient, including potential vitamin K deficiency. A careful occupational history, especially with respect to exposure to radiation, industrial toxins, pesticides, benzene, carbon tetrachloride, lead, or any other potentially marrow-damaging agents should be recorded.

A very careful family history including the birth date, birth place, status of health of the parents or if dead, the age they died, and the cause of death should be recorded. The patient should be asked about any bleeding tendencies in the mother, father, or any siblings. Because many inherited disorders are sex-linked and may skip several generations, a careful history regarding bleeding tendencies in maternal and paternal grandparents, aunts, uncles, and cousins also should be obtained. If the patient is married, the general health of the spouse should be recorded. Of more importance, however, is to inquire regarding the general health of the patient's children, and in this capacity, it is of obvious importance to take a very attentive bleeding history to determine if it may be manifest in any of the children. The patient should be specifically asked if any children have any type of bleeding tendency, including easy or spontaneous bruising, the noting of petechiae or purpura, or any other type of bleeding. In addition, if the bleeding history in children is negative, the patient should be specifically asked if any of the children have been stressed by surgery or trauma. It is again important to ask if any relative, both maternal and paternal, going back to the great grandparents, including grandparents, aunts, uncles, and cousins have had any type of bleeding disorder, real or imagined. A family history of the presence or absence of cerebral vascular disease, hypertension, tuberculosis, diabetes mellitus, thyroid disease, gout, arthritis, coronary artery disease, other heart disease, pulmonary disease, peptic ulcer disease, chronic inflammatory conditions, renal disease, or anemia should be elicited. The clinician should carefully query the patient about any type of bleeding tendency in any immediate or remote family members. After eliciting a complete history, the clinician should summarize by asking the patient if there are any additional points of information that the patient wishes to tell to the physician taking the history.

PHYSICAL EXAMINATION

Once a detailed history has been obtained, a careful and thorough physical examination is performed; often the physical examination will be preferentially directed by points mentioned in the history. First, the vital signs of the patient should be noted and recorded, including the brachial blood pressure, pulse rate and regularity, respiratory rate, temperature, weight, height, and body surface area. During this time, a careful general inspection of the patient is done to obtain clues regarding the general health of the patient. A general inspection of the patient will usually immediately demonstrate changes associated with chronic illness including sallow skin, tenting of the skin, loss of subcutaneous supportive tissue, or symmetrical muscle wasting. An observant examination of the entire integumentary system should occur, carefully searching for petechiae, purpura, ecchymoses, nonpulsatile, pinpoint, or nodular telangiectasia, and other signs of a systemic bleeding disorder. A careful examination of the nail beds (subungual areas and capillary filling), perioral areas, and the sublingual areas are imperative. Examination of the eyes should include a careful inspection of the vasculature and looking for arteriovenous (A-V) fistulae, vascular conjunctival abnormalities, bulbar and palpebral conjunctival erythema, petechiae, purpura, telangiectasia, or the presence of bulbar conjunctival icterus. A careful funduscopic examination also should be performed, looking carefully at the vasculature for signs of hemorrhages, exudates, or the formation of A-V fistulae or other abnormal arterial or venous formations and retinal hemorrhage. The oral and nasal mucosa should be carefully inspected; the nasal mucosa is inspected for signs of localized vascular defects, or the presence of petechiae, purpura, or telangiectasia. The oral mucosa is likewise carefully examined; patients should always be asked to remove dentures. Special attention is directed to searching for petechiae, purpura, telangiectasia, hemorrhagic bullae, or other signs of a platelet defect, vascular defect, or other coagulopathy. It is important to note the presence or absence of lateral papillae and always to look under the tongue for sublingual telangiectasia and to inspect the gums for hyperplasia or the presence of petechiae, purpura, or hemorrhagic bullae. In addition, the circumoral area should be inspected for the presence or absence of perioral telangiectasia. Weber and Rinne tests should be done to assess hearing, and the auditory canals also should be inspected for any signs of blood, vascular malformations, or the presence of petechiae, purpura, or telangiectasia. The presence or absence of supraclavicular, cervical, submental, axillary, epitrochlear, inguinal, and deep iliac adenopathy should next be assessed. After this, the presence or absence of sternal, cervical, thoracic, or lumbosacral spine tenderness, costovertebral angle tenderness, and rib tenderness should be evaluated. The chest is next examined to ascertain whether it is clear to percussion and auscultation, to prove the presence or absence of rhonchi, localized wheezing, or rales, and to document the presence of adequate diaphragmatic excursion bilaterally. Palpation and auscultation of the heart should be performed, listening particularly for murmurs that may be indicative of a chronic underlying anemia secondary to a hemorrhagic tendency. All women older than 25 years should have a careful breast examination. After this, the carotid and femoral arteries and the abdominal aorta should be palpated and auscultated for fullness and bruits. An assessment of carotid pulses, brachial pulses, radial pulses, ulnar pulses, femoral pulses, dorsalis pedis pulses, and posterior tibial pulses also should be done. The abdominal examination should include careful percussion and palpation of the liver and spleen, including an attempt to elicit hepatic or splenic tenderness and to auscultate the left upper quadrant for splenic rubs. In addition, bowel sounds should be recorded, the entire abdomen palpated for evidence of any masses, aortic aneurysm, and the presence or absence of direct or indirect inguinal hernias also should be searched for at this time. After this, an examination of the genitalia should occur. A rectal examination should be done in any adult patient, and the stool examined and tested for occult blood.

The extremities are next carefully evaluated, looking for changes or abnormalities of the integument including petechiae, purpura, or telangiectasia, which may, sometimes, be quite pinpoint and require the use of a magnifying glass. With inspection of the integument, the fingernail beds and toenail beds should be carefully inspected for underlying petechiae (splinter hemorrhages), purpura, and telangiectasia; capillary filling should be noted. Any vascular malformations of the skin should likewise be noted and recorded. While inspecting the extremities and integument, note the presence or absence of muscle wasting, chronic hemosiderin deposits, especially in the lower extremities and around the ankles, or any changes compatible with varicosities or chronic venous insufficiency, including the presence or absence of ankle edema. The presence of chronic hemosiderin deposits should alert one to the potential presence of a chronic long-standing extravasation of blood from the vasculature, suggesting a potential of chronic venous insufficiency, or alternatively, a long-standing quantitative or qualitative platelet defect, or a vascular defect affecting the small or large vessels, or both. The presence or absence of an ashen complexion must be noted. The neurologic examination is usually performed last and should consist of a general assessment of the cerebrum and cerebellum, including evaluation of the biceps, triceps, brachioradialis, patellar, and Achilles tendon reflexes. Vibratory sensation and pinpoint sensation of the lower extremities should be tested. Information regarding function or dysfunction of cranial nerves II through XII would have been gathered in previous parts of the examination.

Often the presence or absence of a disorder of hemostasis can be documented with at least 90% accuracy with the performance of a careful history and physical examination. The history and physical examination, including careful questioning of the patient regarding site and severity of hemorrhage, type of hemorrhage (petechiae, purpura, and ecchymoses vs. deep tissue bleeding, vs. telangiectasia) should allow categorization of the type of defect present in more than 90% of patients; this allows one to subject the patient to *selected* laboratory testing procedures, and shields one from chaotic ordering of innumerable unnecessary laboratory procedures. Once the history and physical and type of bleeding are carefully delineated, the clinician will usually have a specific diagnosis or several diagnoses in mind, and many others will have been ruled out. At this time, the clinician will have a good idea whether this is a hereditary or acquired hemorrhagic disorder.

After the evaluation and the impressions of the clinician, a directed laboratory screening and subsequent definitive laboratory tests usually are ordered. It should be realized that a tremendous amount of time and money can be wasted on laboratory hemostasis testing procedures; therefore, the testing procedures should be strongly directed by the initial clinical impression, which is based on a sound history and physical examination. When the history and physical are completed, the clinician will have developed a strong suspicion that this represents a hereditary or an acquired disorder and whether the disorder involves the vasculature, the platelets, or the blood protein system, or alternatively, is a multiple hemostatic compartment defect [for example, liver dysfunction or a disseminated intravascular coagulation (DIC)-type syndrome] and involves several or all the hemostatic compartments. With this clinical impression, the clinician then orders appropriate laboratory testing modalities to confirm the presence or absence of a suspected defect or defects and to ascertain the severity of the defect suspected to be present.

LABORATORY TESTING

Laboratory testing should always be strongly directed by the initial clinical impression(s). Laboratory tests of hemostasis are not only numerous but also extremely expensive, and a phenomenal amount of time, money, and effort can be wasted unless the laboratory investigation of a bleeding disorder is strongly directed by early clinical impressions and the working diagnosis. Laboratory screening tests for compartmentalizing a specific type of defect into that of the vasculature, the platelets, or the blood proteins, or a combination thereof, can be performed by using simple screening tests. These screening tests of hemostasis are a platelet count, microscopic morphologic evaluation of the peripheral blood smear, a prothrombin time, and a partial thromboplastin time. If a platelet-function defect or vascular defect is suspected, in the presence of a normal platelet count, platelet aggregation will be required. The template bleeding time (TBT) was previously used, but has been found to be notoriously unreliable over time. Often all the screening tests will not be needed, as the clinician will, based on the clinical evaluation, have a strong working diagnosis, which might eliminate defects of the vasculature or platelets and/or coagulation factors, only one compartment will be suspected to be at fault, and only tests appropriate to that particular hemostatic compartment will be necessary. If these are negative, other hemostatic compartments are then evaluated in instances in which the first clinical impression was incorrect. In the vast majority of circumstances, the eliciting of a careful history and the performance of a careful physical examination and then the conceptualization of a working diagnosis, followed by the directed and specific ordering of laboratory tests to confirm or rule out the diagnosis will lead to a correct diagnosis and definition of the severity of the defect suspected.

Thus it is strongly emphasized that the approach to a patient with a potential or real bleeding disorder must be logical and sequential and must be preceded by a careful clinical evaluation of the patient instead of the indiscriminate ordering of numerous laboratory tests of hemostasis. If a strong working diagnosis is not suggested by the history or physical examination, the aforementioned laboratory screening tests, including platelet aggregation studies when indicated, may be needed to define the hemostatic compartment or compartments housing the defect. If a vascular or platelet defect is present, the TBT may be prolonged; exceptions are noted in hereditary hemorrhagic telangiectasia, the allergic vasculitides, and the vascular defects associated with paraprotein disorders, wherein the TBT may be normal despite a significant vascular defect. A normal TBT does not rule out the presence of any platelet function or vascular defect.

The finding of a prolonged TBT in the face of a normal platelet count suggests platelet or vascular dysfunction. The aspirin tolerance test will help distinguish between a questionable or borderline TBT in the face of a strongly suggestive history. A careful examination of the peripheral blood smear, often neglected by clinicians, is paramount and may reveal findings suggestive of an associated blood dyscrasia, such as leukemia, leukocytosis, schistocytosis, reticulocytosis, or other underlying condition to account for the hemostatic defect. In this regard, it must be recalled that up to 50% of patients with acute leukemia may initially have easy and spontaneous bruising, petechiae, and purpura. In addition, during a careful evaluation of the blood smear, platelet morphology and number should be noted. If the TBT is prolonged and the platelet count normal, one cannot differentiate between a platelet-function defect and a vascular defect, and platelet aggregation or lumi-aggregation should be done to differentiate between a platelet-function defect and a vascular defect. Abnormal platelet aggregation or lumi-aggregation will document a clinically significant platelet-function defect; normal aggregation, in the presence of a normal platelet count and petechiae or purpura, is strongly suggestive of a vascular defect.

If a clinically significant coagulation protein abnormality is present, either the prothrombin time, activated partial thromboplastin time, or both, will be prolonged, except, of course, in factor XIII deficiency or α_2-antiplasmin deficiency. In multiple compartment defects, such as DIC with secondary fibrinolysis, many tests of hemostasis may be abnormal, including the prothrombin time, the partial thromboplastin time, the platelet count, and platelet aggregation. Primary fibrinolytic syndromes will demonstrate the same findings, except that platelets may be normal in number. More sophisticated techniques for making a specific differential diagnosis from the laboratory standpoint are found in appropriate chapters in discussions after appropriate disease categories.

Bleeding resulting from a vascular disorder may require a very careful clinical and laboratory evaluation to undercover an underlying primary disease such as Cushing syndrome, scurvy, the allergic vasculitides, or malignant paraprotein disorder. If no primary disease can be found, the TBT, and more specifically, normal platelet-function studies will help to define or suggest the vascular nature of a disorder. In this regard, the TBT should never be performed in the face of obvious bleeding or obvious thrombocytopenia, because unnecessary bleeding may occur. Because the TBT and aspirin tolerance test may be abnormal in other than vascular disorders, further studies are necessary to establish the diagnosis and specifically to diagnose differentially a vascular disorder from a platelet-function defect. When initial screening tests suggest a platelet disorder, a platelet count must be done. If it is low, the bone marrow should next be examined if the cause of thrombocytopenia is not obvious. If the platelet count is normal, however, platelet aggregation or lumi-aggregation studies must be performed to help to define the qualitative abnormalities of platelets that are most probably present.

As previously mentioned, clinically significant coagulation factor abnormalities are almost always diagnosed from the initial prothrombin time and/or partial thromboplastin time; factor XIII deficiency and α_2-antiplasmin deficiency will not, however, be detected by the prothrombin time or partial thromboplastin time. The ability to do these assays by totally automated instrumentation with premeasured small amounts of reagents has greatly enhanced their accuracy and convenience for use by physicians in private practice environments and in outpatient facilities when ambulatory patients require evaluation. Reagents, however, should be carefully chosen. Several recent comparative studies have shown that some commercial reagents do not perform adequately as screening tests of hemostasis. The interpretation of abnormal laboratory parameters is discussed in appropriate chapters, along with each disease category, in this textbook.

SUMMARY

When approaching a patient with a bleeding disorder or a bleeding history, the clinician must have a systematic and logical approach to the clinical and laboratory diagnosis. A simple and workable approach is to think of the hemostasis system as comprising three hemostatic compartments: the vasculature, the platelets, and the coagulation proteins. Generally for normal hemostasis to occur, all three of these compartments must be intact. Platelets must be normal in both number and function, and coagulation proteins must be quantitatively and qualitatively normal. Often a defect in only one hemostatic compartment can be corrected by overcompensation of the other two compartments, and clinically significant bleeding may or may not follow. For example, disruption of the vasculature, as in minor trauma or surgery, may not lead to pathologic bleeding if platelet number and function and coagulation proteins are intact and function to overcome this insult. Commonly, abnormalities in two of the three hemostatic systems must be present for significant pathologic bleeding to occur. It should be recalled that hemophiliacs often do not bleed (coagulation protein abnormality) unless another of the hemostatic compartments is disrupted (for example, interruption of the vasculature by surgery or trauma, thus inducing a defect in two of the three hemostatic compartments). Once one can discern which compartment or combination of compartments contains a defect, a thorough evaluation of this compartment can then be carried out from both the clinical and laboratory standpoints.

In the vast majority of instances, a clinical evaluation of the patient, including a careful history, will compartmentalize a defect of hemostasis with more than 90% accuracy. If the patient has petechiae and purpura, one can assume that the vasculature or platelets (either number or function) are at fault. Petechiae and purpura almost never arise from coagulation protein disorders alone; thus platelet-function defects, thrombocytopenia, and vascular defects are most commonly characterized by petechiae and purpura, easy and spontaneous bruising, gingival bleeding with tooth brushing, and mild to moderate mucosal membrane bleeding. Alternatively, single or multiple coagulation protein abnormalities are usually manifest by deep tissue bleeding, including intramuscular bleeding, intraarticular bleeding, and intracranial bleeding in association with moderate to severe mucosal membrane bleeding and the development of large subcutaneous ecchymoses. A careful history should pinpoint a family history of bleeding, a personal history of bleeding, and the type, site, and severity of bleeding that has occurred. Obviously, patients should be thoroughly questioned about drugs for the detection of drug-induced platelet dysfunction, drug-induced thrombocytopenia, or drug-induced vascular defects. Drugs interfering with the vasculature, interfering with platelet function, or inducing thrombocytopenia are listed in detail in appropriate chapters of this textbook.

Probably no area of laboratory medicine is more confusing to the clinician than hemostasis. Rapid growth in the understanding of hemostasis and blood proteins involved with hemostasis, the superfluity in terminology, the potpourri of techniques claimed to measure the same factors, and the mystique of reagents used, such as "thromboplastin" and "activators," serve to nurture this bewildering state of affairs. Even to the present time, there is still no global agreement on even such a routine procedure as the prothrombin time, despite more than three decades of international committee meetings. Additionally, newer recombinant reagents, primarily developed for use in assessing warfarin therapy [the international normalized ratio (INR)] or intravenous heparin therapy [the activated partial thromboplastin time (aPTT)] have led to flaws in their use as screening tests of hemostasis, the original reason(s) for which these tests were developed! Tables 2.1, 2.2, and 2.3 classify the bleeding disorders according to pathogenic mechanisms and outline laboratory screening procedures that facilitate a systematic approach to the categorization of most bleeding disorders. Although a bleeding disorder can usually be defined without the aid of laboratory screening tests, merely with a meticulous history and physical examination, the diagnosis must be confirmed and the severity of the defect delineated by using appropriate laboratory testing modalities. However, the choice and interpretation of these tests should always be predicated on the major clinical data obtained by performing a careful history and conducting a rigorous physical examination. Although a complete history should be taken, particular emphasis should be directed to the family history and drug ingestion (conspicuous or surreptitious). A history of obstetric and surgical events associated with unusual bleeding calls for a search for defects in hemostasis. Vascular defects are usually associated with easy and spontaneous bruising, petechiae, and purpura, which are usually dependent, and mild to moderate bleeding from mucous membranes. Alternatively, platelet defects, although also associated with easy and spontaneous bruising and mild to moderate mucosal membrane bleeding, are usually associated with symmetric petechiae and purpura (also found on the torso) instead of primarily only dependent. In contrast, the blood protein defects rarely, if ever, are first seen as petechiae and purpura, except von Willebrand syndrome, but are usually associated with large subcutaneous ecchymoses, moderate to severe mucosal membrane hemorrhage, and deep tissue bleeding. Thrombocytopenias, hereditary or acquired, are discussed in the chapter on quantitative platelet defects and may be due to (a) bone marrow failure, (b) maturation/metabolic defects, or (c) peripheral platelet loss. However, it also should be recognized that more commonly, bleeding may be due to hereditary or acquired platelet dysfunction. Coagulation protein abnormalities, whether hereditary or acquired, may result from absent, decreased, or abnormal synthesis of a clotting factor, or the development of antibodies against factors.

In liver disease or suspected drug induced bleeding (particular antibiotics), a therapeutic trial of vitamin K may prove useful in selected patients. In life-threatening situations, specific hemotherapeutic agents may be necessary to establish the diagnosis and to manage hemorrhage (e.g., the

TABLE 2.1. CLASSIFICATION OF HEMORRHAGIC DISORDERS

Vascular compartment
Hereditary
Acquired
Drug-induced
Platelet compartment
Quantitative
Hereditary
Acquired
Drug-induced
Qualitative
Hereditary
Acquired
Drug-induced
Blood (coagulation) protein compartment
Hereditary (quantitative or qualitative)
Single factor (common)
Multiple factors (rare)
Acquired (quantitative or qualitative)
Single factor (rare)
Multiple factors (common)
Multiple-compartment defects
Disseminated intravascular coagulation syndromes
Primary fibrinolytic syndromes

TABLE 2.2. SCREENING TESTS OF HEMOSTASIS

Complete blood and platelet count
Peripheral blood smear evaluation
Template bleeding time[a]
Prothrombin time
Activated partial thromboplastin time
Platelet (lumi)-aggregation[b]

[a]Not reliable.
[b]When clinically indicated.

TABLE 2.3. SCREENING TEST RESULT VERSUS COMPARTMENT CONTAINING THE HEMOSTASIS DEFECT

	Vascular Disorder	Platelet Function	Platelet Number	Blood Proteins
Platelet count	Normal	Normal	Abnormal	Normal
Platelet aggregation	Normal	Abnormal	Abnormal	Normal[a]
Prothrombin time	Normal	Normal	Normal	Abnormal or normal[b]
Partial thromboplastin time	Normal	Normal	Normal	Abnormal or normal[b]
Template bleeding time	Abnormal	Abnormal	Abnormal	Normal

[a]Except von Willebrand syndrome.
[b]Protime and/or PTT will be prolonged depending on factor involved; factor XIII deficiency and alpha-2-α-antiplasmin deficiency are not detected by PT or PTT.
PT, prothrombin time; PTT, partial thromboplastin time.

use of prothrombin complex concentrates in selected clinical situations in which a diagnosis is strongly suspected but not yet confirmed and bleeding is so severe that laboratory confirmatory evidence cannot be awaited).

The recognition of inhibitors to specific clotting factors has increased greatly in recent years, and these are discussed in appropriate sections of this textbook. These may develop in up to 10% of hemophiliacs but also occur in postpartum women, in autoimmune disorders, and in association with other well-defined disease entities. Sometimes circulating anticoagulants occur spontaneously with no obvious associated condition. Most acquired defects, including both DIC-type syndromes and primary fibrinolytic syndromes and in patients with chronic liver disease, will harbor multiple coagulation-factor abnormalities and multiple hemostatic compartment–type defects; after the underlying disease process is known, the laboratory evaluation of such patients should be guided by knowing the types of hemorrhagic syndromes that occur in selected clinical disorders. In our era of unrestrained polypharmacy, drug-induced bleeding must be strongly considered, the classic example being aspirin ingestion. However, a host of other drugs, alone or in combination, may induce bleeding tendencies and not always by the same mechanisms. Drugs should be suspected when one or more defects can be demonstrated, without other obvious cause, and should especially be suspected when the discontinuation of medication causes hemostasis tests to return to normal.

Careful initial clinical evaluation of the patient, including a careful history and a diligently performed physical examination, is the mainstay of diagnosis in the patient with a suspected or real hemorrhagic disorder. After this is performed, an initial clinical impression or working diagnosis is formulated and is most often correct in the vast majority of instances, up to 90% of patients. After the formulation of a working diagnosis or initial impression, laboratory testing procedures, carefully chosen and based on the logical and sequential clinical evaluation of the patient, are selectively ordered to document the presence or absence of the defect and to delineate the severity. In this regard, a simple screening battery to assess all hemostasis compartments consists of a peripheral blood smear evaluation, platelet prothrombin time, activated partial thromboplastin time, and, when clinically justified, platelet-aggregation studies.

3

HEREDITARY AND ACQUIRED VASCULAR THROMBOHEMORRHAGIC DISORDERS

RODGER L. BICK

Disorders of the vasculature are common but often-unappreciated causes of bruising, bleeding, and vasculitis/small vessel thrombosis, and are the topic of this chapter. Petechiae and purpura and other dermal findings, including dermal vascular thrombosis, livido reticularis, and variants such as cutis marmorata, pallor, cyanosis, and dusky cyanosis are hallmark findings of vascular disorders, depending on whether vascular leakage, occlusion, or both are occurring. Most typically patients with vascular disorders complain of mild to moderate mucosal membrane bleeding, often manifest as bilateral epistaxis, gastrointestinal (GI) bleeding (often occult), intrapulmonary bleeding, or genitourinary bleeding. Patients also may have a history of easy and spontaneous bruising or gingival bleeding with tooth brushing. Many normal individuals experience occasional gingival bleeding with tooth brushing; however, if this occurs almost daily, or more than 2 to 3 times a week, a vascular or platelet defect should be considered. Another clinical clue to the presence of a vascular disorder is the finding of dependent petechiae and purpura found primarily on the extremities and usually absent from the torso. This is a characteristic of vascular bleeding, whereas platelet defects are typically associated with symmetrical petechiae and purpura, found on the extremities and torso. If microvascular disorders are manifest by occlusion, likewise, the findings are usually dependent or distal. Common clinical findings of vascular disorders are summarized in Table 3.1 (1–3). When suspecting a vascular disorder, one must first rule out coagulation protein defects (prothrombin time and activated partial thromboplastin time) and thrombocytopenia. If these are normal, in the appropriate setting, the differential diagnosis is, therefore, a vascular defect versus a platelet-function defect. If the distinction cannot be made clinically, the most reliable method of diagnosing a vascular defect is to document normal platelet function. In the past, prolongation of the standardized template bleeding time (TBT) was used to document the presence of vascular or platelet dysfunction; however, this test is very unreliable for this particular use. Thus with suspected vascular dysfunction, the appropriate ways to rule out platelet dysfunction are (a) platelet aggregation or lumi-aggregation studies or use of the newer PFA-100 or Thrombostat 4000 platelet-function analyzers (4–6). Once platelet dysfunction is ruled out, vascular dysfunction is likely.

R. L. Bick: Departments of Medicine and Pathology, University of Texas Southwestern Medical Center; Dallas Thrombosis/Hemostasis Clinical Center; ThromboCare Laboratories, Dallas, Texas.

CLINICAL VASCULAR DISORDERS

Vascular disorders are best categorized as hereditary, acquired, and drug induced. These are summarized in Table 3.2. The hereditary vascular disorders generally are the hereditary collagen vascular diseases, and most are rare clinical oddities. The one exception to rarity is Osler–Weber–Rendu disease [hereditary hemorrhagic telangiectasia (HHT)], which is

TABLE 3.1. CLINICAL FINDINGS IN VASCULAR DISEASES

Petechiae
Purpura
Large ecchymoses
History of easy bruising
History of spontaneous bruising
Gingival bleeding
Mucosal membrane bleeding
Pulmonary
Gastrointestinal
Genitourinary
Epistaxis
Petechiae and purpura usually dependent

TABLE 3.2. CLASSIFICATION OF VASCULAR DISORDERS

Hereditary
Ehlers–Danlos syndrome
Marfan syndrome
Osteogenesis imperfecta
Pseudoxanthoma elasticum
Homocystinemia
Giant cavernous hemangiomata
Hereditary hemorrhagic telangiectasia
Acquired
Collagen (autoimmune) vascular disorders
Cushing syndrome
Amyloidosis
Myeloma
Waldenström macroglobulinemia
Circulating immune complex diseases
Cryoglobulinemia
Allergic purpuras
Autoerythrocytic sensitization
Drug-induced vascular defects/vasculitis

TABLE 3.3. DETERMINANTS OF CLINICAL FINDINGS IN VASCULAR DISORDERS

Potential host response
Allergic reaction
Coagulation activation
Fibrinolytic activation
Kinin activation
Complement activation
Other enzyme activation
Migration of leukocytes
Potential severity of defect
Mild
Serum effusion with bullae and erythema only
Moderate
Serum and blood effusion with bullae, erythema, wheals, petechiae, and purpura
Severe
Effusion of blood and endothelial cell death with petechiae, purpura, gross hemorrhage, and thrombosis

common. Alternatively, the acquired vascular disorders are very common, and all clinicians should be familiar with them. The importance of becoming familiar with acquired vascular disorders is severalfold: when a patient is first seen with dependent petechiae and purpura, and easy or spontaneous bruising or the other clinical manifestations of vascular dysfunction previously discussed, the patient should be evaluated for vascular disorders. If an individual has one of the acquired disorders known to be associated with vascular defects and undergoes surgery or sustains trauma, it should be assumed the patient has a systemic vascular defect that might lead to clinically significant thrombohemorrhagic problems.

Vascular disorders may occur in bizarre and varied ways. The reasons for this are the many complex determinants that may alter clinical findings in individual patients. These determinants accounting for varied clinical presentations are summarized in Table 3.3. There are many potential host responses to a vascular disorder or defect. For example, there may be simply an antigenic response, there may be only activation of the coagulation system, only activation of fibrinolysis, only kinin activation, activation of only complement, or any combination of these activation pathways may be present. There are differing severities of vascular insults, injuries, or diseases. A mild vascular insult (disorder) will usually lead to only serum effusion, which clinically is interpreted as bullae and erythema. However, if the insult (disease) is more pronounced, both serum and blood may effuse from the vasculature, giving rise to bullae, erythema, and wheals in association with petechiae and purpura. If the insult is severe, there will be not only effusion of blood but also endothelial cell death, petechiae, purpura, and gross hemorrhage, often large ecchymoses, and small- or large-vessel thrombosis. In addition, the other dermal manifestations previously discussed may be present. The findings may or may not be consistent on any given examination. When the myriad host responses to a vascular disorder are integrated with severity of the vascular disorder or insult, it becomes obvious how many seemingly similar vascular disorders may demonstrate varied clinical findings, thus taxing the clinical acumen of the clinician.

HEREDITARY VASCULAR DISORDERS

The hereditary vascular disorders are summarized in Table 3.4. These are Ehlers–Danlos syndrome (EDS), Marfan syndrome, osteogenesis imperfecta, pseudoxanthoma elasticum, homocystinuria, giant cavernous hemangiomata, and the Kasabach–Merritt syndrome [the combination of giant cavernous hemangiomata and disseminated intravascular coagulation (DIC)] and hereditary hemorrhagic telangiectasia. Each of these disorders is discussed separately.

Ehlers–Danlos Syndrome

The EDS is a rare connective tissue disorder usually inherited by autosomal dominance (7). Interestingly, one of the earliest descriptions of this syndrome may have concerned the violin virtuoso Paganini; this disorder was thought to contribute to his remarkable dexterity and talent. The EDS is variable in

TABLE 3.4. HEREDITARY VASCULAR DISEASES

Ehlers–Danlos syndrome
Marfan syndrome
Osteogenesis imperfecta
Pseudoxanthoma elasticum
Giant cavernous hemangiomata
Homocystinemia
Hereditary hemorrhagic telangiectasia

inheritance, variable in pathophysiology, and highly variable in phenotypic clinical expression. There are at least nine types of EDS, referred to as EDS types I to IX. In general, EDS is characterized by extreme vascular fragility, skin fragility, hypermobile joints, and molluscoid pseudotumors of the knees and elbows. Joint pain, particularly of the shoulders, hands, and knees, is a prominent feature (8). Bleeding may be highly variable; however, easy and spontaneous bruising is a hallmark. Patients commonly have gingival bleeding with tooth brushing and have severe bleeding after dental extraction. Petechiae, purpura, GI bleeding, and hemoptysis are often present. In some instances, the bleeding may be severe enough to suggest hemophilia. Some patients may have associated platelet dysfunction (4,9). Other characteristics commonly noted in this syndrome are blue sclerae, angioid streaks, and aortic insufficiency. Mitral valve prolapse was once thought to be a significant feature, but recent studies have shown this not to be the case (10). Women with EDS have a high incidence of incontinence, endometriosis, prolapse, and dyspareunia (11). Of particular concern in EDS are vascular aneurysms and vascular rupture; any artery is susceptible; infants with abdominal aortic aneurysms should be suspected of having EDS, especially type IV (12,13). Individuals with childhood aneurysms or any patient with multiple aneurysms should be suspected of harboring EDS; these are most common in type IV. Many individuals with EDS have intracerebral aneurysms. It is thought that about 5% of intracerebral aneurysms are congenital, and EDS type IV is prominent among these (14). Despite the catastrophic vascular consequences of EDS, one investigation failed to demonstrate abnormalities or alterations in vascular wall mechanics in patients with EDS (15). EDS type I is a severe form of the disease (16) and appears to be the result of mutations in the COL5A2 gene on chromosome 9 (17), leading to abnormalities of type V collagen (18,19); this same defect also is thought to account for EDS type II (20). The pathophysiology of EDS types III, V, and VIII are obscure. EDS type IV also is a severe form of the disease, and although patients with this variant have the problems previously depicted, these patients are particularly prone to aneurysms, vascular rupture, and hepatic or colon rupture (21–24). EDS type IV is due to a mutation in the COL3A1 gene, which codes for type III procollagen, leading to abnormal type III collagen (25–28). EDS type VI, unlike the other forms, is inherited as an autosomal recessive and is due to abnormally low lysyl hydrolase activity (29) secondary to a defect of the lysyl hydrolase gene (30–32). EDS type VII is due to a defect in type I collagen; this is brought about by a mutation in the COL1A1 or COL1A2 gene. Those with mutations of the COL1A1 gene have a more severe form of the disease than do those with the COL1A2 mutation (33). As previously noted, the pathophysiology of type VIII remains obscure. EDS type XI is due to unclear abnormalities in copper metabolism; this leads to severe reductions in lysyl oxidase, which, in turn, leads to abnormalities of collagen and elastin cross-linking (34). The common laboratory findings are a prolonged TBT, and sometimes abnormal platelet aggregation if the patient has an associated platelet-function defect. A prolonged TBT is classically present.

Therapy for bleeding depends on the site and severity; however, 1-deamino-8-D-arginine vasopressin (DDAVP) has been successful in controlling not only mucosal surface bleeds but also bleeding associated with surgery or dental extractions (35). If platelet dysfunction is documented to be present, platelet concentrates also should be considered for significant bleeds. The treatment of large aneurysms, colonic rupture, or vascular rupture is obviously surgical. Cerebrovascular aneurysms are either neurosurgical or treated with the modalities discussed in the section on HHT. Characteristics of EDS are summarized in Table 3.5.

Marfan Syndrome

This syndrome is the most popularized of the hereditary collagen vascular disorders. It is inherited as an autosomal dominant trait and is characterized by skeletal defects (marked by long extremities and arachnodactyly), cardiovascular abnormalities (ascending aortic aneurysm or dissection), and ocular defects, usually manifest as ectopia lentis (36,37). Hyperextensible joints also are uniformly present. The basic pathophysiology is poorly defined but involves molecular defects in the glycoprotein fibrillin, which come about through mutations of the fibrillin gene, FBN-1, located on chromosome 15q21.3 (38–40). Of all the hereditary collagen vascular disorders, Marfan syndrome is least characterized clinically by a systemic hemorrhagic diathesis. However, many patients have easy and spontaneous bruising, and some may have a poorly characterized platelet-function defect as well. Among the most devastating clinical manifestations of Marfan syndrome are the aortic and cardiac problems. Recent studies have clearly indicated that early intervention, during childhood, can prolong survival after catastrophic cardiovascular events.

TABLE 3.5. THE EHLERS–DANLOS SYNDROME

Clinical findings
Autosomal dominant trait
Vascular and skin fragility
Easy and spontaneous bruising
Gingival and dental bleeding
Petechiae and purpura
Gastrointestinal bleeding
Hemoptysis
Ocular: blue sclerae and angioid streaks
Molluscoid pseudotumors
Mitral valve prolapse
Aortic insufficiency
Laboratory features
Prolonged template bleeding time
Platelet dysfunction (storage pool type)

The most common surgical indications in children with Marfan syndrome is aortic root dilatation, followed by mitral regurgitation; in addition, aortic dissection is apparently unusual in children, but careful follow-up with new imaging techniques, such as magnetic resonance imaging (MRI), is strongly suggested (41). As with EDS, the finding of an abdominal aortic aneurysm should immediately suggest Marfan syndrome in the differential diagnosis (42). Because aortic dissection and its sequelae are usually progressive in patients with Marfan syndrome, surgical intervention early in the disease is advised and has been shown to be associated with reduced mortality at 8 years (43). In a study assessing outcome of pregnancy in Marfan syndrome, it was noted that aortic dissection is clearly a complication of pregnancy, occurring in 17% of patients without preconception aortic problems. It also was concluded that preconception aortic root dilatation may often, but not always, be a reasonable predictor of this complication (44). Another catastrophic event in Marfan syndrome is retinal detachment; in a recent study, 89% of uncomplicated detachments were successfully repaired, and a 56% success rate was noted with complicated detachments (45). As with other hereditary collagen vascular disorders, cerebral aneurysms are a problem; a recent assessment of autopsy cases revealed 28% of patients to have multiple cerebral aneurysms (46). An additional interesting complication of Marfan syndrome is sleep apnea, presumably due to maxillary constriction, high-arched palate, and faulty, relaxed connective tissue, which leads to this increased upper airway collapsibility (47,48). There are no characteristic hemostasis laboratory characteristics; however, a prolonged TBT may be present (4). The characteristics are summarized in Table 3.6.

Osteogenesis Imperfecta (Brittle Bones and Blue Sclerae Syndrome)

Osteogenesis imperfecta is one of the more common hereditary collagen vascular disorders and is inherited as an autosomal dominant trait. The genetic abnormality appears to reside in mutations of the COL1A1 or COL1A2 gene, leading to abnormalities of type I collagen (49–53). This disorder is characterized by a patchy lack of bone matrix. However, the matrix existing undergoes normal calcification. Osteogenesis imperfecta is clinically manifest as deformed and brittle bones that fracture easily; the primary clinical problems are orthopedic, with many patients requiring intramedullary shaft and nail repairs of the femur and tibia (54, 55). Several recent studies have revealed bisphosphonate therapy, in particular pamidronate and olpadronate to be very helpful for the bone manifestations of osteogenesis imperfecta (56–58). Skin and subcutaneous hemorrhages are characteristic (59). Death often occurs at childbirth, resulting from intracranial hemorrhage caused by an abnormal calvarium, coupled with a vascular hemorrhagic diathesis. Easy and spontaneous bruising, hemoptysis, epistaxis, and intracranial bleeding are common in osteogenesis imperfecta. Major vascular, systemic hemorrhagic and arterial events also may occur (60,61). An abnormal TBT is characteristic (4,62). Many cases have been described with abnormal platelet function, as defined by aggregation studies. The basic pathophysiology of osteogenesis imperfecta is characterized by the inability of reticulin to mature into collagen; the collagen present contains an abnormal amino acid composition. Characteristics of this syndrome are summarized in Table 3.7.

Pseudoxanthoma Elasticum

Pseudoxanthoma elasticum (PE syndrome), unlike the other hereditary vascular diseases, often does not become manifest until the second or third decade of life (4,63). This very rare disorder is usually inherited as an autosomal recessive trait, but autosomal dominant forms also have been described; regardless of mode of inheritance, the genetic defect has been mapped to chromosome 16p13.1 (64). The PE syndrome is commonly characterized by significant hemorrhage, because abnormal elastic fibers involve the entire arterial system. Vascular proteoglycans also are abnormal (65), and elevated levels of markers of endothelial dam-

TABLE 3.6. MARFAN SYNDROME

Clinical findings
Autosomal dominant trait
Easy and spontaneous bruising
Systemic bleeding uncommon
Ectopia lentis
Arachnodactyly
Hyperextensible joints
Ascending aortic aneurysms
Dissecting aortic aneurysms
Laboratory findings
Prolonged template bleeding time
Platelet dysfunction in some

TABLE 3.7. OSTEOGENESIS IMPERFECTA

Clinical findings
Autosomal dominant trait
Easy and spontaneous bruising
Subcutaneous bleeding
Intracranial bleeding
Epistaxis
Hemoptysis
Death at birth due to CNS bleeding
Deformed and brittle bones
Patchy lack of bone matrix
Laboratory findings
Prolonged template bleeding time
Platelet dysfunction in some

CNS, central nervous system.

age, including endothelin 1 and von Willebrand factor, have been described (66). Hemorrhage happens in any organ, but most commonly involves the skin, eyes, kidneys, central nervous system (CNS), and GI tract (67–69). These patients also have a marked tendency to easy and spontaneous bruising and commonly have petechiae and purpura. These individuals also have a marked predisposition to thrombosis, especially cerebral vascular thrombosis, acute myocardial infarction, and peripheral vascular occlusion with resultant gangrene and loss of extremities (70,71). Other clinical characteristics include relaxed, inelastic, and redundant skin in facial, neck, axillary, orbital, and inguinal areas. Hyperkeratotic plaques develop in these areas, and subcutaneous calcinosis also is common. Angioid streaks are characteristic ocular findings (72,73). Death is frequently caused by GI hemorrhage (4). Excessive uterine bleeding and intraarticular bleeding, with formation of characteristic hemarthroses, are common. The basic vascular pathology of this disorder is unclear but is thought to be the result of metabolic (enzyme) defects in elastic fibers (4). This syndrome is summarized in Table 3.8.

Homocystinurea and Hyperhomocystinemia

Homocystinemia may be a hereditary or acquired disorder. The classic hereditary form results in severe clinical symptoms during early childhood. The most common hereditary form is due to deficiency of cystathionine β-synthetase deficiency; the homozygous form is seen in about one in 200,000 to one in 335,000 births, and heterozygous forms, in about one in 70 to one in 200 live births (74,75). The gene responsible is located on chromosome 21q22.3 (74). Patients have decreased levels of cystathionine β-synthetase, leading to characteristic homocystinemia, methioninemia, and homocystinuria. A second inherited form is due to deficiencies of enzymes in the remethylation pathway. The enzyme methylenetetrahydrofolate reductase (MTHFR) is responsible for the conversion of 5,10-methylenetetrahydrofolate to 5-methyltetrahydrofolate; individuals homozygous for this enzyme deficiency are much rarer than those with cystathionine β-synthetase deficiency; the clinical pictures are similar. Heterozygous deficiency of MTHFR results in homocysteine levels that are adequate to protect against neurologic, but not vascular deficiencies. A thermolabile mutant of MTHFR occurs in neurologically normal individuals; this defect may be quite common (76,77). Another very rare other inherited form of homocystinemia may be due to deficiencies or mutations of the cobalamine coenzyme synthesis enzymes (78,79). Patients with the hereditary, particularly homozygous, form of hyperhomocystinemia characteristically have ectopia lentis, varying degrees of mental retardation, and skeletal deformities, including osteoporosis with resultant biconcave vertebrae, scoliosis, and pes cavus (80). Striking and unusual vascular changes are noted. Histologically, significant fibrosis of the intima and frayed muscle fibers in the media of arteries are found. Veins also may show these fibrous changes. Clinically, patients sustain arterial and venous thrombi; carotid artery thrombosis is a common event. In arteries and veins, both large and small vessels may be involved with thrombosis and resultant occlusions. Patients, including children, have venous thrombosis, cerebrovascular thrombosis, peripheral arterial occlusions, and acute coronary artery thrombosis (81). Widespread atheromatous changes happen in patients at an early age (82). Homocysteine-induced endothelial cell damage with resultant patchy endothelial cell sloughing and later platelet-induced intimal proliferation of smooth muscle media cells occurs, leading to widespread atheroma formation. The acquired forms of hyperhomocystinemia come about through deficiencies of cobalamin (B_{12}), folate, or pyridoxine (B_6) deficiencies. These acquired forms also are thought to account for many instances of arterial and venous thrombotic and atherosclerotic/occlusive events. Interestingly, as women become postmenopausal and risks of atherosclerosis increase, so does plasma homocysteine; this is often reversed with estrogen replacement therapy. Elevated levels of homocysteine also are associated with increasing age, male sex, cigarette smoking, elevated cholesterol, hypertension, and sedentary lifestyle. Clearly, epidemiologic and clinical prospective studies have clearly shown hyperhomocystinemia to be associated with a wide variety of thrombotic events, about 50% arterial and 50% venous, or combinations (78). The arterial events range from peripheral arterial thrombosis (79,80), coronary artery thrombosis (79,81), and cerebrovascular thrombosis (79,82). The mechanisms of thrombosis and atherosclerosis induced by hyperhomocysteine appear to be multifaceted. Homocysteine is directly toxic to endothelial cells; homocysteine has been shown to increase endothelial free radical production and

TABLE 3.8. PSEUDOXANTHOMA ELASTICUM SYNDROME

Clinical findings
Autosomal recessive trait
Easy and spontaneous bruising
Petechiae and purpura
Mucosal membrane bleeding
Severe gastrointestinal bleeding
GI bleeds may be fatal
All bleeding may be severe
Intraocular bleeding
Intraarticular bleeding
Relaxed, inelastic, and redundant skin
In axillae, neck, and inguinal areas
Hyperkeratotic plaques
Subcutaneous calcium deposits
Becomes manifest in second or third decades
Laboratory findings
Prolonged template bleeding time
Platelet dysfunction in some

GI, gastrointestinal.

subsequent lipid peroxidation; and the toxic effects on the endothelium appear to interfere with adequate endothelial production of endothelium-derived relaxing factor. Homocysteine has been shown to have a growth-promoting effect on smooth muscle cells and concomitantly an inhibitory effect on endothelial cell growth; this combination may lead to atherosclerotic occlusion. Platelet dysfunction also may arise from elevated homocysteine levels; these changes consist of increased platelet adhesion (83) and increased thromboxane A_2 release (84). Elevated levels of homocysteine have been reported to activate factors XII and V, and to inhibit endothelial thrombomodulin (85–88). Thus multiple mechanisms may lead to thrombus and atheroma formation in hyperhomocystinemia.

Although not all agree, the diagnosis may generally be made by a fasting total (reduced and oxidized forms) homocysteine level (74,78). Some, however, believe that methionine loading should be done because some heterozygotes for cystathionine β-synthetase deficiency have demonstrated normal fasting homocysteine levels (89,90) (in this instance, a methionine load of 100 mg/kg given just after an overnight fast). Homocysteine levels are determined immediately before, and at 2, 4, 6, 8, 12, and 24 hours. It is likely that the majority of clinically significant hyperhomocystinemia will, however, be detected by simple fasting homocysteine levels.

Homocysteine levels may be decreased by the use of pyridoxine (50 mg/day, p.o.), folate (1 mg/day, p.o.), and, at times, vitamin B_{12}. Use of these vitamin supplements is benign, and although they are not always effective, many complications and thrombotic episodes can be reduced by their use. Acute thrombi should be treated as usual, depending on the particular clinical situation and event, but some thrombotic manifestations have been successfully controlled with combination platelet-suppressive therapy consisting of dipyridamole and aspirin (4). Ticlopidine and clopidogrel also may be effective. Several excellent reviews on this complex topic are available (74,78,91,92).

Giant Cavernous Hemangiomata and the Kasabach–Merritt Syndrome

Hemangiomata are usually congenital, although they may not become clinically obvious until several years of age; they are more common in girls and may be of three types: capillary, cavernous, or capillary–cavernous mixtures (93). Cavernous forms are less common than capillary types, but are more often associated with systemic thrombohemorrhagic problems. Cavernous hemangiomata are benign vascular tumors having dilated thin-walled vessels and sinuses lined with abnormal endothelium. The most common sites of involvement are the GI tract, bones, liver, integument of the face and neck, and various mucosal membrane surfaces, including the oral mucosa (4,94–96). Hemangiomata of the extremities may often involve the skin, subcutaneous tissue, and adjacent bone (4). Many thrombi may form in these cavernous hemangiomata, and a local or DIC syndrome may develop. The association of giant cavernous hemangiomata and DIC is called the Kasabach–Merritt syndrome after two investigators who originally noted this association (97). The DIC may be low grade, but frequently progresses to a fulminant form. In some patients, a life-threatening fulminant DIC develops with attempted surgical resection of these hemangiomatous masses (98). In other patients, DIC develops spontaneously. Hepatic hemangiomata have been so excessive in association with DIC that transplant has, in some instances, been performed (99). DIC can often be controlled with heparin or low-molecular-weight (LMW) heparin, usually delivered subcutaneously, or antithrombin concentrate; however, occasionally local radiation therapy or injections of sclerosing agents have been reported to be beneficial (4,98,100). Of particular interest are recent reports of the efficacy of α interferon in treating the Kasabach–Merritt syndrome (101,102). Localized but extensive deep vein thrombosis may develop in association with giant cavernous hemangiomata (103). In patients with giant cavernous hemangiomata, proper laboratory evaluation to determine the presence or absence of DIC should be instituted, as the occurrence of DIC may significantly change morbidity or mortality, and the clinician may wish to consider appropriate prophylactic therapy for low-grade DIC, as low-dose heparin/LMW heparin, antithrombin, or interferon therapy, to abort a more fulminant form. Surely any patient with giant cavernous hemangiomatous lesions considered candidates for corrective surgery should be evaluated for DIC, and the DIC syndrome corrected before surgery is done. Treatment is symptomatic and, as mentioned earlier, steroids also may be of benefit in decreasing the size of hemangiomatous lesions (4).

Hereditary Hemorrhagic Telangiectasia (Osler–Weber–Rendu Disease)

Hereditary hemorrhagic telangiectasia (HHT) is a common disorder and is the most common hereditary vascular disorder leading to a hemorrhagic diathesis (104–106). The disorder is inherited by autosomal dominance, with 70% of afflicted individuals having a family history of the disorder (4). The incidence is between one in 2,000 and one in 3,500, but because the disease is so underdiagnosed, these are probably gross underestimates (107,108). The homozygous state is thought to be lethal. The gene responsible for HHT is somehow linked to blood group O (4). There are at least two forms of the disease: HHT I and HHT II. HHT I is the more common. HHT I has been mapped to abnormalities in chromosome 9q33-34, which codes for the Endoglin gene (109,110). Endoglin is an endothelial glycoprotein membrane receptor for transforming growth factor β (TGF-β), and absence of endoglin receptors is thought to lead to abnormal (although usually local) vascular defects, including proliferation, adhesion, and extracellular matrix composition and organization (111), leading to the telangiectatic lesions. HHT II involves a defect of chromosome 12q13, involving the activin receptor–like kinase 1 gene (ALK-1), a serine–threonine receptor found mainly on vascular endothelial cells (112) and, like endoglin, it binds TGF-β. The defect(s) appear to be due to defects in endothelial cell junctions (113), incomplete formation of vascular elastic fibers and vascular smooth muscle cells (114), or poor perivascular supportive tissue (115). The clinical manifestations of the two forms appear similar, except the incidence of pulmonary arteriovenous fistulae, which appear, in one preliminary report, to be about 30% in HHT I and only 3% in HHT II (116). In both forms of HHT, the vascular lesions may involve almost all sites, including any mucosal surface, the GI and genitourinary tract, the pulmonary circulation, the circulation of the CNS, and almost any other area. Because of this, the clinical manifestations may be highly varied, complex, and taxing to the clinician. The most serious sequelae of HHT are the pulmonary and CNS manifestations. Because significant pulmonary arteriovenous (AV) fistulae or malformations (AVMs) may occur, patients also may demonstrate significant arterial oxygen desaturation, leading to clubbing, abnormal arterial blood gases, polycythemia, cyanosis and, occasionally, frank heart failure. On rare occasions, hepatic cirrhosis and failure may occur. The hallmark characteristic of this disease is epistaxis, which may be profuse and usually begins in early childhood. Epistaxis, if severe enough, can be controlled with electrocauterization (117) or neodymium/yttrium–aluminum–garnet (Nd:YAG) laser ablation (118,119). The classic telangiectatic lesions of HHT may not appear until later in life, commonly the second or third decade. The classic diagnostic triad of HHT is (a) a hereditary basis (70%), (b) telangiectasia, and (c) bleeding from telangiectatic lesions (4). Chronic blood loss, commonly from the GI or genitourinary tract, is often severe enough for patients to have iron deficiency anemia of unknown etiology.

The telangiectatic lesions of HHT may be of three types: pinpoint, nodular, and spider-like (4,120). Although HHT is found in most, if not all, ethnic groups, the lesions may be very difficult to detect in hyperpigmented races such as blacks and Asians. Unlike telangiectasias associated with chronic liver disease, those of HHT are nonpulsatile (4). Telangiectasias and bleeding, especially GI, usually increase with advancing age, although epistaxis often decreases with age (4). The bleeding of HHT may be a covert, but common cause of GI or genitourinary hemorrhage, hemoptysis, or heavy menstrual flow. Successful control of excessive menstrual flow has been noted with use of leuprolide followed by electrocauterization (121). In about 20% to 30% of patients, AV fistulae of the pulmonary vasculature develop (122). Solitary pulmonary fistulae appear to be more common than multiple-site pulmonary fistulae (123) and are much more common in HHT type I. Significant clinical problems resulting from pulmonary fistulae (hemoptysis, shunting, or CNS manifestations) may be treated with photodynamic therapy (124), coil embolization (125), or surgical removal (126). Hepatic AVMs may develop in about 55% of patients, and there is an inordinately high incidence of Laënnec-type cirrhosis in these patients (4,127,128). Hamartomata of the liver and spleen also may be associated with HHT (129). The most serious problem in HHT involves CNS manifestations, which may occur in up to 15% of patients with HHT. Patients with pulmonary AVMs have a high incidence of CNS infections, most commonly abscess formation, but also meningitis (130). These complications arise in at least 5% of patients with pulmonary AVMs. Other CNS manifestations include recurrent transient cerebral ischemic attacks (emboli or small thrombi), overt cerebrovascular thrombosis, intracranial hemorrhage (2% to 3% of all patients with HHT; rupture of telangiectatic lesions or CNS AVMs), and spasms of cerebral vasculature (131,132). Successful treatment for significant cerebral telangiectasias or AVMs has included endovascular embolization (133), surgery, or gamma knife radioneurosurgery (134). Because of the serious pulmonary and CNS sequelae of HHT, all patients should be considered candidates for screening for both pulmonary and CNS AVMs.

There are few characteristic laboratory findings in HHT. The TBT may be normal or abnormal, depending on the integrity of the vasculature in the particular area where the test is done (4). The diagnosis is suggested by a history of recurrent bilateral epistaxis, usually first noted in early years, occult GI bleeding, and the noting of nonpulsatile pinpoint, nodular, or spider-like telangiectasia, most commonly found in the skin, in sublingual and perioral areas, in the buccal mucosa, or under the nails (4).

HHT is often associated with other defects in hemostasis. Abnormal platelet function is present in many patients with HHT (4,135,136). A poorly defined defect in the fibrinolytic system may occur (137,138). Of major importance, and often unappreciated, is an associated DIC syndrome. DIC is often present in a low-grade form but periodically may become fulminant. If looked for, DIC is found in about 50% of patients with HHT; one study, however, did not find DIC in a population of patients with HHT (139,140). In some patients, bleeding may be severe enough that spontaneous intraarticular bleeds, and resultant hemarthroses, develop. HHT may be somewhat similar to the syndrome of giant cavernous hemangiomata and DIC, so a "mini"-Kasabach–Merritt syndrome manifests in some patients, although it is often not recognized (4). When DIC occurs, treatment should be targeted at stopping or blunting the process before a fulminant stage is attained (4,141). Characteristics of HHT are depicted in Table 3.9.

Therapy for uncomplicated HHT depends on the particular clinical situation and age of the patient. Localized epistaxis can often be controlled with local supportive measures and vasoconstrictive nasal sprays. However, electro-

TABLE 3.9. HEREDITARY HEMORRHAGIC TELANGIECTASIA

Clinical findings
Autosomal dominant trait
70% with family history
Epistaxis in early childhood
Easy and spontaneous bruising
Occult mucosal membrane bleeding
Telangiectasia of skin and mucosal surfaces
Pulmonary A-V fistulae
AVMs of central nervous system
Hamartomas and AVMs of liver and spleen
Laennec cirrhosis may occur
Telangiectasia usually increase with age
Bleeding may decrease with age in some
Laboratory findings
Template bleeding time often normal
Platelet dysfunction in 50%
Low-grade DIC findings in 50%

AVM, arteriovenous malformation; DIC, disseminated intravascular coagulation.

TABLE 3.10. ACQUIRED VASCULAR DEFECTS

Cushing syndrome
Diabetes mellitus
Allergic purpuras
Infectious purpuras
Drug-induced purpuras
Collagen (autoimmune) diseases
Systemic lupus erythematosus
Scleroderma
Rheumatoid arthritis
Dermatomyositis
Polyarteritis
Mixed connective tissue disease
Malignant paraprotein disorders
Myeloma
Waldenström
Benign paraprotein disorders
Amyloidosis
Cryoglobulinemia
Essential monoclonal gammopathy

cauterization may become necessary. Some instances of bleeding in HHT, such as gingival bleeding with tooth brushing, spontaneous bruising, and GI/genitourinary bleeding, can sometimes be controlled with adrenosem (142). This agent is usually used as 5 to 10 mg orally every 3 to 4 hours during waking hours and is without significant toxicity. High-dose estrogens may be used to scarify telangiectatic lesions and control bleeding. However, this modality should be used as a last resort, especially in younger patients (143).

Specific therapy for significant bleeding associated with congenital vascular defects, other than HHT, is generally not satisfactory and depends primarily on supportive measures and control of the underlying disease process.

ACQUIRED VASCULAR DEFECTS

The common acquired vascular defects are summarized in Table 3.10. It is important to be familiar with these defects, as they are quite common. Patients with easy and spontaneous bruising, petechiae, and purpura, especially dependent, and other suggestive historical and physical findings should be suspected of having, and be evaluated for, the disorders associated with acquired vascular defects. Alternatively, if an individual has one of these disorders and is going to have surgery or experiences trauma, it can be assumed that a systemic vascular defect is probably present, and significant hemorrhagic or thrombotic problems may follow. The common acquired diseases associated with systemic vascular problems leading to systemic hemorrhagic problems include the acquired collagen vascular disorders, circulating immune complex disorders, multiple myeloma, Waldenström macroglobulinemia, cryoglobulinemia, amyloidosis, Cushing syndrome, diabetes mellitus, the allergic (Henoch–Schönlein) purpuras, many infectious agents, and drug-induced vascular defects (4). Table 3.11 depicts several mechanisms by which these vascular defects develop.

In collagen vascular disorders, the vascular hemorrhagic defect is thought to be because of poor vascular support from intrinsic collagen abnormalities. In Cushing syndrome, it is thought that the vascular disorder and typical hemorrhage are caused by abnormal mucopolysaccharides in perivascular supporting tissue. All the paraproteins, including immunoglobulin A (IgA), IgM, and IgG, have an affinity for attachment to the vascular endothelium and lead to a vascular hemorrhagic problem. This is most commonly noted with IgM and IgG3 paraproteins. Paraproteins also may occlude the vasa vasorum of affected vasculature, again giving rise to hemorrhage (4).

Aspirin is commonly regarded as a platelet-function inhibitor; however, aspirin also is a very effective inhibitor of acetylcholine esterase; this leads to a vascular bleeding

TABLE 3.11. ACQUIRED VASCULAR DISORDERS: PROPOSED MECHANISMS

Cushing syndrome
Loss of mucopolysaccharides in perivascular supporting tissues
Paraprotein diseases
Coating of endothelium by paraprotein and occlusion of vasa vasorum
Allergic, drug, and infectious vasculitis
Immune complex–induced vascular and perivascular injury
Autoimmune diseases
Collagen and connective tissue abnormalities in vascular supportive tissue
Diabetes mellitus
Basement membrane thickening with porosity, decreased proteoglycans, and lipohyaline deposits

problem (144). If a patient is ingesting aspirin, and trauma (or microtrauma in the form of a TBT) ensues, prolonged vascular bleeding may occur. The usual vascular response to trauma is constriction. With vascular trauma, acetylcholine esterase degrades acetylcholine, which keeps the vessel dilated; trauma-induced release of catecholamines will constrict the vessel. If the patient is taking aspirin and the vasculature is severed, acetylcholine esterase is inhibited, acetylcholine cannot be degraded, and inadequate vascular constriction results (4). Prolongation of the TBT after aspirin ingestion may result from the vascular, instead of the platelet, inhibitory effect (4).

Malignant Paraprotein Disorders and Amyloidosis

The many thrombotic and hemorrhagic tendencies in patients with malignant paraprotein disorders and amyloidosis, be they primary or secondary, are well recognized. These disorders can occur with a wide clinical spectrum of hemorrhagic and thrombotic problems, depending on host response, size and site of the vasculature involved, and response of the particular end organ. There have been many proposed mechanisms for the vascular complications of malignant paraprotein disorders, and only the salient features of most of these mechanisms are discussed here. Increased circulating levels of IgG and IgM, which are complement fixing and may lead to histamine release, chemotaxis of leukocytes, and platelet aggregation and release, can lead to increased vascular permeability, serum and blood effusion, and sometimes small vessel thrombosis. Hyperviscosity in the malignant paraprotein disorders is a well-known cause of stasis and resultant ischemia and acidosis. This leads to increased vascular permeability, the consequences of which may be retinal hemorrhage and exudates, epistaxis, petechiae and purpura, and hemorrhage into other organs, including vital organs. Necrotizing vasculitis may happen through unclear mechanisms in malignant paraprotein disorders. Obviously, the clinical manifestations, whether they be thrombosis, hemorrhage, or a combination thereof, will depend on site and severity of the necrotizing vasculitis. When the malignant paraprotein disorders are associated with cryoglobulinemia (IgG and IgM paraprotein disorders), paraprotein is commonly found in the walls of the small vessels, and this may lead to a frank vasculitis; the clinical manifestations range from effusions, bullae, petechiae and purpura, or frank end-organ damage (especially glomerulonephritis) to ischemia, cellular death, and end-organ failure. In malignant paraprotein disorders, there is a high chance of thrombosis, especially manifest as diffuse recurrent deep venous thrombosis, thromboembolism, pulmonary emboli, and renal vein thrombosis (145,146). The mechanisms leading to this are unclear but need not be related to the development of hyperviscosity, except in cases of retinal vein thrombosis (147).

DIC also is seen in patients with malignant paraprotein disorders. Whether this is because of endothelial damage by paraprotein or because of other unexplained mechanisms is unclear. The fibrino(geno)lysis occurring in patients with malignant paraprotein disorders is initiated through unclear mechanisms. This might be fibrinolysis secondary to DIC, fibrinolysis secondary to endothelial damage, or may result from deranged endothelial plasminogen activator activity (148).

Amyloidosis further complicates the vascular changes of malignant paraprotein disorders, and is associated with increased hemorrhage or thrombosis through disruptions of the vasculature. Classically, primary amyloidosis is of unknown etiology or associated with malignant paraprotein disorders. Primary amyloidosis characteristically involves the skin, tongue, heart, and GI tract, whereas secondary amyloidosis is seen with chronic inflammatory/infectious diseases and typically involves the liver, spleen, kidney, and adrenal glands (149). However, many "crossovers" and mixtures of the two are commonly seen, and sometimes one cannot precisely define amyloidosis as primary or secondary (149). Although there are many proposed mechanisms for vasculitis in primary and secondary amyloidosis, precise mechanisms are unclear. Vascular hemorrhage is a hallmark of amyloidosis, and is manifest as petechiae and purpura, ecchymoses, easy and spontaneous bruising, including spontaneous hemorrhage into lymph nodes, recurrent hematuria, and spontaneous hemorrhage into vital organs (4). Several proposed pathophysiologic events leading to generalized vasculitis have included antigen–antibody complex–induced endothelial damage or deposits of amyloid on the endothelium and in the perivascular areas (150). Endothelial and perivascular amyloid deposits are more commonly appreciated in the secondary forms, especially in arterioles. This leads to both a hemorrhagic and a thrombotic tendency. In secondary amyloidosis, amyloid deposits are noted along the endothelium; intimal deposits start in the intima and progress to the media, with amyloid being deposited in parallel with reticulum fibers instead of around the collagen fibers, just as it is in primary amyloidosis. In primary amyloidosis, the deposits are usually seen along the collagen, with progression from the adventitia to the media of arterioles and veins. The same process appears to happen in veins, possibly accounting for the thrombotic tendencies seen in these individuals.

In some patients with systemic amyloidosis, acquired factor X deficiency occurs (151–157). In two patients similarly afflicted, an acquired combined deficiency of factors IX and X was noted (157). Furie et al. (158) explored the mechanisms of factor X deficiency in amyloidosis by using ^{131}I-labeled factor X. A triphasic plasma-clearance pattern was noted; 85% of the labeled factor X cleared in less than 30 seconds, about 10% in less than 90 seconds, and the remaining 5% was absent in 10.5 hours. Subsequent surface scanning of the patients 24 hours after the labeled infusion showed high concentrations in the liver and spleen. This observation, coupled with the rapid clearance of the label on initial transit in the circulation, led these investigators to conclude that the factor X is deposited at prior tissue sites of amyloid. These cases should respond to therapeutic infusions with factor II, VII, IX, and X concentrates; however, only a transient correction by concentrates in factor X–deficient cases of amyloidosis is noted (4). The wide variability of hemorrhagic and thrombotic manifestations in patients with paraprotein disorders and amyloidosis will depend on the particular end organ involved and the degree of vascular permeability and/or occlusion.

In summary, in patients with malignant paraprotein disorders and amyloidosis, a diffuse vascular disease may manifest as hemorrhage, thrombosis, or both. A high variability of end-organ damage may be seen. It is important to appreciate that these patients may experience significant vascular bleeding, and bleeding from obvious other causes, when subjected to surgery or trauma. In evaluation of patients with vascular disorders, malignant paraprotein defects or amyloidosis should be considered in the differential diagnosis. When a selective acquired factor X deficiency in an adult is found, underlying systemic amyloidosis should be strongly suspected.

Autoimmune Disorders and Vascular Defects

Immunologic diseases associated with circulating immune complexes, especially those associated with circulating cryoglobulins, are of paramount importance as disorders associated with a diffuse vasculitis and resultant thrombosis or hemorrhage. At least three potential mechanisms by which circulating immune complexes, circulating cryoglobulins, or circulating antibodies may lead to vasculitis have been described.

1. The production of an antibody directed specifically against the endothelium (159). This is the least common operative mechanism.
2. The production of a nonspecific antibody or immune complex that nonspecifically attacks and damages endothelium and other cellular systems (160).
3. The generation of an antibody or immune complex that attaches to and damages perivascular tissues (including basement membrane), and secondarily causes endothelial damage and increased vascular permeability (161).

The vascular responses and clinical manifestations are variable and depend on severity, duration, and degree of repetition of endothelial or periendothelial insult and damage (162). If the attack is mild, then increased vascular permeability, fibrin deposition, and a fibrinolytic response will occur and leads to minimal hemorrhage and thrombosis (4). If, however, the insult is persistent, there is excessive endothelial damage, depletion of fibrinolytic enzymes and endothelial fibrinolytic activators, increased fibrin and platelet deposition, more pronounced thrombosis or hemorrhage, and more enhanced and perpetuated endothelial damage. In yet more severe insults to the endothelium or surrounding tissue by antibody, immune complex, or cryoglobulins, endothelial death, sloughing, and more severe thrombosis, hemorrhage, and end-organ failure may follow. Antibody directed specifically against the endothelium is a rare mechanism of autoimmune-induced vasculitis and is limited to the allergic purpuras (Henoch–Schönlein, etc.) and polyarteritis nodosum (159). However, future immunologic investigations may define other disorders in this class. The other two mechanisms of immune complex–induced vasculitis are more common and are seen in a wide variety of "autoimmune disorders." In many of these diseases, circulating immune complexes (IgG and IgM) attach to the endothelium, fix complement, and induce migration of leukocytes, which disintegrate and destroy the vessel (163). For example, all are familiar with the results of antistreptococcal antibody attaching to the glomerular endothelium or basement membrane, giving rise to later renal vascular damage (164). An extension of this is Goodpasture syndrome, in which antibody or immune complexes are directed against both renal and pulmonary basement membrane, with associated resultant endothelial damage and thrombohemorrhagic manifestations.

Many infectious agents are known to be associated on rare occasions with vasculitis and the attendant clinical manifestations mentioned earlier. These include many bacterial, viral, and mycoplasma infections. The mechanisms, where known, include the induction of nonspecific antiendothelial antibody by the invading organism, the inducement of specific antiendothelial antibody by the invading microorganism, and the development of circulating immune complexes (165–168). These mechanisms were earlier described. Table 3.12 lists the most common infectious agents associated with a vasculitis.

In most circulating immune complex diseases, the injury is nonspecific, and not only the endothelium but also many other cellular systems are damaged. Diseases with circulating antibody, immune complex, or cryoglobulin-induced vasculitis are many and include collagen vascular disorders, drug reactions, serum sickness, and a large group of seemingly unrelated disorders. Table 3.13 summarizes pathophysiologic mechanisms. Table 3.14 depicts the most common disorders that fit into this category of acquired diseases associated with circulating immune complex, resultant endothelial damage, vasculitis, and clinical thrombohemorrhagic manifestations (4).

Malignant Hypertension, Eclampsia, Cushing Disease, Diabetes Mellitus, and Vascular Defects

Patients with malignant hypertension, advancing age, or diabetes mellitus deposit lipohyaline material (fibrin) in the

TABLE 3.12. COMMON INFECTIOUS AGENTS ASSOCIATED WITH VASCULITIS

Bordatella pertussis
Chlamydia
Clostridium tetani
Coccidioidomycosis
Cornybacterium diphtheriae
Cytomegalovirus
Epstein–Barr virus
Escherichia coli
Hepatitis virus
Human immunodeficiency virus (HIV)
Influenza virus
Leprosy
Malaria
Mycobacteria
Pseudomonas aeruginosa
Salmonella typhi
Staphylococcus
Streptococcus
Subacute bacterial endocarditis
Syphilis
Tuberculosis

subendothelium of arteries and arterioles (4). In malignant hypertension, fibrinoid necrosis is another characteristic feature. As constant unrelenting damage proceeds, the vessels eventually develop increased vascular permeability with plasma seepage and fibrin deposition. This leads to thrombosis and thromboembolism, a common clinical problem in these disorders (169). The resultant downstream capillary stasis leads to the development of chronic purpura and local hyperpigmentation of the skin, resulting from chronic hemosiderin deposits. The reader is referred to authoritative reviews for more complete pathophysiologic events in these disorders (170–172). The findings in eclampsia are similar to those earlier described, with the development of hypertension and localized intravascular coagulation (fibrin deposition) in the placental and renal microcirculation (173,174). Some women have classic findings of either chronic or acute DIC with any or all the clinical manifestations of DIC (98,175).

The vascular changes of Cushing disease are poorly defined, but include loss of subcutaneous elastic tissues, leading to inadequate endothelial cell support, increased vascular permeability and fragility, and loss of elastic tissue in the vascular walls (4). Advanced atherosclerotic changes also occur in larger vessels (176). Easy and spontaneous bruising is seen in most patients with Cushing syndrome, as is a marked increase of thrombosis and thromboembolic disease (4). Many patients with Cushing syndrome experience profuse bleeding, because of a vascular defect, when undergoing surgery or trauma (4).

TABLE 3.13. IMMUNE-ASSOCIATED VASCULAR DISEASE: PROPOSED MECHANISMS

Anti–endothelial cell antibody and endothelial cell destruction
Immune complex (IgG and IgM) attachment to endothelium with complement fixation, migration of leukocytes, and destruction of the vessel
Immune complex (IgG and IgM) attachment to basement membrane or perivascular supportive tissue with increased vascular permeability or other damage

Ig, immunoglobulin.

TABLE 3.14. IMMUNE-MEDIATED DISORDERS ASSOCIATED WITH VASCULAR DEFECTS

Cryoglobulinemia
Sjögren syndrome
Proliferative glomerulonephritis
Lymphoma and lymphoid leukemia
Chronic infection or inflammation
Malignant hypertension
Viral infection
Subacute bacterial endocarditis
Allergic vasculitis
Drug-induced vasculitis
Collagen diseases
Systemic lupus
Mixed connective tissue disease
Scleroderma
Dermatomyositis
Polyarteritis
Rheumatoid arthritis
Behçet syndrome

Behçet Syndrome

Behçet syndrome is most commonly, but certainly not exclusively, seen in people of Mediterranean area and Japan (177) and is typically characterized by a typical triad of aphthous stomatitis, genital ulcerations, and iritis (178–180). In many patients, recurrent deep venous thrombosis of unexplained pathophysiologic origin develops, usually involving large veins, the saphenous veins, sagittal and dural sinus, portal and hepatic veins, and the superior and inferior vena cava (181–183). Many with superior vena cava thrombosis have or develop superior vena cava (SVC) syndrome (184–186). Of patients with thrombosis, about 60% are venous, 30% are arterial events, and about 10% are both arterial and venous (187). Aneurysms also have been reported (188). In many patients, a widespread, poorly defined arteritis develops (189). Patients may show fibrinoid necrosis of the arterial tree (190). Case reports have documented impaired fibrinolysis, and some patients have responded to thrombolytic therapy (191). Except for the finding of impaired endothelial fibrinolytic activity, thus far the pathophysiologic mechanisms responsible for recurrent deep venous thrombosis, arteritis, and hemorrhage, usually manifest as petechiae and purpura, are unclear. Pathological examinations of patients with Behçet syndrome generally reveal perivascular inflammatory changes

(192). Although oral and genital ulcers are the most common mucocutaneous manifestations, many have skin ulcers as well (193). The ocular manifestations are usually white patches of retinitis with hemorrhage, retinal vasculitis, optic neuritis, and cataract formation (194,195). Several reports have related Behçet syndrome to development of myelodysplastic syndromes, but this requires confirmation (196,197). Therapeutic agents suggested to be effective in Behçet syndrome include colchicine, prednisone, other immunosuppressives, dapsone, methotrexate, and thalidomide (198–200).

Vascular Defects Associated with Cardiopulmonary Bypass

Poorly understood defects in the vasculature may occur during or after cardiopulmonary bypass (CPB) surgery. A syndrome of mild to moderate nonthrombocytopenic purpura, accompanied by splenomegaly and atypical lymphocytosis after CPB has been noted (201). In this syndrome, purpura is usually benign, self-limiting, and frequently manifest only after discharge from the hospital. One patient has been reported in whom post-CPB classic glomerulonephritis was found, of the type seen with the allergic vasculitides. Fatal purpura fulminans also may occur after CPB (202). An inflammatory vasculitis may be associated with CPB; however, the mechanisms are unclear.

Drug-induced Vasculitis

Drug-induced vasculitis is common in clinical medicine and very often is neglected as a cause of petechiae and purpura, skin necrosis, or frank gangrene. There are many mechanisms by which drugs may induce vasculitis, and most do not significantly differ from the mechanisms operative in circulating immune complex disorders. Frequently, however, the precise mechanisms by which drugs induce vasculitis are poorly understood. Among the mechanisms by which drugs may induce vascular defects are the development of a specific antivessel antibody (203); the development of circulating immune complexes, sometimes associated with cryoglobulinemia (204); and more rarely, drug-induced independent changes in vascular permeability. A characteristic, catastrophic, and well-characterized vasculitis associated with warfarin anticoagulants should be familiar to all (205–210). This and hemorrhagic skin vasculitis are manifest by hemorrhagic skin infarction, and sometimes have been associated with intravascular coagulation (211,212). Most warfarin derivatives have been incriminated: 90% of cases have been women, and gangrene of the breast has happened in at least 25% of cases reported in the literature. The histologic features of this syndrome have been described quite well and show perivascular accumulations of inflammatory cells involving mainly the venules, with extensive thrombosis of the draining veins with little or no invasion of arterioles (213). Typically the clinical picture develops 3 to 10 days after starting therapy and bears little relation to the prothrombin time. Many patients are deficient in protein C, protein S, or antithrombin III, and it is thought that there is a short period of hypercoagulability, resulting from initial imbalance of the procoagulant and anticoagulant systems of these patients when they start warfarins (214,215). However, some patients with this disorder have normal protein C, protein S, and antithrombin III levels, and in these instances, the mechanism may be that of a direct toxic effect on the endothelium by warfarin. Many patients will respond to heparin/LMW heparin therapy (213–215). However, unfractionated heparin also has been associated with this syndrome in patients with protein C or S defects and in the presence or absence of heparin-induced thrombocytopenia with or without paradoxic thrombosis (216). The most common drugs causing vascular problems are listed in Table 3.15. A complete list of drugs associated with vascular defects/disease is given in Tables 3.16, by generic name, and in Table 3.17, by brand name.

TABLE 3.15. COMMON DRUGS ASSOCIATED WITH VASCULAR DEFECTS

Aspirin	Iodine
Allopurinol	Isoniazid
Arsenicals	Meprobamate
Chloramphenicol	Methyldopa
Chlorothiazide	Piperazine
Chlorpropamide	Quinidine
Digoxin	Quinine
Estrogens	Reserpine
Furosemide	Sulfonamides
Gold	Tolbutamide
Heparin	Warfarins
Indomethacin	

LABORATORY FINDINGS IN VASCULAR DEFECTS

The primary laboratory screening test for a vascular disorder or a platelet function defect is the standardized TBT (217,218). However, the standardized TBT is generally quite unreliable (219,220) and may be abnormal in normal individuals, may be normal in abnormal individuals, and a normal TBT is no assurance that a patient may not bleed at surgery or trauma. However, if the TBT is greater than 15 minutes, it may be assumed that bleeding with trauma or surgery is a likely possibility. A standardized TBT is usually not done in young individuals, especially infants and children younger than 15 years; a normal range has not been established for this age group, and undue scar formation may occur. Prolonged bleeding times in children are common and therefore difficult, if not impossible, to interpret. In these instances, the petechiometer test should be used; the petechiometer is discussed in later sections. If an indi-

TABLE 3.16. DRUGS ASSOCIATED WITH VASCULAR DEFECTS BY GENERIC NAME

Generic Name/Composition	Brand Name	Classification
Allopurinol	Zyloprim	NSAID
Amiloride/hydrochlorothiazide	Moduretic	Diuretic
Amoxapine	Asendin	CNS
Atenolol/chlorothalidone	Tenoretic	Cardiac
Biperiden	Akineton	CNS
Bleomycin	Blenoxane	Antineoplastic
Chlorthalidone	Thalitone	Diuretic
Chlorthiazide	Diuril	Diuretic
Clofazimine	Lamprene	Antibiotic
Clonidine	Combipres	Cardiac
Cromolyn	Intal	Pulmonary
	Nasalcrom	Pulmonary
Dexamethasone	Dalalone	Steroid
Diflunisal	Dolobid	NSAID
Doxorubicin	Doxorubicin	Antineoplastic
Edrophonium	Tensilon	CNS
Fluoxetine	Prozac	CNS
Furosemide	Lasix	Cardiac
Guanethidine/thiazide	Esimil	Diuretic
Hydralazine/thiazide	Apresazide	Cardiac
Hydrochlorothiazide	Esidrix	Diuretic
	Hydrodiuril	Diuretic
Hydroflumethiazide/reserpine	Salutensin	Diuretic
Indomethacin	Indocin	NSAID
	Indomethacin	NSAID
Isoniazid	INH	Antibiotic
Methyldopa/chlorothiazide	Aldoclor	Cardiac
Methyldopa/hydrochlorothiazide	Aldoril	Cardiac
Methylphenidate	Ritalin	CNS
Metolazone	Mykrox	Diuretic
	Zaroxolyn	Diuretic
Neostigmine	Prostigmin	CNS
Penicillamine	Cuprimine	Hematologic
Pentamidine	Nebupent	Antibiotic
	Pentam	Antibiotic
Pergolide	Permax	CNS
Pyridostigmine	Mestinon	CNS
Quinethazone	Hydromox	Diuretic
Reserpine/chlorothiazide	Diupress	Cardiac
Reserpine/hydrochlorothiazide	Hydropres	Cardiac
Reserpine/thiazide	Serpasil-esidrex	Cardiac
Reserpine/thiazide/hydralazine	Ser-Ap-Es	Cardiac
Rifampin/isoniazid	Rifamate	Antibiotic
Streptokinase	Streptase	Cardiac
Sulindac	Clinoril	NSAID
Triamcinolone	Aristocort	Steroid
Triamterene/hydroclorothiazide	Maxzide	Cardiac
Vancomycin	Vancocin	Antibiotic
Verapamil	Isoptin	Cardiac
	Verelan	Cardiac
Warfarin	Coumadin	Cardiac
	Dicumarol	Anticoagulant
	Panwarfin	Anticoagulant

NSAID, nonsteroidal antiinflammatory drug; CNS, central nervous system.

TABLE 3.17. DRUGS ASSOCIATED WITH VASCULAR DEFECTS BY BRAND NAME

Brand Name	Generic Name/Composition	Classification
Akineton	Biperiden	CNS
Aldoclor	Methyldopa/Chlorothiazide	Cardiac
Aldoril	Methyldopa/Hydrochlorothiazide	Cardiac
Apresazide	Hydralazine/Thiazide	Cardiac
Aristocort	Triamcinolone	Steroid
Asendin	Amoxapine	CNS
Blenoxane	Bleomycin	Antineoplastic
Clinoril	Sulindac	NSAID
Combipres	Clonidine	Cardiac
Coumadin	Warfarin	Cardiac
Cuprimine	Penicillamine	Hematologic
Dalalone	Dexamethasone	Steroid
Dicumarol	Warfarin	Anticoagulant
Diupress	Reserpine/Chlorothiazide	Cardiac
Diuril	Chlorothiazide	Diuretic
Dolobid	Diflunisal	NSAID
Doxorubicin	Doxorubicin	Antineoplastic
Esidrix	Hydrochlorothiazide	Diuretic
Esimil	Guanethidine/Thiazide	Diuretic
Hydrodiuril	Hydrochlorothiazide	Diuretic
Hydromox	Quinethazone	Diuretic
Hydropres	Reserpine/Hydrochlorothiazide	Cardiac
Indocin	Indomethacin	NSAID
Indomethacin	Indomethacin	NSAID
INH	Isoniazid	Antibiotic
Intal	Cromolyn	Pulmonary
Isoptin	Verapamil	Cardiac
Lamprene	Clofazimine	Antibiotic
Lasix	Furozemide	Cardiac
Maxzide	Triamterene/Hydroclorothiazide	Cardiac
Mestinon	Pyridostigmine	CNS
Moduretic	Amiloride/Hydrochlorothiazide	Diuretic
Mykrox	Metolazone	Diuretic
Nasalcrom	Cromolyn	Pulmonary
Nebupent	Pentamidine	Antibiotic
Panwarfin	Warfarin	Anticoagulant
Pentam	Pentamidine	Antibiotic
Permax	Pergolide	CNS
Prostigmin	Neostigmine	CNS
Prozac	Fluoxetine	CNS
Rifamate	Rifampin/Isoniazid	Antibiotic
Ritalin	Methylphenidate	CNS
Salutensin	Hydroflumethiazide/Reserpine	Diuretic
Ser-Ap-Es	Reserpine/Thiazide/Hydralazine	Cardiac
Serpasil-Esidrex	Reserpine/Thiazide	Cardiac
Streptase	Streptokinase	Cardiac
Tenoretic	Atenolol/Chlorthalidone	Cardiac
Tensilon	Edrophonium	CNS
Thalitone	Chlorthalidone	Diuretic
Vancocin	Vancomycin	Antibiotic
Verelan	Verapamil	Cardiac
Zaroxolyn	Metolazone	Diuretic
Zyloprim	Allopurinol	NSAID

CNS, central nervous system; NSAID, nonsteroidal antiinflammatory drug.

vidual demonstrates a borderline TBT, in the 10- to 12-minute range, with a positive or suggestive history, the aspirin tolerance test is useful (4,221). The aspirin tolerance test consists of giving 600 mg of aspirin and repeating the TBT in the opposite antecubital fossa 2 hours after the aspirin. Most TBTs will be prolonged by about 2 to 3 minutes; however, the ingestion of 600 mg aspirin will unmask an underlying vascular or platelet-function defect and render the repeated bleeding time about 3 times the baseline TBT, usually 20 to 30 minutes (4). Once an abnormal TBT, abnormal petechiometer test, or aspirin tolerance test has been shown in the appropriate clinical setting, with a normal platelet count, the differential diagnosis is then between a platelet-function and a vascular defect. To make this differential diagnosis, platelet-function testing must next be done. The definitive tests useful to differentiate between vascular and platelet defects is platelet aggregation or lumi-aggregation by densitometry or impedance, use of the newer PFA-100 or use of the Thrombostat 4000; these are discussed in Chapter 4 (Platelet Function Defects). An abnormal TBT and a normal platelet function, as defined by acceptable tests to assess platelet function, define a vascular disorder. Once a vascular defect has been documented, more definitive tests including an evaluation for autoimmune disease, paraprotein disorders, possibly a connective tissue or vascular biopsy, or other similar modalities will often be needed to make a definitive diagnosis (4).

Many tests are now available to the hemostasis laboratory to assess vascular function; these consist of compounds synthesized by or released by the endothelium and include E-selectin, soluble thrombomodulin, endothelin, tissue plasminogen activator, thromboxane derivatives, and others. The presence of an immune component to vascular disease/damage may be accomplished by performing a Raji cell assay and C1q complement level for circulating immune complexes (222–225). The presence of a vascular disorder is usually documented in the hemostasis laboratory; however, once the presence of a vascular disorder has been established, the specific diagnosis usually falls outside the realm of the hemostasis laboratory, and other types of laboratory procedures, including special biopsies and staining, are needed for a definitive diagnosis. Table 3.18 summarizes the laboratory assays for evaluation of vascular defects.

TABLE 3.18. TESTS USEFUL FOR ASSESSING VASCULAR DISORDERS

Template bleeding time[a]
Soluble thrombomodulin
von Willebrand Factor
E-Selectin
Tissue plasminogen activator (t-PA)
Plasminogen activator inhibitor (PAI-1)
Thromboxane B_2
Prostacyclin
Endothelin
Platelet-activating factor (PAF)
Raji cell assay[b]
C1q[b]
Cryoglobulins
Antiphospholipid antibodies
Annexin V
Paraproteins
Cold agglutinins
Vascular biopsy
Test to rule out platelet dysfunction
Platelet (LUMI) aggregation[c]
PFA-100
THROMBOSTAT 4000

[a]Unreliable.
[b]Establishes immune/autoimmune etiology or component.
[c]Densitometry or impedance.

SUMMARY

This chapter summarizes the more important diseases that may be accompanied by or lead to a disorder of hemostasis or thrombosis through alterations of the vasculature. It is to be stressed that the vascular component of hemostasis is often overlooked by clinicians caring for patients with disorders of hemostasis and thrombosis. It should be appreciated that the vasculature is intricately related to the coagulation protein system and to platelets when involved in a thrombohemorrhagic diatheses. Although many vascular disorders themselves may lead to hemorrhage or thrombosis, it must be appreciated that often it is impossible to discriminate between a primary vascular defect/damage and a defect that has been induced by platelet activation/dysfunction or procoagulant abnormalities.

REFERENCES

1. Bick RL. Hereditary and acquired vascular bleeding disorders. In: Bick RL, Bennett JM, Brynes RK, eds. *Hematology: clinical and laboratory practice.* St. Louis: Mosby, 1993:1325.
2. Bick RL. Clinical evaluation of the patient with hemorrhage. In: Bick RL, Bennett JM, Byrnes RK, eds. *Hematology: clinical and laboratory practice.* St. Louis: Mosby, 1993:1317.
3. Bick RL. Vascular disorders associated with thrombohemorrhagic phenomenon. In: *Disorders of hemostasis and thrombosis.* New York: Thieme, 1985:44.
4. Bick RL. Vascular bleeding disorders. In: *Disorders of thrombosis and hemostasis: clinical and laboratory practice* Chicago: ASCP Press, 1992:35.
5. Alshameeri RS, Mammen EF. Clinical experience with the Thrombostat 4000. *Semin Thromb Hemost* 1995;21(suppl 2):1.
6. Kundo SK, Heilmann EJ, Sio R, et al. Description of an in-vitro platelet function analyzer: PFA-100. *Semin Thromb Hemost* 1995;21(suppl 2):106.
7. Johnson SA, Falls EF. Ehlers-Danlos syndrome: a clinical and genetic study. *Arch Dermatol Suppl* 1949;60:82.
8. Sacheti A, Szemere J, Bernstein BJ, et al. Chronic pain is a manifestation of the Ehlers-Danlos syndrome. *J Pain Symptom Manage* 1997;14:88.
9. Roberts HR, Kroncke FG. Tests of platelet activity: application to

clinical diagnosis. In: Brinkhous KM, Shermer RW, Mostofi FK, eds. *The platelet.* Baltimore: Williams & Wilkins, 1971:365.

10. Dolan AL, Mishra MB, Chambers JB, et al. Clinical and echocardiographic survey of the Ehlers-Danlos syndrome. *Br J Rheumatol* 1997;36:459.
11. McIntosh LJ, Mallett VT, Frahm JD, et al. Gynecologic disorders in women with Ehlers-Danlos syndrome. *J Soc Gynecol Invest* 1995;2:559.
12. Millar AJ, Ghilbert RD, Brown RA, et al. Abdominal aortic aneurysms in children. *J Pediatr Surg* 1996;31:1624.
13. Oyen O, Clausen OP, Brekke IB, et al. Spontaneous rupture of the renal artery in a patient with the Ehlers-Danlos syndrome. *Eur J Vasc Endovasc Surg* 1997;13:509.
14. Schievink WI. Genetics of intracranial aneurysms. *Neurosurgery* 1997;40:651.
15. Sonesson B, Hansen F, Lanne T. The mechanical properties of elastic arteries in Ehlers-Danlos syndrome. *Eur J Vasc Endovasc Surg* 1997;14:258.
16. Paradisi M, Guibilie L, Canzona F, et al. Ehlers-Danlos syndrome type I: ultrastructural study. *Minerva Pediatr* 1997;49:215.
17. Greenspan DS, Northrup H, Au KS, et al. COL5A1: fine genetic mapping and exclusion as a candidate gene in families with nail-patella syndrome, tuberous sclerosis 1, hereditary hemorrhagic telangiectasia and Ehlers-Danlos syndrome type II. *Genomics* 1995;25:737.
18. Michalickova K, Susic M, Willing MC, et al. Mutations of the alpha2(V) chain of type V collagen impair matrix assembly and produce Ehlers-Danlos syndrome type I. *Hum Mol Genet* 1998; 7:249.
19. Wenstrup RJ, Langland GT, Willing MC, et al. Splice-junction mutation in the region of COL5A1 that codes for the carboxyl propeptide of pro alpha 1(V) chains results in the gravis form of the Ehlers-Danlos syndrome (type 1). *Hum Mol Genet* 1996;5: 1733.
20. De Paepe A, Nuytinck L, Hausser I, et al. Mutations in the COL5A1 gene are causal in the Ehlers-Danlos syndrome I and II. *Am J Hum Genet* 1997;60:547.
21. Angelsw CH, van Dongen PW, Boers GH, et al. Ehlers-Danlos syndrome type IV: phenotype variation. *Ned Tijdschr Geneeskd* 1997;141:296.
22. Eltchaninoff H, Cribier A, Letac B. Peripheral and coronary artery dissections in a young woman: a rare case of type IV Ehlers-Danlos syndrome. *Arch Mal Coeur Vaiss* 1997;90:841.
23. Gelbmann CM, Kollinger M, Gmeinweiser J, et al. Spontaneous rupture of liver in a patient with Ehlers-Danlos disease, type IV. *Dig Dis Sci* 1997;42:1724.
24. Lauwers G, Nevelsteen A, Daenen G, et al. Ehlers-Danlos syndrome type IV: a heterogenous disease. *Ann Vasc Surg* 1997;11: 178.
25. Schwarze U, Goldstein JA, Byers PH. Splicing defects in the COL3A1 gene: marked preference for 5′ (donor) splice-size mutations in patients with exon-skipping mutations and Ehlers-Danlos syndrome type IV. *Am J Hum Genet* 1997;61:1276.
26. Liu X, Wu H, Byrne M, et al. Type III collagen is crucial for collagen I fibrillogenesis and for normal cardiovascular development. *Proc Natl Acad Sci U S A* 1997;94:1852.
27. Anderson DW, Thakker-Varia S, Tromp G, et al. A glycine (415)-to-serine substitution results in impaired secretion and decreased thermal stability of type III procollagen in a patient with Ehlers-Danlos syndrome type IV. *Hum Mutat* 1997;9:62.
28. Smith LT, Schwarze U, Goldstein J, et al. Mutations in the COL3A1 gene result in the Ehlers-Danlos syndrome type IV and alterations in the size and distribution of the major collagen fibrils of the dermis. *J Invest Dermatol* 1997;108:241.
29. Pajunen L, Soukas M, Hautala T, et al. A slice-site mutation that induces exon skipping and reduction in lysyl hydroxylase mRNA levels but does not create a nonsense codon in Ehlers-Danlos syndrome type IV. *DNA Cell Biol* 1998;17:117.
30. Pousi B, Hautala T, Hyland JC, et al. A compound heterozygote patient with Ehlers-Danlos syndrome type IV has a deletion in one allele and a splicing defect in the other allele of the lysyl hydroxylase gene. *Hum Mutat* 1998;11:55.
31. Yeowell HN, Walker LC, Murad S, et al. A common duplication in the lysyl hydroxylase gene of patients with Ehlers-Danlos syndrome type IV results in preferential stimulation of lysyl hydroxylase activity and mRNA by hydralazine. *Arch Biochem Biophys* 1997;347:126.
32. Yeowell HN, Walker LC. Ehlers-Danlos syndrome type IV results from a nonsense mutation and a splice-site-mediated exon-skipping mutation in the lysyl hydroxylase gene. *Proc Assoc Am Physicians* 1997;109:383.
33. Byers PH, Duvic M, Atkinson M, et al. Ehlers-Danlos syndrome type VIIA and VIIB result from splice-junction mutations or genomic deletions that involve exon 6 in the COL1A1 and COL1A2 genes of type I collagen. *Am J Med Genet* 1997;72:94.
34. Kuivaniemi H, Peltonen L, Kivirikko KI. Type IX Ehlers-Danlos syndrome and Menkes syndrome: the decrease in lysyl oxidase activity is associated with a corresponding deficiency in the enzyme protein. *Am J Hum Genet* 1985;37:798.
35. Stine KC, Becton DL. DDAVP therapy controls bleeding in Ehlers-Danlos syndrome. *J Pediatr Hematol Oncol* 1997;19:156.
36. Anderson M Pratt-Thomas RH. Marfan's syndrome. *Am Heart J* 1953;46:911.
37. Futcher PH, Southworth H. Arachnodactyly and its medical complications. *Arch Intern Med* 1938;61:693.
38. Toriello HV, Glover TW, Takahara K, et al. A translocation interrupts the COL5A1 gene in a patient with Ehlers-Danlos syndrome and hypomelanosis of Ito. *Nat Genet* 1996;13:361.
39. Fleischer KJ, Nousari HC, Anhalt GJ, et al. Immunohistochemical abnormalities of fibrillin in cardiovascular tissues in Marfan's syndrome. *Ann Thorac Surg* 1997;63:1012.
40. Reinhardt DP, Chalberg SC, Sakai LY. The structure and function of fibrillin. *Ciba Found Symp* 1995;192:128.
41. Gillinov AM, Zehr KJ, Redmond JM, et al. Cardiac operations in children with Marfan's syndrome: indications and results. *Ann Thorac Surg* 1997;64:1140.
42. Millar AJ, Gilbert RD, Brown RA, et al. Abdominal aortic aneurysms in children. *J Pediatr Surg* 1996;31:1624.
43. Sekine S, Abe T, Kuribayashi R, et al. Aortic root syndrome. *Cardiovasc Surg* 1996;4:635.
44. Lipscomb KJ, Smith JC, Clarke B, et al. Outcome of pregnancy in women with Marfan's syndrome. *Br J Obstet Gynaecol* 1997; 104:201.
45. Dotrelova D, Karel I, Clupkova E. Retinal detachment in Marfans syndrome: characteristics and surgical results. *Retina* 1997; 17:390.
46. Schievink AU, Parisi WI, Piepgras JE, et al. Intracranial aneurysms in Marfan's syndrome: an autopsy study. *Neurosurgery* 1997;41:866.
47. Sullivan CE. Influence of maxillary constriction on nasal resistance and sleep apnea severity in patients with Marfan's syndrome. *Chest* 1996;110:1184.
48. Cistulli PA, Sullivan CE. Sleep apnea in Marfan's syndrome: increased upper airway collapsibility during sleep. *Chest* 1995; 108:631.
49. Cole WG. The molecular pathology of osteogenesis imperfecta. *Clin Orthop* 1997;343:235.
50. De Paepe A, Nuytinck L, Raes M, et al. Homozygosity by descent for a COL1A2 mutation in two sibs with severe osteogenesis imperfecta and mild clinical expression in the heterozygotes. *Hum Genet* 1997;99:478.
51. Lund AM, Nicholls AC, Schwartz M, et al. Parenteral mosaicism

and autosomal dominant mutations causing structural abnormalities of collagen I are frequent in families with osteogenesis imperfecta type III / IV. *Acta Paediatr* 1997;86:711.
52. Bouvier M, Colson F, Noel E, et al. Two new case reports of reflex sympathetic dystrophy syndrome in patients with osteogenesis imperfecta: review of the literature. *Rev Rhum* 1997;64:202.
53. Korkko J, Ala-Kokko L, De Paepe A, et al. Analysis of the COL1A1 and COL1A2 genes by PCR amplification and scanning by conformation-sensitive gel electrophoresis identifies only COL1A1 mutations in 15 patients with osteogenesis imperfecta type I: identification of common sequences of null-allele mutations. *Am J Hum Genet* 1998;62:98.
54. Forlino A, D'Amato E, Valli M, et al. Phenotypic comparison of an osteogenesis imperfecta type IV proband with a de novo alpha2(I) Gly 922 to Ser substitution in type I collagen and an unrelated patient with an identical mutation. *Biochem Mol Med* 1997;62:26.
55. Williams CJ, Smith RA, Ball RJ, et al. Hypercalcaemia in osteogenesis imperfecta treated with pamidronate. *Arch Dis Child* 1997;76:169.
56. Bembi B, Parma A, Bottega M, et al. Intravenous pamidronate treatment in osteogenesis imperfecta. *J Pediatr* 1997;131:622.
57. Landsmeer-Beker EA, Massa GG, Maaswinkel,-Mooy PD, et al. Treatment of osteogenesis imperfecta with the biphosphanate olpadronate (dimethylaminohydroxypropylidene bisphosphonate). *Eur J Pediatr* 1997;156:792.
58. Williams CJ, Smith RA, Ball RJ, et al. Hypercalcaemia in osteogenesis imperfecta treated with pamidronate *Arch Dis Child* 1997;76:169.
59. Albright JA, Miller AE. Osteogenesis imperfecta. *Clin Orthop* 1981;159:2.
60. Myrmel T, Christensen O, Lunde P. Cardiac manifestations in osteogenesis imperfecta: a case report and therapeutic implications. *Tidsskr Nor Laegeforen* 1997;117:519.
61. Gilbert GJ. Spontaneous dissections. *Neurology* 1997;48:1475.
62. Seibel BM, Briedman IA, Schwartz SO. Hemorrhagic disease in osteogenesis imperfecta: studies of platelet function defect. *Am J Med* 1957;22:315.
63. Polimer IJ. Pseudoxanthoma elasticum and gastrointestinal hemorrhage. *J Maine Med Assoc* 1967;58:76.
64. Struk B, Neldner KH, Rao VS, et al. Mapping of both autosomal recessive and dominant variants of pseudoxanthoma elasticum to chromosome 16p13.1. *Hum Mol Genet* 1997;6:1823.
65. Swart J, Tijmes NT. Proteoglycan alterations in skin fibroblast cultures from patients affected with pseudoxanthoma elasticum. *Cell Biochem Funct* 1996;14:111.
66. Piccoli A, Ricciardi D, Santucci A, et al. Elevated levels of plasma endothelin-1, von Willebrand factor, and urinary albumin excretion in three relatives with pseudoxanthoma elasticum *Thromb Haemost* 1996;76:278.
67. Spinzi G, Strocchi E, Imperiali G, et al. Pseudoxanthoma elasticum: a rare cause of gastrointestinal bleeding. *Am J Gastroenterol* 1996;91:1631.
68. Fred HL, Hariharan R. Hematemesis in a woman with skin, eye, and heart abnormalities. *Hosp Pract* 1995;30:28.
69. Okamura T, Yamamoto M, Ohta K, et al. A case of ruptured cerebral aneurysm associated with fenestrated vertebral artery in osteogenesis imperfecta]. *Neurol Surg* 1995;23:451.
70. Cailleux N, Hachulla E, Perez-Cousin M, et al. Pseudoxanthoma elasticum: a rare cause of leg artery diseases in young adults *J Mal Vasc* 1997;22:51.
71. Hirano T, Hashimoto Y, Kimura K, et al. Lacunar brain infarction in patients with pseudoxanthoma elasticum. *Clin Neurol* 1996;36:633.
72. Gurwood AS, Mastrangelo DL. Understanding angioid streaks. *J Am Optomet Assoc* 1997;68:309.
73. Janotka H, Hess J, Wlodarczyk J. Angioid streaks: pathogenesis and the clinical picture. *Klin Oczna* 1995;97:299.
74. Guba SC, Fink LM, Fonseca V. Hyperhomocysteinemia: an emerging and important risk factor for thromboembolic and cardiovascular disease. *Am J Clin Pathol* 1996;105:709.
75. Rees MM, Rodgers GM. Homocysteinemia: association of a metabolic disorder with vascular disease and thrombosis. *Thromb Res* 1993;71:337.
76. Kang SS, Zhou J, Wong PWK, et al. Intermediate homocysteinemia: a thermolabile variant of methylenetetrahydrofolate reductase. *Am J Hum Genet* 1988;43:414.
77. Frosst P, Blom HJ, Milos R. A candidate genetic risk factor for vascular disease: a common mutation in methylenetetrahydrofolate reductase. *Nat Genet* 1995;10:111.
78. Mudd SH, Levy HL, Skovby F. Disorders of transsulfuration. In: Schriver CR, Beaudet AL, Sly WS, et al., eds. *The metabolic basis of inherited disease.* New York: McGraw-Hill, 1995:1279.
79. Fenton WA, Rosenberg LE. Inherited disorders of cobalamine transport and metabolism. In: Scriver CR, Beaudet AL, Sly WS, et al., eds. *The metabolic basis of inherited disease.* New York: McGraw-Hill, 1995:3129.
80. Valle D, Pai GS, Thomas GH. Homocystinuria due to cystathionine beta-synthetase deficiency: clinical manifestations and therapy. *Johns Hopkins Med J* 1980;146:110.
81. Boers GHJ, Smals AG, Trijbels FJ. Heterozygosity for homocystinuria in premature peripheral and cerebral occlusive arterial disease. *N Engl J Med* 1985;313:709.
82. Carey MC, Donovan DE, Fitzgerald O, et al. Homocystinuria, I: a clinical and pathologic study of nine subjects in six families. *Am J Med* 1968;45:17.
83. Harker LA, Ross R, Slichter SJ, et al. Homocysteine-induced arteriosclerosis: the role of endothelial cell injury and platelet response in its genesis. *J Clin Invest* 1976;58:731.
84. Di Minno G, Davi G, Margaglione M. Abnormally high thromboxane biosynthesis in homozygous homocystinuria: evidence for involvement and probucol-sensitive mechanism. *J Clin Invest* 1993;92:1400.
85. Ratnoff OD, Activation of Hageman factor by L homocystine. *Science* 1968;162:1007.
86. Rodgers GM, Conn MT. Homocysteine: an atherogenic stimulus reduces protein C activation by arterial and venous endothelial cells. *Blood* 1990;75:895.
87. Lentz SR, Sadler JE. Inhibition of thrombomodulin surface expression and protein C activation by the thrombogenic agent homocystine. *J Clin Invest* 1991;88:1906.
88. Harpel PC, Zhang X, Borth W. Homocysteine and hemostasis: pathogenetic mechanisms predisposing to thrombosis. *J Nutr* 1996;126:1285.
89. Anderson A, Isaksson A, Hultberg B. Homocysteine export from erythrocytes and its implication for plasma testing. *Clin Chem* 1992;38:1311.
90. Brenton DP, Cusworth DC, Gaull GE. Homocystinuria: metabolic studies on three patients. *J Pediatr* 1965;67:58.
91. Kottke-Marchant K, Green R, Jacobsen DJ, et al. High plasma homocysteine: a risk factor for arterial and venous thrombosis in patients with normal coagulation profiles. *Clin Appl Thromb Hemost* 1997;3:239.
92. Cocceri S, Palareti G. Premature vascular disease in homocystinaemia. *Haemostasis* 1989;19(suppl 1):4.
93. Burbank MK, Spittell JA. Tumor of blood and lymph vessels. In: Juergens JL, Spittell JA, Fairbairn JF, eds. *Peripheral vascular diseases.* Philadelphia: WB Saunders, 1980:679.
94. Takahashi T, Katoh H, Dohke M, et al. A giant hepatic hemangioma with secondary portal hypertension: a case report of successful surgical treatment. *Hepatogastroenterology* 1997; 44:1212.

95. Greif F, Zifroni A, Madhala OG. Giant cavernous hemangioma of the liver. *Harefuah* 1996;131:471.
96. Allen PW, Enzinger FM. Hemangiomata of skeletal muscle: analysis of 89 cases. *Cancer* 1972;28:8.
97. Kasabach HH, Merritt KK. Capillary hemangioma with extensive purpura. *Am J Dis Child* 1940;59:1016.
98. Bick RL, Arun B, Frenkel EP. Disseminated intravascular coagulation: clinical and pathophysiological mechanisms and manifestations. *Haemostasis* 1999;29:111–134.
99. Valls C, Rene M, Gil M, et al. Giant cavernous hemangioma of the liver: atypical CT and MR findings. *Eur Radiol* 1996;6:448.
100. Edgerton MT. The treatment of hemangiomas: with special reference to the role of steroid therapy. *Ann Surg* 1976;183:517.
101. Castello MA, Ragni G, Antimi A, et al. Successful management with interferon alpha-2a after prednisone therapy failure in an infant with a giant cavernous hemangioma. *Med Pediatr Oncol* 1997;28:213–215.
102. Lobato R, Martinez L, Leal N, et al. Hemangiomas and vascular malformations: review and update. *Cir Pediatr* 1997;10:119.
103. Bick RL, Pegram MD. Giant cavernous hemangioma and deep vein thrombosis: a clinical syndrome. *Blood* 1991;78:493.
104. Hans FM. Multiple hereditary telangiectasia causing hemorrhage (hereditary hemorrhagic telangiectasia). *Bull Johns Hopkins Hosp* 1909;20:63.
105. Osler W. On multiple hereditary telangiectasia with recurrent hemorrhages. *Q J Med* 1907;Oct:53.
106. Osler W. On telangiectasia circumscripta universalis. *Bull Johns Hopkins Hosp* 1901;12:33.
107. Plauchu H, Bideau A. Epidemiologie et constitution d'un registre de population a propos d'une concentration geographique d'une maladie rare. *Population* 1984;4:765.
108. Vase P, Grove O. Gastrointestinal lesions in hereditary hemorrhagic telangiectasia. *Gastroenterology* 1986;91:1079.
109. Shovlin CL, Hughes JMB, Tuddenham EGD. A gene for hereditary hemorrhagic telangiectasia maps to 9q33-34. *Nat Genet* 1994;6:197.
110. Yamashita H, Ichijo H, Grimsby S. Endogulin forms a heterodimeric complex with the signaling receptors for transforming growth factor-β. *J Biol Chem* 1994;269:1995.
111. Marchuk DA. The molecular genetics of hereditary hemorrhagic telangiectasia. *Chest* 1997;111:79s.
112. Berg JN, Gallione CJ, Stenzel TT, et al. The activin receptor-like kinase 1 gene: genomic structure and mutations in hereditary hemorrhagic telangiectasia type 2. *Am J Hum Genet* 1997;61:60.
113. Hashimoto K, Pritzker M. Hereditary hemorrhagic telangiectasia: an electron microscope study. *Oral Surg Oral Med Oral Pathol* 1972;34:751.
114. Jahnke V. Ultrastructure of hereditary telangiectasia. *Otolaryngology* 1970;91:262.
115. Menefee MG, Flessa C, Glueck HI. Hereditary hemorrhagic telangiectasia (Osler-Weber-Rendu disease): an electron microscopic study of the vascular lesions before and after therapy with hormones. *Arch Otolaryngol* 1975;101:246.
116. Berg JN, Guttmacher AE, Marchuk DA. Clinical heterogeneity in hereditary hemorrhagic elangiectasia. *J Med Genet* 1996;33:256.
117. Askin MP, Lewis BS. Push enteroscopic cauterization: long-term follow-up of 83 patients with bleeding small intestinal angiodysplasia. *Gastrointest Endosc* 1996;43:580.
118. Velegrakis GA, Prokopakis EP, Papadakis CE, et al. Nd:YAG laser treatment of recurrent epistaxis in heredity hemorrhagic telangiectasia. *J Otolaryngol* 1997;26:384.
119. Shay SM. Hereditary hemorrhagic telangiectasia: what the otolaryngologist should know. *Am J Rhinol* 1997;11:55.
120. Osler W. On a family form of recurrent epistaxis associated with telangiectasia of the skin and mucous membranes. *Bull Johns Hopkins Hosp* 1901;12:33.
121. Berry DL, DeLeon FD. Endometrial ablation for severe menorrhagia in a patient with hereditary hemorrhagic telangiectasia: a case report. *J Reprod Med* 1996;41:183.
122. Hodgsum CH, Kaye RL. Pulmonary arteriovenous fistula and hereditary hemorrhagic telangiectasia. *Dis Chest* 1963;43:449.
123. Wang HC, Yang PC, Kuo SH, et al. Pulmonary arteriovenous malformation: analysis of 10 cases. *J Formos Med Assoc* 1998; 97:97.
124. McCaughan JS Jr, Hawley PC, LaRosa JC, et al. Photodynamic therapy to control life-threatening hemorrhage from hereditary hemorrhagic telangiectasia. *Lasers Surg Med* 1996;19:492.
125. Dutton JA, Jackson JE, Hughes JM, et al. Pulmonary arteriovenous malformations: results of treatment with coil embolization in 53 patients. *AJR Am J Roentgenol* 1995;165:1119.
126. Tripathy U, Kaul S, Bhosle K, et al. Pulmonary arteriovenous fistula with cerebral arteriovenous malformation without hereditary hemorrhagic telangiectasia: unusual case report and literature review. *J Cardiovasc Surg* 1997;38:677–680.
127. Buscarini E, Buscarini L, Danesino C, et al. Hepatic vascular malformations in hereditary hemorrhagic telangiectasia: Doppler sonographic screening in a large family. *J Hepatol* 1997;26:111.
128. Mukasa C, Nakamura K, Chijiiwa Y, et al. Liver failure caused by hepatic angiodysplasia in hereditary hemorrhagic telangiectasia. *Am J Gastroenterol* 1998;93:471.
129. Fitz-Hugh T. Splenomegaly and hepatic enlargement in hereditary hemorrhagic telangiectasia. *Am J Med Sci* 1931;181:261.
130. Press OW, Ramsey PG. Central nervous system infections associated with hereditary hemorrhagic telangiectasia. *Am J Med* 1984;77:86.
131. Adams HP, Subbiah B, Bosch EP. Neurological manifestations of hereditary hemorrhagic telangiectasia. *Arch Neurol* 1977;34:101.
132. Roman G, Fisher M, Perl DP, et al. Neurological manifestations of hereditary hemorrhagic telangiectasia (Osler-Weber- Rendu disease): report of two cases and review of the literature. *Ann Neurol* 1978;4:130.
133. Baroudet S, Houdart E, Boissonnet H, et al. Cerebromeningeal hemorrhages in Rendu-Osler disease: 2 cases treated by embolization. *Presse Med* 1997;26:1622.
134. Weiner RL. Gamma knife radiosurgery treatment of AVMs. *Clin Appl Thromb Hemost* 1995;1:179.
135. Bick RL, Fekete LF. Hereditary hemorrhagic telangiectasia and associated defects in hemostasis. *Blood* 1978;52:179.
136. Quick AJ. Telangiectasia. In: Quick AJ, ed. *Hemorrhagic diseases and thrombosis.* Philadelphia: Lea & Febiger, 1966:285.
137. McDervitt TJ, Toh AS. Epistaxis: management and prevention. *Laryngoscope* 1967;47:1109.
138. Ryan AJ. Control of bleeding in familial telangiectasia. *Meriden Hosp Bull* 1958;7;1.
139. Bick RL. Hereditary hemorrhagic telangiectasia and disseminated intravascular coagulation: a new clinical syndrome. In: Walz DA, McCoy LE, eds. *Contributions to hemostasis. Ann N Y Acad Sci* 1981;370:851.
140. Steel D, Bovill EG, Golden E. Hereditary hemorrhagic telangiectasia: a family study. *Am J Clin Pathol* 1988;90:274.
141. Bick RL. Disseminated intravascular coagulation: pathophysiological mechanisms and manifestations. *Semin Thromb Hemost* 1998;24:3.
142. Stitch MH. Carbazochrome salicylate therapy in hereditary hemorrhagic telangiectasia. *N Y State J Med* 1959;59:2725..
143. Koch HJ, Escher GL, Lewis JS. Hormonal management of hereditary hemorrhagic telangiectasia. *JAMA* 1952;149:1376.
144. Quick AJ Hemostasis then and now. In: Quick AJ, ed. *The hemorrhagic diseases and the pathology of hemostasis.* Springfield, Ill: Charles C Thomas, 1974:3.
145. Lachner H. Hemostatic abnormalities associated with paraprotein abnormalities. *Semin Hematol* 1973;10:125.

146. Bick RL. Alerations of hemostasis in malignancy. In: Bick RL, Bennett JM, Brynes RK, eds. *Hematology: clinical and laboratory practice.* St. Louis: Mosby, 1993:1583.
147. Glaspy JA. Disturbances in hemostasis in patients with B cell malignancies. *Semin Thromb Hemost* 1992;18:440.
148. Bick RL, Strauss JF, Frenkel EP. Thrombosis and hemorrhage in oncology patients. *Hematol Oncol Clin North Am* 1996;10:875.
149. Gallo G, Picken M, Buxbaum J. The spectrum of monoclonal immunoglobulin deposition disease associated with immunocytic disorders. *Semin Hematol* 1989;26:234.
150. Cawley LP, Minard BJ. Amyloidosis. In: Bick RL, Bennett JM, Brynes RK, eds. *Hematology: clinical and laboratory practice.* St. Louis: Mosby, 1993:729.
151. Kunkel LA. Acquired circulating anticoagulants. *Hematol Oncol Clin North Am 1992;6:1341.*
152. Triplett DA, Bang NU, Harms CS, et al. Mechanisms of acquired factor X deficiency in primary amyloidosis. Blood 1977;50:285.
153. Galbraith PA, Sharma N, Parker WL, et al. Acquired factor X deficiency: altered plasma antithrombin activity and association with amyloidosis. *JAMA* 1974;230:1658.
154. Glenner GG. Factor X deficiency and systemic amyloidosis. *N Engl J Med* 1977;297:108.
155. Howell M. Acquired factor X deficiency associated with systematized amyloidosis: report of a case. *Blood* 1963;21:739.
156. Krause JR. Acquired factor X deficiency and amyloidosis. *Am J Clin Pathol* 1977;67:170.
157. McPherson RA, Onstad JW, Vgoretz RT, et al. Coagulopathy in amyloidosis: combined deficiency of factor IX and X. *Am J Hematol* 1977;3:225.
158. Furie B, Green E, Furie BC. Syndrome of acquired factor X deficiency and systemic amyloidosis. *N Engl J Med* 1977; 297:81.
159. Stefanini M, Mednicoff IB. Demonstration of antivessel antibodies in serum of patients with anaphylactoid purpura and polyarteritis nodosa. *J Clin Invest* 1954;33:967.
160. Dixon FJ, Vazques JJ, Weigle WD, et al. Pathogenesis of serum sickness. *Arch Pathol* 1958;65:18.
161. Pierson KK. Leukocytoclastic vasculitis viewed as a phase of immune-mediated vasculopathy. *Semin Thromb Hemost* 1984; 10:196.
162. Markowitz AS, Lang CF. Streptococcal related glomerulonephritis. *J Immunol* 1964;92:565.
163. Cochrane CG. Mediators of the arthus and related syndromes. *Prog Allergy* 1967;11:1.
164. Freedman P, Meister NP, Lee HJ, et al. The renal response to streptococcal infections. *Medicine* 1970;49:433.
165. Parish WE. Studies on vasculitis: I. immunoglobulins, beta-1-C, C-reactive protein, and bacterial antigens in cutaneous vasculitis lesions. *Clin Allergy* 1971;1:97.
166. Parish WE. Studies on vasculitis: II. some properties of complexes formed of antibacterial antibodies from persons with or without cutaneous vasculitis lesions. *Clin Allergy* 1971;1:111.
167. Tanaseanu S, Purice S. The systemic vasculitides. *Med Interne* 1989;27:167.
168. Bigby M, Stern RS, Arndt KA. Allergic cutaneous reactions to drugs. *Prim Care* 1989;16:713.
169 Ashton N. The eye in malignant hypertension. *Trans Am Acad Ophthalmol Otolaryngol* 1972;76:17.
170. Farber EM, Hines AE, Montgomery H, et al. Arterioles of skin in essential hypertension. *J Invest Dermatol* 1947;9:215.
171. Kazmier FJ, Didisheim P, Fairbanks VF, et al. Intravascular coagulation and arterial disease. *Thromb Diath Haemorrh Suppl* 1969;36:295.
172. Ryan TJ. The investigation of vasculitis. In: Ryan TJ, ed. *Microvascular injury.* Philadelphia: WB Saunders, 1976:333.
173. Morris RN, Vassalli P, Beller FK, et al. Immuno-fluorescent studies of renal biopsies in the diagnosis of toxemia of pregnancy. *Obstet Gynecol* 1964;24:32.
174. Robboy SJ, Mihm MC, Coleman RW, et al. The skin in disseminated intravascular coagulation: prospective analysis of 36 cases. *Br J Dermatol* 1973;88:221.
175. Bick RL. Disseminated intravascular coagulation: objective clinical and laboratory diagnosis, treatment and assessment of therapeutic response. In: Weiss K, Sterz F, eds. *Thrombosis and hemostasis in emergency medicine. Semin Thromb Hemost* 1996;22:69.
176. Bondy PK. Disorders of the adrenal cortex. In: Wilson JD, Foster DW, eds. *Textbook of endocrinology.* Philadelphia:WB Saunders, 1985:816.
177. Kaklamani VG, Vaiopoulos G, Kaklamanis PG. Behçet's disease. *Semin Arthritis Rheum* 1998;27:197.
178. Haim S, Sobel JD, Freidman-Birnbaum F. Thrombophlebitis and a cardinal symptom of Behçets syndrome. *Acta Derm Venereol* 1974;54:299.
179. Lee SK, Lee J. Behçet's disease: a rheumatologic perspective. *Yonsei Med J* 1997;38:395.
180. Zierhut M, Saal J, Pleyer U, et al. Behçet's disease: epidemiology and eye manifestations in German and Mediterranean patients. *Ger J Ophthalmol* 1995;4:246.
181. Nazzarro P. Cutaneous manifestations of Behçets disease: clinical and histological findings. *Proc Int Symp Behcets Dis* Basel: Karger, 1966:15.
182. Farah S, Al-Shubaili A, Montaser A, et al. Behcet's syndrome: a report of 41 patients with emphasis on neurological manifestations. *J Neurol Neurosurg Psychiatry* 1998;64:382.
183. Bayraktar Y, Balkanci F, Bayraktar M, et al. Budd-Chiari syndrome: a common complication of Behcet's disease. *Am J Gastroenterol* 1997;92:858.
184. Roguin A, Edelstein S, Edoute Y. Superior vena cava syndrome as a primary manifestation of Behcet's disease. *Angiology* 1997; 48:365.
185. Kroger K, Ansasy M, Rudofsky G. Postoperative thrombosis of the superior caval vein in a patient with primary asymptomatic Behcet's disease: a case report. *Angiology* 1997;48:649.
186. Han DS, Kim JB, Lee OY, et al. A case of Behcet's syndrome with superior vena cava syndrome. *Korean J Intern Med* 1998;13:72.
187. Sagdic K, Ozer ZG, Saba D, et al. Venous lesions in Behcet's disease. *Eur J Vasc Endovasc Surg* 1996;11:437.
188. Lenk N, Ozet G, Alli N, et al. Protein C and protein S activities in Behcet's disease as risk factors of thrombosis. *Int J Dermatol* 1998;37:124.
189. Hills EA. Behcets syndrome with aortic aneurysms. *Br Med J* 1967;4:152.
190. Sakuri M, Miyaji T. Behcets disease from the point of view of vascular pathology. *Folia Ophthalmol Jpn* 1971;22:903.
191. Chajek T, Fainard M. Behcets disease with decreased fibrinolysis and superior vena caval occlusion. *Br Med J* 1973;1:782.
192. Jorizzo JL, Abernethy JL, White WL, et al. Mucocutaneous criteria for the diagnosis of Behcet's disease: an analysis of clinicopathologic data from multiple international centers. *J Am Acad Dermatol* 1995;32:968.
193. Mangelsdorf HC, White WL, Jorizzo JL. Behcet's disease: report of twenty-five patients from the United States with prominent mucocutaneous involvement. *J Am Acad Dermatol* 1996;34:745.
194. Dominguez LN, Irvine AR. Fundus changes in Behcet's disease. *Trans Am Ophthalmol Soc* 1997;95:367.
195. Ciftci OU, Ozdemir O. Cataract extraction in Behcet's disease. *Acta Ophthalmol Scand* 1996;74:74.
196. Ohno E, Ohtsuka E, Watanabe K, et al. Behcet's disease associated with myelodysplastic syndromes: a case report and a review of the literature. *Cancer* 1997;79:262.
197. Yano K, Seguchi K, Migita K, et al. Behcet's disease complicated

with myelodysplastic syndrome: a report of two cases and review of the literature. *Clin Rheumatol* 1996;15:91.
198. Celik G, Kalaycioglu O, Durmaz G. Colchicine in Behcet's disease with major vessel thrombosis. *Rheumatol Int* 1996;16:43.
199. Kaklamani VG, Vaiopoulos G, Kaklamanis PG. Behcet's disease. *Semin Arthritis Rheum* 1998;27:197.
200. Tseng S, Pak G, Washenik K, et al. Rediscovering thalidomide: a review of its mechanism of action, side effects, and potential uses. *J Am Acad Dermatol* 1996;35:969.
201. Behrendt PM, Epstein SE, Marrow AG. Postperfusion nonthrombocytopenic purpura: an uncommon sequel of open heart surgery. *Am J Cardiol* 1968;22:631.
202. Bick RL. Hemostasis defects in cardiac surgery and use of cardiac devices. In: Piffare R, ed. *Cardiac surgery and principles of practice.* Philadelphia: Belfus Publ, 1999:9.
203. Calabrese LH, Michel BA, Bloch DA. The American College of Rheumatology 1990 criteria for the classification of hypersensitivity vasculitis. *Arthritis Rheum* 1990;33:1108.
204. Criep LH, Cohen CG. Purpura as a manifestation of penicillin sensitivity. *Ann Intern Med* 1951;34:1219.
205. Nalbandian RM, Mader JJ, Barrett JL, et al. Petechiae, ecchymoses, and necrosis of skin induced by coumarin congeners. *JAMA* 1965;192:603.
206. Nalbandian RM, Beller FK, Hamp AK, et al. Coumarin necrosis of the skin treated successfully with heparin. *Gynecology* 1971;38:395.
207. Nudelman HL, Kempson RL. Necrosis of the breast: a rare complication of anticoagulant therapy. *Am J Surg* 1966;111:728.
208. Cole MS, Minifee PK, Wolma FJ. Coumarin necrosis: a review of the literature. *Surgery* 1988;103:271.
209. Becker CG. Oral anticoagulant therapy and skin necrosis. In: Wessler S, Becker CG, Nemerson Y, eds. *The new dimensions of warfarin prophylaxis.* New York: Plenum Press, 1987:217.
210. Triplett DA. Current recommendations for warfarin therapy: use and monitoring. *Med Clin North Am* 1998;82:601.
211. Conrad J, Horellou MH, van Dreden P. Homozygous protein C deficiency with late onset and recurrent coumarin-induced skin necrosis. *Lancet* 1992;339:743.
212. Hyman BT, Landas SK, Ashman RF. Warfarin-related purple toes syndrome and cholesterol microembolization. *Am J Med* 1987;82:1233.
213. Samama MM. Laboratory control of anticoagulant therapy. In: Bick RL, Bennett JM, Brynes RK, eds. *Hematology: clinical and laboratory practice.* St. Louis: Mosby, 1993:729.
214. Francis RB. Acquired purpura fulminans. *Semin Thromb Hemost* 1990;16:310.
215. Adcock DM, Bronza J, Marler RA. Proposed classification and pathologic mechanisms of purpura fulminans and skin necrosis. *Semin Thromb Hemost* 1990;16:333.
216. Walenga J, Bick RL. Heparin associated thrombocytopenia and other adverse effects of heparin therapy. *Cardiol Clin* 1998;2:123.
217. Rodgers RP, Levin J. A critical reappraisal of the bleeding time. *Semin Thromb Hemost* 1990;16:1.
218. Burns ER, Lawrence C. Bleeding time: a guide to its diagnostic and clinical utility. *Arch Pathol Lab Med* 1989;113:1219.
219. Rodgers RPC, Levin J. A critical reappraisal of the bleeding time. *Semin Thromb Hemost* 1990;16:1.
220. Burns ER, Lawrence C. Bleeding time: a guide to its diagnostic and clinical utility. *Arch Pathol Lab Med* 1989;113:1219.
221. Bick RL, Adams T, Schmalhorst WR. Bleeding times, platelet adhesion, and aspirin. *Am J Clin Pathol* 1976;65:65.
222. Davis KA. Complement, immune complexes and systemic lupus erythematosus. *Br J Rheumatol* 1996;35:5.
223. Bentwich Z, Beverley PCL, Hammarstrom L. Laboratory investigations in clinical immunology: methods, pitfalls, and clinical indications. *Clin Immunol Immunopathol* 1988;49:478.
224. Anderson CL, Stillman WS. Raji cell assay for immune complexes: evidence for detection of Raji-directed immunoglobulin G antibody in patients with systemic lupus erythematosus. *J Clin Invest* 1980;66:353.

Disorders of Thrombosis and Hemostasis: Clinical and Laboratory Practice, Third Edition, edited by Rodger L. Bick.
Lippincott Williams & Wilkins, Philadelphia © 2002

4

PLATELET-FUNCTION DEFECTS

RODGER L. BICK

The common clinical findings of qualitative or quantitative platelet defects are petechiae and purpura; mild to moderate mucosal membrane bleeding, including bilateral epistaxis; gastrointestinal, pulmonary, and genitourinary bleeding; and easy and spontaneous bruising (1). Frequent gingival bleeding with tooth brushing also is common (2). Platelet-function defects, or thrombocytopenia, are characteristically accompanied by symmetrical petechiae and purpura, found throughout the skin, including both torso and extremities. This is in contradistinction to dependent petechiae and purpura (extremities only), characteristically seen with vascular disorders (3,4). Clinical findings of platelet defects are summarized in Table 4.1.

TYPES OF PLATELET DEFECTS

Platelet disorders are divided into quantitative and qualitative defects. The qualitative disorders, the platelet-function defects, are further conveniently divided into hereditary or acquired. Quantitative defects consist of (a) thrombocytopenia resulting from decreased production and metabolic/maturation defects; this group includes the hereditary, congenital, and infantile thrombocytopenias associated with decreased platelet production, acquired platelet-production defects, and drug-induced nonimmune thrombocytopenias; (b) acquired thrombocytopenia resulting from increased destruction, increased consumption, or peripheral loss; and (c) thrombocytosis and thrombocythemia. Hyperactive platelets associated with, leading to, or formed as a consequence of hypercoagulability and thrombosis are a special category of abnormal platelet function.

Table 4.2 summarizes platelet defects, divided into qualitative (functional) disorders versus quantitative disorders: thrombocytopenia, thrombocytosis, and thrombocythemia. There is little use in instituting an expensive and laborious platelet-function assessment until normal platelet counts are documented. Attempting to study platelet function in the face of thrombocytopenia is usually fruitless (5). Hereditary platelet-function defects are clinical oddities and extremely rare (5), but the acquired defects are very common, are associated with many often-seen acquired diseases, and frequently lead to clinically significant bleeding problems (5).

Table 4.3 depicts traditional tests of platelet number and function. New methods for assessing molecular markers of platelet reactivity and other modalities to assess platelet function are discussed in later sections. An attentive evaluation of the peripheral blood smear for quantitative estimation of platelet numbers and an evaluation of platelet morphology are of extreme importance in initial assessment. This is an often-neglected simple modality performed in the hemostasis laboratory, and certainly the peripheral blood smear should be evaluated by the physician caring for patients with easy or spontaneous bruising or petechiae and purpura. Important clinical clues may be noted on evaluation of platelet morphology, such as abnormal granularity in the gray platelet syndrome, the large platelets and borderline thrombocytopenia of Bernard–Soulier syndrome, or many large bizarre platelets, or young platelets, indicative of rapid platelet turnover and decreased platelet survival. An examination of the peripheral blood smear may lead to the specific diagnosis accounting for petechiae and purpura or easy bruising (for example, a leukemia). A quantitative platelet count also should always be done. Only in the face of a normal platelet

TABLE 4.1. CLINICAL FINDINGS OF PLATELET DEFECTS

Petechiae
Purpura
Mild to moderate mucosal membrane bleeding
Gastrointestinal
Genitourinary
Pulmonary
Epistaxis
History of easy bruising
History of spontaneous bruising
Frequent gingival bleeding with tooth brushing
Symmetrical petechiae and purpura (usually)

R. L. Bick: Departments of Medicine and Pathology, University of Texas Southwestern Medical Center; Dallas Thrombosis/Hemostasis Clinical Center; ThromboCare Laboratories, Dallas, Texas.

TABLE 4.2. TYPES OF PLATELET DISORDERS

- Qualitative
  - Hereditary
    - Adhesion defects
    - Aggregation defects
    - Factor deficiencies
    - Miscellaneous
  - Acquired
    - Associated with other diseases
    - Drug-induced
- Quantitative
  - Hereditary
    - Megakaryocytic
    - Amegakaryocytic
  - Acquired
    - Megakaryocytic
    - Amegakaryocytic
    - Drug-induced
  - Thrombocytosis and thrombocythemia
    - Benign
    - Malignant
  - Hyperactive and Prethrombotic

count can a platelet-function defect be defined (5). Formerly, platelet adhesion in glass bead columns by varying techniques was advocated to assess platelet function; however, platelet-adhesion testing by glass bead techniques is unreliable and of no clinical relevance (6,7).

The standardized template bleeding time device is the primary screening test for platelet function and vascular function (8,9). Once a normal platelet count is documented with a suggestive or positive history, consisting of petechiae, purpura, and easy and spontaneous bruising, the differential diagnosis is between a vascular defect and a platelet-function defect, both of which will frequently, but not always, cause prolongation of the standardized template bleeding time (3,10–12). A petechiometer, instead of the template bleeding time, is sometimes used in children (5,13). The template bleeding time has not been standardized in children, and the test tends to leave scars. Template bleeding times are used to screen for a platelet function or vascular defect in adults, and the petechiometer test is used to screen for platelet function or vascular defects in children. These two tests are done only with a normal platelet count and positive or suggestive history (3,11). Although the template bleeding time is useful as a simple screening test for platelet function, it is sometimes unreliable, and a normal template bleeding time does not rule out the presence of a clinically significant platelet-function defect (12). If the template bleeding time is normal, and a suggestive history is obtained or platelet dysfunction suspected on clinical grounds, platelet aggregation or lumi-aggregation should immediately be done. These more definitive tests of platelet function are discussed later.

TABLE 4.3. LABORATORY EVALUATION OF PLATELET FUNCTION

- Peripheral smear evaluation
- Quantitative platelet count
- Template bleeding time
- Petechiometer test (children and elderly)
- Platelet aggregation to
  - Adenosine diphosphate
  - Epinephrine
  - Collagen
  - Ristocetin
  - Arachidonate
  - Thrombin
- Platelet lumi-aggregation (release)
- Platelet antibodies (IgG and IgM)
- Platelet membrane glycoproteins (flow cytometry)
- Cyclooxygenase
- Platelet factor 4[a]
- β-Thromboglobulin[a]
- Thromboxanes[a]
- Flow cytometry

[a]For hyperactive/prethrombotic platelets.
Ig, immunoglobulin.

HEREDITARY PLATELET DYSFUNCTION

The hereditary platelet-function defects are summarized in Table 4.4. These are conveniently divided into those of (a) platelet adhesion, such as the Bernard–Soulier syndrome; (b) defects of primary aggregation, characterized by Glanzmann thrombasthenia; and (c) defects of secondary aggregation characterized by storage pool diseases and other rarer defects (14). Also described are patients with an isolated deficiency of platelet factor 3 (PF-3), and patients with very severe plasma coagulation protein deficiencies may have an associated platelet-function defect. This is noted in severe afibrinogenemia and severe hemophilia A or B (5). The accompanying platelet-function defect seen in these patients exemplifies the importance of blood coagulation proteins for normal platelet function. The division of hereditary platelet-function defects into those of adhesion,

TABLE 4.4. HEREDITARY PLATELET-FUNCTION DEFECTS

- Adhesion defects
  - Bernard–Soulier syndrome
  - Impaired adhesion to collagen
- Aggregation defects: primary
  - Glanzmann thrombasthenia
  - Essential athrombia
- Aggregation defects: secondary
  - Storage pool diseases
  - Aspirin-like defect
  - Release reaction defects
- Isolated platelet factor-3 deficiency
- Severe coagulation factor deficiencies
  - Afibrinogenemia
  - Factor VIII:C deficiency
  - Factor IX:C deficiency

primary aggregation, or secondary aggregation is somewhat artificial, but provides a convenient way to categorize the defects and to recall the laboratory manifestations.

The Bernard–Soulier Syndrome

The Bernard–Soulier syndrome is inherited as an autosomal trait and typifies a disorder of platelet adhesion. Bernard–Soulier platelets are missing platelet membrane glycoproteins (PMGPs) Ib, V, and IX. Heterozygous patients often are asymptomatic. The clinical features are those of easy bruising, epistaxis, hypermenorrhagia, and petechiae and purpura (15–17). Patients with Bernard–Soulier syndrome show abnormal adhesion and abnormal ristocetin-induced aggregation, and a peripheral smear usually demonstrates giant platelets and borderline thrombocytopenia in most, but not all patients (17,18). If only adhesion and ristocetin aggregation were performed, one could mistake the patient as having von Willebrand syndrome instead of the Bernard–Soulier syndrome. The difference is noted by thoroughly evaluating the patient, as if von Willebrand disease were suspected; factor VIII coagulation activity (factor VIII:c), factor VIII–related antigen (factor VIII:RAg), and ristocetin cofactor activity (factor VIII:RCo/factor VIII:vW) also would be done to render the correct diagnosis (19). Table 4.5 summarizes characteristics of the Bernard–Soulier syndrome.

Glanzmann Thrombasthenia and Essential Athrombia

Primary aggregation disorders are Glanzmann thrombasthenia and an even rarer syndrome, essential athrombia (20–22). Glanzmann thrombasthenia is extremely rare. The clinical features are those usually expected with platelet dysfunction: easy and spontaneous bruising, subcutaneous hematomata, and petechiae are characteristic (20,23). Rare patients have intraarticular bleeding with resultant hemarthroses; the bleeding tendency tends to decrease in severity with age, as happens with many hereditary hemostasis defects. The clinical and laboratory diagnostic features are depicted in Table 4.6 and consist of a prolonged standardized template bleeding time, totally absent primary aggregation induced by adenosine diphosphate (ADP), thrombin, collagen, or epinephrine, abnormal PF-3 availability, and abnormal clot retraction (5,24,25). The platelets are missing the PMGP IIb/IIIa complex. All of these abnormalities also are noted for the even rarer related disorder, essential athrombia. However, in essential athrombia, clot retraction is normal (22). Therapy for these disorders is the infusion of platelet concentrates as needed for serious or life-threatening bleeding (5,26).

TABLE 4.5. THE BERNARD–SOULIER SYNDROME

Clinical manifestations
Autosomal recessive
Easy bruising
Spontaneous bruising
Epistaxis
Hypermenorrhagia
Petechiae and purpura (moderate)
Laboratory manifestations
Giant platelets
Mild or moderate thrombocytopenia
Abnormal template bleeding time
Abnormal petechiometer test
Abnormal ristocetin aggregation
Other aggregation normal
Absence of PMGPs 1b, V, and IX
Therapy
Platelet concentrates for significant or life-threatening hemorrhage

PGMP, platelet membrane glycoprotein.

TABLE 4.6. GLANZMANN THROMBASTHENIA AND ESSENTIAL ATHROMBIA

Clinical findings
Autosomal recessive
Petechiae and purpura
Easy bruising
Spontaneous bruising
Mucosal membrane bleeding
Large hematomata
Intraarticular bleeding (rare)
Decreasing severity with age
Laboratory findings
Prolonged template bleeding time
Abnormal/absent primary aggregation with
ADP
Epinephrine
Thrombin
Collagen
Abnormal platelet factor-3 release
Clot retraction
Glanzmann: Abnormal
Essential athrombia: Normal
Absence of PMGP IIb/IIIa Complex
Therapy
Platelet concentrates

ADP, adenosine diphosphate; PGMP, platelet membrane glycoprotein.

Hereditary Storage Pool Defect

Secondary aggregation disorders are more common than primary aggregation disorders, and the most common types seen in this category are storage pool diseases (27,28). Secondary aggregation disorders are summarized in Table 4.7. Among all the hereditary platelet-function defects, hereditary storage pool disease–type disorders are by far the most common. In rare instances, storage pool defects are seen in patients with other rare clinical oddities including the Wiskott–Aldrich syndrome (29), the thrombocytopenia absent radii syndrome (TAR syndrome) (30), the Hermansky–Pudlak syndrome (31), and the Chediak–Higashi syndrome (32). Most patients with these rare clinical syndromes have an associated storage pool defect, but most patients with a hereditary storage pool defect have no such

TABLE 4.7. SECONDARY AGGREGATION DEFECTS

Storage pool disease
Isolated defect (most common presentation) associated with (less common)
TAR-baby syndrome
Hermansky–Pudlak syndrome
Chediak–Higashi syndrome
Wiskott–Aldrich syndrome
Aspirin-like defect
Cyclooxygenase deficiency
Thromboxane synthetase deficiency
Release reaction defects
Hereditary collagen disorders
Glycogen storage disease
May–Hegglin anomaly
Hurler syndrome
Hunter syndrome

TAR, thrombocytopenia with absent radii.

TABLE 4.8. HEREDITARY STORAGE POOL DISEASE

Clinical findings
Variable inheritance
Petechiae, uncommon
Purpura, uncommon
Mucosal membrane bleeding
Epistaxis
Easy bruising
Spontaneous bruising
Hematuria, common
Laboratory findings
Abnormal template bleeding time
Abnormal adhesion to collagen
Absent aggregation to collagen
Absent second aggregation curve to
Adenosine diphosphate
Epinephrine
Normal ristocetin aggregation
Normal arachidonate aggregation (usually)
Therapy
Platelet concentrates

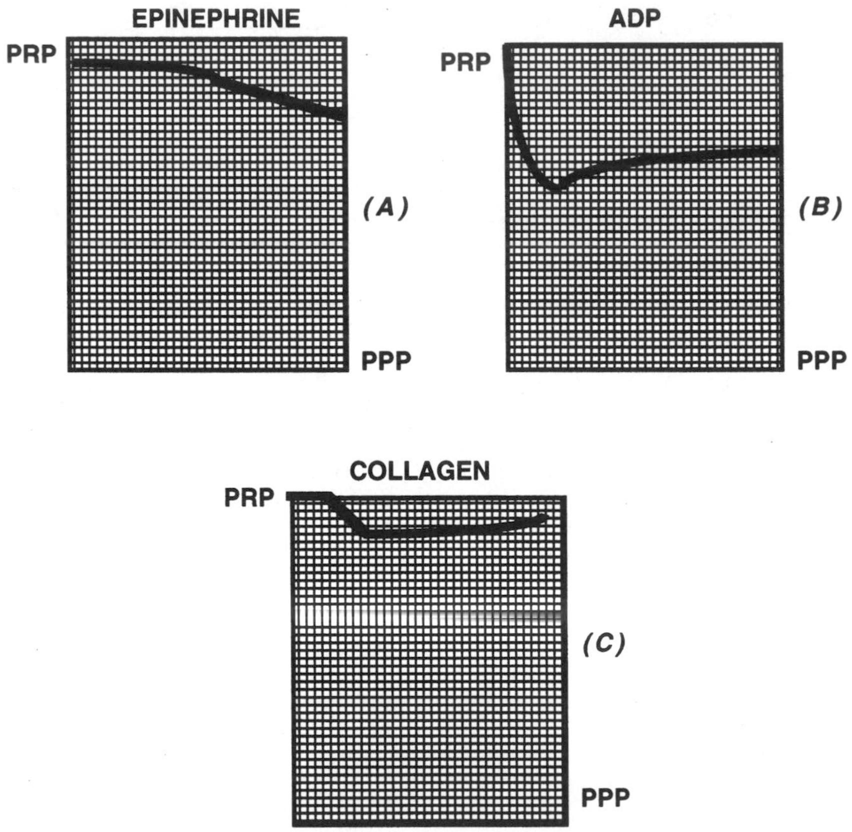

FIGURE 4.1. Hereditary storage pool defect: platelet-aggregation patterns. *ADP*, adenosine diphosphate; *PRP*, platelet-rich plasma; *PPP*, platelet-poor plasma.

associated disease and are otherwise normal (33). The clinical features of secondary aggregation disorders are mucocutaneous hemorrhages, hematuria, and epistaxis (34). Petechiae are less common than in other qualitative platelet disorders. Easy and spontaneous bruising are common complaints. Patients with storage pool defects have absent epinephrine and ADP-induced secondary aggregation waves, although the primary waves are present. Collagen-induced aggregation is absent or markedly blunted, and normal ristocetin-induced aggregation is typically noted

(35,36). A prolonged standardized template bleeding time is usual. The mainstay of therapy is the use of platelet concentrates if the patient bleeds. The clinical and laboratory features of hereditary storage pool disease are summarized in Table 4.8. Figure 4.1 summarizes platelet aggregation findings in hereditary storage pool disease. In this figure is noted a small primary wave induced by epinephrine (Fig. 1A), primary aggregation induced by ADP, followed by disaggregation (Fig. 1B), and a markedly blunted collagen-induced aggregation curve (Fig. 1C). These findings are classic for hereditary storage pool defects (42).

Hereditary Aspirin-like Defects

Another rarer secondary aggregation defect is the aspirin (ASA)-like effect, which is inherited as an autosomal dominant trait (37). This disorder is extremely rare, with very few cases having been described (38–41). The clinical features are similar to those of other platelet-function defects, consisting of easy and spontaneous bruising, occasional spontaneous bleeding from mucosal membranes, epistaxis, hypermenorrhagia, petechiae, and purpura. Patients demonstrate a prolonged template bleeding time, an absent secondary wave to epinephrine, and absent collagen-induced aggregation; therefore they have platelet-aggregation patterns similar to the pattern seen in patients ingesting ASA or other cyclooxygenase inhibitors (4). This defect may be because of a hereditary deficiency of either cyclooxygenase or thromboxane synthetase (43–45). Therapy, when clinically significant bleeding occurs, is platelet concentrate infusion. Some patients have improved with the use of steroids (46). The features of this heterogeneous syndrome are summarized in Table 4.9. Platelet-aggregation findings in the ASA-like effect are seen in Fig. 4.2.

TABLE 4.9. HEREDITARY ASPIRIN-LIKE DEFECT

Clinical findings
Easy bruising
Spontaneous bruising
Mucosal membrane bleeding
Epistaxis
Laboratory findings
Abnormal template bleeding time
Abnormal adhesion to collagen
Absent secondary aggregation curves to
Adenosine diphosphate
Epinephrine
Absent aggregation to collagen
Absent aggregation to arachidonate
Absence of cyclooxygenase or thromboxane synthetase
Therapy
Platelet concentrates
Possibly steroids

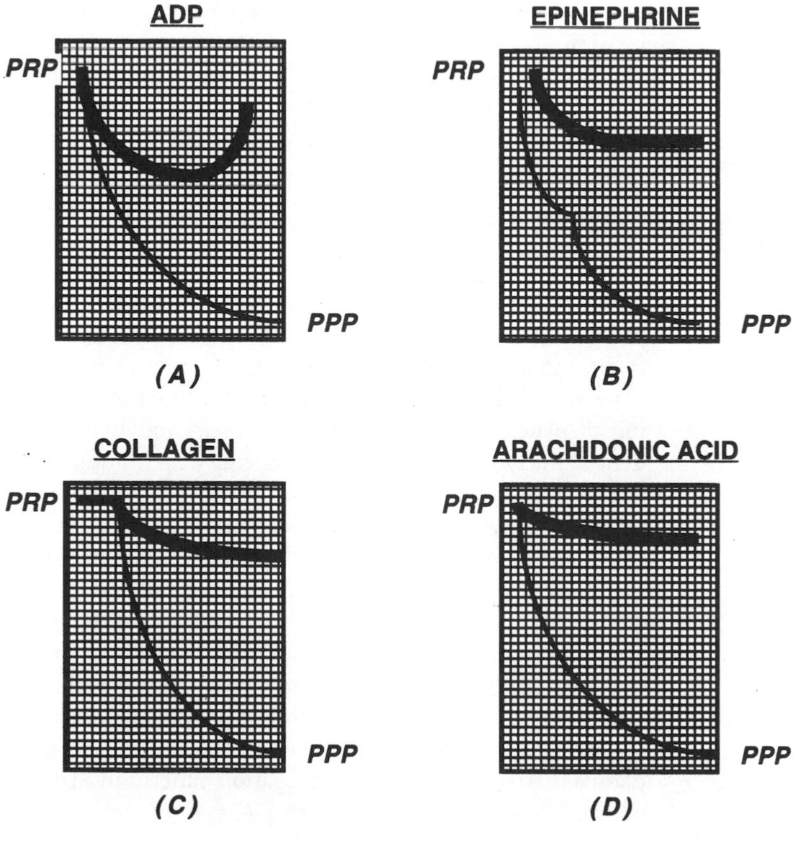

FIGURE 4.2. The aspirin (*ASA*)-like defect. The thin curve indicates normal. The thick curve indicates ASA-like defect. *ADP*, adenosine diphosphate; *PRP*, platelet-rich plasma; *PPP*, platelet-poor plasma.

More recently, a congenital platelet-function defect was described in a bleeding individual demonstrating an inherited impairment of platelet membrane phosphatidylinositol metabolism. The defect was characterized by clinical hemorrhage, delayed platelet aggregation to collagen, an absent epinephrine-induced second wave of platelet aggregation, and normal arachidonic acid–induced platelet aggregation (47). The mode of inheritance and other clinical and laboratory features were not described.

Hereditary storage pool diseases are the most common of the otherwise rare hereditary platelet-function defects and are usually not associated with one of the other rare clinical syndromes such as Chediak–Higashi or Wiskott–Aldrich syndrome. The other hereditary platelet-function defects mentioned are extremely rare and are best classified as true clinical oddities.

ACQUIRED PLATELET DYSFUNCTION

Common acquired platelet defects are summarized in Table 4.10. Acquired platelet-function defects are common causes of bleeding. Many patients having the subsequently discussed underlying disorders are surgical candidates and may bleed profusely with surgery or trauma if an accompanying platelet-function defect is present. If unexplained hemorrhage develops in a patient, resulting from a platelet-function defect, the subsequent evaluation should include a search for the disorders often associated with acquired platelet dysfunction.

TABLE 4.10. ACQUIRED PLATELET FUNCTION DEFECTS

Myeloproliferative syndromes
Essential thrombocythemia
Chronic myelogenous leukemia
Polycythemia vera
Paroxysmal nocturnal hemoglobinuria
Agnogenic myeloid metaplasia
Myelofibrosis
RAEB and other myelodysplastic syndromes
Sideroblastic anemia
Paraprotein disorders
Multiple myeloma
Waldenström macroglobulinemia
Essential monoclonal gammopathy
Autoimmune diseases
Collagen vascular disease
Antiplatelet antibodies
Immune thrombocytopenias
Fibrin(ogen) degradation products
Disseminated intravascular coagulation
Primary fibrinolytic syndromes
Liver disease
Anemia
Severe iron deficiency
Severe B_{12} or folate deficiency
Uremia
Drug induced

RAEB, refractory anemia with excess blasts.

Platelet Dysfunction in Uremia

All are familiar with the almost universal finding of a platelet-function defect in patients who are uremic (48–50). In uremic patients, it is thought that circulating guanidinosuccinic (51,52) and/or hydroxyphenolic acids (53) interfere with platelet function by eradicating PF-3 activity. Both compounds are dialyzable, and dialysis will often correct or improve platelet function. Other mechanisms of altered platelet function in uremia, including altered prostaglandin metabolism, or intraplatelet nucleotides, also have been proposed (54–60). Studies have shown an abnormality in the interaction between von Willebrand factor and the platelet membrane GPIIb/IIIa complex in uremic patients; however, platelet membrane GPIb, IIb, and IIIa are quantitatively normal in uremia (61,62). These findings suggest a functional defect in the von Willebrand factor–IIb/IIIa adhesive interaction. Figure 4.3 shows lumi-aggregation patterns in a uremic patient. However, like the other acquired platelet-function defects, the aggregation-pattern abnormalities are not uniform or characteristic, and essentially any combination of defects may be seen. Platelet concentrates are indicated for most instances of life-threatening bleeding in uremia; however, other modes of therapy that have been noted to correct the prolonged bleeding time in a variety of disorders will not only correct the bleeding time but also often control significant hemorrhage in uremic patients. Modalities used are cryoprecipitate, 1-deamino-8-D-arginine vasopressin (DDAVP; i.v., i.m., or intranasal), and estrogen compounds (63–69). Dialysis also tends to correct the platelet-function defect (70–73), and the degree of correction toward normal appears to correlate with frequency of this procedure (74).

Platelet Dysfunction in Paraprotein Disorders

Many patients with malignant paraprotein disorders including multiple myeloma, Waldenstrom macrogobulinemia, or other monoclonal gammopathies have an accompanying platelet-function defect (75–79). This is caused by the coating of platelet membrane by paraprotein and is independent of the type of paraprotein, occurring with immunoglobulin A (IgA), IgM, or IgG monoclonal proteins. Platelet dysfunction by identical mechanisms may occur with benign monoclonal proteins. Almost all patients with malignant paraprotein disorders will demonstrate significant platelet dysfunction, manifest by clinically significant bleeding, and abnormal platelet function may be noted by aggregation on lumi-aggregation testing. The template bleeding time is notoriously unreliable as a predictor of bleeding secondary to platelet dysfunction in paraprotein disorders. Pre- and post-plasmapheresis therapy lumi-aggregation patterns in a patient with IgA myeloma are depicted in Fig. 4.4.

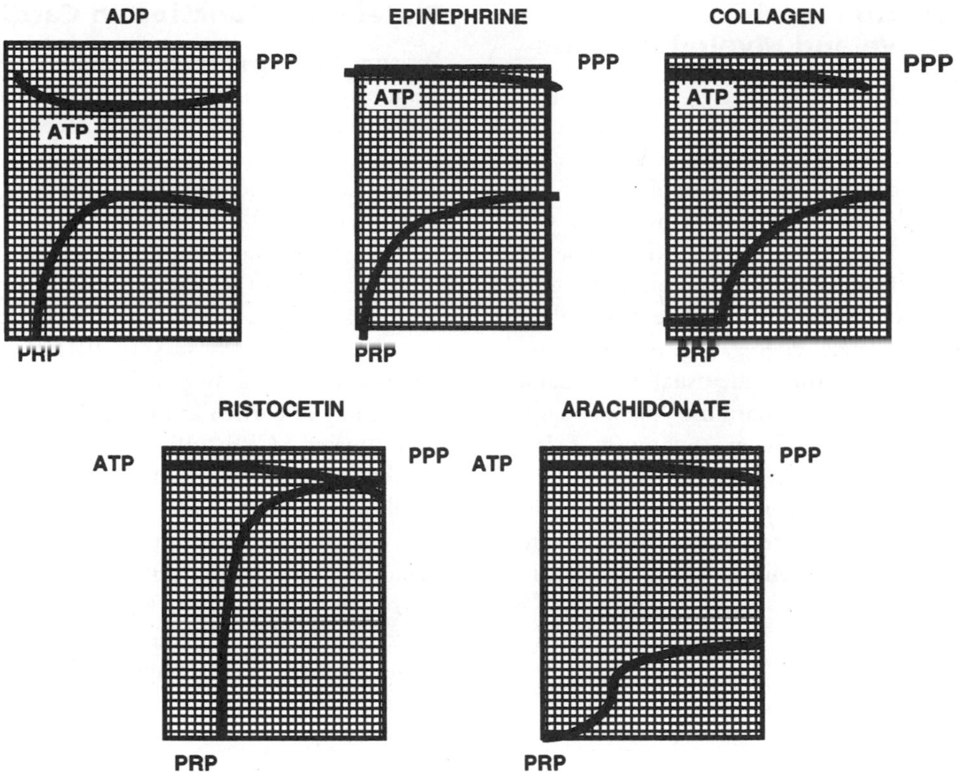

FIGURE 4.3. Platelet function in uremia (lumi-aggregation). *ADP*, adenosine diphosphate; *ATP*, adenosine triphosphate; *PRP*, platelet-rich plasma; *PPP*, platelet-poor plasma.

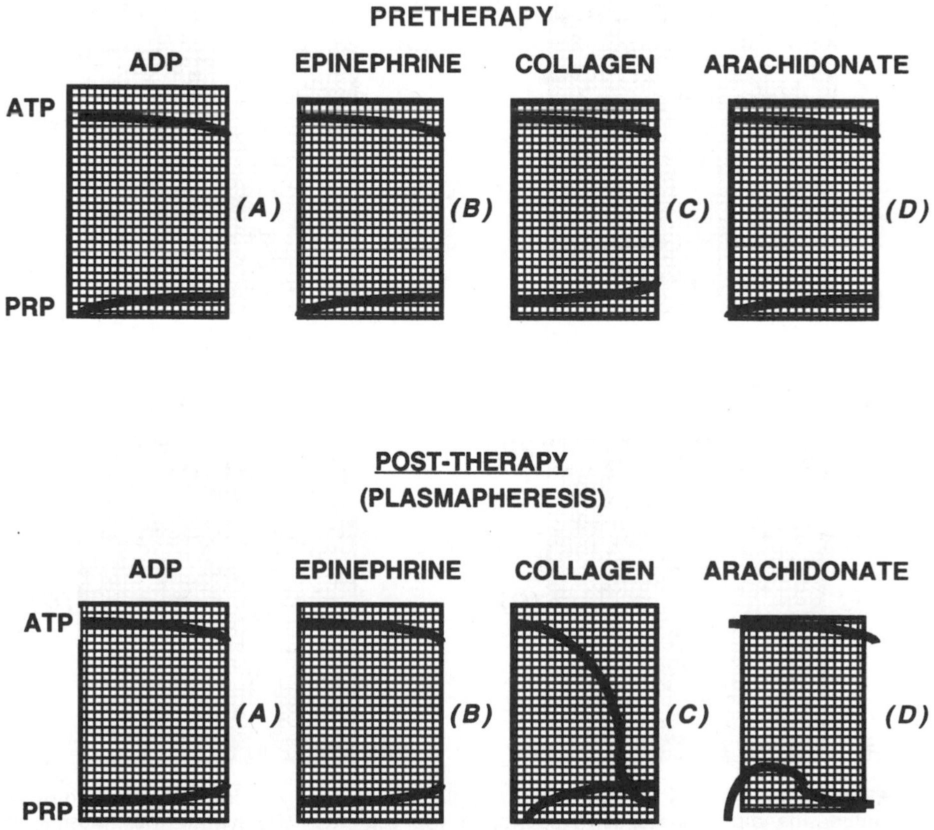

FIGURE 4.4. Platelet dysfunction in multiple myeloma: lumi-aggregation patterns. *ADP*, adenosine diphosphate; *ATP*, adenosine triphosphate; *PRP*, platelet-rich plasma.

Platelet Dysfunction in Myeloproliferative and Myelodysplastic Syndromes

Acquired platelet-function defects are commonly seen in all the myeloproliferative syndromes, especially essential thrombocythemia, agnogenic myeloid metaplasia, paroxysmal nocturnal hemoglobinuria, polycythemia rubra vera, chronic myelogenous leukemia, patients with refractory anemia and excessive blasts (RAEB syndrome), and other of the myelodysplastic syndromes and the sideroblastic anemias (80–83). The platelet-aggregation patterns noted in association with these syndromes are usually not characteristic, and essentially any combination of platelet-aggregation defects may be seen (5). The most common defects are abnormal aggregation and release to epinephrine, followed by abnormalities in collagen and ADP aggregation and release (84–86). The template bleeding time is often abnormal, but may not be a reliable guide to bleeding propensity in patients with myeloproliferative or myelodysplastic syndromes and associated platelet dysfunction (84,85).

Platelet Dysfunction in Cardiac Surgery

Patients undergoing cardiopulmonary bypass (CPB) demonstrate the most severe of platelet-function defects, and this assumes major importance in post-CPB surgical bleeding (87–91). Many factors associated with CPB may affect platelet function; these include (a) pH, (b) absolute platelet count, (c) hematocrit, (d) drugs, (e) the presence of fibrin(ogen) degradation products (FDPs), (f) the type of pump prime, and (g) the type of oxygenation system used (92). Studies have shown selective platelet degranulation to occur during bypass surgery (91). However, no studies reported thus far allow conclusions regarding the contribution of any of particular mechanisms to alter platelet function during CPB. Regardless of the mechanism(s) involved, a significant platelet-function defect is induced in all patients undergoing CPB surgery. The magnitude of this defect may have potential serious consequences for hemostasis during and after bypass. In addition, patients who have ingested drugs known to interfere with platelet function would be expected to have more blood loss than those not ingesting such agents, and drug-induced platelet

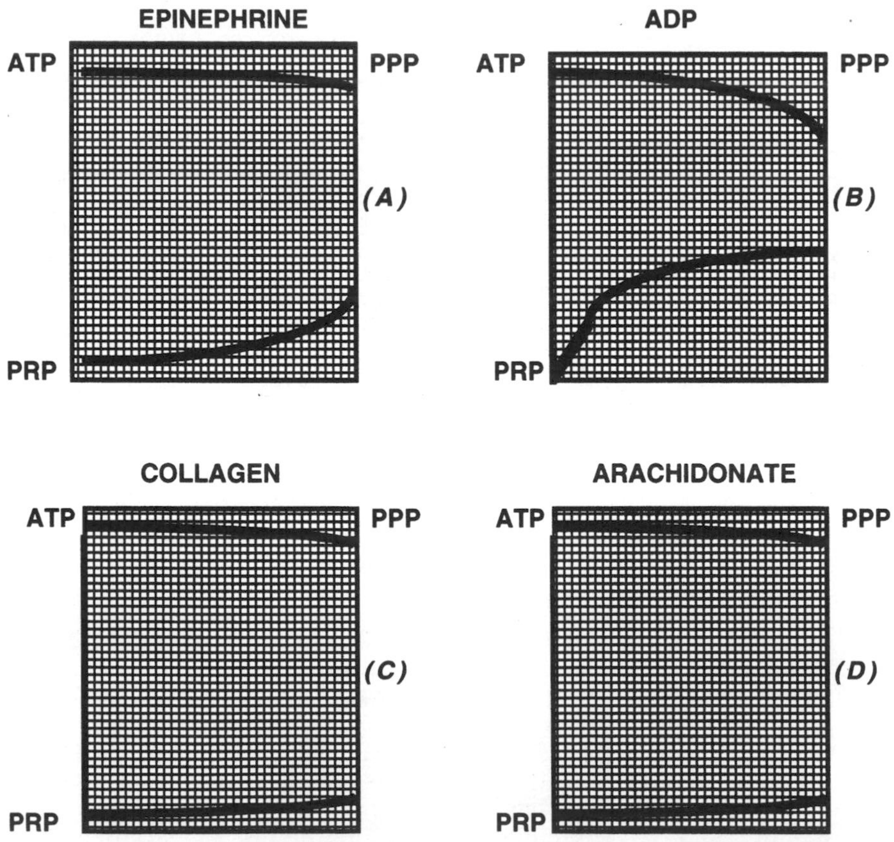

FIGURE 4.5. Cardiopulmonary bypass surgery: platelet lumi-aggregation patterns (mid-bypass). *ADP*, adenosine diphosphate; *ATP*, adenosine triphosphate; *PRP*, platelet-rich plasma; *PPP*, platelet-poor plasma.

dysfunction may compound the defects already induced by CPB and enhance the chances for hemorrhage. Platelet dysfunction is of major significance in post-CPB hemorrhage, and the use of platelet concentrates for CPB bleeding will usually promptly correct or significantly reduce most episodes of CPB or post-CPB hemorrhage. Typical mid-CPB and post-CPB lumi-aggregation patterns are seen in Figs. 4.5 and 4.6.

Platelet Dysfunction in Liver Disease

Significant platelet dysfunction is seen in patients with acute and chronic liver disease, although this hemostatic defect is uncommonly appreciated and often goes unrecognized (93–97). Causes of platelet dysfunction in patients with liver disease are multifactorial. Most patients with chronic liver disease have primary activation of the fibrinolytic system and resultant elevated circulating FDPs (93–95). These circulating FDPs may severely compromise platelet function. Another reason for platelet dysfunction in liver disease is an increase in older platelets, as noted by a decreased mean platelet volume (MPV) in patients with liver disease; these are presumably less hemostatically active platelets (97). Patients with both acute and chronic liver disease often show secondary aggregation defects or storage pool–type aggregation defects manifest as blunted aggregation to collagen, thrombin, and ristocetin, and absent secondary aggregation waves after aggregation with ADP and epinephrine (98,99). PF-3 release is often impaired. Platelet dysfunction in liver disease may be a manifestation of altered platelet membrane palmate and stearate metabolism, may result from coating of platelet membranes by FDPs, or may be a combination of these defects; these defects also may be a manifestation of many as-yet-undefined changes in platelet metabolic pathways (95,96,100).

If the patient with liver disease abuses ethanol, platelet function is further compromised. Ingestion of high doses of ethanol, even without significant liver disease, may induce a storage pool–type defect; decreased storage pool ADP and adenosine triphosphate (ATP) are induced by ethanol alone, and cyclic adenosine monophosphate (AMP) levels also are reduced by ethanol-induced inhibition of adenylate cyclase (98,99,101). As another insult, ethanol inhibits thromboxane A_2 synthesis (98,99). Ethanol also inhibits monoamine oxidase but causes a 50% to 100% increase in intraplatelet serotonin; the significance of this is unknown (98,102–104). Ethanol induces significant changes in intraplatelet metabolism of adenine nucleotides, cyclic AMP, prostaglandins, and thromboxanes, and impairs PF-3 availability. Folate deficiency also may accompany heavy ethanol ingestion without significant liver disease, and this

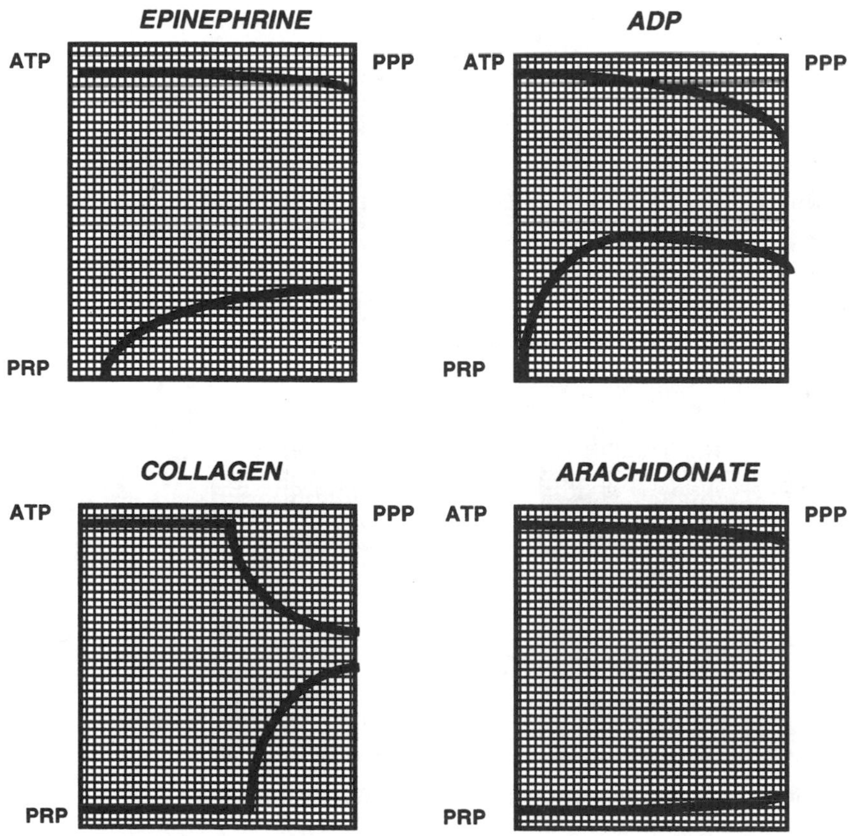

FIGURE 4.6. Cardiopulmonary bypass surgery: platelet lumi-aggregation patterns (1 hour after bypass). *ADP*, adenosine diphosphate; *ATP*, adenosine triphosphate; *PRP*, platelet-rich plasma; *PPP*, platelet-poor plasma.

also may induce a platelet-function defect, independent of folate-associated thrombocytopenia (96,98,105). Morphologic changes of platelets induced by ethanol, and presumably associated with defects in platelet function, include vacuolization of both platelets and megakaryocytes, abnormal platelet granules, microtubular fragmentation, and the presence of giant platelets (98,99). Platelet-function defects, like thrombocytopenia, also are noted in association with liver transplantation (106). This is probably because of coating of platelets by FDPs, resulting from a disseminated intravascular coagulation (DIC)-type syndrome. As with thrombocytopenia associated with transplantation rejection and resultant circulating immune complexes, these immune complexes also compromise platelet function, as they are potent inducers of a platelet-release reaction.

In summary, acute and chronic liver disease is often associated with a severe and clinically significant platelet-function defect. This defect is multifactorial and may result from altered intraplatelet metabolism of the compounds earlier discussed and from the presence of FDPs. If the patient also is an ethanol abuser, these defects are compounded, and ethanol alone, without significant liver disease, may induce significant platelet dysfunction. It is important to recall that most patients with acute and chronic liver disease do have significant platelet dysfunction; clinicians cannot assume a false sense of security when seeing a patient with liver disease, hemorrhage, and a normal or near-normal platelet count, as the platelets circulating, although normal in number, may be significantly dysfunctional and contribute to hemorrhage that has remained unresponsive to infusions of fresh frozen plasma. In patients with liver disease and hemorrhage, platelet dysfunction should be recalled, its presence or absence documented by aggregation or lumi-aggregation, and if present, treated with DDAVP or proper numbers of platelet concentrates despite the platelet count (93,107,108).

MISCELLANEOUS DISORDERS AND PLATELET DYSFUNCTION

Acquired platelet dysfunction is seen in autoimmune disorders including systemic lupus erythematosus, rheumatoid arthritis, scleroderma, and others (109,110). Patients with immune-mediated thrombocytopenia commonly have associated severe platelet dysfunction resulting from coating of the platelet membrane by immunoglobulin; thus assessment of bleeding tendency in patients with immune-mediated thrombocytopenias such as immune/idiopathic thrombocytopenia purpura (ITP) must be made by evaluation of not only the absolute platelet count but also the associated platelet function (111,112). Figure 4.7 demonstrates platelet dysfunction in a patient with ITP.

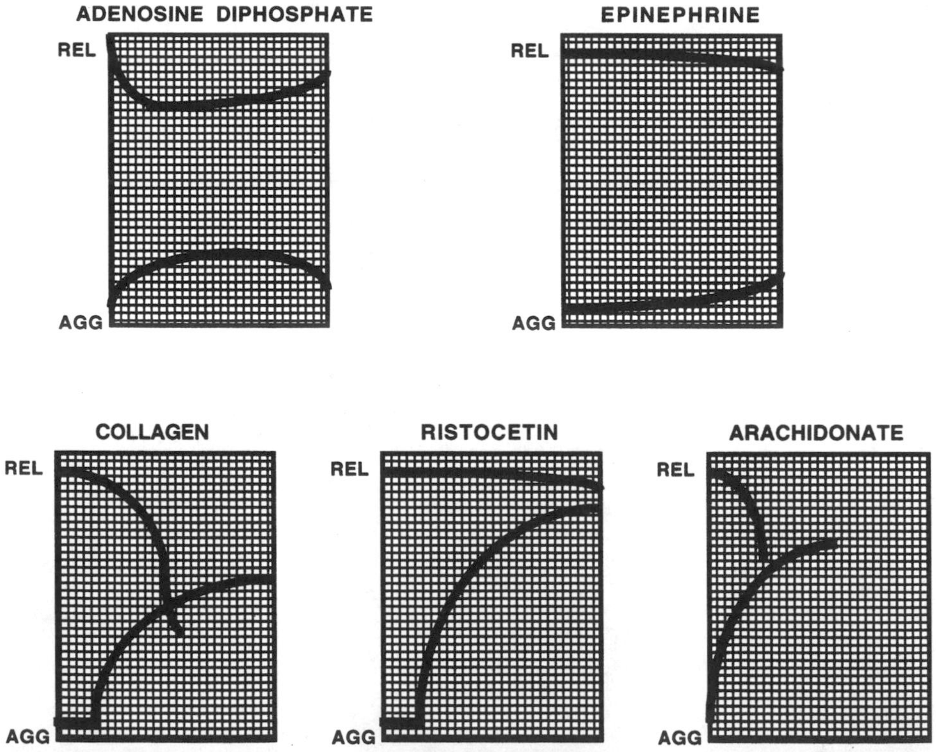

FIGURE 4.7. Platelet dysfunction in immune thrombocytopenia purpura. *AGG*, aggregation; *REL*, release reaction (adenosine triphosphate).

The presence of FDPs very often induces a clinically significant platelet-function defect (95,113,114). The fibrinogen/fibrin degradation products can be of any origin including DIC or primary hyperfibrino(geno)lytic syndromes (94,115–117). The later degradation products, especially fragment D and fragment E, have a high affinity for platelet membranes, attach to the membrane, and cause a severe and clinically significant acquired platelet-function defect. Patients with severe iron deficiency or severe folate or vitamin B_{12} deficiency also may have platelet dysfunction, which may sometimes lead to clinically significant hemorrhage (118,119). Drug-induced platelet-function defects are very commonly noted and are a common cause of easy and spontaneous bruising, petechiae and purpura, and bleeding associated with surgery or trauma (5,120). Drug-induced defects are discussed subsequently. Unlike the rare hereditary platelet-function defects, the acquired platelet-function defects do not show typical platelet-aggregation abnormalities when patterns are studied. For example, one can study many patients with chronic myelogenous leukemia, and all will probably have abnormal aggregation patterns. However, many different varieties of abnormalities will often be seen.

Drug-induced Platelet Dysfunction

Common clinical drugs causing clinically significant platelet dysfunction and hemorrhage are numerous. The number of drugs interfering with platelet function, as defined by laboratory tests (aggregation or lumi-aggregation), is much more extensive. This review is limited to commonly used drugs reported to cause clinically significant hemorrhage in patients. The three most common mechanisms by which drugs interfere with platelet function, in descending order of prevalence, are (a) drug interference with the platelet membrane or membrane receptor sites, (b) drug interference with prostaglandin biosynthetic pathways, and (c) drug interference with phosphodiesterase activity (121,122).

Drugs Interfering with Platelet Membrane Receptors

The most common drugs interfering with platelet membrane function or receptors are amitriptyline (Elavil) (123), imipramine (Tofranil) (124), doxepin (Sinequan) (125), chlorpromazine (Thorazine) (126), cocaine (127), lidocaine (Xylocaine) (128), isoproterenol (Isuprel) (129), propranolol (130), cephalothin (Keflin) (131), ampicillin (132), carbenicillin (133), penicillin (134), diphenhydramine (Benadryl) (135), promethazine (Phenergan) (136), and alcohol (98). Other drugs inducing platelet dysfunction by this mechanism are phentolamine (Regitine) (137), phenoxylbenzamine (Dibenzyline) (137), reserpine (138), dihydroergotamine (139), morpramine (124), nortriptyline (Aventyl) (124), trifluoperazine (Stelazine) (140), procaine (140), dibucaine (Nupercaine) (141), nitrofurantoin (Furadantin) (142), nafcillin (143), moxalactam (144), ticarcillin (145), dextran (146), and hydroxyethyl starch (147).

Drug Inhibition of Prostaglandin Pathways

The most common drugs interfering with platelet prostaglandin synthetic pathways are ASA (148), indomethacin (149), phenylbutazone (150), ibuprofen (Motrin) (151), naproxen (Naprosyn) (109), sulfinpyrazone (152), furosemide (153), and verapamil (154). Less commonly used drugs that share this mechanism of inducing platelet dysfunction are hydralazine (155), quinacrine (156), fenoprofen (Nalfon) (121), mefenamic acid (Ponstel) (157), tocopherol (158), hydrocortisone (159), methylprednisolone (160), and cyclosporine (161).

Drugs Inhibiting Platelet Phosphodiesterase Activity

The most common drugs interfering with platelet phosphodiesterase activity and inducing platelet dysfunction are caffeine (162), dipyridamole (163), aminophylline, theophylline, and papaverine (164–166). Vinblastine, vincristine (167), and colchicine (168) interfere with the platelet contractile protein, thrombosthenin.

Drugs with Unknown Mechanisms of Action on Platelet Function

Acetazolamide (169), ethacrynic acid (169), Areomycin (170), hydroxychloroquine (Plaquenil) (171), dicoumarol (172), nitroprusside (173), cyproheptadine (Periactin) (174), glycerol guaiacolate (175), and heparin (176–179) interfere with platelet function by unclear mechanisms. Nitroglycerin induces platelet dysfunction by interference with platelet cyclic AMP (180).

Classification of Drugs Inducing Platelet Dysfunction

Antiinflammatory drugs are very common offenders; ASA, colchicine, ibuprofen (Motrin), indomethacin (Indocin), and sulfinpyrazone are the most common. Any nonsteroidal antiinflammatory drug (NSAID) can induce significant platelet dysfunction, and all inhibit prostaglandin pathways (109). Sulfinpyrazone and ASA are used pharmacologically to suppress platelet function and have the same mode of action; both drugs inhibit cyclooxygenase, therefore inhibiting the eventual platelet synthesis of thromboxane A_2. Of course, these drugs also, therefore, inhibit endothelial cell synthesis of prostacyclin; however, it is thought that the inhibitory selectivity of these drugs is about 70% against platelet cyclooxygenase and 30% against endothelial cyclooxygenase, thus accounting for the antithrombotic instead of prothrombotic action of these agents (181–185). Psychiatric drugs also may inhibit platelet function. The phenothiazine-related drugs including chlorpromazine (Thorazine) and trifluoperazine (Stelazine) may induce clinically significant platelet dysfunction. The tricyclic amines interfere with platelet function. Many cardiovascular drugs interfere with platelet function including clofibrate, dipyridamole (Persantine), nicotinic acid, papaverine, propranolol, and the newer calcium channel–blocking drugs, including verapamil. Newer agents such as the new generation β-blocking drugs and diltiazem inhibit platelet function (186). Sodium nitroprusside and trimethorphan (Arfonad) induce platelet dysfunction (187,188). This category is of particular importance, as many candidates for CPB surgery may be ingesting one or several of these agents such as papaverine, propranolol, theophylline, or a calcium channel–blocking agent and may have enhanced bleeding risk with CPB surgery because of a drug-induced platelet dysfunction (189). Antibiotics also are common inducers of platelet dysfunction. Most of the penicillin derivatives including nafcillin, ampicillin, carbenicillin, and ticarcillin can interfere with platelet function; this is most commonly seen with carbenicillin. Gentamicin and other aminoglycosides also are capable of interfering with platelet function. Various anesthetics including the local anesthetics, cocaine, and procaine, as well as gaseous anesthetics, may interfere with platelet function and lead to hemorrhage. Miscellaneous drugs interfering with platelet function are the antihistamines [the most common offenders are diphenhydramine (Benadryl) and Actifed (a combination)], the dextrans, furosemide (Lasix), glycerol guaiacolate (the base of many common cough syrups), nitroprusside, and vincristine or vinblastine.

Categories of common clinical drugs capable of causing a clinically significant platelet-function defect are listed in Tables 4.11, 4.12, and 4.13. The mechanism of action, where known, also is depicted. Table 4.14 lists common drugs containing ASA (190,191).

A "compendium" of drugs capable of altering platelet function is listed in Table 4.15 (alphabetical by brand) and Table 4.16 (alphabetical by generic name).

TABLE 4.11. DRUG-INDUCED PLATELET DYSFUNCTION: CARDIOVASCULAR/RESPIRATORY AND ANTIBIOTICS

Cardiovascular/Respiratory	Antibiotics
Aminophylline (PD)	Ampicillin (MEM)
Clofibrate (MEM)	Aureomycin (UK)
Dibenzyline (MEM)	Carbenicillin (MEM)
Dicoumarol (UK)	Nitrofuradantin (Furadantin) (MEM)
Dihydroergotamine (MEM)	Gentamicin (MEM)
Dipyridamole (PD)	Cephalothin (Keflin) (MEM)
Heparin (UK)	Moxalactam (MEM)
Hydralazine (PG)	Nafcillin (MEM)
Isoproterenol (Isuprel) (MEM)	Piperacillin (MEM)
Nitroglycerine (AMP)	Hydroxychloroquine (Plaquenil) (UK)
Nitroprusside (UK)	Quinacrine (PG)
Papaverine (PD)	
Propranolol (MEM)	
Phentolamine (Regitine) (MEM)	
Reserpine (MEM)	
Theophylline (PD)	
Verapamil (PG)	

MEM, interference with membrane or membrane receptors; PG, interference with prostaglandin synthesis; PD, interference with phosphodiesterase; AMP, interference with platelet cyclic AMP; UK, unknown mechanism of action.

Hyperactive "Prethrombotic" Platelets

Hereditary and acquired hyperactive platelets are responsible for a significant number of arterial and thrombotic events, although clinicians still often fail to be familiar with these defects, fail to assess appropriate patients for these defects, and often fail to render appropriate therapy. Less commonly appreciated is that platelet defects also may be responsible for many arterial and venous thrombotic events and are thus responsible for significant morbidity and mortality in the United States population. One such defect, the Wein–Penzing defect, was first described in 1991, but appears to be extremely rare (192). However, another platelet defect that (a) appears quite common, (b) accounts for many episodes of arterial and venous thrombosis and significant morbidity and mortality, (c) is easy to diagnose, and (d) is easy to treat, is sticky platelet syndrome (SPS). SPS was first described by Mammen et al. (193) in 1983 at the Ninth International Joint Conference on Stroke and Cerebral Circulation. Subsequently Mammen et al. (194) described 41 patients with coronary artery disease and SPS; this was followed by a report in 1986 delineating this syndrome in a number of individuals with cerebrovascular disease; the inheritance was noted to be autosomal dominant (195). Finally in 1995, more than 200 families, with a wide variety of arterial and venous thrombotic events due to SPS, were described (196). Although these publications have clearly delineated SPS as a common inherited and easily diagnosed and treated syndrome leading to significant, and often preventable, arterial and venous thrombosis, most clinicians and laboratory scientists are still unfamiliar with the prevalence of SPS and fail to consider this diagnosis in appropriate patient populations. In additional, the actual prevalence remains unclear, especially as relates to venous versus arterial events. A more recent study (197) assessed the prevalence of SPS in a wide variety of patients with various types of arterial and venous events referred to the Dallas Thrombosis Hemostasis Clinical Center over a 2-

TABLE 4.12. DRUG-INDUCED PLATELET DYSFUNCTION: PSYCHIATRIC, ANESTHETIC, ANTIINFLAMMATORY, AND DIURETIC DRUGS

Psychiatric Drugs	Antiinflammatory Drugs
Nortriptyline (Aventyl) (MEM)	Sulfinpyrazone (Anturane) (PG)
Amitriptyline (Elavil) (MEM)	Acetylsalicylic acid (Aspirin) (PG)
Desipramine (Norpramine) (MEM)	Colchicine (TS)
Doxepin (Sinequan) (MEM)	Ibuprofen (PG)
Trifluoperazine (Stelazine) (MEM)	Indomethacin (PG)
Chlorpromazine (Thorazine) (MEM)	Fenoprufen (Nalfon) (PG)
Imipramine (Tofranil) (MEM)	Naprozen (Naprosyn) (PG)
	Phenylbutazone (PG)
	Mefenamic acid (Ponstel) (PG)
Anesthetics	Diuretics
Cocaine (MEM)	Acetazolamide (UK)
Dibucaine (Nupercaine) (MEM)	Ethacrynic acid (UK)
Procaine (MEM)	Furosemide (PG)
Lidocaine (Xylocaine) (MEM)	

MEM, interference with membrane or membrane receptors; PG, interference with prostaglandin synthesis; TS, interference with thrombosthenin; UK, unknown mechanism of action.

year period; the results of these findings and recommendations for diagnosis and management are discussed.

One hundred fifty patients were referred for evaluation to determine the etiology, if possible, of unexplained arterial or venous events; 78 had had venous events consisting of deep vein thrombosis (DVT) with or without pulmonary embolus (PE). Seventy-five patients were referred for evaluation of arterial events; these patients had coronary artery thrombosis (21%), cerebrovascular thrombosis (50.6%), transient cerebral ischemic attacks (TIAs; 13.3%), retinal vascular thrombosis (6.6%), or peripheral arterial thrombosis (8%). Peripheral arterial thrombotic events consisted of unexplained thrombosis of renal (two), radial (one), popliteal (one), and mesenteric (one) arteries. All patients referred for determining the etiology of an unexplained thrombotic event were subjected to a complete history and physical examination and then were studied for hypercoagulability syndromes, including SPS.

SPS evaluations were performed according to the method of Mammen et al. Normal controls were first assessed, and the normal ranges were found to be similar

(text continues on page 75)

TABLE 4.13. DRUG-INDUCED PLATELET DYSFUNCTION: MISCELLANEOUS DRUGS

Alcohol	(MEM)
Diphenhydramine (Benadryl)	(MEM)
Caffeine	(PD)
Cyclosporine	(PG)
Dextran	(MEM)
Glycerol guaiacolate	(UK)
Hydroxyethyl starch	(MEM)
Hydrocortisone	(PG)
Methylprednisolone	(PG)
Ciproheptadine (Periactin)	(UK)
Promethazine (Phenergan)	(MEM)
Methysergide (Sansert)	(UK)
Tocopherol	(PG)
Vinblastine	(TS)
Vincristine	(TS)

MEM, interference with membrane or membrane receptors; PG, interference with prostaglandin synthesis; PD, interference with phosphodiesterase; TS, interference with thrombosthenin; UK, unknown mechanism of action.

TABLE 4.14. DRUG-INDUCED PLATELET DYSFUNCTION: BRAND NAMES OF COMMON DRUGS CONTAINING ASPIRIN

Alka Seltzer	Empiral
Anacin	Empirin
Anahist	Empirin w/codeine
APC	Emprazil
APC w/codeine	Emprazil-C
APC w/demerol	Equagesic
ASA	Excedrin
ASA compound	Excedrin PM
ASA compound w/codeine	Florinal
Aspergum	Florinal w/codeine
Aspirin (USP)	Fizrin
Aspirin-children's	4-way cold tablets
Bayer	Liquiprin
Bayer-children's	Measurin
Bayer timed-release	Midol
Bufferin	Norgesic
Calurin	PAC Compound
Cama Inlay	PAC Compound
w/codeine	
Cope	Percodan
Coricidin	Robaxisal
Coricidin "D"	Robaxisal-PH
Coricidin demilets	Sine-Off
Coricidin medilets	St. Joseph's
Darvon w/ASA	St. Joseph's for children
Darvon-N w/ASA	Super-Anahist
Darvon compound	Synalgos
Dolene	Synalgos-DC
Dristan	Triaminicin
Ecotrin	Vanquish

TABLE 4.15. DRUGS ASSOCIATED WITH PLATELET DYSFUNCTION BY BRAND NAME

Brand Name	Generic Name/Composition	Classification
4-Way cold tabs	Clorpheniramine	Decongestant
4-Way nasal spray	Phenylephrine	Decongestant
Achromycin	Tetracycline	Antibiotic
Actibine	Yohimbine	CNS
Actifed	Pseudoephedrine	Decongestant
Activase	Alteplase	Cardiac
Adapin	Doxepin	CNS
Adipex	Phentermine	Gastric
Aerobid	Flunisolide	NSAID
Aerolate	Theophylline	Pulmonary
Akineton	Biperiden	CNS
Alupent	Metaproterenol	Pulmonary
Ambenyl	Codeine/Bromodiphenhydramine	Decongestant
Amicar	Aminocaproic acid	Hematology
Amikin	Amikacin	Antibiotic
Amoxil	Amoxicillin	Antibiotic
Anafranil	Clomipramine	CNS
Anatuss	Guaifenesin/Pseudoephedrine	Decongestant
Anturane	Sulfinpyrazone	NSAID
Apresazide	Hydralazine/Thiazide	Cardiac
Apresoline	Hydralazine	Cardiac
Aramine	Metaraminol	Cardiac
Aristocort	Triamcinolone	Steroid
Asendin	Amoxapine	CNS
Atrohist	Brompheniramine	Decongestant
Augmentin	Amoxicillin	Antibiotic
Azdone	Hydrocodone/ASA	Analgesic
Biphetamine	Amphetamine	CNS
Blocadren	Timolol	Cardiac
Bontril	Phendimetrazine	Obesity
Brethaire	Terbutaline	Pulmonary
Brethine	Terbutaline	Pulmonary
Brevibloc	Esmolol	Cardiac
Bricanyl	Terbutaline	Pulmonary
Bufferin	Aspirin	NSAID
Butazolidine	Phenylbutazone	NSAID
Calciparine	Heparin	Anticoagulant
Carbamazepine USP	Carbamazepine	CNS
Cardizem	Diltiazem	Cardiac
Cartrol	Carteolol	Cardiac
Catapres	Clonidine	Cardiac
Ceclor	Cefaclor	Antibiotic
Cefizox	Ceftizoxime	Antibiotic
Ceftin	Cefuroxime	Antibiotic
Claforan	Cefotaxime	Antibiotic
Clinoril	Sulindac	Antiinflammatory
Codimal	Hydrocodone/Phenylephrine	Decongestant
Colbenemid	Probenecid/Colchicine	Uricosuric
Combipres	Clonidine	Cardiac
Comtrex	Pseudoephedrine	Decongestant
Congess	Pseudoephedrine	Decongestant
Constant-T	Theophylline	Pulmonary
Corgard	Nadolol	Cardiac
Cortone	Cortisone	Steroid
Corzide	Nadolol	Cardiac
Coumadin	Warfarin	Cardiac
Dalalone	Dexamethasone	Steroid
Damason-P	Hydrocodone/ASA	Analgesic
Darvon compound	Propoxyphene/ASA	Analgesic
Decadron	Dexamethasone	Hormone

(continued)

TABLE 4.15. *(continued)*

Brand Name	Generic Name/Composition	Classification
Declomycin	Demeclocycline	Antibiotic
Deconamine	Chlorpheniramine	Decongestant
Deconsal	Pseudoephedrine	Decongestant
Depakene	Valproic acid	Psychiatric
Depakote	Valproic acid	Psychiatric
Desoxyn	Methamphetamine	Psychiatric
Dicumarol	Warfarin	Anticoagulant
Diethylstilbestrol	Diethylstilbestrol	Hormone
Disalcid	Salsalate	Antiinflammatory
Diupress	Reserpine/Chlorothiazide	Cardiac
Dolobid	Diflunisal	NSAID
Doral	Quazepam	CNS
Duricef	Cefadroxil	Antibiotic
Edecrin	Ethacrynic acid	Diuretic
Elixophyllin	Theophylline	Pulmonary
Empirin	ASA/Codeine	Analgesic
Enduron	Methylclothiazide	Diuretic
Enduronyl	Methylclothiazide	Diuretic
Enkaid	Encainide	Cardiac
Ergomar	Ergotamine	CNS
Esgic	Butalbital/Acetaminophen/Caffeine	CNS
Esidrix	Hydrochlorothiazide	Diuretic
Esimil	Guanethidine/Thiazide	Diuretic
Estrace	Estradiol	Hormone
Ethamolin	Ethanolamine	Vascular
Ethmozine	Moricizine	Cardiac
Ethrane	Enflurane	Anesthetic
Excedrin-sinus	Pseudoephedrine	Decongestant
Extendryl	Phenylephrine	Decongestant
Flexeril	Cyclobenzaprine	Muscular
Forane	Isoflurane	Anesthetic
Fortaz	Ceftazidime	Antibiotic
Gris-PEG	Griseofulvin	Antibiotic
Heparin	Heparin	Anticoagulant
Hespan	Hetastarch	Cardiac
Humibid	Guiafenesin	Respiratory
Hycomine	Hydrocodone/Phenylpropanolamine	Decongestant
Hycomine CMPD	Hydrocodone/Chlopheniramine	Decongestant
Hydeltra-T.B.A.	Prednisolone	Hormone
Hydeltrasol	Prednisolone	Hormone
Hydrocortone	Hydrocortisone	Hormone
Hydromox	Quinethazone	Diuretic
Hydropres	Reserpine/Hydrochlorothiazide	Cardiac
Hylorel	Guanadrel	Cardiac
Indocin	Indomethacin	NSAID
Indomethacin	Indomethacin	NSAID
Innovar	Fentanyl/Droperidol	Anesthetic
Intropin	Dopamine	Cardiac
Ionamin	Phentermine	Gastric
Isoptin	Verapamil	Cardiac
Kabikinase	Streptokinase	Cardiac
Keflex	Cephalexin	Antibiotic
Keftab	Cephalexin	Antibiotic
Kefurox	Cefuroxime	Antibiotic
Kefzol	Cefazolin	Antibiotic
Lasix	Furoxemide	Cardiac
Lidocaine HCL	Lidocaine	Anesthetic
Lopressor	Metoprolol	Cardiac
Loxitane	Loxapine	CNS
Ludiomil	Maprotiline	CNS
Mandole	Cefamandole	Antibiotic

(continued)

TABLE 4.15. *(continued)*

Brand Name	Generic Name/Composition	Classification
Maxair	Pirbuterol	Pulmonary
Maxzide	Triamterene/Hydrochlorothiazide	Cardiac
Medipren	Ibuprofen	NSAID
Mefoxin	Cefoxitin	Antibiotic
Midrin	Mixed	CNS
Minitran	Nitroglycerin	Cardiac
Minocin	Minocycline	Antibiotic
Monogesic	ASA	NSAID
Mykrox	Metolazone	Diuretic
Myleran	Busulfan	Antineoplastic
Naldecon	Mixed	Decongestant
Nalfon	Fenoprofen	NSAID
Nitro-BID	Nitroglycerin	Cardiac
Nitrogard	Nitroglycerin	Cardiac
No-Doz	Caffeine	Stimulant
Nocofed	Pseudoephedrine	Decongestant
Nolahist	Phenindamine	Decongestant
Nolamine	Mixed	Decongestant
Nolex-LA	Phenylpropanolamine	Decongestant
Norpramine	Desipramine	CNS
Novafed	Pseudoephedrine/Chlorpheniramine	Decongestant
Novahistine	Pseudoephedrine/Chlorpheniramine	Decongestant
Nuprin	Ibuprofen	NSAID
Octamide	Metoclopramide	Gastric
Oncovin	Vincristine	Antineoplastic
Oretic	Hydroclorothiazide	Diuretic
Oreticyl	Hydroclorothiazide	Diuretic
Ovcon	Norethindrone/Estradiol	Hormone
Panwarfin	Warfarin	Anticoagulant
Papaverine	Papaverine	Cardiac
Pavabid	Papaverine	Cardiac
PBZ	Tripelennamine	Decongestant
PBZ-SR	Tripelennamine	Decongestant
Pediacare	Chlorpheniramine	Decongestant
Pediapred	Prednisolone	Steroid
Pediaprofen	Ibuprofen	NSAID
Pentaspan	Pentastarch	Cardiac
Percodan	Oxycodone/ASA	Analgesic
Permax	Pergolide	CNS
Persantine	Dipyridamole	Cardiac
Pipracil	Piperacillin	Antibiotic
Precef	Ceforanide	Antibiotic
Prelu-2	Phendimetrazine	Gastric
Preludin	Phenmetrazine	Gastric
Prescoline	Tolazoline	Cardiac
Propagest	Phenylpropanolamine	Decongestant
Propranolol USP	Propranolol	Cardiac
Prozac	Fluoxetine	CNS
Quadrinal	Ephedrine/Phenobarbital/Theophylline	Pulmonary
Quelidrine	Mixed	Pulmonary
Quibron	Theophylline	Pulmonary
Quinaglute	Quinidine	Cardiac
Regitine	Phentolamine	Cardiac
Respbid	Theophylline	Pulmonary
Ru-Tuss	Phenylpropanolamine	Decongestant
Rufen	Ibuprofen	NSAID
Rythmol	Propafenone	Cardiac
Saluron	Hydroflumethiazide	Diuretic
Salutensin	Hydroflumethiazide/Reserpine	Diuretic
Ser-Ap-Es	Reserpine/Thiazide/Hydralazine	Cardiac
Serentil	Mesoridazine	CNS

(continued)

TABLE 4.15. *(continued)*

Brand Name	Generic Name/Composition	Classification
Serpasil	Reserpine	Cardiac
Serpasil-Apresoline	Reserpine/Hydralazine	Cardiac
Serpasil-Esidrex	Reserpine/Thiazide	Cardiac
Sine-Aid	Pseudoephedrine/Acetaminophen	Decongestant
Sinemet	Carbidopa/Levodopa	CNS
Sinulin	Phenylpropanolamine	Decongestant
Soophyllin	Aminophylline	Pulmonary
Streptase	Streptokinase	Cardiac
Sudafed	Pseudoephedrine	Decongestant
Suprax	Cefixime	Antibiotic
Sus-phrine	Epinephrine	Pulmonary
Tace	Chlorotrianisene	Antineoplastic
Tambocor	Flecainide	Cardiac
Tazidime	Ceftazidime	Antibiotic
Tegretol	Carbamazepine	CNS
Temaril	Trimeprazine	Dermatology
Tenoretic	Atenolol/Chlorothalidone	Cardiac
Tenormin	Atenolol	Cardiac
Tenuate	Diethylpropion	CNS/Obesity
Thalitone	Chlorothalidone	Diuretic
Theo-dur	Theophylline	Pulmonary
Theochron	Theophylline	Pulmonary
Ticar	Ticarcillin	Antibiotic
Tigan	Trimethobenzamine	Antiemetic
Timentin	Ticarcillin	Antibiotic
Tofranil	Imipramine	CNS
Tolectin	Tolmetin	NSAID
Trandate	Labetalol	Cardiac
Trandate HCT	Labetalol/HCT	Cardiac
Trental	Pentoxifylline	Cardiac
Tridil	Nitroglycerin	Cardiac
Tussionex	Hydrocodone/Chlorpheniramine	Decongestant
Ultracef	Cefadroxil	Antibiotic
Vasoxyl	Methoxamine	Cardiac
Velban	Vinblastine	Antineoplastic
Ventolin	Albuterol	Pulmonary
Verelan	Verapamil	Cardiac
Voltaren	Diclofenac	NSAID
Wellbutrin	Bupropion	CNS
Xylocaine	Lidocaine	Analgesic
Yohimex	Yohimbine	CNS
Yutopar	Ritodrine	Obstetric
Zantac	Ranitidine	Gastric
Zaroxolyn	Metolazone	Diuretic
Zinacef	Cefuroxime	Antibiotic
Zorprin	Aspirin	NSAID

CNS, central nervous system; NSAID, nonsteroidal antiinflammatory drug.

(continued from page 71)
to those previously reported by Mammen et al. The assay for SPS, using the method of Mammen et al., consists of collecting blood in 3.2% sodium citrate by clean venipuncture with butterfly needles. The first 5.0 mL is discarded, and then 18 mL is aspirated into a 20-mL syringe containing the sodium citrate in a ratio of 9:1. The anticoagulated blood is then centrifuged for 10 minutes at 100 *g*. The resultant platelet-rich plasma (PRP) is then carefully placed into a plastic tube. Aggregation is performed by using ADP and epinephrine (EPI) as follows: ADP stock solution of 0.5 mL reagent (BioData) is diluted to obtain three initial working solutions of 2.34×10^{-5} *M*, 1.17×10^{-5} *M*, and 5.8×10^{-5} *M*. EPI (BioData) stock solution of 0.5 mL reagent was diluted to the three initial working solutions of 11×10^{-5} *M*, 1.1×10^{-5} *M*, and 0.55×10^{-5} *M*. The equipment used was a Payton Scientific Aggregometer, Omniscribe recorders, siliconized glass cuvettes, and siliconized glass stir bars. The recorders

(text continues on page 79)

TABLE 4.16. DRUGS ASSOCIATED WITH PLATELET DYSFUNCTION BY GENERIC NAME

Generic Name/Composition	Brand Name	Classification
Albuterol	Ventolin	Pulmonary
Alteplase	Activase	Cardiac
Amikacin	Amikin	Antibiotic
Aminocaproic acid	Amicar	Hematology
Aminophylline	Soophyllin	Pulmonary
Amoxapine	Asendin	CNS
Amoxicillin	Amoxil	Antibiotic
	Augmentin	Antibiotic
Amphetamine	Biphetamine	CNS
ASA	Monogesic	NSAID
ASA/Codeine	Empirin	Analgesic
Aspirin	Bufferin	NSAID
	Zorprin	NSAID
Atenolol/Chlorthalidone	Tenoretic	Cardiac
Atenolol	Tenormin	Cardiac
Biperiden	Akineton	CNS
Brompheniramine	Atrohist	Decongestant
Bupropion	Wellbutrin	CNS
Busulfan	Myleran	Antineoplastic
Butalbital/Acetaminophen/ Caffeine	Esgic	CNS
Caffeine	No-Doz	Stimulant
Carbamazepine	Tegretol	CNS
	Carbamazepine USP	CNS
Carbidopa/Levodopa	Sinemet	CNS
Carterolol	Cartrol	Cardiac
Cefaclor	Ceclor	Antibiotic
Cefadroxil	Duricef	Antibiotic
	Ultracef	Antibiotic
Cefamandole	Mandol	Antibiotic
Cefazolin	Kefzol	Antibiotic
Cefixime	Suprax	Antibiotic
Ceforanide	Precef	Antibiotic
Cefotaxime	Claforan	Antibiotic
Cefoxitin	Mefoxin	Antibiotic
Ceftazidime	Fortaz	Antibiotic
Ceftazidime	Tazidime	Antibiotic
Ceftizoxime	Cefizox	Antibiotic
Cefuroxime	Ceftin	Antibiotic
	Kefurox	Antibiotic
	Zinacef	Antibiotic
Cephalexin	Keflex	Antibiotic
	Keftab	Antibiotic
Chlorotrianisene	Tace	Antineoplastic
Chlorpheniramine	Deconamine	Decongestant
	Pediacare	Decongestant
Chlorthalidone	Thalitone	Diuretic
Clomipramine	Anafranil	CNS
Clonidine	Catapres	Cardiac
Clonidine	Combipres	Cardiac
Clorpheniramine	4-Way cold tabs	Decongestant
Codeine/Bromodiphenhydramine	Ambenyl	Decongestant
Cortisone	Cortone	Steroid
Cyclobenzaprine	Flexeril	Muscular
Demeclocycline	Declomycin	Antibiotic
Desipramine	Norpramine	CNS
Dexamethasone	Dalalone	Steroid
Dexamethasone	Decadron	Hormone
Diclofenac	Voltaren	NSAID
Diethylpropion	Tenuate	CNS/Obesity

(continued)

TABLE 4.16. ***(continued)***

Generic Name/Composition	Brand Name	Classification
Diethylstilbestrol	Diethylstilbestrol	Hormone
Diflunisal	Dolobid	NSAID
Diltiazem	Cardizem	Cardiac
Dipyridamole	Persantine	Cardiac
Dopamine	Intropin	Cardiac
Doxepin	Adapin	CNS
Encainide	Enkaid	Cardiac
Enflurane	Ethrane	Anesthetic
Ephedrine/Phenobarbital/Theophylline	Quadrinal	Pulmonary
Epinephrine	Sus-Phrine	Pulmonary
Ergotamine	Ergomar	CNS
Esmolol	Brevibloc	Cardiac
Estradiol	Estrace	Hormone
Ethacrynic acid	Edecrin	Diuretic
Ethanolamine	Ethamolin	Vascular
Fenoprofen	Nalfon	NSAID
Fentanyl/Droperidol	Innovar	Anesthetic
Flecainide	Tambocor	Cardiac
Flunisolide	Aerobid	NSAID
Fluoxetine	Prozac	CNS
Furosemide	Lasix	Cardiac
Griseofulvin	Gris-Peg	Antibiotic
Guaifenesin/Pseudoephedrine	Anatuss	Decongestant
Guanadrel	Hylorel	Cardiac
Guanethidine/Thiazide	Esimil	Diuretic
Guiafenesin	Humibid	Respiratory
Heparin	Calciparine	Anticoagulant
	Heparin	Anticoagulant
Hetastarch	Hespan	Cardiac
Hydralazine	Apresoline	Cardiac
Hydralazine/Thiazide	Apresazide	Cardiac
Hydrochlorothiazide	Esidrix	Diuretic
	Oretic	Diuretic
	Oreticyl	Diuretic
Hydrocodone/ASA	Azdone	Analgesic
	Damason-P	Analgesic
Hydrocodone/Chlopheniramine	Hycomine CMPD	Decongestant
	Tussionex	Decongestant
Hydrocodone/Phenylephrine	Codimal	Decongestant
Hydrocodone/Phenylpropanolamine	Hycomine	Decongestant
Hydrocortisone	Hydrocortone	Hormone
Hydroflumethiazide	Saluron	Diuretic
Hydroflumethiazide/Reserpine	Salutensin	Diuretic
Ibuprofen	Medipren	NSAID
	Pediaprofen	NSAID
	Rufen	NSAID
	Nuprin	NSAID
Imipramine	Tofranil	CNS
Indomethacin	Indocin	NSAID
	Indomethacin	NSAID
Isoflurane	Forane	Anesthetic
Labetalol	Trandate	Cardiac
Labetalol/HCT	Trandate HCT	Cardiac
Lidocaine	Lidocaine HCL	Anesthetic
	Xylocaine	Analgesic
Loxapine	Loxitane	CNS
Maprotiline	Ludiomil	CNS
Mesoridazine	Serentil	CNS
Metaproterenol	Alupent	Pulmonary
Metaraminol	Aramine	Cardiac

(continued)

TABLE 4.16. ***(continued)***

Generic Name/Composition	Brand Name	Classification
Methamphetamine	Desoxyn	Psychiatric
Methoxamine	Vasoxyl	Cardiac
Methylclothiazide	Enduron	Diuretic
	Enduronyl	Diuretic
Metoclopramide	Octamide	Gastric
Metolazone	Mykrox	Diuretic
	Zaroxolyn	Diuretic
Metoprolol	Lopressor	Cardiac
Minocycline	Minocin	Antibiotic
Mixed	Midrin	CNS
	Naldecon	Decongestant
	Nolamine	Decongestant
	Quelidrine	Pulmonary
Moricizine	Ethmozine	Cardiac
Nadolol	Corgard	Cardiac
	Corzide	Cardiac
Nitroglycerin	Minitran	Cardiac
	Nitro-BID	Cardiac
	Nitrogard	Cardiac
	Tridil	Cardiac
Norethindrone/Estradiol	Ovcon	Hormone
Oxycodone/ASA	Percodan	Analgesic
Papaverine	Papaverine	Cardiac
	Pavabid	Cardiac
Pentastarch	Pentaspan	Cardiac
Pentoxifylline	Trenta	Cardiac
Pergolide	Permax	CNS
Phendimetrazine	Bontril	Obesity
	Prelu-2	Gastric
Phenindamine	Nolahist	Decongestant
Phenmetrazine	Preludin	Gastric
Phentermine	Adipex	Gastric
	Ionamin	Gastric
Phentolamine	Regitine	Cardiac
Phenylbutazone	Butazolidin	NSAID
Phenylephrine	4-Way-nasal spray	Decongestant
	Extendryl	Decongestant
Phenylpropanolamine	Nolex-LA	Decongestant
	Propagest	Decongestant
	Ru-Tuss	Decongestant
	Sinulin	Decongestant
Piperacillin	Pipracil	Antibiotic
Pirbuterol	Maxair	Pulmonary
Prednisolone	Hydeltra-T.B.A.	Hormone
	Hydeltrasol	Hormone
	Pediapred	Steroid
Probenecid/Colchicine	Colbenemid	Uricosuric
Propafenone	Rythmol	Cardiac
Propranolol	Propranolol USP	Cardiac
Propoxyphene/ASA	Darvon compound	Analgesic
Pseudoephedrine	Actifed	Decongestant
	Comtrex	Decongestant
	Congess	Decongestant
	Deconsal	Decongestant
	Excedrin-Sinus	Decongestant
	Nocofed	Decongestant
	Sudafed	Decongestant
Pseudoephedrine/Acetaminophen	Sine-Aid	Decongestant
Pseudoephedrine/Chlorpheniramine	Novafed	Decongestant
	Novahistine	Decongestant

(continued)

TABLE 4.16. *(continued)*

Generic Name/Composition	Brand Name	Classification
Quazepam	Doral	CNS
Quinethazone	Hydromox	Diuretic
Quinidine	Quinaglute	Cardiac
Ranitidine	Zantac	Gastric
Reserpine	Serpasil	Cardiac
Reserpine/Chlorothiazide	Diupress	Cardiac
Reserpine/Hydralazine	Serpasil-Apresoline	Cardiac
Reserpine/Hydrochlorothiazide	Hydropres	Cardiac
Reserpine/Thiazide	Serpasil-Esidrex	Cardiac
Reserpine/Thiazide/Hydralazine	Ser-Ap-Es	Cardiac
Ritodrine	Yutopar	Obstetric
Salsalate	Disalcid	Antiinflammatory
Streptokinase	Kabikinase	Cardiac
	Streptase	Cardiac
Sulfinpyrazone	Anturane	NSAID
Sulindac	Clinoril	Antiinflammatory
Terbutaline	Brethaire	Pulmonary
	Brethine	Pulmonary
	Bricanyl	Pulmonary
Tetracycline	Achromycin	Antibiotic
Theophylline	Elixophyllin	Pulmonary
	Aerolate	Pulmonary
	Constant-T	Pulmonary
	Quibron	Pulmonary
	Respbid	Pulmonary
	Theo-dur	Pulmonary
	Theochron	Pulmonary
Ticarcillin	Ticar	Antibiotic
	Timentin	Antibiotic
Timolol	Blocadren	Cardiac
Tolazoline	Prescoline	Cardiac
Tolmetin	Tolectin	NSAID
Triamcinolone	Aristocort	Steroid
Triamterine/Hydroclorothiazide	Maxzide	Cardiac
Trimeprazine	Temaril	Dermatology
Trimethobenzamine	Tigan	Antiemetic
Tripelennamine	PBZ	Decongestant
	PBZ-SR	Decongestant
Valproic acid	Depakene	Psychiatric
	Depakote	Psychiatric
Verapamil	Isoptin	Cardiac
	Verelan	Cardiac
Vinblastine	Velban	Antineoplastic
Vincristine	Oncovin	Antineoplastic
Warfarin	Coumadin	Cardiac
	Dicumarol	Anticoagulant
	Panwarfin	Anticoagulant
Yohimbine	Actibine	CNS
	Yohimex	CNS

CNS, central nervous system; NSAID, nonsteroidal antiinflammatory drug.

(continued from page 75)

were adjusted to detect 100% aggregation and no aggregation. Quality control is achieved by determining the levels in a normal control individual each day. The aggregation procedure is performed by pipetting 450 µL of patient PRP into the glass siliconized cuvette, the cuvette placed into the testing chamber, and at the same time placing a cuvette with 500 µL of platelet-poor plasma (PPP) into the blank chamber. The cuvettes are allowed to incubate for 3 minutes at 37°C, and then 50 µL of one of the working solutions is added; this is repeated for all three working solutions of ADP and of EPI. The final (second) aggregation reagent concentrations for EPI are 11×10^{-6} *M*, 1.1×10^{-6} *M*, and 0.55×10^{-6} *M*, and for ADP, are 2.34×10^{-6} *M*, 1.17×10^{-6} *M*, and 0.58×10^{-6} *M*. The resul-

TABLE 4.17. NORMAL RANGES FOR STICKY PLATELET SYNDROME

Reagent	Normal Range (% aggregation)
EPI: 11×10^{-6} *M*	39%–80%
EPI: 1.1×10^{-6} *M*	15%–27%
EPI: 0.55×10^{-6} *M*	9%–20%
ADP: 2.34×10^{-6} *M*	7.5%–55%
ADP: 1.17×10^{-6} *M*	2%–36%
ADP: 0.58×10^{-6} *M*	0%–12%

EPI, epinephrine; ADP, adenosine diphosphate.

tant aggregation graphs are removed from the recorder and interpreted. The results are reported as percentage aggregation, with 100% being complete aggregation, and 0% being no aggregation. Normal ranges are depicted in Table 4.17. The procedure works equally well with the BioData aggregometer and PRP instead of whole blood. If a patient is referred while taking ASA, any drug known to contain ASA, or any drug known to be capable of cyclooxygenase inhibition, the study is delayed until the patient has been without the drug for a full 10 days before study. Interpretation is as follows: if the patient demonstrated only one hyperaggregable pattern to only one reagent, the interpretation was "suggestive, but not diagnostic of SPS," and repeated testing is performed. If a repeat demonstrates the same pattern, a diagnosis of SPS is made, and the patient treated. If a patient demonstrates hyperaggregable responses to at least two concentrations of one reagent or at least one hyperaggregable response to both reagents, a firm diagnosis of SPS may be made. Those demonstrating abnormalities to both EPI and ADP are classified as type I SPS, and those demonstrating hyperaggregable abnormalities to only EPI are classified as type II SPS. Although Mammen et al. (195) did not find patients demonstrating thrombosis and hyperaggregability to only ADP, this study did find several such patients and classified these as type III SPS. The classification system and criteria for diagnosis are depicted in Table 4.18. Treatment for all patients diagnosed with SPS initially consisted of low-dose ASA at 81 mg/day.

Of the 78 patients with DVT, 14.1% (11 patients) were found to have SPS as the cause of their thrombosis. Of 75 patients with arterial thrombotic events, 18.7% of those with coronary artery thrombosis had SPS, and SPS was found in 26.3% of those with cerebrovascular thrombosis, in 33.3% of those with TIAs, in 50.0% of those with retinal vascular thrombosis, and in 12% of those with peripheral arterial thrombosis. The results are summarized in Table 4.19. No correlation was noted between type of thrombosis (arterial vs. venous) and type of SPS (I, II, or III).

All patients were treated with ASA at 81 mg/day. Seven to 10 days after therapy was initiated, all patients were reassessed with SPS evaluation. In all but two patients, the SPS aggregation patterns normalized. In the two patients

TABLE 4.18. STICKY PLATELET SYNDROME: DIAGNOSTIC CRITERIA

Type I
 Hyperaggregability to both EPI and ADP
Type II
 Hyperaggregability to EPI only
Type III
 Hyperaggregability to ADP only
Suggestive diagnosis of SPS
 Hyperaggregability to only one concentration of only one reagent and history of thrombosis
 A firm diagnosis is made if repeated testing is again abnormal
Firm diagnosis of SPS
 (1) History of thrombosis and hyperaggregability to two concentrations of one reagent, or
 (2) History of thrombosis and hyperaggregability to one concentration of both reagents, or
 (3) History of thrombosis and hyperaggregability to only one concentration of one reagent and repeated testing demonstrates same/similar results

EPI, epinephrine; ADP, adenosine diphosphate; SPS, sticky platelet syndrome.

still demonstrating hyperaggregability to the SPS assay, one normalized with a larger dose of ASA (325 mg/day), and the other, after failing to normalize with ASA at 325 mg/day, normalized with ticlopidine. No patient had another thrombotic event or TIA while in the study.

Based on these results, it appears that SPS is a common cause of both arterial and venous events. A similar study was performed by Anderson et al. (198); this also was a prospective study wherein 195 patients with arterial, venous, or arterial plus venous thrombosis were assessed for hypercoagulability. SPS was the singular most common defect found, being detected in 28% of the entire population. The authors also concluded, as in the previous study, that SPS is a common inherited prothrombotic disorder leading to arterial and venous thrombosis. The association of SPS as a cause of young age cerebrovascular thrombosis also was recently noted by German investigators (199). Given that it appears that SPS accounts for about 14% of unexplained venous thrombotic events and between 12% (peripheral arterial thrombo-

TABLE 4.19. INCIDENCE OF SPS IN THROMBOSIS

Diagnosis	Percentage with SPS (%)
Deep vein thrombosis-PE	14.10
Cerebrovascular thrombosis	26.30
Transient cerebral ischemia (TIA)	33.30
Acute coronary thrombosis	18.70
Retinal vascular thrombosis	50.00
Peripheral artery thrombosis	12.00
Fetal wastage syndrome	16.20

SPS, sticky platelet syndrome; PE, pulmonary embolism.

sis) and 33% (TIAs) of arterial events, this hereditary platelet-function defect should be strongly suspected, and searched for, in any individual with an otherwise unexplained arterial or venous event. If one assumes, based on prevalence studies, that the congenital blood-coagulation protein defects, including antithrombin defects, protein S, protein C, and other rare defects account for about 20% of all venous events, and activated protein C (APC) resistance (factor V Leiden) accounts for another 20% of unexplained venous events, then with SPS (at 14%), it may be concluded that congenital defects account for about 50% to 60% of unexplained venous events. If it is then considered that antiphospholipid syndrome, based on prevalence studies, accounts for another 25% of venous events, it may reasonably be concluded that about 80% to 90% of venous events, and a somewhat lesser number of arterial events, can be defined as to cause. Because the treatment(s) for these disorders may differ and because about half are hereditary, it is important to define the presence of hereditary and acquired coagulation protein or platelet defects whenever possible. This leads to the inescapable conclusion that a diagnosis of thrombosis, like a diagnosis of anemia, is only a partial diagnosis, and the precise nature and cause must next be defined. In the case of SPS, warfarin or heparin therapy would not generally be indicated, and ASA appears to be the treatment of choice.

Large "bizarre" platelets are commonly seen in hypercoagulable patients and in patients undergoing frank clinical or subclinical thrombotic episodes. Large platelets represent the young and presumably hemostatically more active platelets (200,201). Therefore in individuals undergoing thrombotic disorders manifest as increased fibrin deposition with the entrapment of platelets, one would expect concomitant consumption of platelets, a rapid platelet turnover, and decreased platelet survival (203,204) and a greater than usual number of young platelets or large platelets, or hemostatically more active platelets, in the peripheral blood (200–202). Thus in a patient undergoing a thrombotic event, be it subclinical or an obvious thrombotic event, an increase in the percentage of young or large platelets in the peripheral smear is expected in the presence of a normal bone marrow and absence of hypersplenism (204,205). Platelet indices, including the platelet crit, the platelet distribution width (PDW) and MPV of platelets circulating in a patient may be of potential diagnostic benefit for assessing response to antiplatelet therapy in hypercoagulable or thrombosing patients. These parameters are now readily available on many automated platelet particle counters (206–208).

With the current trend of using antiplatelet agents as prophylaxis for thrombotic events, modalities to assess the efficacy of antiplatelet therapy are needed; platelet indices and platelet size distributions may give a reasonable clinical indication of response to antiplatelet therapy (209–211).

As platelets become activated, there is release of PF-4, β-thromboglobulin (β-TG), and thromboxane A_2, and as platelets are consumed, subsequent to activation, large young platelets are anticipated in the peripheral blood. Thus platelet activation is associated with elevated PF-4, β-TG, the degradation product of thromboxane A_2, thromboxane B_2, and an increase in MPV. These parameters, in varying combinations, have been assessed in a variety of prethrombotic and thrombotic conditions. Generally these parameters are elevated in DVT and PE (209,212) and in patients with unstable angina or acute myocardial infarction (213–217). Some studies also have shown these parameters to decrease during antithrombotic therapy. These molecular markers of platelet reactivity are commonly elevated in patients with a variety of peripheral arterial disease including acute myocardial infarction, cerebrovascular thrombosis, TIAs, diabetic microangiopathy, and in patients with atherosclerotic peripheral vascular disease (218–225).

Disorders associated with prethrombotic states often associated with arterial or venous thrombosis also are often noted to be accompanied by these elevated markers of platelet reactivity, including term delivery, preeclampsia, eclampsia, inflammatory bowel disease, early DIC, orthopedic surgery, and use of estrogens (226–230). These molecular markers of platelet reactivity, including PF-4, β-TG, thromboxane derivatives, and MPV, may be useful clinical indices of early thrombotic or thromboembolic events, and some studies have suggested that correction of these parameters is associated with effective antithrombotic therapy. Noting decreases in PF-4 levels or β-TG levels after the institution of antiplatelet therapy also may be indicative of clinical efficacy for stopping or blunting increased fibrin deposition (231–233). Some investigations, however, have failed to show decreases in PF-4 or β-TG levels in patients with arterial occlusive disease being treated with antiplatelet drugs (234).

Newer methods available to assess platelet hyperactivity and "consumption,"most of which are amenable to full automation, are summarized in Table 4.20 and consist of MPV and molecular markers of platelet reactivity, including CD markers by flow cytometry or similar methods. The diagnostic roles of these appear promising, but remain to be established.

The "Wein–Penzing" defect is characterized by a deficiency of the lipoxygenase metabolic pathway and con-

TABLE 4.20. EVALUATION OF PLATELET HYPERACTIVITY AND ANTIPLATELET THERAPY

Peripheral blood smear
Mean platelet volume (MPV)
Platelet distribution width (PDW)
Platelet crit
Platelet factor 4
β-Thromboglobulin
Thromboxane B_2
P-selectin
Flow cytometry

comitant compensatory increases in cyclooxygenase pathway products, including thromboxane, PGE_2, and PGD_2. Both patients reported had precocious myocardial infarction (192).

LABORATORY EVALUATION OF PLATELET DYSFUNCTION

The laboratory evaluation of platelet function is summarized in Table 4.21. The platelet count is fundamental to rule out thrombocytopenia in patients with petechiae and purpura, mucosal membrane bleeding, and other suggestive historic findings. The usual methods available to assess platelet function have been the standardized template bleeding time, the aggregating agents ADP, EPI, thrombin, collagen, ristocetin, and arachidonic acid, and lumi-aggregation, to study simultaneous platelet aggregation and ATP release (lumi-aggregation). Examination of the peripheral blood smear for platelet number and morphology is critical, as many clinical clues may be obtained from an evaluation of platelet morphology. A quantitative platelet count should always be done, as only with a normal platelet count can a platelet-function defect be defined. If a normal platelet count is documented with a suggestive history, the differential diagnosis is between a vascular defect and a platelet-function defect; both often cause prolongation of the standardized template bleeding time. A petechiometer may be used in children to avoid scar formation. Although the template bleeding time is useful as a simple screening test for platelet function, it is unreliable, and a normal template bleeding time does not rule out the presence of a clinically significant platelet-function defect. If the template bleeding time is normal, and a suggestive history is obtained or platelet dysfunction suspected on clinical grounds, platelet aggregation or lumi-aggregation should be done.

TABLE 4.21. LABORATORY EVALUATION OF PLATELET FUNCTION

Peripheral smear evaluation
Quantitative platelet count
Template bleeding time
Petechiometer test (children and elderly)
Platelet aggregation[a] to
Adenosine diphosphate
Epinephrine
Collagen
Ristocetin
Arachidonate
Thrombin
Platelet lumi-aggregation (release)[a]
Platelet antibodies (IgG and IgM)
Platelet membrane glycoproteins (flow cytometry)
Cyclooxygenase
Platelet factor 4[b]
β-Thromboglobulin[b]
Thromboxanes[b]
P-selectin
Flow cytometry

[a]Platelet-rich plasma (PRP) or whole blood.
[b]For hyperactive/prethrombotic platelets.
Ig, immunoglobulin.

The aggregometer is a standardized spectrophotometer; PRP is added to a spectrophotometric well, and various aggregating reagents are then added to the PRP (235–238). One aggregation agent at a time is studied. As platelets aggregate, increasing amounts of light are able to pass through the spectrophotometric chamber; the change in light density (percentage transmission) is then recorded on a strip recorder, giving rise to typical platelet-aggregation "patterns" (5,239). Figure 4.8 summarizes normal platelet-aggregation patterns as seen on a standardized platelet aggregometer. The usual aggregating agents used are ADP, EPI, ristocetin, collagen, and arachidonic acid. Serotonin, or 5-hydroxytryptamine, was commonly used formerly but appears now to be an uncommonly used platelet-aggregating reagent. EPI is usually used at two doses [a final concentration of 2.5×10^{-5} (high-dose "EPI") and a final concentration of 2.5×10^{-6} (low-dose EPI)]; similarly, ADP is characteristically used at two concentrations [2.0×10^{-5} (high dose ADP) and 2.5×10^{-6} (low-dose ADP)]; collagen is used at a final concentration of 0.19 mg/mL; ristocetin is used at a final concentration of 1.5 mg/mL; and arachidonic acid is most often used at a final concentration of 0.5 mg/mL. The patterns depicted in Fig. 4.8 are normal patterns elicited by the addition of each of these reagents, individually, to PRP in the aggregometer. It will be noted that a monophasic (all-or-none) curve is elicited with ADP (Fig. 4.8A); the top of the curve represents PRP, and the bottom of the curve represents PPP after aggregation has occurred. A biphasic curve is usually elicited with epinephrine (Fig. 4.8B). Ristocetin also usually induces a monophasic curve, with the change in light density going from the very top, PRP, to the very bottom, representing PPP (Fig. 4.8C). This also is true for arachidonic acid (Fig. 4.8E) (184). Collagen characteristically shows a lag-phase, which is seen in the bottom of Fig. 4.8 on the left corner, followed by complete aggregation to PPP (Fig. 4.8D). The slight curve seen with 5-hydroxytryptamine is a normal serotonin-induced platelet-aggregation curve (Fig. 4.8F).

A subsequent refinement of aggregation to assess platelet function is lumi-aggregation (240–244). The lumi-aggregometer has two wells, a photometric and a fluorometric well. The use of firefly luciferase (ATPase) in the fluorometric well allows the measurement of simultaneous ATP release and aggregation in the photometric well. The final concentrations of the aggregating agents are the same as described previously; the final concentration of luciferase (ATPase) used in the fluorometric well to assess the release reaction is 3.0 mg/mL. Figure 4.9 summarizes normal lumi-aggregation patterns generated by the aggregating reagents depicted. The aggregation curves are now read upside down

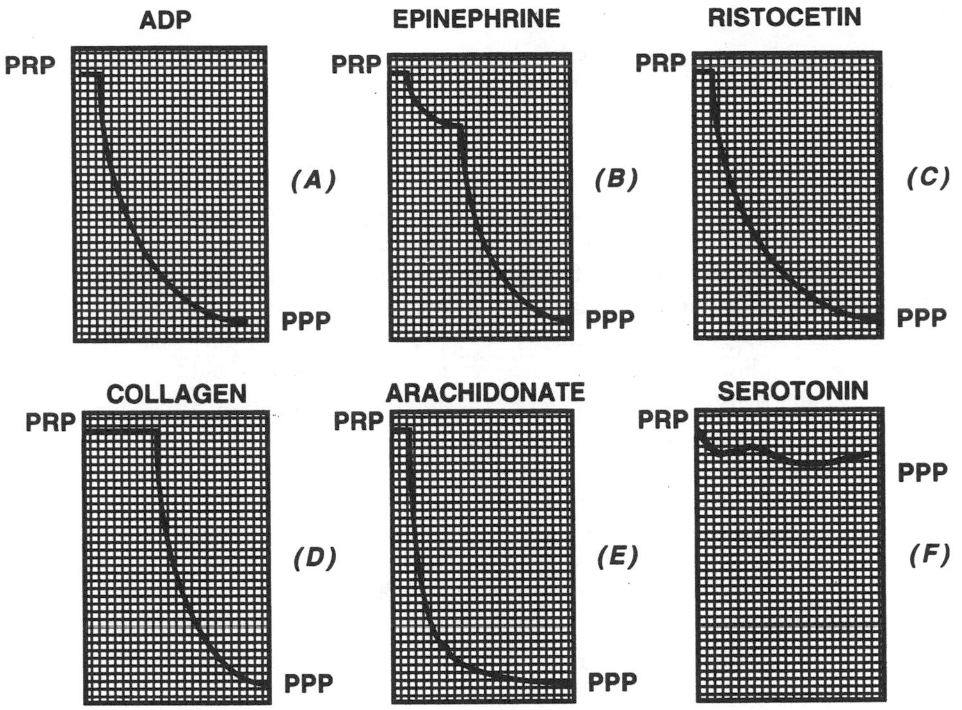

FIGURE 4.8. Normal platelet-aggregation patterns. *ADP*, adenosine diphosphate; *PRP*, platelet-rich plasma; *PPP*, platelet-poor plasma.

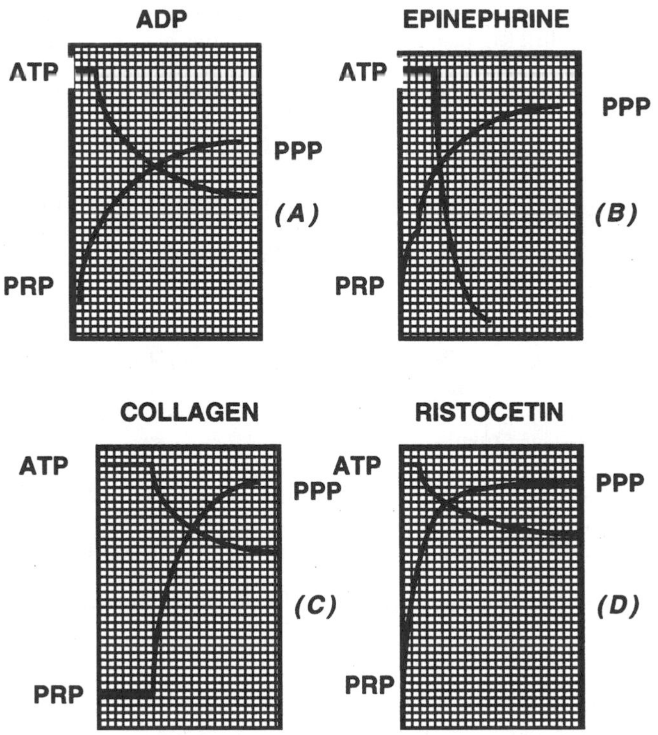

FIGURE 4.9. Normal platelet lumi-aggregation patterns. *ADP*, adenosine diphosphate; *ATP*, adenosine triphosphate; *PRP*, platelet-rich plasma; *PPP*, platelet-poor plasma.

as compared with the aggregation curves seen in Fig. 4.8. The aggregation pattern, for example, on the bottom of the top left box in Fig. 4.9E is the lag-phase characteristically seen with collagen, going from PRP on the bottom to PPP on the top; simultaneous ATP release is seen from top to bottom (Fig. 4.9C). The right upper box shows ATP release with epinephrine; the typical biphasic epinephrine curve goes from PRP on the bottom to PPP at the end of the curve (Fig. 9B). Ristocetin commonly causes only partial ATP release, usually about 35% (Fig. 9D) (245). On the bottom right of Fig. 4.9 is a normal lumi-aggregation pattern induced by ADP (Fig. 9A). Thus lumi-aggregation has added a significant new dimension to assessment of platelet function, allowing observation of simultaneous platelet-release reaction and platelet aggregation.

Another method of performing platelet aggregation is that of impedance (electrical resistance), which is a nonoptical method. Using this method, two metal probes are immersed into the platelet-containing sample, and electronic voltage is applied to the probe circuit, thus measuring the electrical resistance, or impedance, between the two immersed probe wires. During aggregation, a monolayer of platelets, forms on the exposed portions of the probe wires, resulting in a stable impedance value. This is a baseline and is assigned a value of 0 ohms resistance. After this, an aggregating agent is added, and stimulated platelets aggregate to the platelet monolayer on the wire probes, thus adding electrical resistance to the circuit. The changes in electrical resistance are measured and, therefore, quantified in ohms—the measurement of electrical resistance. The increase in the impedance is directly proportional to the platelet aggregate mass. It is thought that impedance aggregation to ristocetin is more sensitive to von Willebrand disease than is optical density, and thus potentially a better method for ristocetin cofactor (von Willebrand factor) activity. It also is thought that sensitivity may also be increased to antiaggregating agents (aggregation inhibitory medications), as compared with photometric or optical determinations. It also is likely that optical/impedance aggregation is more sensitive to hyperaggregable platelets; in addition, impedance aggregation is less likely to be influenced by lipemic blood and mild to moderate thrombocytopenia. Typical impedance lumi-aggregation patterns are similar to those seen with photometric (lumi)-aggregation patterns (246–252).

With the general availability of flow cytometry, many monoclonal antibodies to various platelet constituents have been developed and may be useful for assessing platelet dysfunction. Monoclonal antibodies are available for assessing both hypofunctional platelet function defects and "hyperactive" platelets. As previously discussed, the platelet membrane GPIIb/IIIa complex is defective in Glanzmann thrombasthenia; a monoclonal antibody: CD41/61 is available. In Bernard–Soulier syndrome, previously discussed, the defect(s) are in platelet membrane GPIIb, V, and IX; the monoclonal antibodies available to assess these are CD42b + CD42c/CD42a/CD32d. Platelet membrane GPIV may be assessed by CD36 (253–255). The absence or decrease of dense body material in storage pool disease may be assessed by CD63, and α-granule diseases (or release) can be assessed by CD62P, which is specific for P-selectin. Monoclonal antibodies, such as those for dense body constituents (CD63) or α-granule constituents (CD62P) also may be useful for assessing platelet activation in hyperaggregable states (256–258). Assessing platelet-release markers in hyperaggregable states may be useful in monitoring efficacy of therapy, but this remains to be determined. Several recent excellent reviews of this rapidly evolving topic are recommended (259,260), as, although the efficacy of using flow-cytometric analysis of platelet function for clinical diagnosis and treatment is still a new approach, additional experience, specific clinical situations, and future development may reveal this modality to be an excellent clinical and diagnostic tool.

SUMMARY

Platelet dysfunctions, especially acquired forms, are common causes of hemorrhage, especially in association with trauma and surgery. Although the hereditary platelet-function defects are generally quite rare, hereditary storage pool disease is common enough to be suspected in an individual, usually a child, with characteristic historic and clinical findings. The acquired platelet-function defects, especially those resulting from drugs, are very common and should promptly be suspected in patients with easy and spontaneous bruising, mild to moderate mucosal membrane hemorrhage, or unexplained bleeding associated with trauma or surgery. The template bleeding time is generally useful as a screening test of platelet function, but a normal template bleeding time, with a suggestive history, suggestive clinical findings, or in the patient frankly bleeding, is not reliable, and platelet aggregation or lumi-aggregation should be done in appropriate clinical situations. The mainstay of therapy for essentially all these defects, if bleeding is significant, is the liberal infusion of appropriate numbers of platelet concentrates. The acquired platelet-function defects, of course, also should be managed by attempts to treat and/or control the underlying disease, if possible, and offending drugs or potentially offending drugs should promptly be discontinued. Antiplatelet agents are the therapy of choice for clinical thrombosis seen in platelet hyperaggregability syndromes.

REFERENCES

1. Bick RL. Clinical evaluation of the patient with hemorrhage. In: Bick RL, Bennett J, Brynes R, et al., eds. *Hematology: clinical and laboratory practice.* St. Louis: Mosby, 1993:1317.
2. Bick RL. Assessment of patients with hemorrhage. In: *Disorders of thrombosis and hemostasis.* Chicago: ASCP Press, 1992:7.
3. Bick RL. Hereditary and acquired vascular bleeding disorders. In: Bick RL, Bennett J, Byrnes R, eds. *Hematology: clinical and laboratory practice.* St. Louis: Mosby, 1993:1325.
4. Kitchens CS. The purpuric disorders. *Semin Thromb Hemost* 1984;10:173.
5. Bick RL. Platelet function defects. *Semin Thromb Hemost* 1992; 18:167–185.
6. Hirsh J. Laboratory diagnosis of thrombosis. In: Colman RW, Hirsh J, Marder VJ, et al., eds. *Hemostasis and thrombosis: basic principles and clinical practice.* Philadelphia: JB Lippincott, 1982:789.
7. Meyer D, Zimmerman TS. von Willebrand's disease. In: Coleman RW, Hirsh J, Marder VJ, et al., eds. *Hemostasis and thrombosis: basic principles and clinical practice.* Philadelphia: JB Lippincott, 1982:64.
8. Mieschner PA, Graf J. Drug-induced thrombocytopenia. *Clin Haematol* 1980;9:505.
9. Bick RL, Adams T, Schmalhorst WL. Bleeding times, platelet adhesion, and aspirin. *Am J Clin Pathol* 1976;65:65.
10. Mielke CH, Kaneshiro MM, Maer LA. The standardized normal ivy bleeding time and its prolongation by aspirin. *Blood* 1969;34:204.
11. Bick RL. Vascular bleeding disorders. In: *Disorders of thrombosis and homeostasis.* Chicago: ASCP Press, 1992:5.
12. Rodgers RP, Levin J. A critical reappraisal of the bleeding time. *Semin Thromb Hemost* 1990;16:1.
13. Sienco. *The petechiometer.* Package insert. Morrison, Colo: Sienco Inc, 1980:1.
14. Lusher JM, Barnhart MI. Congenital disorders affecting platelets. *Semin Thromb Hemost* 1977;4:123.
15. Bernard J, Soulier JP. Sur une nouvelle variete dystrophic

thrombocytaire hemorrhagipase congenitale. *Semin Hopitaux Paris* 1948;24:3217.

16. White JG. Inherited abnormalities of the platelet membrane and secretory granules. *Hum Pathol* 1987;18:123.
17. Bithel TC, Parokh SJ, Strong RR. Platelet function in the Bernard-Soulier syndrome. *Ann N Y Acad Sci* 1972;201:145.
18. Howard MA, Hutton RA, Hardisty RM. Hereditary giant platelet syndrome: a new disorder of platelet function. *Br Med J* 1973;2:586.
19. Bick RL. Hereditary coagulation protein defects. In: *Disorders of thrombosis and hemostasis.* Chicago: ASCP Press, 1992:6.
20. Glanzmann E. Hereditare hamorrhagische thrombasthenic. *Beitr Pathol Blutplatt Jahrb Kinderheilkd* 1918;88:1.
21. Fonio A, Schwendener J. *Die thrombocyten des menschlichen clutes.* Bern: Huber, 1942.
22. Inceman S, Tangun V. Essential athrombia. *Thromb Diath Haemorrh* 1975;33:278.
23. Cronberg S, Nilsson IM. Investigators in a family with thrombasthenia of moderately severe type with 16 affected family members. *Scand J Haematol* 1968;5:17.
24. Caen JP, Castaldi PA, Leclerc JC. Congenital bleeding disorders with long bleeding time and normal platelet count, I: Glanzmann's thrombasthenia (report of 15 patients). *Am J Med* 1966; 41:4.
25. Caen JP. Glanzmann's thrombasthenia. *Clin Haematol* 1972;1: 383.
26. Bick R, Murano L. Physiology of hemostasis. *Clin Lab Med* 1994;14:677.
27. Holmawn H, Weiss WH. Further evidence for a deficient storage pool of adenine nucleotides in platelets from some patients with thrombocytopathia: "storage pool disease." *Blood* 1972;39:197.
28. Pareti FI, Mannucci L, Capitanio L, et al. Heterogeneity of storage pool deficiency. *Thromb Haemost* 1977;38:3.
29. Grottum KA, Hovig T, Holmsen H, et al. Wiskott-Aldrich syndrome: qualitative platelet defects and short platelet survival. *Br J Haematol* 1969;17:373.
30. Day HJ, Holmsen H. Platelet adenine nucleotide "storage pool deficiency" in thrombocytopenic absent radii syndrome. *JAMA* 1972;221:1053.
31. Rendu F, Breton-Gorius J, Trutlnan G, et al. Studies on a new variant of the Hermansky-Pudlak syndrome: qualitative ultrastructural bodies associated with a phospholipase A defect. *Am J Hematol* 1978;4:387.
32. Buchanon GR, Handin RI. Platelet function in the Chediak-Higashi syndrome. *Blood* 1976;47:941.
33. Weiss HJ. Pathophysiology and detection of clinically significant platelet dysfunction. In: Baldini MG, Ebbe S, eds. *Platelets: production, function, transfusion, and storage.* New York: Grune & Stratton, 1974:253.
34. Weiss HJ, Lages BA, Witte LD, et al. Storage pool disease: evidence for clinical and biochemical heterogeneity. *Thromb Haemost* 1977;38:3.
35. Minkes MS, Joist JN, Needleham P. Arachidonic acid-induced platelet aggregation independent of ADP-release in a patient with a bleeding disorder due to platelet storage pool disease. *Thromb Res* 1979;15:169.
36. Weiss HJ. Platelet aggregation, adhesion, and adenosine diphosphate release in thrombopathia (platelet factor-3 deficiency): a comparison with Glanzmann's thrombasthenia and von Willebrand's disease. *Am J Med* 1967;43:570.
37. Stuart MJ. Inherited defects of platelet function. *Semin Hematol* 1975;12:233.
38. Arkel YS. Evaluation of platelet aggregation in disorders of hemostasis. *Med Clin North Am* 1976;60:881.
39. Weiss HJ, Ames RP. Ultrastructural findings in storage pool disease and aspirin-like defects of platelets. *Am J Pathol* 1973;71:447.
40. Adashi E, Farber M, Mitchell GW. Congenital release thrombocytopathy, pathophysiology and management. *Obstet Gynecol* 1976;48:403.
41. Scheck R, Rasche H, Queiber W, et al. Platelet dysfunction as a result of inhibition of a release (aspirin-like defect) in two identical twins. *Dtsch Med Wochenschr* 1975;100:1842.
42. Weiss HJ, Rogers J. Thrombocytopathia due to abnormalities in platelet release reaction: studies on six unrelated patients. *Blood* 1972;39:187.
43. Malmsten C, Hamberg M, Svensson J, et al. Physiological role of an endoperoxide in human platelets: hemostatic defect due to platelet cyclo-oxygenase deficiency. *Proc Natl Acad Sci U S A* 1975;72:1446.
44. Horellou MH, LeCompte T, LeCruber C, et al. Familial and constitutional bleeding disorder due to platelet cyclo-oxygenase deficiency. *Am J Hematol* 1983;14:1.
45. Lagard M, Byron PA, Vargaftig BB, et al. Impairment of platelet thromboxane A_2 generation and of the platelet release reaction in two patients with congenital deficiency of platelet cyclo-oxygenase. *Br J Haematol* 1978;38:251.
46. Zucker S, Mielke H, Durocher JR, et al. Oozing and bruising due to abnormal platelet function. *Ann Intern Med* 1971;76:725.
47. Lages B, Weiss HJ. Impairment of phosphatidylinositol metabolism in a patient with a bleeding disorder associated with defects of the initial platelet response. *Thromb Haemost* 1988; 59:175.
48. Rabiner SF. Uremic bleeding. *Prog Hemost Thromb* 1972;1:233.
49. Schetz MRC. Coagulation disorders in acute renal failure. *Kidney Int* 1998;53(suppl 66):96.
50. Saito H. Alterations of hemostasis in renal disease. In: Ratnoff OD, Forbes CD, eds. *Disorders of hemostasis.* 3rd ed. Philadelphia: WB Saunders, 1996:43.
51. Horowitz HI, Cohen DB, Martinez P, et al. Defective ADP-induced platelet factor 3 activation in uremia. *Blood* 1967;30: 331.
52. Horowitz HI, Stein IM, Cohen BD, et al. Further studies on the platelet-inhibiting effect of guanidino-succinic acid and its role in uremic bleeding. *Am J Med* 1970;49:339.
53. Rabiner SF, Molinas F. The role of phenol and phenolic acids on the thrombocytopathy and defective platelet aggregation of patients with renal failure. *Am J Med* 1970;49:346.
54. Evans EP, Jones GR, Bloom AL. Abnormal breakdown of adenosine diphosphate in uraemic plasma and its possible relationship to defective platelet aggregation. *Thromb Res* 1972;1:323.
55. Schondorf TH, Hey D. Platelet function tests in uraemia and under acetylsalicylic acid administration. *Haemostasis* 1974;3: 129.
56. Remuzzi G, Livio M, Cavenagh AE, et al. Unbalanced prostaglandin synthesis and plasma factors in uraemic bleeding: a hypothesis. *Thromb Res* 1978;13:531.
57. Kamoun P, Kleinknecht D, Duerot H, et al. Platelet-serotonin in uraemia. *Lancet* 1970;1:782.
58. Remuzil G, Cavenaghe AE, Mecca G, et al. Prostacyclin (PGI_2) and bleeding time in uremic patients. *Thromb Res* 1977;11:919.
59. Albertazzi A, Spisni C, Palmieri PF. Nucleotide deficit and functional platelet alterations in patients on regular dialysis treatment. *Life Support Syst* 1985;3:77.
60. Ware JA, Clark BA, Smith M. Abnormalities of cytoplasmic Ca++ in platelets from patients with uremia. *Blood* 1989;73: 172.
61. Escolar G, Casa A, Bastidi E. Uremic platelets have a functional defect affecting the interaction of von Willebrand factor with glycoprotein IIb-IIIa. *Blood* 1990;76:1336.
62. Komarnicki M, Twardowski T. Platelet glycoprotein concentrations in patients with chronic uraemia. *Folia Haematol* 1987; 114:642.

63. Jubelirer SJ. Hemostatic abnormalities in renal disease. *Am J Kidney Dis* 1985;5:219.
64. Rydzewski A, Rowinski M, Mysiwiec M. Shortening of bleeding time after intranasal administration of 1-deamino-8-arginine vasopressin to patients with chronic uremia. *Folia Haematol* 1986;113:823.
65. Mannucci PM. Desmopressin (DDAVP) for treatment of disorders of hemostasis. *Prog Hemost Thromb* 1986;8:19.
66. Gotti E, Mecca G, Valentino C, et al. Renal biopsy in patients with acute renal failure and prolonged bleeding time: a preliminary report. *Am J Kidney Dis* 1985;6:397.
67. Livio M, Mannucci P, Vigano G, et al. Conjugated estrogens for the management of bleeding associated with renal failure. *N Engl J Med* 1986;315:731.
68. Vigano GL, Mannucci PM, Lattuada A. Subcutaneous desmopressin (DDAVP) shortens the bleeding time in uremia. *Am J Hematol* 1989;31:32.
69. Rydzewski A, Rowinski M, Mysliwiec M. Shortening of bleeding time after intranasal administration of 1-deamino-8-D-arginine vasopressin to patients with chronic uremia. *Folia Haematol* 1986;113:823.
70. Vigano G, Gaspari F, Locatelli M. Dose-effect and pharmacokinetics of estrogens given to correct bleeding time in uremia. *Kidney Int* 1988;34:853.
71. Harker LA. Acquired disorders of platelet function. *Ann N Y Acad Sci* 1987;509:188.
72. Carvalho AC. Acquired platelet dysfunction in patients with uremia. *Hematol Oncol Clin North Am* 1990;4:129.
73. Gordge MP, Faint RW, Rylance PB. Platelet function and the bleeding time in progressive renal failure. *Thromb Haemost* 1988; 60:83.
74. Lindsay RM, Moorthy AV, Koens F. Platelet function in dialyzed and non-dialyzed patients with chronic renal failure. *Clin Nephrol* 1975;4:52.
75. Bick RL. Clinical aspects of acquired circulating anticoagulants. In: Bick RL, Bennett J, Brynes R, et al., eds. *Hematology: clinical and laboratory practice.* St. Louis: Mosby, 1993:1533.
76. Bick RL, Strauss JF, Rutherford CJ, et al. Thrombosis and hemorrhage in oncology patients. *Hematol Oncol Clin North Am* 1996;10:875.
77. Frenkel UP, Bick RL. Issues of thrombosis and hemorrhagic events in patients with cancer. *Anticancer Res* 1998;18:1–4.
78. Lachner H. Hemostatic abnormalities associated with dysproteinemias. *Semin Hematol* 1973;10:125.
79. Lisiewicz J. Plasma cell myeloma. In: *Hemorrhage in leukemias.* Warsaw: Polish Medical Publishers, 1976:153.
80. Adams TL, Schultz L, Goldberg L. Platelet function abnormalities in myeloproliferative disorders. *Scand J Haematol* 1974;13:215.
81. Tangun Y. Platelet aggregation and platelet factor 3 activity in myeloproliferative syndromes. *Thromb Diath Haemorrh* 1971; 25:241.
82. Bick RL. Alterations of hemostasis in malignancy. In: Bick RL, Bennett J, Byrnes R, eds. *Hematology: clinical and laboratory practice.* St. Louis: Mosby, 1993:1583.
83. Frenkel EP, Bick RL. Prothrombin G202010A gene mutation: heparin cofactor II defects, primary (essential) thrombocythemia and thrombohemorrhagic manifestations. *Semin Thromb Hemost* 1999;25:375–386.
84. Lovenberg E, Nilsson TK. Qualitative platelet defects in chronic myeloproliferative disorders: evidence for reduced ATP secretion. *Eur J Haematol* 1989;43:435.
85. Raman BK, Van-Slyck EJ, Riddle J. Platelet function and structure in myeloproliferative disease, myelodysplastic syndrome, and secondary thrombocytosis. *Am J Clin Pathol* 1989;91:647.
86. Pfliegler G, Boda Z, Udvardy M. Platelet function studies in myeloproliferative disorders. *Folia Haematol* 1986;113:655.
87. Bick RL. Pathology of hemostasis in cardiac surgery and cardiovascular prosthetic devices. In: Piffare R, ed. *Anticoagulants in cardiac medicine.* Philadelphia: Belfus Press, 1996:551.
88. Bick RL. Hemostasis defects in cardiac surgery and use of cardiac devices. In: Piffare R, ed. *Cardiac surgery: principles and practice.* Philadelphia: Belfus Press, 1999.
89. Bick RL, Schmalhorst WR, Arbegast NR. Alterations of hemostasis associated with cardiopulmonary bypass. *Thromb Res* 1976;8:285.
90. Bick RL. Alterations of hemostasis associated with cardiac surgery, prosthetic devices and transplantation. In: Ratnoff OD, Forbes CD, eds. *Disorders of hemostasis.* Philadelphia: WB Saunders, 1991:2
91. Harker LA, Malpass TW, Bronson NE. Mechanisms of abnormal bleeding in patients undergoing cardiopulmonary bypass: acquired transient platelet dysfunction associated with selective alpha-granule release. *Blood* 1980;56:824.
92. Bick RL. Physiology and pathophysiology of coagulation during heart surgery. In: Piffare R, ed. *Cardiac surgery: state of the art.* St. Louis: CV Mosby, 1993.
93. Mammen EF. Coagulopathies of liver disease. *Clin Lab Med* 1994;14:769.
94. Bick RL. Syndromes associated with hyperfibrino(geno)lysis. In: *Disseminated intravascular coagulation and related syndromes.* Boca Raton, Fla: CRC Press, 1983:105.
95. Bick RL. The clinical significance of fibrinogen degradation products. *Semin Thromb Hemost* 1982;8:302.
96. Ratnoff OD. Hemostatic defects in liver and biliary tract disease and disorders of vitamin K metabolism. In: Ratnoff OD, Forbes CD, eds. *Disorders of hemostasis.* Philadelphia: WB Saunders, 1991:459.
97. Ashud MA. Platelet size and number in alcoholic thrombocytopenia. *N Engl J Med* 1972;286:355.
98. Cowan DH. Effect of alcoholism on hemostasis. *Semin Hematol* 1980;17:137.
99. Cowan DH, Graham RC Jr. Studies on the platelet defect in alcoholism. *Thromb Diath Haemorrh* 1975;33:310.
100. Thomas DP, Ream VJ, Stuart RK. Platelet aggregation patients with cirrhosis of the liver. *N Engl J Med* 1967;276:1344.
101. Cowan DH, Kikta M, Baunach D. Alteration of platelet cyclic AMP (cAMP) by ethanol. *Thromb Haemost* 1977;38:270.
102. Brown JB. Platelet MAO and alcoholism. *Am J Psychiatry* 1977;134:206.
103. Major LF, Murphy DL. Platelet and plasma amine oxidase activity in alcoholic individuals. *Br J Psychiatry* 1978;132:548.
104. Cowan DH, Shook P. Effects of ethanol on platelet serotonin metabolism. *Thromb Haemost* 1977;38:33.
105. Jandl JH, Lear AA. The metabolism of folic acid in cirrhosis. *Ann Intern Med* 1956;45:1027.
106. Owen CA, Rettke SR, Bowie EJW. Hemostatic evaluation of patients undergoing liver transplantation. *Mayo Clin Proc* 1987; 62:761.
107. Cramer SC, Schiller CS. Platelet function in liver disease. *N Engl J Med* 1991;324:1670.
108. Mannucci PM, Vicente V, Vianello L. Controlled trial of desmopressin in liver cirrhosis and other conditions associated with a prolonged bleeding time. *Blood* 1986;67:1148.
109. Rao AK, Walsh PN. Acquired qualitative platelet disorders. *Clin Haematol* 1983;12:201.
110. Zahavi J. Acquired "storage pool disease" of platelets. *Thromb Haemost* 1976;35:501.
111. Bick RL. Laboratory evaluation of platelet dysfunction. *Clin Lab Med* 1995;15:1.
112. Parquet-Gernez A, Mazurier C, Goudemand J. Acquired thrombasthenia induced by platelet autoantibodies. *Thromb Haemost* 1991;65:1104.

113. Bick RL. Primary fibrino(geno)lytic syndromes. In: Murano G, Bick RL, eds. *Basic concepts of hemostasis and thrombosis.* Boca Raton, Fla: CRC Press, 1980:181.
114. Kowalski E. Fibrinogen derivatives and their biological activities. *Semin Hematol* 1968;5:45.
115. Bick RL, Arun B, Frenkel EP. Disseminated intravascular coagulation: clinical and pathophysiological mechanisms and manifestations. *Haemostasis* 1999;29:111–134.
116. Bick RL, Kunkel L. Disseminated intravascular coagulation syndromes. *Int J Haematol* 1992;55:1–26.
117. Bick RL. Disseminated intravascular coagulation: objective criteria for diagnosis and management. *Med Clin North Am* 1994; 70:511–544.
118. Levine PH. A qualitative platelet defect in severe vitamin B_{12} deficiency: response, hyper-response, and thrombosis after vitamin B_{12} therapy. *Ann Intern Med* 1973;78:533.
119. Ingeberg S, Stofferson E. Platelet dysfunction in patients with vitamin B_{12} deficiency. *Acta Haematol* 1979;61:75.
120. Bick RL. Platelet function defects. *Biomed Prog* 1999;12:41.
121. Weiss HJ. Antiplatelet drugs: pharmacological aspects. In: *Platelets: pathophysiology and antiplatelet drug therapy.* New York: Alan R. Liss, 1982:45.
122. Triplett DA. Appendix C: miscellaneous lists and forms. In: Triplett DA, ed. *Platelet function evaluation: laboratory evaluation and clinical application.* Chicago: ASCP Press, 1978:291.
123. Mills DCB, Robb IA, Roberts GCK. The release of nucleotides, 5-hydroxytryptamine and enzymes from blood platelets during aggregation. *J Physiol* 1968;195:715.
124. Rysanek R, Suehla C, Spankova H, et al. The effect of tricyclic antidepressive drugs on adrenaline and adenosine diphosphate induced platelet aggregation. *J Pharm Pharmacol* 1966;18:616.
125. Weiss HJ. Pharmacology of platelet inhibition. *Prog Hemost Thromb* 1972;1:199.
126. Mills DCB, Roberts GCK. Membrane active drugs and the aggregation of human blood platelets. *Nature* 1967;213:35.
127. Stacy RS. Uptake of 5-hydroxytryptamine by platelets. *Br J Pharmacol* 1961;16:284.
128. O'Brien JR. Platelet aggregation, Part 1: some effects of the adenosine phosphates, thrombin and cocaine upon platelet adhesiveness. *J Clin Pathol* 1962;15:446.
129. O'Brien JR. Some effects of adrenaline and anti-adrenaline compounds on platelets in vitro and in vivo. *Nature* 1973;200: 763.
130. Weksler BB, Gillik M, Pink J. Effect of propanolol on platelet function. *Blood* 1977;49:185.
131. Natelson EA, Brown CH, Bradshaw MW. Influence of cephalosporin antibiotics on blood coagulation and platelet function. *Antimicrob Agents Chemother* 1976;9:91.
132. Cazenave JP, Guccione MA, Packham MA, et al. Effects of cephalothin and penicillin G on platelet function in vitro. *Br J Haematol* 1977;35:135.
133. Brown CH, Natelson EA, Bradshaw MW, et al. The hemostatic defect produced by carbenicillin. *N Engl J Med* 1974;291:265.
134. Brown CN, Bradshaw MW, Natelson EA, et al. Defective platelet function following the administration of penicillin compounds. *Blood* 1976;47:949.
135. O'Brien JRL. The adhesiveness of native platelets and its prevention. *J Clin Pathol* 1961;14:140.
136. Seeman PM. Membrane stabilization of drugs: tranquilizers, steroids, and anesthetics. *Int Rev Neurobiol* 1966;9:145.
137. Bygdeman S, Johnson I. Studies on the effect of adrenergic blocking agents on catecholamine-induced platelet aggregation and uptake of noradrenaline and 5-hydroxytryptamine. *Acta Physiol Scand* 1969;75:129.
138. Born GVR, Bricknell J. The uptake of 5-hydroxytryptamine by blood platelets in the cold. J Physiol 1959;147:153.
139. Mills DCB, Roberts GCK. Effects of adrenaline on human blood platelets. *J Physiol* 1967;193:443.
140. White JG, Raynor ST. The effects of trifluoroperazine, an inhibitor of calmodulin on platelet function. *Thromb Res* 1980; 18:279.
141. Anderson ER, Foulkes JG, Godin DV. The effect of local anaesthetics and antiarrhythmic agents on the responses of rabbit platelets to ADP and thrombin. *Thromb Haemost* 1981;45:81.
142. Rossie EC, Levin NW. Inhibition of primary ADP-induced platelet aggregation in normal subjects after administration of nitrofurantoin (Furadantin). *Clin Invest* 1973;52:2457.
143. Alexander DP, Russo ME, Gohram DE, et al. Nafcillin-induced platelet dysfunction and bleeding. *Antimicrob Agents Chemother* 1983;23:59.
144. Bang NU, Tessler SS, Heidenreich RO, et al. Effects of moxalactam on blood coagulation and platelet function. *Rev Infect Dis* 1982;4:546.
145. Brown CN, Natelson EA, Bradshaw MW. A study of the effects of ticarcillin on blood coagulation and platelet function. *Antimicrob Agents Chemother* 1975;7:652.
146. Ewald RA, Eichelberger JW, Young AA, et al. The effect of dextran on platelet factor 3. *Transfusion* 1965;5:109.
147. Gollub S, Shafer C, Squitieri A. The bleeding tendency associated with plasma expanders. *Surg Gynecol Obstet* 1967;124:1203.
148. Cohen LS. The pharmacology of acetylsalic acid. *Semin Thromb Hemost* 1976;2:146.
149. Kocsis JJ, Hernadovich J, Silver MJ, et al. Duration of inhibition of platelet prostaglandin formation and aggregation by ingested aspirin or indomethacin. *Prostaglandins* 1973;3:141.
150. Zucker MB, Peterson J. Effect of acetylsalicylic acid, other nonsteroidal anti-inflammatory agents, and dipyridamole on human blood platelets. *J Lab Clin Med* 1970;76:66.
151. Nishizawa EE, Wynalda DJ. Inhibitory effect of ibuprofen (Motrin) on platelet function. *Thromb Res* 1981;21:347.
152. Wiley JS, Chesterman CN, Morgan FJ, et al. The effect of sulfinpyrazone on the aggregation and release reactions of human platelets. *Thromb Res* 1979;14:23.
153. Rossie EC, Levin NW. Inhibition of ADP-induced platelet aggregation by furosemide. *J Lab Clin Med* 1973;81:140.
154. Addonizio VP, Fisher CA, Strauss JF, et al. Inhibition of human platelet function by verapamil. *Thromb Res* 1982;28:545.
155. Burns TS, Saunders RN. Antiplatelet activity of hydralazine. *Thromb Res* 1979;16:837.
156. Winocour PD, Kinlough-Rathbone RL, Mustard JF. The effect of the phospholipase inhibitor mepacrine on platelet release reaction, and fibrinogen binding to the platelet surface. *Thromb Haemost* 1981;45:257.
157. O'Brien JR. Effect of anti-inflammatory agents on platelets. *Lancet* 1968;1:894.
158. Steiner M, Anastasi J. Vitamin E: an inhibitor of the platelet release reaction. *J Clin Invest* 1976;57:732.
159. Glass F, Lippon H, Kadowitz PJ. Effects of methyl-prednisolone and hydrocortisone on aggregation of rabbit platelets induced by arachidonic acid and other aggregating substances. *Thromb Haemost* 1981;46:676.
160. Pierce CH, Oshiro G, Nickerson M. Effect of methyl-prednisone sodium succinate (MP) on platelet aggregation. *Circulation* 1974;49(suppl 111):289.
161. Neild GH, Rocchi G, Imberti L, et al. Effect of cyclosporin A on prostacyclin synthesis by vascular tree. *Thromb Res* 1983;32:373.
162. Michel H, Caen JP, Born GVR. Relation between the inhibition of aggregation and the concentration of cAMP in human and rat platelets. *Br J Haematol* 1976;33:27.
163. Rajah SM, Crow MJ, Perry AF, et al. The effects of dipyridamole on platelet function: correlation with blood levels in man. *Br J Clin Pharmacol* 1979;4:129.

164. Ardlie NG, Glew G, Shultz BG, et al. Inhibition and reversal of platelet aggregation by methylxanthines. *Thromb Diath Haemorrh* 1968;18:670.
165. Wolf SM, Shulman NR. Inhibition of platelet energy production and release reaction by PGE_1, theophylline and cAMP. *Biochem Biophys Res Commun* 1970;41:128.
166. Ball G, Brereton GG, Fulwood M, et al. Effect of prostaglandin E, alone and in combination with theophylline or aspirin on collagen-induced platelet aggregation and on platelet nucleotides including adenosine 3′:5′-cyclic monophosphate. *Biochem J* 1970;120:709.
167. White JG. Effects of colchicine and vinca alkaloids on human platelets, I: influence on platelet microtubules and contractile function. *Am J Pathol* 1968;53:281.
168. Soppitt GD, Mitchell JRA. The effect of colchicine on human platelet behavior. *J Atheroscler Res* 1969;10:247.
169. Zieve PD, Solomon HM. Effects of diuretics on the human platelet. *Am J Physiol* 1968;215:650.
170. Murer EH, Siojo E. Inhibition of thrombin-induced secretion from platelets by chlortetracycline and its analogs. *Thromb Haemost* 1982;47:62.
171. Carter AE, Eban R, Perrett RD. Prevention of post-operative deep venous thrombosis and pulmonary embolism. *Br Med* 1971;1:312.
172. Spooner M, Meyers OO. The effect of dicumerol (3.3-methylenebis) (4-hydroxy-coumarin) on platelet adhesiveness. *Am J Physiol* 1944;142:279.
173. Saxon A, Kattlove H. Platelet inhibition by sodium nitroprusside, a smooth muscle inhibitor. *Blood* 1976;47:957.
174. Rattazzi L, Haimov MN. Role of the platelet in the obliterative vascular transplant rejection phenomenon. *Surg Forum* 1970; 21:243.
175. Silverman JL, Wurzel HA. The effect of glycerol guaiacolate on platelet function and other coagulation factors in vivo. *Am J Clin Pathol* 1969;51:35.
176. O'Brien JR, Shoobridge SM, Finch WJ. Comparison of the effect of heparin and citrate on platelet aggregation. *J Clin Pathol* 1969;22:28.
177. Salzman EW, Rosenberg RD, Smith HJ, et al. Effect of heparin and heparin fractions on platelet aggregation. *J Clin Invest* 1980;65:621.
178. Zucker MB. Effect of heparin on platelet function. *Thromb Diath Haemorrh* 1975;33:63.
179. Wessler S, Gitel SN. Heparin: new concepts relevant to clinical use. *Blood* 1979;53:525.
180. Schafer AJ, Alexander RW, Handin RT. Inhibition of platelet function by organic nitrate vasodilators. *Blood* 1980;55:649.
181. Amezcua JL, Parsons M, Moncada S. Unstable metabolites of arachidonic acid, aspirin and the formation of the haemostatic plug. *Thromb Res* 1978;13:477.
182. Altman R, Scaziotta A, Funes JC. Why single daily dose of aspirin may not prevent platelet aggregation. *Thromb Res* 1988; 51:259.
183. Weksler BB, Pett SB, Alnoso D, et al. Inhibition by aspirin of vascular and platelet prostaglandin synthesis in atherosclerotic patients. *N Engl J Med* 1983;308:800.
184. Patrignani P, Filabozzi P, Patrono C. Selective cumulative inhibition of platelet thromboxane production by low-dose aspirin in healthy subjects. *J Clin Invest* 1982;69:1366.
185. Preston FE, Greaves M, Jackson CA. Cumulative inhibitory effect of daily 40 mg aspirin on prostacyclin synthesis. *Lancet* 1981;1:1211.
186. Yamauchi K, Furui H, Taniguchi N. Effects of diltiazem hydrochloride on cardiovascular response, platelet aggregation, and coagulation activity during exercise testing in systemic hypertension. *Am J Cardiol* 1986;57:609.
187. Hines R, Barash PG. Infusion of sodium nitroprusside induces platelet dysfunction in vitro. *Anesthesiology* 1989;70:611.
188. Hines R. Preservation of platelet function during trimethaphan infusion. *Anesthesiology* 1990;72:834.
189. Bick RL, Fekete LF. Cardiopulmonary bypass hemorrhage: aggravation by pre-op ingestion of antiplatelet agents. *Vasc Surg* 1979;13:277.
190. Leist ER, Banwell JG. Products containing aspirin. *N Engl J Med* 1974;291:710.
191. Selner JC. More aspirin-containing drugs. *N Engl J Med* 1975; 292:372.
192. Sinzinger H, Kaliman J, O'Grady J. Platelet lipoxygenase defect (Wien-Penzing defect) in two patients with myocardial infarction. *Am J Hematol* 1991;36:202.
193. Holliday PL, Mammen E, Gilroy J. Sticky platelet syndrome and cerebral infarction in young adults. In: *9th International Joint Conference on Stroke and Cerebral Circulation.* Phoenix: 1983(abst).
194. Rubenfire M, Blevins RD, Barnhart MI, et al. Platelet hyperaggregability in patients with chest pain and angiographically normal coronary arteries. *Am J Cardiol* 1986;57:657.
195. Mammen EF, Barnhart MI, Selik NR, et al. "Sticky platelet syndrome": a congenital platelet abnormality predisposing to thrombosis. *Folia Haematol* 1988;115:361.
196. Mammen EF. Ten year's experience with the "sticky platelet syndrome." *Clin Appl Thromb Hemost* 1995;1:66.
197. Bick RL. Sticky platelet syndrome: a common cause of arterial and venous thrombosis. *J Clin Appl Thromb Hemost* 1998;4: 77–81.
198. Anderson JC, Lachant NA, Haggood AS. Sticky platelet syndrome: clinical manifestations and modulation by coexisting conditions in patients with thrombosis. *Blood* 1998;92:188a.
199. Berg-Dammer E, Henkes H, Trobisch H, et al. Sticky platelet syndrome: a cause of neurovascular thrombosis and thromboembolism. *Intervent Neuroradiol* 1997;3:145.
200. Karpatkin S, Khan O, Freedman M. Heterogeneity of platelet function: correlation with platelet volume. *Am J Med* 1978; 64:542.
201. Kraytman M. Platelet size in thrombocytopenias and thrombocytosis of various origin. *Blood* 1973;41:587.
202. Martin JF. Megakaryocytes and thrombopoiesis in vascular disease. *Prog Clin Biol Res* 1990;356:319.
203. Harker LA. Platelet survival time: its measurement and use. *Prog Hemost Thromb* 1978;4:321.
204. Karpatkin S, Charmatz A. Heterogeneity of human platelets, 1: metabolic and kinetic evidence suggestive of young and old platelets. *J Clin Invest* 1969;48:1073.
205. Penington DG, Lee NLY, Roxburgh AE, et al. Platelet density and size: the interpretation of heterogeneity. *Br J Haematol* 1976;34:365.
206. Roper-Drewinko P, Drewinko B, Corrigan G, et al. Standardization of platelet function tests. *Am J Hematol* 1981;11:183.
207. Rowan RM, Fraser C, Gray JH. Comparison of Channelyser and model S plus determined platelet size measurements. *Clin Lab Haematol* 1981;3:165.
208. Corash L, Shafter B, Weinberg D, et al. Platelet sizing in whole blood total platelet populations. In: Day NJ, Holmsen H, Zucker MB, eds. *Platelet function testing.* DHEW publishing no (NIH) 78-1087. Bethesda: DHEW, 1978:315.
209. Bick RL, McClain BJ. Platelet indices as markers of acute thrombosis and response to antithrombotic study. *Thromb Haemost* 1983;50:153.
210. Weiss HJ. Antiplatelet drugs in clinical medicine. In: *Platelets: pathophysiology and antiplatelet drug therapy.* New York: Alan R. Liss, 1982:75.
211. Renney JTG, O'Sullivan EF, Burke PF. Prevention of post-oper-

ative deep vein thrombosis with dipyridamole and aspirin. *Br Med J* 1976;2:992.
212. Blanke H, Praetorius G, Leschke M. Significance of the thrombin-antithrombin III complex in the diagnosis of pulmonary embolus and deep venous thrombosis: a comparison with fibrinopeptide A, platelet factor 4 and beta-thromboglobulin. *Klin Wochenschr* 1987;65:757.
213. Grande P, Grauholt AM, Madsen JK. Unstable angina pectoris: platelet behavior and prognosis in progressive angina and intermediate coronary syndrome. *Circulation* 1990;81:16.
214. Rapold HJ, Haeberli A, Kuemmerli H. Fibrin formation and platelet activation in patients with myocardial infarction and normal coronary arteries. *Eur Heart J* 1989;10:323.
215. von Reucker A, Hufnagel P, Dickerhoff R. Qualitative and quantitative changes in platelets after coronary artery bypass surgery may help identify thrombotic complications and infections. *Klin Wochenschr* 1989;67:1042.
216. Dalby-Kristensen S, Milner PC, Martin JF. Bleeding time and platelet volume in acute myocardial infarction: a 2 year followup study. *Thromb Haemost* 1988;59:353.
217. Erne P, Wardle J, Sanders K. Mean platelet volume and size distribution and their sensitivity to agonists in patients with coronary artery disease and congestive heart failure. *Thromb Haemost* 1988;59:259.
218. Cortellaro M, Cofrancesco E, Vicari A. High heparin released platelet factor 4 in uncomplicated type 1 diabetes mellitus. *Thromb Res* 1990;58:571.
219. Sinzinger H, Virgolini I, Fitscha P. Platelet kinetics in patients with atherosclerosis. *Thromb Res* 1990;57:507.
220. Arusio E, Lechi C, Pancera P. Usefulness of several laboratory tests on prethrombotic status in arterial vascular pathology. *Recent Prog Med (Italy)* 1989;80:18.
221. Tohgi H, Suzuki H, Tamura K. Platelet volume, aggregation, and adenosine triphosphate release in cerebral thrombosis. *Stroke* 1991;22:17.
222. Catalano M, Russo U, Belletti S. Beta-TG and plasma catecholamines levels after sympathetic stimuli in hypertensives and patients with peripheral vascular disease. *Thromb Haemost* 1990;63:383.
223. Wilson J, Orchard MA, Spencer AA. Anti-hypertensive drugs non-specifically reduce "spontaneous" activation of blood platelets. *Thromb Haemost* 1989;62:776.
224. Uchiyama S, Tsutsumi Y, Nagayama T. Antiplatelet effects of combination therapy with low-dose aspirin and ticlopidine in cerebral ischemia. *Rinsho Shink Clin Neurol (Japan)* 1989; 29:579.
225. Minar E, Ehringer H. Influence of acetylsalicylic acid (1.0 g/day) on platelet survival time, beta-thromboglobulin and platelet factor 4 in patients with peripheral arterial occlusive disease. *Thromb Res* 1987;45:791.
226. Gerbasi FR, Bottoms S, Farag A. Changes in hemostasis activity during delivery and the immediate postpartum period. *Am J Obstet Gynecol* 1990;162:1158.
227. Rao AK, Schapira M, Clements ML. A prospective study of platelets and plasma proteolytic systems during the early stages of Rocky Mountain spotted fever. *N Engl J Med* 1988;318: 1021.
228. Gilabert J, Estelles A, Anzar J. Contribution of platelets to increased plasminogen activator inhibitor type 1 in severe preeclampsia. *Thromb Haemost* 1990;63:361.
229. Hgevold HE, Mundal HH, Norman N. Platelet release reaction and plasma catecholamines during total hip replacement. *Thromb Res* 1990;57:21.
230. Paramo JA, Rocha E. Deep vein thrombosis and related platelet changes after total hip replacement. *Haemostasis* 1985; 15:389.
231. Dumoulin-Lagrange M, Capelle C. Evaluation of automated platelet counters for the enumeration and sizing of platelets in the diagnosis and management of hemostatic problems. *Semin Thromb Hemost* 1983;9:235.
232. Fareed J, Walenga JM, Bick RL, et al. Impact of automation on the quantitation of low molecular weight markers of hemostatic defects. *Semin Thromb Hemost* 1983;9:355.
233. Fareed J, Walenga JM. Current trends in hemostatic testing. *Semin Thromb Hemost* 1983;9:380.
234. Minar E, Ehringer H, Jung M, et al. Lack of influence of low-dose acetylsalicylic acid (100 mg/day) on platelet survival time, beta-thromboglobulin and platelet factor 4 in patients with peripheral arterial occlusive disease. *Thromb Res* 1988; 52:219.
235. Adams GA. In vivo and in vitro platelet function testing. *Plasma Ther Transfusion Technol* 1982;3:265.
236. Henry RL. Platelet function. *Semin Thromb Hemost* 1977;4:93.
237. Harms C. Laboratory evaluation of platelet function. In: Triplett DA, ed. *Platelet function.* Chicago: ASCP Press, 1978:35.
238. Born GVR. Aggregation of blood platelets by adenosine diphosphate and its reversal. *Nature* 1962;194:927.
239. Packham MA, Kinlough-Rathbone RL, Mustard JF. Aggregation and agglutination. In: Day HD, Holmsen H, Zucker MB, eds. *Platelet function testing.* HEW Publication (NIH) 78-1087. Bethesda: HEW, 1978:66.
240. Feinman RD, Zabinski MP, Lubowsky J. Simultaneous measurement of aggregation and secretion. In: Day HJ, Holmsen H, Zucker MB, eds. *Platelet function testing.* DHEW Publication (NIH) 78-1087. Bethesda: HEW, 1978:133.
241. Miller JL. Platelet function testing: an improved approach utilizing lumi-aggregation and an interactive computer. *Am J Clin Pathol* 1984;81:471.
242. Feinman RD, Lubowsky J, Charo I, et al. The lumi-aggregometer: a new instrument for simultaneous measurement of secretion and aggregation. *J Lab Clin Med* 1977;90:125.
243. Sweeney JD, Labuzetta JW, Fitzpatrick JE. The effect of the platelet count on the aggregation response and adenosine triphosphate release in an impedance lumi-aggregometer. *Am J Clin Pathol* 1988;89:655.
244. Malmgren R. ATP secretion occurs as an initial response in collagen induced platelet activation. *Thromb Res* 1986;43:445.
245. Rick M. Laboratory diagnosis of von Willebrand's disease. *Clin Lab Med* 1994;14:781.
246. Ingerman-Wojenski CM, Silver MJ. A quick method for screening platelet dysfunctions using the whole blood lumi-aggregometer. *Thromb Haemost* 1984;51:154.
247. Gresele P, Zoja C, Deckmyn H, et al. Dipyridamole inhibits platelet aggregations in whole blood. *Thromb Haemost* 1983; 50:852.
248. Nieuwenhuis HK, Akkerman JW, Sixma JJ. Patients with a prolonged bleeding time and normal aggregation tests may have storage pool deficiency: a study of one hundred six patients. *Blood* 1987;70:620.
249. Swart SS, Pearson D, Wood JK, et al. Effects of adrenaline and alpha adrenergic antagonists on platelet aggregation in whole blood: evaluation of electrical impedance aggregometry. *Thromb Res* 1984;36:411.
250. Sweeney JD, Hoernig LA, Fitzpatrick JE. Whole blood aggregation in von Willebrand disease. *Am J Hematol* 1989;32:190.
251. Mannucci P, Redaelli R, Tremoli E. Effects of aggregating agents and of blood cells on the aggregation of whole blood by the impedance technique. *Thromb Res* 1988;52:143.
252. Sweeney JD, Hoernig LA, Michnik A, et al. Whole blood aggregometry: influence of sample collection and delay in study performance on test results. *Am J Clin Pathol* 1989;92:676.
253. Fabris F, Casotato A, Randi ML, et al. The use of fluorescence

flow cytometry in the characterization of Bernard-Soulier syndrome and Glanzmann's thrombasthenia. *Haematologica* 1989; 74:39.

254. Gordon N, Thom J, Baker C. Rapid detection of hereditary and acquired storage pool deficiency by flow cytometry. *Br J Haematol* 1995;89:117.
255. Michelson AD. Platelet activation by thrombin can be directly measured in whole blood through the use of the peptide GPRP and flow cytometry: methods and clinical studies. *Blood Coagul Fibrinolysis* 1994;5:121.
256. Schlossman SF, Boumsell L, Gilks W, et al. CD antigens. *Blood* 1994;83:879.
257. Gerrard JM, Limt D, Sims PJ, et al. Identification of a dense-granule membrane protein that is deficient in a patient with Hermansky-Pudlak syndrome. *Blood* 1991;77:101.
258. Isreals SJ, Gerrard JM, Jaques YV, et al. Platelet dense granule membranes contain both granulophysin and P-selectin (GMP-140). *Blood* 1992;80:143.
259. Michelson AD. Flow cytometry: a clinical test of platelet function. *Blood* 1996;87:4925.
260. Schmitz G, Rothe G, Ruf A, et al. European Working Group on Clinical Cell Analysis: consensus protocol for the flow cytometric characterization of platelet function. *Thromb Haemost* 1998; 79:885.

Disorders of Thrombosis and Hemostasis: Clinical and Laboratory Practice, Third Edition, edited by Rodger L. Bick.
Lippincott Williams & Wilkins, Philadelphia © 2002

5

THROMBOCYTOPENIA AND THROMBOCYTOSIS

EUGENE P. FRENKEL

QUANTITATIVE PLATELET DEFECTS

Thrombocytopenia, Thrombocytosis, and Thrombocythemia

Clinical Features

Significant alterations in platelet numbers, whether thrombocytopenia or thrombocythemia, result in similar clinical expression. Very often the numeric alterations in platelets also are associated with functional platelet defects (see Chapter 4), resulting in more clinical findings than expected from the measured platelet count.

Cutaneous and mucosal petechiae and purpura are commonly seen in patients with either decreased or increased platelet numbers. Thus epistaxis and gastrointestinal and genitourinary bleeding are common (1). A particularly important clinical aspect of patients with increased platelet numbers is that thrombotic symptoms and signs usually predominate; thus the clinical presentation is commonly termed "thrombohemorrhagic."

In patients with thrombocytopenia who do not have an associated platelet functional defect, increased bleeding with trauma or surgery is uncommon unless the platelet count is less than 50,000/μL. Spontaneous bleeding is not usually seen unless the platelet count is less than 10,000 to 15,0000/μL (2). Unfortunately, similar numeric correlations in circumstances of increased platelet numbers cannot be made because of the highly variable relations.

Laboratory Assessment

The diagnostic hallmark is the quantitative platelet count. With automated counting, the average platelet size is expressed as the mean platelet volume (MPV). The MPV is elevated when platelet turnover is increased and younger platelets are released. By contrast, the MPV is reduced when platelet production is decreased.

Examination of the peripheral blood smear provides recognition of pseudothrombocytopenia or pseudothrombocythemia. In addition, identification of abnormal platelet architecture often provides the diagnostic clue to congenital disorders of platelet production.

Platelet functional evaluation (see Chapter 4) has relevance because associated dysfunction compounds the clinical findings of altered numbers. In general, template bleeding times are abnormal when platelet counts are less than 60,000 to 70,000/μL, and their performance is therefore not useful. The recent development of the PFA-100 (Dade-Behring Inc., Miami, FL, U.S.A.) analytic system for platelet function does not appear to depend critically on the number of platelets and therefore appears capable of defining platelet dysfunction in the presence of altered platelet numbers (3).

Thrombopoietin (TPO) serum levels have now been shown to help differentiate thrombocytopenias due to increased destruction from those due to production failure (4–6). Although an inverse relation between circulating platelet numbers and TPO levels has been seen, the current evidence is that the megakaryocyte mass is the significant regulator of circulating TPO levels (5,6). Thus absent or suppressed megakaryocytopoiesis results in increased levels of TPO in the blood (5,7). Another measure of megakaryocyte–platelet body mass is the assay of glycocalicin (GC), which is the soluble portion of GPI shed from mature megakaryocytes and platelets. It can serve as a reflection of increased platelet turnover (8); reduced levels reflect a decreased megakaryocyte–platelet body mass.

Examination of the thrombopoietic receptor, Mpl, provides another approach to the characterization of changes in megakaryopoiesis and the pathophysiology of alterations of circulating numbers of platelets (9). Two cytokine domains are present on Mpl; the first receptor domain encoded by exons 2–5 is critical for TPO binding (10). Exon 12 encoding is required for transduction of proliferation and differentiation signals (11). Thus with these techniques, congen-

E. P. Frenkel: Departments of Medicine and Radiology, University of Texas Southwestern Medical Center; Simmons Cancer Center, Zale–Lipshy University Hospital, Dallas, Texas.

ital amegakaryocyte thrombocytopenia has been shown to be due to mutations in the Mpl gene (12).

Pseudothrombocytopenia

Because thrombocytopenia is found by the platelet count, it is important to recognize that platelet aggregates are commonly pulse edited by electronic cell counters (13). Therefore it is absolutely essential to determine whether true thrombocytopenia exists or whether the reported platelet count is in error because of platelet clumping, agglutination, or platelet satellitism (around granulocytes). These changes, termed pseudothrombocytopenia (13,14), can be quickly identified by the examination of peripheral blood smears for this in vitro event and eliminate the diagnostic concern that true thrombocytopenia is present.

Platelet autoagglutinins are usually immunoglobulin G (IgG) and/or IgM (15). These may induce spontaneous autoagglutination of platelets, which is enhanced by the anticoagulant ethylenediaminetetraacetic acid (EDTA) (16). Additionally, adherence of platelets to granulocytes (platelet satellitism) also may be mediated by EDTA and/or platelet membrane IgG (17,18). Pseudothrombocytopenia also may be seen if a small platelet-trapping clot forms in the collection tube (14). EDTA-induced clumping of platelets is the most common cause of pseudothrombocytopenia (19,20).

Dilutional Thrombocytopenia

Thrombocytopenia can be seen on a simple dilutional basis after massive transfusions of packed red blood cells or in circumstances of marked fluid overload. These transient events can be expected when 10 or more units is given in a 24-hour period. A common approach is to administer platelet concentrates when 12 or more units of packed red cells is replaced rapidly.

THROMBOCYTOPENIA

Three basic etiologic mechanisms exist for thrombocytopenia, and the framework of differential diagnosis can be related to these, either individually or in combination: diminished platelet production, altered platelet distribution, and increased platelet destruction.

Thrombocytopenia Due to Decreased Platelet Production

Congenital and Neonatal Platelet-production Defects

Fanconi Syndrome

Fanconi syndrome is a rare disorder inherited as an autosomal recessive and comprising congenital aplastic anemia with multiple congenital abnormalities (1,21,22). The salient features are summarized in Table 5.1. Thrombocytopenia may precede the development of granulocytopenia and anemia; however, macrocytic anemia is the most pronounced hematologic feature noted. Bone marrow hypoplasia is almost always seen. In addition, congenital heart disease may be present. The hematologic abnormalities usually occur after age 4 years. Fanconi anemia is actually a clinical circumstance of a progressive marrow hypoplastic state. The genetic lesions are now known to be heterogeneous, and several complementation groups have been identified by somatic cell hybridization. The present evidence suggests that lesions occurring on different chromosomes and different genes can all result in the same characteristic clinical phenotype (23). Splenectomy may increase the platelet count to nonbleeding levels; however, the most common cause of death in patients with Fanconi syndrome is intracranial or gastrointestinal hemorrhage. Life-threatening hemorrhages should be treated with appropriate numbers of platelet transfusions; single-donor platelets are preferable, as these patients are candidates for numerous platelet transfusions throughout their lifetimes. Presently, allogeneic bone marrow transplantation is the only definitive therapy.

TABLE 5.1. FANCONI SYNDROME

Clinical Findings	Laboratory Findings
Autosomal recessive	Bone marrow hypoplasia
Usually manifested after age 4 yr	Aplastic anemia
Petechiae and purpura	Macrocytic anemia
Gastrointestinal hemorrhage	Granulocytopenia
Intracranial hemorrhage	Thrombocytopenia
Hypermelanosis	
Microcephaly	
Mental retardation	
Hyperactive deep tendon reflexes	
Deafness	
Ocular ptosis	
Skeletal deformities	
Dwarfism	
Congenital heart defects	

TAR-Baby Syndrome

The TAR-baby syndrome (thrombocytopenia and absent radii) is an autosomal recessive trait associated with severe thrombocytopenia due to marked deficiency of marrow megakaryocytes (23). The basis for this congenital lesion is not understood, although in utero infections with rubella have been implicated in some cases (24). Studies exploring the pathophysiologic mechanisms of the thrombocytopenia have shown that TPO secretion is appropriately increased, and that the TPO receptor, Mpl, on the platelet surface is normally expressed and has a normal molecular weight, supporting the view that the basis for the lesion is a lack of response to TPO in the signal-transduction pathway of Mpl (25,26). Bilateral aplasia of the radii is the most common associated abnormality, but cardiac and renal abnormalities also may be present. More than 50% of patients die of intracranial hemorrhage before reaching age 1 year (23). The syndrome is differentiated from Fanconi syndrome by the earlier onset and the absence of granulocytopenia and anemia. When life-threatening bleeding occurs, platelet concentrates, preferably from a single donor, should be infused to control bleeding. Single-donor platelets are preferable because long-term platelet concentrate use can usually be anticipated.

Wiskott–Aldrich Syndrome

Wiskott–Aldrich syndrome is a rare sex-linked recessive disorder characterized by severe eczema, increased susceptibility to infections, and severe thrombocytopenia (27,28). Circulating platelets are classically small and demonstrate a decreased MPV. Severe bleeding usually becomes manifest in the first 6 months of life and then may, like many other hereditary hemostasis defects, tend to improve. However, patients who survive bleeding episodes in their early childhood commonly die of overwhelming pyogenic infections or a malignancy, usually lymphoma. Cellular and humoral immune defects are noted (29). Patients usually demonstrate decreased IgM levels with normal IgG and IgA levels. Splenectomy has been successful in selected patients, but this places them at an even greater risk of infection because of the already compromised cellular and humoral immune defects (29,30).

May–Hegglin Anomaly

The May–Hegglin anomaly is a rare inherited autosomal dominant lesion, and approximately 50% of the patients have significant thrombocytopenia (31). Bleeding is generally modest. The lesion is characterized by giant hypergranular platelets with an increased MPV and Döhle body inclusions in circulating granulocytes (31,32). In spite of the thrombocytopenia, marrow megakaryocytes are normal in number. The locus for the disease has been mapped to chromosome 22 at 12.3 to 13.2; and recent evidence indicates the gene encodes nonmuscle myosin heavy chain-A (NMMHC-A) and is mutated in this disorder (32).

Alport Syndrome

Alport syndrome is a rare autosomal dominant lesion clinically characterized by proliferative and sclerosing glomerulonephritis with associated interstitial nephritis with sclerosis (32,33). Deafness is usually present. Thrombocytopenia with an increased MPV is characteristic, and platelets display a poorly defined platelet functional defect (34). Clinical hemorrhage is usually manifest as microscopic or gross hematuria; however, rarely nonrenal hemorrhage may occur. Significant or life-threatening hemorrhage should be treated with platelet concentrates.

Gray Platelet Syndrome

The gray platelet syndrome is a rare disorder that is inherited as an autosomal dominant trait and is characterized by large platelets and an increased MPV (35). The platelets are either markedly hypogranular or agranular, hence the name "gray platelet." The decreased granularity is due to an absence or marked reduction of α granules; thus, although adenine nucleotide pools remain normal, these platelets lack β-thromboglobulin and platelet factor 4. Nevertheless, platelet function is usually normal. The thrombocytopenia is usually severe, and significant bleeding can occur. Platelet concentrates can be used to control life-threatening hemorrhage. In addition, the thrombocytopenia can usually be corrected by splenectomy.

Bernard–Soulier Syndrome

The Bernard–Soulier syndrome (see Chapter 4) is an autosomal recessive trait, with markedly enlarged platelets, an elevated MPV, and shortened platelet survival. The degree of thrombocytopenia is moderate to severe, although in some, thrombocytopenia is periodic or absent. Because the Bernard–Soulier platelet classically does not aggregate to ristocetin, the disorder can be confused with the von Willebrand variant associated with thrombocytopenia (36), unless platelet morphology is carefully examined and appropriate tests performed.

Congenital Marrow Infiltrative Disorders

Congenital marrow infiltrative lesions can result in significant thrombocytopenia. Thrombocytopenia with and without associated myeloid and erythroid depression occurs in children with numerous infiltrative disorders including leukemia, lymphoma, solid tumors, myelofibrosis, Gaucher disease, Neimann–Pick disease, and the mucopolysaccharidoses. A leukoerythroblastic pattern with thrombocytopenia in some neonates and infants should suggest that the thrombocytopenia was caused by a marrow infiltrative process.

Congenital Thrombocytopenia Associated with Maternal Disorders

The maternal ingestion of ethanol, thiazides, and tolbutamide may lead to significant thrombocytopenia in the newborn. In addition, if the mother is receiving cytotoxic chemotherapeutic drugs that are capable of crossing the placenta, neonatal thrombocytopenia may result. Maternal infections with cytomegalovirus, hepatitis, varicella, or rubella may lead to congenital thrombocytopenia in the newborn; additionally, recent maternal vaccinations (rubella or rubeola) may lead to neonatal thrombocytopenia (37).

Acquired Platelet Production Defects

The common acquired causes of defective platelet production are shown in Table 5.2.

TABLE 5.2. ACQUIRED CAUSES OF PLATELET PRODUCTION DEFECTS

Aplastic anemia	Drug-induced marrow suppression
Isolated megakaryocyte aplasia	Cytotoxic chemotherapy
Marrow infiltrative diseases	Thiazides
Leukemia	Ethanol
Lymphoma	Gold antiinflammatory drugs
Hodgkin disease	Tranquilizers
Metastatic carcinoma	Anticonvulsants
Myelofibrosis	Cyclic thrombocytopenia
Myelosclerosis	Renal failure
Gaucher disease	Myeloproliferative syndromes
Niemann–Pick disease	Maturation: metabolic defects
Mucopolysaccharidoses	B_{12} deficiency
Infiltrative infections	Folate deficiency
Coccidioidomycosis	
Tuberculosis	
Toxoplasmosis	
Histoplasmosis	
Various bacteria	
Various viruses	

Aplastic Anemia

Aplastic anemia is often associated with severe thrombocytopenia (38). The thrombocytopenia may precede the myeloid and erythroid decreases by weeks to months in patients in whom aplastic anemia is developing, and a bone marrow examination may demonstrate an absence of only megakaryocytes (39,40). In addition, during the recovery phase, the thrombocytopenia may persist for months and even years after myeloid and erythroid recovery.

Megakaryocytic Marrow Aplasia

Isolated selective megakaryocyte marrow aplasia is an extremely rare condition (39), although this finding may herald the development of an autoimmune disorder [e.g., systemic lupus erythematosus (SLE)], a myelodysplasia, or represent toxicity from a drug, toxin, or infectious agent. The finding of vacuolated megakaryocytes suggests such an event. One unusual presentation of thrombocytopenia associated with decreased megakaryocytes has on rare occasions been seen during pregnancy (40,41). The aplastic state can develop during pregnancy, and in some who have had prior aplasia with clinical recovery, relapse has been seen. It is of interest that after delivery, about one third of patients spontaneously recover (42).

Marrow Infiltrative Disorders

Any widespread infiltrative lesion in the bone marrow can result in decreased platelet production as a result of reduced megakaryocyte mass. In general terms, this results from marrow infiltration and replacement by hematopoietic neoplasms (i.e., leukemias, lymphomas, and plasma cell malignancies), metastatic carcinoma (e.g., especially breast, prostate, and lung), infectious granulomatous diseases, lipid storage and mucopolysaccharidoses states, and myelofibrosis and myelosclerosis. These infiltrative processes are often associated with evidence of leukoerythroblastic changes, and large platelets on the examination of the peripheral blood smear commonly provides the diagnostic clue to marrow replacement. This is most commonly seen in metastatic carcinoma or myelofibrosis, perhaps because these lesions produce the most remarkable changes in the marrow sinusoids, thereby allowing premature release of marrow elements to the circulating blood.

Thrombocytopenia Caused by Marrow Suppression with Drugs

A wide variety of drugs and chemicals can cause megakaryocyte injury and resultant thrombocytopenia (Table 5.3). Cytoreductive chemotherapy is presently the most common mechanism for marrow suppression and resultant cytope-

TABLE 5.3. COMMON DRUGS AND CHEMICALS CAUSING DECREASED PLATELET PRODUCTION

Acetaminophen	Furosemide
Acetazolamide	Gold indomethacin
Allopurinol	Mephenytoin
Amphotericin	Meprobamate
Aspirin	Oxyphenbutazone
Benzene	Phenylbutazone
Chloramphenicol	Prednisone
Chlordiazepoxide	Primidone
Chlorpropamide	Pyrimethamine
Chlorthalidone	Quinacrine
Cimetidine	Streptomycin
Colchicine	Sulfamethoxazole
Diazepam	Sulfisoxazole
Diethylstilbestrol	Sulfonamides
Diphenylhydantoin	Thiazides
Estrogens	Tolbutamide
Ethanol	

nias, including thrombocytopenia. In general, chemotherapy is not selective for megakaryocytes and actually induces more significant granulocytopenia and anemia than thrombocytopenia. The degree of induced thrombocytopenia is most severe when drugs are used to induce specifically marrow aplasia in leukemia or lymphoma, in which the agents further injure an already reduced megakaryocyte mass. For most drugs, a dose–intensity relation exists, so that high-dose chemotherapy (as in myeloablative therapy in bone marrow transplantation) is more likely to result in thrombocytopenia than standard dose therapy. Multidrug chemotherapy or chemotherapy given with radiation therapy similarly provides a potential setting for resultant thrombocytopenia. In developing multiagent chemotherapy programs, an attempt is usually made to incorporate agents with differing patterns of toxicity. As a result, some attempt has been made to define the potential for the severity of induced thrombocytopenia with standard doses of chemotherapy agents, and such a categorization is shown in Table 5.4.

Many other drugs and chemicals (Table 5.3) are capable of inducing severe and uncommonly, irreversible thrombocytopenia by nonimmune marrow-suppression mechanisms (1). The agent may act at the promegakaryocyte stem cell stage, or directly on the megakaryocyte, or more rarely, on the circulating platelet. Thiazide diuretics are common causes, as are ethanol, antiinflammatory drugs, tranquilizers, and anticonvulsants. Unlike drug or chemical immune-mediated thrombocytopenia, the thrombocytopenia associated with drug/chemical-induced marrow suppression is gradual in onset, requiring from weeks to several months to become manifest, and megakaryocytes are usually decreased rather than increased, as in immune-induced thrombocytopenia. When the offending drug is removed, the platelet count is slow to return to normal in comparison to most instances of immune-mediated drug-induced thrombocytopenia, in which recovery is usually rapid. If the drug or chemical exposure is continued for a long period, irreversible thrombocytopenia and even aplastic anemia may ensue.

TABLE 5.4. INTENSITY OF THROMBOCYTOPENIA WITH ANTINEOPLASTIC THERAPY

Mild thrombocytopenia	**Severe thrombocytopenia**
L-Asparaginase	Busulfan
Bleomycin	Chlorambucil
Cisplatin	Cytosine arabinoside
Vincristine	Melphalan
Diethylstilbestrol	Nitrogen mustard
Prednisone	Nitrosourea compounds
Tamoxifen	Vinblastine
Moderate thrombocytopenia	
Actinomycin D	
Cyclophosphamide	
5-Fluorouracil	
6-Mercaptopurine	
Methotrexate	
Procarbazine	

Cyclic Thrombocytopenia

Cyclic thrombocytopenia by unclear mechanisms has been noted, primarily in women (43–45). The average cycle or nadir of thrombocytopenia is approximately 30 days. Thrombocytopenia may be severe enough that significant or life-threatening hemorrhage may occur. Splenectomy and prednisone therapy have been without significant benefit. Thus platelet transfusions, preferably single-donor platelets, remain the treatment of choice (1).

Infections Associated with Decreased Platelet Production

Infections associated with decreased production of platelets include those caused by numerous viral, bacterial, and fungal agents. Disseminated tuberculosis, coccidioidomycosis, brucellosis, and toxoplasmosis are most prominent. The megakaryocytes provide an ideal cell for bacterial and viral invasion and replication, thereafter interfering with platelet production. When this occurs, morphologic changes in the megakaryocytes can often be noted in the marrow with cytoplasmic vacuolization and nuclear degeneration; in addition, megakaryocytes may be decreased in number. Viral invasion of megakaryocytes, with resultant viral replication and subsequent megakaryocyte degeneration and decreased platelet production, occurs in measles, including individuals receiving live measles vaccinations, as well as in infectious mononucleosis, herpes simplex, herpes zoster, cytomegalovirus infection, and hepatitis (46–51). Common viruses known to be associated with thrombocytopenia due to marrow-suppressive mechanisms are shown in Table 5.5.

Bacterial infections, especially septicemia, are often associated with thrombocytopenia (52); however, it is often difficult, if not impossible, to incriminate marrow suppression alone as the mechanism. In many instances, disseminated intravascular coagulation (DIC) secondary to sepsis may be

TABLE 5.5. COMMON VIRUSES CAUSING DECREASED PLATELET PRODUCTION

Adenoviruses
Cytomegalovirus
Enteroviruses
Epstein–Barr virus
Hepatitis virus
Herpes simplex virus
Herpes zoster virus
Human immunodeficiency virus
Mumps virus
Rubella
Rubeola
Variola

involved, bacteria–platelet complexes may cause splenic removal of platelets (peripheral loss), and antibiotic use also may contribute to thrombocytopenia through several mechanisms. In gram-negative sepsis, endotoxin may induce platelet release and subsequent thrombocytopenia. Thus, in patients with bacterial infections, especially with septicemia, the often-associated thrombocytopenia is a clinical summation of numerous pathophysiologic mechanisms. Because the mechanisms are unclear and often impossible to define clinically, significant or life-threatening hemorrhage is wisely treated with platelet concentrates.

Miscellaneous Production Problems

Renal failure may be associated with defective platelet production; the mechanism(s) remain unclear. Generally, the recognized thrombocytopenia is multifactorial and includes immune complex–mediated platelet destruction (53,54,56, 57). The platelet-function defect seen in renal failure is a much more common cause of significant bleeding in patients with renal disease than is thrombocytopenia. Effective treatment of the underlying disease process leading to renal failure or vigorous hemodialysis will usually correct, or partially correct, both the quantitative and qualitative platelet defects seen in these patients.

Unexplained thrombocytopenia can be the presenting feature of paroxysmal nocturnal hemoglobinemia (PNH) (55, 56). PNH, generally characterized by the triad of hemolytic anemia, pancytopenia secondary to marrow failure, and thrombosis, is the result of a somatic mutation of the X-linked phosphatidyl inositol glycan (complementation group A) gene, now commonly labeled PIG-A gene (57–59). This clonal mutation results in alterations in the hematopoietic stem cell with deficiency of glycosylphosphatidylinositol (GPI) membrane-linked proteins related to the loss of the GPI "anchoring" capacity. The complexity of the molecular change is emphasized by current evidence of more than 174 somatic mutations identified to date (60). The exact basis for the phenotypic expression of the marrow aplasia is not yet clear; and, as would be anticipated, why some express greater suppression of one cell line over the other is not known. In general, bleeding is quite rare in PNH; rather it is the risk of thrombosis that largely propels the clinical picture. When thrombocytopenia-related bleeding is seen, the treatment of choice is platelet transfusions.

Maturation/Metabolic Defects

Severe iron deficiency may be associated with thrombocytosis or thrombocytopenia (61). The mechanisms of decreased platelet production remain unclear, but may be related to the need for iron in platelet production by megakaryocytes. Iron therapy will usually induce prompt correction of the thrombocytopenia. Significant bleeding and the need for platelet transfusions are extremely rare in severe iron-deficiency anemia.

Patients with severe B_{12} or folate deficiency may have hemorrhage due to thrombocytopenia (62,63). Thrombocytopenia may be quite pronounced and is primarily due to ineffective megakaryocytopoiesis; however, other mechanisms also are operative, including absence of megakaryocytes in the marrow and reduced platelet survival. The thrombocytopenia in severe folate or severe B_{12} deficiency usually is corrected promptly with appropriate hematonic therapy (64).

General Issues in Therapy for Thrombocytopenia Secondary to Decreased Production

Three general approaches have been used to manage life-threatening or severe bleeding associated with clinical states that result in decreased platelet production. The most common has been the transfusion of platelets. In general, platelets from a unit of blood will increase the recipients' platelet count approximately 12,000/μL/m^2. Because the goal is approximately 50,000/μL, thus platelets from 4 units of blood can be expected to produce that increment per meter body surface area (m^2). A common practice for transfusion programs is to supply platelets in a "six-pack," because most adults are in the range of 1.5 m^2. For larger individuals and for continued bleeding, this common six-pack approach may not be adequate, and repeated transfusions are required. To determine therapeutic adequacy, a repeated platelet count should be done 20 to 30 minutes after the transfusion. If the "recovery" (i.e., increment) is inadequate, repeated transfusions may be needed, and platelet refractoriness must be considered. Refractoriness is commonly defined as a lack of adequate posttransfusion platelet increment after two or more consecutive transfusions. Although refractoriness can be due to nonimmune causes (especially massive splenomegaly, microangiopathic platelet destruction, DIC, sepsis, or veno-occlusive disease after bone marrow transplantation), most often alloimmune mechanisms [i.e., human leukocyte antigen (HLA), HPA, or ABO antibodies) are the basis (65, 66). Single-donor HLA-matched platelet acquisition is the common approach to circumvent this problem. In some circumstances, even further manipulation is required, such as the use of HLA-stripped platelets or intravenous immunoglobulin (IVIG).

A second approach has been the use of recombinant human interleukin-11 (Neumega), now approved for use after chemotherapy (67–70). Isolation of interleukin-11 (IL-11) led to the characterization of its role as a hematopoietic cytokine with thrombopoietic activity (67). IL-11 has been shown to act synergistically with IL-3, thrombopoietin, and stem cell factor to stimulate multiple stages of megakaryocytopoiesis and result in platelet production (67). Recombinant IL-11 has now demonstrated efficacy in enhancing platelet recovery after major chemotherapeutic suppression (67,68,70). It is of note that the activity of IL-11 is actually not lineage specific within the hematopoietic system, but rather is pleiotropic and interacts with other cytokines at multiple sites of cellular differentiation and maturation. That these interactions are complex is suggested by the evidence in megakaryocytic differentiation that IL-11 appears important in early differentiation from progenitor cells, whereas maturation and platelet production appear more dependent in thrombopoietin.

Finally, although the initial studies of recombinant thrombopoietin and clinical trials were very promising, the development of platelet-directed antibodies has limited its introduction as a clinical modality. Resolution of this side effect is certain, and it will likely join the therapeutic profile.

Thrombocytopenia Secondary to Altered Platelet Distribution

Circulating thrombocytopenia can result from an altered distribution of platelets. In that event, the platelet count decreased by the total body platelet numbers is normal.

Congestive Splenomegaly (Hypersplenism)

Congestive splenomegaly is commonly associated with decreased numbers of circulating platelets. Such congestion has been termed "hypersplenism" to characterize the clinical and laboratory findings of splenic enlargement, circulating cytopenias (especially thrombocytopenia), and a bone marrow with hyperplasia of the cellular elements found to be decreased in the blood (71). More than 200 etiologic mechanisms have been described as causes of hypersplenism, the most common of which are listed in Table 5.6.

Several clinical features characterize the thrombocytopenia in congestive splenomegaly. First, the decrease in platelets is almost always associated with significant splenic enlargement, making the presence of a palpable spleen a specific diagnostic criterion. Second, the degree of thrombocytopenia is modest and rarely is less than 50,000/μL. Consistent with that is the absence of clinical bleeding, thereby defining a laboratory event rather than a clinical problem in these patients. When bleeding is present, a second defect (e.g., platelet functional defect) or a vascular abnormality (e.g., varices) is usually superimposed on the thrombocytopenia.

TABLE 5.6. COMMON CAUSES OF HYPERSPLENISM

Amyloidosis
Autoimmune disorders
Systemic lupus erythematosus
Rheumatoid arthritis
Gaucher disease
Hemolytic anemias
Hodgkin disease
Idiopathic splenomegaly
Infections
Inflammatory diseases
Leukemia
Lymphoma
Metastatic carcinoma
Multiple myeloma
Myeloproliferative syndromes
Niemann–Pick disease
Portal hypertension
Thalassemia
Waldenström macroglobulinemia

The laboratory features that help confirm congestive splenomegaly as the basis for the thrombocytopenia include the modest decrease in platelet numbers with a normal MPV; thus there is little evidence of a significant increase in platelet turnover. Commonly in patients with congestive splenomegaly, other cellular elements (white blood cells or red blood cells or both) are also decreased because of splenic sequestration.

The characteristics of the thrombocytopenia in congestive splenomegaly are of interest and define platelet sequestration (72,73). The platelet survival (half-life) is normal, the spleen can be induced to release sequestered platelets, and examination of the bone marrow demonstrates adequate megakaryocytes with a normal platelet production. A bone marrow examination is rarely needed. The lesion is one of platelet sequestration in an enlarged spleen (69,70). Splenic trapping of cells is different for red cells and white cells. It merits emphasis that increased platelet destruction (in the spleen) does not occur in congestive splenomegaly, in contrast to red cell sequestration in which increased red cell destruction (i.e., true hemolysis) occurs. Further evidence of splenic platelet pooling comes from the decreased "recovery" of platelets after their transfusion into the patient with congestive splenomegaly. Circulating platelet numbers an hour after platelet transfusion are in the range of 80% to 95% of the calculated dose; in contrast, in congestive splenomegaly, the 1-hour platelet count is decreased to 20% to 40% of expected values because of the sequestration.

Because the total body platelet pool is normal in congestive splenomegaly and mobilization of platelets can occur with stress, there is little indication for specific therapeutic intervention in patients with thrombocytopenia. Specifically, splenectomy is virtually never a required approach in such patients. However, absorbable gelatin foam (Gelfoam) embolization of the splenic artery has been used successfully in highly selected patients in whom the clinical concept was that increased platelet numbers would enhance hemostasis (74).

Hypothermia

Transient thrombocytopenia has been observed in experimental animals and in patients who have had procedures carried out during a hypothermic state. Significant reduction in body temperatures to well below 25°C appears to be required to produce this event. Because rewarming is associated with a return of platelet numbers to normal, this represents another phenomenon of platelet sequestration.

Thrombocytopenia Due to Increased Consumption or Destruction

Neonatal Increased Platelet Destruction or Consumption

Maternal ingestion of drugs or agents known to induce immune-mediated thrombocytopenia may induce it in the newborn in response to agents capable of crossing the placenta. Thus the maternal ingestion of quinine, quinidine, hydralazine, or selected antibiotics known to induce immune-mediated thrombocytopenia may induce congenital immune-mediated thrombocytopenia (75). Thrombocytopenia in these neonates usually abates rapidly, and significant hemorrhage is rare.

A more serious neonatal thrombocytopenia can arise from a maternal immune reaction to fetal platelet antigens that have been inherited from the father (76). Transplacental passage of the maternal antibody (usually an IgG) may create a severe thrombocytopenia in the neonate in utero (76). This usually occurs when the mother has PLA1-negative platelets, and the fetus has inherited PLA1-positive platelets from the father (77,78). In other instances, anti-HLA antibodies have been incriminated. Infants with this type of alloimmune neonatal thrombocytopenia may be covered with petechiae and purpura or may demonstrate more severe hemorrhage at the time of birth, or may appear normal at delivery and then manifest severe bleeding within the first week after birth. The thrombocytopenia usually abates within 1 month. Because approximately 30% of these individuals may die of central nervous system (CNS) hemorrhage, cesarean sections have been advocated to avoid the trauma of childbirth if a prenatal diagnosis has been made (79). Other successful therapy includes platelet transfusions, exchange transfusions, and steroids in the severely thrombocytopenic infant (80). Prenatal administration of corticosteroids to the mother also may be of benefit. Splenectomy is not appropriate, because the disorder is self-limiting. Neonatal infection with toxoplasmosis, rubella, cytomegalovirus, herpes, or syphilis may cause an immune-mediated increased platelet destruction. The mechanisms are poorly understood and poorly defined.

Other causes of neonatal thrombocytopenia due to increased platelet consumption or destruction include neonatal thrombocytopenia in association with maternal immune thrombocytopenia purpura (ITP). In addition, neonatal thrombocytopenia may occur in women who have preeclampsia or toxemia of pregnancy (see Chapter 7.). Infants born of mothers with lupus or other autoimmune diseases, especially if the mother has a lupus anticoagulant and/or anticardiolipin antibodies, may be born with immune-mediated thrombocytopenia.

Acquired Increased Platelet Destruction or Consumption

Nonimmune Mechanisms

Disseminated Intravascular Coagulation. This is clearly the most common acquired mechanism for thrombocytopenia; it is separately reviewed in Chapter 10.

Hemolytic–uremic Syndrome. Hemolytic–uremic syndrome (HUS) is a poorly understood platelet consumptive disease first described in 1955 (81). It has been related to thrombotic thrombocytopenic purpura (TTP) with respect to its pathophysiology. However, unlike TTP or DIC, this disease has a high degree of organ specificity (i.e., kidney) with respect to endothelial damage and thrombus formation. The disorder may be seen at any age; however, it is much more common in children (82). Many of the clinical and laboratory findings seen in childhood and adult HUS are similar, although some striking differences exist. The common clinical features are moderate to severe thrombocytopenia, a microangiopathic hemolytic anemia, renal failure, and hypertension (83,84). In children, boys and girls are equally affected, but in adults, women develop the syndrome 3 times as commonly as men (85). In childhood HUS, there is commonly a prodrome of a viral or bacterial febrile illness, often associated with gastroenteritis or pneumonia. One agent has been particularly implicated in HUS; that is a verocytotoxin produced by several different serotypes of *Escherichia coli* (86), but in particular, 0157:H7. An interesting physiologic correlate has been posed by the recognition of the verotoxin receptor glycolipid in the kidneys (87). These relations have suggested that the common unifying basis for the syndrome is a mechanism inducing renal endothelial cell injury (88–91). Adult HUS, however, is almost never preceded by this type of clinical pattern. It is often associated with a variety of complications of pregnancy (89). Adult HUS also may be associated with renal transplantation rejection or the use of oral contraceptives (90,91). An almost uniformly fatal form of HUS has been noted to develop after bone marrow transplantation (92–95).

Children and adults demonstrate the usual clinical findings of anemia, petechiae, purpura, and at times, severe bleeding. Hematuria, renal failure, hypertension, and neurologic symptoms also are seen. The neurologic symptoms may be mild, including slurred speech and dull mentation, or may be very severe, including coma and frank seizures; however, neurologic complaints are less common than in TTP or DIC. The neurologic symptoms may be due to renal failure and severe hypertension or may be due to CNS microvascular damage, thrombosis, or intracranial hemorrhage. A definite familial tendency has been noted in both children and adults with HUS, and some have suggested this to be due to an inherited deficiency of a plasma prostacyclin-stimulating factor (96). Tissue examination reveals platelet and fibrin-like material in renal afferent arterioles, glomerular capillaries, and subendothelial spaces. These same findings may be noted in multiple end organs.

Laboratory findings are those of a microangiopathic hemolytic anemia, with histocytes and thrombocytopenia with "large bizarre platelets." Azotemia with hematuria and proteinuria are common (97). Coagulation abnormalities, besides thrombocytopenia, are usually limited to an expected universal elevation of fibrinogen/fibrin degradation products (FDPs). In occasional cases, typical laboratory findings of DIC also may be present.

Steroids, heparin, and antiplatelet agents are usually ineffective in childhood HUS. However, the use of washed packed red blood cells, plasma exchange, and prompt dialysis have reduced the mortality to around 10%, and only 10% to 15% of surviving patients have impaired renal function. Unlike children, adults may respond to heparin or the use of antiplatelet agents (aspirin plus dipyridamole) in conjunction with dialysis, prompt control of hypertension, and infusion of washed packed red cells to control anemia (96,97).

In addition, plasma exchange appears helpful (94,96, 98). The mortality in adults is much higher than that in children and approaches 50% in spite of vigorous therapy. The clinical features and laboratory findings of HUS are shown in Table 5.7.

Thrombotic Thrombocytopenia Purpura. TTP is a thrombotic microangiopathy with many findings similar to those of HUS. First described by Moschcowitz in 1924 (99), the pattern that has evolved is one of intravascular platelet aggregation at microvascular sites with microthrombic thrombocytopenia, neurologic and renal lesions, and intravascular hemolysis secondary to red cell fragmentation at sites of aggregation where flow rates result in shear. TTP has been seen in conjunction with a wide variety of clinical events ranging from pregnancy (100,101), hemolysis, elevated liver enzymes, and low platelet count (HELLP) syndrome, acquired immunodeficiency syndrome (AIDS), and cancer. In addition, several drugs have clearly been implicated including cyclosporine, mitomycin, and the antiplatelets drugs ticlopidine and cloipidogrel (102–105).

This clinical heterogeneity has made the delineation of pathogenetic mechanisms elusive. Recent evidence that unusually large von Willebrand factor (vWF) multimers are found in the plasma of patients with recurrent TTP suggests that these highly adhesive vWF multimers could produce agglutination of platelets, particularly in the microcirculation (106). Normally, vascular endothelial cells synthesize vWF peptides and then assemble them into varying molecule-sized multimers. The larger molecular multimers are particularly important in supporting platelet adhesion and aggregation (106,107). Normally, these large multimers undergo proteolytic cleavage and degradation in the circulation (107). A unique protease from normal plasma specifically cleaves the vWF submit at the peptide bond between Ty 842 and Met 843, the expected site of degradation of the vWF (108,109). The recognition of this unique physiologic protease led to the study of several patients with TTP, and deficiency of this vWF cleaving protease was found (110). This protease appears in the pathophysiology of TTP. Normal protease activity has been seen in normal controls, and both constitutional and acquired deficiency of the vWF-clearing protease has been found in patients with TTP; in some, a circulating IgG inhibitor of

TABLE 5.7. HEMOLYTIC–UREMIC SYNDROME: CLINICAL

Common Clinical Findings	**Common Laboratory Findings**
Anemia	Microangiopathic hemolytic anemia
Thrombocytopenia	Schizocytes
Petechiae and purpura	Thrombocytopenia
Hypertension	Large "young" platelets
Renal failure	Elevated fibrin–fibrinogen degradation products
Hematuria	DIC-type laboratory findings rare
Neurologic findings	Hematuria
Familial tendency	Microscopic
	Gross
	Proteinuria
	Azotemia
Pediatric differences	**Adult differences**
More common than in adults	Less common than in children
Prodome of fever or infection	Prodome of
Female/male ratio, 1:1	Eclampsia
	Obstetric accidents
	Oral contraceptive use
	Renal transplant rejection
	Normal postpartum state
	Female/male ratio, 3:1

DIC, disseminated intravascular coagulation.

the enzyme also has been seen (111). Of interest, virtually all patients studied with acute TTP have severe deficiency of vWF-cleaving protease; when clinical remission occurs, the enzyme level is normal (112,114). This suggests that vWF-cleaving protease deficiency is an important factor in the pathogenesis of TTP, perhaps by triggering endothelial release of the high-molecular-weight multimers of vWF capable of inducing platelet clumping in the microcirculation under high shear stress (106,109,113). This provides an explanation for the complex and multiple triggers to an episode of TTP. It appears that most cases of protease deficiency and TTP are the result of antibodies, whereas the familial forms have a constitutional enzyme deficiency. The roles of such antibodies help explain cases of relapsing TTP, and the observations that immunosuppressive therapy and splenectomy sometimes resulted in clinical response. Most remarkable has been the observation that patients with classic HUS have normal protease activity. Thus, although clinical similarities exist between HUS and TTP, it is very likely that the pathophysiologic mechanisms are different (111, 112); and, heterogeneity of causes is likely.

Clinically, TTP has often been defined as a triad, with microangiopathic hemolytic anemia, thrombocytopenia, and fluctuating neurologic abnormalities (99,102,115). When defined as a pentad or quintad, fever and renal abnormalities are added. Sixty percent of patients with TTP are females between the ages of 10 and 40 years, with a peak incidence occurring in the third decade. Previously, within 2 to 3 months of the onset of TTP, 80% of patients were dead. There is almost always evidence of hemorrhage. The signs, symptoms, and physical findings of TTP and laboratory findings are in Table 5.8. The classic laboratory findings of DIC are usually absent in patients with TTP, although a red cell fragmentation is classic. The one consistent finding in TTP, which is reminiscent of DIC and is often confusing, is elevated FDP levels.

Therapy for TTP remained controversial and confusing for many years, as the pathophysiology remained unknown. Early therapeutic approaches were empirical and included corticosteroids, antiplatelet agents, splenectomy, and/or trials of immunosuppressive chemotherapeutic agents. The overall response rate to high-dose corticosteroids is around 10%. The general response rate to antiplatelet agents is similar, although studies are limited. These treatments had modest success, and a mortality rate of approximately 30% was seen in those patients with classic TTP, without neurologic signs or symptoms. For those patients with clinical evidence of neurologic involvement, the mortality rate was approximately 90% in spite of all these therapeutic approaches.

A remarkable advance in the treatment of TTP occurred with the introduction of plasma therapy and exchange by Bukowski et al. (116–122). Although plasma infusion was thought to have efficacy equal to that of exchange, a multiinstitutional study demonstrated superiority of plasma exchange (123). With exchange, survival rates in excess of 90% are seen (124). The potential role of antiplatelet therapy is still not clear (125,126). The success of plasma exchange has limited the likelihood of a well-executed randomized trial. The observations of the pivotal role of the protease have now helped to explain a potential role for splenectomy as well as immunosuppressive therapy (127–129).

Infections and Drugs Directly Toxic to Platelets

Thrombocytopenia can occur with numerous bacterial, viral, fungal, and protozoan infections. The mechanisms are complex, and the thrombocytopenia noted is often a clinical summation of many pathophysiologic events in the patient with infection. Nonimmunologic mechanisms of thrombocytopenia in the patient with infection may include direct platelet destruction by interaction of the infectious agent with platelets, in vivo platelet aggregation induced by bacteria or bacterial products, the development of infection-induced DIC with resultant consumption of platelets, the release of thromboxane A_2 by infectious agents or their products, or the interaction of platelets with endothelium that has sustained significant damage by the infectious agent.

TABLE 5.8. THROMBOTIC THROMBOCYTOPENIA PURPURA

Signs and Symptoms	Laboratory Findings
Prodome of fatigue, pallor, and nausea	Schizocytes
Petechiae, purpura, and ecchymoses	Anemia
Epistaxis	Thrombocytopenia
Retinal hemorrhages	Reticulocytosis
Gastrointestinal bleeding	Hematuria
Fever	Leukocytosis
Jaundice	Elevated fibrin–fibrinogen degradation products
Neurologic deficits	DIC-type laboratory findings usually negative
Abdominal pain	Proteinuria
Hepatomegaly	Azotemia
Splenomegaly	Indirect hyperbilirubinemia

DIC, disseminated intravascular coagulation.

Thrombocytopenia often occurs early in the course of septicemia, and the noting of thrombocytopenia in a febrile patient should prompt early suspicion of the development of septicemia, commonly due to meningococci, other gram-negative organisms (especially those that produce endotoxin), or staphylococcal organisms (130,131). Thrombocytopenia is seen much more commonly in gram-negative septicemia than in gram-positive septicemia. Up to 60% of patients with sepsis will have some degree of thrombocytopenia.

A variety of drugs can be directly toxic to platelets, causing increased platelet destruction by nonimmunologic mechanisms. Two currently used drugs, gold and valproic acid, are the most serious agents. Gold used in the treatment of rheumatoid arthritis can induce thrombocytopenia. Although the most serious side effect of gold therapy is aplastic anemia, thrombocytopenia is the single most common hematologic complication, occurring in 3% of patients (132). The exact mechanism is unclear, but the early onset of thrombocytopenia, decreased platelet survival, and normal or increased megakaryocytes in the marrow suggests that peripheral platelet destruction is operative. Treatment is immediate discontinuation of gold; other therapy of benefit is the use of chelating agents and prednisone (132,133). In spite of these therapeutic modalities, many patients remain persistently thrombocytopenic after discontinuation of gold. Valproic acid has become popular as an antiepileptic agent and is associated with thrombocytopenia. The mechanism is thought to be due to valproic acid interaction with platelets, leading to increased peripheral destruction; however, immunologic mechanisms also have been suggested.

Cardiovascular Diseases And Increased Platelet Consumption And Destruction

Aortic and mitral valvular diseases, especially the types seen in association with rheumatic fever, have been associated with increased platelet consumption/destruction (116,134). Mild thrombocytopenia commonly occurs in patients with severe aortic stenosis; in addition, patients with mitral disease associated with left atrial thrombosis or peripheral vascular embolization may have thrombocytopenia. (134–136). Thrombus formation and associated platelet consumption is common in patients with prosthetic valves; the incidence of platelet consumption is significantly lower in patients with tissue valves than in those with nontissue valves; however, porcine valves have been associated with platelet consumption and thrombocytopenia (136,137). Peripheral arterial disease, especially if associated with significant claudication and gangrene or thromboembolism, also may be associated with increased consumption and thrombocytopenia. Extensive deep venous thrombosis, especially involving the inferior vena cava or iliofemoral system, may be associated with thrombocytopenia (137,138).

Immune-Induced Platelet Destruction

Immune Thrombocytopenic Purpura

Acute Immune Thrombocytopenic Purpura. Acute ITP occurs primarily in children, but may be seen in adults (139,140). In acute ITP, there is commonly a prodrome of an acute viral illness a few weeks before the rapid onset of thrombocytopenia (141). The most common viral illnesses implicated are chickenpox, rubeola, rubella, and nonspecific upper respiratory infections (139,141,142). However, acute ITP also has been noted after vaccination with live virus for measles, mumps, chickenpox, and smallpox. In many children, spontaneous recovery will occur in days to a few weeks. The mechanisms thought to be responsible for the abrupt onset of thrombocytopenia is the binding of a virus-induced immune complex to platelets and megakaryocytes (143). Platelets are thus removed by the reticuloendothelial system, primarily in the spleen but also the liver and in part the bone marrow. In addition, megakaryocytopoiesis is compromised because of immune complex binding. Because the disease usually occurs well after the viremia has abated, the immune response against the virus produces an immune complex, which then binds to platelet membrane Fc receptors (143,144). It is noteworthy that immune complexes isolated from patients with ITP will not bind to platelets of patients with Glanzmann thrombasthenia; thus the immune complexes may be directed toward Fc receptors on platelet membrane GPs IIb or IIIa, missing from Glanzmann platelets (145). Significantly increased levels of platelet-associated IgG (PLAIgG) are noted to be present in the vast majority of cases (143). Infusions of IVIG will block the Fc receptors of phagocytic cells and subsequently reverse the thrombocytopenia, suggesting that viral antigens may be absorbed onto the platelet membrane surface, followed by immune complex formation (146).

Acute ITP commonly occurs in children and young adults. Clinical symptoms of petechiae, purpura, ecchymoses, and mucosal membrane bleeding from the gastrointestinal tract, genitourinary tract, gingiva, or epistaxis usually begin abruptly (139–143). Hemorrhagic bullae may be seen on the oral mucosa. Shotty adenopathy is common, but hepatosplenomegaly is found in fewer than 10% of patients with acute ITP. Recovery occurs in the vast majority of patients despite the mode of therapy. Recovery is usually within 2 months; but some patients may not recover for 6 to 12 months. Very few patients have recurrences, if recovery occurs. Because there is a high spontaneous remission rate in acute ITP, it is difficult to evaluate efficacy of any therapy.

Recent analysis of the approach to therapy has confirmed that existing guidelines for treatment are based on opinion rather than on level 1 evidence (147,148). Careful analysis of practice patterns have shown that the projected guidelines are not followed (149), and clinical practice is strongly propelled by the fear of intracranial hemorrhage and death, especially in pediatric practice (150). As a result, the decision to treat depends on clinical judgment of the projected risk of serious hemorrhage, often emphasized by platelet counts less than 10,000/μL. Because most therapeutic trials use the rate of increase of the platelet count, it is noteworthy that the median time to reach a platelet count more than 20,000/μL appears similar, that is approximately 3 to 5 days, whether the initial therapy is corticosteroids or IVIG (150–153). These observations led to the view that a short sharp course of steroid therapy appears a reasonable option at the initial approach to the patient (150) because the risk of significant hemorrhage is greatest at the onset. Prednisone has been found to inhibit prostacyclin (PGI_2) synthesis by the endothelium, and its rapid effect may reduce platelet inhibition and vasodilatation and provide improved "capillary integrity." Certainly, IVIG is an excellent alternative and may provide a more rapid response than prednisone. The recommended dose is a single infusion of 0.8 g/kg (152,153). Platelet transfusions are of minimal efficacy, as transfused donor platelets also are affected by the immune complex–containing recipient blood and are rapidly consumed. They should be used to abort intracranial or life-threatening hemorrhage. For those children whose thrombocytopenia does not improve, splenectomy should be considered after proper immunization.

Chronic Immune Thrombocytopenic Purpura. Chronic ITP usually occurs in adults; and women predominate 3:1. A prodrome of viral illness is absent. Chronic ITP is an immune-mediated disorder in which the immune complex attaches to platelets, leading to destruction by the spleen, bone marrow, or liver, in descending order of importance; immune-complex attachment to the megakaryocyte leading to ineffective platelet production also is operative in chronic ITP. In addition, women with chronic ITP give birth to thrombocytopenic children in 50% to 80% of cases (154).

The immunologic characterization and definition of the mechanism of the platelet destruction in ITP has lacked the benefit of good assays. PPLAIgG is elevated in 90% of patients, and serum tests for this same antibody are positive in 50% of patients (143). All four classes of IgG are found, but IgG1 has been the predominant type. It has been speculated that chronic ITP is a disorder of immunoregulation. Decreased T-suppressor cell activity has been seen. The often rapid increase in platelet counts and decrease in PAIgG after splenectomy have suggested the spleen to be both the primary site of platelet destruction, as well as the major organ of pathologic immunoglobulin synthesis in chronic ITP. In those patients failing to respond to splenectomy, the IgG may originate from the bone marrow or possibly the liver. As in acute ITP, the Fc receptor mechanism appears important; platelet destruction in ITP may occur through splenic (or other reticuloendothelial) phagocytosis with or without complement activation. The role of complement activation in platelet destruction remains unclear. Blockade of Fc receptors can result in a rapid increase in platelet counts.

A clinical and laboratory picture of ITP is well recognized in SLE, hepatitis and chronic liver disease, and in infections with human immunodeficiency virus (HIV)-1. Because these lesions have clinical and therapeutic implications somewhat different from those seen in chronic "idiopathic" (immune) thrombocytopenia, the use of an "immunologic profile" has been suggested to separate classic ITP from these other more clearly immune complex–mediated mechanisms of ITP (155). Such profile analysis showed that PAIgG, platelet C3/C4, and platelet IgM were all significantly higher in patients with diseases associated with immune complex production than were those with classic ITP. In addition, serum PEG-IC levels were similarly increased. When an immunologic panel was generated, there was no overlap between the 75th percentile for classic ITP and the 25th percentile for all immune-complex patients (155). These observations provide an infrastructure for further clarification of the immunologic mechanisms involved in the various types of ITP.

Unlike acute ITP, chronic ITP usually begins insidiously, with easy and spontaneous bruising usually preceding more serious hemorrhagic manifestations (156,157). Epistaxis and gingival bleeding are common, and petechiae and ecchymoses are usually noted. Mild splenomegaly is noted in approximately 30% of cases (156,157). The finding of marked hepatosplenomegaly should cause the consideration of a malignant lymphoma or infectious granulomatous disease.

Bone marrow examination in the presence of the classic clinical complex of ITP is rarely needed. In children, it is done in those with persistent thrombocytopenia (i.e., lasting more than 6 to 12 months) and in those unresponsive to IVIG. In adults it is recommended in those older than 60 years or in those for whom a splenectomy is planned (145).

The current practice recommendations for therapy of adults have been well defined by a panel of the American Society of Hematology; these are, however, not true evidence-based guidelines, but rather opinion derived (148). The recommendations argue against hospitalization for patients with platelet counts more than 20,000/μL who are asymptomatic or have only minor purpura. They believe that most patients with a platelet count more than 50,000/μL need no therapy. Initial therapy for patients with platelet counts less than 20,000/μL or with significant bleeding should be prednisone (1 to 2 mg/kg/day) for approximately 21 days. In general, one can anticipate that the median time to achieve a platelet count of 50,000/μL is approximately 4 days. Between 70% and 90% of patients can be expected to achieve normal platelet values in 10 to 20 days; then the steroids can be tapered over the next 2 to 4 weeks. After cessation of steroids, platelet stability is seen in 45% to 55%. Unfortunately, late recurrences (months to even years) may be seen. Patients with life-threatening bleeding should be considered candidates for IVIG therapy. Although a variety of dosage schedules have been used (148,152,153), the current recommendation is for 1 g/kg given on day 1 (and repeated on day 2 if necessary) rather than smaller doses administered over a 2- to 5-day period. In children, IVIG is considered the initial therapy of choice (148,152,153). Although the mechanism of the efficacy of IVIG in ITP is still not certain (158), durable remissions are commonly seen in children, and less commonly in adults.

Splenectomy is recommended for patients after steroids and IVIG therapy with subsequent lack of effect or relapse. A general parameter is that the patient has bleeding symptoms and platelet counts much less than 50,000/μL (preferably less than 30,000/μL) after such medical therapy. At least 2 weeks before splenectomy, the patient should be immunized with polyvalent pneumococcal vaccine, *Haemophilus influenzae* b vaccine, and quadrivalent meningococcal polysaccharide vaccine (159). Steroids should be continued to the day of surgery and continued twice daily until oral medication can be given and promptly tapered. Alternatively, IVIG can be given on the day before surgery. Approximately 80% of patients will have a sustained platelet response after surgery.

Patients for whom splenectomy fails have been considered "refractory" and have been treated with a variety of chemotherapeutic agents (e.g., azathioprine, cyclophosphamide, *Vinca* alkaloids), danazol, protein A immunoadsorption columns, plasma exchange, cyclosporine, and interferon α. In a careful review of efficacy, virtually all fall at level V evidence or less (148,160); in addition, some of these (e.g. danazol, interferon) can result in thrombocytopenia. The goal of treatment should be a safe platelet count, not a normal count (160). Because the platelets are younger than those in normal individuals, these patients commonly have a better hemostatic mechanism than expected from the count.

Recently, an anti-D polyclonal antibody (Win Rho SDF), a Rho (D) immune globulin, has been approved for treatment of acute childhood ITP, chronic adult and childhood ITP, and ITP secondary to HIV infection in nonsplenectomized Rho (D)-positive patients. Current experience in children (148) suggests the results are comparable to those with IVIG. Data in adults are still too incomplete; nevertheless, we have seen excellent durable responses; and some of these have been in splenectomized patients. An important adverse effect has been the development of alloimmune hemolysis related to the positive direct antiglobulin test, which results from treatment (148). Fc-receptor blockade may be the basis of its action; however, its long-term mechanisms may be antiidiotypic or cytokine related.

The role of thrombopoietin (TPO) in therapy is not certain. TPO levels are reduced in ITP; it is possible that such therapy could significantly increase platelet production to restore satisfactory numbers. Finally, the monoclonal antibody rituximab (Rituxan) has shown therapeutic promise, particularly in postsplenectomy failures. Its mechanism of action is unclear.

ITP in pregnancy is a complex clinical problem and merits special emphasis. Thrombocytopenia in pregnancy has multiple mechanisms, which include incidental thrombocytopenia of pregnancy (often termed gestational or pregnancy-associated thrombocytopenia); thrombocytopenia related to a hypertensive disorder during pregnancy, such as preeclampsia of HELLP syndrome; DIC; folate deficiency; HUS/TTP, as well as classic ITP (148,161–165). The term incidental thrombocytopenia of pregnancy has been applied to the occurrences of thrombocytopenia in approximately 7% of all women during otherwise normal pregnancies (161–164). The platelet count rarely is less than 70,000/μL, and most have only a slight decrease from the normal value. Actually, all women have a slight (10%) decline in their platelet counts during pregnancy, but the diagnostic label applies to that group whose values are below normal. The MPV is normal, and no hemostatic problems exist. In large part, it is a diagnosis made after excluding other biologically significant mechanisms. Its prevalence is emphasized by the fact that in a large study of patients with thrombocytopenia in pregnancy, it represented 74% of the patients. It requires no therapy, it does not produce parturitional complications, and the infants do not have thrombocytopenia. The second most common clinical event in pregnant patients with thrombocytopenia are the hypertensive disorders of pregnancy, accounting for nearly 20% of cases (158); these and related mechanisms are reviewed in Chapter 7.

True ITP accounts for 3% of all cases of thrombocytopenia at delivery (162). The lack of evidence-based data has led to opinion-based decisions relative to the care of the pregnant patient with ITP. Most use the rules used for the nonpregnant, although IVIG has been more commonly selected as first line of therapy because it does not affect the fetus (148). The route of delivery of the baby has been widely debated, but the current view is that the babies should be managed as they would for any pregnancy; the approach dictated by the obstetrical findings (163–165). This changes from the earlier era when cesarean sections were recommended (148).

The management of the newborn is a separate and important issue. A cord platelet count should be done at delivery. If it is low, the neonate should have repeated counts for at least 3 to 4 days or until resolution of the thrombocytopenia. Alloimmune neonatal thrombocytopenia can complicate ITP, producing severe thrombocytopenia requiring immediate therapy (148,164,165). It is not possible to predict which infants are likely to have severe thrombocytopenia, although it does appear that mothers with the most severe ITP are the most likely to have a severely affected infant (166–168).

Drugs and Immune-mediated Thrombocytopenia. Drugs constitute a major cause of immune thrombocytopenia. Unfortunately the list of drugs capable of pro-

TABLE 5.9. COMMON DRUGS CAUSING IMMUNE THROMBOCYTOPENIA[a]

Heparin	Chlorpropamide
Gold	Oxypenbutazone
Quinidine	Phenylbutazone
Quinine	α-Methyldopa
Sulfonamides	Bleomycin
Indomethacin	Acetazolamide
Arsenicals	Ampicillin
Aspirin	Isoniazid
Heroin	Mercurial diuretics
Valproic acid	Nitrofurantoin
Chlorothiazide	Pertussis vaccine
Chlorthalidone	Tolbutamide
Furosemide	Trimethoprim
Rifampicin	Cephalothins
Digitalis derivatives	Sulindac (Clinoril)
Diphenylhydantoin	Penicillin
Cimetidine	Procainamide
Acetaminophen	

[a]In descending order of incidence.

ducing decreased platelet numbers is very long, and most commonly when the thrombocytopenia is recognized, the patient is usually taking several possible agents, making the specific etiologic diagnosis difficult (169–172). Laboratory delineation of the drug-dependent antibodies is difficult and generally not available. As a result, clinical judgment relative to the drug is important; then the resolution of the thrombocytopenia after drug removal has been used as the diagnostic approach. A recent careful review of the published case reports provides the best current analysis of drugs with level I and level II evidence (173) (Table 5.9).

Drug-induced ITP is suggested by a rapid onset of petechiae and purpura and profound thrombocytopenia. The patient may have been ingesting the drug for a very variable duration, even years. This is in distinction to nonimmune drug-induced thrombocytopenia, in which the platelet count decreases very slowly and returns to normal slowly after discontinuation of the offending drug. Catastrophic intracranial hemorrhage is rare. Many patients have constitutional symptoms of fever, chills, headaches, generalized malaise, nausea, and emesis as the bleeding occurs. Unlike nonimmune drug-induced thrombocytopenia, immune-mediated drug-induced thrombocytopenia usually, but not always, abates rapidly after removing the offending drug; the response is usually seen in weeks to a few months.

The diagnosis is made by the sudden onset of petechiae and purpura associated with thrombocytopenia in a patient ingesting one or more drugs, providing the need for a careful drug history. Laboratory confirmation can be pursued by documenting the presence of PAIgG and agglutination of normal platelets when incubated with the patient's serum and the offending drug.

Therapy for drug-induced immune thrombocytopenia consists of discontinuation of all suspected drugs, hospitalization of the patient if the platelet count is less than $50,000/cm^2$ or significant hemorrhage is present, avoidance of any drug or compound known to interfere with platelet function, and careful observation for suggestions of the potential for significant hemorrhage. IVIG and steroids are of benefit in life-threatening hemorrhage. Platelet transfusions have a shortened platelet life span, but can be used in intracranial or massive hemorrhage.

Heparin-induced Thrombocytopenia and Thrombosis Currently the most common cause of immune thrombocytopenia is heparin (174). Two clinical forms of heparin-induced thrombocytopenia (HIT) are now recognized. The first, now commonly termed HIT-I, is nonidiosyncratic and nonimmune (Table 5.10). As shown in Table 5.10, the thrombocytopenia occurs early in the exposure, within the first few days of therapy in the heparin naïve, and within hours in the patient previously exposed to heparin. The decline in platelet numbers is modest (10% to 30%), and it is not associated with any clinical manifestations. The thrombocytopenia is the result of platelet aggregation by uncertain mechanism(s). High(er)-molecular-weight heparins have the greatest likelihood of producing this change. The episodes are transient, and platelet counts normalize, in spite of continued exposure to heparin. There is no evidence that this clinical labora-

TABLE 5.10. HEPARIN-INDUCED THROMBOCYTOPENIA TYPE I (NONIMMUNE; NONIDIOSYNCRATIC)

Episode of thrombocytopenia occurs early in exposure: generally in first few days in naïve and in first hours in previously exposed
Mild thrombocytopenia: 10%–30% decrease in platelet numbers
Clinical manifestations: None
Mechanism: Heparin-induced platelet aggregation
Incidence: Uncertain but common
Biologic issues: Counts normalize even with continued therapy
Therapy: None
Relationship to HIT type II: Unclear; but probably none

HIT, heparin-induced thrombocytopenia.

TABLE 5.11. CLINICAL FEATURES OF HEPARIN-INDUCED THROMBOCYTOPENIA II

Usual onset at day 3–14 (median, day 10)
Nadir platelet count: usually 30–60,000, but may be as low as 5,000. The most appropriate defination is a 50% decrease in platelet numbers from the baseline values
Risk factors:
- Occurs with all methods of administration:
  - Most common: continuous infusion of unfractionated heparin
  - Amount not critical; can even be seen with heparin flushes: 500/U/d or heparin-coated catheters: 3/U/h
  - More frequent with i.v. than s.c. administration
  - Greater: bovine > porcine > LMW heparins
- Can occur within hours in previously treated patients
- Increased incidence with recent surgery (primarily venous problems)
- Increased incidence with preexisting cardiovascular disease (primarily arterial)
- Absent risks:
  - Equal in men and women
  - Age not a factor
  - No relation to inherited deficiency or founder defects of clotting factors

i.v., intravenous; LMW, low molecular weight; s.c., subcutaneous.

tory event is related to the more serious immune form of HIT-II (175).

In contrast, HIT-II is an immune-mediated lesion with serious clinical sequelae and significant morbidity and mortality (174–182). The common clinical characteristics are shown in Table 5.11. The usual recognition of the decreased number of platelets is generally at 3 to 14 days (median, day 10); however, prior exposure to heparin can result in precipitate declines in circulating platelet numbers, even within hours.

Historically, the diagnosis was based on a decrease in platelets to fewer than 1000,000/μL. It is now clear that clinical sequelae can occur when a significant decline in platelet numbers occurs, even when the usual parameter of true thrombocytopenia is not present (183,184). Currently the best working rule is that the diagnosis must be considered when platelet numbers have declined to 50% of their baseline levels (174). This implies that the thrombocytopenia may be relative rather than absolute. Postoperative patients who have undergone cardiac surgery (particularly bypass procedures) have special criteria, because most such patients have platelet counts in the 100,000 to 150,000/μL range in the first postoperative day. For them the diagnosis of HIT-II should be based on a platelet count that is reduced 50% from the postoperative day 1 platelet count (174).

A very important clinical rule is that HIT-II can occur with any amount of heparin administered by any route. Although it is most common with the continuous infusion of unfractionated heparin, it has occurred with heparin flushes as low as 500 U per day, and even with heparin-coated catheters with which the delivery can be as low as 3 U per hour (174,176,181,182,185,186).

An important component of HIT-II is the development of thrombotic lesions. This is ominous and is associated with a significant morbidity and mortality. Its threat, therapeutic urgency, and treatment complexities are such that the term heparin-induced thrombocytopenia–thrombosis has been applied to highlight this sequence. Even with very severe thrombocytopenia (counts less than 10,000/μL), thrombosis is a more common sequel than is bleeding. Vascular thrombosis had been correlated with large-vessel arterial occlusions, and the term "white clot syndrome" was popular to describe a massive extremity arterial occlusion (187–189). We now know that thrombotic events occur in both the arterial and venous circulation (174–176). Unfortunately, we cannot predict either the subsequent advent of thrombosis as HIT develops or its site.

The common diagnostic criteria for HIT-II are shown in Table 5.12. Other causes of thrombocytopenia should be excluded. Unfortunately the onset of symptoms and signs

TABLE 5.12. HEPARIN-INDUCED THROMBOCYTOPENIA TYPE II (IMMUNE–IDIOSYNCRATIC)

Common diagnostic criteria are:
- Thrombocytopenia: decrease of ≥50% from baseline platelet numbers
- Absence of other cause
- Confirmation by a heparin-associated antibody assay
- Return to normal platelet numbers when heparin stopped

may be very abrupt; a long, agonizing clinical evaluation of other potential mechanisms is not appropriate. Prompt clinical judgment must be exercised. Similarly, a delay in diagnosis and therapy to await a serologic confirmation is not reasonable. From the studies of Walenga et al. (184,185,190), it is now evident that no one test for its presence can serve as the diagnostic "gold standard," further emphasizing the importance of clinical judgment. This is particularly important in that as many as 45% of the thrombotic episodes in HIT-II occur in the first 48 hours after identification of the thrombocytopenia (189,190). A delay in diagnosis to await laboratory confirmation can therefore result in serious clinical risk.

Comorbid diseases are particularly important in HIT. Concurrent illness can alter the pattern and severity of onset of HIT-II. Another difficult aspect of HIT-II is the circumstance of "delayed onset of HIT-II." Clinical features and thrombocytopenia have been seen to develop 7 to 14 days after discontinuing the heparin therapy (174,175). Although it is uncommon, the clinician must be aware of such potential; this further complicates the role of confirmatory testing.

The true incidence of HIT-II is not certain, although an occurrence in 1% to 5% of all heparin-treated individuals is a reasonable figure (174–183). Determination of incidence has been hampered by the specific diagnostic criteria (i.e., what platelet change or absolute platelet count should serve as the diagnostic marker, are positive serologic tests required for the diagnosis, and how does one vector in comorbid diseases in the determination (191–193).

Several controversies exist in the emerging clinical understanding of HIT-II. First the level of platelet numbers or change of platelet numbers from the baseline level to serve as the clinical parameter of diagnosis and thereby provide the parameter to perform other laboratory studies and alter therapy is not yet absolutely established. Second, the issue of whether incidence can be defined only by a specific serologic assay continues to be controversial and will probably always be so, as long as no single absolute assay defines all cases. The clinical evidence that up to 45% of the thrombotic episodes occur in the first 48 hours after the recognition of HIT-II strongly interdicts "waiting for laboratory confirmation" before a therapeutic action, particularly now, when excellent alternatives to heparin are available. Third, the exact incidence of thrombosis is not well defined in HIT-II. Fourth, whether an HIT-II thrombosis is clinically more dangerous in circumstances in which the patient is being treated with heparin for a thrombosis, and the true role of comorbid conditions are not settled issues. Fifth, the relation of an uncommonly described event, that of the paradoxical thrombotic complication of venous limb gangrene in patients taking heparin during their transition to oral anticoagulant therapy with coumadin is not fully clarified.

Therapy for HIT demands immediate cessation of heparin therapy and resolute avoidance of platelet transfusions. Effective alternatives to heparin are now available and should be instituted. The direct thrombin inhibitors argatroban, lepirudin, bivaliruden and melagatran, are now excellent choices. Presently bivaliruden is approved only after angioplasty; melagatran is being formulated as a prodrug in an oral preparation (H376/95), which should have great potential. Argatroban is our current drug of choice because it is partially reversibly bound to thrombin, it can be used in patients with decreased renal function, and dose adjustments are not needed (174,194–196).

Posttransfusion Purpura

Posttransfusion purpura is a rare event and occurs approximately 1 week after transfusions in a patient who is PLA1 negative. Ninety-eight percent of the population is PLA1 positive; thus the transfused patient who is PLA1 negative has a high risk of receiving incompatible (PLA1-positive) platelets. The vast majority of cases are seen in women who are PLA1 negative and have been previously sensitized by either transfusion or pregnancy (197). A few cases have occurred in PLA1-positive patients and some in nonsensitized individuals, suggesting that in rare instances, other platelet antibodies must be involved (198). Patients with Glanzmann thrombasthenia are lacking platelet GPIIb/IIIa and are PLA1 negative (199); thus it appears that the PLA1 antigen site may be associated with platelet membrane GPIIIa or the IIb/IIIa complex. The clinical course is typically that of a sudden onset of petechiae, purpura, and mucosal membrane hemorrhage in association with thrombocytopenia during the first week after transfusions. Some described a mild transfusion reaction consisting of chills and fever at the time of their transfusion (200). In most cases, anti-PLA1 antibody can be easily demonstrated in the laboratory. In the majority of patients, the thrombocytopenia will spontaneously abate in 2 weeks to 2 months, but in rare instances, a protracted course occurs. Platelet transfusions should not be used, as further isoimmunization of the patient may occur (200,201). Steroids are of uncertain benefit. If severe thrombocytopenia is present (platelet count less than 10,000/mL) or if significant hemorrhage is seen or suspected, the patient should be treated with plasma exchange to remove the anti-PLA1 antibody (202). This mode of therapy has almost always been successful and is the treatment of choice in high-risk patients.

THROMBOCYTOSIS AND THROMBOCYTHEMIA

Thrombocytosis refers to a benign secondary reactive increase in the platelet count. Thrombocytosis is usually associated with increased platelet production or interference with splenic pooling of platelets, such as postsplenectomy thrombocytosis, thrombocytosis after epinephrine infusion, or the use of large doses of steroids. *Thrombocythemia,* on the other hand, refers to a primary, uncontrolled (malignant) increase in platelet counts; this may accompany any of the myeloproliferative syndromes, especially polycythemia vera and chronic myelogenous leukemia, or may represent a malignant transformation of the megakaryocyte or stem cell precursor of the megakaryocyte; this latter myeloproliferative disorder is referred to as essential or primary thrombocythemia.

Pseudothrombocytosis

This is an uncommon event that can be seen in any form of cryoglobulinemia. It is due to protein precipitates that are misidentified by electronic counters as "platelet-sized" particles; examination of the blood smear will correct this error. Alternatively the clinician must be aware that because current automated blood cell counting is based on impedance, large platelets are often counted as white cells, thereby underestimating the platelet numbers, particularly in thrombocythemia.

Thrombocytosis

Thrombocytosis is benign and asymptomatic and is commonly associated with acute or chronic inflammatory disorders, infections, and cancer (203). The common clinical circumstances associated with thrombocytosis are shown in Table 5.13. In thrombocytosis, platelets display normal morphologic features and function normally; this is in contrast to thrombocythemia, in which platelet morphology and platelet function are commonly abnormal.

Patients with thrombocytosis are asymptomatic and require no therapy. An increased risk of thrombosis is seen in two selected instances of reactive thrombocytosis; the first instance is seen in postsplenectomy thrombocytosis in the presence of anemia of any etiology (1,203). Very rarely thrombocytosis associated with severe iron deficiency may have an increased risk of thrombosis. The reactive thrombocytosis associated with iron-deficiency anemia will usually promptly cease within 1 week of initiating appropriate iron therapy.

Reactive thrombocytosis may be associated with laboratory findings of hyperkalemia, hypercalcemia, and, occasionally, decreased pO_2 levels due to increased platelet consumption by the increased platelet population. These laboratory findings are in vitro events, and can be corrected by proper and prompt handling of the phlebotomy tubes.

Primary (Essential) Thrombocythemia

Thrombohemorrhagic events are the clinical hallmarks of primary thrombocythemia, commonly termed "essential" thrombocythemia in the United States, and recently entitled thrombocythemia vera in Europe (204). Primary thrombocythemia is a clonal disorder of the multipotent stem cell (205), and it is clinically grouped as a myeloproliferative lesion (e.g., chronic myelogenous leukemia, polycythemia vera, myelofibrosis with myeloid metaplasia, and primary thrombocythemia). These clinical entities are interrelated because of their pattern of clonal expansion, the evidence of transition of one form to another during their course, and the uncertainty of the basic pathophysiologic mechanism for the specific lineage amplification and proliferation that each expresses.

It is now evident that many patients with primary thrombocythemia may have a clinically silent presentation and even a prolonged stable uneventful clinical status. This has provided significant hesitation in labeling a disease

TABLE 5.13. CLINICAL CIRCUMSTANCES ASSOCIATED WITH THROMBOCYTOSIS (REACTIVE THROMBOCYTOSIS)

- Acute and transient:
  - Persisting minutes to hours
    - Epinephrine
    - Exercise
  - Persisting hours to a few days
    - Acute blood loss
    - Recovery from acute infection
    - After (rebound) thrombocytopenia
      - Post immune
      - After cytoreductive chemotherapy (especially methotrexate and *Vinca* agents)
      - After megaloblastic anemia
      - After alcohol-associated thrombocytopenia
- Chronic
  - Persisting during a significant duration of
    - Chronic blood loss with iron deficiency
    - Chronic inflammatory disease
    - Chronic infectious disease
    - Cancer
    - Hemolytic anemia
  - Potential life-long: after splenectomy (auto or surgical)

process in an asymptomatic patient. In addition, the absence of a specific cytogenetic or molecular marker has led to the misconception that definite diagnostic parameters do not exist. That these are real dilemmas is emphasized by the changing criteria for diagnosis over the past 20-year period (204,206).

The defining clinical laboratory feature of primary thrombocythemia is the recognition of an elevated platelet count, to which correlative clinical findings and relations are related. Therefore, the initial clinical consideration must be certain that true thrombocythemia is present, and that the laboratory report of elevated circulating platelets is not due to pseudothrombocytosis or due to (reactive) thrombocytosis.

The diagnostic criteria for primary thrombocythemia have slowly evolved, over recent decades, and these continue to be refined as new biologic data have become available. The Polycythemia Vera Study Group (PVSG) developed criteria in 1975 that used platelet counts greater than 1,000,000/μL as the essential diagnostic parameter (207–209). These "platelet millionaires" (210) frequently manifested hemorrhagic clinical features on presentation. As the disease process became better understood and the sometime subtle thrombotic features were recognized, the specific criterion of a given platelet number was progressively modified downward, and the correlated clinical findings better defined (206,211–214). Recently the European Working Group on Myeloproliferative Disorders proposed new diagnostic criteria in light of the growing evidence that bone marrow morphologic findings have become more specific, splenomegaly more commonly recognized with the newer imaging technology, and in vitro culture of hematopoietic progenitors more informative (204,215). This criterion does imply that any elevated platelet count is abnormal; their number is 400,000/μL. They believe that the previous use of significantly higher platelet counts as the initial parameter of diagnosis failed to recognize that the clinical symptom complex often seen in patients with primary thrombocythemia has an inexact correlation with specific platelet numbers. In a similar mode, the criteria we have been using (Table 5.14) acknowledges that an elevated platelet count is the primary initial clinical recognition unit, that the only reasonable line of demarcation is that of a count elevated beyond that which is normal for that laboratory, and that the increased number is confirmed by a repeated analysis. Because most laboratories in the United States use 440,000/μL as the upper limit of normal, our number is admittedly different from that in Europe. Further confirmation of the wisdom of these parameters is emphasized by long-term study of patients receiving therapy who developed thrombohemorrhagic complications; all occurred at platelet counts greater than 400,000/μL (216), although some continue to emphasize only the marrow findings (217).

Because the differential diagnostic confusion in the past related to those cases of thrombocythemia associated with a myelodysplastic or other myeloproliferative state, these lesions should be eliminated from the diagnostic consideration by appropriate evaluation. Morphologic examination of the peripheral blood and bone marrow material has confirmed architectural changes that help define the disease. Abnormal platelets and aggregation are commonly seen in the peripheral blood. Increased mature, often hyperploid, megakaryocytes are seen in the marrow and, in the absence of a significant increase in fibrosis or proliferative erythroid or myeloid changes, serve to clarify the nature of these changes. Evaluation of leukocyte alkaline phosphate activity and erythrocyte sedimentation rates used by our European colleagues has largely disappeared from clinical practice in the United States, because these are nonspecific parameters. Finally, it merits comment that some degree of splenomegaly, albeit it usually less than 4 cm, often identified only by imaging methods, does commonly occur in primary thrombocythemia.

Historically Epstein and Goedel (218) are credited with the description, in 1934, of a hemorrhagic disorder associated with increased numbers of circulating platelets. This may well have been a case of "reactive thrombocytosis," because postmortem examination in this 56-year-old man identified an atrophic spleen weighing 7 g. In 1960, Fred Gunz (219) carefully reviewed five of his own cases and 50 previously reported patients and delineated the clinical features of primary ("hemorrhagic" or "essential") thrombocythemia, establishing this syndrome with the unusual presentation of either a thrombotic or hemorrhagic or

TABLE 5.14. DIAGNOSTIC CRITERIA FOR PRIMARY (ESSENTIAL) THROMBOCYTHEMIA

Platelet count >4,500,000 per μL (confirmed on more than one occasion)
Absence of an identifiable cause for the increased platelet counts
Absence of a myelodysplastic syndrome or other myeloproliferative state
Bone marrow with
Megakaryocytic hyperplasia
Fibrosis less than 1/3 of marrow cross section
Ancillary supportive criteria
Spenomegaly
In vitro: spontaneous megakaryocyte colony formation

thrombohemorrhagic diathesis, in the presence of increased numbers of platelets (216–225). The clinical features have been well defined (220–227).

The usual patient is older than 50 years, although cases have been seen in those as young as 2 years (225). Bleeding is generally mild and primarily involves mucous membranes, skin, or retina. Thrombotic lesions, especially of the microvessel bed, are the most common and serious clinical problem. Their multiplicity often provides the evidence to support the clinical recognition of the disease. One especially interesting microvascular lesion is that of erythromelalgia; the occurrence of painful, burning, itching palms and soles.

This is nearly a pathognomonic finding in patients with primary thrombocythemia, although the same findings do occur in polycythemia vera with associated thrombocythemia (228,229). Erythromelalgia has a very characteristic clinical pattern that often provides an immediate diagnosis simply by eliciting the history. It commonly begins as acroparethesias or itching sensations of the feet. Promptly the balls of the feet become painful and burning. Often the feet and toes appear red and congested. The pain can be severe and is sometimes precipitated by exercise or heat (229). These episodes have occurred with even only marginal elevations in circulatory platelet numbers. Significant histopathologic changes have been characterized by arteriolar vascular changes with swollen endothelial cells and fibromuscular internal proliferation (229). The remarkable feature of this lesion is the prompt and immediate response of the entire symptom complex with the administration of aspirin.

Griesshammer et al. (230) reviewed 11 retrospective clinical studies of 809 patients and identified cerebral artery, portal venous (with associated Budd–Chiari syndrome), and coronary atherothrombosis in a surprisingly high number of cases. Thus although the past focus was on changes in the microcirculation, it is clear that large-vessel involvement occurs. One intermediate vessel-bed thrombosis does provide a special clinical presentation, that of priapism.

A high incidence of obstetrical complications occurs in women with thrombocythemia. Placental vessel thrombosis with infarction and related spontaneous abortions are common events. It is of note that spontaneous declines in platelet numbers often occur during the course of the pregnancy, and these patients have successful term pregnancies. Similarly, in those patients whose platelet aggregation is controlled with aspirin, and platelet numbers reduced with interferon, successful pregnancies can be expected.

Two other clinical findings include splenomegaly of a slight degree (1 to 4 cm), as seen in nearly 70% of patients. In addition, hypertension is seen in nearly one third of patients and may represent a comorbid condition that increases the risk of an occlusive vascular lesion.

The pathophysiology of primary (essential) thrombocythemia is not completely clear. Although initially considered a clonal disorder with potential neoplastic implications, it is now evident that it is a heterogeneous disorder. Hereditary thrombocythemia has been identified in several families as an autosomal dominant pattern, but their findings have been variable with mutations in the thrombopoietin gene (231), as well as upstream gene abnormalities (232). In the common nonhereditary patients, thrombopoietin levels are not appropriately downregulated as one would expect with the increased platelet number, suggesting dysregulation of the megakaryocyte pool (233); although reduced expression of the Mpl receptor has been seen (234).

The endovascular changes have been well defined. These include swollen large cellular nuclei, lumen narrowing due to proliferation of smooth muscle cells with vacuolization and swelling of the cytoplasm and deposition of intercellular material, and fragmentation of the internal elastic lamina (228,235). Changes in platelet architecture and function have been related to both clinical symptoms and the endothelial changes described. These changes include platelet-size heterogeneity and ultrastructural changes, as well as elevated levels of platelet-specific proteins, increased thromboxane generation, and the expression of activation-dependent epitopes on the platelet surface (236). Finally, an inverse relation has been seen in patients with thrombocythemia between high platelet counts and large von Willebrand multimers. The increased platelets are thought to be caused by increased degradation of platelet-bound von Willebrand multimers (237). These effects have been considered an additional factor for hemostatic problems in thrombocythemia.

The therapy for patients with primary thrombocythemia has focused on the use of antiaggregating agents and the reduction of circulating platelet numbers. Traditionally, concern regarding the use of platelet antiaggregating agents has focused on the evidence that platelet dysfunction is commonly seen in primary thrombocythemia. Some of the hemorrhagic phenomena have been ascribed to such defective platelet function. These findings led to a fear of any agent that could further affect platelet function. This thesis was perturbed by evidence that aspirin could reverse vascular lesions and even incipient gangrene (238). More recently, aspirin has been shown to improve neurologic function, even in the continued presence of increased platelet numbers (239). It is now quite clear that aspirin is effective at reducing clinical symptoms and signs in patients with vascular occlusive lesions (230,240–243). The use of aspirin has become an important therapeutic agent during pregnancy (241,243–246). Aspirin has been effective in helping patients carry a pregnancy to successful term.

The major therapeutic focus has been on the reduction of platelet numbers. Virtually every cytoreductive chemotherapeutic agent has been explored in therapy. Most are successful, but the side effects are prohibitive. Hydroxyurea, a ribonucleoside reductase inhibitor (247,248) has emerged as the cytoreductive agent of choice. It has been easy to use, with few side effects; daily oral doses beginning at 500 to 1,000 mg can subsequently be titrated for continued control (203,206). It had been considered a very safe agent, but recent reports of myelodysplasia and leukemia (249–251) suggest that care be expressed in its long-term use.

The biologic response modifier, interferon-α, has been shown to lower platelet counts in patients with primary and secondary thrombocythemia (252–256). Its mechanism of action appears to be mediated by an inhibitory effect of the interferon on megakaryocytopoiesis, as discussed earlier. The usual therapeutic dose is 25 million units subcutaneously per week, given in divided (four to six) doses per week. Unfortunately, only approximately 50% of patients achieve a stable state of remission with interferon therapy. In addition, on cessation of the therapy, recurrence of the clinical and laboratory findings is usual.

After almost a decade of clinical trials anagrelide has become an important addition to the therapeutic armamentarium for patients with thrombocythemia, regardless of the underlying form of myeloproliferative disease. It was originally introduced because it had anti–cyclic adenosine monophosphate (AMP) phosphodiesterase activity that inhibited platelet aggregation (257). Evidence of a dose-dependent reduction in platelet numbers in normal individuals (258) and in patients with thrombocythemia (259–261) has led to use as an important therapeutic modality. The exact mechanism of action is not completely defined, but in vitro and in vivo studies have shown that it altered the maturation of megakaryocytes, with a resultant decrease in their size and morphologic abnormalities (262). It is of note that other studies of platelet survival and proliferation of the megakaryocyte committed progenitor pool were normal. In general, initial starting doses can be 0.5 mg, given 2 to 4 times per day. A significant decline in platelet numbers is usually evident in 7 to 14 days, and dose adjustments can then be done. Anagrelide does have a vasodilatory effect, and headaches, postural hypotension, and fluid retention have been seen as side effects. Palpitations and tachycardia are seen in nearly a fourth of patients; these seem to be significantly worse in patients who ingest coffee close to the time of a dose of the drug. These symptoms generally disappear after 4 to 8 weeks of therapy.

REFERENCES

1. Bick RL. Quantitative platelet defects. In: *Hematology: clinical and laboratory practice* St. Louis: Mosby, 1993:1337.
2. Rutherford CJ, Frenkel EP. Thrombocytopenia: issues in diagnosis and therapy. *Med Clin North Am* 1994;78:55.
3. Mammen EF, Comp PC, Gosselin R, et al. PFA-100 system: a new method for assessment of platelet dysfunction. *Semin Thromb Hemost* 1998;24:195.
4. Broudy VC, Kaushansky K. Thrombopoietin, the C-mpl ligand is a major regulator of platelet production. *J Leukoc Biol* 1995; 57:719.
5. Emmons RVB, Reid DM, Cohen RL, et al. Human thrombopoietin levels are high when thrombocytopenia is due to megakaryocyte deficiency and low when due to increased platelet destruction. *Blood* 1996;87:4068.
6. Engel C, Loeffler M, Franke H, et al. Endogenous thrombopoietin serum levels during multicycle chemotherapy. *Br J Heme* 1999;105:832.
7. Porcelijn L, Folman CC, Bossers B, et al. The diagnostic value of thrombopoietin levels measurements in thrombocytopenia. *Thromb Haemost* 1998;79:1101.
8. Beer JH, Buchi L, Steiner B. Glycocalicin: a new assay: the normal plasma levels and its potential usefulness in selected diseases. *Blood* 1994;3:691.
9. Alexander WS, Roberts AW, Nicola NA, et al. Deficiencies in progenitor cells of multiple hematopoietic lineages and defective megakaryocytopoiesis in mice lacking the thrombopoietin receptor c-mpl. *Blood* 1996;87:2162.
10. Sabath DE, Kaushansky K, Broydy VC. Deletion of the extracellular membrane-distal cytokine receptor homology module of Mpl results in constitutive cell growth and loss of thrombopoietin binding. *Blood* 1999;94:365.
11. Drachman JG, Kauskansky K. Dissecting the thrombopoietin receptor: functional elements of the Mpl domain. *Proc Natl Acad Sci U S A* 1997;94:2350.
12. Oudenrijn SVD, Bruin M, Folmon CC, et al. Mutations in the thrombopoietin receptor, Mpl, in children with congenital a megakaryocytic thrombocytopenia. *Br J Heme* 2000;110:441.
13. Watkins SP Jr, Shulman NR. Platelet cold agglutinins. *Blood* 1970;36:153.
14. Shreiner DP, Bell WR. Pseudothrombocytopenia: manifestation of a new type of platelet agglutinin. *Blood* 1973; 42:541.
15. Veenhoven WA. Pseudothrombocytopenia due to agglutinins. *Am J Clin Pathol* 1979;72:1005.
16. Onder O, Weinstein A, CW Hoyer. Pseudothrombocytopenia caused by platelet agglutinins that are reactive in blood anticoagulated by chelating agents. *Blood* 1980;56:177.
17. Zeigler Z. In vitro granulocyte-platelet rosette formation mediated by an IgG immunoglobulin. *Haemostasis* 1974;3:282.
18. Kjeldsberg CR, Swanson J. Platelet satellitism. *Blood* 1974;43:831.
19. Payne BA, Pierre RV. Pseudothrombocytopenia: laboratory artifact with potentially serious consequences. *Mayo Clin Proc* 1984;59:123.
20. Lombarts AJ, de Kieviet W. Recognition and prevention of pseudo-thrombocytopenia and concomitant pseudoleukocytosis. *Am J Clin Pathol* 1988;89:634.
21. O'Neill EM, Varadi S. Neonatal aplastic anaemia and Fanconi's anaemia. *Arch Dis Child* 1963;38:92.
22. Nilsson LR. Chronic pancytopenia with multiple congenital abnormalities. *Acta Paediatr* 1960;49:518.
23. Faivre L, Guardiola P, Lewis C, et al. Association of complementation group and mutation type with clinical outcome in Fanconi anemia. *Blood* 2000;96:4064.
24. Hall JG, Levin J, Kuhn JP, et al. Thrombocytopenia with absent radius (TAR). *Medicine* 1969;78:411.
25. Berge T, Brunnhage F, Nisson LR. Congenital thrombocytopenia in rubella embryopathy. *Acta Paediatr Scand* 1963;52:349.
26. Ballmaier M, Schulze H, Straub G, et al. Thrombopoietin inpatients with congenital thrombopoietin and absent radii: elevated serum levels, normal receptor expression, but defective reactivity to thrombopoietin. *Blood* 1997;90:612.
27. Perry GS. The Wiskott-Aldrich syndrome in the United States and Canada (1892-1979). *J Pediatr* 1980;97:72.
28. Aldrich RA, Steinberg AG, Campbell DC. Pedigree demonstrating a sex-linked recessive condition characterized by draining ears, eczematoid dermatitis, and bloody diarrhea. *Pediatrics* 1954;3:133.

29. Ochs ND, Slichter SJ, Harker LA, et al. The Wiskott-Aldrich syndrome: studies of lymphocytes, granulocytes and platelets. *Blood* 1980;55:243.
30. Lum LG, Tubergen DG, Corash L, et al. Splenectomy in the management of the thrombocytopenia of Wiskott-Aldrich syndrome. *N Engl J Med* 1980;302:892.
31. Godwin NA, Ginsburg AD. May-Hegglin anomaly: a defect in megakaryocyte fragmentation. *Br J Haematol* 1974;26:117.
32. Kunishima S, Kujima T, Matsushita T, et al. Mutations in the NMMHC-A gene cause autosomal dominant macrothrombocytopenia with leukocyte inclusions (May-Hegglin anomaly/Sebastian syndrome). *Blood* 2001;97:117.
33. Gardner F, Bessman JD. Thrombocytopenia due to defective platelet production. *Clin Haematol* 1983;12:23.
34. Bernheim J, Dechavanne M, Bryon PA, et al. Thrombocytopenia, macrothrombocytopathia, nephritis, and deafness. *Am J Med* 1976;61:145.
35. Clare NM, Montiel MM, Lifschitz MD, et al. Alport's syndrome associated with macrothrombopathic thrombocytopenia. *Am J Clin Pathol* 1979;72:111.
36. Raccuglia G. Gray platelet syndrome: a variety of qualitative platelet disorders. *Am J Med* 1971;51:818.
37. Takahashi N, Nagayama R, Hattori A, et al. Von Willebrand disease associated with familial thrombocytopenia and increased ristocetin-induced platelet aggregation. *Am J Hematol* 1981; 10:89.
38. Gale RP, Champlin RE, Feig SA. Aplastic anemia: biology and treatment. *Ann Intern Med* 1981;95:477.
39. Lewis SM, Gordon-Smith EC. Aplastic and dysplastic anaemias. In: Hardisty RM, Weatherall DJ, eds. *Blood and its disorders.* Oxford: Blackwell Scientific, 1982:1229.
40. Stoll DB, Blum S, Pasquale B, et al. Thrombocytopenia with decreased megakaryocytes: evaluation and prognosis. *Ann Intern Med* 1980;94:170.
41. Atchinson RGM, Marsh JCW, Hows JM. Pregnancy associated aplastic anemia: a report of 5 cases and review of current management. *Br J Haematol* 1989;73:541.
42. Fleming AF. Hypoplastic anemia in pregnancy. *Br Med J* 1973; 3:166.
43. Cohen T, Cooney DP. Cyclic thrombocytopenia: case report and review of the literature. *Scand J Haematol* 1974;12:9.
44. Skoog WA, Lawrence JS, Adams WS. A metabolic study of a patient with idiopathic cyclical thrombocytopenic purpura. *Blood* 1957;12:844.
45. Engstrom E, Lundquist A, Soderstrom N. Periodic thrombocytopenia or tidal platelet dysgenesis in a man. *Scand J Haematol* 1966;3:290.
46. Clawson CC, White JG, Nerzberg MC. Platelet interaction with bacteria: contrasting the role of fibrinogen and fibronectin. *Am J Hematol* 1980;9:43.
47. Espinoza C, Kuhn C. Viral infection of megakaryocytes in varicella with purpura. *Am J Clin Pathol* 1974;61:203.
48. Alter HJ, Scanlon RT, Schechter GP. Thrombocytopenic purpura following vaccination with attenuated measles virus. *Am J Dis Child* 1968;115:111.
49. Osborn JE, Shahadi NT. Thrombocytopenia in murine cytomegalovirus infection. *J Lab Clin Med* 1973;81:53.
50. Chesney PJ, Shahidi NT. Acute viral-induced thrombocytopenia: a review of human disease, animal models, and in vitro studies. In: Lusher AJM, Barnhart MI, eds. *Acquired bleeding disorders of children.* New York: Masson Publishers, 1981:65.
51. Carter RL. Platelet levels in infectious mononucleosis. *Blood* 1965;25:817.
52. Cohen P, Gardner FH. Thrombocytopenia as a laboratory sign and complication of gram negative bacteremic infection. *Arch Intern Med* 1966;117:113.
53. Lewis JH, Zucker MB, Ferguson JH. Bleeding tendency in uremia. *Blood* 1956;11:1073.
54. Rabiner SF. Uremic bleeding. *Prog Hemost Thromb* 1972;1:233.
55. Hartmann RC, Jonkins DE. Paroxysmal nocturnal hemoglobinuria: current concepts of certain pathophysiological features. *Blood* 1965; 25:850.
56. Dacie JV. Paroxysmal nocturnal hemoglobinuria. *Proc R Soc Med* 1963;56:587.
57. Bessler M, Mason PJ, Hillmen P, et al. Somatic mutations and cellular selection in paroxysmal nocturnal hemoglobinuria. *Lancet* 1994;343:951.
58. Bessler M, Mason PF, Hillmen P, et al. Mutations in the PIG-A gene causing partial deficiency of GP linked surface proteins (PNH II) in patients with paroxysmal nocturnal hemoglobinuria. *Br J Hematol* 1994;87:863.
59. Ware RE, Rosse WF, Howard TA. Mutations within the PIGA gene in patients with paroxysmal nocturnal hemoglobinuria. *Blood* 1994;83:2418.
60. Luzzatto L, Nafa K. Genetics of PNII. In: Young NS, Moss J, eds. *Paroxysmal nocturnal hemoglobinuria and the GPI linked proteins.* New York: Academic Press, 2000:21.
61. Murphy S. Thrombocytosis and thrombocythaemia. *Clin Haematol* 1983;12:89.
62. Smith MD, DA Smith, Fletcher M. Hemorrhage associated with thrombocytopenia in megaloblastic anemia. *Br Med J* 1962;1:982.
63. Levine PH. A qualitative platelet defect in severe vitamin B12 deficiency: response, hyperresponse, and thrombosis after vitamin B12 therapy. *Ann Intern Med* 1973;78:533.
64. Frenkel EP, Yardley DA. Clinical and laboratory features and sequelae of deficiency of folic acid (folate) and vitamin B_{12} (cobalamin) in pregnancy and gynecology. *HematolOncol Clin North Am* 2000;14:1079.
65. Novotny VMJ. Prevention and management of platelet transfusion refractoriness. *Vox San* 1999;76:1.
66. Delaflor-Weiss E, Mintz P. The evaluation and management of platelet refractoriness and alloimmunization. *Transfus Med Rev* 2000;14:180.
67. Holmberg L. The biology and currently approved uses of interleukin-11. *Res Pract* 2000;2:4–11.
68. Kaye JA. The clinical development of recombinant human interleukin 11 (Neumega ih IL-11 growth factor). *Stem Cell* 1996;14:256.
69. Cairo MS. Dose reductions and delays: limitations of myelosuppressive chemotherapy. *Oncology* 2000;14(suppl 8):21.
70. Tepler I, Elias I, Smith JW, et al. A randomized placebo controlled study of recombinant human interleukin-11 in cancer patients with severe thrombocytopenia due to chemotherapy. *Blood* 1996;87:3607.
71. Rutherford CJ, Frenkel EP. Thrombocytopenia: issues in diagnosis and therapy. *Med Clin North Am* 1994;78:555.
72. Aster RH. Pooling of platelets in the spleen: role in the pathogenesis of "hypersplenic" thrombocytopenia. *J Clin Invest* 1964; 45:645.
73. Penny R, Rozenberg MC, Firkin BG. The splenic platelet pool. *Blood* 1966;27:1.
74. Sangro B, Bilbo I, Herrero C. Partial splenic embolization for the treatment of hypersplenism in cirrhosis. *Hepatology* 1993; 18:309.
75. Pearson HA, McIntosh S. Neonatal thrombocytopenia. *Clin Hematol* 1978;7:111.
76. Pearson HA, Shulman NR, Marder VJ, et al. Isoimmune neonatal thrombocytopenic purpura: clinical and therapeutic considerations. *Blood* 1964;23:154.
77. von dem Borne AEG, van Leeuwen EF, von Risez LE, et al. Neonatal alloimmune thrombocytopenia: detection and charac-

terization of the responsible antibodies by the platelet immunofluorescence test. *Blood* 1981;57:649.
78. Murphy MF. Neonatal alloimmune thrombocytopenia. *Haematologica* 1999;84:110.
79. Kelton JG, Blanch HE VS, Wilson WE, et al. Neonatal thrombocytopenia due to passive immunization: prenatal diagnosis and distinction between maternal platelet alloantibodies and autoantibodies. *N Engl J Med* 1980;302:1401.
80. Andrew M, Barr RD. Increased platelet destruction in infancy and childhood. *Semin Thromb Hemost* 1982;8:248.
81. Gasser C, Gautier E, Steck A, et al. Hamolytisch-uramische syndrome: bilaterale nierenrendennekrosen bei akuten erwerbenen haemolytischen anamien. *Schweiz Med Wochenschr* 1955; 85:905.
82. Harlan JM. Thrombocytopenia due to non-immune platelet destruction, *Clin Haematol* 1983;12:39.
83. Goldstein MH, Churq J, Strauss I, et al. Hemolytic-uremic syndrome. *Nephron* 1979;23:263.
84. Neild G. The hemolytic uremic syndrome: a review. *Q J Med* 1985;63:116.
85. Kaplan BS, Proesmans W. The hemolytic-uremic syndrome of childhood and its variant. *Semin Hematol* 1987;24:148.
86. Karmali MA, Petrie M, Lim C, et al. The association between idiopathic hemolytic-uremic syndrome and infection by verotoxin-producing *Escherichia coli. J Infect Dis* 1985;151:775.
87. Boyd B, Lingwood CA. Verotoxin receptor glycolipid in human renal tissue. *Nephron* 1989;51:207.
88. Hofmann SL. Southwestern Internal Medicine Conference: Shiga-like toxins in hemolytic-uremic syndrome and thrombotic thrombocytopenia purpura. *Am J Med Sci* 1993;306:6.
89. Dolislager D, Tune B. The hemolytic-uremic syndrome: spectrum of severity and significance of prodrome. *Am J Dis Child* 1978;132:55.
90. Clarkson AR, Lawrence JR, Meadows R. The hemolytic-uremic syndrome in adults. *Q J Med* 1970;39:227.
91. Morel-Maroger L. Adult hemolytic-uremic syndrome. *Kidney Int* 1980;18:125.
92. Herbert D, Sibley RK, Mauer SM. Recurrence of hemolytic-uremic syndrome in renal transplant recipients. *Kidney Int* 1986;30:551.
93. Arends MJ, Harrison DJ. Novel histopathologic findings in a surviving case of hemolytic uremic syndrome after bone marrow transplantation. *Hum Pathol* 1989;20:89.
94. Marshall RI, Sweny P. Haemolytic uremic syndrome in recipients of bone marrow transplants not treated with cyclosporin A. *Histopathology* 1986;10:953.
95. Craig JIO, Sheehan T, Bell K. The hemolytic uremic syndrome and bone marrow transplantation. *Br Med J* 1987;295:887
96. Jurgensen KA, Pedersen RS. Familial deficiency of prostacyclin production stimulating factor in the hemolytic-uremic syndrome of childhood. *Thromb Res* 1981;21:311.
97. Brain MC, Neame PB. Thrombotic thrombocytopenia purpura and the hemolytic uremic syndrome. *Semin Thromb Hemost* 1982;8:186.
98. Remuzzi G. Treatment of the hemolytic-uremic syndrome with plasma. *Clin Nephrol* 1979;12:279.
99. Moschcowitz E. Hyaline thromboses of the terminal arterials and capillaries: a hitherto undescribed disease. *Proc N Y Pathol Soc* 1924;24:21.
100. Nalbandian RM, Henry RL, Bick RL. Thrombotic thrombocytopenic purpura. *Semin Thromb Hemost* 1979;5:216.
101. Weiner CP. Thrombotic microangiopathy in pregnancy and the postpartum period. *Semin Hematol* 1987;24:119.
102. Kwaan HC. Clinicopathologic features of thrombotic thrombocytopenic purpura. *Semin Hematol* 1987;24:71.
103. Gordon LI, Kwaan HC. Cancer and drug associated thrombotic thrombocytopenic purpura and hemolytic uremic syndrome. *Semin Hematol* 1997;34:140.
104. Bennett CL, Weinberg PD, Rozenberg-Ben-Dror K, et al. Thrombotic thrombocytopenic purpura associated with ticlopidine: a review of 60 cases. *Ann Intern Med* 1998;128:541.
105. Bennett CL, Connors JM, Carivile JM. Thrombotic thrombocytopenic purpura associated with clopidogrel. *N Engl J Med* 2000;342:1773.
106. Moake JL, Turner NA, Stathopoulos NA, et al. Involvement of large plasma von Willebrand factor (vWF) multimers and unusually large vWF forms derived from endothelial cells in shear stress-induced platelet aggregation. *J Clin Invest* 1986;78: 1456.
107. Kelton JG, Moore J, Santos A, et al. Detection of a platelet-agglutinating factor in thrombotic thrombocytopenic purpura. *Am Intern Med* 1984;101:559.
108. Dent JA, Gal Busera M, Ruggeri ZM. Heterogeneity of plasma von Willebrand factor multimers resulting from proteolyses of the constituent subunit. *J Clin Invest* 1991;88:774.
109. Furlan M, Robles R, Lammle B. Partial purification and characterization of a protease from human plasma cleaving von Willebrand factor to fragments produced by in vivo proteolyses. *Blood* 1996;87:4223.
110. Tsai HM. Physiologic cleavage of von Willebrand factor by a plasma protease is dependent on its confirmation and requires calcium ion. *Blood* 1996;87:4235.
111. Furlan M, Robles R, Solenthaler M, et al. Acquired deficiency of van Willebrand factor cleaving protease in a patient with thrombotic thrombocytopenic purpura. *Blood* 1998;91:2839.
112. Lammle B, Furlan M. New insights into the pathogenesis of thrombotic thrombocytopenic purpura. In: *Hematology educational program.* Washington, DC: American Society of Hematology, 1999:243–248.
113. Furlan M, Robles R, Galbusera M, et al. Von Willebrand factor-cleaving protease in thrombotic thrombocytopenic purpura. *N Engl J Med* 1998;339:1578.
114. Tsai, Lian ECY. Antibodies to von Willebrand factor cleaving protease in acute thrombotic thrombocytopenic purpura. *N Engl J Med* 1998;339:1585.
115. Amorosi EL, Ultmann JE. Thrombotic thrombocytopenic purpura: report of 16 cases and review of the literature. *Medicine* 1966;45:139.
116. Bick RL. Disseminated intravascular coagulation and related syndromes: a clinical review. *Semin Thromb Hemost* 1988;14:229.
117. Bukowski RM, King JW, Hewlett JS. Plasmapheresis in the treatment of thrombotic thrombocytopenic purpura. *Blood* 1977;50:413.
118. Byrnes JJ, Lian ECY. Recent therapeutic advances in thrombotic thrombocytopenic purpura. *Semin Thromb Hemost* 1979; 5:199.
119. Bukowski RM, Hewlett JS, Reimer RR, et al. Therapy of thrombotic thrombocytopenic purpura: an overview. *Semin Thromb Hemost* 1981;7:1.
120. Gandolfo GM, Afeltra A, Fern GM. Plasmapheresis for thrombocytopenia. *Lancet* 1978;1:1095.
121. Shepard KV, Bukowski RM. The treatment of thrombotic thrombocytopenic purpura with exchange transfusions, plasma infusions, and plasma exchange. *Semin Hematol* 1987;24:178.
122. Taft EG, Baldwin ST. Plasma exchange transfusion. *Semin Thromb Hemost* 1981;7:15.
123. Rock GA, Shumak KR, Buskard NA, et al. Comparison of plasma exchange with plasma infusion in the treatment of thrombotic thrombocytopenic purpura. *N Engl J Med* 1991; 325:393.
124. Bukowski RM. Thrombotic thrombocytopenic purpura: a review. *Prog Hemost* Thromb 1982;6:287.

125. Bell WR, Braine HG, Ness PM, et al. Improved survival in thrombotic thrombocytopenic purpura hemolytic uremic syndrome. *N Engl J Med* 1991;325:398.
126. Amorosi EL, Karpatkin S. Antiplatelet treatment of thrombotic thrombocytopenic purpura. *Ann Intern Med* 1977;86:102.
127. Crowther MA, Heddle N, Haywood CPM, et al. Splenectomy done during hematologic remission to prevent relapse in patients with thrombotic thrombocytopenic purpura. *Ann Intern Med* 1996;125:294.
128. Rose M, Row JM, Eldor A. The changing course of thrombotic thrombocytopenic purpura and modern therapy. *Blood Rev* 1993;7:94.
129. Kolodziej M. High dose intravenous immunoglobulin as therapy for thrombotic thrombocytopenic purpura. *Am J Med Sci* 1993;305:101.
130. Wilson JJ, Neame PB, Kelton JG. Infection-induced thrombocytopenia. *Semin Thromb Hemost* 1982;8:217.
131. Baker WF. Clinical aspects of disseminated intravascular coagulation: a clinician's point of view. *Semin Thromb Hemost* 1989; 15:1.
132. Kay AGL. Myelotoxicity of gold. *Br Med J* 1976;1:1266.
133. Stafford BT, Crosby WH. Late onset of gold-induced thrombocytopenia: with a practical note on the injections of dimercaprol. *JAMA* 1978;239:50.
134. Jacobson RI, Rath CE, Perloff JK. Intravascular hemolysis and thrombocytopenia in left ventricular outflow obstruction. *Br Heart J* 1973;35:849.
135. Roberts WC, Bulkley BH, Morrow AG. Pathologic anatomy of cardiac valve replacement: a study of 224 necropsy patients. *Prog Cardiovasc Dis* 1973;15:539.
136. Bick RL. Hemostasis defects associated with cardiac surgery, prosthetic devices, and other extracorporeal circuits. *Semin Thromb Hemost* 1985;11:249.
137. Bick RL, McClain BJ. Deep venous thrombosis: a laboratory evaluation of 118 consecutive patients. *Thromb Haemost* 1983; 50:305.
138. Turpie AGG, de Boer AC, Genton E. Platelet consumption in cardiovascular disease. *Semin Thromb Hemost* 1982,8.161.
139. Lusher JM, Iyer R. Idiopathic thrombocytopenic purpura in children. *Semin Thromb Hemost* 1977;3:175.
140. McWilliams NB, Mauer HM. Acute idiopathic thrombocytopenic purpura in children. *Am J Hematol* 1979;7:87.
141. Cohn J. Thrombocytopenia in childhood: an evaluation of 433 patients. *Scand J Haematol* 1976;16:226.
142. McClure J. Idiopathic thrombocytopenic purpura in children: diagnosis and management. *Pediatrics* 1975;55:68.
143. Kelton JG, Gibbons S. Autoimmune platelet destruction: idiopathic thrombocytopenic purpura. *Semin Thromb Hemost* 1982;8:83.
144. Pfueller SL, Cosgrove U. Activation of human platelets in PRP via their Fc-receptor by antigen-antibody complexes or immunoglobulin G: requirement for particle bound fibrinogen. *Thromb Res* 1980;20:97.
145. Klein CA, Blajchman MA. Alloantibodies and platelet destruction. *Semin Thromb Hemost* 1982;8:105.
146. Carroll RR, Noyes WD, Kitchens CS. High-dose intravenous immunoglobulin therapy in patients with immune thrombocytopenic purpura. *JAMA* 1983;249:1748.
147. Eden OB, Lilleyman JS. Guidelines for management of idiopathic thrombocytopenic purpura. *Arch Dis Child* 1992;67: 1056.
148. George JN, Woolf SH, Raskob GE, et al. Idiopathic thrombocytopenic purpura: a practice guideline developed by explicit methods for the American Society of Hematology. *Blood* 1996; 88:3.
149. Bolton-Maggs P, Moon I. Assessment of UK practice for management of acute childhood idiopathic thrombocytopenic purpura against published guidelines. *Lancet* 1997;350:620.
150. Lilleyman JS. Management of childhood idiopathic thrombocytopenic purpura. *Br J Haematol* 1999;105:871.
151. Buchanon G, Holtkamp C. Prednisone therapy for children with newly diagnosed idiopathic thrombocytopenic purpura: a randomized clinical trial. *Am J Pediatr HematolOncol* 1984; 6:355.
152. Blanchette VS, Luke B, Andrew M, et al. A prospective randomized trial of high dose intravenous immunoglobulin G therapy, oral prednisone and no therapy in childhood acute immune thrombocytopenic purpura. *J Pediatr* 1993;123:989.
153. Blanchette V, Imbach P, Andrew M, et al. Randomized trial of intravenous immunoglobulin G, intravenous anti-D, and oral prednisone in childhood acute immune thrombocytopenic purpura. *Lancet* 1994;344:703.
154. Hathaway WE. The bleeding newborn. *Semin Hematol* 1975; 12:175.
155. Samuel H, Nardi M, Karpatkin M, et al. Differentiation of autoimmune thrombocytopenia from thrombocytopenia associated with immune complex disease: systemic lupus erythematosus, hepatitis-thromboses, and HIV-1 infection by platelet and serum immunologic measurements. *J Haematol* 1999; 105:1086.
156. McMillan R. Chronic idiopathic thrombocytopenic purpura. *N Engl J Med* 1981;304:1135.
157. McMillin R. Immune thrombocytopenia. *Clin Haematol* 1983; 12:69.
158. Yu Z, Lennon VA. Mechanism of intravenous immune globulin therapy in antibody-mediated autoimmune diseases. *N Engl J Med* 1999;340:227.
159. Centers for Disease Control and Prevention. Recommendations of the Advisory Committee on Immunization Practices: use of vaccines and immune globulins in persons with altered immunocompetence. *MMWR Morbid Mortal Wkly Rep* 1993;42:1.
160. George IN, Kojouri K, Perdue JJ, et al. Management of patients with chronic refractory idiopathic thrombocytopenic purpura. *Semin Hematol* 2000;37:290.
161. Matthews JH, Benjamin S, Gill DS, et al. Pregnancy-associated thrombocytopenia: definition, incidence, and natural history. *Acta Haematol* 1990;84:24.
162. Burrows RF, Kelton JG. Fetal thrombocytopenia and its relation to maternal thrombocytopenia. *N Engl J Med* 1993;329:1463.
163. McCrae KR, Samules P, Schneiber AD. Pregnancy-associated thrombocytopenia: pathogenesis and management. *Blood* 1992;80:2697.
164. Letsky EA, Greaves M. Guidelines on the investigation and management of thrombocytopenia and neonatal alloimmune thrombocytopenia. *Br J Haematol* 1996;95:21.
165. Kelton JG. Thrombocytopenia in pregnancy. In: *Hematology education program.* Washington, DC: American Society of Hematology, 1999:490–497.
166. Bussel TB, Zabusky MR, Berkowitz RL, et al. Fetal alloimmune thrombocytopenia. *N Engl J Med* 1997;337:22.
167. Christiaens GCML, Nieuwenhuis HK, Bussel JB. Comparison of platelet counts in first and second newborns of mothers with immune thrombocytopenic purpura. *Obstet Gynecol* 1997;90:546.
168. Ajzenberg N, Dreyfus M, Kaplan C, et al. Pregnancy-associated thrombocytopenia revisited: assessment and follow-up of 50 cases. *Blood* 1998;92:4573.
169. Hackett T, Kelton JG, Powers P. Drug-induced platelet destruction. *Semin Thromb Hemost* 1982;8:116.
170. Mieschner PA, Graf J. Drug-induced thrombocytopenia. *Clin Haematol* 1980;9:505.
171. Mieshner PA. Drug-induced thrombocytopenia. *Semin Hematol* 1973;10:311.

172. Horowitz HI, Nachman RL. Drug purpura. *Semin Hematol* 1965;2:287.
173. George TN, Raskob GE, Shah SR, et al. Drug-induced thrombocytopenia: a systematic review of published case reports. *Ann Intern Med* 1998;129:886.
174. Bick RL, Frenkel EP. Clinical aspects of heparin-induced thrombocytopenia on thromboses and other side effects of heparin therapy. *Clin Appl Thromb Hemost* 1999;5:(suppl 1):57.
175. King DJ, Kelton JG. Heparin associated thrombocytopenia. *Ann Intern Med* 1984;100:535.
176. Warkentin TE, Kelton JG. Heparin and platelets. *Hematol Oncol Clin North Am* 1990;4:243.
177. Chong BH. Heparin induced thrombocytopenia. *Br J Haematol* 1995;89:431.
178. Aster RH. Heparin-induced thrombocytopenia and thrombosis. *N Engl J Med* 1995;332:1374.
179. Kelton JG, Warkentin TE. Diagnosis of heparin-induced thrombocytopenia: still a journey, not yet a destination [editorial]. *Am J Clin Pathol* 1995;104:611.
180. Schmitt BP, Adelman B. Heparin associated thrombocytopenia: a critical review and pooled analysis. *Am J Med Sci* 1993;305:208.
181. Shorten GD, Comunale ME. Heparin induced thrombocytopenia. *J Cardiothorac Vasc Anesth* 1996;10:521.
182. Kibbe MR, Rhee RY. Heparin induced thrombocytopenia: pathophysiology. *Semin Vasc Surg* 1996;9:284.
183. Warkentin TE, Kelton JG. A 14 year study of heparin induced thrombocytopenia. *Am J Med* 1996;101:502.
184. Walenga JM, Bick RL. Heparin-induced thrombocytopenia, paradoxical thromboembolism, and other side effects of heparin therapy. *Cardiol Clin Annu Drug Ther* 1998;2:123.
185. Walenga JM, Bick RL. Heparin-induced thrombocytopenia, paradoxical thromboembolism, and other side effects of heparin therapy. *Med Clin North Am* 1998;82:635.
186. Molberg P, Geary V, Sheikh M. Heparin-induced thrombocytopenia: a possible complication of heparin-coated pulmonary artery catheters. *J Cardiothorac Anesth* 1990;4:266.
187. Weismann RE, Tobin RW. Arterial embolism occurring during systemic heparin therapy. *Arch Surg* 1958;76:219.
188. Towne JB, Bernhard VM, Hussey C, et al. White clot syndrome: peripheral vascular complications of heparin therapy. *Arch Surg* 1979;114:372.
189. Stanton PE Jr, Evans JR, Lefemine AA, et al. White clot syndrome. *South Med J* 1988;81:616.
190. Wallis DE, Lewis BE, Messmore HL, et al. Inadequacy of current prevention strategies for heparin-induced thrombocytopenia. *Clin Appl Thromb Hemost* 1999;5:S16–S20.
191. Powers PJ, Kelton JG, Carter CJ. Studies on the frequency of heparin associated thrombocytopenia. *Thromb Res* 1984;33:439.
192. Ansell JE, Price JM, Beckner RR. Heparin induced thrombocytopenia: what is its real frequency? *Chest* 1985;88:878.
193. Warkentin TE. Clinical presentation of heparin-induced thrombocytopenia. *Semin Hematol* 1998;35(suppl):9.
194. Jackson MR, Krishnamurti C, Aylesworth CA. Diagnosis of heparin induced thrombocytopenia in the vascular surgery patient. *Surgery* 1997;121:419.
195. Warkentin TE. Limitations of conventional treatment options for heparin-induced thrombocytopenia. *Semin Hematol* 1998; 35(suppl):17.
196. Neverre DR, Digiovanni A. Hypercoagulability and the management of anticoagulant therapy in surgical patients: review and recommendations. *J Endovasc Surg* 1998;5:282.
197. Zeigler Z, Murphy S, Gardner FH. Post-transfusion: a heterogeneous syndrome. *Blood* 1975;45:529.
198. Vaughn-Neil EF, Ardeman S, Bevan G, et al. Post-transfusion purpura associated with unusual platelet antibody (anti-PLB1). *Br Med J* 1975;1:436.
199. Solum NO. Platelet membrane proteins. *Semin Hematol* 1985; 22:289.
200. Abramson N, Eisenberg PD, Aster RH. Post-transfusion purpura: immunologic aspects and therapy. *N Engl J Med* 1974; 291:1163.
201. Phadke KP, Isbister JP. Post-transfusion purpura. *Med J Austr* 1980;1:430.
202. Vogelsang G, Kickler TS, Bell WR. Post-transfusion purpura: a report of five patients and a review of the pathogenesis and management. *Am J Hematol* 1986;21:259.
203. Frenkel EP. The clinical spectrum of thrombocytosis and thrombocythemia. *Am J Med Sci* 1991;301:69.
204. Michiels JJ, Juvonen E. Proposal for revised diagnostic criteria of essential thrombocythemia and polycythemia vera by the thrombocythemia vera study group. *Semin Thromb Hemost* 1997;23:339.
205. Fialkow PJ, Faquet GB, Jacobson RI. Evidence that essential thrombocythemia is a clonal disorder with origin in a multipatient stem cell. *Blood* 1981;58:916.
206. Frenkel EP, Bick RL. Prothrombin G20210A gene mutation, heparin cofactor II defects, primary (essential) thrombocythemia, and thrombohemorrhagic manifestations. *Semin Thromb Hemost* 1999;25:375.
207. Laszlo J. Myeloproliferative disorders (MPD): myelofibrosis, myelosclerosis, extramedullary hematopoiesis, undifferentiated MPD, and hemorrhagic thrombocythemia. *Semin Hematol* 1975;12:409.
208. Iland HJ, Laszlo J, Peterson P, et al. Essential thrombocythemia: clinical and laboratory characteristics at presentation. *Trans Assoc Am Physicians* 1983;96:165.
209. Iland HJ, Laszlo J, Case DC Jr, et al. Differentiation between essential thrombocythemia and polycythemia vera with marked thrombocytosis. *Am J Heme* 1987;25:191.
210. Schilling RF. Platelet millionaires. *Lancet* 1980;230:828.
211. Murphy S. Thrombocytosis and thrombocythemia. *Clin Hematol* 1983;12:89.
212. Schafer AI. Bleeding and thrombosis in the myeloproliferative disorders. *Blood* 1984;64:1.
213. Mitus AJ, Schafer AL. Thrombocytosis and thrombocythemia. *Hematol Oncol Clin North Am* 1990;4:157.
214. Frenkel EP. Polycythemia vera, myelofibrosis, and primary (essential) thrombocythemia. In: Calabresse P, Schein P, eds. *Medical oncology: basic principles and clinical management.* 2nd ed. New York: McGraw-Hill, 1993:503–515.
215. Michiels JJ, Kutti J, Stark M, et al. Diagnosis, pathogenesis and treatment of the myeloproliferative disorders: essential thrombocythemia, polycythemia vera and essential megakaryocytic granulocytic metaplasia and myelofibrosis. *Proc Rotterdam MPD–Work Shop* 1998:1–21.
216. Tefferi A, Fonseca R, Pereira DL, et al. A long term retrospective study of young women with essential thrombocythemia. *Mayo Clin Proc* 2001;76:22.
217. Lengfelder E, Hochhaus A, Kronawitter U, et al. Should a platelet count of 600 × 10^9/L be used as a diagnostic criterion in essential thrombocythemia? An analysis of the natural course including early stages. *Br J Haematol* 1998;100:15.
218. Epstein E, Goedel A. Hamorrhagische thrombocythemia bei vascular schrumpfmelz. *Virchows Arch (Pathol Anat)* 1934;293:233.
219. Gunz, FW. Hemorrhagic thrombocythemia: a critical review. *Blood* 1960;15:706.
220. Ozer FL, Truax WE, Miesch DC, et al. Primary hemorrhagic thrombocythemia. *Am J Med* 1960;28:807.
221. Silverstein MN. Primary or hemorrhagic thrombocythemia. *Arch Int Med* 1968;122:18.
222. Lewis SM, Szur L, Hoffbrand AV. Thrombocythemia. *Clin Heme* 1972;1:339.

223. Sceats EJ, Baition D. Primary thrombocythemia in a child. *Clin Pediatr* 1980;19:298.
224. Eyster ME, Saletan SL, Rabellino EM, et al. Familial essential thrombocythemia. *Am J Med* 1986;80:497.
225. Hoagland HC, Silverstein MN. Primary thrombocythemia in the young patient. *Mayo Clin Proc* 1978;53:578.
226. Millard FE, Hunter CS, Anderson M, et al. Clinical manifestations of essential thrombocythemia in young adults. *Am J Heme* 1980;33:27.
227. Mitus AJ, Barbui T, Shulmar LN, et al. Hemostatic complications in young patients with essential thrombocythemia. *Am J Med* 1990;88:371.
228. Michiels JJ, Abels J, Stekette J, et al. Erythromelalgia caused by platelet-mediated arteriolar inflammation and thrombosis in thrombocythemia. *Ann Int Med* 1985;102:466.
229. Van Genderen PJJ, Michiels JJ. Erythromelalgia: a pathognomic microvascular thrombotic complication in essential thrombocythemia and polycythemia vera. *Semin Thromb Hemost* 1997;23:357.
230. Griesshammer M, Bongerter M, Van Vliet HH, et al. Aspirin in essential thrombocythemia: status quo and quo vadis. *Semin Thromb Hemost* 1997;23:371.
231. Ghilardi N, Wiestner A, Kikuchi M, et al. Hereditary thrombocythemia in a Japanese family is caused by a novel point mutation in the thrombopoietin gene. *Br J Hematol* 1999; 107:310.
232. Wiestner A, Padosch SA, Ghilardi N, et al. Hereditary thrombocythemia is a genetically heterogenous disorder: exclusion of TPO and MPL in two families with hereditary thrombocythemia! *Br J Hematol* 2000;110:104.
233. Pitcher L, Taylor K, Nichol J, et al. Thrombopoietin measurement in thrombocytosis: dysregulation and lack of feedback inhibition in essential thrombocythemia. *Br J Hematol* 1997; 99:929.
234. Horikawa Y, Matsumura I, Hashimoto K, et al. Markedly reduced expression of platelet C-MPL receptor in essential thrombocythemia. *Blood* 1997;90:4031.
235. Michiels JJ, tenKate FWJ, Vuzeuski VD, et al. Histopathology of erythromelalgia in thrombocythemia. *Histopathology* 1984; 8:669.
236. Wehmeier A, Sudhoff T, Meierkord F. Relation of platelet abnormalities to thrombosis and hemorrhage in chronic myeloproliferative disorders. *Semin Thromb Hemost* 1997;23:391.
237. Budde U, von Genderen PJJ. Acquired von Willebrand disease in patients with high platelet counts. *Semin Thromb Hemost* 1997;23:425.
238. Preston FE, Emmanuel IG, Winfield DA, et al. Essential thrombocythemia and peripheral gangrene. *Br J Haematol* 1974;50:157.
239. Koudstaal PJ, Koudstaal A. Neurologic and visual symptoms in essential thrombocythemia: efficacy of low-dose aspirin. *Semin Thromb Hemost* 1997;23:365.
240. Millard FE, Hunter CS, Anderson M, et al. Clinical manifestations of essential thrombocythemia in young adults. *Am J Hematol* 1990;33:27.
241. Bellucci S, Janvier M, Tobelem G, et al. Essential thrombocythemia. *Cancer* 1986;58:2440.
242. Schror K. Aspirin and platelets: the antiplatelet action of aspirin and its role in thrombosis treatment and prophylaxis. *Semin Thromb Hemost* 1997;23:349.
243. Frenkel EP. Myeloproliferative disorders: polycythemia vera, thrombocythemia and myelofibrosis. In: Kelley W, ed. *Textbook of internal medicine.* 3rd ed. Philadelphia: Lippincott, 1997: 1388–1392.
244. Snethlage W, Tencate JW. Thrombocythemia and recurrent late abortions: normal outcome of pregnancies after anti-aggregatory treatment. *Br J Obstet Gynaecol* 1986;93:386.
245. Falconer J, Pineo G, Blahey W. Essential thrombocythemia associated with recurrent abortions and fetal growth retardation. *Am J Hematol* 1987;25:345.
246. Mercer B, Drovin J, Jolly E, et al. Primary thrombocythemia in pregnancy: a report of two cases. *Am J Obstet Gynecol* 1988; 159:127.
247. Frenkel EP, Skinner W, Smilay JD. Studies on the metabolic defect induced by hydroxyurea and its relationship to megaloblastosis. *Cancer Res* 1967;27:1016.
248. Bergsagel DE, Frenkel EP, Alfrey CP, et al. Megaloblastic erythropoiesis induced by hydroxyurea. *Cancer Chemother Rep* 1964;40:15.
249. Anker-Lugtenberg PJ. Myelodysplastic syndrome and secondary acute leukemia after treatment of essential thrombocythemia with hydroxyurea. *Am J Hematol* 1990;33:152.
250. Sterkers Y, Preudhomme C, Lai JL, et al. Acute myeloid leukemia and myelodysplastic syndromes following essential thrombocythemia treated with hydroxyurea: high proportion of cases with 17 p deletion. *Blood* 1998;91:616.
251. Finazzi G, Ruqqeri M, Rodeghiero F, et al. Second malignancies in patients with essential thrombocythemia treated with busulfan and hydroxyurea: long-term follow-up of a randomized clinical trial. *Br J Hematol* 2000;110:577.
252. Giles FJ, Singer CRJ, Gray AG, et al. Alpha-interferon therapy for essential thrombocythemia. *Lancet* 1988;2:70.
253. Chott A, Gisslinger H, Thiele J, et al. Interferon-alpha-induced morphological changes of megakaryocytes: a histomorphometric study on bone marrow biopsies in chronic myeloproliferative disorders with excessive thrombocytosis. *Br J Haematol* 1990; 74:10.
254. Gisslinger H, Linkesch W, Fritz E, et al. Long term interferon therapy for thrombocytosis in myeloproliferative diseases. *Lancet* 1989;1:634.
255. Elliott MA, Tefferi A. Interferon therapy in polycythemia vera and essential thrombocythemia. *Semin Thromb Hemost* 1997; 23:463.
256. Petit JJ, Callis M, deSevilla AF. Normal pregnancy in a patient with essential thrombocythemia treated with interferon. *Am J. Hematol* 1992;40:80.
257. Gillespie E. Anagrelide: a potent and selective inhibitor of platelet cyclic AMP phosphodiesterase enzyme activity. *Biochem Pharmacol* 1988;37:2866–2868.
258. Andes WA, Noveck RJ, Fleming JS. Inhibition of platelet production induced by an antiplatelet drug, anagrelide, in normal volunteers. *Thromb Haemost* 1984;52:325.
259. Silverstein MN, Petitt RM, Solberg LA Jr, et al. Anagrelide: a new drug for treating thrombocytosis. *N Engl J Med* 1988; 318:129.
260. Anagrelide Study Group. Anagrelide: a therapy for thrombocythemic states: experience in 577 patients. *Am J Med* 1992; 92:69.
261. Solberg LA Jr, Teffer A, Oles KJ. The effects of anagrelide on human megakaryocytopoiesis. *Br J Haematol* 1997;99:174.
262. Tefferi A, Silverstein MN, Petitt RM, et al. *Semin Thromb Hemost* 1997;23:379.

Lippincott, Williams & Wilkins Philadelphia © 2002

6

HEREDITARY COAGULATION PROTEIN DEFECTS

FRANK A. NIZZI, JR.
SUNEETI SAPATNEKAR
RODGER L. BICK

Hereditary defects of the blood proteins leading to hemorrhagic diseases and associated disease states are the topic of this chapter. Inherited hereditary coagulation protein defects may be secondary to the production of an abnormal protein or lack of production of a coagulation protein.

Clinical manifestations of coagulation factor disorders are different from those disorders of the vessel or platelets. With the exception von Willebrand disease (vWD), coagulation factor disorders are characterized by deep tissue bleeding, including intraarticular bleeding, deep intramuscular bleeding, and sometimes intracranial bleeding. Conversely, vWD is characterized by decreased or abnormal production of von Willebrand factor (vWF), which plays an important role in endothelium–platelet interaction, and therefore these patients have symptoms characteristic of "platelet-type" bleeding characterized by petechiae, purpura, and mucosal bleeding. However, severe forms of vWD may be seen similarly with severe bleeding typical of classic coagulation factor deficiencies.

Most clinically significant coagulation protein disorders may be detected by global tests of coagulation that depend on the conversion of fibrinogen to fibrin. These tests include the prothrombin time (PT), the activated partial thromboplastin time (aPTT), thrombin time, whole blood clotting time, and other specialized assays. Any one or several of these may be prolonged in clinically significant protein defects. Exceptions to this are α_2-antiplasmin deficiency, plasminogen activator inhibitor, and factor XIII deficiency, which require specialized assays for detection. Other in vitro assays for hemostasis including the platelet count, the appearance of the peripheral blood smear, and template bleeding time are normal in patients with isolated coagulation protein problems. The specific and definitive diagnosis of a particular coagulation factor defect or defects is usually achieved by a specific functional factor assay that will detect both the decreased presence of a coagulation protein or the presence of abnormal protein.

The hereditary coagulation protein disorders are summarized in Table 6.1. Most specific factor deficiency states are quite rare, with the exception of vWD and the hemophilias. vWD may be seen in 1% to 4% of the population, and the hemophilias account for about 1 in 8,000 to 10,000 births in the United States.

FIBRINOGEN DEFECTS

The fibrinogen molecule is a 340-kDa dimeric glycoprotein composed of three pairs of nonidentical polypeptide chains connected by disulfide bonds and hydrophobic interactions. Fibrinogen is synthesized by hepatocytes and circu-

TABLE 6.1. HEREDITARY COAGULATION FACTOR DEFICIENCIES

Afibrinogenemia, hypofibrinogenemia, dysfibrinogenemia
Factor II defects
Factor V defects
Factor VII defects
Factor VIII defects (hemophilia A)
Factor IX defects (hemophilia B)
Factor X defects
Factor XI defects
Factor XII (Hageman factor) defects
Factor XIII defects
Prekallikrein (Fletcher factor) defects
Kininogen defects (Williams, Fitzgerald, Reid, Flaujeac, Fujiwara factors)
Fibrinolytic system defects
von Willebrand factor defects

F. A. Nizzi, Jr.: Department of Pathology, University of Texas Southwestern Medical Center, Dallas, Texas; Medical Services, Carter BloodCare, Bedford, Texas.

S. Sapatnekar: American Red Cross Blood Services, Northern Ohio Region, Cleveland, Ohio.

R. L. Bick: Departments of Medicine and Pathology, University of Texas Southwestern Medical Center; Dallas Thrombosis/Hemostasis Clinical Center; ThromboCare Laboratories, Dallas, Texas.

lates in the plasma at a concentration of 150 to 350 mg/dL. It has an important role not only in blood coagulation, fibrinolysis, and platelet function, but also in tissue repair and cell proliferation (1).

Congenital defects of fibrinogen may be classified as quantitative defects, which usually have autosomal recessive inheritance, and qualitative defects, or dysfibrinogenemia, which are usually autosomal dominant disorders. Quantitative defects of fibrinogen synthesis may result in complete absence of fibrinogen (afibrinogenemia, the homozygous state) or decreased levels of fibrinogen (hypofibrinogenemia, the heterozygous state). Such defects are caused by defective synthesis, secretion, or intracellular transport of the fibrinogen molecule (1,2). The molecular basis of some of these defects has been characterized (1,3,4). The dysfibrinogenemias are a heterogeneous group of disorders resulting from abnormalities in the fibrinogen molecule. They are named for the city of origin of the patient first described, and are characterized by a defect in one or more steps in the conversion of soluble fibrinogen into an insoluble fibrin clot, such as abnormal fibrinopeptide release, polymerization defects, or alterations of cross-linking (1,4). Dysfibrinogenemia may coexist with hypofibrinogenemia.

Congenital afibrinogenemia and hypofibrinogenemia are uncommon disorders. Approximately 200 cases are reported in the literature. Clinical manifestations are generally mild and are related to the plasma fibrinogen concentration. Bleeding usually occurs in response to trauma or surgery, and spontaneous bleeding is rare at fibrinogen levels greater than 50 mg/dL (Table 6.2). Mucosal bleeding of variable severity is more common than deep tissue bleeding, and includes epistaxis, gum bleeding, menorrhagia, and gastrointestinal bleeding (2,3). Serious intracranial hemorrhage has been described (5). There is an increased incidence of spontaneous abortion and abruptio placentae. Neonates may have bleeding from the umbilical stump (6). Rare instances of thrombosis, rather than hemorrhage, have been described (7,8). Some patients with hypofibrinogenemia also may have a coexistent congenital thrombophilia (7,9).

Patients with congenital dysfibrinogenemia are frequently asymptomatic (Table 6.3). About half of the patients have a mild bleeding tendency and a history of easy and spontaneous bruising or menorrhagia. Bleeding may follow trauma or surgery, especially in homozygous patients, but is rarely life threatening (3,6). Approximately 10% of patients with congenital dysfibrinogenemia have a thrombotic tendency. These are discussed in Chapter 13.

The aPTT, PT, thrombin time, and reptilase time are usually moderately prolonged in hypofibrinogenemic patients and markedly prolonged or not clottable in afibrinogenemic patients. These tests are also abnormally and variably prolonged in dysfibrinogenemia. When plasma fibrinogen is measured by a clot-based (functional) assay, the level is low or absent in both afibrinogenemia/hypofibrinogenemia and dysfibrinogenemia. The fibrinogen concentration is approximately 50% of normal in hypofibrinogenemia and less than 20 mg/dL in afibrinogenemia. To distinguish hypofibrinogenemia/afibrinogenemia from dysfibrinogenemia, an immunologic assay for fibrinogen is required. Plasma fibrinogen measured by an immunologic assay, or by a protein precipitation technique, is low or absent in hypofibrinogenemia/afibrinogenemia, but near normal in dysfibrinogenemia. Occasional patients with afibrinogenemia may have trace levels of fibrinogen, and this may represent cross-reactivity with nonfibrinogen material, possibly fibronectin. A significant discrepancy between the concentration of fibrinogen detected by clot-based and immunologic assays is characteristic of dysfibrinogenemia (3,6). Some patients may have mild to moderate thrombocytopenia (2,3). Because fibrinogen has an important role in platelet aggregation, patients with fibrinogen defects have a prolonged bleeding time and abnormal platelet aggregation (10).

TABLE 6.2. AFIBRINOGENEMIA AND HYPOFIBRINOGENEMIA

Clinical presentation
Usually autosomal recessive inheritance
Bleeding tendency at plasma fibrinogen <50 mg/dL
Mucosal bleeding, excessive bleeding after trauma
Spontaneous abortion, abruptio placentae
Umbilical stump bleeding, intracranial bleeding in neonate
Laboratory evaluation
PT prolonged
aPTT prolonged
Thrombin time, reptilase time prolonged
Plasma fibrinogen, functional assay: low
Plasma fibrinogen, immunologic assay, or protein precipitation: near normal
Abnormal platelet aggregation
Management
Cryoprecipitate, 2–3 bags/10 kg body weight

PT, prothrombin time; aPTT, activated partial thromboplastin time.

TABLE 6.3. DYSFIBRINOGENEMIA

Clinical presentation
Usually autosomal dominant inheritance
Frequently asymptomatic
Mild bleeding in 50% of patients: easy bruising, or menorrhagia, bleeding after trauma. Thrombotic tendency in 10% of patients
Laboratory evaluation
PT prolonged
aPTT prolonged
Thrombin time, reptilase time prolonged
Plasma fibrinogen low or absent
Abnormal platelet aggregation
Management
Cryoprecipitate, 2–3 bags/10 kg body weight

PT, prothrombin time; aPTT, activated partial thromboplastin time.

Most patients with afibrinogenemia/hypofibrinogenemia or dysfibrinogenemia do not require specific therapy. Patients with menorrhagia may be treated with oral contraceptive pills (11,12). Specific replacement therapy is required only to control bleeding episodes or in preparation for surgery. Cryoprecipitate is the mainstay of such treatment. Each bag of cryoprecipitate contains approximately 200 mg of fibrinogen in approximately 15 mL of plasma. Support of normal hemostasis during surgery requires a plasma fibrinogen concentration of approximately 100 mg/dL (1,2). A loading dose of two to three bags of cryoprecipitate for every 10 kg of body weight is recommended, followed by a daily maintenance dose equivalent to a third of the starting dose for as long as treatment is necessary (1,6,13). Thrombotic complications may occur in some patients after cryoprecipitate administration, particularly with concomitant use of antifibrinolytic agents or oral contraceptives (12,14,15). Prophylactic treatment to maintain the plasma fibrinogen at >60 mg/dL is used in pregnant patients to prevent spontaneous abortion. Antifibrinogen antibodies may develop after cryoprecipitate therapy.

PROTHROMBIN DEFECTS

Congenital defects of prothrombin (factor II) are very rare and are inherited as autosomal recessive traits. The defect may be a true deficiency of prothrombin, or hypoprothrombinemia, or dysprothrombinemia resulting from an abnormal, nonfunctional prothrombin molecule (16). Some dysprothrombinemias, such as the Habana, Houston, Metz, Molise, and Quick variants, are associated with hypoprothrombinemia. Prothrombin deficiency results in decreased thrombin activity and consequent defects in both clot formation and platelet aggregation.

Patients with hypoprothrombinemia have a hemorrhagic diathesis that may range from mild to severe. The most common presentation is prolonged bleeding after trauma (Table 6.4). Other manifestations are easy bruising, epistaxis, soft tissue hemorrhage, and menorrhagia (16–18). Affected neonates may have bleeding from the umbilical stump. Significant bleeding is seen only with prothrombin levels less than 2%. However, the extent of prothrombin deficiency does not necessarily correlate with clinical bleeding (16,17).

Patients with prothrombin defects have a prolonged PT and aPTT, and a normal thrombin time. The prothrombin level is low in both hypoprothrombinemia and dysprothrombinemia, when measured with a functional, clot-based assay. Most homozygotes have prothrombin activity levels of approximately 10%. To differentiate between the two conditions, prothrombin levels must be measured by using an immunologic assay. Patients with hypoprothrombinemia have concordant results with functional

TABLE 6.4. PROTHROMBIN DEFICIENCY

Clinical presentation	
	Very rare
	Autosomal recessive inheritance
	Hypoprothrombinemia or dysprothrombinemia
	Prolonged bleeding after trauma
	Easy bruising, epistaxis, menorrhagia
Laboratory evaluation	
	PT prolonged
	aPTT prolonged
	Prothrombin assay, functional = immunologic: hypoprothrombinemia
	Prothrombin assay, functional < immunologic: dysprothrombinemia
Management	
	FFP at 15–20 mL/kg loading dose, 5 mL/kg daily maintenance dose
	Target prothrombin level about 20% to 40%
	Factor IX complex concentrate

PT, prothrombin time; aPTT, activated partial thromboplastin time; FFP, fresh frozen plasma.

and immunologic assays. In contrast, patients with dysprothrombinemia show prothrombin antigen levels, detected with the immunologic assay, far in excess of prothrombin activity levels, as detected with the functional assay (16,18).

Hypoprothrombinemia and dysprothrombinemia are treated with fresh frozen plasma (FFP) at a loading dose of 15 to 20 mL/kg, followed by 5 mL/kg every 24 hours. Prothrombin has a half-life of approximately 72 hours, and levels of about 20% to 40% are required for normal hemostasis. Alternatively, prothrombin complex concentrate may be used (6,13,18). Mucosal bleeding can be treated with topical thrombin or antifibrinolytic agents (17).

FACTOR V DEFECTS

Factor V is a plasma protein that acts in the final common pathway of coagulation as a part of the prothrombinase complex, which catalyzes the conversion of prothrombin to thrombin. About 20% of total factor V is present in platelet α-granules in association with the carrier protein, multimerin. Platelet factor V is released into the plasma when platelets are activated.

Congenital factor V deficiency, also known as parahemophilia, is extremely rare. The defect is inherited as an autosomal recessive trait that manifests clinically only in homozygous individuals. Some cases are associated with congenital factor VIII deficiency or vWD. Most patients have a complete absence of factor V in the plasma, although their platelets may contain variable amounts of factor V. A few patients have detectable factor V in the plasma, but the molecule is dysfunctional. One such variant, factor V Quebec, results from a deficiency of platelet multimerin, and is characterized by low levels of factor V in both plasma and platelets (16).

The bleeding diathesis in patients with factor V defects varies greatly. Heterozygous individuals are usually asymptomatic. Most patients have a mild bleeding disorder with epistaxis, easy bruising, menorrhagia, and excessive bleeding after trauma, dental extraction, or surgery (Table 6.5) (16,19). However, severe spontaneous bleeding, soft tissue hematomas, and central nervous system hemorrhage may occur (20,21). A few cases of factor V deficiency associated with thrombotic, rather than hemorrhagic, manifestations have been described (22,23). Bleeding symptoms correlate poorly with plasma factor V levels and may correlate better with the factor V content of platelets. Factor V deficiency is associated with a high incidence of other congenital abnormalities, such as cleft palate, dwarfism, microcephaly, and cardiac anomalies (19).

The PT and aPTT are prolonged. The diagnosis of factor V deficiency depends on a quantitative factor V assay. The factor V activity level in homozygotes is less than 10%, and in heterozygotes is approximately 50%. Specific assays for factor VIII should be performed to exclude the rare combined deficiency. The bleeding time is prolonged in approximately one third of patients (6).

Factor-replacement therapy is generally required only for surgical prophylaxis or surgical bleeding. Adequate levels of factor V can be delivered with infusion of FFP at 15 to 20 mL/kg as a loading dose. The half-life of factor V shows individual variation, ranging from 5 to 36 hours. However, a daily maintenance dose of approximately 5 mL/kg is usually adequate (6,13,20). The factor V level should be kept at 25% to 30% for hemostasis during surgery and maintained at more than 15% for several days after surgery (19). Platelet transfusions are not recommended for factor V replacement because of the risk of platelet antibody formation (16).

TABLE 6.5. FACTOR V DEFICIENCY

- Clinical presentation
  - Extremely rare
  - Autosomal recessive inheritance
  - Mild to severe bleeding diathesis
  - Easy bruising, epistaxis, menorrhagia
  - Excessive bleeding after surgery or trauma
  - Occasionally, soft-tissue hematomas, intracranial bleeding
- Laboratory evaluation
  - PT prolonged
  - aPTT prolonged
  - Factor V activity <10% in homozygotes
  - Bleeding time may be prolonged
  - Concomitant factor VIII deficiency may be present
- Management
  - FFP at 15–20 mL/kg loading dose, 5 mL/kg daily maintenance dose
  - Target factor V level of 30%

PT, prothrombin time; aPTT, activated partial thromboplastin time; FFP, fresh frozen plasma.

FACTOR VII DEFECTS

Factor VII (proconvertin) is a vitamin K–dependent factor synthesized in the liver as a single-chain glycoprotein (MW, 47,000). After vascular injury, factor VII binds tissue factor (TF) exposed on the disrupted cells to form a TF-FVIIa complex. This complex then activates factors IX and X as well as itself (autocatalytically). The first description of the rare factor VII deficiency state was by Alexander et al. in 1951 (24). Since then, more than 80 mutations in the factor VII gene have been described (25). Factor VII deficiency is inherited in an autosomal recessive manner and, like most factor deficiency states, may be due to an absence of the protein [cross-reacting material (CRM)−] or a dysfunctional protein (CRM+ or CRMR) (26). The severity of the deficiency state is quite variable and does not always correlate with plasma levels. However, the clinical features are similar to those of other single coagulation factor defects and may consist of intraarticular bleeding with hemarthrosis, epistaxis, and mucosal bleeding (including gastrointestinal, genitourinary, and intrapulmonary bleeding) (27). Patients may have life-threatening hemorrhage with surgery or trauma. In the neonate, umbilical stump bleeding may occur, although they may have more severe symptoms of cephalohematoma or intracranial hemorrhage. The clinical and laboratory features of factor VII deficiency are summarized in Table 6.6.

TABLE 6.6. FACTOR VII DEFECTS

- Clinical manifestations
  - Autosomal recessive trait
  - Rare defect
  - Absence form and dysfunctional form
  - Intraarticular bleeding
  - Severe epistaxis
  - Umbilical stump bleeding occasionally
  - Mucosal membrane hemorrhage common
    - Gastrointestinal
    - Genitourinary
    - Intrapulmonary
  - Profuse bleeding with surgery or trauma
  - Heterozygous patients rarely bleed spontaneously
  - Heterozygous patients bleed with surgery or trauma
- Laboratory manifestations
  - Prolonged PT
  - Normal aPTT
  - Normal Russell's viper venom time
  - Normal template bleeding time
  - Normal platelet function (aggregation)
  - Definitive diagnosis requires quantitative factor VII assay
- Therapy
  - Increase factor VII to >30%
  - Fresh frozen plasma
  - Some prothrombin complex concentrates
  - Recombinant factor VII concentrate

PT, prothrombin time; aPTT, activated partial thromboplastin time.

Two curious variants of dysfunctional factor VII are Padua I and Padua II. Padua I factor VII–deficient patients demonstrate prolonged PT with rabbit thromboplastin but not ox-brain thromboplastin, and the opposite is seen in those with factor VII Padua II (28,29). Several other dysfunctional factor VII variants have been described according to sensitivity to thromboplastin preparations of differing origin. Examples of other dysfunctional factor VII defects are noted in Table 6.7.

Deficiency of factor VII is manifest as a prolonged PT with a normal aPTT. Heterozygotes will typically demonstrate a prolongation of a few seconds over the upper limits of the reference range, whereas severe deficiency states may be more than double the upper limit. The confirmation of factor VII deficiency is accomplished with factor VII–specific assays. Ideally, at least one other vitamin K–dependent factor assay should be included in the evaluation to ensure that vitamin K deficiency or other production abnormality is not the culprit. Given the short half-life of factor VII as compared with other vitamin K–dependent factors, deficiency states may appear within the extrinsic pathway first.

Because of the short half-life of factor VII of only 4 to 6 hours, treatment is challenging. The goal of episodic treatment is to increase the factor VII level to above homeostatic levels, minimally 15% to ideally near 30%. This can be achieved with 10 to 30 mL/kg of FFP. However, volume considerations limit the utility of FFP for ongoing treatment, and factor concentrates must be used. The characteristics of the factor concentrate being used should be known to prevent untoward effects such as thrombosis. Prothrombin complex concentrates (PCCs) have little factor VII activity; however, a plasma-derived, virally inactivated concentrate (Provertin; Immuno, Vienna, Austria) and recombinant factor VIIa (rVIIa) (NovoSeven; NovoNordisk, Princeton, NJ, U.S.A.) concentrate are available. rVIIa has shown efficacy in factor VII–deficient patients in the treatment of bleeding episodes, as well as in those undergoing surgical challenge. Doses range from 15 to 30 mg/kg body weight, and the PT should be monitored during treatment (30). Some responses to 1-deamino-8-D-arginine vasopressin (Desmopressin, DDAVP) also have been noted (31).

TABLE 6.7. EXAMPLES OF DYSFUNCTIONAL FACTOR VII

Briet	1976
Croze	1982
Denson	1972
Girolami	1977
Girolami	1978
Girolami	1979
Goodnight	1971
Kernoff	1981
Mazzucconi	1977

FACTOR VIII:C DEFECTS

Activated factor VIII is part of the "tenase" complex that accelerates factor Xa generation. Therefore, deficiency of factor VIII, or hemophilia A, results in insufficient generation of thrombin and a bleeding tendency (32–34).

Hemophilia A is an X-linked recessive disease with an incidence of about 1 in 5,000 male births. The factor VIII gene is located at the tip of the long arm of the X chromosome. Multiple different mutations have been described throughout the factor VIII gene, but nearly half of severe hemophilia A results from inversion of a portion of intron 22. Approximately 30% of cases represent spontaneous mutations without any family history of a bleeding disorder (34–36). Hemophilia A affects males almost exclusively. Female carriers of hemophilia A are asymptomatic because they have sufficient levels of factor VIII to prevent bleeding. Rare exceptions include females with unequal lyonization of the factor VIII alleles or with hemizygosity for part or all of the X chromosome (37). Combined deficiency of factors V and VIII has been described (34,38).

According to the standard nomenclature for factor VIII proposed by the International Committee on Thrombosis and Haemostasis, the plasma property that corrects the coagulation defect of patients with hemophilia A, is referred to as factor VIII:c (6,39). Factor VIII:c is made in the hepatocyte, and this moiety is measured in the aPTT test system and the traditional aPTT-derived factor VIII coagulant assay. The antigenic expression of factor VIII:c is called factor VIII:Ag. Generally, Factor VIII:c and Factor VIII:Ag levels parallel each other in normal persons and in most, but not all hemophilic patients. The carrier protein for factor VIII in the plasma is vWF. The antigenic expression of vWF is called vWF:Ag. About 90% of patients with hemophilia A have a deficiency of both factors VIII:c and VIII:Ag. The remaining 10% are missing factor VIII:c activity but have normal factor VIII:Ag; these patients have dysfunctional factor VIII:c.

The clinical manifestations of hemophilia A vary in severity depending on the plasma concentration of factor VIII (Table 6.8). In general, all affected members of a kindred have the same severity of bleeding. Patients with mild disease (factor VIII:c, 5% to 30%) do not bleed spontaneously, but have prolonged bleeding after surgery or significant trauma. Patients with moderate disease (factor VIII:c, 1% to 5%) may have occasional spontaneous bleed-

TABLE 6.8. SEVERITY OF HEMOPHILIA A

	Factor VIIIc Activity	Spontaneous Bleeding	Bleeding After Trauma
Mild	5%–30%	No	Yes
Moderate	1%–5%	Occasional	Yes
Severe	<1%	Frequent	Yes

ing episodes, but bleed profusely with surgery or trauma. Patients with severe disease (factor VIII:c, fewer than 1%), who account for approximately two thirds of hemophiliacs, are usually diagnosed in early childhood, and have frequent spontaneous bleeding episodes (6,40). Co-inheritance of a prothrombotic mutation may decrease the severity of hemophilia A (41).

The hallmark of hemophilia A is bleeding into joints, or hemarthrosis (Table 6.9) (6,32,33,37). Acute hemarthrosis is preceded by a tingling or burning sensation, and is accompanied by intense pain and swelling of the joint. The joints most commonly affected are the knees, elbows, and ankles. Recurrent hemarthrosis leads to chronic synovial inflammation and joint damage, and may ultimately result in permanent joint deformity (chronic hemophilic arthropathy). Spontaneous hemarthrosis is rare before age 9 months because of limited ambulation before this age. Another common clinical presentation in hemophiliacs is soft tissue bleeding, which can result in extensive, possibly life-threatening, blood loss. Hemorrhage into a closed space, such as a muscular compartment in the extremities, can cause compartment syndrome with resultant vascular and peripheral nerve compromise. Such an event may occur after antecubital venipuncture. Other sites of bleeding in hemophilic patients are the gastrointestinal and urinary tracts and the retroperitoneum. Intracranial bleeding may occur and is the leading cause of death from hemorrhage (6,32,33,37).

Alloantibodies against factor VIII:c, also known as factor VIII inhibitors, develop in about 15% of patients with severe hemophilia treated with factor VIII concentrates. The development of such inhibitors is unrelated to the source of factor VIII:c concentrate used to treat the patient. In the presence of factor VIII inhibitors, bleeding episodes fail to respond to adequate doses of factor VIII concentrate (6,40,42).

The whole blood clotting time and aPTT are generally prolonged in patients with hemophilia A. The PT is normal. The elevated aPTT can be corrected by mixing the patient's plasma with an equal volume of normal pooled plasma. In some patients with mild disease, the aPTT may lie within the normal range. Therefore, it is essential to use sensitive and reliable reagents for the aPTT when this test is used as a presurgical screening procedure or to evaluate a bleeding patient for potential hemophilia (37,40). Some patients have a thrombocytosis even in the absence of bleeding. Some others may have a prolonged bleeding time (37).

Quantitative factor VIII:c measurement, by means of a one- or two-stage aPTT assay, or a chromogenic assay, is required for the diagnosis of hemophilia A. If borderline values are obtained, the assay must be repeated. Factor VIII levels in the individual patient are generally stable over time, with the exception of acute-phase increases in factor VIII levels and Heckathorn syndrome, a rare condition associated with dramatic variation in factor VIII levels over time (37,43). Factor VIII:Ag levels usually parallel the levels of factor VIII:c. In patients with a dysfunctional factor VIII molecule, factor VIII:Ag is detectable, and the VIII:c-to-VIII:Ag ratio is low.

Factor VIII inhibitors are typically temperature and time dependent (i.e., they progressively neutralize over time the factor VIII:c present in normal pooled plasma). To detect such an inhibitor, the aPTT mixing study includes incubation of the test system for 60 minutes at 37°C. Neutralization of the factor VIII:c in the test system over time results in a prolonged aPTT after the hour-long incubation. Factor VIII inhibitors are quantitated by the Bethesda assay. Serial dilutions of patient plasma are incubated with normal pooled plasma for 2 hours at 37°C, and the residual factor VIII activity is measured. One Bethesda unit (BU) is the amount of inhibitor that neutralizes 50% of factor VIII in the test system. High-titer inhibitors have levels greater than 10 BU and show an anamnestic response after exposure to factor VIII:Ag. Low-titer inhibitors have levels less than 5 BU and show no anamnestic response.

The diagnosis of hemophilia A is not difficult in patients with severe disease. However, mild cases may be significantly underrecognized. Other bleeding disorders with a clinical presentation similar to that of hemophilia A are factor IX deficiency (hemophilia B) and vWD, particularly the 2N variant, which is characterized by a lack of binding of vWF to factor VIII.

Purified factor VIII products, either plasma derived or recombinant, are the treatment of choice for hemophilia A. The risk of viral transmission due to plasma-derived factor VIII concentrates is extremely low because these are sub-

TABLE 6.9. HEMOPHILIA A

Clinical presentation
X-linked recessive inheritance
Almost exclusively in males
Severity parallels factor VIII_c levels
Deep tissue hemorrhage: joints, soft tissue, intracranial
Severe bleeding with surgery or trauma
Laboratory evaluation
Bleeding time normal; rarely prolonged
PT normal
aPTT prolonged
Factor VIII_c activity decreased
Time-dependent factor VIII inhibitor in 15%
Management of uncomplicated case
Factor VIII concentrate, usually 15 U/kg, depending on severity of bleeding
Maintenance dose every 8–12 h
Monitor with factor VIII_c assay
Target factor VIII level: 30% for mild bleeding, 50% to 100% for severe bleeding
Supportive care: joint immobilization, pain relief
Management of case with factor VIII inhibitors
Low-titer inhibitor: high doses of factor VIII concentrate
High-titer inhibitor: factor IX complex concentrate, porcine factor VIII concentrate

PT, prothrombin time; aPTT, activated partial thromboplastin time.

jected to virus-inactivation procedures and polymerase chain reaction (PCR) tested for the non–lipid-enveloped viruses, hepatitis A virus and human parvovirus B19. Recombinant factor VIII concentrates of varying degrees of purity also are available.

Therapy for hemophilia A is dependent on site and severity of hemorrhage. For the treatment of a minor bleeding episode, such as epistaxis, or oral mucosal bleeding, local treatment in the form of local pressure, cold compresses, topical thrombin, and antifibrinolytic agents and desmopressin may be sufficient to stop bleeding. In some cases, factor VIII:c replacement therapy may be necessary. One unit of factor VIII concentrate per kilogram of body weight will increase the plasma factor VIII:c by approximately 2 U/dL. Therefore, a 70-kg man with severe hemophilia and a desired factor VIII:c increment of 100% would require a loading dose of 3,500 U of factor VIII concentrate (Table 6.10). In minor bleeding episodes, a single dose of factor VIII concentrate at 15 U/kg is usually sufficient. The aim of factor replacement is to increase factor VIII:c levels to approximately 30%. For more serious bleeding, such as hematomas in critical locations, higher levels of factor VIII:c (about 50%) are recommended. This may be achieved with factor VIII concentrate at 30 to 40 U/kg. For surgical prophylaxis, surgical bleeding, or intracranial bleeding, it is essential to maintain factor VIII:c levels at 80% to 100% (6,37,40).

It is critical to monitor factor VIII:c levels during replacement therapy. The aPTT is not sufficiently sensitive for monitoring adequacy of therapy. In accordance with the biologic half-life of factor VIII:c, maintenance doses of factor VIII concentrate may be administered every 8 to 12 hours. The duration of treatment depends on the severity of bleeding. For minor episodes, treatment may be continued for 1 to 2 days, but for major bleeding, factor replacement may be necessary for as long as 2 weeks (40).

When factor VIII:c levels fail to increase after an adequate replacement dose of factor VIII concentrate, the patient should be tested for a factor VIII inhibitor. Treatment of the patient with a factor VIII inhibitor depends on the inhibitor titer. Low-titer inhibitors (less than 5 BU) can be overcome and treated with high doses of factor VIII concentrates. High-titer inhibitors (more than 10 BU) may be treated with factor IX complex concentrates at an empiric dose of 75 U/kg, repeated every 8 to 12 hours (34). Alternatively, porcine factor VIII concentrate may be used as a bolus of 100 U/kg, with subsequent dosing guided by factor VIII:c assays. The rapid development of antibodies against the porcine protein generally limits its use to a single bleeding episode. Other treatment options include recombinant factor VIIa, extracorporeal immunoadsorption using a *Staphylococcus aureus* protein A column, and plasma exchange (37,40,43).

TABLE 6.10. FACTOR VIII$_C$ REPLACEMENT THERAPY BASED ON PLASMA VOLUME

Dose of factor VIII concentrate (U) = 0.5 × [% desired increase in factor VIII$_C$ level] × [weight in kg]
Example: A severely hemophiliac man weighing 70 kg, scheduled for major surgery:
Desired increase in factor VIII$_C$ level = (Target level – Present level) % = (100 – 0) = 100%
Dose of factor VIII concentrate = 0.5 × 100 × 70 = 3,500 U

Pain relief is an important part of the supportive treatment of hemophiliac patients during an acute bleeding episode. Nonsteroidal antiinflammatory agents, acetaminophen/codeine, or nonacetylated choline magnesium trisalicylate may be used (37). Aspirin is contraindicated because of the risk of fresh bleeding and potentiation of existing hemorrhage. Narcotics also may be necessary. Acute hemarthrosis is treated additionally with joint immobilization, and with arthrocentesis in selected cases with severely distended joints. As soon as the acute bleed has resolved, careful physiotherapy should be instituted to restore full mobility of the affected joint. Chronic hemophiliac arthropathy may require supportive orthopedic devices or joint reconstruction. Hemophiliac patients and their caregivers can be trained to administer factor VIII concentrates in the home at the first sign of bleeding. Such home-treatment programs allow the patient to receive prompt replacement therapy, thus minimizing morbidity such as joint damage resulting from hemarthrosis, and permit the patient to lead a more active and independent life (6).

Carrier status of hemophilia A can be assessed by measuring plasma levels of factor VIII:c and vWF for a decrease in the ratio of factor VIII:c to vWF, or by Southern blotting of genomic DNA for detection of the factor VIII gene inversion that is responsible for nearly 50% of cases of hemophilia A. Prenatal testing for hemophilia A can be achieved by fetal blood sampling for factor VIII:c activity, or by chorionic villus sampling for DNA analysis for inheritance of the defective allele (34). The delivery of a neonate with suspected hemophilia requires special care. Factor VIII does not cross the placenta, but the risk of intracranial bleeding with an uncomplicated vaginal delivery is reported to be low (37). Prolonged labor, vacuum extraction, and forceps application must be avoided because of the risk of serious intracranial hemorrhage. Hemorrhage in the neonate must be treated promptly with factor replacement.

FACTOR IX DEFECTS

Factor IX deficiency also is known as hemophilia B, Christmas disease, or plasma thromboplastin component (PTC) deficiency (44–46). This disorder, like hemophilia A, also is inherited as a sex-linked recessive trait. The clinical features are identical to those of hemophilia A: deep tissue bleeding including intraarticular bleeding with hemarthroses, intramuscular bleeding, intracranial bleeding, and potentially severe mucosal membrane hemorrhages (44,47). Factor IX is a vitamin K–dependent protein with a molecular weight of 57,000 that circulates as a proenzyme and is converted to the active form (IXa) by factor XIa or factor VIIa tissue factor complex. Factor IX then rapidly converts factor X to Xa. The deficiency states can be clinically divided into patients who have mild (5% to 30% factor IX), moderate (1% to 5% factor IX), or severe (less than 1% factor IX) disease/deficiency (44). Correlation between factor IX:c and severity of the disease is the same as that noted with factor VIII deficiency. Seventy to ninety percent of patients are truly deficient in factor IX:c and are CRM–. However, 10% to 30% of patients are CRM+ (44,48,49). As another variable, some CRM+ patients have prolonged ox-brain thromboplastin times, and others are normal; several variants of hemophilia B exist. One variant is hemophilia B Leyden; in this variant, the factor IX:c levels increase with age, and these patients convert from CRM– to CRM+. The basis for this change is a mutation in the factor IX promoter region, which contains an androgen response element. With increasing age, factor IX gene transcription and subsequent protein production are stimulated (50–53). Other named variants are factor IX Chapel Hill, factor IX Alabama, Deventer, Kashihara, Zutphen, Eindhoven, Elsinore, Long Beach, Los Angeles, Nagoya, Cambridge, and Niigata (44). Variants of hemophilia B are summarized in Table 6.11.

The clinical features of hemophilia B are summarized in Table 6.12. About 60% to 70% of patients have a family history of the disorder. Patients characteristically have a prolonged aPTT and a normal PT (44). The diagnosis is usually made when a patient with an appropriate history, family history, or appropriate bleeding history presents with a prolonged aPTT and a normal PT, and the factor VIII:c assay is normal. In this circumstance, the next logical assay to be done would be a factor IX assay. Management, like that for hemophilia A, depends on the clinical significance of hemorrhage. Mild mucosal or cutaneous bleeding may be controlled with local supportive measures including cold compresses and, when appropriate, antifibrinolytic agents or topical thrombin. More significant bleeding or preparation for surgery is managed with factor IX concentrates or prothrombin complex concentrates. Replacement therapy for factor IX deficiency is more variable than that for factor VIII because of the factor IX extravascular as well as intravascular distribution. Factor IX has a half-life of 12 to 24 hours, and one unit will increase factor IX levels 1 to 1.5 U/dL (13). One of the primary hazards of using prothrombin complex concentrates is thrombogenicity, including the initiation of disseminated intravascular coagulation (DIC)-type syndromes in recipients (44,54,55). Alternatively, recombinant factor IX concentrates are available and provide a product free of human blood-borne pathogens. In about 5% to 7% of patients with factor IX deficiency, anti-factor IX antibodies develop (44). Further to complicate treatment, anaphylaxis also has been reported in children with inhibitors receiving factor concentrates. Historically, therapy for this complication is to neutralize the antibody with prothrombin complex concentrate, followed by increasing the factor IX:c level to the desired range to achieve hemostasis. There has been success using recombinant factor VIIa (NovoSeven; Novo Nordisk, Princeton, NJ) in the treatment of hemophilia B with inhibitors (56–61). Like factor VIII antibodies, factor IX antibodies in hemophilia B patients also respond poorly to immunosuppressive therapy; however, some patients, even those who experience anaphylaxis with therapy, can achieve long-lasting immune tolerance (62). DNA techniques are available for detection of carriers.

TABLE 6.11. VARIANTS OF HEMOPHILIA B

Factor IX Protein	Ox-brain Thromboplastin Time	Term Used
CRM+	Normal	Hemophilia B+
CRM+	Long	Hemophilia B–$_{M}$
CRM–	Normal	Hemophilia B–
CRM–	Long	Hemophilia B–$_{M}$

TABLE 6.12. HEMOPHILIA B

- Clinical manifestations
  - Sex-linked recessive
  - Absence of factor IX in 70% to 90%
  - Presence of dysfunctional factor IX in 10% to 30%
  - Deep tissue hemorrhage
    - Intraarticular
    - Intracranial
    - Intramuscular
    - Compartment compression syndromes
  - Clinical course parallels factor IX level
    - Severe, 0% to 5%, many spontaneous bleeds
    - Moderate, 5% to 10%, occasional spontaneous bleeds
    - Mild, 10% to 40%, rare spontaneous bleeds
  - Severe bleeding with surgery or trauma
  - Anti–factor IX antibody in 7% to 10% (usually IgG λ)
  - Hemophilia B accounts for 10% to 15% of hemophiliac patients
  - Most patients are male (sex-linked recessive)
- Laboratory manifestations
  - Prolonged partial thromboplastin time
  - Normal prothrombin time
  - Normal template bleeding time
  - Platelet dysfunction (aggregation) may be seen in very severe conditions

Ig, immunoglobulin.

FACTOR X DEFECTS

Activated factor X forms a part of the prothrombinase complex that converts prothrombin to thrombin in the final common pathway of blood coagulation. Congenital factor X deficiency is a rare and heterogeneous disorder with approximately 50 cases reported in the literature. The disorder has an autosomal recessive inheritance. Deficiency occurs as a result of decreased synthesis of normal factor X or synthesis of a variant factor X, as in factor X Friuli, factor X Roma, factor X San Antonio, and factor X Padua (6,16).

The clinical features of homozygous factor X deficiency are similar to those seen with factor VII deficiency. Patients tend to be first seen early in life with moderate or severe bleeding. The most common clinical presentation is mucosal bleeding, particularly epistaxis and menorrhagia. Severe bleeding often follows surgery or trauma (Table 6.13) (63). Intracranial hemorrhage is a frequent presentation, with serious consequences, particularly in the fetus and infant (64–68). Patients with moderate or severe deficiency (factor X levels less than 5%) may have spontaneous soft tissue hematomas and recurrent hemarthroses. In neonates, there may be delayed bleeding from the umbilical cord stump, as is seen in factor XIII deficiency. Pregnancy in patients with factor X deficiency is complicated by repeated abortion and preterm delivery. Individuals with heterozygous factor X deficiency are usually asymptomatic (63).

The aPTT and PT are markedly prolonged in homozygous patients and mildly prolonged or normal in heterozygous individuals. Russell viper venom (RVV) directly activates factor X in vitro; therefore, the RVV test is usually prolonged, but may be normal in patients with factor X Friuli (6,16,63,69). Although factor X deficiency affects the final common pathway of coagulation, the PT and aPTT are often unequally prolonged, particularly in patients with factor X variants. A quantitative factor X assay is required for a definitive diagnosis. Homozygous individuals have low or absent levels of factor X; heterozygous individuals have low or low-normal factor X activity.

Factor levels of approximately 15% to 20% levels are usually sufficient for clinical hemostasis, although higher levels may be required for severe hemorrhage or surgical prophylaxis (69). Factor X replacement is achieved by the use of FFP infusion at a loading dose of 15 to 20 mL/kg, followed by a daily maintenance dose of 5 to 10 mL/kg. Severe hemorrhage may be treated with factor IX complex concentrates at a loading dose of 15 U/kg, followed by a 10 U/kg daily maintenance dose. However, such products contain significant amounts of activated coagulation factors, and are potentially thrombogenic. Therefore, their use should be limited to major bleeding episodes or major surgery. Antifibrinolytic agents should not be used in patients receiving factor IX complex concentrates. Pregnant patients are managed with early and aggressive factor replacement as prophylaxis against bleeding (6,13,16).

TABLE 6.13. FACTOR X DEFICIENCY

Clinical presentation
Autosomal recessive inheritance
Moderate or severe bleeding: mucosa, soft tissue, joints, intracranial
Severe bleeding after surgery or trauma
Repeated abortion and preterm delivery
Bleeding from the umbilical cord stump in neonates
Laboratory evaluation
PT prolonged
aPTT prolonged
Russell viper venom time prolonged
Factor X levels low or absent
Management
FFP at 15–20 mL/kg loading dose, 5 mL/kg daily maintenance dose
Target factor X level, 15% to 20%
Factor IX complex concentrates

PT, prothrombin time; aPTT, activated partial thromboplastin time; FFP, fresh frozen plasma.

FACTOR XI DEFICIENCY

Factor XI is a component of the intrinsic pathway of blood coagulation. Deficiency of this factor was first described by Rosenthal et al. in 1953 (69a). The disease has a high incidence among Ashkenazi Jews, in whom the gene frequency is 4% (16,70). Factor XI deficiency is inherited as an autosomal recessive trait. Three different mutations of the factor XI gene, designated types I, II, and III, account for most cases of deficiency. Type II (a nonsense mutation) and type III (a missense mutation) are most commonly identified in population studies.

The clinical features of factor XI deficiency are variable. Patients with major deficiency (factor XI level less than 20%) are usually homozygotes or compound heterozygotes. They often have excessive bleeding after trauma or surgery (Table 6.14) (16,70). Tissues with high intrinsic fibrinolytic activity, such as the oral cavity and urinary tract, are particularly prone to such bleeding (71). Other hemorrhagic manifestations, such as epistaxis and soft tissue hemorrhage, may occur. Some affected women have menorrhagia and excessive postpartum bleeding (72,73). Patients with minor deficiency (factor XI level, 30% to 65%) are usually heterozygotes and have little or no bleeding (6,16). Some patients with very low levels of factor XI deficiency do not exhibit a bleeding tendency (70,71). It is possible that factor XI–like activity on platelet membranes may partly compensate for deficiency of the plasma factor (16). Mild factor XI deficiency may be associated with Noonan syndrome and Gaucher disease.

Patients with factor XI deficiency usually have a prolonged aPTT and normal PT, although heterozygotes with mild deficiency may have normal aPTT (6,74). There is often little correlation between the severity of bleeding symptoms and the

TABLE 6.14. FACTOR XI DEFICIENCY

Clinical presentation
Autosomal recessive inheritance
Common in Ashkenazi Jews
Excessive bleeding after trauma or surgery
Severe bleeding in oral cavity and urinary tract
Epistaxis, soft-tissue bleeding, menorrhagia, postpartum hemorrhage
Laboratory evaluation
PT normal
aPTT usually prolonged
Plasma factor XI, low
Management
FFP at 15–20 mL/kg loading dose, 5 mL/kg daily maintenance dose
Target factor XI level, 20%
Antifibrinolytic agents

PT, prothrombin time; aPTT, activated partial thromboplastin time; FFP, fresh frozen plasma.

degree of prolongation of the aPTT. Factor XI deficiency must be suspected in any patient with a prolonged aPTT, especially if the family history is suggestive of an autosomal recessive inheritance (16). Diagnosis is established by measuring the level of plasma factor XI. Factor XI deficiency has been associated with deficiency of other clotting factors (6).

Replacement therapy is indicated for significant bleeding episodes and consists of FFP infused at a loading dose of 15 to 20 mL/kg, followed by 5 mL/kg every 12 hours. The half-life of factor XI is about 80 hours. The level should be increased to 30% to 40% of normal to achieve hemostasis (6,13,16,70). Preoperative FFP infusion to increase the factor XI level is recommended, although not all factor XI–deficient patients bleed during surgery. Antifibrinolytic agents may be used as adjunctive therapy (75). Bleeding after prostatectomy may be severe enough to require plasma exchange to achieve factor XI levels adequate for hemostasis (16).

FACTOR XII DEFECTS

Congenital factor XII deficiency was first described by Ratnoff and Colopy in 1955 (76,77). Since then, several hundred cases have been reported (76,78). The name of the first patient studied by Ratnoff and Colopy was John Hageman, and the disorder also is commonly called Hageman trait (77). Factor XII or Hageman factor has a molecular weight of 80,000 and is a serine protease glycoprotein. Usually the disorder is inherited as an autosomal recessive, but instances of autosomal dominant inheritance also have been described. Homozygous patients of the autosomal recessive variety have very low levels of factor XII, frequently less than 1%; heterozygotes can be quite variable, but tend to have around 50% of normal factor XII activity, usually between 17% and 80%. As is the case with most factor deficiency, the disorder may exist in the absence of the protein, factor XII:c–, or present in a dysfunctional form, factor XII:c+ (CRM+) (79–81). However, the absence form appears to be more common than the dysfunctional variety.

Factor XII deficiency is usually an incidental finding when a screening PTT is noted to be markedly prolonged, often in a routine presurgical patient (78). Because this is the manner in which many patients are seen, it has been assumed that patients with factor XII deficiency have no bleeding diathesis. Some patients do have a mild bleeding tendency, and rarely even life-threatening bleeding may occur (77). Uncommonly, fatal hemorrhage has been reported (82). Of particular interest, patients with factor XII deficiency have defective surface-mediated activation of fibrinolysis, and many patients dying with factor XII deficiency have died of thrombosis or thromboembolism (83–86). John Hageman, a railroad worker, died of a pulmonary embolus after hip fracture (87). Historically, it appeared that an inordinately large number of patients with factor XII deficiency have died of a myocardial infarction or pulmonary embolus and have an increased risk of deep vein thrombosis. However, several subsequent studies have not found an association between factor XII deficiency and thrombosis (88–90). In addition, patients may have defects in neutrophil/macrophage chemotaxis (91).

The diagnosis of factor XII deficiency comes to light in noting a prolonged PTT and normal PT in an asymptomatic patient, usually on routine presurgical screening, as is the case with other contact factors without a lupus anticoagulant (77,78). A definitive diagnosis requires specific quantitative factor XII assay by a functional assay (92). Because hemorrhage is rare, replacement therapy is generally not needed. In those exceptionally rare patients with significant hemorrhage, replacement should be with FFP. Certainly, when thrombosis or thromboembolism occurs, it should be treated appropriately. Findings of factor XII defects are shown in Table 6.15.

TABLE 6.15. FACTOR XII DEFECTS

Clinical manifestations
Autosomal recessive trait in most patients
Autosomal dominant trait in few patients
Absence form (CRM–) and dysfunctional form (CRM+) exist
Incidental finding via prolonged PTT
May have defective surface-mediated fibrinolytic activation
Historically considered to have incidence of thrombosis/thromboembolism
Laboratory manifestations
Markedly prolonged aPTT
Normal PT
Normal template bleeding time
Normal platelet function (aggregation)
Definitive diagnosis requires factor XII assay
Therapy
FFP replacement for hemorrhage
Anticoagulants for thrombosis/thromboembolus

PT, prothrombin time; aPTT, activated partial thromboplastin time; FFP, fresh frozen plasma.

PREKALLIKREIN DEFECTS

Prekallikrein (PK) deficiency was first noted by Hathaway et al. (93) in 1965, when children from a consanguineous marriage had frostbite after a fire in their rural Kentucky home in winter. After treatment of their injuries, tonsillectomies were planned. Preoperative PTTs were markedly prolonged in four of 14 children. The defect was noted to be corrected with factor XII–deficient plasma, and the new disorder was called Fletcher trait, after the surname of the family. Later in 1972, Wuepper et al. (93a) demonstrated that PK and Fletcher factor were one and the same. The mode of inheritance is unclear or variable; some have described autosomal recessive characteristics, but others have noted autosomal dominance (94). Although most patients yet studied have a true deficiency (CRM–), several instances of a dysfunctional form (CRM+) also have been described (95,96). Patients with PK deficiency are usually of African ancestry and have no bleeding tendency, although these patients, like those with factor XII deficiency, also have defects of in vitro activation of the fibrinolytic system (97,98). However, there are no discernible clinical effects. The diagnosis is suggested usually during presurgical screening procedures when a markedly prolonged PTT and a normal PT and thrombin time are noted in an asymptomatic individual in the absence of a lupus anticoagulant (78,94). The diagnosis is confirmed by performing a specific PK assay by clot-based or synthetic substrate–based techniques; both types of assays are readily available. A characteristic of PK deficiency is the noting of correction of the PTT when incubating the PTT system for 10 minutes with kaolin, diatomaceous earth, or silica (93, 99). This test should not be used for a diagnosis because the same phenomena may be observed with Passovoy deficiency; an erroneous interpretation could lead to a missed diagnosis of Passovoy defect and a potential bleeding problem. The features of PK deficiency are summarized in Table 6.16.

TABLE 6.16. PREKALLIKREIN DEFICIENCY

Clinical manifestations	
Autosomal recessive and dominant cases described	
Majority have absence of protein (CRM–)	
Some have dysfunctional protein (CRM+)	
No hemorrhagic tendency yet described	
Defective surface-mediated activation of fibrinolysis	
Laboratory manifestations	
Prolonged aPTT	
Normal PT	
Normal template bleeding time	
Normal platelet function (aggregation)	
Definitive diagnosis requires prekallikrein assay	
Correction of PTT with long incubation (10 min) is characteristic but should not be used as diagnostic tool. The same findings may be seen in passovoy defect	

PT, prothrombin time; aPTT, activated partial thromboplastin time; FFP, fresh frozen plasma.

KININOGEN DEFECTS

High-molecular-weight kininogen (HMWK) deficiency is known by a variety of surnames, including the most common, Fitzgerald trait (100); however, the defect also is known as Williams trait, Fleaujac trait, Fujiwara trait, and Reid trait (101–104). Kallikrein cleaves HMWK, which then binds to anionic surfaces and functions to bring factor XI and PK in close proximity to facilitate the generation of factor XIIa. The disorder is inherited as an autosomal recessive trait. Patients do not have a hemorrhagic tendency, but do have abnormal surface-mediated activation of fibrinolysis, as noted by a long euglobulin clot-lysis time (98). All patients thus far studied have a true deficiency of HMWK. Fitzgerald and Reid traits represent a deficiency of HMWK; however, Williams trait, Fleaujac trait, and Fujiwara trait represent a deficiency of both HMWK and low-molecular-weight kininogen. These last three forms of deficiency also are deficient in PK. The diagnosis is suspected by noting a prolonged PTT and a normal PT and thrombin time, noncorrecting of the aPTT with prolonged incubation in an asymptomatic individual, usually during a routine preoperative screening workup (78,94). A presumptive diagnosis may be made by using a functional assay with normal and HMWK-deficient plasma; however, definitive diagnosis is made by immunologic assay for HMWK (94,105). Individuals are asymptomatic but have abnormal surface-activated fibrinolysis and defective neutrophil/macrophage chemotaxis. In one individual, abnormal inflammatory responses were noted (100). The features of HMWK deficiency are summarized in Table 6.17.

TABLE 6.17. HIGH-MOLECULAR-WEIGHT KININOGEN DEFICIENCY

Clinical manifestations	
Autosomal recessive trait	
No hemorrhagic tendency	
Abnormal surface-mediated activation of fibrinolysis	
Variety of synonyms	
Name	Deficiency
Fitzgerald trait	High-molecular-weight kininogen only
Reid trait	High-molecular-weight kininogen only
Williams trait	High- and low-molecular-weight kininogen
Flaujeac trait	High- and low-molecular-weight kininogen
Fujiwara trait	High- and low-molecular-weight kininogen
Laboratory manifestations	
Prolonged aPTT	
Normal PT	
Normal template bleeding time	
Normal platelet function (aggregation)	
Definitive diagnosis requires immunologic assay for high molecular-weight kininogen	

PT, prothrombin time; aPTT, activated partial thromboplastin time.

α_2-ANTIPLASMIN DEFECTS

α_2-Antiplasmin, or α_2-plasmin inhibitor, is the plasma protein primarily responsible for inhibiting the fibrinolytic activity of plasmin (106,107). Small amounts of this enzyme also are found in platelets. Deficiency of α_2-antiplasmin results in a bleeding tendency because of the unopposed activity of plasmin on the fibrin clot. The disorder is inherited in an autosomal recessive manner and appears to be very rare. α_2-Antiplasmin deficiency may occur as a result of decreased enzyme synthesis, or the synthesis of a nonfunctional molecule, such as α_2-antiplasmin Enschede and α_2-antiplasmin Bakersfield (107,108).

Homozygous patients have a severe bleeding tendency, with easy bruising, mucosal bleeding, hemarthrosis, intramedullary hematomas in long bones, and prolonged bleeding after minor trauma (Table 6.18) (106,107, 109–113). A typical feature is rebleeding from wounds some time after initial hemorrhage has ceased, consistent with rapid lysis of the hemostatic fibrin clot. Bleeding from the umbilical stump in neonates is reported in some patients (107). Heterozygous individuals are asymptomatic or may have a mild bleeding tendency (106).

The standard screening tests for patients with a hemorrhagic disorder, including whole blood clotting time, bleeding time, PT, PTT, bleeding time, platelet count, von Willebrand profile, and platelet-function tests, are generally normal. Clotting factor levels are normal. The whole blood clot-lysis time and euglobulin lysis time are markedly prolonged. Occasionally, elevated fibrin(ogen) degradation products are seen. Quantitation of α_2-antiplasmin is required for diagnosis. The level of this enzyme is markedly decreased in homozygotes (less than 10%) and mildly decreased in heterozygotes (around 50%) (106,107,109).

Patients are treated with oral or intravenous antifibrinolytic agents, such as ε-aminocaproic acid, or tranexamic acid (106). Invasive procedures at the bedside have been performed with a tranexamic acid drip (114).

TABLE 6.18. α_2-ANTIPLASMIN DEFICIENCY

Clinical presentation
- Autosomal recessive inheritance
- Severe bleeding tendency in homozygotes: mucosa, joints, long bones
- Rebleeding from wounds

Laboratory evaluation
- Clotting time, PT, aPTT normal
- Platelet count and function normal
- von Willebrand profile normal
- α_2-antiplasmin level <10% in homozygotes

Management
- Antifibrinolytics: ε-aminocaproic acid (εACA), transexamic acid

PT, prothrombin time; aPTT, activated partial thromboplastin time.

PLASMINOGEN ACTIVATOR INHIBITOR DEFECTS

Plasminogen activator inhibitor (PAI-1) is a serine protease inhibitor that functions, as its name implies, to inhibit production of plasmin by tissue plasminogen activator (t-PA). In the deficiency of PAI-1, increased amounts of plasmin are produced by t-PA, initiating excessive fibrinolysis with resultant hemorrhage. Congenital deficiency results in a lifelong bleeding disorder, similar to that seen in factor XIII and α_2-antiplamsin deficiency, characterized by mucosal bleeding, including epistaxis, postsurgical hemorrhage, and delayed hematomas after injury (Table 6.19) (115,116). The euglobin clot-lysis time is abnormally shortened, and the diagnosis may be definitively assessed with functional and quantitative assays (116). PAI-1 is an acute-phase reactant; therefore, studies should be performed in the absence of illness if deficiency is suspected clinically. Patients with PAI-1 deficiency undergoing dental extractions have been successfully treated with antifibrinolytic agents (117).

FACTOR XIII DEFECTS

Congenital factor XIII deficiency has been described in more than 100 families and is inherited as an autosomal recessive trait (118–120) and has been associated with consanguinity. Factor XIII is a dimeric protein consisting of an α and a β chain, and the complex circulates as a dimer (A2B2) in plasma (120,121) and as two A subunits within platelets. Congenital deficiency states may be due to decreased A and B subunits (type I), or deficiency of either A (type II) or B subunits (type III) (122,123). Most severely affected patients have defects of the α chain, con-

TABLE 6.19. PLASMINOGEN ACTIVATOR INHIBITOR DEFECTS

Clinical manifestations
- Very rare
- Epistaxis
- Gastrointestinal bleeding
- Postsurgical hemorrhage
- Delayed hematomas after injury

Laboratory manifestations
- Normal PT
- Normal aPTT
- Normal template bleeding time
- Normal platelet function (aggregation)
- Abnormal Euglobin lysis time
- Definitive diagnisis requires assay for PAI-1

Therapy
- Epsilon aminocaproic acid
- Tranexamic acid

PAI, plasminogen activator inhibitor; PT, prothrombin time; aPTT, activated partial thromboplastin time.

taining the activation site. Additionally, an acquired deficiency state has been described as due to an inhibitor of factor XIII (124). If immunologic techniques are used to assay factor XIII, anti–α-chain and anti–β-chain antibodies must be used, and such techniques are available (118,120,121,123, 125,126).

The clinical manifestations of factor XIII deficiency usually occur only in homozygous individuals, typically with less than 1% factor XIII, as greater than 1% of normal factor XIII levels are necessary for normal fibrin monomer cross-linking to occur (118–120). Ninety percent of patients demonstrate delayed umbilical stump bleeding at childbirth, and this finding should immediately prompt a strong suspicion of factor XIII deficiency, or less probably, afibrinogenemia, homozygous dysfibrinogenemia, or factor X deficiency (78,118–120). Patients with homozygous factor XIII deficiency also characteristically have significant deep tissue hemorrhages, especially into muscle and muscle compartments; these most commonly develop several days after minor trauma but may happen spontaneously (119). In many patients, later destruction of bone and pseudocysts may be especially prominent in the thigh and gluteal areas (119). The most common cause of death is intracranial hemorrhage, which occurs in factor XIII deficiency more commonly than in other congenital coagulation protein defects; these intracranial bleeds also are commonly preceded by minor trauma occurring several days earlier (118,119). Although deep tissue bleeding is common, intraarticular bleeds are rare. In addition, although patients have delayed posttraumatic bleeding, postsurgical bleeding is less commonly a problem. Most homozygous men are sterile, and a high incidence of spontaneous abortion is seen in homozygous women (119). It has been suggested that factor XIII is involved not only in adequate wound healing, by possibly cross-linking collagen as well as fibrin, but also may be necessary for normal implantation of a fertilized ovum into the uterine decidua (119).

A screening test for the presence or absence of factor XIII consists of observing for clot solubility or insolubility in 5 M urea or 1% monochloroacetic acid, two agents that will disrupt hydrophobic bonds, but not the γ-glutamyl–lysine bonds created by factor XIIIa (78,118). Therefore normal clots will not lyse, but those clots produced by factor XIII–deficient patients will dissolve, typically after a few minutes. These solubility tests are, however, limited screening techniques and may rarely miss a symptomatic individual with slightly more than 1% activity (118). More specific techniques are available including assays for γ-γ dimer (cross-linked by factor XIII), radioactive amine incorporation tests, latex agglutination inhibition tests, or radioimmunoassay (120,125,126). The goal of therapy for factor XIII deficiency is to maintain factor XIII activity at 2% to 3% and may be achieved by infusion of cryoprecipitate (one bag/10 kg) or FFP (2 to 3 mL/kg) every 4 to 6 weeks (13). Characteristic findings of factor XIII defects are noted in Table 6.20.

TABLE 6.20. FACTOR XIII DEFECTS

Clinical manifestations
Autosomal recessive trait
Most patients have absence of α chain (CRM–)
Umbilical stump bleeding in 90%
Delayed deep tissue hemorrhage is typical
Intramuscular
Intracranial
Pseudocysts often develop
Most common cause of death is intracranial bleeding
Most homozygous men are sterile
Most homozygous women have miscarriages
Heterozygous patients are usually asymptomatic
Laboratory manifestations
Clot solubility in urea or monochloracetic acid
Definitive diagnosis requires specific assay for factor XIII cross-linking activity
Therapy
Fresh frozen plasma or cryoprecipitate every few weeks

VON WILLEBRAND DISEASE

von Willebrand disease (vWD) is a quantitative or qualitative defect of vWF that was first described in 1926 by Erik von Willebrand in a family on the Åland Islands off the coast of Sweden (127). In 1953, Ben Alexander, Armand J. Quick, and Professor Larrieu simultaneously discovered a new characteristic of vWD, that of low factor VIII levels (128–130). This important discovery acted as a catalyst to launch investigations that have subsequently led to a more complete understanding of the biology of the factor VIII macromolecular complex, classic hemophilia, and vWD. In 1971 Zimmerman et al. (131) developed an antibody to factor VIII and were able to demonstrate that the presence of an antigen, factor VIII:RAg (now called vWF:Ag), in normal and hemophiliac plasma but not in von Willebrand plasma; this discovery began the era of molecular biology of hemophilia, vWD, and factor VIII moieties, and supplied a tool for the discovery and defining of von Willebrand types and the separately recognized portions/activities of the factor VIII macromolecular complex.

vWD is now known to be the most common heritable coagulopathy in the world, with an incidence between 1% and 4% (132–133), without apparent racial or ethnic predilection (134). This disorder is the most common, clinically significant, congenital bleeding disorder in humans. The diagnosis is not always straightforward and ideally requires three prerequisites: history of bleeding, documentation of decreased or abnormal vWF, and demonstration of inheritance (135). The diagnosis is further complicated by many variables such as age and blood group, which may require appropriately adjusted reference ranges (136).

Clinical presentation of vWD is quite variable among individuals but generally consistent among families and is characteristic of "platelet-type" bleeding (that is, easy bruising, mucocutaneous bleeding, menorrhagia, postpartum bleeding and hemorrhage with minor surgical procedures) (127,137,138). Individuals with mild disease may be asymptomatic except in situations of severe hemostatic challenge. Bleeding that does occur in affected patients typically begins in early childhood when the child begins to ambulate. Severe types of vWD may appear clinically identical to hemophilia (Table 6.21).

vWF is a 270-kDa monomer that assembles into variably sized multimers (600 to 20,000 kDa). vWF functions by binding primarily to subendothelial collagen, thereby acting as molecular "glue" for platelet adhesion via the glycoprotein (GP)Ib and GPIIb/IIIa receptors and facilitating platelet–platelet adhesion (139). The largest vWF multimers that are the most active in facilitating primary hemostasis. vWF also plays a crucial role in hemostasis by protecting coagulation factor VIII:c from proteolytic cleavage by activated protein C, thereby markedly increasing the half-life of factor VIII in the circulation (140). This close and necessary relation of factor VIII and vWF explains why vWF has historically been referred to as factor VIII:c–related antigen (factor VIII:R). vWF is produced in endothelial cells and megakaryocytes. Endothelial cell–produced vWF is stored in the endothelial Weibel–Palade bodies and is subsequently constitutively secreted into the plasma. Endothelial vWF also may be released by a variety of stimuli including endothelial injury, products of secondary hemostasis (thrombin and fibrin), complement components, and others. vWF produced in megakaryocytes is stored within the platelet granules. Platelet vWF functions mostly in binding to the GPIIb-IIIa receptors (141).

TABLE 6.21. VON WILLEBRAND SYNDROME

- Clinical manifestations
  - Variable inheritance
  - Easy and spontaneous bruising
  - Petechiae and purpura
  - Mucosal membrane hemorrhage
    - Genitourinary
    - Gastrointestinal
    - Intrapulmonary
    - Gingival bleeding
  - Bilateral epistaxis in early childhood
  - Deep tissue bleeding rare
  - Hemorrhage may be severe with surgery or trauma
- Therapy
  - Antifibrinolytic agents (ε-aminocaproic acid transexamic acid)
  - Useful adjunct in mild bleeding, especially mucosal
  - Desmopressin (DDAVP)
    - Useful in type I and selected other types
    - Avoid use in type 2B due to thrombocytopenia
    - Monitor for side effects (mainly hyponatremia)
  - Moderately pure factor VIII concentrates (Humate-P)
    - Useful in all types
    - 20–30 U/kg every 12 h
    - Monitor vWF levels (keep >50%)
  - Cryoprecipitate, 1 to 3 bags per 10 kg of body weight
  - Fresh frozen plasma to factor VIII:C >75%
  - Inhibitors have been treated with intravenous immunoglobulin or protein A columns

vWF, von Willebrand factor.

The vWF gene is very large, spans 180 kb on chromosome 12, and contains 52 exons. The primary protein is 2,813 amino acids and consists of several repeated areas that correspond roughly to functional domains of the protein-like binding to collagen and platelet GPIb(A-repeats), binding to factor VIII(D-repeat), binding to platelet GPIIb-IIIa complex (C-repeat). The N-terminal two D-repeats are important for multimer formation but are cleaved off the mature form of the protein (142). The large size of the vWF gene increases not only the likelihood of accumulating mutations but also the difficulty of finding and characterizing new mutations and/or polymorphisms.

vWD may be conveniently divided into disorders that are mainly quantitative and disorders that are predominantly qualitative (i.e., with vWF activity relatively decreased in proportion to the quantity of vWF antigen). For our purposes, vWD may be divided into three main types (143). Type 1 is a quantitative deficiency of all vWF multimer sizes, type 2 is a qualitative and quantitative deficiency that lacks only high-molecular-weight (HMW) multimers (in most subtypes), and type 3, which is characterized by an almost complete absence of vWF. Each type (and most important for the type 2 deficiency states) contains several subtypes (Table 6.22).

The assessment of vWD requires a combination of in vivo and in vitro tests (144). As is the case with all bleeding disorders, the primary assessment is a complete history and physical examination. A bleeding time is frequently used to assess primary hemostasis; however, this in vivo assay lacks sensitivity in mild cases and has poor reproducibility. A new in vitro assay of primary hemostasis, the PFA-100 (Dade-Behring, Miami, FL) uses whole blood forced through an aperture in a epinephrine/collagen-coated or adenosine diphosphate (ADP)/collagen–coated membrane with a resultant "closure time" as platelets occlude the lumen of the aperture. This assay has shown promise as a replacement for the uncomfortable and somewhat subjective bleeding time measurement in individuals suspected of having a disorder of primary hemostasis (145–148). The vWF ristocetin cofactor (vWFR:Co) activity measures the functional activity of vWF (149). This assay uses ristocetin to induce a conformational change in the vWF present in the patient's plasma and allows vWF to aggregate platelets through the GPIb receptor. The vWF antigen (vWF:Ag) assay is a quantitative measure of vWF, usually performed by immunologic means. Multimer analysis is performed by agarose gel electrophoresis for the characterization of multimer size and quantity. Assays are used to evaluate factor VIII activity, and

TABLE 6.22. COMMON FORMS OF VON WILLEBRAND SYNDROME

Type I
- von Willebrand syndrome type 1A
  - Autosomal dominant trait
  - Concordant decreases in factor VIII:C, factor VIII:CAg, vW factor, vW factor:Ag
  - vWF multimer analysis reveals decrease in normal structure and distribution
  - A quantitative defect in entire factor VIII complex
- von Willebrand syndrome type 1B
  - Same findings as in type 1A, but a disproportionate decrease in large vWF multimers

Type II
- von Willebrand syndrome type IIA
  - Autosomal dominant trait
  - Discordant decreases in factor VIII:C (reduced), factor VIII:CAg (reduced), vW factor:Ag (reduced), vW factor (very reduced)
  - Depolymerization of vWF complex with many monomeric "fast" forms
- von Willebrand syndrome type IIB
  - Autosomal dominant trait
  - Discordant findings as in type IIA
  - Factor VIII:C near normal
  - vWF factor:Ag moderately reduced
  - Enhanced platelet agglutination to ristocetin
  - Depolymerization of vWF complex but fewer monomeric forms than IIA

Type III
- von Willebrand syndrome type III/IS
  - Severe hemorrhage of many sites
  - High incidence of consanguinity
  - Very prolonged template bleeding time
  - Very reduced vWF (ristocetin cofactor)
  - Very reduced vWF:Ag

an immunologic assay, usually enzyme-linked immunosorbent assay (ELISA), may be used to quantitate factor VIII antigen (Table 6.23).

Type 1 von Willebrand Disease

Type I vWD is defined as a quantitative deficiency of all sizes of vWF multimers and accounts for approximately 70% of all patients with vWD. This abnormality appears to be inherited in an autosomal dominant manner with incomplete penetrance.

On the molecular level, vWD type 1 is a very heterogeneous disorder that may include some hemorrhagic diatheses that are not caused primarily by vWF gene mutations but by alterations in some other, unidentified gene that modifies vWF levels. However, the lack of expression of one of the vWF genes is usually compensated for by the second, normally functioning gene (150). It has been proposed that many patients with autosomal dominant type 1 vWD actually have additional, undetected mutations in their second vWF allele if they are symptomatic, or that these patients show other confounding factors like blood group O or female sex, both of which are associated with significantly lower vWF levels. Testing of individuals with type IA vWD usually reveals a prolonged bleeding time, decreased von Willebrand antigen with a concomitant decrease in vWF ristocetin activity, and a proportional decrease in factor VIII activity that is expected to occur in the absence of vWF "protection." Agarose gel electrophoresis reveals a decrease in all sizes of multimers. A subtype of type 1, type 1B, is similar to type 1A, except there is disproportionate decrease in large vWF multimers.

TABLE 6.23. COMPARISON OF LABORATORY ASSAYS IN COMMON FORMS OF VON WILLEBRAND DISEASE

Trait	Type I	Type 2A	Type 2B	Type 3
Autosomal inheritance	Dominant/not known	Dominant	Dominant	Recessive
vWF:Ag	Decreased	Normal/decreased	Normal/decreased	Markedly decreased
vWF R:Co	Decreased	Decreased	Increased to low-dose ristocetin	Markedly decreased
Factor VIII activity	Decreased	Normal	Normal	Markedly decreased
vWF multimer analysis	All multimers decreased	Loss of HMW multimers	Loss of HMW multimers	Virtual absence of all multimers

HMW, high molecular weight.

Treatment of vWD type 1, if not severe, constitutes the use of the vasopressin analogue, desmopressin (DDAVP). DDAVP increases the release of vWF from the storage sites in endothelial cells, thereby increasing plasma concentrations from two- to sixfold (151). This therapy is most useful in mild to moderate type I vWD, because such patients possess qualitatively normal but quantitatively deficient vWF. DDAVP may be administered either intravenously or intranasally. Tachyphylaxis may develop with repeated administration. Patients with severe type I disease or those experiencing bleeding unresponsive to DDAVP may require use of moderately pure factor VIII concentrates, which have been shown to be safe and effective (152), or alternatively, cryoprecipitate may be used.

Type 2 von Willebrand Disease

Type 2 vWD may be thought of as a predominantly qualitative vWF disorder, although HMW multimers also are lacking. This type accounts for 20% to 30% of individuals with vWD. Because vWF serves many functions, numerous subtypes have been described. In contrast to vWD type 1, genetics and molecular causation of type 2 vWD are well understood.

Type 2A von Willebrand Disease

Type 2A is characterized by loss of the most active vWF forms, the high- and intermediate-molecular-weight multimers, and manifests clinically by decreased platelet function. This loss of the HMW multimers may be due to increased proteolysis after secretion from the endothelial cells (153) or to abnormal intracellular processing (154). Laboratory analysis of individuals with vWD type 2A reveals a prolonged bleeding time, decreased vWF:RCo activity, and normal or near-normal vWF antigen and factor VIII:c activity. The agarose gel electrophoresis will demonstrate a lack of high- to intermediate-molecular-weight multimers and normal quantities of lower-molecular-weight multimers.

vWD type 2A is inherited in an autosomal dominant manner. On the molecular level, type 2A shows a variety of missense mutations, changing just a single amino acid. Most of these mutations are located in a relatively short domain of the protein, encompassing amino acids 742 to 875 (155).

Type 2B von Willebrand Disease

Type 2B is defined by a "gain of function" exhibited by enhanced platelet aggregation to low concentrations of ristocetin that would not aggregate normal platelets. Again, HMW multimers are lacking, and there is normal to slightly decreased antigen.

Patients with vWD 2B may demonstrate variable thrombocytopenia (156,157). Occasionally, even severe thrombocytopenia has been described (158). The etiology of this thrombocytopenia is consumption secondary to increased vWF affinity for platelet GPIb receptors and their subsequent aggregation. Several different point mutations causing single amino acid replacements of vWF have been proven to cause the increased affinity in the platelet GPIb binding area of vWF.

Moderately pure factor VIII concentrates have been successfully used to treat vWD 2B individuals with or without thrombocytopenia. Cryoprecipitate also may be considered, generally as a second choice or when concentrates are not available because no viral or pathogen inactivation is currently performed on cryoprecipitate. The use of DDAVP in these individuals is controversial but should generally be avoided because of reported cases of thrombocytopenia and/or thrombosis associated with its use in this subtype (159).

Type 2N von Willebrand Disease

vWD Normandy is a rare variant of vWD defined by a defect in the factor VIII binding site of vWF. This molecular defect prevents factor VIII from binding to the vWF (142). Without the protection from proteolysis by vWF, the intravascular half-life of factor VIII:c is dramatically decreased. These patients may experience more severe bleeding episodes than is typically associated with most subtypes of vWD, and the disease may mimic mild hemophilia A.

Inheritance of vWD type 2N is autosomal recessive. In patients with this rare type of vWD, both vWF genes carry a mutation that changes either one of six amino acids in the N-terminal D repeat of the mature vWF protein. This N-terminal D repeat constitutes the factor VIII binding domain of vWF (155).

Laboratory evaluation reveals markedly decreased factor VIII activity with normal or near-normal vWF:Ag, vWF:RCo, and a normal multimer pattern on electrophoresis. Treatment of type 2N patients is achieved with moderately pure factor VIII concentrates or cryoprecipitate.

Type 2M von Willebrand Disease

This qualitative defect is different in that HMW multimers are present; however, there is a defect in platelet adhesion. This type of vWD is very rare and clinically less important. It is caused by small deletions or specific missense mutations in the GPIb binding domain. Type 2M mutations seem to disrupt the affinity of vWF to platelet GPIb. This can be demonstrated in vitro by the absence of ristocetin-induced platelet binding with conservation of botrocetin-induced binding (160).

von Willebrand Disease Type 3

Type 3 vWD is rare, occurring in approximately one in a million individuals and is characterized by severe bleeding and clinical behavior similar to that seen in hemophiliacs. This severe phenotype is due to the virtual absence of vWF and concomitantly decreased factor VIII:c activity. This type of vWD is inherited in an autosomal recessive manner; therefore both parents may appear normal clinically and in laboratory evaluation. This phenotype also has been described in type 1/type 3 compound heterozygotes. Type 3 vWD is characterized by the absence of functional vWF and is usually caused by complete deletion, frameshift mutation, or premature termination codons in both vWF alleles of the patient. In patients with total lack of vWF expression, alloantibodies to vWF frequently develop, presenting a challenge to replacement therapy.

The primary treatment in these individuals is factor replacement or cryoprecipitate. Occasionally platelet concentrates may be required for hemostasis.

Pseudo–von Willebrand Disease

Pseudo-vWD also is known as platelet-type vWD and is an autosomal dominant platelet, not a vWF, defect. This disorder is characterized by dysfunction of platelet membrane GPIb, the binding site for vWF activity (161,162). Although this is a platelet-function defect, the clinical and routine laboratory features are similar to those of vWD IIb. The mutation in the platelet GP1b receptor for vWF produces increased affinity for vWF and, therefore, may result in consumption of large vWF multimers, thrombocytopenia, and account for increased ristocetin-induced platelet aggregation (161). A diagnosis of this disorder is confirmed by adding vWF (cryoprecipitate) to the patient's platelet-rich plasma in aggregation studies. This will induce platelet aggregation in platelet-type vWD, whereas aggregation will not occur in true vWD (161).

OTHER RARE DEFECTS

Other rare solitary and combined hereditary protein defects characterized by a bleeding diathesis have been described. One such disorder, Passovoy deficiency, is typified by moderate bleeding including mucosal bleeding and easy bruising. Passovoy deficiency is transmitted in an autosomal dominant manner. The aPTT is prolonged but will shorten with incubation (similar to that of PK deficiency). Other routine coagulation studies, including the PT and thrombin time are unremarkable. Treatment for hemorrhage or for prophylactic treatment before surgery consists of FFP infusions (163–165).

Congenital deficiencies of protein C inhibitor have led to bleeding diathesis secondary to subsequent deficiencies of factors V and VIII because of proteolytic cleavage of activated protein C (166,167).

REFERENCES

1. Martinez J. Quantitative and qualitative disorders of fibrinogen. In: Hoffman R, Benz EJ, Shattil SJ, et al., eds. *Hematology: basic principles and practice.* New York: Churchill Livingstone, 2000: 1925.
2. Al-Mondhiry H, Ehmann WC. Congenital afibrinogenemia. *Am J Hematol* 1994;46:343.
3. Mammen E. Fibrinogen abnormalities. *Semin Thromb Hemost* 1983;9:1.
4. Galanakis DK. Inherited dysfibrinogenemia: emerging abnormal structure associations with pathologic and nonpathologic dysfunctions. *Semin Thromb Hemost* 1993;19:386.
5. Henselmans JML, Meijer K, Haaxma R, et al. Recurrent spontaneous intracerebral hemorrhage in a congenitally afibrinogenemic patient: diagnostic pitfalls and therapeutic options. *Stroke* 1999;30:2479.
6. Rodgers GM, Greenberg CS. Inherited coagulation disorders. In: Lee GR, Foerster J, Lukens J, et al., eds. *Wintrobe's clinical hematology.* Baltimore: Williams & Wilkins, 1999:1682.
7. Hanano M, Takahashi H, Itoh M, et al. Coexistence of congenital afibrinogenemia and protein C deficiency in a patient. *Am J Hematol* 1992;41:57.
8. Chafa O, Chellali T, Sternberg C, et al. Severe hypofibrinogenemia associated with bilateral ischemic necrosis of toes and fingers. *Blood Coagul Fibrinolysis* 1995;6:549.
9. Funai EF, Klein SA, Lockwood CJ. Successful pregnancy outcome in a patient with both congenital hypofibrinogenemia and protein S deficiency. *Obstet Gynecol* 1997;89:858.
10. Rao AK. Congenital disorders of platelet function: disorders of signal transduction and secretion. *Am J Med Sci* 1998;316:69.
11. Castaman G, Ruggeri M, Rodeghiero F. Congenital afibrinogenemia: successful prevention of recurrent hemoperitoneum during ovulation by oral contraceptive. *Am J Hematol* 1995;49:363.
12. Rizk DEE, Kumar RM. Congenital afibrinogenemia: treatment of excessive menstrual bleeding with continuous oral contraceptive. *Am J Hematol* 1996;52:237.
13. Alving BA. Beyond hemophilia and von Willebrand disease: treatment of patients with other inherited coagulation factor and inhibitor deficiencies. In: Alving B, ed. *Blood components and pharmacological agents in the treatment of congenital and acquired bleeding disorders.* Bethesda: AABB Press, 2000:341.
14. Cronin C, Fitzpatrick D, Temperley I. Multiple pulmonary emboli in a patient with afibrinogenemia. *Acta Haematol* 1988; 79:53.
15. MacKinnon HH, Fekete JF. Congenital afibrinogenemia: vascular changes and multiple thromboses induced by fibrinogen infusions and contraceptive medication. *Can Med Assoc J* 1971; 104:597.
16. Roberts HR, Hoffman M. Other clotting factor deficiencies. In: Hoffman R, Benz EJ, Shattil SJ, et al., eds. *Hematology: basic principles and practice.* New York: Churchill Livingstone, 2000: 1912.
17. Gill FM, Shapiro SS, Schwartz E. Severe congenital hypoprothrombinemia. *J Pediatr* 1978;93:264.
18. Mammen E. Factor II abnormalities. *Semin Thromb Hemost* 1983;9:13.

19. Tsuda H, Mizuno Y, Hara T, et al. A case of congenital factor V deficiency combined with multiple congenital anomalies: successful management of palatoplasty. *Acta Haematol* 1990;83:49.
20. Schultz SC, Breall J, Hannan R. Acute cardiac tamponade secondary to congenital factor V deficiency. *Cardiology* 1997;88:48.
21. Totan M, Albayrak D. Intracranial haemorrhage due to factor V deficiency. *Acta Paediatr* 1999;88:342.
22. Manotti C, Quintavalla R, Pini M, et al. Thromboembolic manifestations and congenital factor V deficiency: a family study. *Haemostasis* 1989;19:331.
23. Petiot P, Croisile B, Confavreux C, et al. Thalamic stroke and congenital factor V deficiency. *Stroke* 1991;22:1606.
24. Alexander B, Goldstein R, Landwehr G, et al. Congenital SPCA deficiency: a hitherto unrecognized coagulation defect with hemorrhage rectified by serum and serum fractions. *J Clin Invest* 1951;30:596.
25. McVey J, Boswell E, Mumford A, et al. Factor VII deficiency and the FVII mutation database. *Hum Mutat* 2001;17:3–17.
26. Triplett D, Brandt J, McGann Batard M, et al. Hereditary factor VII deficiency: heterogeneity defined by combined functional and immunochemical analysis. *Blood* 1985;66: 1284–1287
27. Mammen EF. Factor VII abnormalities. *Semin Thromb Hemost* 1983;9:19.
28. Girolami A, Fabris F, Zamon Dal Bo R. Factor VII Padura: a congenital coagulation disorder due to abnormal factor VII with a peculiar activation problem. *J Lab Clin Med* 1978;91: 387.
29. Girolami A, Cattorozzi G, Zamon Dal Bo R. Factor VII Padura 2: another factor VII abnormality with defective ox-brain thromboplastin activation and a complex hereditary pattern. *Blood* 1979;54:46.
30. Bauer K. Treatment of factor VII deficiency with recombinant factor VIIa. *Haemostasis* 1996;26(suppl 1):155–158.
31. Berrettini M, De Ceunto M, Agnelli G. DDAVP increases factor XII and factor VII activity in normal subjects and in patients with congenital FVII deficiency. *Thromb Haemost* 1983;50:12.
32. Mammen EF. Factor VIII abnormalities. *Semin Thromb Hemost* 1983;9:22.
33. Hoyer LW. Hemophilia A. *N Engl J Med* 1994;330:38.
34. Kaufman RJ, Antonarakis SE. Structure, biology, and genetics of factor VIII. In: Hoffman R, Benz EJ, Shattil SJ, et al., eds. *Hematology: basic principles and practice.* New York: Churchill Livingstone, 2000:1851.
35. Gitschier J, Kogan S, Diamond C, et al. Genetic basis of hemophilia A. *Thromb Haemost* 1991;66:37–39.
36. Tuddenham EGD, Schwaab R, Seehafer J, et al. Hemophilia A: database of nucleotide substitutions, deletions, insertions, and rearrangements of the factor VIII gene. *Nucleic Acids Res* 1994; 22:4851.
37. Lozier JN, Kessler CM. Clinical aspects and therapy of hemophilia. In: Hoffman R, Benz EJ, Shattil SJ, et al., eds. *Hematology: basic principles and practice.* New York: Churchill Livingstone, 2000:1883.
38. Fischer RR, Giddings JC, Rosenberg I. Hereditary combined deficiency of clotting factor V and factor VIII with involvement of von Willebrand factor. *Clin Lab Haematol* 1988;10:53.
39. Marder VJ, Mannucci PM, Firkin BG, et al. Standard nomenclature for factor VIII and von Willebrand factor: a recommendation by the International Committee on Thrombosis and Haemostasis. *Thromb Haemost* 1985;54:871–872.
40. Konkle BA, Crescenzo R. Treatment choices in hemophilia A and B. In: Alving B, ed. *Blood components and pharmacological agents in the treatment of congenital and acquired bleeding disorders.* Bethesda: AABB Press, 2000:309.
41. Nichols WC, Seligsohn U, Zivelin A, et al. Linkage of combined factors V and VIII deficiency to chromosome 18q by homozygosity mapping. *J Clin Invest* 1997;99:596.
42. Briet E, Rosendaal FR. Inhibitors in hemophilia A: are some products safer? *Semin Hematol* 1994;31:11.
43. Ratnoff OD, Lewis JH. Heckathorn's disease: variable functional deficiency of antihemophilic factor (factor VIII). *Blood* 1975;46:161.
44. Mammen EF. Factor IX abnormalities. *Semin Thromb Hemost* 1983;9:28.
45. Aggeler PM, White SG, Glendening MB, et al. Plasma thromboplastin component (PTC) deficiency: a new disease resembling hemophilia. *Proc Soc Exp Biol Med* 1952;79:692.
46. Biggs R, Douglas AM, Macfarlane RA, et al. Christmas disease: a condition previously mistaken for haemophilia. *Br Med J* 1952;2:1378.
47. Ahlberg A. Haemophilia in Sweden: incidence, treatment and prophylaxis of arthropathy and other musculoskeletal manifestations of haemophilia A and B. *Acta Orthop Scand* 1965;77:1.
48. Denson KWE, Biggs R, Mannucci PM. An investigation of three patients with Christmas disease due to an abnormal type of factor IX. *J Clin Pathol* 1968;21:160.
49. Roberts HR, Grizzle JE, McLester WD. Genetic variants of hemophilia B: detection by means of a specific inhibitor. *J Clin Invest* 1968;47:360.
50. Veltkamp JJ, Meilof J, Remmelts HG, et al. Another genetic variant of haemophilia B: haemophilia B-Leyden. *Scand J Haematol* 1970;7:82.
51. Crossley M, Ludwig M, Stowell KM, et al. Recovery from hemophilia B Leyden: an androgen-responsive element in the factor IX promoter. *Science* 1992;257:377–379.
52. Kurachi S, Furukawa M, Salier JP, et al. Regulatory mechanism of human factor IX gene: protein binding at the Leyden specific region. *Biochemistry* 1994;33:1580–1591.
53. Morgan GE, Rowley G, Green PM, et al. Further evidence for the importance of an androgen response element in the factor IX promoter. *Br J Haematol* 1997;98:79–85.
54. Blatt PM, Lundblad RL, Kingdon HS. Thrombogenic materials in prothrobmin complex concentrates. *Ann Intern Med* 1974;81:766.
55. White GC, Roberts HR, Kingdon HS, et al. Prothrombin complex concentrates: potentially thrombogenic materials and clues to the mechanism of thrombosis in vivo. *Blood* 1977;49:159.
56. Warrier I. Management of haemophilia B patients with inhibitors and anaphylaxis. *Haemophilia* 1998;4:574–576.
57. Ingerslev J. Efficacy and safety of recombinant factor VIIa in the prophylaxis of bleeding in various surgical procedures in hemophilic patients with factor VIII and factor IX inhibitors. *Semin Thromb Hemost* 2000;26:425.
58. Negrier C, Hay CR. The treatment of bleeding in hemophilic patients with inhibitors with recombinant factor VIIa. *Semin Thromb Hemost* 2000;26:407.
59. Hedner U. Recombinant coagulation factor VIIa: from the concept to clinical application in hemophilia treatment in 2000. *Semin Thromb Hemost* 2000;26:363.
60. Johannessen M, Andreasen RB, Nordfang O. Decline of factor VIII and factor IX inhibitors during long term treatment with NovoSeven. *Blood Coagul Fibrinolysis* 2000;11:239.
61. Hedner U. Treatment of patients with factor VIII and factor IX inhibitors with special focus on the use of recombinant factor VIIa. *Thromb Haemost* 1999;82:531.
62. Barnes C, Rudzki Z, Ekert H. Induction of immune tolerance and suppression of anaphylaxis in a child with haemolphilia B by simple plasmapheresis and antigen exposure. *Haemophilia* 2000;6:693.
63. Mammen E. Factor X abnormalities. *Semin Thromb Hemost* 1983;9:31.

64. Peyvandi F, Mannucci PM, Lak M, et al. Congenital factor X deficiency: spectrum of bleeding symptoms in 32 Iranian patients. *Br J Haematol* 1998;102:626.
65. Fujimoto Y, Aguiar PH, Carneiro JD, et al. Spontaneous epidural hematoma following a shunt in an infant with congenital factor X deficiency: case report and literature review. *Neurosurg Rev* 1999;22:226.
66. de Sousa C, Clark T, Bradshaw A. Antenatally diagnosed subdural haemorrhage in congenital factor X deficiency. *Arch Dis Child* 1988;63:1168.
67. El Kalla S, Menon NS. Neonatal congenital factor X deficiency. *Am J Pediatr Hematol Oncol* 1993;15:135.
68. Kumar M, Mehta P. Congenital coagulopathies and pregnancy: report of four pregnancies in a factor X-deficient woman. *Am J Hematol* 1994;46:241.
69. el Kallas, Menon NS. Neonatal congenital factor X deficiency. *Pediatr Hematol Oncol* 1991;8:347.
69a. Rosenthal RL, Dreskin OH, Rosenthal N. New hemophilia-like disease caused by deficiency of a third plama thromboplastin factor. *Proc Soc Exp Biol Med* 1953;82:171.
70. Mammen EF. Factor XI deficiency. *Semin Thromb Hemost* 1983; 9:34.
71. Gailani D. Advances and dilemmas in factor XI. *Curr Opin Hematol* 1994;1:347.
72. Bolton-Maggs PH. Bleeding problems in factor XI deficient women. *Haemophilia* 1999;5:155.
73. Kadir RA, Economides DL, Lee CA. Factor XI deficiency in women. *Am J Hematol* 1999;60:48.
74. Seligsohn U, Modan M. Definition of the population at risk of bleeding due to factor XI deficiency in ashkenazic Jews and the value of activated partial thromboplastin time in its detection. *Isr J Med Sci* 1981;17:413.
75. Franchini M, de Gironcoli M, Lippi G, et al. Prophylactic use of desmopressin in surgery of six patients with symptomatic heterozygous factor XI deficiency. *Haematologica* 2000;85: 106.
76. Meier HL, Pierce JV, Colemand RW. Activation and function of human Hageman factor: the role of high molecular weight kininogen and prekallikrein. *J Clin Invest* 1977;60:18.
77. Ratnoff OK, Colopy JE. A familial hemorrhagic trait associated with a deficiency of clot-promoting fraction of plasma. *J Clin Invest* 1955;34:602.
78. Bick RL. Congenital coagulation factor defects and von Willebrand's disease. In: *Disorders of hemostasis and thrombosis: principles of clinical practice.* New York: Thieme, 1985:127.
79. Saito H, Scott JG, Movat HZ, et al. Molecular heterogeneity of Hageman trait (factor XII deficiency): evidence that two of 49 subjects are cross-reacting material positive (CRM+). *J Lab Clin* Med 1979;94:256.
80. Miyata T, Kawabata SI, Iwanaga S. Coagulation factor XII (Hageman factor) Washington, DC: inactive factor XIIa results from Cys-571-Ser substitution. *Proc Natl Acad Sci U S A* 1989; 86:8319.
81. Saito H, Scialla SJ. Isolation and properties of an abnormal Hageman factor (factor XII) molecule in a cross-reaction material-positive Hageman trait plasma. *J Clin Invest* 1981;68:1028.
82. Kovalainen S, Myllyla VV, Tolonen U, et al. Recurrent subarachnoid haemorrhages in patient with Hageman factor deficiency. *Lancet* 1979;1:1035.
83. McPherson RA. Thromboembolism in Hageman trait. *Am J Clin Pathol* 1977;68:240.
84. Azner J, Fernandez Pavnon J. Thromboembolic accident in patients with congenital deficiency of factor XII. *Thromb Diath Haemorrh* 1974;31:525.
85. Hoak JC, Swanson LW, Warner ED, et al. Myocardial infarction associated with severe factor XII deficiency. *Lancet* 1966;2:884.
86. Glueck HI, Roehll W. Myocardial infarction in a patient with a Hageman (factor XII) defect. *Ann Intern Med* 1966;64:390.
87. Ratnoff OD, Busse RJ, Sehon RP. The demise of John Hageman. *N Engl J Med* 1968;297:760.
88. Goodnough LT, Saito H, Ratnoff OD. Thrombosis or myocardial infarction in congenital clotting factor abnormalities and chronic thrombocytopenias: a report of 21 patients and a review of 50 previously reported cases. *Medicine* 1983;62:248.
89. von Kanel R, Wuillemin WA, Furlan M, et al. Factor XII clotting activity and antigen levels in patients with thromboembolic disease. *Blood Coagul Fibrinolysis* 1992;3:555–561.
90. Zeerleder S, Schloesser M, Redondo M, et al. Reevaluation of the incidence of thromboembolic complications in congenital factor XII deficiency: a study on 73 subjects from 14 Swiss families. *Thromb Haemost* 1999;82:1240–1246.
91. Coleman REW, Wong PY. Participation of Hageman factor-dependent pathways in human disease states. *Thromb Haemost* 1977;38:751.
92. Schmaier AH, Silverberb M, Kaplan AP. Contact activation and its abnormalities. In: Colman RW, Hirsh J, Marder VJ, eds. *Hemostasis and thrombosis.* Philadelphia: JB Lippincott, 1987:18.
93. Hathaway WE, Belhasen LP, Hathaway HS. Evidence for a new plasma thromboplastin factor, I: case report, coagulation studies and physicochemical properties. *Blood* 1965;26:521.
93a. Wuepper RD, Cochran CG. Plasma prekallikrein: isolation, characterization, and mechanism of activation. *J Exp Med* 1972; 135:1.
94. Mammen EF. Contact factor abnormalities. *Semin Thromb Hemost* 1983;9:36.
95. Saito H, Goonough LT, Soria J, et al. Heterogeneity of human prekallikrein deficiency (Fletcher trait): evidence that five of 18 cases are positive for cross reacting material. *N Engl J Med* 1981; 305:910.
96. Bouma BN, Kerbiriou DM, Baker J. Characterization of a variant of prekallikrein, prekallikrein Long Beach, from a family with mixed cross-reacting material-positive and cross-reacting material negative prekallikrein deficiency. *J Clin Invest* 1986; 78:170.
97. Estelles A, Aznar J, Espana F. The absence of release of plasminogen activator after venous occlusion in a Fletcher trait patient. *Thromb Haemost* 1983;49:66.
98. Sollo DG, Saleem A. Prekallikrein (Fletcher factor) deficiency. *Ann Clin Lab Sci* 1985;15:279.
99. Entes K, LaDuca FM, Tourbaf KD. Fletcher factor deficiency, source of variation of the activated partial thromboplastin time. *Am J Clin Pathol* 1981;75:626.
100. Saito H, Ratnoff OD, Waldmann R. Fitzgerald trait: deficiency of a hitherto unrecognized agent, Fitzgerald factor, participation in surface-mediated reaction of clotting, fibrinolysis, generation of kinins and the property of diluted plasma enhancing vascular permeability (PF/DIL). *J Clin Invest* 1975;55:1082.
101. Coleman RW, Bagdasarian, A, Talamo RC. Williams trait: human kininogen efficiency with diminished levels of plasminogen proactivator and prekallikrein associated with abnormalities of the Hageman factor-dependent pathways. *J Clin Invest* 1975;56:1650.
102. Lacombe MJ, Varet B, Levy JP. A hitherto undescribed plasma factor acting at the contact phase of blood coagulation (Flaujeac factor): case report and coagulation studies. *Blood* 1975; 46:761.
103. Oh-Ishi S, Ueno A, Uchida Y. Abnormalities in the contact activation through factor XII in Fujiwara trait: a deficiency in both high and low molecular weight kininogens with low level of prekallikrein. *Tohoku J Exp Med* 1981;133:67.
104. Lutcher CL. Reid trait: a new expression of high molecular

weight kininogen (HMW kininogen) deficiency. *Clin Res* 1976; 24:47.

105. Stormorken H, Briseid K, Hellum B. A new case of total kininogen deficiency. *Thromb Res* 1990;60:457.
106. Mammen EF. Alpha-2 antiplasmin deficiency. *Semin Thromb Hemost* 1983;9:52.
107. Saito H. Alpha2-plasmin inhibitor and its deficiency states. *J Lab Clin Med* 1988;112:671.
108. Bick RL, Wheeler A. Alpha-2-antiplasmin deficiency: a dysfunctional protein leading to hemorrhage in afflicted family members. *Thromb Haemost* 1991;65:1261.
109. Griffin GC, Mammen EF, Sokol RJ, et al. Alpha-2-antiplasmin deficiency: an overlooked cause of hemorrhage. *Am J Pediatr Hematol Oncol* 1993;15:328.
110. Miyauchi Y, Mii Y, Aoki M, et al. Operative treatment of intramedullary hematoma associated with congenital deficiency of alpha-2-plasmin inhibitor: a report of three cases. *J Bone Joint Surg Am* 1996;78:1409.
111. Paqueron X, Favier R, Richard P, et al. Severe postadenoidectomy bleeding revealing congenital alpha-2-antiplasmin deficiency in a child. *Anesth Analg* 1997;84:1147.
112. Devaussuzenet VMP, Ducou le Pointe HA, Doco AM, et al. A case of intramedullary haematoma associated with congenital alpha-2-plasmin inhibitor deficiency. *Pediatr Radiol* 1998;28: 978.
113. Lind B, Thorsen S. A novel missense mutation in the human plasmin inhibitor (alpha2 antiplasmin) gene associated with a bleeding tendency. *Br J Haematol* 1999;107:317.
114. Tatematsu M, Higa A, Sunagawa H, et al. Dialysis for a patient who had congenital deficiency of alpha2 plasmin inhibitor. *Clin Nephrol* 1998;49:335.
115. Dieval J, Nguyen G, Gross S, et al. A lifelong bleeding disorder associated with a deficiency of plasminogen activator inhibitor type 1. *Blood* 1991;77:528.
116. Schleef RR, Higgins DL, Pillemer E, et al. Bleeding diathesis due to decreased functional activity of type 1 plasminogen activator inhibitor. *J Clin Invest* 1989;83:1747.
117. Tanimura LK, Weddell JA, McKown CG, et al. Oral management of a patient with a plasminogen activator inhibitor (PAI-1) deficiency: case report. *Pediatr Dent* 1994;16:133.
118. Mammen EF. Factor XIII deficiency. *Semin Thromb Hemost* 1983;9:10.
119. Kitchens CS, Newcomb TF. Factor XIII. *Medicine* 1979;58:413.
120. Lorand L, Losowsky MS, Miloszewski K. Human factor XIII: fibrin-stabilizing factor. *Prog Hemost Thromb* 1980;5:245.
121. McDonagh J. Structure and function of factor XIII. In: Coleman RW, Hirsch J, Marder VJ, et al., eds. *Hemostasis and thrombosis*. Philadelphia: JB Lippincott, 1987:289.
122. Girolami A, Capellato MG, Lazzaro AR. Type I and type II disease in congenital factor XIII deficiency: a further demonstration of the correctness of the classification. *Blut* 53:411:1986.
123. Girolami A, Sartoli MT, Simioni P. An updated classification of factor XIII defect. *Br J Haematol* 1991;77:565.
124. Daly HM, Carson PJ, Smith JK. Intracerebral haemorrhage due to acquired factor XIII inhibitor: successful response to factor XIII concentrate. *Blood Coagul Fibrinolysis* 1991;2:507.
125. Isreals ED, Paraskevus F, Isreals LG. Immunological studies of coagulation factor XIII. *J Clin Invest* 1973;52:2398.
126. Ikematsu S, McDonagh RP, Reisner HM. Immunochemical studies of human factor XIIII: radioimmunoassay for the carrier subunit of the zymogen. *J Lab Clin Med* 198;97:662.
127. von Willebrand E. Hereditary pseudohaumofilie. *Fin Lakaresallsk Handl* 1926;68:87.
128. Alexander B, Goldstein R. Dual hemostatic defect in pseudohemophilia. *J Clin Invest* 1953;32:551.
129. Larrieu MJ, Soulier, JP. Deficit en facteur anti-hemophilique a chez une fille associe a un trouble du saignement. *Rev Haematol* 1953;8:361.
130. Quick AJ, Hussey CV, Hussey. Hemophilic condition in the female. *J Lab Clin Med* 1953;42:929.
131. Zimmerman TS, Ratnoff OD, Powell AE. Immunologic differentiation of classic hemophilia (factor VIII deficiency) and von Willebrand's disease. *J Clin Invest* 1971;50:244.
132. Miller C, Lenzi R, Breen C. Prevalence of von Willebrand's disease among US adults. *Blood* 1987;70:377a.
133. Rodeghiero F, Castman G, Dini E. Epidemiological investigation of the prevalence of von Willebrand's disease. *Blood* 1987; 69:454.
134. Werner E, Broxson E, Tucker E, et al. Prevalence of von Willebrand disease in children: a multiethnic study. *J Pediatr* 1993; 123:893.
135. Batlle J, Torea J, Rendal E, et al. The problem of diagnosing von Willebrand's disease. *J Intern Med* 1997;242(suppl 740):121.
136. Gill J, Brooks J, Bauer P, et al. The effect of ABO blood group on the diagnosis of von Willebrand disease. *Blood* 1987;69:1691.
137. Quick A. Menstruation in hereditary bleeding disorders. *Obstet Gynecol* 1966;28:37.
138. Bowie E, Didisheim P, Thompson J, et al. Von Willebrand's disease: a critical review. *Hematol Rev* 1968;1:1.
139. Weiss H, Hawiger J. Ruggeri Z, et al. Fibrinogen-independent platelet adhesion and thrombus formation on subendothelium mediated by glycoprotein IIb-IIIa complex at high shear rate. *J Clin Invest* 1989;83:288.
140. Koedam JA, Meijers JC, Sixma JJ, et al. Inactivation of human factor VIII by activated protein C: cofactor activity of protein S and protective of von Willebrand factor. *J Clin Invest* 1988; 82:1236.
141. Parker R, Gralnick HR. Identification of platelet glycoprotein IIb/IIIa as the major binding site for released platelet-von Willebrand factor. *Blood* 1986;68:732.
142. Nishino M, Girma J, Rothschild C. New variant of von Willebrand disease with defective binding to factor VII. *Blood* 1989; 74:1591–1599.
143. Sadler J. A revised classification of von Willebrand disease: for the subcommittee on von Willebrand factor of the Scientific and Standardization Committee of the International Society on Thrombosis and Haemostasis. *Thromb Haemost* 1994;71:520.
144. Triplett D. Laboratory diagnosis of von Willebrand's disease. *Mayo Clin Proc* 1991;66:832.
145. Fressinaud E, Veyradier A, Truchaud F, et al. Screening for von Willebrand disease with a new analyzer using high shear stress: a study of 60 cases. *Blood* 1998;91:1325.
146. Carcao M, Blanchette V, Dean J, et al. The platelet function analyzer (PFA-100): a novel in-vitro system for evaluation of primary haemostasis in children. *Br J Haemetol* 1998;101:70.
147. Mammen E, Comp P, Gosselin R, et al. PFA-100 system: a new method for assessment of platelet dysfunction. *Semin Thromb Hemost* 1998;24:195.
148. Favaloro E, Facey D, Henniker A. Use of a novel platelet function analyzer (PFA-100) with high sensitivity to disturbances in von Willebrand factor to screen for von Willebrand's disease and other disorders. *Am J Hematol* 1999;62:165.
149. Wiess H, Hoyer L, Rickles F, et al. Quantitative assay of a plasma factor deficient in von Willebrand's disease that is necessary for platelet aggregation. *J Clin Invest* 1973;52:2708.
150. Eikenboom J, Castman G, Vos H, et al. Characterization of the genetic defects in recessive type 1 and type 3 von Willebrand disease patients of Italian origin. *Thromb Haemost* 1998;79:709.
151. Cash JD, Gader AMA, Da Costa J. The release of plasminogen activator and factor VIII by LVP, AVP, DDAVP, AT III and OT in man. *Br J Haematol* 1974;24:363.
152. Lubetsky A, Schulman S, Varon D, et al. Safety and efficacy of

continuous infusion of a combined factor VIII-von Willebrand factor (vWF) concentrate (Haemate-P) in patients with von Willebrand disease. *Thromb Haemost* 1999;81:229.

153. Zimmerman TS, Dent JA, Ruggeri Zm, et al. Subunit composition of plasma in von Willebrand factor: cleavage is present in normal individuals, increased in IIA and IIB von Willebrand disease, but minimal in variants with aberrant structure of individual oligomers (types IIC, IID, and IIE). *J Clin Invest* 1986; 77:947.
154. Lyons SE, Bruch ME, Bowie EJ, et al: Impaired intracellular transport produced by a subset of type IIA von Willebrand disease mutations. *J Biol Chem* 1992;267:4424.
155. Nichols W, Ginsburg D. Reviews in molecular medicine. *Medicine* (Baltimore) 1997;76:1.
156. Rick M, Williams S, Sacher R, et al. Thrombocytopenia associated with pregnancy in a patient with type IIB von Willebrand's disease. *Blood* 1987;69:786.
157. Ruggeri ZM, Pareti FI, Manucci PM, et al. Heightened interaction between platelets and factor VIII/von Willebrand factor in a new subtype of von Willebrand's disease. *N Engl J Med* 1980; 302:1047.
158. Valster F, Feijen H, Hutten J. Severe thrombocytopenia in a pregnant patient with platelet-associated IgM, and known von Willebrand's disease: a case report. *Eur J Obstet Gynecol Reprod Biol* 1990;36:197.
159. Holmberg L, Nilsson I, Borge L, et al. Platelet aggregation induced by 1-desamino-8-D-arginine vasopressin (DDAVP) in type IIB von Willebrand's disease. *N Engl J Med* 1983;309:816.
160. Hillery C, Mancuso D, Sadler J, et al. Type 2M von Willebrand disease: F6061 and I662F mutation in the glycoprotein Ib binding domain selectively impair ristocetin—but not botrocetin—mediated binding of von Willebrand factor to platelets. *Blood* 1998;91:1572.
161. Miller JL, Castella A. Platelet-type von Willebrand's disease: characterization of a new bleeding disorder. *Blood* 1982;60:794.
162. Bryckaert MC, Pietu G, Ruan C, et al. Abnormality of glycoprotein Ib in two cases of "pseudo"-von Willebrand's disease. *J Lab Clin Med* 1985;106:393.
163. Hougie C, McPherson RA, Aronson L. Passovoy factor: a hitherto unrecognized factor necessary for haemostasis. *Lancet* 1975;2:290.
164. Hougie C, McPherson RA, Brown JE. The Passovoy defect: further characterization of a hereditary hemorrhagic diathesis. *N Engl J Med* 1978;298:1045.
165. Jackson JM, Marshall LR, Herrmann RP. Passovoy factor deficiency in five western Australian kindreds. *Pathology* 1981; 13:517.
166. Giddings JC, Sugrue A, Bloom AL. Quantitation of coagulant antigens and inhibition of activated protein C in combined factor V and VIII deficiency. *Br J Haematol* 1982;52:495.
167. Marlaer RA, Griffin JH. Deficiency of protein C inhibitor in combine factor V/VIII deficiency disease. *J Clin Invest*

Disorders of Thrombosis and Hemostasis: Clinical and Laboratory Practice, Third Edition, edited by Rodger L. Bick.
Lippincott Williams & Wilkins, Philadelphia © 2002

7

DISSEMINATED INTRAVASCULAR COAGULATION

RODGER L. BICK

Disseminated intravascular coagulation (DIC) is a complex disorder, with pathophysiology that is variable and highly dependent on the triggering event(s), host response(s), and comorbid conditions. As a result of these complicated interactions, the clinical expression and laboratory findings are varied, thereby affecting the specifics of diagnosis and therapeutic approaches. The highly complex and variable pathophysiology of DIC often results in a lack of uniformity in clinical manifestations, a lack of consensus in the specific appropriate laboratory criteria for diagnosis, and a lack of specific therapeutic modalities. Indeed, recommendations for therapy and the evaluation of the efficacy of the management regimens is often difficult because the morbidity and survival are more dependent on the specific cause of DIC and because the generally used specific therapeutic approaches, which include heparin, low-molecular-weight heparin (LMWH), antithrombin concentrate, protein C concentrate, and so on, have never been subjected to objective prospective randomized trials, except antithrombin concentrates.

DIC is an intermediary mechanism of disease usually seen in association with well-defined clinical disorders (1–5). The pathophysiology of DIC serves as an intermediary mechanism in many disease processes, which sometimes remain organ specific. This catastrophic syndrome spans all areas of medicine and presents a broad clinical spectrum that is confusing to many. DIC was called "consumptive coagulopathy" in early literature (6,7); this is not a proper description, as very little is consumed in DIC; most factors and plasma constituents are plasmin biodegraded. Terminology after use of this phrase was "defibrination syndrome" (8,9); however, a more suitable term would be "defibrinogenation syndrome." The contemporary term is disseminated intravascular coagulation; this is a useful descriptive pathophysiologic term if one accepts the concept that "coagulation" is expressed as both hemorrhage and thrombosis (2–5). Most physicians consider DIC to be a systemic hemorrhagic syndrome; however, this is only because hemorrhage is evident and often impressive. Less commonly appreciated is the occurrence of profound microvascular thrombosis and, sometimes, large vessel thrombosis. The hemorrhage is often simple to contend with in patients with fulminant DIC, but it is the small and large vessel thrombosis, with impairment of blood flow, ischemia, and associated end-organ damage that usually leads to irreversible morbidity and mortality. Throughout this review, fulminant DIC versus "low-grade" compensated DIC and the attendant differences in clinical manifestations, laboratory findings, and treatment are discussed. However, these are often pure and theoretical clinical spectrums of a disease continuum; patients may belong anywhere in this continuum and may lapse from one end of the spectrum into another. A clear definition of DIC is outlined in Table 7.1.

R. L. Bick: Departments of Medicine and Pathology, University of Texas Southwestern Medical Center; Dallas Thrombosis/Hemostasis Clinical Center; ThromboCare Laboratories, Dallas, Texas.

ETIOLOGY

DIC is usually seen in association with well-defined clinical entities. Those clinical disorders and circumstances most commonly associated with DIC are summarized in Table 7.2.

DIC Syndromes Unique to Pregnancy and Obstetrics

Obstetrical accidents are common events leading to DIC. Amniotic fluid embolism with DIC is the most catastrophic and common of the life-threatening obstetrical accidents (6–10).

The syndrome of amniotic fluid embolism (AFE) is manifest by the acute onset of respiratory failure, circulatory collapse, shock, and the serious thrombohemorrhagic syndrome of DIC. The first careful description of this syndrome was by Steiner and Lushbaugh in 1941 (11); in this landmark article, these authors described the clinical histo-

TABLE 7.1. DEFINITION OF DISSEMINATED INTRAVASCULAR COAGULATION (MINIMAL ACCEPTABLE CRITERIA)

A systemic thrombohemorrhagic disorder seen in association with well-defined clinical situations
AND
Laboratory evidence of (a) procoagulant activation, (b) fibrinolytic activation, (c) inhibitor consumption, and (d) biochemical evidence of end-organ damage or failure

ries of eight obstetrical patients and demonstrated that these patients formed a distinct group with a unique pathophysiologic basis for the constellation of symptoms now associated with this syndrome. These authors also were able to duplicate this syndrome in animal models and demonstrated that AFE is a relatively common cause of sudden death during labor or in the immediate postlabor period. These eight patients came from 4,000 consecutive autopsies performed over a period of 15 years, representing an incidence of 0.2% of deaths in this autopsy series. In this study, it was noted that these eight cases were among a total of 24,200 deliveries, representing an incidence of one in 8,000 of their obstetrical cases. When analyzing their obstetrical deaths, these authors were the first to show that AFE was the most common cause of maternal death in the period during labor and within the first 9 hours after labor.

TABLE 7.2. THE ACCEPTED DISEASE ENTITIES GENERALLY ASSOCIATED WITH DIC

Fulminant DIC	Low-grade DIC
Obstetric accidents	Cardiovascular diseases
Amniotic fluid embolism	Autoimmune diseases
Placental abruption	Renal vascular disorders
Retained fetus syndrome	Hematologic disorders
Eclampsia	Inflammatory disorders
Abortion	
Intravascular hemolysis	
Hemolytic transfusion reactions	
Minor hemolysis	
Massive transfusions	
Septicemia	
Gram-negative (endotoxin)	
Gram-positive (mucopolysaccharides)	
Viremias	
HIV	
Hepatitis	
Varicella	
Cytomegalovirus	
Metastatic malignancy	
Leukemia	
Acute promyelocytic (M-3)	
Acute myelomonocytic (M-4)	
Many others	
Burns	
Crush injuries and tissue necrosis	
Trauma	
Acute liver disease	
Obstructive jaundice	
Acute hepatic failure	
Prosthetic devices	
Leveen or denver shunts	
Aortic balloon assist devices	
Vascular disorders	

HIV, human immunodeficiency virus;

Etiology of AFE

The common etiologic factor in the syndrome of AFE is the entrance, by various proposed mechanisms and routes, of amniotic fluid, with or without meconium, into the systemic maternal circulation, followed by embolization of amniotic fluid and its contents to the lungs; subsequently, circulatory collapse and the development of DIC occurs almost uniformly and instantaneously (12). The incidence has been reported to be between one in 8,000 and one and 30,000 births (11,13). The syndrome is commonly fatal for both the mother and child (13). The mortality for the mother is generally 60% to 80%, and 50% of survivors have permanent neurologic damage (14,15). One recent series, however, reported a 26.4% mortality (16). Of those surviving AFE, thrombotic stroke is a major sequel (14,17,18). Whereas the finding of amniotic fluid in maternal blood is not physiologic, there have been rare instances in which amniotic fluid may enter the systemic maternal circulation without any significant manifestations of this catastrophic syndrome (12). In 1970, it was noted that the syndrome of AFE represented 10% of all maternal deaths, and a study in Sweden from 1965 to 1974 demonstrated that the syndrome of AFE accounted for 22% of all maternal deaths (19,20). Asner et al. (21) described AFE to account for DIC in only one of six patients with clinically obvious DIC and in none of 35 obstetrical patients with laboratory evidence of DIC (21). However, it also was been noted in a combined retrospective and prospective study of DIC taken from the records of Massachusetts General Hospital, consisting of 60 prospectively studied patients and 15 retrospectively studied patients, that not one of these patients had DIC in association with AFE (22). However, of these 75 DIC patients, three were associated with various other obstetrical accidents. Thus, in assessment of the etiologic "triggers" of patients with DIC as a group, AFE is quite rare. The risk factors associated with development of AFE (Table 7.3) consist of older age, multiparity, marked exaggeration of uterine contraction after rupture of the uterine membranes, or markedly exaggerated uterine contraction due to the use of oxytocin (Pitocin) or other uterine stimulatory agents, cesarean section, uterine rupture, high cervical laceration, premature separation of the placenta, and intrauterine fetal death (2,23,24). Other factors have been spontaneous rupture of the fetal membranes and blunt trauma to the abdomen (25,26). The syndrome can, on rare occasions, occur late in pregnancy but most commonly occurs during labor in 80% of patients; in only up to 20% of

TABLE 7.3. AMNIOTIC FLUID EMBOLISM: RISK FACTORS

Older age
Multiparity
Physiologic intense uterine contractions
Drug-induced intense uterine contractions
Caesarian section
Uterine rupture
High cervical tear
Premature placental separation
Intrauterine fetal death
Placental abruption
Trauma to abdomen
80% of cases develop during labor
20% may develop before or after labor

patients does the syndrome occur before labor begins and before rupture of the amniotic sac (27,28). Twenty-five percent of women die within 1 hour of developing this syndrome and up to 80% will die within the first 9 hours (29,30). It is of interest that in 10% of women, the syndrome develops without warning, usually during delivery, as amniotic fluid enters the systemic maternal circulation during an apparently normal labor and delivery, unassociated with predelivery complications.

There is generally rapid onset of signs and symptoms of pulmonary failure and circulatory collapse; in at least 50% of patients, this is followed by systemic bleeding. Fifty percent of fetuses die or develop intrauterine asphyxia/distress before the sudden maternal onset of acute respiratory failure and circulatory collapse. In one series of 30,000 deliveries described by Graeff (12), there were six cases of AFE; two patients died, and four recovered. The syndrome also has been described to occur immediately after delivery but almost always occurs during delivery. Typically, the patient is in active delivery with the amnion intact and suddenly develops respiratory failure and circulatory collapse, followed by a systemic thrombohemorrhagic disorder. The cause is only partially understood, but the common etiologic event is entrance into the systemic maternal circulation of amniotic fluid, which then causes extensive pulmonary microcirculatory occlusion and local pulmonary activation of the procoagulant system; in addition, there is systemic activation of the procoagulant system. This occurs in conjunction with intense induction of pulmonary fibrinolytic activity, presumably through release of pulmonary endothelial plasminogen activator activity in the lungs (31,32).

Because this is a life-threatening and not uncommon syndrome, all clinicians involved with obstetrics and care during delivery should be familiar with the potential of this syndrome when a patient has the risk factors depicted in Table 7.3, and when a patient immediately preceding, during, or immediately after delivery suddenly develops respiratory distress, shock, and uncontrolled bleeding. The general characteristics of AFE are presented in Table 7.4.

TABLE 7.4. AMNIOTIC FLUID EMBOLISM: GENERAL CHARACTERISTICS

1 in 8,000 to 1 in 30,000 deliveries
10% of all maternal deaths in United States
22% of all maternal deaths in Sweden
80% overall mortality
25% will die within 1 h
50% fetal death or distress before symptoms

Pathophysiology of Amniotic Fluid Embolism

Amniotic fluid contains much cellular material including vernix caseosa, squamous epithelial cells, and debris from the fetus (11,33). The lipid content, cellular content, fetal debris, procoagulant activity, and viscosity of amniotic fluid increase with duration of pregnancy and are at a maximum at the time of delivery (12,34,35). In most instances, the actual mechanism(s) and site of entry of amniotic fluid into the uterine and, subsequently, the systemic maternal circulation remain unclear. Indeed, several investigators examining pathologic specimens of patients with AFE have, in most incidences, been unable to define clearly the portals of entry (36,37). Thus the mechanism(s) by which amniotic fluid enters the maternal circulation in general often remains undefined. However, lacerations of the membrane and placenta may be portals of entry to the maternal venous sinuses in the uterus (12). Entrance may be via a tear in the membranes at the placental margin with compression–injection of fluid into the maternal vessels or lacerated veins in the posterior vaginal wall, or the entrance of amniotic fluid into the systemic maternal circulation may occur with a defect in the fetal membranes if this defect is in proximity to areas of maternal venous vessels (12). In general, the site of entry is thought to be the area of the placental insertion or the area of the lower uterus or cervix (12). It is possible that the cervical veins that open during labor permit entry of amniotic fluid after rupture of the membranes when the fetal head obstructs the intracervical canal, therefore blocking drainage and causing retrograde (upward) hydrostatic pressure, thereby injecting amniotic fluid into open cervical veins and thus allowing entrance into the systemic returning circulation (99). It is clear that amniotic fluid may enter the maternal circulation via a rupture of the uterus or through an abnormal placental placement site or as a part of the placental abruption syndrome. If meconium accompanies the amniotic fluid, the syndrome is accompanied by more intense DIC than occurs without meconium (38). There appear to be many possible mechanisms by which amniotic fluid may enter the uterine and subsequently the systemic maternal circulation; however, these mechanisms are rarely documented on pathologic analysis (36,37). It was recently demonstrated that the monoclonal antibody THK-2 may be a specific pathological marker for AFE (39,40). Another suggestion is that finding fetal megakaryocytes and syncytiotrophoblastic cells in the maternal pulmonary circulation by monoclonal antibodies [CD 61–glycoprotein (GP)IIIa, β-human chorionic gonadotropin (HCG), and factor VIII–von Willebrand (vW) hPL antibodies] may be diagnostic (41).

On entering the systemic maternal circulation, amniotic fluid simultaneously activates the procoagulant system leading to profound DIC, and in addition, causes intense and extensive pulmonary microembolization via not only activation of the coagulation system, but also hyperviscous amniotic fluid and amniotic fluid debris. As noted, this process appears more pronounced in the presence of meconium contamination (38).

Pulmonary Pathophysiology in Amniotic Fluid Embolism

The severity of the pulmonary manifestations is highly dependent on the contents, amount, and viscosity of amniotic fluid reaching the maternal pulmonary circulation. Of course, the higher the content of cellular elements, the more viscous the material will be, with cellular elements being vernix, caseosa, fetal squamous epithelial cells, and complexes of squamous cellular material (11,12). Amniotic fluid itself, as well as amniotic fluid content, will mechanically obstruct the pulmonary circulation, occluding both large and small vessels, with the subsequent usual manifestations of severe pulmonary embolization. This then leads to defective perfusion, defective diffusion capacity, and intense vasoconstriction, which, in turn, is accompanied by right heart failure and the findings of acute cor pulmonale, increased pulmonary artery pressure with subsequent decreased left ventricular filling, decreased cardiac output and resultant tissue hypoxia and ischemia, metabolic acidosis, and eventually, cardiogenic shock.

Hemostasis Pathophysiology in Amniotic Fluid Embolism

Amniotic fluid contains a highly potent total thromboplastin-like activity; this procoagulant activity increases with time of gestation (34,35). In addition, amniotic fluid contains a relatively strong antifibrinolytic activity and, as such, causes a nonspecific inhibition of fibrinolytic system; this activity of amniotic fluid also increases during gestation (21). The fibrinolytic inhibition activity may predispose a patient to DIC and diffuse thrombotic phenomenon by inhibiting or dampening the usual secondary fibrinolytic response seen in DIC patients (42,43). The secondary fibrinolytic response that usually occurs in DIC is responsible for hemorrhage due to plasmin digestion of numerous clotting factors; however, this secondary fibrinolytic response also serves to help keep the circulation free of thrombi. It remains controversial whether amniotic fluid itself has a direct effect on the vasculature or if this a secondary effect of procoagulant/platelet activation (44). However, endothelin-1, a potent vasoconstrictor and bronchoconstrictor, appears to be released, systemically, from circulating fetal squamous cells and may intensify the severe hemodynamic alterations noted in AFE (45).

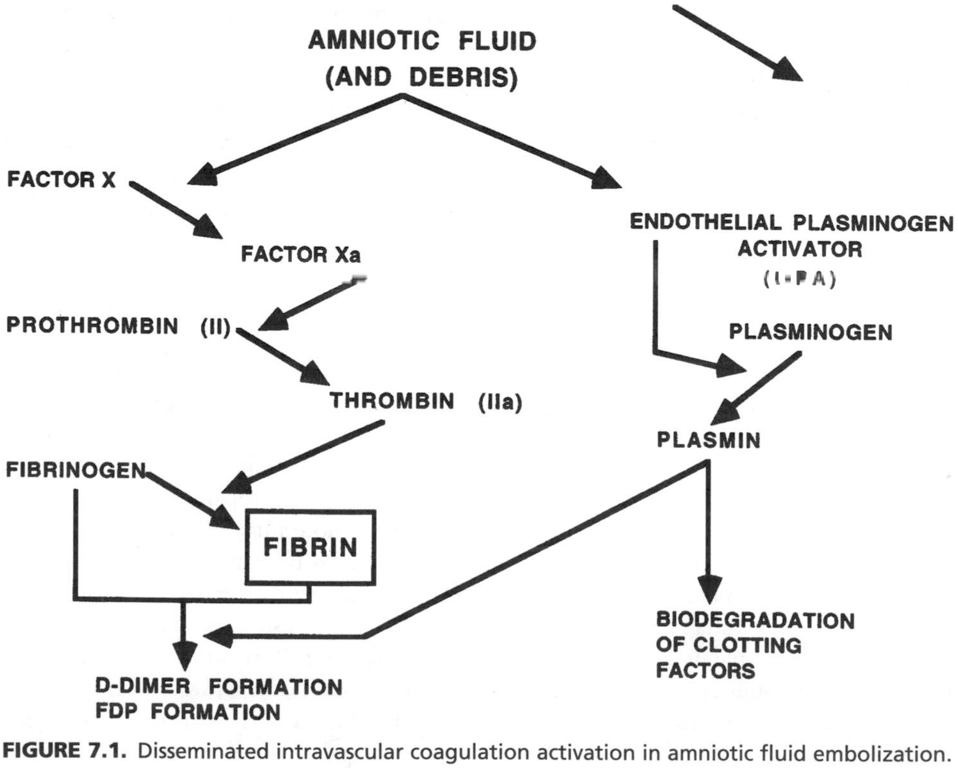

FIGURE 7.1. Disseminated intravascular coagulation activation in amniotic fluid embolization.

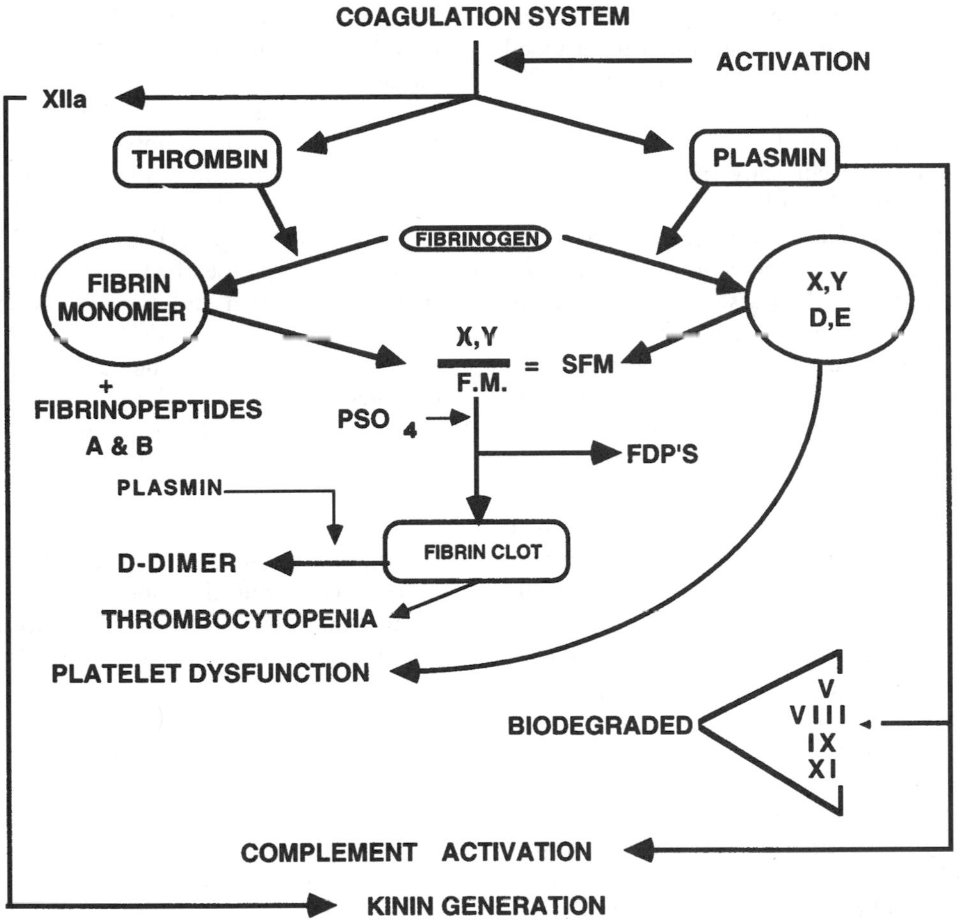

FIGURE 7.2. Pathophysiology of disseminated intravascular coagulation. *FDPs,* fibrin(ogen) degradation products; *PSO,* protamine sulfate; *SFM,* soluble fibrin monomer.

The procoagulant activity of amniotic fluid correlates very well with lecithin/sphingomyelin (LS) ratio during gestation (46). Amniotic fluid, in vitro, will accelerate the prothrombin time, the activated partial thromboplastin time (PTT), the Russell's viper venom time, and will accelerate the clotting of factor VII–deficient plasma (47). Thus amniotic fluid acts not only as a "total thromboplastin," but also as a substitute for "tissue phase activation." The mechanism(s) by which amniotic fluid activates the procoagulant system is the direct activation of factor X, in the presence of calcium ions, to factor Xa (48). Factor Xa is one of the most thrombogenic substances known. Factor Xa, in the presence of factor V and additional phospholipid (including amniotic fluid and platelet surfaces) will rapidly convert prothrombin to thrombin. Once thrombin is formed, fibrinogen is converted to fibrin (49). Thus in patients with AFE, platelet–fibrin microthrombi develop throughout the systemic and pulmonary circulations. This DIC syndrome is therefore associated with microcirculatory thrombosis, thromboembolism, and hemorrhage. The pathophysiology of activation in AFE is depicted in Fig. 7.1. The pathophysiology of DIC, associated with hemorrhage and thrombosis throughout the circulation, is depicted in Fig. 7.2.

DIAGNOSIS OF AMNIOTIC FLUID EMBOLISM

The diagnosis of AFE should be strongly suspected when there is a sudden development of acute respiratory failure in an otherwise normal delivery. The acute respiratory failure occurs from occlusion of pulmonary vessels by amniotic fluid, intense vasoconstriction of pulmonary vessels, and then further occlusion by platelet–fibrin thrombi. This initial event is usually followed by cardiogenic shock and systemic cardiovascular and pulmonary collapse. The usual clinical findings of acute pulmonary insufficiency are the sudden onset of tachypnea, dyspnea, and peripheral cyanosis due to the abrupt development of abnormal perfusion and diffusion. These findings are usually accompanied by acute cor pulmonale with resultant right-sided failure with subsequent decreased filling of the left ventricle and low-output failure with subsequent peripheral end-organ hypoxia, ischemia, and metabolic acidosis. Arterial blood gases will reveal decreased Po_2 and Pco_2. Abnormal diffusion capacity, metabolic acidosis, and elevated central venous pressure also will be noted.

These events typically occur early in delivery and are usually without any clinical warning. After the development of acute respiratory failure, cardiogenic shock, and peripheral circulatory collapse, there will usually be excessive uterine bleeding, followed by systemic bleeding from multiple sites. As DIC develops, the sites of bleeding can be numerous and unpredictable; however, the most common bleeding sites noted will be oozing from intravenous (i.v.) puncture sites, hematuria, hemoptysis, and at times, intracranial bleeding (42). In addition, the development of petechiae and purpura usually are rapidly noted throughout the skin and mucosal membranes. As DIC progresses, there will be additional systemic microcirculatory occlusion by platelet–fibrin thrombi in multiple end organs, especially the renal system, hepatic system, and central nervous system (CNS). This will further compromise adequate end-organ perfusion and thus lead to even more compromised end-organ hypoxia, ischemia, and failure. The most reliable laboratory tests to evaluate the development of DIC are the antithrombin (AT) III level, fibrinopeptide A level, D-dimer level, prothrombin fragment 1.2 (PF 1.2), thrombin precursor protein [soluble fibrin monomer by enzyme-linked immunosorbent assay (ELISA)], and platelet count. More global tests, including the PT, PTT, and fibrinogen level are helpful if abnormal; however, these tests may frequently be normal in DIC (discussed in detail in Laboratory Diagnosis of DIC section).

MANAGEMENT OF AMNIOTIC FLUID EMBOLISM

The approach to management of acute respiratory failure is straightforward and consists of immediate establishment of an airway by use of an oropharyngeal tube, an endotracheal tube, or tracheostomy. Oxygen should be started immediately via nasal cannula or prongs, Venturi mask, or a reservoir mask. A mechanical ventilator will probably be needed. Circulatory collapse must be managed immediately with the use of vasoconstrictive agents, usually dopamine. A central venous line should immediately be established, and the central venous pressure carefully monitored. The patient should be digitalized if the central venous pressure is elevated. There should also be immediate institution of measures to induce uterine contraction and thus reduce bleeding from the placental site and uterus. Circulatory collapse is further managed with volume replacement. Those surviving AFE have been treated with large amounts of blood and blood components (50,51). One report suggests that aerosolized prostacyclin may be highly effective (52). Management of DIC in AFE should be through immediate consideration of heparinization to stop quickly the further deposition of platelet–fibrin thrombi and to stop the further generation of activated coagulation factors (42,53). I choose to use AT concentrate or subcutaneous unfractionated (UF) heparin at 100 units per kilogram, every 6 hours, in this clinical setting or LMW heparin at 100 to 150 units/kg every 12 to 24 hours. After heparinization or AT infusion, DIC should be further managed with the use of component therapy in the form of fresh frozen plasma and platelets, depending on the prothrombin time, PTT, platelet count, and sites and severity of hemorrhage. If there is enough time, and if available, AT concentrates should be used to control DIC (54–56). The neonate, if it survives birth, will usually require resuscitation and assessment for DIC (57). The sequential management of AFE is summarized in Table 7.5.

Placental abruption may induce DIC. In placental abruption with DIC, placental enzymes or tissues including procoagulants and thromboplastin-like material may be released into the uterine and next into the systemic maternal circulation and lead to activation of the coagulation system. Rapid initiation of delivery will almost always cause cessation of DIC, and only rarely are other treatment modalities needed (6–9,58–61).

In the retained-fetus syndrome, the incidence of DIC approaches 50% if the woman retains a dead fetus in utero for longer than 5 weeks. The first findings are usually those of a low-grade compensated DIC, which then progresses into a fulminant thrombohemorrhagic form. In this instance, necrotic fetal tissue, including enzymes derived from necrotic fetal tissue, are released into the uterine and then the systemic maternal circulation and act at diverse sites to activate the procoagulant and fibrinolytic systems and trigger fulminant DIC (6,8–10,58–63).

TABLE 7.5. MANAGEMENT OF AMNIOTIC FLUID EMBOLISM

I. Treat respiratory failure
   - Airway
   - Mechanical ventilator
II. Treat shock and heart failure
   - Vasopressors
   - Digitalis preparations
   - Fluids and electrolytes
   - Establish central line
III. Treat hemorrhage and DIC
   - Subcutaneous heparin or subcutaneous LMW heparin
   - Antithrombin concentrate
   - Packed red cells as needed
   - Plasma as needed
   - Platelets as needed
   - Evacuate uterus
   - Uterine contraction as needed
   - Prostacyclin ??

DIC, disseminated intravascular coagulation; LMW, low molecular weight.

Toxemia of pregnancy is referred to as preeclampsia or eclampsia. Preeclampsia, usually occurring in the third trimester, is characterized by hypertension, edema, proteinuria, sodium retention, hyperreflexia, and DIC. When frank convulsions occur in preeclampsia, the term eclampsia is used to define the syndrome (64). Preeclampsia, eclampsia, and HELLP syndrome (hemolysis, elevated liver enzymes, and low platelet count; discussed subsequently) appear to constitute a progressive spectrum of the same pathophysiologic processes. Unfortunately, the pathophysiology remains elusive. It remains unclear whether the process starts as one of endothelial damage, which then activates procoagulant proteins and platelets, or if the process starts as a procoagulant/platelet problem that then damages endothelium; most likely, the former is at play. If eclampsia develops, the chances of developing isolated thrombocytopenia are about 18%, the chances of developing DIC are about 11%, and the chances of developing HELLP syndrome are about 15% (65,66). In preeclampsia/eclampsia, if a coagulation defect develops (thrombocytopenia, HELLP, and/or DIC), the maternal mortality is between 16% (65) and more than 50% (66), and the perinatal mortality may be greater than 40% (67). In addition, in about 16% of patients with preeclampsia/eclampsia, placental abruption will develop, thus enhancing the probability of DIC and maternal/fetal death (66). In eclampsia, DIC often remains of low grade and specific to the renal and placental microcirculation; however, in at least 10% to 15% of women, the process becomes systemic and fulminant (42,68). Laboratory monitoring of hemostasis parameters has been found useful for assessing potential progression from mild preeclampsia to more catastrophic syndromes of HELLP and DIC; these include the D-dimer level, thrombin–antithrombin (TAT) complex, plasminogen activator inhibitor type-1 (PAI-1), soluble fibrin monomer (thrombin precursor protein by ELISA), and PF 1.2, all of which will progressively increase while fibrinogen, AT, and PAI-2 will decrease (69,70). Characteristics of eclampsia and complications are summarized in Table 7.6.

HELLP syndrome is generally thought to be a progression or complication of preeclampsia/eclampsia and comprises (a) microangiopathic *H*emolytic anemia, (b) *E*levated *L*iver enzymes, and (c) *L*ow *P*latelet count. HELLP syndrome occurs in about 0.5% to 0.9% of all pregnancies (71,72) and between 15% and 26% of preeclampsia/eclampsia patients (65,73). The maternal mortality varies between 1.0% and 4% (74), and the perinatal mortality may be as high as 40% (74,75). In some patients, a prodrome of weakness and fatigue, nausea and vomiting, abdominal pain (particularly in the right upper quadrant), headache, visual changes, and shoulder or neck pain develops (75). In some women, the syndrome occurs after delivery (72). The pathophysiology is poorly understood, but is thought to be the result of initial inadequate placental vasculature, with placental ischemia leading to systemic release of thromboxanes, angiotensin, procoagulant prostaglandins, endothelin-1, and tumor necrosis factor-α (TNF-α) (72,76). The subsequent DIC leads micro- and macrothrombi, with the placental, ovarian, renal, hepatic, and cerebral vasculature being the most vulnerable. The thrombi then lead to endothelial damage, microangiopathic hemolytic anemia, and of course, varying degrees of end-organ failure in the organs involved with micro/macrothrombi. This includes not only hepatic failure, but also renal and pulmonary failure and cerebral edema and/or infarct (77,78). Hepatic rupture is a catastrophic event in HELLP syndrome (79,80). Laboratory monitoring for early DIC, as discussed earlier for preeclampsia, is recommended. Therapy is usually prompt delivery, control of hypertension, and control of DIC; many have demonstrated the efficacy of steroid therapy (81–84), and plasma exchange/plasmapheresis has been beneficial in some cases (85,86). Maternal death is most commonly due to manifestations of uncontrolled DIC (87).

TABLE 7.6. FEATURES OF PREECLAMPSIA/ECLAMPSIA

1. Usually begins in third trimester
2. Usually occurs in primigravidas
3. Hypertension
4. Proteinuria
5. Edema
6. Oliguria ±
7. Sodium retention
8. Hyperreflexia (preeclampsia)
9. Seizures (eclampsia)
10. Disseminated intravascular coagulation

In many patients undergoing hypertonic saline-induced abortion, a DIC-type process develops, which sometimes becomes fulminant and at other times remains compensated until the abortion is completed (88).

Obstetrical patients with other complications not unique to obstetrics also may develop DIC; these conditions are discussed subsequently.

Disseminated Intravascular Coagulation Syndromes Unique to Gynecology

The most common setting for DIC in gynecologic patients is malignancy; however, as in obstetric patients, medical and surgical complications not limited to gynecology also may provide a triggering of DIC.

DIC is commonly seen with ovarian carcinoma, with or without complicating hemolytic anemia (89–93) and may be seen with metastatic uterine carcinoma. Breast cancer also may be complicated by DIC (89–92,94). Although thrombosis is more commonly the abnormality of hemostasis manifest with gynecologic malignancies, and hemorrhage is more commonly associated with acute leukemias, hemorrhage may be a significant clinical problem in patients with solid tumors as well (92,94,95). Intravascular coagulation is present in many patients with malignancy and manifests varying clinical expressions, the most extreme form being acute fulminant DIC with catastrophic hemorrhage and thrombosis (60,92,94,96). DIC in cancer patients may be low grade or fulminant. Patients with fulminant DIC will manifest oozing from intravenous sites or sites of other invasive procedures, such as intraarterial lines, subclavian catheters, and hepatic artery catheters (58, 59,96–100). Although these are the most common bleeding manifestations, more life-threatening bleeding, such as intracranial and intrapulmonary hemorrhage with massive hemoptysis, also may occur. Fulminant DIC may be noted in association with carcinoma of the uterus, breast, and ovary. Initiation of chemotherapy has occasionally been associated with triggering or acceleration of DIC (94, 101–104). Most patients with disseminated solid malignancy have some laboratory or clinical evidence of DIC; in many patients with malignancy, clinical manifestations of DIC never develop, but if one looks for laboratory findings of DIC, these are usually present. If present, molecular markers of activation should be monitored for evidence of progression to overt DIC and treatment instituted, when warranted. The patient with disseminated malignancy is a special problem because DIC may be manifest in a fulminant, subacute, or low-grade form, and may, therefore, be manifest as local thrombosis, diffuse thrombosis, thromboembolism, minor hemorrhage, diffuse hemorrhage, or any combination thereof (58,59,94,98–100).

In patients with adenocarcinoma of gynecologic sites, the mechanism for DIC may be multifaceted. However, the sialic acid moiety of secreted mucin from adenocarcinomatous tissue can invoke the nonenzymatic activation of factor X to factor Xa (105,106). This can easily provide a trigger for systemic thrombin generation and a later course of fulminant or subacute DIC (58,107). This sequence also may lead to thrombosis alone (58,96,98,108). It is probable that other less clearly defined mechanisms exist for initiating DIC in these malignancies. The systemic release of necrotic tumor tissue and/or enzymes with procoagulant or phospholipoprotein-like activity may activate the early phases of coagulation and/or platelet release. Many tumors undergo neovascularization; this process could potentially produce abnormal endothelial cell lining, which may either cause a platelet release or generation of factor XIIa and XIa with subsequent procoagulant activation and the development of a fulminant, subacute, or low-grade DIC process. Another not uncommon trigger for DIC in the patient with malignancy is the use of LeVeen or Denver shunts for malignant ascites, commonly used in gynecologic malignancies. Patients with malignant ascites must be carefully chosen for this procedure; if ascitic fluid is positive for malignant cells, the placement of a LeVeen shunt is usually not successful, does not lead to significant prolongation of quality of life, and is commonly associated with the development of DIC (42,58,59,109–111). DIC may be blunted or aborted by removal of ascitic fluid at the time of shunt placement (112). In this clinical setting, a less common although significant complication of LeVeen shunting in the patient with malignant ascites is that of thromboembolism (112).

Intravascular hemolysis of any etiology is a common cause of DIC. A frank hemolytic transfusion reaction is a triggering event for DIC; however, hemolysis of any etiology, even though minor, may trigger intravascular coagulation. During hemolysis, the release of red cell adenosine diphosphate (ADP) or red cell membrane phospholipoprotein activates the procoagulant system, and a combination of these may account for DIC associated with major or minor hemolysis (113–118).

Septicemia is often associated with DIC. An early organism to be associated with DIC was meningococcus (119). Later, other gram-negative organisms also were associated with DIC (120–122). The triggering mechanisms consist of the initiation of coagulation by endotoxin: bacterial coat lipopolysaccharide (123,124). Endotoxin activates factor XII to factor XIIa, induces a platelet-release reaction, causes endothelial sloughing with later activation of XII to XIIa or XI to XIa, and releases granulocyte procoagulant materials, any of which might independently trigger DIC. Endotoxin also induces release of tumor necrosis factor-α (TNF-α), interleukin-1 (IL-1), and complement activation, all leading to endothelial damage and disruption and endothelial permeability and multiple end-organ damage. What is most common is a clinical summation of several or all of these activation events. Later, many gram-positive organisms also were noted to be associated with DIC, and the mechanisms have been aptly described (113,114,125–128). Bacterial coat mucopolysaccharides induce DIC by the same mechanisms noted with endotoxin. However, as with gram-negative endotoxemia, what is seen clinically is probably a summation of several or all of these activation events (113,114, 125,126,129).

Many viremias, including human immunodeficiency virus (HIV), are associated with DIC; the most common are varicella, hepatitis, or cytomegalovirus infections (130, 131). Many other acute viremias also induce DIC (113, 114,125,126,129). The triggering mechanisms are unclear but may represent antigen–antibody-associated activation of factor XII, a platelet-release reaction, or endothelial sloughing with subsequent exposure of subendothelial collagen and basement membrane (132).

Severe viral hepatitis and acute hepatic failure of any etiology, including drug, toxin, or infection, can lead to DIC, which can be difficult to separate from the myriad other coagulation abnormalities associated with severe hepatic dysfunction. Intrahepatic or extrahepatic cholestasis, especially when present for longer than 5 days, also may be accompanied by DIC (113,114,125,126,129).

DIC is common in malignancy, and most patients with disseminated solid malignancy will have at least laboratory evidence of DIC that may or may not become clinically manifested (133–138).

Many hematologic disorders also are associated with DIC. Angiogenic myeloid metaplasia has been associated with DIC, and many patients with polycythemia rubra vera have clinical and laboratory findings of an underlying compensated DIC process (113,114,126,132,133,136,137). There is an increased tendency for thrombosis or thromboembolization in patients with paroxysmal nocturnal hemoglobinuria, representing DIC that is clinically manifest primarily as thrombosis (138,139). Metabolic abnormalities, particularly acidosis, have been implicated as "triggers" for DIC (113,114,125,126,129).

Acidosis has been commonly noted as a triggering event, with the conceptual construct that endothelial sloughing with activation of XII to XIIa, activation of XI to XIa, and platelet release provide the bases for activation of the procoagulant system. Several problems exist in characterizing the metabolic changes as causal in DIC, because almost all of the clinical circumstances that produced the acidosis also are causal in the complex pathophysiology of DIC. Recent evidence has implicated cytokine release as an important mediator of the initiation and propagation of DIC, and it is likely that the metabolic changes are secondary events to such release. Certainly release of TNF, IL-1, IL-6, and interferon-γ have been shown to participate in the activation of the coagulation sequence with resultant local fibrin deposition (140,141). The pathophysiologic events that result from TNF administration mimic those seen in shock and associated DIC (140–145). Acidosis, along with IL-1, IL-6, endotoxin, and TNF, inhibits endothelial and soluble thrombomodulin activity, leading to inhibition of thrombin-mediated activities, some of which are antithrombotic in nature, such as activation of the protein C and S system, thus providing more propensity for thrombus formation in DIC (146,147). Decreased levels of thrombomodulin also are associated with elevation of TNF-α, which also leads to further endothelial damage and disruption, creating a vicious loop, the end point of which is enhanced end-organ damage (148).

DIC often develops in patients with extensive burns, and several mechanisms exist (149,150). Microhemolysis, with release of red cell membrane phospholipid and/or red cell ADP may provide the trigger (113,114,126). Necrotic burn tissue also may release tissue materials and/or cellular enzymes into the systemic circulation and initiate DIC. In any patient with a large crush injury and attendant tissue necrosis, DIC also may develop because of the release of tissue enzymes and/or phospholipoprotein-like materials into the systemic circulation (119,151,152). In patients with open head wounds or undergoing craniotomy, DIC may be relatively local or systemic from the brain phospholipid released into the surrounding area or systemic circulation; this complication is usually catastrophic and often fatal (153,154).

Selected vascular disorders and other miscellaneous disorders can be associated with DIC (113,125,126,155). The Kasabach–Merritt syndrome is the association of giant cavernous hemangiomata and DIC (156,157). In about 25% of patients with giant cavernous hemangiomata, a low-grade, "compensated" DIC may accelerate into fulminant DIC; the transformation into a fulminant form may happen without identifiable reasons. About 50% of patients with hereditary hemorrhagic telangiectasia will have a low-grade DIC, which occasionally becomes fulminant (113,125,126,155). In individuals with systemic small vessel disease such as vasospastic phenomena, including Raynaud syndrome, severe diabetic angiopathy, or angiopathy associated with autoimmune disorders or Leriche syndrome, compensated DIC may develop and often becomes fulminant. Collagen vascular diseases may be associated with DIC, and in any patient with a collagen vascular disorder, especially when associated with significant small vessel involvement, DIC may develop. This DIC, usually in a compensated form, may be seen in patients with severe rheumatoid arthritis, systemic lupus erythematosus, Sjögren syndrome, dermatomyositis, and scleroderma (113, 125,126,156). Hemolytic–uremic syndrome (HUS), like eclampsia, shares similar pathophysiology with DIC. However, HUS often remains organ specific and localized to the renal microcirculation (113,114,126). In about 10% of individuals with HUS, the syndrome becomes systemic (113,114,126). Chronic inflammatory disorders including sarcoidosis, Crohn disease, and ulcerative colitis can be associated with compensated or fulminant DIC (113,114, 125,126,157–159).

Cardiovascular diseases also may be associated with low-grade DIC, and occasionally in patients with acute myocardial infarction, a compensated or fulminant DIC process develops (113,114,125,126,160). The mechanisms are unclear but may include shock, hypoxia, and acidosis with resultant endothelial sloughing and/or activation of the contact activation system through stasis. Various prosthetic devices may trigger DIC. Exposure of the blood to foreign surfaces is often linked with activation of the procoagulant system and provides a major obstacle to the use of certain prosthetic devices (161). The hemostatic complications that accompany the insertion of prosthetic devices include activation of coagulation factors, "consumption" of coagulation factors and other plasma proteins and platelets, and the generation of microthrombi. Life-threatening thrombosis or thromboembolism also may develop in those with prosthetic devices (113,114,125,162). Intraaortic balloon assist devices may activate the coagulation system with an attendant low-grade DIC, which may become fulminant (113). LeVeen or Denver valve shunting for peritoneovenous or pleurovenous shunting is a common palliative procedure, and generalized DIC is often seen with the use of these shunts (113,125,162,163). The removal of ascitic fluid at the time of LeVeen or Denver valve implantation and the use of low-dose heparin may abort DIC (113,114,125, 126). In an acute situation, simply placing the patient with a LeVeen shunt and DIC in a sitting position will usually blunt shunt function and temporarily abort the DIC process (113).

Many other disorders are associated with DIC, including the allergic vasculitides, such as Henoch–Schönlein purpura and the other allergic purpuras, sarcoidosis, amyloidosis, and the acquired immune deficiency syndrome (AIDS) (113,114,125,126,129). Compensated DIC also may occur in patients who have hyperlipoproteinemias (113,125). On very rare occasions, DIC may develop in patients with no apparent etiology defined (113,114,125,126).

Figure 7.3 illustrates the mechanisms by which a broad spectrum of unrelated pathophysiologic insults can give rise to the same common ultimate pathway, the syndrome of DIC. Many disorders are associated with endothelial damage, circulating antigen–antibody complexes, endotoxemia, tissue damage, platelet damage or release, and red cell damage (113,114,126,164). When one of these insults happens, there are many potential activation pathways by which systemically circulating plasmin and circulating thrombin may arise; when these two enzymes are circulating systemically, DIC is the usual result (113,114,126,164). Conversely, both enzymes must be present for development of DIC. Often the pathways leading from the first pathophysiologic insult to the generation of systemic thrombin and plasmin are different; despite the differences in initiating the activation pathway, once triggered, the resultant pathophysiology of DIC is the same (113,114,126). Only recently has the important contribution of cytokines and vasoactive peptides in leading to end-organ damage and necrosis in DIC become appreciated (165).

PATHOPHYSIOLOGIC EVENTS

The pathophysiology of DIC, once a triggering event is provided, is summarized in Fig. 7.2. After the coagulation system has been activated and both thrombin and plasmin circulate systemically, the pathophysiology of DIC is similar in all disorders.

Consequences of Systemic Thrombin Activity

When thrombin circulates systemically, fibrinopeptides A and B are cleaved from fibrinogen, leaving behind fibrin monomer, which polymerizes into fibrin (clot), leading to microvascular and macrovascular thrombosis and interference with blood flow, peripheral ischemia, and end-organ damage (164,166). As fibrin is deposited in the microcirculation, platelets become trapped, and thrombocytopenia follows (167). On the other side of the "circle" depicted in Fig. 7.3, plasmin also circulates systemically and cleaves the carboxy-terminal end of fibrinogen into fibrin(ogen) degradation products (FDPs), creating the clinically recognized X, Y, D, and E fragments (164,168–170). Plasmin also rapidly releases specific peptides, the B-β 15-42 and related peptides, which serve as diagnostic molecular markers.

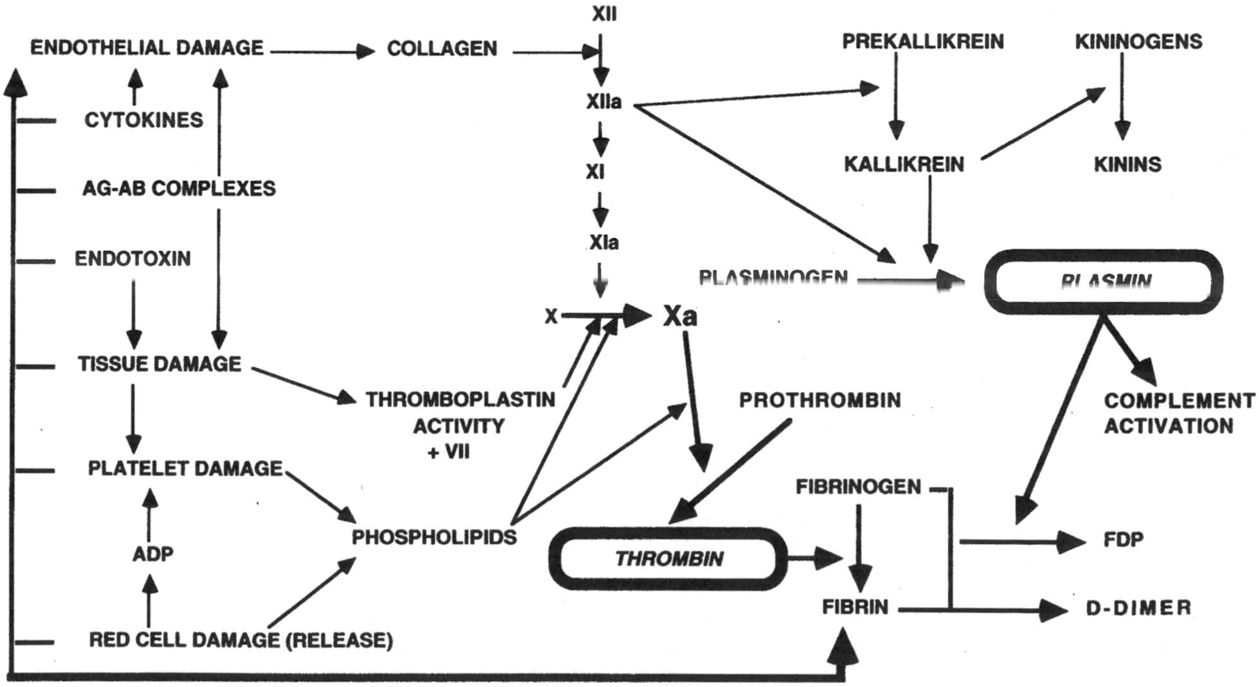

FIGURE 7.3. Triggering mechanisms for disseminated intravascular coagulation. *ADP,* adenosine diphosphate; *FDP,* fibrin(ogen) degradation products.

FDPs may combine with circulating fibrin monomer before polymerization, and the fibrin monomer becomes "solubilized." This complex of FDPs and fibrin monomer is called soluble fibrin monomer; the presence of soluble fibrin monomer forms the basis of the "paracoagulation" reactions, the ethanol gelation and protamine sulfate tests (171–174). The systemically circulating FDPs interfere with fibrin monomer polymerization; this further impairs hemostasis and may lead to hemorrhage (113,114). The subsequent fragments (D and E) have a high affinity for platelet membranes and induce a profound platelet function defect, which may contribute to clinically significant hemorrhage (113,114,175–177). FDPs and D-dimer, discussed later, induce synthesis and release of monocyte/macrophage-derived IL-1, IL-6, and PAI-1; IL-1 and IL-6 induce additional vascular endothelial damage and disruption, thus more end-organ damage, and elevated PAI-1 inhibits fibrinolysis, leading to accelerated thrombus formation (172). Thrombin also induces monocyte release of TNF, IL-1, IL-6, and may induce endothelial release of soluble thrombomodulin and endothelin and selectin (178, 179). The endothelin release can produce intense vasoconstriction, vasospasm, and subsequent thrombus and vascular occlusion, leading to further end-organ damage and failure (180). The selectin E (ELAM-1) released binds to granulocytes, lymphocytes, and monocytes/macrophages inducing further cytokine release and release of platelet activating factor (PAF). PAF induces further thrombocytopenia (179–181). Additionally, FDPs may induce monocyte release of monocyte-derived IL-1 and tissue factor (TF) (178), both of which enhance thrombosis (176). The binding of granulocytes to endothelium also induces release of granulocyte cathepsins and elastases, which can produce end-organ damage and further cytokine release (182,183).

Plasmin, unlike thrombin, is a global proteolytic enzyme and has equal affinity for fibrinogen and fibrin (113,114). Plasmin also effectively biodegrades factors V, VIII:c, IX, XI, and other plasma proteins, including growth hormone, adrenocorticotropic hormone (ACTH), insulin, and many more (113,114,164,184,185). As plasmin degrades cross-linked fibrin, specific FDPs appear in the circulation; one of these is D-dimer. Plasmin free in the circulation also may activate the complement sequence (113,114,164,186). Complement also is activated by TNF, through thrombin-mediated release of TNF from the monocyte/macrophage system (148,187). Red cell lysis releases red cell ADP and red cell membrane phospholipids, supplying more procoagulant material. Complement-induced platelet lysis also prompts further thrombocytopenia and provides more platelet procoagulant material. Of added clinical importance, activation of the complement system will increase vascular permeability, leading to hypotension and shock (113,114,163). Elevated levels of PAI-1 in DIC may blunt some of these activities and clearly leads to hypoactivity of overall fibrinolysis and fibrinogenolysis, thus enhancing fibrin precipitation (188).

Activation of the kinin system also is an important pathophysiologic event with serious clinical consequences in DIC. With generation of factor XIIa in DIC, there is subsequent conversion of prekallikrein to kallikrein and later conversion of high-molecular-weight kininogen into circulating kinins (189–191). This also leads to increased vascular permeability, hypotension, and shock (113).

In summary, as thrombin circulates systemically, the consequences are mainly thrombosis with deposition of fibrin monomer and polymerized (cross-linked) fibrin in the microcirculation and, occasionally, large vessels. Many of these consequences of thrombin are mediated by both the procoagulant system and consequences of other thrombin-activated systems and by thrombin-induced release of cytokines. Many of these adverse actions in DIC also are mediated by subsequent endothelial damage/disruption, release of endothelium-derived products and cytokines, and endothelial interactions with granulocytes, lymphocytes, and monocyte/macrophage cells. Concomitantly, plasmin also circulates systemically and is primarily responsible for the hemorrhage seen in DIC because of the creation of FDPs and the interference of FDPs with fibrin monomer polymerization and platelet function. Plasmin-induced lysis of many aforementioned clotting factors also leads to hemorrhage. With appreciation of this circular concept of pathophysiology, it is understandable why most patients with DIC experience both hemorrhage and thrombosis. Clinicians are repeatedly misguided by appreciating only the hemorrhage evolving in DIC patients, as this is the most obvious physical finding. However, of greater importance is the substantial microvascular and large vessel thromboses that occur, because these can lead to irreversible end-organ damage. It is important to recognize that most patients with DIC not only have hemorrhage but also have significant and often diffuse thrombosis (113,114,192, 193). Understanding and appreciating the extraordinarily complex pathophysiology of DIC provides the dictum that DIC is always accompanied by (a) procoagulant system activation, (b) fibrinolytic system activation, (c) inhibitor consumption, (d) cytokine release, (e) cellular activation, and resultant (f) end-organ damage.

CLINICAL FINDINGS

The systemic signs and symptoms of DIC are variable, but the specific signs, which include petechiae and purpura (found in most patients), hemorrhagic bullae, acral cyanosis, and sometimes, frank gangrene, should immediately forewarn one of the probable diagnosis of DIC (113, 114,163,194,195). Other symptoms include fever, hypotension, acidosis, proteinuria, hypoxia, and wound bleeding; oozing from a surgical or traumatic wound is common in patients who have undergone surgery or had trauma. Oozing from venipuncture sites or intraarterial lines is

TABLE 7.7. MINIMAL CLINICAL FINDINGS REQUIRED FOR A DIAGNOSIS OF DISSEMINATED INTRAVASCULAR COAGULATION

The usual clinical manifestations of DIC and the minimal criteria required for the clinical diagnosis of DIC:

1. Clinical evidence of hemorrhage, thrombosis, or both should be present

AND

2. Should occur in the appropriate clinical setting as defined in the text

another common finding. Large subcutaneous hematomas and deep tissue bleeding also are often seen (113). The average patient with DIC usually bleeds from at least three unrelated sites, and any combination may be seen (113, 114). A remarkable volume of microvascular and large vessel thrombosis may not be clinically obvious, unless and until looked for. Those organ systems having a high chance of microvascular thrombosis associated with dysfunction include cardiac, pulmonary, renal system, hepatic system, and CNS (196). Thrombotic thrombocytopenic purpura (TTP) is commonly associated with CNS dysfunction; however, it should be realized that this is observed just as commonly in DIC (113,114).

Patients with low-grade DIC, also termed "compensated DIC," present with subacute bleeding and diffuse thromboses instead of acute fulminant life-threatening hemorrhage (197). In this instance, there is usually an increased turnover and decreased survival of many components of the hemostasis system, including the platelets, fibrinogen, and factors V and VIII:c; because of this, most global coagulation laboratory tests are near normal or normal (197). Patients with low-grade DIC, however, uniformly have elevated FDPs, leading to impairment of fibrin monomer polymerization and a clinically significant platelet-function defect resulting from the coating of platelet membranes by FDPs. Molecular markers of hemostatic activation also are typically abnormal in low-grade DIC.

The minimal clinical findings required for a diagnosis of fulminant or low-grade DIC are summarized in Table 7.7.

MORPHOLOGIC FINDINGS IN DISSEMINATED INTRAVASCULAR COAGULATION

Morphologic findings in DIC consist of characteristic peripheral smear findings and hemorrhage or thrombosis in any organ(s) (113,114,198,199). Early morphologic findings are platelet-rich microthrombi (113,198,199). These are usually seen in association with intense vasoconstriction, resulting from compounds released from platelets including biogenic amines, adenine nucleotides, thromboxanes, and kinins (113,114,200). These are later replaced by fibrin-rich microthrombi (198,199). Another early finding is fibrin monomer deposition, occurring primarily in the reticuloendothelial system (113,114,201). The precipitation of fibrin monomer may cause end-organ damage because of both primary parenchymal damage and microvascular occlusion. This also may impair reticuloendothelial clearance of FDPs, activated clotting factors, and circulating soluble fibrin monomer. Later findings are the typical fibrin-rich hyaline microthrombi thought to replace earlier deposited platelet-rich microthrombi (197). In patients with DIC, pulmonary hyaline membranes may account, in part, for significant pulmonary dysfunction and hypoxemia. Schistocytes are seen in about 50% of individuals with fulminant DIC (113,114, 163,202–204). Most patients with fulminant DIC will present with a mild reticulocytosis and a mild leukocytosis, usually associated with a mild to moderate shift to immature forms. Thrombocytopenia is usually present and often obvious by examination of the peripheral blood smear (113, 114,205). Large platelets are usually seen on the peripheral smear, representing an increased population of young platelets resulting from increased platelet turnover and decreased platelet survival, because of platelet entrapment in microthrombi (113,114,206–208).

The platelet-rich microthrombi are later replaced by hyaline (fibrin) microthrombi (209). Hyaline microthrombi cause three types of end-organ damage: (a) globular hyaline microthrombi, which may be seen on periodic acid–Schiff (PAS)-stained peripheral blood smears and are polymerized complexes of fibrinogen, fibrin, their degradation products and many intermediates; (b) intravascular hyaline microthrombi, which are typically seen by pathologists at postmortem examination in DIC patients; these intravascular hyaline microthrombi are homogeneous, compact, intravascular hyaline structures oriented parallel to the blood flow, which occasionally contain platelets or white cell fragments, are easily seen by PAS staining, trichrome staining, tryptophan staining, and fluorescein-labeled antifibrinogen antiserum staining and by electron microscopy (210,211); and (c)pulmonary hyaline membranes, which also are a form of hyaline microthrombus and are highly polymerized complexes of fibrinogen, fibrin, their degradation products, and all types of intermediates (212,213). They are usually seen to cover the alveolar epithelium, with a preference for areas denuded of epithelial cells. The interalveolar capillaries beneath these hyaline membranes also typically exhibit abnormal vascular permeability with the circulation of endothelial cells, plasma protein precipitation between endothelial borders, and the formation of interstitial edema. In many patients with DIC, pulmonary hyaline membranes develop, leading to overt respiratory failure, abnormal arterial blood gases, or abnormal pulmonary-function tests [especially altered diffusion capacity (DCO)].

DIC is a process associated with hemorrhage and thrombosis, although thrombosis is less clinically evident and less commonly appreciated by the clinician until late in a course of DIC or until autopsy. Hemorrhage can often be successfully treated in patients with DIC, whereas thrombosis in the microcirculation and macrocirculation often leads to end-organ damage with irreversible ischemic changes that lead to morbidity and death. The parameters that accelerate or precipitate microthrombi and macrothrombi in patients with DIC are vasomotor reactions, including elevated catecholamines, acidosis, and progressive vasoconstriction (208, 214–216); use of exogenous glucocorticoids or endogenous ACTH; therefore careful thought must accompany use of steroids in these patients; although often steroid use is desirable and warranted (113,114,217); and impairment of reticuloendothelial clearance, resulting from fibrin monomer precipitation or use of steroids, of FDPs, circulating soluble fibrin monomer, or activated coagulation factors. These mechanisms and interplays between them lead to accelerated fibrin monomer precipitation in the circulation, resulting in severe end-organ damage that may be irreversible and often is associated with significant morbidity and mortality.

LABORATORY DIAGNOSIS

Because of the complex pathophysiology depicted earlier, many laboratory findings of DIC may be quite variable, complex, and difficult to interpret unless the pathophysiology is clearly understood and appropriate tests are performed. Fortunately, many newer modalities have become available to the routine clinical laboratory for easily assessing patients with DIC (218–221).

Global Coagulation Tests in Disseminated Intravascular Coagulation

The prothrombin time should be abnormal in DIC for multiple reasons, but often is normal and therefore is an unreliable test in this setting (113,114,221). The prothrombin time is prolonged in about 50% to 75% of patients with DIC, and in up to 50% of patients, it is normal or short. The reasons for normal or short times are the presence of circulating activated clotting factor(s), such as thrombin or factor Xa, which may accelerate the formation of fibrin, and early degradation products that may be rapidly clottable by thrombin and quickly "gel" the test system, giving a normal or fast prothrombin time.

The activated (aPTT) also should be prolonged in fulminant DIC for a variety of reasons, but is more unreliable than the prothrombin time. There is plasmin-induced biodegradation of factors V, VIII:c, IX, and XI, which should prolong the aPTT. The aPTT, like the prothrombin time, is prolonged by fibrinogen levels less than 100 mg/dL. The aPTT may be prolonged because of FDP inhibition of fibrin monomer polymerization. However, the aPTT is prolonged in only 50% to 60% of patients with DIC, and a normal PTT can certainly not be used to rule out the diagnosis. The reasons for a fast or normal PTT in 40% to 50% of patients are the same as for the prothrombin time (221). Like the prothrombin time, the aPTT is of minimal usefulness in DIC (221).

A prolonged thrombin or reptilase time is expected in DIC. Both tests should be prolonged by the presence of circulating FDPs and interference with fibrin monomer polymerization and from the hypofibrinogenemia commonly present (113,114,221), but for reasons earlier mentioned, these tests may sometimes be normal or fast. A "bonus test" of the thrombin or reptilase time is to observe the resultant clot for presence or absence of clot lysis. This simple nonquantitative tool may provide significant clinical information; if the clot is not dissolving in 10 minutes, clinically significant fibrinolysis is unlikely to be present. However, if the clot begins to lyse within this period, a clinically significant amount of plasmin is probably present.

Coagulation factor assays provide little, if any, meaningful information in patients with DIC (221). In most patients with fulminant DIC, systemically circulating activated clotting factor(s), especially factors Xa, IXa, and thrombin, are present (113,114,221). Coagulation factor assays done by the standard aPTT or prothrombin time–derived laboratory techniques using deficient substrates will give uninterpretable results in DIC patients. The reasons for this are obvious; for example, if a factor VIII:c assay is attempted in the presence of circulating factor Xa in a patient with DIC, a high level of factor VIII:c is recorded, because factor Xa "bypasses" the requirement for factor VIII:c in the test system (113,114,221,222), and a rapid conversion of fibrinogen to fibrin occurs; a rapid time will be recorded on the typical "standard curve," and this will be interpreted as a high factor VIII:c level when there may be no factor VIII:c present.

FDPs are elevated in 85% to 100% of patients with DIC (113,209,221–224). These degradation products are "diagnostic" only of plasmin biodegradation of fibrinogen or fibrin, and are therefore indicative only of the presence of plasmin (113,114,209). The protamine sulfate or ethanol gelation tests for circulating soluble fibrin monomer are usually positive (113,114,225–227). Like the FDP titer, however, these are not diagnostic, as both elevated FDPs and circulating soluble fibrin monomer may be seen in other clinical situations, including women using oral contraceptives, patients with pulmonary emboli, some patients with myocardial infarction, patients with certain renal diseases, and patients with arterial or venous thrombotic or thromboembolic events (113,228). Sometimes the protamine sulfate test or ethanol gelation test may be negative. A quantitative assay for fibrin monomer, the FM test (KABI) has been shown to be a sensitive marker in the management of chronic DIC in cancer patients (229).

A newer test for DIC is the D-dimer assay. D-dimer is a neoantigen formed when thrombin initiates the transition of fibrinogen to fibrin and activates factor XIII to cross-link the fibrin formed; this neoantigen is formed as a result of plasmin digestion of cross-linked fibrin (230,231). The D-dimer test is, therefore, specific for *fibrin* degradation products, whereas the formation of fibrinolytic degradation products (FDPs), the X, Y, D, and E fragments, discussed earlier, may be either fibrinogen or fibrin derived, after plasmin digestion. Monoclonal antibodies have been harvested against the D-dimer neoantigen DD-3B6/22 that are specific for cross-linked fibrin derivatives containing the D-dimer configuration (232,233). After the harvesting of monoclonal antibodies, a latex agglutination assay was developed for the clinical laboratory. Of the common tests used in assessing DIC patients, the D-dimer assay appears to be the most reliable test for the probability of being abnormal in patients with confirmed DIC. With our battery of DIC tests, in the appropriate clinical setting, the reliability of tests used, in descending order of reliability, are the prothrombin fragment 1+2 (PF 1+2), D-dimer assay (abnormal in 93%), the antithrombin level (abnormal in 89%), the fibrinopeptide A level (abnormal in 88%), and FDP titer, which is usually abnormal in 75% of patients (234,235). Lane et al. (236) studied the D-dimer fragment in nine patients with DIC and found the levels to be elevated in eight of the nine. Elms et al. (237) found elevated D-dimer levels in all patients with DIC. Many newer D-dimer assays commercially available do not use the DD-3B6/22 monoclonal antibody and have recently been found to be inadequate, as they are not specific for *fibrin* degradation products (238–240).

Sometimes, FDP titers and paracoagulation reactions may be negative in DIC. The available FDP determinations use latex particles that are "antifibrinogen," and because they are antifibrinogen, thrombin clot tubes are supplied to clot out fibrinogen, so latex particles will not react with fibrinogen and erroneously measure fibrinogen instead of its degradation products (113,221,209). However, fibrinogen and its degradation products have common antigenic determinants (241). When these thrombin clot-tubes are used, not only is fibrinogen removed from the system but also fragment X and fragment Y. Commonly available FDP methodologies measure fragments D and E, and in some cases of DIC, there may be minimal secondary fibrinolytic response and minimal plasmin circulating; thus there may only be degradation to the X fragment stage or some intermediate between fibrin(ogen) and fragment X. In this instance, there will be nothing for the test to measure, because fragment X and its intermediates will be removed from the test system by the thrombin clot tubes used. Alternatively, in instances of acute DIC in which there is a massive secondary fibrinolytic activation and overwhelming amounts of plasmin circulating, degradation past the D and E stage may happen. Fragments D and E are the last degradation products retaining antigenic determinants capable of being detected by the available commercial FDP titer kits. Another problem is that of overwhelming release of granulocyte proteases, collagenases, and elastases, which also may degrade all available D and E fragments, and again, render false-negative FDP titers in patients with acute DIC. Therefore, the presence of a negative FDP titer does not rule out a diagnosis of DIC. Despite these difficulties, FDP titers are elevated in most DIC patients. However, with general availability of the D-dimer assay, there is only limited use for the FDP titer and the protamine sulfate test in DIC patients.

Molecular Markers for the Diagnosis of Disseminated Intravascular Coagulation

The conversion of prothrombin to thrombin is a key event in the normal coagulation of blood; this activation results in the release of an inactive prothrombin fragment 1.2 (F1+2) from the amino terminus of the prothrombin molecule, thus generating an intermediate species, prethrombin 2. The prethrombin 2 can be internally scissioned to yield thrombin; once produced, this serine protease can either proteolyze fibrinogen with the liberation of fibrinopeptide A (FPA) or combine with its major antagonist, antithrombin, to form a stable inactive enzyme–inhibitor complex, the TAT complex (242). Approved ELISA assays are now generally available to quantitate the levels of prothrombin fragment PF1+2 and TAT within the circulation to provide evidence of excessive factor Xa and thrombin generation (243). The PF1+2 assay is an easily performed reliable molecular marker for factor Xa generation (244–250), whereas the FPA assay is an easily performed reliable marker for thrombin generation. Unfortunately, some commercially available prothrombin fragment assays do not provide reliable results in DIC patients, so our laboratories prefer the Behringwerke assay (145). These activation sequences are depicted in Fig. 7.3. Another new assay, highly sensitive to early procoagulant activation, is the assay of thrombin precursor protein (TPP) performed by ELISA; this assay detects circulating soluble fibrin polymer and must be further assessed in DIC patients, but preliminarily appears useful (251,252).

The AT determination is a key test for the diagnosis and monitoring of therapy in DIC (113,114,221,253–255). During activation of DIC, there is irreversible complexing of thrombin and circulating activated clotting factors with AT, leading to considerable decreases of functional AT. Several studies have compared the clinical applicability of various AT methodologies and, based on these studies, synthetic substrate assays are clearly the method of choice (256,257). Immunologic assays for AT ignore biologic function and may be low or normal in DIC; therefore they should not be used (114,209,254). There has been at least one exception to the generalization that functional AT levels decrease in DIC. In patients with acute promyelocytic leukemia (APL-M-3), a severe coagulopathy is usually attributed to DIC. However, it has been reported that even though TAT complexes were significantly higher in cases of M-3 and other cases of DIC compared with those in normal subjects, the functional level of AT remained normal in some APL patients. It is unclear at this time why some APL patients retain a normal AT level, but this does support the possibility that the coagulopathy in a subset of APL (subtype M-3m) patients is not caused by DIC but by primary fibrinolysis (258). FPA is usually elevated in patients with DIC and provides a general assessment of hemostasis activation, much as PF-4 and β-thromboglobulin levels provide for platelets. The presence of FPA is "diagnostic" of the presence of thrombin acting on fibrinogen. FPA determinations also may be of help in assessing efficacy of therapy in DIC (209,221,259,260). The FPA level may be elevated in a wide variety of other micro- or macrovascular thrombotic events and increases generally as a function of age (261). A newer modality, available by radioimmunoassay, is that of B-β 15–42 and related peptide determinations (262,263). Plasmin rapidly cleaves B-β peptides 1 through 118, 1 through 42, and 15 through 42 (after thrombin has cleaved fibrinopeptide B or amino acid sequence 1 through 14) from the B-β chain of fibrinogen. The findings of elevated B-β 15–42 and related peptides may, when done in conjunction with FPA levels, add to the differential diagnosis of DIC versus primary lysis (113). The elevation of B-β 15–42 and related peptides without FPA elevation is strong evidence for primary fibrinolysis, whereas the elevation of both FPA and B-β 15-42–related peptides is strong evidence of DIC. The B-βe 15–42 assays are not routinely recommended, as they are difficult to perform and have a long turnaround time.

To summarize, the PF1+2, TPP, and FPA elevation provide direct evidence of procoagulant activation, decreased AT levels provide indirect evidence of both procoagulant activation and inhibitor consumption, and elevated TAT complex is direct evidence of procoagulant activation and inhibitor consumption.

Fibrinolytic system assays are now readily available in the clinical laboratory and provide useful information in DIC. Typically, plasminogen is decreased, and circulating plasmin is present. Intensity of the secondary fibrinolytic response is of clinical consequence for predicting potential microvascular thrombosis and resultant irreversible end-organ damage in patients with DIC. If there is impaired activation of the fibrinolytic system, morbidity and mortality resulting from end-organ damage may be even greater than expected. Fibrinolytic system activation can be assessed by measuring plasminogen and plasmin levels by commonly available synthetic substrate techniques (264–266). The euglobulin lysis time provides little or no clinically useful information for assessing the fibrinolytic system in clinical disorders, including DIC (267,268). Direct measurement of plasmin in plasma can be difficult because it is rapidly inactivated by complexing with fast-acting α_2-antiplasmin, also termed α_2-plasmin inhibitor (α_2PI), and slow acting α_2-macroglobulin (269–271). If these two fibrinolytic system inhibitors are markedly elevated, there may be an ineffective fibrinolytic response with resultant enhanced fibrin monomer precipitation, fibrin deposition, and vascular thrombosis. The plasmin–α_2-plasmin inhibitor (PAP) complex is measured by crossed immunoelectrophoresis, ELISA, and radioimmunoassays (271–273). α_2-Macroglobulin–plasmin complexes also can be measured with ELISA. The presence of these complexes is, therefore, a direct indicator of in vivo plasmin generation. The PAP complex has been shown to be markedly elevated in DIC at the time of presentation and changes in parallel with the course of DIC, with levels decreasing in clinical remission (274). The PAP complex is useful in DIC because elevation suggests fibrinolytic system activation (plasmin) and inhibitor (α_2-PI) consumption. Recently, assays for tissue (endothelial) plasminogen activator and tissue plasminogen activator inhibitor have become available; their potential role in DIC is unclear at present.

In summary, elevated plasmin and decreased plasminogen provide direct evidence of fibrinolytic activation, decreased α_2-PI provides indirect evidence of fibrinolytic activation and inhibitor consumption, and elevated PAP complex provides direct evidence of both fibrinolytic activation and inhibitor consumption.

The platelet count is typically decreased in DIC; however, the range may be variable, from as low as 20 to 30 × 10^9/L to greater than 100 × 10^9/L. Most tests of platelet function including the template bleeding time, platelet aggregation, and platelet lumi-aggregation are abnormal in patients with DIC. This is caused by FDP coating of platelet membranes or partial release of platelet procoagulant materials. There is no reason to perform tests of platelet function. Increased platelet turnover and decreased platelet survival is usual in patients with DIC; PF-4 levels and β-thromboglobulin levels are markers of general platelet reactivity and release and are usually elevated in DIC patients. It has been suggested that either of these may be worthwhile in DIC and for monitoring efficacy of therapy of the intravascular clotting process (275,276). PF-4 and β-thromboglobulin are elevated in most DIC patients; however, neither of these modalities is diagnostic of DIC and may be elevated with pulmonary emboli, acute myocardial infarction, deep venous thrombosis, and in disorders associated with microvascular disease, such as diabetes and autoimmunity. However, if elevated in DIC and then decreased after therapy, this suggests that therapy has been successful in either blunting or stopping the intravascular clotting process. Elevation of either PF-4 or β-thromboglobulin provides indirect evidence of procoagulant activation.

Tests useful for aiding in a diagnosis of DIC are depicted in Table 7.8 (277–279). The differential diagnosis of DIC

TABLE 7.8. RELIABILITY OF LABORATORY TESTS IN DISSEMINATED INTRAVASCULAR COAGULATION IN DESCENDING ORDER OF RELIABILITY

Profragment 1 + 2
D-Dimer
AT-III
Fibrinopeptide A
Platelet factor 4
FDP
Platelet count
Protamine test
Thrombin time
Fibrinogen
Prothrombin time
Activated PTT
Reptilase time

FDP, fibrin degradation product; AT, angiotensin; PTT, partial thromboplastin time.

versus primary fibrinolysis versus TTP by molecular-marker profiling is shown in Table 7.9 (277–280). Most molecular markers discussed are very sensitive to hemostasis activation and careful phlebotomies are necessary.

In summary, the laboratory diagnosis of DIC requires documentation of procoagulant system activation (group I tests), fibrinolytic system activation (group II tests), inhibitor consumption (group III tests), and end-organ damage (group IV tests). The manner in which these tests are used to provide documentation of these four requirements is summarized in Table 7.10 (280).

TABLE 7.9. MOLECULAR MARKERS USEFUL FOR THE DIFFERENTIAL DIAGNOSIS OF DIC, PRIMARY LYSIS, AND THROMBOTIC THROMBOCYTOPENIC PURPURA

Marker	DIC	Primary Lysis	TTP
Fibrinopeptide A	Elevated	Normal	Normal
Fibrinopeptide B	Elevated	Normal	Normal
B-β 15–42 peptide	Elevated	Normal	Normal
B-β 1–42 peptide	Elevated	Elevated	Normal
B-β 1–118 peptide	Elevated	Elevated	Normal
Platelet factor 4	Elevated	Normal	Elevated
β-Thromboglobulin	Elevated	Normal	Elevated
D-Dimer	Elevated	Normal	
Normal/Elevated			
Fibronectin	Decreased	Normal	Normal
Plasminogen activator	NL/Elevated	Elevated	Decreased
Thromboxanes	Elevated	Normal	Elevated
6-Keto-PGF 1-α	Normal	Normal	Decreased
Profragment 1 + 2	Elevated	Normal	Normal
SFM/TPP-ELISA	Normal	Normal	Normal

PG, prostaglandin; DIC, disseminated intravascular coagulation; TTP, thrombotic thrombocytopenic purpura; SFM, serum-free medium; ELISA, enzyme-linked immunosorbent assay.

TABLE 7.10. LABORATORY DIAGNOSTIC CRITERIA[a]

Tests currently suitable for evidence of procoagulant activation (group I tests)
- Elevated prothrombin fragment 1 + 2
- Elevated fibrinopeptide A
- Elevated thrombin–antithrombin complex (TAT)
- Elevated D-dimer[b]
- Elevated soluble fibrin monomer (TPP) ELISA

Tests currently suitable as evidence for fibrinolytic activation (*group II tests*)
- Elevated D-dimer
- Elevated FDP
- Elevated PLASMIN
- Elevated plasmin–antiplasmin complex (PAP)
- Elevated soluble fibrin monomer (TPP) ELISA

Tests currently suitable as evidence for inhibitor consumption (*group III tests*)
- Decreased AT-III
- Decreased α-2-antiplasmin
- Decreased heparin cofactor II
- Decreased protein C or S
- Elevated T.A.T. complex
- Elevated P.A.P. complex

Tests currently suitable as evidence for end-organ damage or failure (*group IV tests*) are:
- Elevated LDH
- Elevated creatinine
- Decreased pH
- Decreased $pA{O_2}$

[a]Only one abnormality each is needed in group I, II, and III and at least two abnormalities are needed in group IV tests to satisfy criteria for a laboratory diagnosis of DIC.
[b]The D-dimer is reliable only for this purpose if using the correct assay and monoclonal antibody, as discussed in the text.
FDP, fibrin degradation product; LDH, lactate dehydrogenase; ELISA, enzyme-linked immunosorbent assay.

THERAPY FOR DISSEMINATED INTRAVASCULAR COAGULATION

Fulminant Disseminated Intravascular Coagulation

The treatment of DIC is confusing and sometimes controversial (1–5,96,281). Concomitant with controversy and confusion is the global perception that therapy is often futile, and most patients die of the disease process. However, most published comments about therapy are based on tradition instead of fact and emotion instead of clinical judgment (1–5). This is because very few objective series of DIC patients, for therapy given, morbidity, mortality, and survival, have been published. Difficulties in therapeutic clinical trials result because of the diverse etiologies and clinical manifestations associated with DIC; a given therapeutic approach may be proper for one particular etiology, but not necessarily another, and one therapeutic approach may be suitable for various types of hemorrhage, but not thrombosis. Thus therapy must be highly individualized. Many individuals vehemently oppose the use of heparin in either fulminant or low-grade DIC, despite the amazing lack of published information regarding the adverse effects of heparin in DIC. Similarly, many individuals strongly urge the use of heparin in DIC; however, there also is a shortage of published reports documenting positive benefits from heparin in DIC patients. If logical, aggressive, and sequential therapy is undertaken, morbidity and mortality rates are not so dismal as suspected (3–5,96,281,282). Clinicians should synthesize judgment with respect to therapy, formulated on experience and published series of patients and documentation instead of dogma and mythology. It is hoped that the future will offer more guidelines than are available now with respect to successes and failures with various forms of potential therapy.

An acceptable approach to therapy in fulminant DIC is somewhat vigorous and is summarized in Table 7.11. Although this approach is aggressive, it is associated with a high survival rate and low morbidity in patients with classic, fulminant DIC (2–5,96,282). As a guiding principle, therapy must be individualized for each patient depending on clinical findings and manifestations of the process (3,96).

TABLE 7.11. LOGICAL AND SEQUENTIAL THERAPY RECOMMENDED FOR DISSEMINATED INTRAVASCULAR COAGULATION

Individualize therapy	
	Site(s) and severity of hemorrhage
	Site(s) and severity of thrombosis
	Precipitating disease state
	Hemodynamic status
	Age
	Other clinical considerations
Treat or remove the triggering process	
	Evacuate/remove uterus
	Antibiotics
	Control shock
	Volume replacement
	Maintain blood pressure
	Airway if needed
	Steroids ?
	Antineoplastic therapy (GYN)
	Other indicated therapy
Stop intravascular clotting process	
	Subcutaneous heparin
	LMW heparin
	Antithrombin concentrate
	Antiplatelet agents
	Intravenous heparin ?
	Hirudin ?
Component therapy as indicated	
	Platelet concentrates
	Packed red cells (washed)
	Antithrombin concentrate
	Fresh frozen plasma
	Prothrombin complex
	Cryoprecipitate
Inhibit residual fibrino(geno)lysis	
	Aminocaproic acid
	Tranexamic acid

Therapy should be based on etiology of the DIC, age, hemodynamic status, site and severity of hemorrhage, site and severity of thrombosis, and other relevant clinical factors. The essential therapeutic modality to be delivered to a patient with fulminant DIC is that of an aggressive but reasonable therapeutic approach to eliminate or treat the triggering disease process thought to be responsible for DIC (2—5,281,282). Treatments that remove or blunt the underlying disease process may in themselves significantly blunt the intravascular clotting process. If, however, control of the triggering event and pathophysiology is not achieved, later attempts at anticoagulant therapy, including heparin, will rarely alleviate the DIC process (2–5,281). Sometimes it is impossible or unlikely that the underlying disease can be alleviated. However, often the removal of the triggering pathophysiology will stop the DIC process; the classic example of this is an obstetric accident, and another is septicemia. In cases of obstetric accidents of any type (except AFE), anticoagulant therapy, especially heparin, is rarely needed. Simply evacuating the uterus, or in rare instances, hysterectomy will usually rapidly stop the intravascular clotting process (3–5,283–285). Although it is often difficult to persuade the obstetrician/gynecologist to take a hemorrhaging hypofibrinogenemic patient to the operating room, the results are usually immediate and dramatic (3–5, 6). In septicemia, specific antibiotic therapy, alleviation of shock, volume replacement, possibly high-dose glucocorticoids, and other specific therapy to stabilize hemodynamics will often cause significant blunting of the intravascular clotting process and sometimes may stop the DIC process altogether. Each case must be evaluated on its own merits, depending on the clinical situation and the clinician's assessment of the dominant triggering event. The crucial point is that an attempt to treat the triggering event is the essential therapeutic modality that must be administered to the patient with DIC. Concomitant with therapy for the triggering or underlying event, indicated supportive therapy must be aggressively started. The particular supportive therapy needed will depend on the clinical situation of the individual patient.

The second principle is to treat the intravascular clotting process, recalling that thrombosis, usually of small vessels, is the process that most affects morbidity and mortality in patients, not hemorrhage! Most patients, except those with DIC secondary to obstetric accidents or massive liver failure, will next usually need anticoagulant therapy of some form to stop the intravascular clotting process. The use of subcutaneous low-dose heparin appears to be highly effective in mild and (sometimes) moderate DIC (3–5,96,282). Anticoagulant therapy is indicated if the patient continues to bleed or clot significantly for about 4 to 6 hours after the initiation of supportive therapy and therapy to stop or blunt the triggering pathophysiologic event. This time period is somewhat empirical and depends on the sites and severity of bleeding and thrombosis; the thromboses usually manifest as progressive end-organ failure. When the patient continues to bleed in this situation, subcutaneous porcine heparin at 80 to 100 units/kg, every 4 to 6 hours, as the clinical situation, site and severity of bleeding and thrombosis, and patient size dictate, is begun. Low-dose subcutaneous heparin appears to be as effective as or possibly more effective than larger doses of intravenous heparin in DIC (1,3–5,96,286,287). With this approach, one often notes cessation of AT consumption, lowering of FDPs, increases in fibrinogen levels, and slow or rapid correction of other abnormal laboratory modalities of acute DIC in 3 to 4 hours, followed shortly by blunting or cessation of clinically significant hemorrhage and thrombosis. The use of subcutaneous low-dose heparin, instead of intravenous heparin, appears reasonable for several reasons: (a) if the patient does not respond, larger doses of heparin can always be administered if thought applicable; (b) unlike fears with larger intravenous doses of heparin, low-dose subcutaneous heparin therapy is associated with minimal chances of increasing the patient's risk of hemorrhage; and (c) most important, the use of low-dose subcutaneous heparin has been as efficacious as large-dose heparin therapy and is associated with a high percentage of patient survival when used with other therapeutic modalities (3–5). Other anticoagulant modalities available, depending on the clinician's experience, are intravenous heparin, combination antiplatelet agents, or antithrombin concentrates. Those clinicians using intravenous heparin therapy for acute DIC usually deliver between 20,000 and 30,000 units per 24 hours by constant infusion, and this may be associated with significant blunting or cessation of the intravascular clotting process; however, aggravation of hemorrhage is a potential risk. The contraindications for subcutaneous heparin, or heparin in any dose, would be in patients with fulminant DIC and CNS insults of any type, DIC associated with fulminant liver failure, and usually obstetric accidents (3–5,96). Combination antiplatelet agents are far less effective, but on occasion may be called for as the specific clinical situation dictates (3–5). Fulminant DIC has been successfully treated with AT concentrates in small groups of patients and in randomized trials (3–5,54–56,285,288, 289), and evidence would suggest these to be quite effective. AT concentrates have become my treatment of choice for most patients with fulminant moderate and severe DIC. The dose needed is calculated as follows: total units needed = (Desired level − Initial level) × 0.6 × Total body weight (kg) (96). The desired level should always be 125% or greater, and the aforementioned calculation should be performed and the derived AT dose delivered every 8 hours. Although I find AT to be highly effective in fulminant DIC, AT concentrate has not yet been subjected to objective prospective clinical trials to clearly establish efficacy. Newer agents of potential therapeutic benefit for fulminant DIC are recombinant hirudin (288,290), defibrotide, and gabexate (291–293). Extensive clinical experience with these newer agents in DIC is limited. About 75% of patients will respond to the two earlier outlined sequential therapeutic steps (96).

If patients continue to bleed after beginning reasonable attempts to treat the triggering pathophysiology responsible for DIC, and anticoagulant therapy has been initiated, the most probable cause of continued bleeding is component depletion. In this instance, the precise components missing and thought to be contributing to hemorrhage should be defined and administered. The delivery of certain components is associated with potential hazards in patients with *ongoing* DIC, and as a general guideline, only concentrates and components void of fibrinogen should be delivered to a patient with ongoing DIC, especially if manifested by a continued severe depression of the AT level. If, however, the AT level, or another specific monitoring modality that the clinician chooses to follow is returning to normal, and it can be assumed that the intravascular clotting process has been controlled, then any component or concentrate thought to be important can safely be given. Generally, the only components considered safe in patients with active, uncontrolled DIC are *washed* packed red cells, platelet concentrates, AT concentrates, and nonclotting protein containing volume expanders, such as plasma protein fraction, albumin, and hydroxyethyl starch. Components containing clotting factors and/or fibrinogen may be associated with enhanced hemorrhage and especially thrombosis in a patient with active DIC, to whom these components are unwisely delivered (98,145, 146,294,295). As would be expected from an understanding of the pathophysiology of DIC, when whole blood, fresh frozen plasma, or cryoprecipitate is given to a patient with ongoing DIC, plasmin will rapidly biodegrade most, if not all, of the coagulation factors supplied (3–5,295). This may not be particularly harmful but is surely not helpful (3). Of greater importance is that these components contain fibrinogen and are associated with a potential for the creation of even higher levels of FDPs that will further impair hemostasis by interference with fibrin monomer polymerization, further decrease already compromised platelet function, and lead to enhanced microvascular deposition of fibrin thrombi and subsequent thrombocytopenia (3–5,98,295). A reasonable approach is to assess the patient after initiation of anticoagulant therapy. If bleeding continues and the AT level, or other selected monitoring modality, has returned to normal or near normal, any component thought significantly depleted and probably be contributing to continued hemorrhage is reasonable to replace. Alternatively, if the patient continues to bleed after anticoagulant therapy has been delivered, the AT level and other modalities used to monitor the patient remain abnormal, and progressive end-organ damage (thrombosis) or deterioration in hemodynamic status is noted, it is highly likely in this situation that the intravascular clotting process has not been controlled. In this instance, the component(s) should be restricted to washed packed red cells, platelets, volume expanders, and, if available, AT (3–5).

After these three sequential aggressive steps, most patients will stop hemorrhaging if they are going to survive.

In those rare instances in which bleeding continues after these three sequential steps are instituted, in conjunction with aggressive supportive therapy, the fourth step in the therapy of fulminant DIC is to consider inhibition of the fibrinolytic system. This is rarely needed and is called for in only about 3% of patients. An exception to this generalization is in the treatment of the acute promyelocytic leukemia (APL) patient in whom primary activation of the fibrinolytic system may coexist with DIC. Addition of ε-aminocaproic acid or tranexamic acid to heparin anticoagulation in some patients with APL (those with functional α_2-plasmin inhibitor levels less than 30%) may result in less hemorrhage and lower transfusion requirements (296,297). There are rare instances of DIC not associated with APL in which the intravascular coagulation process and fibrin deposition have been alleviated, and the patient continues to bleed because, for unexplained reasons, secondary fibrinolysis has continued with the concomitant biodegradation of the usual plasma protein targets of plasmin. In this rare instance, antifibrinolytic therapy may be indicated and should be considered as the clinical situation dictates. Antifibrinolytic therapy should not be routinely delivered to patients with ongoing DIC, as these patients need the fibrinolytic system to render the microcirculation clear of microthrombi (3–5). Antifibrinolytic therapy is not delivered unless the first three sequential steps described have been initiated and it has been established from the clinical and laboratory standpoints that the intravascular coagulation process has been eliminated by noting correction of biologic AT levels or other modalities used by the clinician to monitor the event. Antifibrinolytic therapy should never be used unless significant amounts of circulating plasmin have been documented by laboratory modalities, such as a decrease in functional plasminogen or α_2-plasmin inhibitor and an increase in plasmin. In those rare instances in which antifibrinolytic therapy is indicated, ε-aminocaproic acid is given as an initial 5- to 10-g slow intravenous push followed by 2 to 4 g per hour for 24 hours or until bleeding stops. This agent may cause ventricular arrhythmias, severe hypotension, and severe hypokalemia. A newer antifibrinolytic is tranexamic acid; this agent is more potent and may be associated with fewer undesirable side effects (98). If a fibrinolytic inhibitor is used in a patient with *ongoing* DIC, it may cause enhanced precipitation of fibrin in the microcirculation and macrocirculation and lead to fatal disseminated thrombosis (3–5,98).

"Low-grade" Disseminated Intravascular Coagulation

Therapy for low-grade DIC is often approached differently from that for fulminant DIC. Most patients with compensated DIC do not have life-threatening hemorrhage but have bothersome bleeding and local or diffuse superficial or deep venous thrombosis and thromboembolus (3–5,192,298). The essential therapy for low-grade DIC is treatment for the underlying disease process; frequently this will produce cessation of the intravascular clotting process and alleviation of hemorrhage or thrombosis. As with fulminant DIC, indicated supportive therapy must be given. If this first step is accomplished and hemorrhage and/or thrombosis and/or thromboembolus continues, then anticoagulant therapy is indicated to stop the intravascular clotting process. However, because low-grade DIC patients usually do not have life-threatening hemorrhage, anticoagulant therapy need not necessarily be vigorous. Aggressive anticoagulant therapy may be contraindicated in some instances of malignancy, especially those with intracranial metastases (3–5,92,98). Combination antiplatelet therapy is often successful in stopping a compensated DIC process after attempts to treat the triggering pathophysiology also have been started. Commonly, a combination of acetylsalicylic acid plus dipyridamole will stop a low-grade intravascular coagulation process within 24 to 30 hours, as manifest by correction of coagulation laboratory parameters and the cessation of bleeding or thrombosis. Low-dose subcutaneous calcium heparin therapy should be considered in patients with low-grade DIC who appear to be evolving into a fulminant process or in whom significant thrombotic or thromboembolic problems are developing. Replacement therapy is rarely indicated in compensated DIC. Inhibition of the fibrinolytic system also is rarely, if ever, indicated in low-grade DIC.

SUMMARY

The pathophysiologic mechanisms and clinical and laboratory manifestations of DIC are complex in part because of interrelations within the hemostasis system. Only by clearly understanding these extraordinarily complex pathophysiologic interrelations can the clinician and laboratory scientist appreciate the divergent and wide spectrum of often confusing clinical and laboratory findings in patients with DIC. Many therapeutic decisions to be made are controversial and lack validation. Nevertheless, newer antithrombotic agents and agents that can block, blunt, or modify cytokine activity and the activity of vasoactive substances appear to be of value. The complexity and variable degree of clinical expression suggests that therapy should be individualized depending on the nature of DIC, age, etiology of DIC, site and severity of hemorrhage or thrombosis, hemodynamics, and other appropriate clinical parameters. Treatment of the triggering event, low-dose heparin or AT concentrate, and wise choice of components when indicated now appear to be the most effective modes of therapy.

REFERENCES

1. Bick RL. Disseminated intravascular coagulation: objective criteria for clinical and laboratory diagnosis and assessment of therapeutic response. *Clin Appl Thromb Hemost* 1995;1:3–23.
2. Baker WF. Clinical aspects of disseminated intravascular coagulation: a clinician's point of view. *Semin Thromb Hemost* 1989; 15:1–57.
3. Bick RL. Disseminated intravascular coagulation and related syndromes: a clinical review. *Semin Thromb Hemost* 1988;14: 299–338.
4. Bick RL. Disseminated intravascular coagulation: objective clinical and laboratory diagnosis, treatment and assessment of therapeutic response. *Semin Thromb Hemost* 1996;22:69–88.
5. Bick RL, Baker WF. Disseminated intravascular coagulation. *Hematol Pathol* 1992;6:1–24.
6. Baker WF. Clinical aspects of disseminated intravascular coagulation: a clinician's point of view. *Semin Thromb Hemost* 1989;15:1.
7. Bick RL. Disseminated intravascular coagulation: pathophysiological mechanisms and manifestations. *Semin Thromb Hemost* 1998;24:3.
8. Bick RL. Disseminated intravascular coagulation: objective laboratory diagnostic criteria and guidelines for management. *Clin Lab Med* 1994;14:729.
9. Bick RL, WF Baker. Disseminated intravascular coagulation. *Hematol Pathol* 1992;6:1.
10. Lasch HG, Henne DL, Huth K, et al. Pathophysiology, clinical manifestations, and therapy of consumptive coagulopathy. *Am J Cardiol* 1967;20:381.
11. Steiner PE, Lushbough CC. Maternal pulmonary embolism by amniotic fluid as a cause of shock and unexplained deaths in obstetrics. *JAMA* 1941;117:1245.
12. Graeff N, Kuhn W. The amniotic infection syndrome. In: Hathaway W, ed. *Coagulation disorders in obstetrics.* Philadelphia: WB Saunders, 1980:91–95.
13. Sperry K. Amniotic fluid embolism: to understand an enigma. *JAMA* 1986;255:2183.
14. Locksmith GJ. Amniotic fluid embolism. *Obstet Gynecol Clin North Am* 1999;26:435.
15. Nadesan K, Jayalakshmi P. Sudden maternal deaths from amniotic fluid embolism. *Ceylon Med J* 1997;42:185.
16. Gilbert WM, Danielsen B. Amniotic fluid embolism: decreased mortality in a population-based study. *Obstet Gynecol* 1999;93: 973.
17. Lamy C, Sharshar T, Mas JL. Cerebrovascular diseases in pregnancy and puerperium. *Rev Neurol* 1996;152:422.
18. Mas JL, Lamy C. Stroke in pregnancy and the puerperium [Review]. *J Neurol* 1998;245:305.
19. Fiana S. Maternal mortality in Sweden: 1955-1974. *Acta Obstet Gynecol Scand* 1978;57:129.
20. Peterson EP, Taylor HB. Amniotic fluid embolism: an analysis of 40 cases. *Obstet Gynecol* 1970;35:787.
21. Aznar J, Gilabert J, Estelles A, et al. Evaluation of the soluble fibrin monomer complexes and other coagulation parameters in obstetric patients. *Thromb Res* 1982;27:691.
22. Minna JD, Robboy SJ, Coleman RW. *Disseminated intravascular coagulation in man.* Springfield, Ill: Charles C Thomas, 1974:12–15, 156–157.
23. Aguillon A, Andrus T, Grayson A, et al. Amniotic fluid embolism: a review. *Obstet Gynecol Surv* 1962;17:619.
24. Cortney LD. Amniotic fluid embolism. *Obstet Gynecol Surv* 1974;29:169.
25. D'Addato F, Repinto A, Angeli G. Amniotic fluid embolism in trial of labor: a case report. *Minerva Ginecol* 1997;49:217.
26. Judich A. Kuriansky J, Engelberg I, et al. Amniotic fluid embolism following blunt abdominal trauma in pregnancy. *Injury* 1998;29:475.
27. Morgan M. Amniotic fluid embolism. *Anesthesia* 1979;34:20.
28. Price T, Baker VV, Cefalo RL. Amniotic fluid embolism: three case reports with a review of the literature. *Obstet Gynecol Surv* 1985;40:462.
29. Albrechtsen OK. Hemorrhagic disorders following amniotic fluid embolism. *Clin Obstet Gynecol* 1964;7:361.
30. Russell WS, Jones WH. Amniotic fluid embolism: a review of the syndrome with a report of 4 cases. *Obstet Gynecol* 1965;26:476.
31. Aznar J, Gilabert J, Estelles A, et al. Evaluation of plasminogen and other fibrinolytic parameters in the amniotic fluid [Letter]. *Thromb Haemost* 1980;43:182.
32. Beller FK, Douglas AW, Debrovnet CH, et al. The fibrinolytic system in amniotic fluid embolism. *Am J Obstet Gynecol* 1963; 87:48.
33. Atwood HD. The histological diagnosis of amniotic fluid embolism. *J Pathol Bacteriol* 1958;76:211.
34. Yaffe H, Eldor A, Hornshtein E, et al. Thromboplastic activity in amniotic fluid during pregnancy. *Obstet Gynecol* 1977;50:454.
35. Yaffe H, Hay-am E, Sadovsky E. Thromboplastic activity of amniotic fluid in term and postmature gestations. *Obstet Gynecol* 1981;57:490.
36. Liban E, Raz S. A clinicopathologic study of fourteen cases of amniotic fluid embolism. *Am J Clin Pathol* 1969;51:477.
37. Sparr RA, Prichard JA. Studies to detect the escape of amniotic fluid into the maternal circulation during parturition. *Surg Gynecol Obstet* 1958;107:560.
38. Petroianu GA, Altmannsberger SH, Maleck WH, et al. Meconium and amniotic fluid embolism: effects on coagulation in pregnant mini-pigs. *Crit Care Med* 1999;27:348.
39. Kobayashi H, Oi H, Hayakawa H, et al. Histological diagnosis of amniotic fluid embolism by monoclonal antibody TKH-2 that recognizes NeuAc alpha 2-6GalNAc epitope. *Hum Pathol* 1997;28:428.
40. Oi H, Kobayashi H, Hirashima Y, et al. Serological and immunohistochemical diagnosis of amniotic fluid embolism. *Semin Thromb Hemost* 1998;24:479.
41. Lunetta P, Penttila A. Immunohistochemical identification of syncytiotrophoblastic cells and megakaryocytes in pulmonary vessels in a fatal case of amniotic fluid embolism. *Int J Legal Med* 1996;108:210.
42. Bick RL. Disseminated intravascular coagulation: objective criteria for diagnosis and management. *Med Clin North Am* 1994; 78:511.
43. Gross P, Benz EJ. Pulmonary embolism by amniotic fluid: report of three cases with a new diagnostic procedure. *Surg Gynecol Obstet* 1947;85:315
44. Vedernikov YP, Saade GR, Zlatnik M, et al. The effect of amniotic fluid on the human omental artery in vitro. *Am J Obstet Gynecol* 1999;180:454.
45. Khong TY. Expression of endothelin-1 in amniotic fluid embolism and possible pathophysiological mechanism. *Br J Obstet Gynaecol* 1998;105:802.
46. English CJ, Poller L, Burslem RW. A study of the procoagulant properties of amniotic fluid and their correlation with the lecithin/sphingomyelin ratio. *Br J Obstet Gynecol* 1981;88:133.
47. Pusey ML, Mende TJ. Studies on the procoagulant activity of human amniotic fluid, I: stability and coagulation factor requirements. *Thromb Res* 1985;39:355.
48. Pusey ML, Mende TJ. Studies on the procoagulant activity of human amniotic fluid, II: the role of factor VII. *Thromb Res* 1985;39:571.
49. Bick RL, Murano G. Physiology of hemostasis. *Clin Lab Med* 1994;14:677.
50. Bussen S, Schwarzmann G, Steck T. Clinical aspects and ther-

apy of amniotic fluid embolism: illustration based on a case report. *Z Geburtshilfe Neonatol* 1997;201:95.
51. Davies S. Amniotic fluid embolism and isolated disseminated intravascular coagulation. *Can J Anaesth* 1999;46:456.
52. Van Heerden PV, Webb SA, Hee G, et al. Inhaled aerosolized prostacyclin as a selective pulmonary vasodilator for the treatment of severe hypoxaemia. *Anaesth Intens Care* 1996;24:87.
53. Strickland MA, Bates AW, Whitworth HS, et al. Amniotic fluid embolism: prophylaxis with heparin and aspirin. *South Med J* 1985;78:377.
54. Bick RL, Fekete LF, Wilson WL. Treatment of disseminated intravascular coagulation with antithrombin III. *Trans Am Soc Hematol* 1976:167.
55. Vinazzer H. Antithrombin III in shock and disseminated intravascular coagulation. *Clin Appl Thromb Hemost* 1995;1:62.
56. Vinazzer H. Hereditary and acquired antithrombin deficiency. *Semin Thromb Hemost* 1999;25:257.
57. Suzuki S, Morishita S. Hypercoagulability and DIC in high-risk infants. *Semin Thromb Hemost* 1998;24:463.
58. Bick RL. Disseminated intravascular coagulation: objective criteria for clinical and laboratory diagnosis and assessment of therapeutic response. *Clin Appl Thromb Hemost* 1995;1:3.
59. Bick RL. Syndromes of disseminated intravascular coagulation. In: *Disseminated intravascular coagulation and related syndromes.* Boca Raton, Fla: CRC Press, 1982.
60. Bick RL, Arun B, Frenkel EP. Disseminated intravascular coagulation: clinical and pathophysiological mechanisms and manifestations. *Haemostasis* 1999;29:111.
61. Bick RL. Disseminated intravascular coagulation: objective clinical and laboratory diagnosis, treatment and assessment of therapeutic response. *Semin Thromb Hemost* 1996;22:69.
62. Hafter R, Graeff H. Molecular aspects of defibrination in a reptilase-treated case of "dead-fetus syndrome." *Thromb Res* 1975;7:391.
63. Steichele DF. Consumptive coagulopathy in obstetrics and gynecology. *Thromb Diath Haemorrh Suppl* 1969;36:177.
64. Brenner BM. Vascular injury to the kidney. In: Fauci AS, Braunwakd E, Isselbacher KJ, et al., eds. *Internal medicine.* 14th ed. St. Louis: McGraw–Hill, 1998:1558.
65. Mjahed K, Hammamouchi B, Hammoudi D, et al. Critical analysis of hemostasis disorders in the course of eclampsia: report of 106 cases. *J Gynecol Obstet Biol Reprod* 1998;27:607.
66. Porozhanova V, Bozhinova S, Khristova V. The perinatal outcome in adolescents with eclampsia and the HELLP syndrome. *Akush Ginekol (Mosk)* 1996;35:14.
67. Yao T, Yao H, Wang H. Diagnosis and treatment of nephrotic syndrome during pregnancy. *Chin Med J* 1996;109:471.
68. Bonnar J, McNicol GP, Douglas AS. Coagulation and fibrinolytic systems in pre-eclampsia and eclampsia. *Br Med J* 1971;1:12.
69. Schjetlein R, Haugen G, Wisloff F. Markers of intravascular coagulation and fibrinolysis in preeclampsia: association with intrauterine growth retardation. *Acta Obstet Gynecol Scand* 1997;76:541.
70. Verduzco Rodriguez L, Gonzalez Puebla E, Manffrini Madrid F, et al. D-dimer in different stages of pregnancy toxemia: a pilot study. *Ginecol Obstet Mex* 1998;66:77.
71. Ishibashi M, Ito N, Fujita M, et al. Endothelin-1 as an aggravating factor of disseminated intravascular coagulation associated with malignant neoplasms. *Cancer* 1994;73:191.
72. Jones SL. HELLP: a cry for laboratory assistance: a comprehensive review of the HELLP syndrome highlighting the role of the laboratory. *Hematopathol Mol Hematol* 1998;11:147.
73. Cincotta R, Ross A. A review of eclampsia in Melbourne: 1978-1992. *Aust N Z J Obstet Gynaecol* 1996;36:264.
74. D'Anna R. The HELLP syndrome: notes on its pathogenesis and treatment. *Minerva Ginecol* 1996;48:147.
75. Portis R, Jacobs MA, Skerman JH, et al. HELLP syndrome (hemolysis, elevated liver enzymes, and low platelets) pathophysiology and anesthetic considerations. *AANA J* 1997;65:37.
76. Stone JH. HELLP syndrome: hemolysis, elevated liver enzymes, and low platelets. *JAMA* 1998;280:559.
77. Debette M, Samuel D, Ichai P, et al. Labor complications of the HELLP syndrome without any predictive factors. *Gastroenterol Clin Biol* 1999;23:264.
78. Paternoster DM, Rodi J, Santarossa C, et al. Acute pancreatitis and deep vein thrombosis associated with the HELLP syndrome. *Minerva Ginecol* 1999;51:31.
79. Sheikh RA, Yasmeen S, Pauly MP, et al. Spontaneous intrahepatic hemorrhage and hepatic rupture in the HELLP syndrome: four cases and a review. *J Clin Gastroenterol* 1999;28:323.
80. Weemhoff RA, van Loon AJ, Aarnoudse JG. Liver rupture in pregnancy: a life-threatening complication of the HELLP syndrome. *Ned Tijdschr Geneeskd* 1996;140:2140.
81. Magann EF, Martin JN. Twelve steps to optimal management of HELLP syndrome. *Clin Obstet Gynecol* 1999;42:532.
82. O'Boyle JD, Magann EF, Waxman E, et al. Dexamethasone-facilitated postponement of delivery of an extremely preterm pregnancy complicated by the syndrome of hemolysis, elevated liver enzymes, and low platelets. *Milit Med* 1999;164:316.
83. Vigil-De Gracia P, Garcia-Caceres E. Dexamethasone in the post-partum treatment of HELLP syndrome. *Int J Gynaecol Obstet* 1997;59:217.
84. Yalcin OT, Sener T, Hassa H, et al. Effects of postpartum corticosteroids in patients with HELLP syndrome. *Int J Gynaecol Obstet* 1998;61:141.
85. Hamada S, Takishita Y, Tamura T, et al. Plasma exchange in a patient with postpartum HELLP syndrome. *J Obstet Gynaecol Res* 1996;22:371.
86. Owen CA, Bowie EJW, Cooper HA. Turnover of fibrinogen and platelets in dogs undergoing induced intravascular coagulation. *Thromb Res* 1973;2:251.
87. Rath W. Aggressive versus conservative management of HELLP syndrome: a status assessment. *Geburtshilfe Frauenheilkd* 1996;56:265.
88. Spivack JL, Sprangler DB, Bell WR. Defibrination after intra-amniotic injection of hypertonic saline. *N Engl J Med* 1972;287:321.
89. Bick RL. Alterations of hemostasis associated with malignancy: etiology, pathophysiology, diagnosis and management. *Semin Thromb Hemost* 1978;5:1.
90. Bick RL. Alterations of hemostasis associated with malignancy. In: Murano G, Bick RL, eds. *Basic concepts of hemostasis and thrombosis.* Boca Raton, Fla: CRC Press, 1980:213.
91. Bick RL. Hemostasis in malignancy. In: Bick RL*Disorders of thrombosis and hemostasis: clinical and laboratory practice.* Chicago: ASCP Press, 1992:239.
92. Bick RL, Strauss JF, Rutherford CJ, et al. Thrombosis and hemorrhage in oncology patients. *Hematol Oncol Clin North Am* 1996;10: 875.
93. Cafagna D, Ponte E. Pulmonary embolism of paraneoplastic origin. *Minerva Med* 1997;88:523.
94. Frenkel UP, Bick RL. Issues of thrombosis and hemorrhagic events in patients with cancer. *Anticancer Res* 1998;18:1–4.
95. Bick RL. Coagulation abnormalities in malignancy. *Semin Thromb Hemost* 1992;18:353.
96. Bick RL. Disseminated intravascular coagulation. *Hematol Oncol Clin North Am* 1992;6:1259.
97. Bick RL. Disseminated intravascular coagulation: a clinical review. *Semin Thromb Hemost* 1988;14:299.
98. Bick RL, Kunkel L. Disseminated intravascular coagulation. *Int J Hematol* 1992;55:1.

99. Bick RL, Scates S. Disseminated intravascular coagulation. *Lab Med* 1992;23:161.
100. Bick RL. Disseminated intravascular coagulation and related syndromes: a review. *Am J Hematol* 1978;5:265.
102. Goodnight SH. Bleeding and intravascular clotting in malignancy: a review. *Ann N Y Acad Sci* 1974;230:271.
103. Gralnick HR, Tan HK. Acute promyelocytic leukemia: a model for understanding the role of the malignant cells in hemostasis. *Hum Pathol* 1974;5:661.
104. Leavy RA, Kahn SB, Brodsky I. Disseminated intravascular coagulation: a complication of chemotherapy in acute promyelocytic leukemia. *Cancer* 1970;26:142.
105. Pineo GF, Brain MC, Gallus AS. Tumors, mucus production, and hypercoagulability. *Ann N Y Acad Sci* 1974;230:262.
106. Pineo GF, Regorczi F, Hatton MWC. The activation of coagulation by extracts of mucin: a possible pathway of intravascular coagulation accompanying adenocarcinomas. *J Lab Clin Med* 1973;82:255.
107. Bick RL. Basic mechanisms of hemostasis pertaining to DIC. In: *Disseminated intravascular coagulation and related syndromes.* Boca Raton, Fla: CRC Press, 1983:1.
108. Bick RL. Disseminated intravascular coagulation. In: Bick RL. *Disorders of thrombosis and hemostasis: clinical and laboratory practice.* Chicago: ASCP Press, 1992:137.
109. Frenkel EP, Bick RL. Issues of thrombosis and hemorrhagic events in patients with cancer. *In Vivo* 1998;12:625.
110. Lerner RG, Nelson JN, Corines P, et al. Disseminated intravascular coagulation: complication of LeVeen peritoneovenous shunts. *JAMA* 1984;240:2064.
111. Stein SF, Fulenwider JT, Ansley JD. Accelerated fibrinogen and platelet destruction after peritoneovenous shunting. *Arch Intern Med* 1981;141:1149.
112. Bick RL, Tse N. Hemostasis abnormalities associated with prosthetic devices and organ transplantation. *Lab Med* 1992;23:462.
113. Bick RL. Disseminated intravascular coagulation and related syndromes: a clinical review. *Semin Thromb Hemost* 1988;14:299.
114. Bick RL, Baker WF. Disseminated intravascular coagulation. *Hematol Pathol* 1992;6:1.
115. Egeberg O. Blood coagulation and intravascular hemolysis. *Scand J Clin Lab Invest* 1962;14:217.
116. Krevins JR, Jackson DP, Cowley CL, et al. The nature of the hemorrhagic disorder accompanying hemolytic transfusion reactions in man. *Blood* 1957;12:834.
117. Langdell RD, Hedgpeth EM. A study of the role of hemolysis in the hemostatic defect of transfusion reactions. *Thromb Diath Haemorrh* 1959;3:566.
118. Surgenor DM. Erythrocytes and blood coagulation. *Thromb Diath Haemorrh* 1974;32:247.
119. Abildgaard CF, Corrigan JJ, Seeler RA, et al. Meningococcemia associated with intravascular coagulation. *Pediatrics* 1967;40:78.
120. McKay DG, Muller-Berghous G. Therapeutic implications if disseminated intravascular coagulation. *Am J Cardiol* 1967;20:392.
121. Corrigan JJ. Changes in the blood coagulation system associated with septicemia. *N Engl J Med* 1968;279:851.
122. Yoshikawa T, Tanaka R, Guze LB. Infection and disseminated intravascular coagulation. *Medicine (Baltimore)* 1971;50:237.
123. Cline MJ, Melmon KL, Davis WC, et al. Mechanism of endotoxin interaction with leukocytes. *Br J Haematol* 1968;15:539.
124. McKay DG, Shapiro SS. Alterations in the blood coagulation system induced by bacterial endotoxin I: in vitro (generalized Schwartzman reaction). *J Exp Med* 1958;107:353.
125. Baker WF. Clinical aspects of disseminated intravascular coagulation: a clinician's point of view. *Semin Thromb Hemost* 1989;15:1.
126. Bick RL. Disseminated intravascular coagulation: objective clinical and laboratory diagnosis, treatment and assessment of therapeutic response. *Semin Thromb Hemost* 1996;22:69.
127. Cronberg S, Skansberg P, Nivenios-Larsson K. Disseminated intravascular coagulation in septicemia caused by beta-hemolytic streptococci. *Thromb Res* 1973;3:405.
128. Rubenberg WL, Baker LR, McBride JA, et al. Brain: intravascular coagulation in a case of *Clostridium perfringens* septicemia: treatment by exchange transfusion and heparin. *Br Med J* 1967; 3:271.
129. Bick RL. Disseminated intravascular coagulation: objective criteria for clinical and laboratory diagnosis and assessment of therapeutic response. *Clin Appl Thromb Hemost* 1995;1:3.
130. Gagel C, Linder M, Muller-Berghous G, et al. Virus infection and blood coagulation. *Thromb Diath Haemorrh* 1970;23:1.
131. McKay DG, Margaretten W. Disseminted intravascular coagulation in virus diseases. *Arch Intern Med* 1967;120:129.
132. Salmon SJ, Lambert PH, Louis J. Pathogenesis of the intravascular coagulation syndrome induced by immunological reactions. *Thromb Diath Haemorrh* 1971;45:161.
133. Bick RL. Hemostasis in malignancy. In: Bick RL, ed. *Disorders of thrombosis and hemostasis: clinical and laboratory practice.* Chicago: ASCP Press, 1992:239.
134. Bick RL. Coagulation abnormalities in malignancy. *Semin Thromb Hemost* 1992;18:353.
135. Bick RL. Alterations of hemostasis in malignancy. In: Bick RL, Bennett JM, Byrnes RK, eds. *Hematology: clinical and laboratory practice.* St. Louis: Mosby, 1993:1583.
136. Brown RC, Campbell D, Thompson J. Increased fibrinolysis with malignant disease. *Arch Intern Med* 1962;109:128.
137. Silverstein MH. *Agnogenic myeloid metaplasia.* Acton, Mass: Publishing Sciences Group, 1975:10.
138. Mersky C. Altered blood coagulability in patients with malignant tumors. *Ann N Y Acad Sci* 1974;23:289.
139. Hartman RC, Jenkins DE. Paroxysmal nocturnal hemoglobinuria: current concepts of certain pathophysiological features. *Blood* 1965;25:850.
140. Bouchama A, Hammami M, Haq A, et al. Evidence for endothelial cell activation/injury in heat stroke. *Crit Care Med* 1996; 24:1173.
141. Tang GJ. Similarity and synergy of trauma and sepsis: role of tumor necrosis factor-alpha and interleukin-6. *Acta Anaesthesiol Sin* 1996;34:141.
142. Gando S, Kameue T, Nanzaki S, et al. Cytokines, soluble thrombomodulin and disseminated intravascular coagulation in patients with systemic inflammatory response syndrome. *Thromb Res* 1995;80:519.
143. Holder LA, Malin LL, Fox CL. Hypercoagulability after thermal injuries. *Surgery* 1963;54:316.
144. Saliba MJ, Demsey WL, Kruggel JL. Large burns in humans: treatment with heparin. *JAMA* 1973;225:261.
145. Al-Mondhiry H. Disseminated intravascular coagulation: experience in a major cancer center. *Thromb Diath Haemorrh* 1975;34:181.
146. Aoki N, Moroi M, Matsuda M. The behavior of alpha-2-plasmin inhibitor in fibrinolytic states. *J Clin Invest* 1977;60:361.
147. Olson JD, Kaufman H, Moake J, et al. The incidence and significance of hemostatic abnormalities in patients with head injuries. *Neurosurgery* 1989;24:825.
148. Touho H, Hirakawa K, Hino A, et al. Relationship between abnormalities of coagulation and fibrinolysis and postoperative intracranial hemorrhage in head injury. *Neurosurgery* 1986;19: 523.
149. Bick RL. Hereditary hemorrhagic telangiectasia and disseminated intravascular coagulation: a new clinical syndrome. *Ann N Y Acad Sci* 1981;370:851.
150. Inceman S, Tangun Y. Chronic defibrination syndrome due to a giant hemangioma associated with microangiopathic hemolytic anemia. *Am J Med* 1969;46:997.

151. Kasabach HH, Merritt KK. Capillary hemangioma with extensive purpura: report of a case. *Am J Dis Child* 1940;59:1063.
152. Kaxmier FJ, Didisheim VK, Fairbanks J, et al. Intravascular coagulation and arterial disease. *Thromb Diath Haemorrh Suppl* 1969;36:295.
153. Schnetzer GW, Penner JA. Chronic intravascular coagulation syndrome associated with atherosclerotic aortic aneurysm. *South Med J* 1973;66:264.
154. Owen CA, Bowie EJW. Chronic intravascular coagulation fibrinolysis (ICF) syndromes (DIC). *Semin Thromb Hemost* 1977;3:268.
155. Bick RL, Tse N. Hemostasis abnormalities associated with prosthetic devices and organ transplantation. *Lab Med* 1992;23:462.
156. Bick RL. Alterations of hemostasis associated with surgery, cardiopulmonary bypass surgery, and prosthetic devices. In: Ratnoff OD, Forbes C, eds. *Disorders of hemostasis.* Philadelphia: WB Saunders, 1991:382.
157. Bick RL. Disseminated intravascular coagulation. *Hematol Oncol Clin North Am* 1992;6:1259.
158. Muller-Berghaus G. Pathophysiologic and biochemical events in disseminated intravascular coagulation: dysregulation of procoagulant and anticoagulant pathways. *Semin Thromb Hemost* 1989;15:58.
159. Mammen EF. Perspectives for the future. *Intens Care Med Suppl* 1993;1:s29.
160. McKay DG, Margaretten W, Csavossy I. An electron microscope study of the effects of bacterial endotoxin on the blood-vascular system. *Lab Invest* 1966;15:1815.
161. Owen CA, Bowie EJW, Cooper HA. Turnover of fibrinogen and platelets in dogs undergoing induced intravascular coagulation. *Thromb Res* 1973;2:251.
162. Latallo ZS. Products of fibrin(ogen) proteolysis. *Thromb Diath Haemorrh Suppl* 1973;24:145.
163. Marder VJ, Shulman HR, Carroll WR. High molecular weight derivatives of human fibrinogen produced by plasmin, I: physico-chemical and immunological characterization. *J Biol Chem* 1969;244:2111.
164. Marder VJ, Budzynski AZ, James HL. High molecular weight derivatives of human fibrinogen produced by plasmin, III: their NH_2-terminal amino acids and comparison of the "NH_2-terminal amino disulfide knot." *J Biol Chem* 1972;247:4775.
165. Bang NU, Chang M. Soluble fibrin complexes. *Semin Thromb Hemost* 1974;1:91.
166. Breen FA, Tullis JZ. Ethanol gelation, a rapid screening test for intravascular coagulation. *Ann Intern Med* 1968;69:111.
167. Fletcher AP, Alkjaersig N, Fisher S, et al. The proteolysis of fibrinogen by plasmin: the identification of thrombin-clottable fibrinogen derivatives which polymerize abnormally. *J Lab Clin Med* 1966;68:780.
168. Gurewich V, Hutchinson E. Detection of intravascular coagulation by protamine sulfate and ethanol gelation tests. *Thromb Res* 1973;2:539.
169. Bick RL. The clinical significance of fibrinogen degradation products. *Semin Thromb Hemost* 1982;8:302.
170. Kopec M, Wegrzynowiczy Z, Budzynski A, et al. Interaction of fibrinogen degradation products with platelets. *Exp Biol Med* 1968;3:73.
171. Niewiarowski S, Regoeczi E, Stewart G, et al. Platelet interaction with polymerizing fibrin. *J Clin Invest* 1972;51:685.
172. Robson S, Shephard E, Kirsch R. Fibrin degradation product D-dimer induces the synthesis and release of biologically active IL-1 beta, IL-6 and plasminogen activator inhibitors from monocytes in vitro. *Br J Haematol* 1994;86:322.
173. Okajima K, Uchiba M, Murakami K, et al. Plasma levels of soluble E-selectin in patients with disseminated intravascular coagulation. *Am J Hematol* 1997;54:219.
174. Ishibashi M, Ito N, Fujita M, et al. Endothelin-1 as an aggravating factor of disseminated intravascular coagulation associated with malignant neoplasms. *Cancer* 1994;73:191.
175. Ono S, Mochizuki H, Tamakuma S. A clinical study on the significance of platelet-activating factor in the pathophysiology of septic disseminated intravascular coagulation in surgery. *Am J Surg* 1996;171:409.
176. Elsayed Y, Nakagawa K, Ichikawa K, et al. Expression of tissue factor and interleukin-1 beta in a novel rabbit model of disseminated intravascular coagulation induced by carrageenan and lipopolysaccharide. *Pathobiology* 1995;63:328.
177. Hoffman M, Cooper ST. Thrombin enhances monocyte secretion of tumor necrosis factor and interleukin-1 by two distinct mechanisms. *Blood Cell Mol Dis* 1995;21:156.
178. Okajima K, Fujise R, Motosato Y, et al. Plasma levels of granulocyte elastase-alpha 1-proteinase inhibitor complex in patients with disseminated intravascular coagulation: pathophysiologic implications. *Am J Hematol* 1994;47:82.
179. Nilsson IM. Local fibrinolysis as a mechanism for haemorrhage. *Thromb Diath Haemorh* 1975;34:623.
180. Stormorken H. Relation of the fibrinolytic to other biological systems. *Thromb Diath Haemorrh* 1975;34:378.
181. Schreiber AD, Austen KF. Interrelationships of the fibrinolytic, coagulation, kinin generation, and complement systems. *Semin Hematol* 1973;6:593.
182. Collins P, Noble K, Reittie J, et al. Induction of tumor factor expression in human monocyte/endothelium cocultures. *Br J Haematol* 1995;91:963.
183. Gando S, Nakanishi Y, Tedo I. Cytokines and plasminogen activator inhibitor-1 in post-trauma disseminated intravascular coagulation: relationship to multiple organ dysfunction. *Crit Care Med* 1995;23:1835.
184. Kaplan A, Meier H, Mandel R. The Hageman factor dependent pathways of coagulation, fibrinolysis, and kinin generation. *Semin Thromb Hemost* 1976;3:6.
185. Bick RL, Murano G. Physiology of hemostasis. In: Bick RL, Bennett JM, Byrnes RK, eds. *Hematology: clinical and laboratory practice.* St. Louis: Mosby, 1993:1285.
186. van Iwaarden F, Bouma B. Role of high molecular weight kininogen in contact activation. *Semin Thromb Hemost* 1987;13:15.
187. Beller FK, Theiss W. Fibrin derivatives, plasma hemoglobin and glomerular fibrin deposition in experimental intravascular coagulation. Thromb Diath Haemorrh 1973;29:363.
188. McKay DG, Linder MM, Cruse VK. Mechanisms of thrombosis of the microcirculation. *Am J Pathol* 1971;63:231.
189. Lerner RG. The defibrination syndrome. *Med Clin North Am* 1976;60:871.
190. Robboy SJ, Coleman RW, Minna JD. Pathology of disseminated intravascular coagulation (DIC): analysis of 26 cases. *Hum Pathol* 1972;3:327.
191. Muller-Berghous G. Pathophysiology of generalized intravascular coagulation. *Semin Thromb Hemost* 1977;3:209.
192. Owen CA, Bowie EJW. Chronic intravascular syndromes. *Mayo Clin Pract* 1974;49:673.
193. Bleyl U. Morphologic diagnosis of disseminated intravascular coagulation: histologic, histochemical, and electron-microscopic studies. *Semin Thromb Hemost* 1977;3:247.
194. Skjorten F. Hyaline microthrombi in an autopsy material: a quantitative study with discussion of the relationship to small vessel thrombosis. *Acta Pathol Microbiol Scand* 1969;76:361.
195. Morris JA, Smith RW, Assali NS. Hemodynamic action of vasopressor and vaso-depressor agents in endotoxin shock. *Am J Obstet Gynecol* 1965;91:491.
196. Bleyl U, Kuhn W, Graeff H. Reticulo-endotheliale clearance intravascaler: fibrinmonere in der milz. *Thromb Diath Haemorrh* 1969;22:87.

197. Boyd JF. Disseminated fibrin-thromboembolism among neonates dying within 48 hours of birth. *Arch Dis Child* 1967;42:401.
198. Bull B, Kuhn IN. The production of schistocytes by fibrin strands (a scanning electron microscope study). *Blood* 1970;35:104.
199. Heyes H, Kohle W, Slijerpcevic B. The appearance of schistocytes in the peripheral blood in correlation to degree of disseminated intravascular coagulation. *Haemostasis* 1976;5:66.
200. Bull B, Rubenberg M, Dacie J, et al. Microangiopathic hemolytic anemia: mechanisms of red-cell fragmentation. *Br J Haematol* 1968;14:643.
201. Slaastad RA, Godal NC. Coagulation profile and ethanol gelation test with special reference to components consumed during coagulation. *Scand J Haematol* 1976;16:25.
202. Bull B, Kuhn IN. The production of schistocytes by fibrin strands (a scanning electron microscope study). *Blood* 1970; 35:104–111.
203. Heyes H, Kohle W, Slijerpcevic B. The appearance of schistocytes in the peripheral blood in correlation to degree of disseminated intravascular coagulation. *Haemostasis* 1976;5:66–73.
204. Bull B, Rubenberg M, Dacie J, et al. Microangiopathic hemolytic anemia: mechanisms of red-cell fragmentation. *Br J Haematol* 1968;14:643–652.
205. Slaastad RA, Godal NC. Coagulation profile and ethanol gelation test with special reference to components consumed during coagulation. *Scand J Haematol* 1976;16:25–32.
206. Bick RL. Platelet defects. In: *Disorders of hemostasis and thrombosis: principles of clinical practice.* New York: Thieme, 1985:65.
207. Karpatkin S. Heterogeneity of human platelets, VI: correlation of platelet function with platelet volume. *Blood* 1978;51:307–316.
208. Eckhardt T, Muller-Berghous G. The role of blood platelets in the precipitation of soluble fibrin endotoxin. *Scand J Haematol* 1975;14:181–189.
209. Bick RL. The clinical significance of fibrinogen degradation products. *Semin Thromb Hemost* 1982;8:302–330.
210. Blaisdell FW, Stallone RJ. The mechanism of pulmonary damage following traumatic shock. *Surg Gynecol Obstet* 1970;130: 15–22.
211. Bleyl U. Comparative studies in adults and newborn infants on the pathogenesis of pulmonary hyaline membranes. *Verh Dtsch Ges Pathol* 1970;54:340–348.
212. Martin AM, Soloway HB, Simmons RL. Pathologic anatomy of the lungs following shock and trauma. *J Trauma* 1968;8: 687–699.
213. Soloway HB, Castillo Y, Martin AM. Adult hyaline membrane disease. *Ann Surg* 1968;168:937–945.
214. Hardaway RM, Adams WH. Blood clotting problems in acute care. *Acute Care* 1989;14/15:138–207.
215. Hardaway RM, Dixon RS, Foster FF, et al. The effect of hemorrhagic shock on disseminated intravascular coagulation. *Ann Surg* 1976;184:43–45.
216. Muller-Berghous G, Mann B. Precipitation of ancrod-induced soluble fibrin by aprotinin and norepinephrine. *Thromb Res* 1973;2:305–322.
217. Bick RL. Disseminated intravascular coagulation: objective clinical and laboratory diagnosis, treatment and assessment of therapeutic response. *Semin Thromb Hemost* 1996;22:69–88.
218. Bick RL. Clinical hemostasis practice: the major impact of laboratory automation. *Semin Thromb Hemost* 1983;9:139–171.
219. Fareed J. New methods in hemostatic testing. In: Fareed J, Messmore HL, Fenton J, et al., eds. *Perspectives in hemostasis.* New York: Pergamon Press, 1981:310.
220. Messmore HL. Automation in coagulation testing: clinical applications. *Semin Thromb Hemost* 1983;9:335–339.
221. Bick RL. Disseminated intravascular coagulation: clinical/laboratory correlations. *Am J Clin Pathol* 1982;77:244(abst).
222. Bick RL. Disseminated intravascular coagulation: objective laboratory diagnostic criteria and guidelines for management. *Clin Lab Med* 1994;14:729–768.
223. Marder VJ, Matchett MO, Sherry S. Detection of serum fibrinogen and fibrin degradation products: comparison of six techniques using purified products and application in clinical studies. *Am J Med* 1971;51:71–82.
224. Thomas DP, Niewiarowski S, Myers AR, et al. A comparative study of four methods for detecting fibrinogen degradation products in patients with various diseases. *N Engl J Med* 1970; 283:663–668.
225. Bick RL. Disseminated intravascular coagulation and related syndromes. In: Bick R, Bennett J, Brynes R, eds. *Hematology: clinical and laboratory practice.* St. Louis: Mosby, 1993:1463.
226. Gurewich V, Lipinsky B. Semiquantitative determination of soluble fibrin monomer complexes by chromatography and serial dilution protamine sulfate test. *Am J Clin Pathol* 1976;65: 397–401.
227. Hedner U, Nilsson IM. Parallel determinations of FDP and fibrin monomers with various methods. *Thromb Diath Haemorrh* 1972;28:268–279.
228. Sonnabend D, Cooper D, Fiddes P, et al. Fibrin degradation products in thromboembolic disease. *Pathology* 1972;4:47–51.
229. Stibbe J, Gomes M, de Ouda A. Management of chronic CID: evaluation of separate measurements of fibrin (FbDP) and fibrinogen (FgDP) degradation products concomitant with fibrin monomers. *Thromb Haemost* 1989;62(suppl 1):373(abst).
230. Francis CW, Marder VJ. A molecular model of plasmic degradation of cross-linked fibrin. *Semin Thromb. Hemost* 1982;8: 25–35.
231. Plow EF, Edgington TS. Surface markers of fibrinogen and its physiologic derivatives related by antibody probes. *Semin Thromb Hemost* 1982;8:36–56.
232. Matsumoto T, Nishijima Y, Teramura Y, et al. Monoclonal antibodies to fibrinogen-fibrin degradation products which contain D-domain. *Thromb Res* 1985;38:297–302.
233. Rylatt DB, Blake AS, Cottis LE, et al. An immunoassay for human D-dimer using monoclonal antibodies. *Thromb Res* 1983; 31:767–778.
234. Bick RL. Disseminated intravascular coagulation. In: Brubaker DB, Simpson MB, eds. *Dynamics of hemostasis and thrombosis.* Bethesda: American Association of Blood Banks (AABB), 1995:133.
235. Bick RL, Baker W. Diagnostic efficacy of the D-dimer assay in DIC and related disorders. *Thromb Res* 1992;65:785–790.
236. Lane DA, Preston FE, Van Ross ME, et al. Characterization of serum fibrinogen and fibrin fragments produced during disseminated intravascular coagulation. *Br J Haematol* 1978;40:609–615.
237. Elms MJ, Bunce IH, Bundesen PG, et al. Measurement of crosslinked fibrin degradation products: an immunoassay using monoclonal antibodies. *Thromb Haemost* 1983;50:591–594.
238. Ellis DR, Eaton AS, Plank MC, et al. A comparative evaluation of ELISAs for D-dimer and related fibrin(ogen) degradation products. *Blood Coagul Fibrinol* 1993;4:537–549.
239. Elias A, Aptel I, Huc B, et al. D-dimer test and diagnosis of deep vein thrombosis: a comparative study of 7 assays. *Thromb Haemost* 1996;76:518–522.
240. Charles L, Edwards T, Macik B. Evaluation of sensitivity and specificity of six D-dimer latex assays. *Arch Pathol Lab Med* 1994;118:1102–1105.
241. Murano G. The molecular structure of fibrinogen. *Semin Thromb Hemost* 1974;1:1–32.
242. Rosenberg JS, Beeler DL, Rosenberg RD. Activation of human prothrombin by highly purified human factors V and Xa in the presence of human antithrombin. *J Biol Chem* 1975;250:1607–1617.
243. Tietel JM, Bauer KA, Lau HK, et al. Studies of the prothrom-

bin activation pathway utilizing radioimmunoassays for the F2/F1+2 fragment and thrombin-antithrombin complex. *Blood* 1982;59:1086–1097.
244. Boneu B, Bes G, Pelzer H, et al. D-dimers, thrombin antithrombin complexes and prothrombin fragments 1+2: diagnostic value in clinically suspected deep vein thrombosis. *Thromb Haemost* 1991;65:28–31.
245. Bruhn HD, Conard J, Mannucci M, et al. Multicentric evaluation of a new assay for prothrombin fragment F 1+2 determination. *Thromb Haemost* 1992;68:413–417.
246. Ceriello A, Giacomello R, Colatutto A, et al. Increased prothrombin fragment 1+2 in type I diabetic patients. *Haemostasis* 1992;22:50–51.
247. Demers C, Ginsberg JS, Henderson P, et al. Measurements of markers of activated coagulation in antithrombin III deficient patients. *Thromb Haemost* 1992;67:542–544.
248. Okamoto K, Takaki A, Takeda S, et al. Coagulopathy in disseminated intravascular coagulation due to abdominal sepsis: determination of prothrombin fragment 1+2 and other markers. *Haemostasis* 1992;22:17–24.
249. Pelzer H, Schwarz A, Stuber W. Determination of human prothrombin activation fragment 1+2 in plasma with an antibody against a synthetic peptide. *Thromb Haemost* 1991;65:153–159.
250. Sorensen JV, Jensen HP, Rahr HR, et al. F 1+2 and FPA in urine from patients with multiple trauma and healthy individuals: a pilot study. *Thromb Res* 1992;67:429–434.
251. Laurino JP, Pelletier TF, Eadry R, et al. Thrombus precursor protein and the measurement of thrombosis in patients with acute chest pain syndrome. *Ann Clin Lab Sci* 1997;27:338–345.
252. Carville DG, Dimitrijevec N, Walsh M, et al. Thrombus precursor protein: marker of thrombosis early in the pathogenesis of myocardial infarction. *Clin Chem* 1996;42:1537–1541.
253. Bick RL, Dukes ML, Wilson WL, et al. Antithrombin III (AT-III) as a diagnostic aid in disseminated intravascular coagulation. *Thromb Res* 1977;10:721–730.
254. Bick RL. Clinical relevance of antithrombin III. *Semin Thromb Hemost* 1982;8:276–287.
255. Okajima K. Clinical relevance of determination of plasma AT-III and alpha 2 PI activities in patients with DIC: applications of the molecular markers for the pathophysiology of DIC. *Jpn J Clin Pathol* 1994;42:45–55.
256. Bick RL, McClain BJ. A clinical comparison of chromogenic, fluorometric, and natural (fibrinogen) substrates for determination of antithrombin-III. *Thromb Haemost* 1981;46:364(abst).
257. Fareed J, Messmore HL, Walenga JM, et al. Laboratory evaluation of antithrombin III: a critical overview of currently available methods for antithrombin III measurements. *Semin Thromb Hemost* 1982;8:288–301.
258. Asakura H, Saito M, Ito K, et al. Levels of thrombin-antithrombin III complex in plasma in cases of acute promyelocytic leukemia. *Thromb Res* 1988;50:895–900.
259. Cronlund M, Hardin J, Burton J, et al. Fibrinopeptide-A in plasma of normal subjects and patients with disseminated intravascular coagulation and systemic lupus erythematosus. *J Clin Invest* 1976;58:142–151.
260. Douglas JT, Shah M, Lowe GDO, et al. Fibrinopeptide-A and beta-thromboglobulin levels in pre-eclampsia and hypertensive pregnancy. *Thromb Haemost* 1982;47:54–55.
261. Bauer KA, Weiss LM, Sparrow D, et al. Aging-associated changes in indices of thrombin generation and protein C activation in humans: normative aging study. *J Clin Invest* 1987; 80:1527–1534.
262. Walenga JM, Fareed J, Mariani G, et al. Diagnostic efficacy of a simple radioimmunoassay test for fibrinogen/fibrin fragments containing the B beta 15-42 sequence. *Semin Thromb Hemost* 1984;10:252–263.
263. Fareed J, Bick RL, Squillaci G, et al. Molecular markers of hemostatic disorders: implications in the diagnosis and therapeutic management of thrombotic and bleeding disorders. *Clin Chem* 1983;29:1641–1658(abst).
264. Harpel PC. Alpha-2-plasmin inhibitor and alpha-2-macroglobulin-plasmin complexes in plasma. *J Clin Invest* 1981;68:46–55.
265. Clavin SA, Bobbitt JL, Shuman RT, et al. Use of peptidyl-4-methoxy-2-naphthylamides to assay plasmin. *Analyt Biochem* 1977;80:355–365.
266. Banez EI, Triplett DA, Harms C. A clinical study on the use of a fluorogenic substrate assay of plasminogen. *Thromb Res* 1983; 31:845–853.
267. Menon IS, Martin A, Weightman D. Estimation of euglobulin lysis time using a time-saving recorder. *Lab Pract* 1969;18: 1186–1187.
268. Menon IS. A study of the possible correlation of euglobulin lysis time and dilute blood clot lysis time in the determination of fibrinolytic activity. *Lab Pract* 1968;17:334–335.
269. Aoki N, Moroi M, Matsuda M. The behavior of alpha-2-plasmin inhibitor in fibrinolytic states. *J Clin Invest* 1977;60:361–369.
270. Collen D, Wiman B. Turnover of antiplasmin, the fast-acting plasmin inhibitor of plasma. *Blood* 1979:53:313–324.
271. Bick RL, Murano G. Physiology of hemostasis. *Clin Lab Med* 1994;14:677–708.
272. Takahashi H, Koike T, Yoshida N, et al. Excessive fibrinolysis in suspected amyloidosis: demonstration of plasmin-alpha-2 plasmin inhibitor complex and von Willebrand factor fragment in plasma. *Am J Hematol* 1986;23:153–166.
273. Wiman B, Jacobsson L, Andersson M, et al. Determination of plasmin-alpha-2-plasmin inhibitor complex in plasma samples by means of a radioimmunoassay. *Scand J Clin Lab Invest* 1983; 43:27–33.
274. Takahashi H, Hanano M, Takizawa S, et al. Plasmin-alpha-2-plasmin inhibitor complex in plasma of patients with disseminated intravascular coagulation. *Am J Hematol* 1988;28:162–166.
275. Matsuda T, Seki T, Ogawara M, et al. Levels of beta-thromboglobulin and platelet factor 4 in various diseases. *Acta Hematol Jpn* 1980;43:871–878.
276. Zahavi J, Kakkar VV. B-thromboglobulin: a specific marker of in vivo platelet release reaction. *Thromb Haemost* 1980;44:23–29.
277. Kwaan HC. Disseminated intravascular coagulation. *Med Clin North Am* 1972;56:177–191.
278. Bick RL. Disseminated intravascular coagulation: objective criteria for diagnosis and management. *Med Clin North Am* 1994; 78:511–544.
279. Bick RL. Clinical implications of molecular markers in hemostasis and thrombosis. *Semin Thromb Hemost* 1984;10:290–293.
280. Bick RL. Disseminated intravascular coagulation: pathophysiological mechanisms and manifestations. *Semin Thromb Hemost* 1998;24:3–18.
281. Feinstein DI. Treatment of disseminated intravascular coagulation. *Semin Thromb Hemost* 1988;14:351.
282. Bick RL. Disseminated intravascular coagulation: a clinical/laboratory study of 48 patients. *Ann NY Acad Sci* 1981;370:843.
283. Kuhn W, Graeft H. *Gerinnungsstorungen in der Geburtshilfe.* Stuttgart: Theime Verlag, 1977:90.
284. Minna JD, Robboy S, Coleman RW. Clinical approach to a patient with suspected DIC. In: Minna JD, Robboy S, Coleman RW, eds. *Disseminated intravascular coagulation.* Springfield, Ill: Charles C Thomas, 1974:167.
285. Thaler E, Lechner K. Antithrombin III deficiency and thromboembolism. *Clin Haematol* 1981;10:369.
286. Bentley PG, Kakkar VV, Scully MF, et al. An objective study of alternative methods of heparin administration. *Thromb Res* 1980;18:177.
287. Bick RL. Heparin therapy and monitoring: guidelines and prac-

tice parameters for clinical and laboratory approaches. *Clin Appl Thromb Hemost* 1996;2:12.
288. Markwardt F. Development of hirudin as an antithrombotic agent. *Semin Thromb Hemost* 1989;15:269.
289. Fourrier F, Chopin C, Huart J, et al. Double-blind, placebo-controlled trial of antithrombin III concentrates in septic shock with disseminated intravascular coagulation. *Chest* 1993;104:882.
290. Talbot M. Biology of recombinant Hirudin (CGP 39393): a new prospect in the treatment of thrombosis. *Semin Thromb Hemost* 1989;15:293.
291. Niada R, Prota R, Pescador R, et al. Thrombolytic activity of defibrotide against old venous thrombi. *Semin Thromb Hemost* 1989;15:474.
292. Ulutin ON. Clinical effectiveness of defibrotide in vaso-occlusive disorders and its mode of action. *Semin Thromb Hemost* 1988;14:58.
293. Umeki S, Adachi M, Watanabe M, et al. Gabexate as a therapy for disseminated intravascular coagulation. *Arch Intern Med* 1988;148:1409.
294. Abildgaard CF, Corrigan JJ, Seeler RA, et al. Meningococcemia associated with intravascular coagulation. *Pediatrics* 1967;40:78.
295. Bick RL, Schmalhorst WR, Fekete LF. Disseminated intravascular coagulation and blood component therapy. *Transfusion (Phila)* 1976;16:361.
296. Avvisati G, Buller HR, Wouter J, et al. Tranexamic acid for control of haemorrhage in acute promyelocytic leukemia. *Lancet* 1989;ii:122.
297. Schwartz BS, Williams EC, Conlan MG, et al. Epsilon-aminocaproic acid in the treatment of acute promyelocytic leukemia and acquired alpha-2-plasmin inhibitor deficiency. *Ann Intern Med* 1986;105:873.
298. Patterson WP, Ringenberg QS. The pathophysiology of thrombosis in cancer. *Semin Oncol* 1990;17:140.
299. Arkel YS. Thrombosis and cancer. *Semin Oncol* 2000;27:362.

Disorders of Thrombosis and Hemostasis: Clinical and Laboratory Practice, Third Edition, edited by Rodger L. Bick.
Lippincott Williams & Wilkins, Philadelphia © 2002

8

THROMBOHEMORRHAGIC DEFECTS IN LIVER AND RENAL DISEASES

EBERHARD F. MAMMEN

HEMOSTASIS DEFECTS WITH LIVER DISEASES

The liver is intimately involved in the physiology of hemostasis. Most clotting and fibrinolysis-related procoagulant and profibrinolytic factors are synthesized in liver parenchymal cells. Exceptions are von Willebrand factor (vWF), which is produced by endothelial cells and by megakaryocytes, tissue-type plasminogen activator (t-PA), which also is predominantly released from endothelial cells, and urokinase-type plasminogen activator (u-PA), which is produced mainly by renal cells. Most anticoagulant factors [antithrombin, protein C, protein S, and tissue factor pathway inhibitor (TFPI)] also are produced by liver parenchymal cells, as is α_2-plasmin inhibitor (α_2-antiplasmin). In contrast, plasminogen activator inhibitor 1 (PAI-1), the main regulator of plasminogen-to-plasmin conversion, is produced mainly by endothelial cells (1,2).

In addition, the liver regulates hemostasis by clearing activated factors or complexes from the circulation and thus helps maintain the physiologic state of equilibrium within and between the systems (2,3).

It, therefore, follows that liver dysfunction may affect hemostasis, and the supervening outcome is usually bleeding. The bleeding also can stem from quantitative and qualitative platelet abnormalities that frequently accompany severe liver dysfunction, from the production of dysfunctional factors, most notably fibrinogen, from vitamin K unavailability, and from superimposed disseminated intravascular coagulation (DIC) with secondary fibrinolysis (1,2). Thrombosis is relatively uncommon unless additional acquired or congenital risk factors are present.

The extent of bleeding in patients with liver-function impairment depends to a great degree on the severity of the dysfunction. The most serious problem is encountered with chronic hepatocellular disease or liver cirrhosis.

E. F. Mammen: Department of Obstetrics/Gynecology, Wayne State University School of Medicine, C.S. Mott Center, Detroit, Michigan.

LIVER CIRRHOSIS

Bleeding Manifestations

Patients with liver cirrhosis frequently present with spontaneous and injury-related bleeding. Spontaneous hemorrhage may be in the form of epistaxis, purpura, ecchymosis, gingival bleeding, gastrointestinal hemorrhage, or menorrhagia. Minor or major trauma, especially surgical interventions, can lead to severe bleeding complications. This is notably found in areas of high levels of local fibrinolysis, such as oral mucosa or the urogenital tract. Bleeding also can ensue from soft-tissue trauma and head trauma (1,2). A high association between spontaneous intracerebral hemorrhage and liver dysfunction has been reported (4). Surgery and anesthesia increase morbidity and mortality markedly in cirrhotic patients (5), and postoperative bleeding, renal failure, and sepsis are major contributors to mortality (6).

Pathogenesis

Several mechanisms lead in cirrhotic patients to the well-recognized coagulopathy (Table 8.1).

TABLE 8.1. MECHANISMS LEADING TO THE COAGULOPATHY IN PATIENTS WITH LIVER CIRRHOSIS

Impaired factor synthesis
Procoagulants
Vitamin K–dependent factors
Other factors
Anticoagulant factors
Profibrinolytic factors
Antifibrinolytic factors
Increased factor consumption
DIC
Primary fibrinolysis
Abnormal factor production
Prothrombin
Fibrinogen
Thrombocytopenia
Thrombocytopathy

DIC, disseminated intravascular coagulation.

Impaired Synthesis

With progressive loss of liver parenchymal cell function, most clotting and fibrinolytic factors can no longer be synthesized. Most sensitive in this respect are the vitamin K–dependent pro- and anticoagulants (factors II, VII, IX, X, protein C, and protein S). Among these, factor VII and protein C levels will decrease early in this process, followed by factors II, X, protein S and, to a lesser extent, factor IX (7). In addition to the limited synthesis capacity, there may be reduced vitamin K availability because of diminished intestinal absorption, by cholestasis, malnutrition, and prolonged gut sterilization by antibiotics (2). Reduced vitamin K availability leads to impaired γ-carboxylation of the vitamin K–dependent proteins (8,9). Hypocarboxylated prothrombin molecules and decreased ratios of prothrombin activity and antigen have been described in patients with liver cirrhosis (10). This would be consistent with diminished vitamin K use.

Over time, other non–vitamin K–dependent factors also will be affected. Decreases in factor V levels appear to correlate best with the extent of liver parenchymal cell dysfunction (7,11). Plasma fibrinogen levels decrease only with advanced liver damage (11,12) or when DIC is present. Factor VIII and vWF levels are frequently elevated, for reasons not fully understood (12–14). Some of the reductions in factors may be due to increased destruction by a variety of enzymes. This has been shown for antithrombin, which is readily destroyed by elastase released from polymorphonuclear (PMN) granulocytes (15) and for high- and low-molecular-weight kininogens (16). vWF, although normal in quantity, may be deficient in the high-molecular-weight multimers because of destruction by proteases (14).

Increased Factor Consumption

This can be related to DIC (consumptive coagulopathy, consumptive thrombohemorrhagic syndrome). Patients with cirrhosis are prone to develop this serious complication (17). The trigger mechanisms discussed include release of tissue factor (TF) from necrotic cells, release of interleukins, especially tumor necrosis factor (TNF)-α and interleukin-1 (18) and possibly endotoxin. Once the systems are activated, the DIC process is enhanced by the reduced levels of the physiologic inhibitors (antithrombin, protein C, protein S and TFPI), by the diminished capacity of the liver to clear activated factors and factor complexes, and by the diminished capacity of liver parenchymal cells to resynthesize the hemostasis-related proteins.

The existence of DIC in patients with cirrhosis is supported by findings of shortened fibrinogen (18) and shortened antithrombin survival (19), by elevated levels of markers of in vivo hemostasis activation, such as thrombin–antithrombin (TAT) complex, prothrombin fragment 1+2 (F 1+2), plasmin–antiplasmin (PAP) complex, fibrin(ogen) degradation products (FDPs), and D-dimer (20). Others have questioned the occurrence of DIC in cirrhotic patients (21,22) because most changes supporting DIC also can be explained by the complex defects caused by the cirrhosis itself (20). It is conceivable that DIC is *a priori* rare, but that it can be triggered when outside factors, especially endotoxemia, become operational (1). Because fibrinogen and factor VIII levels are near normal or even increased in cirrhotic patients, a decline of these two factors would support the concept that increased consumption, or DIC, is operational (2,20).

Fibrinolysis

Activation of fibrinolysis may occur in conjunction with DIC (secondary fibrinolysis) or without concomitant activation of the clotting system (primary fibrinolysis). The increased fibrinolysis (primary) is basically related to an impaired control of the system. Levels of t-PA and u-PA are frequently elevated in cirrhotics (23), because none is produced by liver parenchymal cells, whereas the synthesis of α_2-plasmin inhibitor is impaired (24). For reasons not fully understood, PAI-1 levels also are decreased in cirrhotics (2,20), although this protein is not produced by liver cells. Elastase released from activated PMN neutrophils also activates fibrinolysis (25). Enhanced secondary fibrinolysis is especially noted when endotoxins serve as the trigger for DIC (2). In some patients, fibrinolysis could be reduced by the administration of heparin (26), again supporting the concept of secondary fibrinolysis.

Abnormal Factor Production

This relates especially to fibrinogen and to prothrombin. The prothrombin defect primarily involves abnormal γ-carboxylation (9). Dysfunctional fibrinogen molecules (dysfibrinogenemia) lead to impaired fibrin polymerization (27). The basic defect in the fibrinogen molecules relates to an increased sialic acid content (28), and removal of the sialic acid by neuraminidase normalizes abnormal fibrin monomer polymerization (2). Dysfibrinogenemia is especially encountered in patients with hepatomas (29). These patients also may have abnormal vitamin K–dependent factors (30,31).

Thrombocytopenia

The main reason for thrombocytopenia in patients with liver cirrhosis is splenomegaly or "hypersplenism" due to portal hypertension. Whereas a normal spleen contains about 33% of the body's platelet mass, up to 90% may be stored in a massively enlarged spleen (32). Shortened platelet survival also has been reported in patients with chronic liver disease (33). In addition, thrombocytopenia can be due to an autoimmune mechanism. It was reported that patients with primary biliary cirrhosis (*not* alcoholic cirrhosis) had antibodies to the glycoprotein (GP) complex Ib/IX and against GPIIb/IIIa (34). Additional causes of thrombocytopenia are DIC, folic acid deficiency, and decreased megakaryopoiesis (35).

Thrombocytopathy

The presence of thrombocytopathy in cirrhotic patients is controversially reported in the literature. One study on 60 patients found no evidence for thrombocytopathy (33), whereas others reported storage pool defects (36), impaired signal transduction (37), reduced thromboxane A_2 synthesis (38), and diminished platelet adhesion under flow conditions (39). The relation between GPIb/IX-receptor complex and vWF also has yielded divergent results. One group of investigators found a reduced number of GPIb/IX receptors on platelets, decreased binding of vWF, and reduced ristocetin-induced platelet agglutination (40), whereas another group found the opposite (41). Increased levels of vWF antigen and activity have been described (41,42), albeit with a reduction in the high-molecular-weight (HMW) vWF multimers, which are hemostatically most active (41). Enhanced proteolysis may be the cause of the decrease in the large vWF multimers, as has been shown in patients subjected to orthotopic liver transplantation (43). Additional mechanisms leading to platelet dysfunction in cirrhotic patients are elevated FDPs (44) that interfere with platelet aggregation, and adverse effects of ethanol in cases of alcoholic cirrhosis (35). The role of thrombocytopathy as a cause of bleeding in cirrhotics is at this time not clear.

Laboratory Tests

The complex hemostasis abnormalities encountered in patients with liver cirrhosis find their reflections in laboratory parameters that are summarized in Table 8.2. The extent of the changes depends on the degree of liver dysfunction. As expected, all screening tests for clotting are prolonged. Thrombin clotting times (TCTs) are abnormal because of either the presence of FDPs, dysfunctional fibrinogen molecules, or low fibrinogen levels. For diagnostic considerations, screening tests [activated partial thromboplastin time (aPTT), prothrombin time (PT), TCT], platelet counts, fibrinogen, D-dimer, and fibrin split products (FSPs) levels should be available. The results allow a reasonably good assessment of whether deficiencies of clotting factors, DIC, primary fibrinolysis, or thrombocytopenia is present. Individual factor assays can give information on the extent of liver dysfunction, most notably factor V determinations (11). Factor VIII levels, which are usually elevated in cirrhotics, may herald DIC when their plasma levels decline. Molecular markers of in vivo activation of hemostasis, such as TAT complex, prothrombin fragment 1+2 (F 1+2), or PAP complex are usually elevated in chronic liver disease patients. They may reflect a state of in vivo activation of hemostasis, but could also be due, or at least in part due to improper clearance from the circulation (1,2). The assay of these markers does not routinely add to the diagnosis of liver dysfunction.

TABLE 8.2. HEMOSTASIS PARAMETERS IN PATIENTS WITH CHRONIC HEPATOCELLULAR DISEASE (CIRRHOSIS)

Clotting System	Fibrinolytic System	Platelets
APTT ↑	ELT ↓	Bleeding time ↑
PT ↑	Plasminogen ↓	Counts ↓
TCT ↑	α_2-Antiplasmin ↓	Adhesion ↓
Reptilase time ↑	t-PA N	Aggregation ↓
	u-PA N	
Vitamin K–dependent factors ↓	PAI-1 N-↓	
Factor V ↓	FDP ↑	
Factor VIII:c N-↑		
vWF N-↑	D-dimer ↑	
Fibrinogen N-↓	PAP complex ↑	
Antithrombin ↓		
Protein C ↓		
Protein S ↓		
TFPI N-↓		
TAT complex ↑		
F1 + 2 ↑		
Fibrinopeptide A ↑		

↑, prolonged or elevated; ↓, shortened or decreased; N, normal; aPTT, activated partial thromboplastin time; PT, prothrombin time; TCT, thrombin clotting time; vFW, von Willebrand factor; TFPI, tissue factor pathway inhibitor; TAT, thrombin/antithrombin; F1 + 2, prothrombin fragment 1 + 2; ELF, euglobulin lysis time; t-PA, tissue-type plasminogen activator; u-PA, urokinase-type plasminogen activator; PAI-1, plasminogen activator inhibitor 1; FDP, fibrin(ogen) degradation product; PAP, plasmin/antiplasmin.

Management

Treatment of the hemostasis defects in cirrhotics depends on the patient's clinical presentation. Without any bleeding evidence, no treatment should be undertaken, unless a major interventional procedure is contemplated. In the presence of bleeding, the cause and source must be considered. In cases of bleeding from esophageal varices, sclerotherapy or treatment to decrease portal hypertension should be the primary target; attempts to correct the hemostasis abnormalities are secondary. In contrast, in patients with spontaneous bleeding, or with posttraumatic or postoperative hemorrhage, correction of the hemostasis defect is the primary focus. Several options are available in these situations:

Fresh frozen plasma (FFP) replenishes all of the deficient clotting and fibrinolytic factors. However, because of the variable half-lives of these proteins (factor VII has the shortest), repeated transfusions are required. This can lead to fluid overload, which can become a serious limiting factor. Another problem is the potential risk of viral transmission, such as hepatitis B and C and human immunodeficiency virus (HIV), although this risk can be reduced by using solvent-detergent–treated plasmas. In extreme cases, plasma exchange can be considered.

Prothrombin complex concentrates contain only the vitamin K–dependent pro- and anticoagulants, but no other factors. Although these proteins are always decreased in patients with severe hepatic dysfunction, they do not, for example, provide factor V, which is closely linked to bleeding in these patients (11). Therefore, FFP may be needed in addition to fully complement the broad hemostasis defect. These complex concentrates also may be thrombogenic (45,46), because some contain "activated" enzymes that are only poorly cleared in these patients. Another caution relates to the potential contamination of these preparations with hepatitis A virus or parvovirus (47).

In some special cases, *cryoprecipitate* may be considered. It is a rich source of fibrinogen, which ordinarily is not so much decreased as to cause bleeding. However, when DIC or primary fibrinolysis dominates the clinical picture, cryoprecipitate may be helpful.

Platelet concentrates can be helpful if counts are very low, especially when invasive procedures are contemplated. Peripheral platelet counts of greater than 75×10^9/L should be obtained to accomplish satisfactory efficacy. This may be difficult to achieve in patients with hypersplenism because the extent of sequestration in the enlarged spleen is unpredictable. If platelets are administered, peripheral counts about 1 hour after completion of the transfusion will give a clue as to the extent of the loss.

Vitamin K administration is of limited usefulness unless a true deficiency is present. Mild cases of hepatocellular damage may profit when the levels of the vitamin K–dependent proteins, especially factor VII, are decreased, and other non–vitamin K–dependent factor levels, especially factor V, are still in normal range. Vitamin K_1 (10 mg) given intravenously may improve or even correct the PT and aPTT.

Antifibrinolytic agents have been successfully used in cirrhotic patients who underwent dental extractions (48). Because hyperfibrinolysis is frequently encountered, ε-aminocaproic acid, tranexamic acid, or aprotinin, where available, can be considered. However, the presence of DIC *must* be ruled out because those patients would be irreparably harmed by the widespread deposition of fibrin in the microvasculature. The differential diagnosis between primary and secondary (DIC-associated) fibrinolysis is extremely difficult to establish under these circumstances, so that from this point of view, antifibrinolytic agents should be considered only with extreme caution.

Other agents may be indicated in specific situations. 1-Deamino-8-D-arginine vasopressin (DDAVP), for example, may be considered when thrombocytopathy seems prevalent (49). As outlined before, this hemostatic disturbance is controversial in the etiology of bleeding in patients with advanced liver disease. Estrogen–progesterone treatment was recently found to be of potential usefulness in patients with chronic bleeding from gastric vascular ectasia and cirrhosis (50).

MILD TO MODERATE LIVER DISEASE

Hemostatic derailment is less severe in patients with mild to moderate liver-function impairment (20). Patients with viral hepatitis may have no alterations at all; others may have slightly prolonged PT due to a slight decrease in factor VII, the most sensitive vitamin K–dependent procoagulant (20). In general, the extent of the hemostatic defects encountered relates directly to the degree of the liver parenchymal cell damage (1,2), unless other complications arise, such as sepsis (Table 8.3). The diagnosis and management must, therefore, be individualized, and no general guidelines seem to be in order.

HEMOSTASIS DEFECTS WITH LIVER TRANSPLANTATION

Orthotopic liver transplantation is associated with severe hemostatic derailments (51), leading to excessive bleeding during the procedure (52). The transplant patient is already hemostatically compromised before surgery, the surgical trauma is extensive, there is an obligatory anhepatic phase in which no factors are produced and no clearance takes place, and excessive fibrinolysis is generated during the anhepatic phase and during the immediate reperfusion phase (53).

Most surgical centers do not address the preoperative defects because the poorly functioning liver will be replaced. Little can be done to affect the extensive surgical procedure itself. However, the excessive fibrinolysis during the anhepatic and postperfusion phases requires careful attention.

TABLE 8.3. HEMOSTASIS DEFECTS WITH MILD TO MODERATE HEPATOCELLULAR DISEASE

Mild forms (viral hepatitis)
No changes
↑ PT
↓ Factor VII
Moderate forms
↑ PT and APTT
↓ Vitamin K–dependent factors
↑ Fibrinolytic activity
↓ Platelet counts
Severe forms (hepatic failure)
Values similar to cirrhosis
(See Table 8.2)

↑, prolonged or increased; ↓, decreased. Other abbreviations, see Table 8.2.

In both instances, a massive release of t-PA accounts for the accelerated activation of the fibrinolytic system (20). During the anhepatic phase, t-PA is released from endothelial cells, and its clearance from the circulation is impaired. Because PAI-1 levels are low, t-PA can massively convert plasminogen to plasmin (54), which can act relatively unopposed because of the low plasma levels of α_2-plasmin inhibitor (α_2-antiplasmin) (55).

The second fibrinolytic "burst" is due to t-PA release from the stored organ (51,56). This is associated with a liberation of other proteolytic enzymes, such as trypsin, elastase, and cathepsin B (57). These also contribute to the proteolytic state and to the severe hemorrhagic tendency. A proteolytic cleavage of vWF also seems to contribute to the bleeding (43).

Monitoring of these events during the procedure can be accomplished by a Thrombelastograph, which gives quick information on clot formation and stability (58). The obtained data allow surgeons and anesthesiologists in the operating room to monitor efficacy of replacement therapy and antifibrinolytic agents (59).

The use of antifibrinolytic agents during orthotopic liver transplantation has greatly reduced the bleeding tendency and therefore the need for blood replacement (60). Much experience has been gained with the use of aprotinin, a broad-spectrum serine protease inhibitor. In most studies, the administration of aprotinin not only reduced need for blood replacement (60), but also decreased plasma levels of t-PA and D-dimer and increased α_2-plasmin inhibitor levels (61–63). ε-Aminocaproic acid and tranexamic acid administrations have principally shown benefits similar to those seen with aprotinin in reducing transfusion needs (64).

Initial concerns about the use of antifibrinolytics in orthotopic liver transplantation centered around the issue of DIC with secondary fibrinolysis or primary fibrinolysis. Because of the uncertainty of the differential diagnosis, antithrombin concentrates were advocated before antifibrinolytic agents were given. It was found, however, that these concentrates did not yield any benefits in patients with terminal chronic liver diseases (65). It thus seems that the fibrinolysis is overwhelmingly primary in nature.

SHUNT PLACEMENT IN LIVER CIRRHOSIS

Medically intractable ascites often requires placement of a portocaval or mesocaval shunt in patients with chronic hepatic diseases. These procedures are frequently associated with a severe bleeding tendency that is not only due to an exacerbation of the previously existing hemostasis defects, but also may be related to a rapidly developing DIC with secondary fibrinolysis (66,67). Cellular and soluble procoagulant material in the ascites fluid (68,69) as well as activators of platelets (70) have been discussed as possible triggers for the DIC. This complication can be largely avoided by removing much of the ascites fluid from the abdominal cavity before the shunt is opened (71).

THROMBOSIS OF THE PORTAL CIRCULATION

Hepatic artery thrombosis is occasionally encountered after orthotopic liver transplantation. This is conceivably due to a transient hypercoagulable state, when procoagulant factors recover more quickly than anticoagulant proteins, most notably antithrombin, protein C, and protein S (72). Heparinization of the patient plus transfusion of FFP have reduced this complication (73). A better option than FFP would likely be antithrombin concentrates or protein C concentrates and should be tried in risk patients.

Portal vein thrombosis is another complication in patients with liver cirrhosis. It was demonstrated that blood from the portal circulation had higher levels of F 1+2 and D-dimer and lower fibrinogen levels than did peripheral blood (74). There is thus, *a priori*, a hypercoagulable state in the portal circulation that could lead to thrombosis when other risk factors, most notably endotoxins, are present (74). A more recent study revealed that about 70% of cirrhotic patients with portal vein thrombosis had an acquired or congenital thrombophilic condition (75). Clinicians should be encouraged to identify such conditions and, if present, protect these patients with appropriate anticoagulant measures.

HEMOSTASIS DEFECTS WITH VITAMIN K DEFICIENCY

Vitamin K is required for the final synthesis of the vitamin K–dependent procoagulants (factors II, VII, IX, and X) and anticoagulants (protein C and protein S). Each of these proteins has a defined number of glutamic acid residues in the N-terminal region that are required for binding to phospholipid surfaces to form activation complexes (tenase, prothrombinase, extrinsic complex) by calcium bridges. Before being able to participate in these complex formations, the glutamic acid residues must be converted to their γ-carboxy form (76). This requires vitamin K in its epoxide form. Vitamin K thus plays a pivotal role in the formation of activation complexes during clotting and an important role in the regulation of clotting.

Much of the daily vitamin K supply is obtained from ingested food, but bacterial synthesis in the gastrointestinal tract also plays a great role. Vitamin K is a fat-soluble vitamin that requires pancreatic lipases, bile, and the absorptive ability of the intestinal wall to be taken up by the organism. Inappropriate diet, biliary diseases, pancreatic disorders, malabsorption, and long-term antibiotic therapy, especially in children and in the geriatric population, can lead to vitamin K deficiency (1,20). Oral anticoagulants have similar effects because these compounds primarily interfere with the vitamin K reductase system (76), preventing efficient recycling of vitamin K to its active form.

Patients with vitamin K deficiency have a bleeding tendency in the form of ecchymoses, hematoma formation, hematuria, and gastrointestinal or genitourinary bleeding.

The *laboratory* investigations reveal prolonged PT and aPTT, but normal TCT. Factor analysis shows decreased levels of factors II, VII, IX, and X, as well as decreased levels of protein C and S. Factor VII and protein C plasma levels are most sensitive to these defects. All other clotting factors are normal; there is no thrombocytopenia or thrombocytopathy and no DIC or fibrinolysis (Table 8.4).

The diagnosis can be confirmed by the administration of vitamin K, in response to which PT and aPTT should normalize, with the corresponding correction of the vitamin K–dependent factor levels.

Treatment should entail correction of the underlying disorder and vitamin K_1 administration. In cases of severe bleeding, FFP can be administered as well, but the use of prothrombin complex concentrates must be exercised with caution because of the potential thrombogenicity, as outlined earlier. Vitamin K_1 is usually given orally, but it can be given parenterally when bleeding is severe or when surgeries are contemplated. It must be kept in mind, however, that it takes about 7 hours or longer after vitamin K_1 administration for the PT to partially improve. This relates to the half-life of the factors (factor VII, 4 to 7 hours; factor II, 3 days; factor X, 1 day; and factor IX, 2 days). Generally, the PT and aPTT should be normal within 3 days.

These considerations are especially important for managing patients with an overdose of oral anticoagulants where the risk of intracerebral bleeding is very high, or when orally anticoagulated patients require surgical interventions or when they sustained major trauma. Here the emphasis must be on an immediate correction of the defects, and thus FFP is the best choice (20). The amount must be sufficient to correct both PT and aPTT. Vitamin K_1 is most certainly also given, but its effect is delayed.

TABLE 8.4. LABORATORY FINDINGS IN PATIENTS WITH VITAMIN K DEFICIENCY

APTT	↑	Antithrombin	N
PT	↑	Protein C	↓
TCT	N	Protein S	↓
		TFPI	N
Factors II, VII, IX, X	↓		
Other factors	N	Platelets	N

aPTT, activated partial thromboplastin time; PT, prothrombin time; TCT, thrombin clotting time; TFPI, tissue factor pathway inhibitor; ↑, prolonged; ↓, decreased; N, normal.

HEMOSTASIS DEFECTS WITH RENAL DISEASE

Although the kidneys are involved in hemostasis only as a source of u-PA, bleeding and thromboses are encountered with different renal disorders (1,77,78). Patients with chronic renal failure and uremia do have a bleeding tendency, whereas those with nephrotic syndrome and glomerulonephritis have a predisposition to thromboembolic complications.

Chronic Renal Failure and Uremia

Bleeding Manifestations

Clinically patients with these problems have mucous membrane hemorrhages, gastrointestinal bleeding, petechiae, purpura, ecchymoses, postoperative bleeding, and occasionally intracerebral hemorrhages. In renal failure patients, occasionally DIC, hemolytic–uremic syndrome (HUS), and thrombotic thrombocytopenic purpura (TTP) may be encountered (78).

Pathogenesis

Although several hemostasis defects have been reported in uremic patients (Table 8.5), the overwhelming underlying defect is a thrombocytopathy. About half of the patients may have, in addition, a mild to moderate thrombocytopenia (77). Because the platelet dysfunction can be corrected by hemodialysis (79) and because normal platelets added to uremic plasma become dysfunctional (78), it appears that the platelet defect is caused by retained metabolites, and creatinine, urea, phenol, and guanidine compounds and guanidinosuccinic acid have been suggested (1,77,78). There is, however, only a poor correlation between prolonged bleeding times, as a reflection of the thrombocytopathy, clinical bleeding, and levels of many of the retained metabolites (1). Best correlations were found between clinical parameters and serum levels of guanidinosuccinic acid (77). When this compound was added to normal plasma in vitro, abnormal platelet function, similar to that found in uremic patients, could consistently be produced (80). Strong evidence was then presented that guanidinosuccinic acid produces nitric oxide (NO) in uremic vessels and that

TABLE 8.5. HEMOSTASIS DEFECTS REPORTED IN PATIENTS WITH UREMIA

Thrombocytopathy
Thrombocytopenia (< 50% of patients)
Clotting defects
Fibrinolytic abnormalities

NO is very likely responsible for the platelet dysfunction and thus the uremia-associated bleeding (81).

Two additional factors contribute to the bleeding tendency in uremic patients: the use of medications that keep patent the shunts for hemodialysis and the uremia-associated anemia. Because the vascular accesses needed for hemodialysis easily thrombose, acetylsalicylic acid (82) or other nonsteroidal antiinflammatory medications (83) often are prescribed. The use of these medications frequently leads to gastrointestinal hemorrhage (84,85). β-Lactam antibiotics exacerbate the bleeding tendency (70).

Because there is an integral relation between red cell mass and platelet function (1), anemia associated with uremia, or of other causes, prolongs bleeding times (86). There is an inverse relation between hematocrit and bleeding times (87). Partial correction of the anemia by red cell transfusions or by erythropoietin administration improves bleeding times in uremic patients (88,89).

Laboratory Tests in Uremic Patients

Besides the complex thrombocytopathy and the thrombocytopenia, several other hemostatic defects have been described (Table 8.6).

Local vascular defects in the form of angiodysplasia, especially in the upper gastrointestinal tract, appear to be common in uremic patients, and these may contribute to bleeding (84). Plasma and platelet vWF levels seem to be increased in uremic patients (1), and there is evidence for a dysfunctional vWF molecule (90).

Platelet dysfunction is rather complex in nature and involves adhesion as well as aggregation defects with multiple agonists (1,77). More recently, defective glycoprotein receptors were described (78). Most bleeding is likely caused by the abnormality in platelet function and is reversible by hemodialysis.

The observed thrombocytopenia is mild to moderate, and the defects described in the clotting and fibrinolytic systems may or may not contribute to the hemorrhagic tendency in uremic patients.

TABLE 8.6. LABORATORY FINDINGS IN PATIENTS WITH UREMIA

Vascular abnormalities
↑ Synthesis of prostacyclin (PGI_2)
↑ von Willebrand factor (vWF)
Abnormal plasma and platelet vWF
Thrombocytopathy
↑ Bleeding time
↓ Platelet adhesion
↓ Platelet aggregation (ADP, collagen, epinephrine, thrombin)
↓ Platelet factor 3 availability
↓ Thromboxane A_2 synthesis
↓ Clot retraction
↓ Glycoprotein (GP) Ib and GPIIb/IIIa
Thrombocytopenia
Clotting defects
↑ Fibrinogen
↑ Factor VIII:c
↓ Protein C
↓ Protein S
Fibrinolytic defects
↓ t-PA
↑ α_2-Antiplasmin
↑ PAI-1

↑, increased or prolonged; ↓, decreased or shortened; t-PA, tissue-type plasminogen activator; PAI-1, plasminogen activator inhibitor 1; ADP, adenosine diphosphate.

Management of Patients with Uremic Bleeding

Because the thrombocytopathy is caused by substances retained in uremic blood, *hemodialysis* will correct not only prolonged bleeding times but also many of the adhesion and aggregation defects (1). Initially, however, cerebrovascular bleeding, gastrointestinal hemorrhage, and hemopericardium may be encountered (78), which may, at least in part, be related to the systemic heparinization. During hemodialysis, platelets become activated because of their contact with "foreign surfaces" of the dialysis membranes (77), leading to decreases in counts and release of substances normally present in platelets. Activation of protein C with decreasing plasma levels and increased levels of tissue factor and PAI-1 also have been described during hemodialysis (91,92). These may be related to some of the thrombotic complications occasionally seen during or immediately after hemodialysis.

Unfractionated *heparin* (UFH) is most widely used as an anticoagulant during hemodialysis, but low-molecular-weight (LMW) heparins have been used. In a prospective, randomized, crossover study comparing an LMW heparin with UFH, less clot formation, but slightly more bleeding was found (93). Similar data were reported for another LMW heparin (94). The increased bleeding tendency is likely due to the accumulation of LMW heparin, which is exclusively eliminated by the kidneys. Patients with renal insufficiency had a greater bleeding tendency when treated with LMW heparin than did patients without renal disease (95). When LMW heparins are used for hemodialysis, plasma levels should probably be monitored to prevent undue hemorrhages. In patients with heparin-induced thrombocytopenia and need for hemodialysis, recombinant hirudin was found to be an effective and safe alternate anticoagulant (96).

DDAVP has been used to treat bleeding in uremic patients (1,77). DDAVP shortened bleeding times in most patients, and the effects lasted for about 4 hours. DDAVP releases factor VIII/vWF macromolecular complexes from endothelial cells, so that its beneficial effects are likely due to the correction of the reported abnormal vWF molecules in uremic patients (90). The same corrections can be achieved by the transfusion of large quantities of FFP or cryoprecipitate, which also contain substantial amounts of factor VIII/vWF complexes (97).

Correction of Anemia

Because red cell mass and platelet function are closely related, and because there is a direct relation between severity of anemia in uremic patients and prolonged bleeding times and clinical hemorrhage (88), it is important to correct the anemia in these patients. Several studies showed improvement in bleeding times and clinical bleeding tendency when red cell concentrates were administered (hematocrit, greater than 26%) (88,98) or when recombinant erythropoietin was given to yield hematocrits greater than 27% to 32% (89,99,100). Improvements in platelet function were inconsistent (1).

NEPHROTIC SYNDROME

Patients with nephrotic syndrome, without uremia, have a tendency to develop thromboembolic complications (1,77), especially renal vein thrombosis (1,101). Platelet hyperaggregability and shortened platelet survival have been described (102) and have been attributed to hypoalbuminemia (103). Increased levels of fibrinogen, factor VIII, and vWF also have been demonstrated (102,104). Most prominent, however, is the loss of antithrombin in the urine (105). This natural inhibitor of the clotting system has a molecular weight similar to that of albumin and is thus subject to urinary loss. Protein C and free protein S may be unchanged (106), and so is TFPI (107). The latter may even be increased in these patients. The fibrinolytic system is basically normal in patients with nephrotic syndrome (1).

GLOMERULONEPHRITIS

There is ample evidence to suggest that platelets are involved in the pathogenesis of glomerulonephritis (1), and a hypercoagulable state has been proposed (108). There is increased platelet consumption that can be reduced by administering platelet antiaggregating medications (109). It has been suggested that platelet-derived growth factor might be related to the proliferation of the membranous changes in this disorder (110). The intraglomerular fibrin deposits could be a result of increased release of TF (111), decreased production of u-PA (112), and upregulation of PAI-1 (113). There is thus little doubt that hypercoagulability plays an important role in the pathogenesis of glomerulonephritis.

REFERENCES

1. Joist JH, George JN. Hemostatic abnormalities in liver and renal disease. In: Coleman RW, Hirsh J, Marder VJ, et al., eds. *Hemostasis and thrombosis: basic principles and clinical practice.* 4th ed. Philadelphia: Lippincott Williams & Wilkins, 2001; 955–973.
2. Mammen EF. Hemostatic dysfunction related to liver diseases and liver transplantation. In: Beutler E, Lichtman MA, Coller BS, et al., eds. *Williams hematology. 6th ed.* New York: McGraw-Hill, 2001:1673–1676.
3. Wells MJ, Sheffield WP, Blajchman MA. The clearance of thrombin–antithrombin and related serpin-enzyme complexes from the circulation: role of various hepatocyte receptors. *Thromb Haemost* 1999;81:325–337.
4. Fujii Y, Takeuchi S, Tanaka R, et al. Liver dysfunction in spontaneous intracerebral hemorrhage. *Neurosurgery* 1994;35: 592–596.
5. Ziser A, Plevak DJ, Wiesner RH, et al. Morbidity and mortality in cirrhotic patients undergoing anesthesia and surgery. *Anesthesiology* 1999;90:42–53.
6. Aranha GV, Sontag SJ, Greenlee HB. Cholecystectomy in cirrhotic patients: a formidable operation. *Am J Surg* 1982;143: 55–60.
7. Lechner K, Niessner H, Thaler E. Coagulation abnormalities in liver disease. *Semin Thromb Hemost* 1977;4:40–56.
8. Blanchard RA, Furie BC, Jørgensen M, et al. Acquired vitamin K-dependent carboxylation deficiency in liver disease. *N Engl J Med* 1981;305:242–249.
9. Uras F, Uras AR, Yardimic T, et al. Determination of the N-terminal amino acid sequence of the purified prothrombin from a patient with liver cirrhosis. *Thromb Res* 2000;99:277–283.
10. Corrigan JJ, Jeter M, Earnest DL. Prothrombin antigen and coagulant activity in patients with liver disease. *JAMA* 1982; 248:1736–1742.
11. Dymock IW, Tucker JS, Wolf IL, et al. Coagulation studies as a prognostic index in acute liver failure. *Br J Haematol* 1975;29: 385–391.
12. Spector I, Corn M. Laboratory tests of hemostasis: the relation to hemorrhage in liver disease. *Arch Intern Med* 1967;119: 577–586.
13. Castillo R, Maragall S, Rodes J, et al. Increased factor VIII complex and defective ristocetin-induced platelet aggregation in liver disease. *Thromb Res* 1977;11:899–906.
14. Maisonneuve P, Sultan Y. Modification of factor VIII complex properties in patients with liver disease. *J Clin Pathol* 1977;30: 221–229.
15. Mammen EF. Antithrombin: its physiological importance and role in DIC. *Semin Thromb Hemost* 1998;24:19–25.
16. Cugmo N, Scott CF, Salerno F, et al. Parallel reduction of plasma levels of high and low molecular weight kininogen in patients with cirrhosis. *Thromb Haemost* 1999;82:1428–1432.
17. Tytgat GN, Collen D, Verstraete M. Metabolism of fibrinogen in cirrhosis of the liver. *J Lab Clin Med* 1974;50:1690–1702.
18. Hanck C, Glatzel M, Singer MV, et al. Gene expression of TNF-receptors in blood mononuclear cells of patients with alcoholic cirrhosis. *J Hepatol* 2000;32:51–57.
19. Schipper HG, ten Cate JW. Antithrombin III transfusion in patients with hepatic cirrhosis. Br J Haematol 1982;52:25–31.
20. Mammen EF. Coagulopathies of liver disease. *Clin Lab Med* 1994;14:769–780.
21. Ben Ari Z, Osman E, Hutton RA, et al. Disseminated intravascular coagulation in liver cirrhosis: fact or fiction? *Am J Gastroenterol* 1999;94:2977–2982.

22. Straub PW. Diffuse intravascular coagulation in liver disease? *Semin Thromb Hemost* 1977;4:29–39.
23. Tytgat G, Collen J, de Vreker RR, et al. Investigations of the fibrinolytic system in liver cirrhosis. *Acta Haematol* 1968;40: 265–276.
24. Hersch SL, Kunelis T, Francis RB. The pathogenesis of accelerated fibrinolysis in liver cirrhosis: a critical role for tissue plasminogen activator. *Blood* 1987;69:1315–1319.
25. Song KS, Kim HK, Kim HS, et al. Plasma granulocyte elastase levels and its relation to D-dimer in liver cirrhosis. *Fibrinol Proteol* 2000;14:300–304.
26. Collen D, Bouvier J, Chamone DAF, et al. Turnover of radiolabeled plasminogen and prothrombin in cirrhosis of the liver. *Eur J Clin Invest* 1978;8:185–198.
27. Green G, Thompson JM, Dymock IW, et al. Abnormal fibrin polymerization in liver disease. *Br J Haematol* 1976;30: 427–435.
28. Martinez J, MacDonald KA, Palascak JE. The role of sialic acid in the dysfibrinogenemia associated with liver disease: distribution of sialic acid on the constituent chain. *Blood* 1983;61: 1196–1202.
29. Green G, Thompson JM, Dymock IW, et al. Abnormal fibrin. I. polymerization in liver disease. *Br J Haematol* 1970;24:425–433.
30. Yoshikawa Y, Sakata Y, Toda G, et al. The acquired vitamin K-dependent gamma carboxylation deficiency in hepatocellular carcinoma involves not only prothrombin, but also protein C. *Hepatology* 1988;8:524–531.
31. Shimada M, Yamashita Y, Halmatsu T, et al. The role of des-γ-carboxy prothrombin levels in hepatocellular carcinoma and liver tissues. *Cancer Lett* 2000;159:87–94.
32. Schmidt KG, Rasmussen J, Bekker C, et al. Kinetics and in vitro distribution of iridium-III labeled autologous platelets in chronic hepatic disease: mechanisms of thrombocytopenia. *Scand J Haematol* 1985;34:39–48.
33. Stein SF, Harker LA. Kinetic and functional studies of platelets, fibrinogen, and plasminogen in patients with hepatic cirrhosis. *J Lab Clin Med* 1986;99:217–229.
34. Feistauer SM, Penner E, Mayr WR, et al. Target platelet antigens of autoantibodies in patients with primary biliary cirrhosis. *Hepatology* 1997;25:1343–1351.
35. Cowan DH. Effect of alcoholism on hemostasis. *Semin Hematol* 1980;17:137–149.
36. Laffi G, Marra F, Gresele P, et al. Evidence for a storage pool defect in the platelets from cirrhotic patients with defective aggregation. *Gastroenterology* 1992;103:641–649.
37. Laffi G, Marra F, Ruggiero M, et al. Defective signal transduction in platelets from cirrhotics is associated with increased cyclic nucleotides. *Gastroenterology* 1993;105:148–157.
38. Laffi G, Cominelli F, Ruggiero M, et al. Altered platelet function in cirrhosis of the liver: impairment of inositol lipid and arachidonic acid metabolism in response to agonists. *Hepatology* 1988;8:1620–1632.
39. Ordinas A, Escolar G, Cirera I, et al. Existence of a platelet-adhesion defect in patients with cirrhosis independent of hematocrit: studies under flow conditions. *Hepatology* 1996;24: 1137–1151.
40. Sanchez-Roig MJ, Rivera J, Moraleda JM, et al. Quantitative defects of glycoprotein Ib in severe cirrhotic patients. *Am J Hematol* 1994;46:812–819.
41. Beer JH, Clerici N, Baillod P, et al. Quantitative and qualitative analysis of platelet GPIb and von Willebrand factor in liver cirrhosis. *Thromb Haemost* 1995;73:601–609.
42. Green AJ, Ratnoff OD. Elevated antihemophilic factor (AHF, factor VIII) procoagulant activity and AHF-like antigen in alcoholic cirrhosis of the liver. *J Lab Clin Med* 1974;83:189–202.
43. Lattuade A, Mannucci PM, Chen C, et al. Transfusion requirements are correlated with the degree of proteolysis of von Willebrand factor during orthotopic liver transplantation. *Thromb Haemost* 1997;78:813–819.
44. Thomas DP, Ream VJ, Stuart RK. Platelet aggregation in patients with Laennec's cirrhosis of the liver. *N Engl J Med* 1967;276:1342–1348.
45. Hultin MB. Activated clotting factors in factor IX concentrates. *Blood* 1979;54:1028–1038.
46. Lusher JM. Thrombogenicity associated with factor IX complex concentrates. *Semin Hematol* 1991;28:3–17.
47. Seligsohn U, White GL II. Inherited deficiencies of coagulation factors II, V, VII, XI and XIII and the combined deficiencies of factors V and VIII and of the vitamin K-dependent factors. In: Beutler K, Lichtman MA, Coller BS, et al., eds. *Williams hematology. 6th ed.* New York: McGraw-Hill, 2001:1617–1638.
48. Francis RB, Feinstein DI. Clinical significance of accelerated fibrinolysis in liver disease. *Haemostasis* 1984;14:460–472.
49. Mannucci PM, Vicente V, Vianello L, et al. Controlled trial of desmopressin in liver cirrhosis and other conditions associated with prolonged bleeding time. *Blood* 1986;67:1148–1153.
50. Tran A, Villeneuve J-P, Bilodean M, et al. Treatment of chronic bleeding from gastric antral vascular ectasia (GAVE) with estrogen-progesterone in cirrhotic patients: an open pilot study. *Am J Gastroenterol* 1999;94:2909–2911.
51. Porte RJ. Coagulation and fibrinolysis in orthotopic liver transplantation: current views and insights. *Semin Thromb Hemost* 1993;19:191–196.
52. Neuhaus P. Hemostasis in liver transplantation: the surgeon's view (Editorial]. *Semin Thromb Hemost* 1993;19:183.
53. Mammen EF. Coagulation defects in liver disease. *Med Clin North Am* 1994;78:545–554.
54. Dzik WH, Arkin CF, Jenkins RL, et al. Fibrinolysis during liver transplantation in humans: role of tissue-type plasminogen activator. *Blood* 1988;71:1090–1095.
55. Porte RJ, Knot EA, Bontempo FA. Hemostasis in liver transplantation. *Gastroenterology* 1989;97:488–496.
56. Porte RJ, Bontempo FA, Knot EA, et al. Systemic effects of tissue plasminogen activator-associated fibrinolysis and its relation to thrombin generation in orthotopic liver transplantation. *Transplantation* 1989;47:478–491.
57. Legnani C, Palareti G, Rodorigo G, et al. Protease activities, as well as plasminogen activators, contribute to the "lytic" state during orthotopic liver transplantation. *Transplantation* 1993; 56:568–582.
58. Kang YG, Martin DJ, Marquez J, et al. Intraoperative changes in blood coagulation and thromboelastographic monitoring in liver transplantation. *Anesth Analg* 1985;64:888–899.
59. McNicol PL, Liu G, Harely ID, et al. Patterns of coagulopathy during liver transplantation: experience with the first 75 cases using thromboelastography. *Anesth Crit Care* 1994;22:659–663.
60. Scudamore CH, Randall TE, Jewesson PJ, et al. Aprotinin reduces the need for blood products during liver transplantation. *Am J Surg* 1995;169:546–558.
61. Llamas P, Cabrera R, Gomez-Arnau J, et al. Hemostasis and blood requirements in orthotopic liver transplantation with and without high-dose aprotinin. *Haematologica* 1998;83:338–346.
62. Porte RJ, Molenaar IQ, Begliomini B, et al. Aprotinin and transfusion requirements in orthotopic liver transplantation: a multicenter randomized double-blind study. *Lancet* 2000;355: 1303–1309.
63. Kufner RP. Use of antifibrinolytics in orthotopic liver transplantation. *Transplant Proc* 2000;32:636–637.
64. Boylan JK, Klinck JR, Sandler AN, et al. Tranexamic acid reduces blood loss, transfusion requirements and coagulation

factor use in primary orthotopic liver transplantation. *Anesthesiology* 1996;85:1043–1056.

65. Scherer R, Kabatnik M, Erhard J, et al. The influence of antithrombin III (AT III) substitution to supranormal activities on systematic procoagulant turnover in patients with end-stage chronic liver disease. *Intens Care Med* 1997;23: 1150–1158.
66. Harmon DC, Demirjan Z, Ellman L, et al. Disseminated intravascular coagulation in the peritoneovenous shunt. *Ann Intern Med* 1979;90:774–786.
67. Lerner RG, Nelson JC, Corines P, et al. Disseminated intravascular coagulation: complications of peritoneovenous shunts. *JAMA* 1978;240:2064–2069.
68. Baele G, Rasquin K, Barbier F. Coagulant, fibrinolytic and aggregating activity in ascites fluid. *Am J Gastroenterol* 1986; 81:440–451.
69. Schölmerich P, Zimmermann U, Kottgen E, et al. Proteases and antiproteases related to the coagulation system in plasma and ascites: prediction of coagulation disorders in ascites retransfusion. *J Hepatol* 1988;6:359–369.
70. Salem HH, Koutts J, Handley C, et al. The aggregation of human platelets by ascitic fluid: a possible mechanism for disseminated intravascular coagulation complicating LeVeen shunts. *Am J Hematol* 1981;11:153–157.
71. Holm A, Halpern NB, Aldrete JS. Peritoneovenous shunt for intractable ascites of hepatic, nephrogenic, and malignant causes. *Am J Surg* 1989;158:162–178.
72. Harper PL, Edgar PF, Luddington RJ, et al. Protein C deficiency and portal thrombosis in liver transplantation in children. *Lancet* 1988;2:924–925.
73. Stahl RL, Duncan A, Hooks MA, et al. A hypercoagulable state follows orthotopic liver transplantation. *Hepatology* 1990;12: 553–560.
74. Voili F, Ferro D, Basili S, et al. Ongoing prothrombotic state in the portal circulation of cirrhotic patients. *Thromb Haemost* 1997;77:44–47.
75. Amitrano L, Brancaccio V, Guardascione MA, et al. Inherited coagulation disorders in cirrhotic patients with portal vein thrombosis. *Hepatology* 2000;31:345–348.
76. Roberts HR, Monroe DM III, Hoffman M. Molecular biology and biochemistry of the coagulation factors and pathways of hemostasis. In: Beutler E, Lichtman MA, Coller BS, et al., eds. *Williams hematology. 6th ed.* New York: McGraw-Hill, 2001: 1409–1434.
77. Mammen EF. Acquired coagulation protein defects. In: Bick RL, ed. *Hematology: clinical and laboratory practice. Vol 2.* St. Louis: Mosby, 1993:1449–1461.
78. Andrassy K. Hämostaseologische Störungen in der Urämie und während der Dialyse: Pathogenese, Diagnose und Therapie. In: Müller-Berghaus G, Pötzsch B, eds. *Hämostaseologie*. Berlin: Springer, 1999:489–492.
79. Stewardt JH, Castaldi PA. Uremic bleeding: a reversible platelet defect corrected by dialysis. *Q J Med* 1967;36:409–419.
80. Horowitz HI, Stein IM, Cohen BD, et al. Further studies on the platelet-inhibitory effect of guanidinosuccinic acid and its role in uremic bleeding. *Am J Med* 1970;49:336–345.
81. Noris M, Remuzzi G. Uremic bleeding: closing the circle after 30 years of controversies? *Blood* 1999;94:2569–2574.
82. Harter HR, Burch JW, Majerus PW, et al. Prevention of thrombosis in patients on hemodialysis by low-dose aspirin. *N Engl J Med* 1979;301:577–579.
83. Domoto DT, Bauman JE, Joist JH. Combined aspirin and sulfinpyrazone in the prevention of recurrent hemodialysis vascular access thrombosis. *Thromb Res* 1991;62:737–743.
84. Zuckerman GR, Cornette GL, Clouse RE, et al. Upper gastrointestinal bleeding in patients with chronic renal failure. *Ann Intern Med* 1985;103:588–592.
85. Gabriel SF, Jaakkimainen L, Bombardier C. Risk for serious gastrointestinal complications related to the use of nonsteroidal anti-inflammatory drugs: a meta-analysis. *Ann Intern Med* 1991;115:787–794.
86. Eknoyam G, Waksman SJ, Glueck HI, et al. Platelet function in renal failure. *N Engl J Med* 1969;280:677–681.
87. Gordge MP, Faint RW, Rylance PB, et al. Platelet function and the bleeding time in progressive renal failure. *Thromb Haemost* 1988;60:83–87.
88. Fernandez F, Goudable C, Sie P, et al. Low hematocrit and prolonged bleeding time in uraemic patients: effect of red cell transfusions. *Br J Haematol* 1985;59:139–148.
89. Moia M, Vizzotto L, Cattaneo M, et al. Improvement in the haemostatic defect of uraemia after treatment with recombinant human erythropoietin. *Lancet* 1987;2:1227–1229.
90. Casonato A, Pontara E, Vertolli UP, et al. Plasma and platelet von Willebrand factor abnormalities in patients with uremia: lack of correlation with uremic bleeding. *Clin Appl Thromb Hemost* 2001;7:81–86.
91. Tagaki M, Wada H, Mukai K, et al. Increased activated protein C:protein C inhibitor complex and decreased protein C inhibitor levels in patients with chronic renal failure on maintenance hemodialysis. *Clin Appl Thromb Hemost* 1999;5: 113–116.
92. Inoue A, Wada H, Tagaki M, et al. Hemostatic abnormalities in patients with thrombotic complications on maintenance hemodialysis. *Clin Appl Thromb Hemost* 2000;6:100–103.
93. Saltissi D, Morgan C, Werthuyzen T, et al. Comparison of low-molecular weight heparin (enoxaparin sodium) and standard unfractionated heparin for hemodialysis anticoagulation. *Nephrol Dial Transplant* 1999;14:2698–2703.
94. Sagedal S, Hartmann A, Sundstrom K, et al. A single dose of dalteparin effectively prevents clotting during hemodialysis. *Nephrol Dial Transplant* 1999;14:1943–1947.
95. Gerlach AT, Pickworth KK, Seth SK, et al. Enoxaparin and bleeding complications: a review of patients with and without renal insufficiency. *Pharmacotherapy* 2000;20:771–775.
96. Bucha E, Nowak G, Czerwinski R, et al. r-Hirudin as anticoagulant in regular hemodialysis therapy: finding of therapeutic r-hirudin blood/plasma concentrations and respective dosages. *Clin Appl Thromb Hemost* 1999;5:164–170.
97. Janson PA, Jubelirer SJ, Weinstein MS, et al. Treatment of bleeding tendency in uremia with cryoprecipitate. *N Engl J Med* 1980;303:1318–1322.
98. Livio M, Gotti E, Marchesi D, et al. Uraemic bleeding: role of anaemia and beneficial effect of red cell transfusions. *Lancet* 1982;2:1013–1015.
99. Vigano G, Benigni A, Mendogni D, et al. Recombinant human erythropoietin to correct uremic bleeding. *Am J Kidney Dis* 1991;18:44–50.
100. Van Geet C, Hauglustaine D, Vanrusselt M, et al. Haemostatic effects of recombinant human erythropoietin in chronic hemodialysis patients. *Thromb Haemost* 1989;61:117–121.
101. Llach F. Hypercoagulability, renal vein thrombosis and other complications of nephrotic syndrome. *Kidney Int* 1985;28: 424–436.
102. Remuzzi G, Mecca G, Marchesi D, et al. Platelet hyperaggregability and the nephrotic syndrome. *Thromb Res* 1979;16: 345–351.
103. Jackson CA, Greaves M, Patterson AD, et al. Relationship between platelet aggregation, thromboxane synthesis and albumin concentration in nephrotic syndrome. *Br J Haematol* 1982; 52:67–72.

104. Vaiziri ND. Nephrotic syndrome and coagulation and fibrinolytic abnormalities. *Am J Nephrol* 1983;3:1–10.
105. Kauffman RH, Veltkamp JJ, van Tilburg NH, et al. Acquired antithrombin III deficiency and thrombosis in the nephrotic syndrome. *Am J Med* 1978;65:607–612.
106. Cosio FG, Harker C, Batard MA, et al. Plasma concentrations of the natural anticoagulants protein C and protein S in patients with proteinuria. *J Lab Clin Med* 1985;106:218–224.
107. Ariëns RAS, Moia M, Rivolto E, et al. High levels of tissue factor pathway inhibitor in patients with nephrotic proteinuria. *Thromb Haemost* 1999;82:1020–1023.
108. Salem HH, Whitworth JA, Koutts J. Hypercoagulation in glomerulonephritis. *Br Med J* 1981;282:2083–2086.
109. Domadio JV Jr, Anderson CF, Mitchel JCI, et al. Membranoproliferative glomerulonephritis: a prospective clinical trial of platelet-inhibitor therapy. *N Engl J Med* 1984;310:1421–1427.
110. Cameron JS. Platelets in glomerular disease. *Annu Rev Med* 1984;35:175–192.
111. Tipping PG, Dowling JP, Haldsworth SR. Glomerular procoagulant activity in human proliferative glomerulonephritis. *J Clin Invest* 1988;81:119–124.
112. Colucci M, Semeraro N, Montmurro P, et al. Urinary procoagulant and fibrinolytic activity in human glomerulonephritis: relationship with renal function. *Kidney Int* 1991;69:1213–1218.
113. Grandaliano G, Cesualdo L, Ranieri E, et al. Tissue factor, plasminogen activator inhibitor-1, and thrombin receptor expression in human crescentic glomerulonephritis. *Am J Kidney Dis* 2000;35:726–738.

Disorders of Thrombosis and Hemostasis: Clinical and Laboratory Practice, Third Edition, edited by Rodger L. Bick.
Lippincott Williams & Wilkins, Philadelphia © 2002

9

THROMBOTIC AND HEMORRHAGIC PROBLEMS DURING CARDIOVASCULAR BYPASS SURGERY AND CARDIOVASCULAR PROCEDURES

RODGER L. BICK

PHYSIOLOGY OF HEMOSTASIS

The characteristic of the circulation by which blood remains fluid within the vasculature and the ability of the system to prevent excessive blood loss on injury is *hemostasis*. Three anatomic compartments, *tissues* (vasculature), *blood cells* (platelets), and *plasma* (proteins), are involved in a series of delicately orchestrated biochemical interactions that, under normal conditions, modulate responses in a manner able to maintain a delicately tuned equilibrium of hemostasis.

The three specific hemostatic compartments are (a) the platelets, which must be normal in both number and function; (b) the plasma proteins, which include procoagulants, anticoagulants, and fibrinolytic proteins; and (c) the vasculature (1).

During injury, vessels constrict and generate compounds that activate platelets and plasma proteins. Platelets adhere and cohere at sites of injury, initiating a complex process that promotes further platelet aggregation, vascular constriction, and activation of coagulation components, resulting in fibrin formation. Many chemical signals designed to initiate or terminate various events serve as a system of checks and balances. Disturbances (inherited or acquired) are reflected in inappropriate responses predisposing to either thrombosis or hemorrhage, and sometimes both (1).

To appreciate the complexity of the inter- and intracompartmental interactions, the normal hemostatic aspects of the vasculature, platelets and plasma proteins are discussed separately. The reader is encouraged, however, to maintain a perspective of integrated function because this is the basis for efficient diagnosis of hemostatic dysfunction and the mainstay for the development of targeted pharmacologic (therapeutic) agents (1).

R. L. Bick: Department of Medicine and Pathology, University of Texas Southwestern Medical Center; Dallas Thrombosis/Hemostasis Clinical Center; ThromboCare Laboratories, Dallas, Texas.

Vascular Function

Normal vascular morphology comprises three discrete layers: the intima, the media, and the adventitia. The intima consists of a monolayer of nonthrombogenic endothelial cells and an internal elastic membrane. The media consists of smooth muscle cells; the size of the media will vary depending on the type (arterial/venous) and size of the vasculature. The adventitia comprises an external elastic lamina or membrane and supportive connective tissue.

Figure 9.1 illustrates the first event occurring when endothelial sloughing occurs (induced by a variety of insults—triggers—including acidosis, hypoxia, endotoxin, circulating antigen–antibody complexes, etc.) with the subsequent exposure of subendothelial collagen and basement membrane. Platelets are immediately recruited to fill this endothelial gap (1–5), with the goal of forming a primary hemostatic plug, thereby stopping blood from leaving the vascular compartment. Subsequent reparative events include smooth muscle or other cells from the media migrating through the internal elastic membrane, and differentiating into new nonthrombogenic endothelial cells. If this is a one-time event, the reparative process is completed. However, sometimes forming the primary hemostatic plug may constitute an overwhelming event leading to a large platelet/fibrin thrombus, and impedance of blood flow with resultant end-organ damage through ischemia. This is particularly alarming when the process evolves repeatedly in the same area over a protracted period. As smooth muscle or other cells differentiate and migrate into the intima, compounds are released, attracting macrophages, which, in turn, ingest cholesterol and other materials, the fundamental construct of an atherosclerotic plaque (6–9). Potential

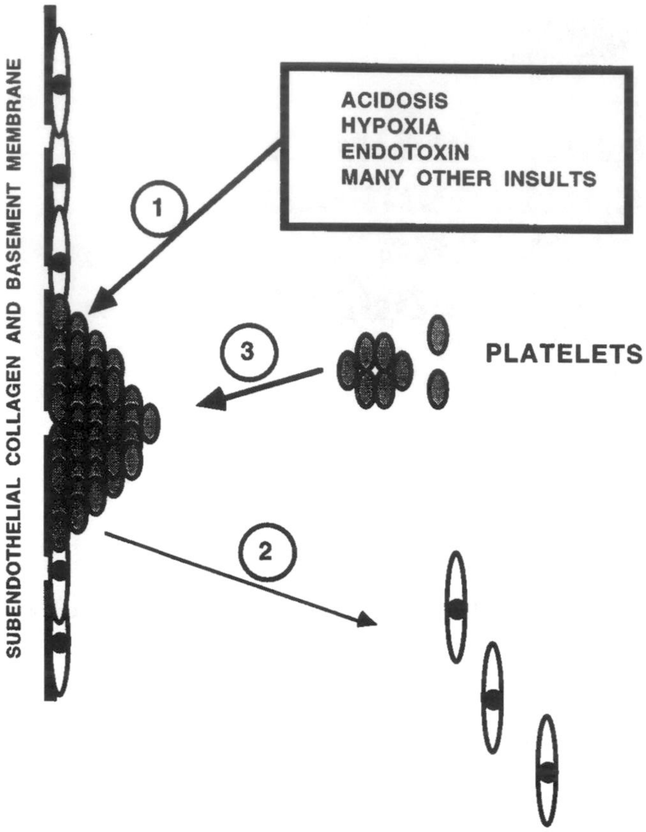

FIGURE 9.1. Platelets filling endothelial gaps.

events consequent to vascular injury are summarized in Fig. 9.2. *Permeability*, *fragility*, and *vasoconstriction* are properties of the vasculature. Increased permeability results in blood leaving the vessel and will manifest as petechiae and purpura or, sometimes, large ecchymoses. Increased fragility results in rupture of the vasculature with ensuing petechiae, purpura (especially in the integument and mucous membranes), and large ecchymoses with potential serious deep-tissue hemorrhage. *Vasoconstriction* is under local, neural, and humoral control. Most important is humoral control effected primarily by compounds released from platelets including epinephrine, norepinephrine, adenosine diphosphate (ADP), kinins, and thromboxanes. Fibrin(ogen) degradation products (FDPs) also modulate vasoconstriction (10,11).

Endothelial cells are contractile, responding when stimulated by histamine, serotonin, kinins, or thromboxanes. The endothelial cell has been identified as a primary site of the biosynthesis of critical hemostatic proteins, specifically von Willebrand factor, plasminogen activator, thrombomodulin inhibitor of active protein C, and prostaglandins (12–16). Platelet attraction and subsequent activation happens when subendothelial basement membrane or collagen is exposed. This also can directly activate factor XII to factor XIIa as well as factor XI to factor Xia (17,18). Clearly, any of these processes, if left unmodulated, can give rise to a generalized activation of the coagulation system (19–23).

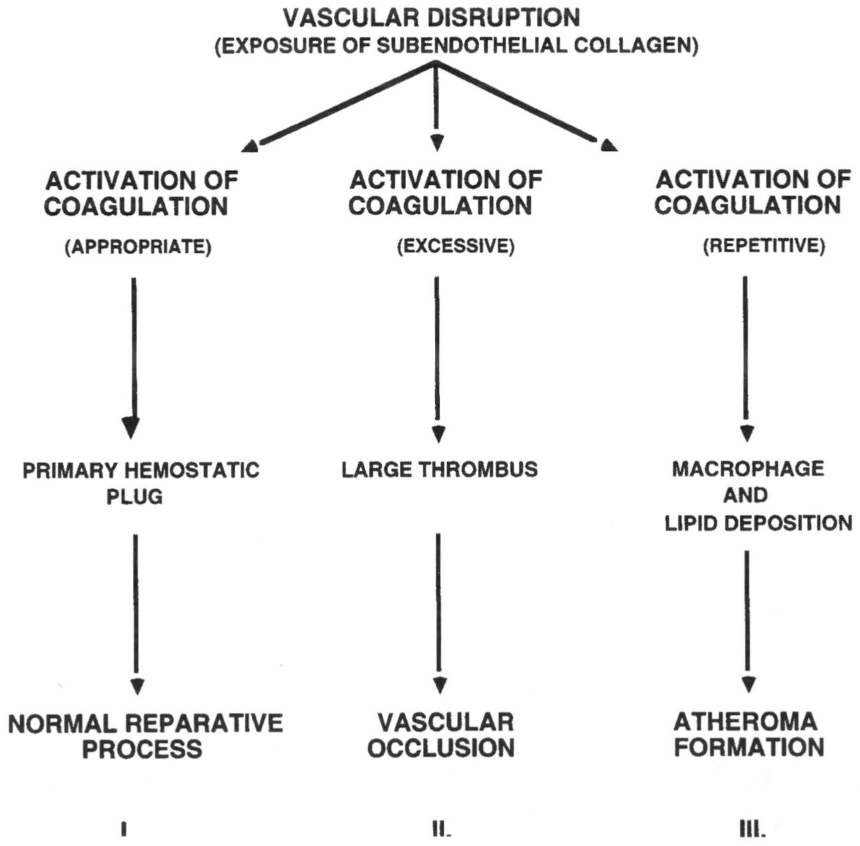

FIGURE 9.2. Vascular damage and consequences (endothelial cell sloughing).

Platelet Function

Morphologically, the platelet can be envisioned as comprising three primary zones: (a) peripheral zone, (b) sol–gel zone, and (c) organelle zone (1,10). The peripheral zone comprises an extramembranous glycocalyx, inside of which is a plasma membrane, similar to other trilamellar cellular plasma membranes. Under this membrane is an open canalicular system. The sol–gel zone comprises microtubules and microfilaments, a dense tubular system that contains primarily adenine nucleotides and calcium ions. In the sol–gel zone also is the contractile protein, thrombosthenin, which is similar to actomyosin. The organelle zone comprises dense bodies, α granules, mitochondria, and the usual array of organelles found in other cellular systems, including lysosomes and endoplasmic reticulum. The α granules contain and release fibrinogen and lysosomal enzymes, whereas dense bodies contain and release adenine nucleotides, serotonin, catecholamines, and platelet factor 4 (1,24–26).

An adequate number of platelets must be present for normal platelet function, in vivo and in vitro. This is usually defined as approximately 100×10^9/L. With a platelet count of less than 100×10^9/L, abnormal laboratory test results are noted; for example, prolonged template bleeding times and abnormal platelet-aggregation profiles. For normal function, platelets require (a) adequate energy metabolism; (b) an adequate number of (and contents of) storage granules, capable of releasing their contents when appropriate stimuli are presented; (c) cationic proteins, such as thrombosthenin; (d) membrane receptors responsive to appropriate stimuli; (e) divalent cations, the most important of which is calcium; and of course, (f) adequate physical conditions, such as pH and temperature (1).

Table 9.1 summarizes the common platelet proteins. Some are not platelet specific and include many plasma proteins found in or on the surface of platelets; these include clotting factors II, V, VII, VIII, IX, X, XI, XII, and XIII (27). Sometimes these proteins are found in a slightly different molecular form in platelets when compared with the molecular species found in plasma (for example, factor XIII). Platelet-specific proteins also are present, including thrombosthenin, platelet factor 4, β-thromboglobulin, and cathepsin A (1).

Table 9.2 lists the seven platelet-specific factors that have been identified and characterized. The essential of these are platelet factor 3 (platelet thromboplastin/phospholipid) and platelet factor 4 (antiheparin factor), which has become an important molecular marker of platelet reactivity (1,28–30).

Compounds released from platelets include the biogenic amines serotonin, catecholamines, and histamine; the adenine nucleotides cyclic adenosine monophosphate (AMP), adenosine diphosphate (ADP), and adenosine triphosphate (ATP); various enzyme activities including acid hydrolases; specific ions including calcium, magnesium, and potassium; and platelet factors, including platelet factor 4, β-thromboglobulin, and platelet factor 3. Other proteins including fibrinogen, other clotting factors, and albumin also are released from platelets during activation.

Multiple stimuli induce platelet activation (1,31,32). Potent inducers of a platelet-release reaction, besides subendothelial collagen and basement membrane, are thrombin, soluble fibrin monomer, some FDPs (especially fragment X), endotoxin, circulating antigen–antibody complexes, γ-globulin–coated surfaces, various viruses, ADP, catecholamines, and free fatty acids (1,33–36). Many proteolytic enzymes including trypsin, snake venoms, papain, and elastase are used in vitro to induce platelet release. Other in vitro release reaction techniques include the use of centrifugation, cold fracture, latex particles, carbon particles, kaolin, and celite (1).

With activation, platelets contract and form pseudopods. During contraction, the numerous intraplatelet compounds and granules are concentrated at the center of the platelet, where organelle membranes are disrupted, and their contents are released and subsequently transported outside the platelet via the open canalicular system. These compounds then interact with neighboring platelet membrane receptors or adjacent endothelium, causing further platelet activation, thereby amplifying the process. Pseudopod formation enhances platelet–surface interactions (adhesion) and platelet–platelet interaction (cohesion) (1).

A summary of platelet function is presented in Fig. 9.3 (1). The process of platelet adhesion refers to a platelet

TABLE 9.1. PLATELET PROTEINS

Nonspecific (plasma) proteins
Fibrinogen
Factors II, V, VII, VIII, IX, X, XII, and XIII
Albumin
Plasminogen
Complement components
Specific platelet proteins
Thrombosthenin
Platelet glycoproteins
Platelet factors 2 and 4
Platelet antiplasmin
Cathepsin A
β-Thromboglobulin

TABLE 9.2. NAMED PLATELET FACTORS

Platelet factor 1: Coagulation factor V
Platelet factor 2: Thromboplastic material
Platelet factor 3: Platelet thromboplastin (phospholipid)
Platelet factor 4: Antiheparin factor
Platelet factor 5: Fibrinogen coagulant factor
Platelet factor 6: Antifibrinolytic factor
Platelet factor 7: Platelet cothromboplastin

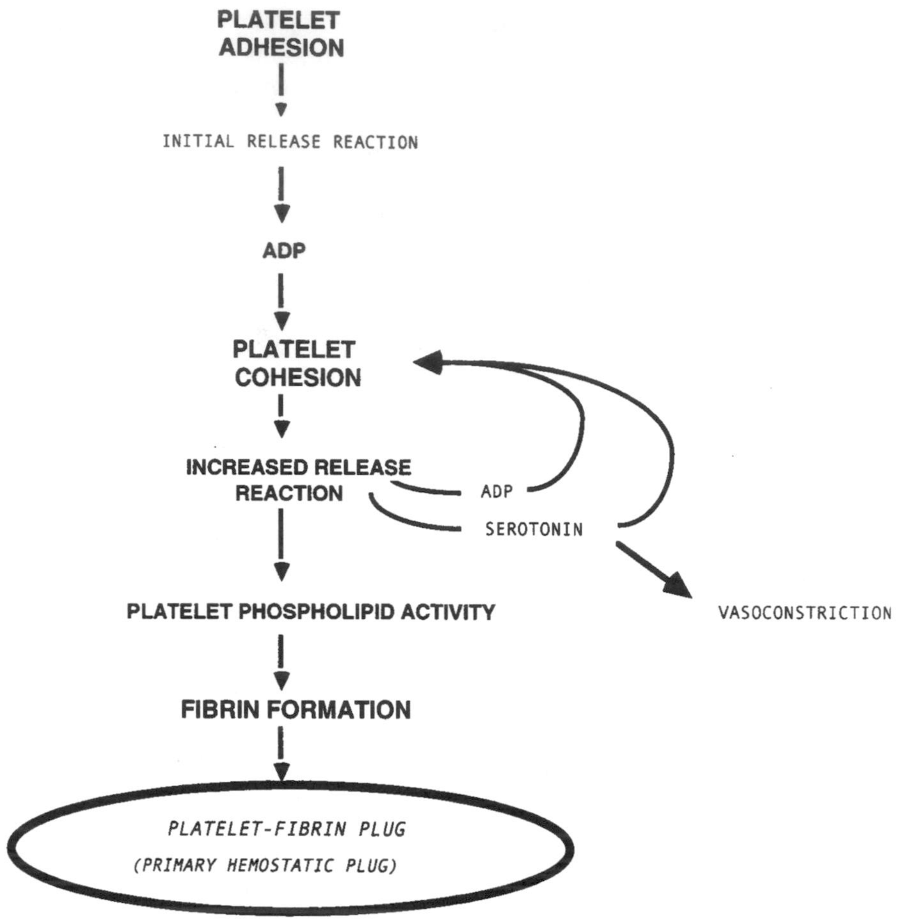

FIGURE 9.3. Simplified platelet function.

adhering to something other than another platelet (for example, an artificial surface, or collagen/basement membrane exposed on injury). This results in an initial release reaction generating ADP. This is a reversible process and accounts for the primary wave on an aggregation pattern ("primary reversible aggregation"). As the concentration of ADP increases, platelet cohesion happens. This refers to platelets sticking to each other. As the process continues, released compounds (including serotonin) not only activate adjacent platelets but also induce vascular constriction. In this advanced phase of activation, there follows an irreversible conformational change in the platelet membrane, making available platelet factor 3 (platelet membrane phospholipid) activity. This material serves as a primary "surface" mediating the formation of complexes in the coagulation protein sequence. This irreversible process accounts for the secondary wave seen in a platelet-aggregation pattern. In vivo, the result is the eventual formation of a platelet/fibrin thrombus or "primary hemostatic plug," the function and integrity of which is facilitated by vasoconstriction (1).

Abbreviated intraplatelet functional biochemical sequences are outlined in Fig. 9.4. The key modulator of intraplatelet function is cyclic AMP (1,37,38). The role of this compound is to combine with a cyclic AMP–dependent protein to generate a kinase activity, the role of which is to phosphorylate a receptor protein, which then binds (sequesters) calcium ions, rendering the platelet hypoaggregable and hypoadhesable. Epinephrine, thrombin, collagen, and serotonin inhibit the enzyme adenylate cyclase, which is responsible for the conversion of ATP to cyclic AMP. This inhibition results in a decrease in kinase concentration, a decrease in phosphorylated receptor protein, and an increase in ionized (free) calcium, which renders the platelet hyperaggregable (1).

Balancing this biochemical sequence is the enzyme phosphodiesterase (39,40), responsible for destroying cyclic AMP. Agents such as dipyridamole, caffeine, and papaverine inhibit this enzyme, resulting in decreased free calcium, making the platelet hypofunctional. Yet another mechanism for regulating the availability of ionized calcium may relate to the activity of membrane-bound alkaline phosphatase, which is responsible for dephosphorylation of the receptor protein–Ca^{2+} complex (1).

The roles of prostaglandins and derivatives in platelet function are summarized in Fig. 9.5. Platelet and endothelial cell membrane phospholipids are converted into arachidonic acid by the enzyme phospholipase A_2 (41), which is activated by both thrombin and collagen. Arachidonic acid

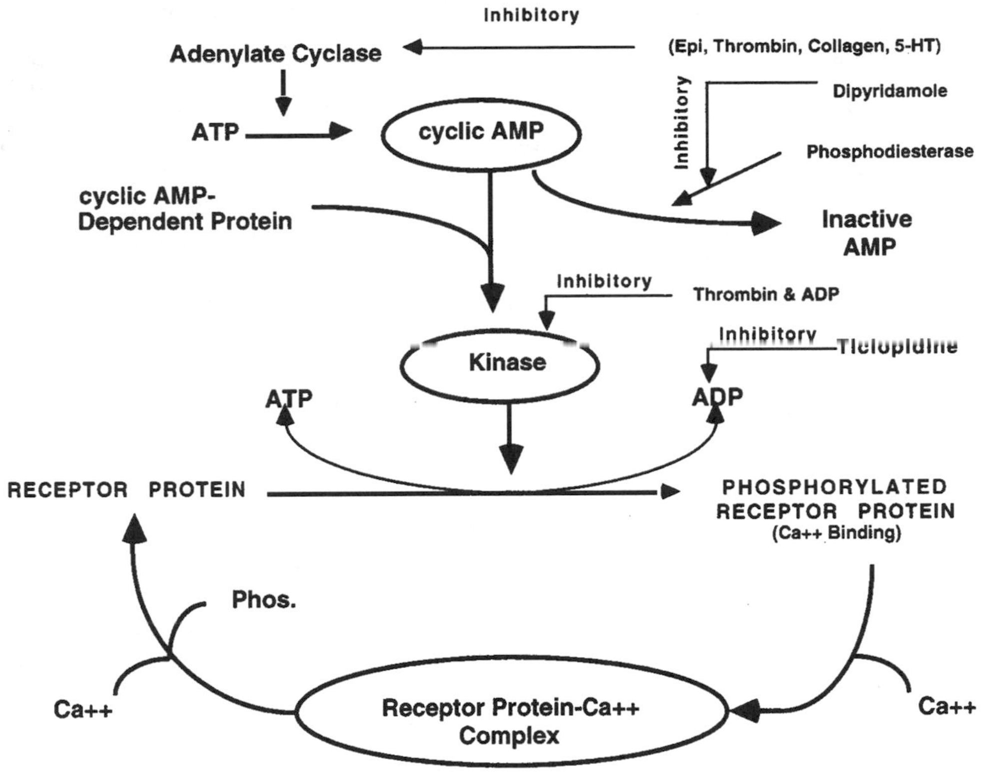

FIGURE 9.4. Intraplatelet biochemistry.

is converted into prostaglandin intermediates, prostaglandin G_2 (PGG_2), and prostaglandin H_2 (PGH_2) by the enzyme cyclooxygenase (1). In the platelet membrane, thromboxane synthetase converts PGH_2 into thromboxane A_2, a potent inhibitor of adenylate cyclase, therefore one of the most potent aggregating agents yet described (1). Thromboxane A_2 also has very potent vasoconstricting activity. In the endothelial cell, and in some subendothelial muscle cells, prostacyclin synthetase converts PGH_2 into prostacyclin, which is a potent stimulator of adenylate

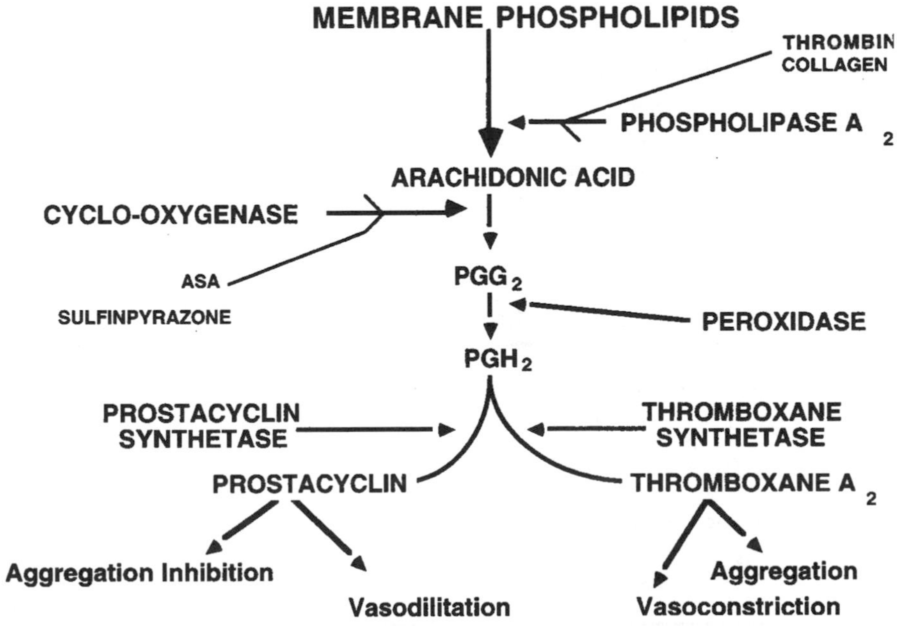

FIGURE 9.5. Prostaglandins in platelet/endothelial function.

cyclase, and therefore a very potent aggregation inhibitor and a potent vasodilator (42,43).

This represents an exquisitely balanced biologic system whereby platelets are synthesizing and releasing into the adjacent milieu a compound (thromboxane A_2) that promotes platelet function, and the adjacent endothelium is synthesizing and releasing prostacyclin, which inhibits platelet function (1). Therefore the predisposition to bleeding or thrombosis may depend on the relative equilibrium between these two compounds (1).

Cyclooxygenase is inhibited by aspirin and sulfinpyrazone, two popular antiplatelet agents (44). Evidence suggests that these two antiplatelet agents function selectively because their activity is directed primarily toward platelets. In their presence, endothelium also continues to synthesize prostaglandins, but platelets do not. The precise mechanisms for this selectivity have not yet been elucidated.

Platelet interactions with the vasculature (adhesion), with other platelets (cohesion), and with plasma proteins occur at the platelet membrane surface, mediated by various platelet membrane glycoproteins (PMGPs) (1,45). The major PMGPs and their functions, where known, are summarized in Table 9.3. PMGP Ia is complexed to PMGP IIa and functions to help platelets adhere to subendothelial collagen, independent of von Willebrand factor (46,47). PMGP Ib has been associated with multiple functions. It has a molecular weight of about 170,000 and comprises an α and a β subunit, one of which fixes it to the platelet membrane. PMGP Ib exists in complex with PMGP IX and V (48). PMGP Ib and IX are absent from platelets in Bernard–Soulier syndrome (49). PMGP Ib serves as a receptor for von Willebrand factor, the first step in platelet adhesion to subendothelial surfaces (47,50,51). PMGP Ib also is the receptor for quinine and quinidine drug-dependent antibody, which is present in quinine and quinidine-induced thrombocytopenia (52). PMGP Ib also is a part of the thrombin-receptor complex of platelets and, although its role is not clearly defined, PMGP V is of vital importance in this mechanism of platelet activation (53). PMGP IIb/IIIa complex is found in platelet α granules, as well as on the membrane (54). PMGP IIb has a molecular weight of about 125,000, and PMGP IIIa, about 93,000. Both appear to be subunits of a single glycoprotein, heavily dependent on calcium for binding of the complex (55). PMGP IIb/IIIa is absent or markedly reduced in Glanzmann thrombasthenia, is the binding site for fibrinogen, and serves as the apparent binding site for platelet antigen 1 antibody (56,57). The binding of fibrinogen to PMGP IIb/IIIa is needed for optimal ADP-induced platelet aggregation. Glycoprotein G, also called thrombospondin, has a molecular weight of about 180,000 and is partly responsible for thrombin- and collagen-induced aggregation (58,59). PMGPs Ic and IIa have been identified but are without known function in hemostasis.

Plasma Protein Function

Plasma protein function in hemostasis comprises multiple interactive systems: (a) coagulation, (b) fibrino(geno)lysis, (c) kinin generation, (d) complement activation, and (e) inhibitors for these systems. Although normally not considered an integral part of "hemostasis" pathophysiologically, kinin generation and complement activation assume considerable importance, especially in syndromes of disseminated intravascular coagulation (DIC) (1,60).

The Coagulation Protein System

Coagulation proteins and some synonyms are listed in Table 9.4 (1). The Roman numeral system is most widely used and is preferred. The chromosome location containing genetic information for synthesis of almost all the coagulation factors is known (1,61) and is summarized in Table 9.5. The formation of a fibrin clot is best thought of as consisting of four key reactions involving the generation of several proteolytic enzymes (serine proteases): (a) formation of factor IXa, (b) formation of factor Xa, (c) formation of thrombin, and (d) formation of fibrin (1).

Formation of Factor IXa

The "contact activation" phase of coagulation begins with the generation of active Hageman factor (factor XIIa). "Sur-

TABLE 9.3. PLATELET MEMBRANE GLYCOPROTEINS

Glycoprotein	Function	Characteristic
Ia	von Willebrand–independent receptor for subendothelium	
Ib	von Willebrand receptor	Missing in Bernard–Soulier quinidine-Ab receptor
IIa		
IIb / IIIa	von Willebrand and fibrinogen receptor	Missing in Glanzmann PlA-1 Ab receptor
V	Thrombin receptor	Missing in Bernard–Soulier
IX	Thrombin receptor ?	Missing in Bernard–Soulier

Ab, antibody; PlA-1, platelet antibody type 1.

TABLE 9.4. COAGULATION FACTORS AND SYNONYMS

Factor	Synonym
I	Fibrinogen
II	Prothrombin
V	AC-Globulin
VII	Prothrombin conversion accelerator
VIII:c	Antihemophilic factor
IX	Christmas factor (PTC)
X	Stuart–Prower factor
XI	Thromboplastin antecedent (PTA)
XII	Hageman (contact) factor
XIII	Profibrinoligase
Fletcher factor	Prekallikrein
Fitzgerald factor	HMW Kininogen
Protein C	Xa Inhibitor
Protein S	None

HMW, high molecular weight.

faces" (phospholipids, subendothelial collagen) and kallikrein can convert factor XII to factor XIIa, which in turn converts factor XI into factor XIa (1,62,63). This reaction happens quickly in the presence of high-molecular-weight kininogen (a significantly prolonged activated partial thromboplastin time is noted in its absence) (64). The role of factor XIa, is to convert inactive factor IX (in the presence of calcium ions) to the active form, factor IXa, which is the enzyme responsible for the second key reaction, the generation of factor Xa. Factor XIIa itself converts prekallikrein into kallikrein, which further enhances the generation of more factor XIIa (1,65).

Formation of Factor Xa

The second key reaction involves two major pathways: "intrinsic and extrinsic." Intrinsic formation of factor Xa involves a five-component system: (a) substrate (factor X), (b) enzyme (factor IXa), (c) determiner or cofactor (factor VIII:c), (d) surface (platelet factor 3), and (e) calcium ions (1,66). The complex formed is mediated by calcium ions. The enzyme factor IXa cleaves a peptide from the substrate (factor X), with resultant exposure of an active serine site. Factor Xa is the product of this reaction. Factor VIII:c is modified and rendered dysfunctional in the process (1).

The extrinsic pathway of factor Xa formation involves the participation of "thromboplastin" (tissue factor), factor VII, and calcium ions. Tissue factor is a membrane-bound protein (lipoprotein) existing in a protected state within the plasma membrane of endothelial cells. On injury, it is released into the circulation, where it forms a complex with coagulation factor VII in the presence of calcium ions. The activity of the complex seems to be largely dependent on the concentration of tissue factor. However, the enzymatic activity responsible for the proteolytic activation of factor Xa resides in the factor VII molecule (1,67,68). Aprotinin, commonly used in cardiac surgery, has been shown to inhibit the factor VIIa–tissue factor complex (69).

TABLE 9.5. CHROMOSOMAL LOCATION CONTAINING COAGULATION FACTOR INFORMATION

Factor	Inheritance	Chromosome	Region
I	A.D.	4	q26–31
II	A.D	11	p11–q12
V	A.R.	1	q21–25
VII	A.R.	13	q34
VIII:c	S.L.R.	X	q28
vWF	A.D.	12	p12–13
IX	S.L.R.	X	q27
X	A.R.	13	q34
XI	A.R.	4	q35
XII	A.R.	5	q33
XIII	A.D.	6	p24–25
AT-III	A.D.	1	p23
Protein C	A.D.	2	q13–14
Protein S	A.D.	3	p21
Plasminogen	A.D.	6	q26–27
t-PA	A.D.	8	p12
t-PA-I-1	A.D.	7	q21–22
t-PA-I-2	A.D.	18	q21–22
Antiplasmin	A.R.	18	?
Fletcher	A.R.	?	?
Fitzgerald	A.R.	?	?
Heparin cofactor-II	A.D.	22	?

Inheritance, usual mode of inheritance; A.D., autosomal dominant; A.R., autosomal recessive; S.L.R., sex-linked recessive; t-PA, tissue plasminogen activators; AT, antithrombin; vWF, von Willebrand factor.

Factor VII exists in plasma as a single-chain glycoprotein with close structural homology to prothrombin, factor IX, and factor X. Contrary to its analogues, however, factor VII is not a zymogen in the true sense, because it has proteolytic activity, although to a limited extent. In the presence of thrombin or factor Xa and lipids and calcium ions, this activity may be increased as much as 400-fold and is accompanied by the formation of a two-polypeptide-chain molecule (1). On further incubation, the two-chain form of factor VII becomes inactive, and the rate of inactivation is dependent on the concentration of factor Xa. It has been proposed that in the activation of factor X by factor VII, the continuing generation of factor Xa results in a "pulse of factor X–converting activity that can quickly disappear" (1,67,68).

Formation of Thrombin

The third key reaction is the formation of thrombin. Similar to the generation of factor Xa (intrinsic), a five-component system is involved: (a) substrate (prothrombin), (b) enzyme (factor Xa), (c) determiner/cofactor (factor V), (d) platelet factor 3, and (e) calcium ions (1,70). These components form a complex on the phospholipid surface and a product [thrombin (factor IIa)], the new enzyme, is generated. Factor V, like factor VIII:c in the previous reaction, is modified and loses biologic activity. The role of the determiner/cofactor in both reactions is to ensure that the correct enzyme and substrate enter into complex formation. The enzymes (thrombin, factor Xa, factor IXa, factor VIIa, and others, such as protein C and protein S) are synthesized in liver parenchymal cells in precursor forms, by a vitamin K–dependent process, which involves the postribosomal attachment of calcium-binding prosthetic groups to the N-terminal region of each of these proteins. The process involves the introduction of an extra carboxyl group on the side chain (γ position) of several glutamic acid residues, forming γ-carboxyglutamic acid (1,71). In the absence of vitamin K, for example, in a patient receiving vitamin K–antagonist therapy (72), although a protein is synthesized, it is dysfunctional. These abnormal vitamin K–dependent factors are called PIVKAs or proteins induced by vitamin K absence/antagonists (1,73).

Formation of Fibrin

The fourth key reaction is the formation of fibrin (1,74). Figure 9.6 summarizes the sequence in the conversion of fibrinogen to fibrin. Thrombin specifically removes fibrinopeptide A and fibrinopeptide B from fibrinogen, a dimeric structure composed of six covalently linked polypeptide chains (two A-α, two B-β, and two γ chains) leaving fibrin monomer (75,76). Fibrin monomer (fibrinogen minus peptides A and B) polymerizes by aggregating end to end and side to side; these aggregates are stabilized by noncovalent bonds. This fibrin is called soluble fibrin because it dissolves in 5 *M* urea or 1% monochloroacetic acid. This is polymerization I. Thrombin, in its multiple roles as a pivotal enzyme in hemostasis (1,74), also activates factor XIII to factor XIIIa. This enzyme, functioning as a transpeptidase, in the presence of calcium ions, introduces isopeptide bonds between the ε-amino groups of certain lysine residues and the γ-carboxyamide groups of certain glutamines in neighboring γ and α chains of the fibrin polymer. This renders the fibrin more elastic and less amenable to lysis (77,78). This is called polymerization II, yielding insoluble fibrin. Figure 9.7 summarizes the pathways of activation for the four key reactions in coagulation (1).

The Fibrinolytic System

With fibrin deposition considered a fundamental mechanism of injured tissue repair, fibrinolysis may be viewed as its physiologic antithesis: the destruction of a fibrin clot (1,79,80). Hemorrhage or thrombosis thus may depend on a delicate balance between the procoagulant system and the fibrinolytic system. Figure 9.8 summarizes the biology of the fibrinolytic system. It consists of a proenzyme, plasminogen, which is converted by many pathways into the active enzyme, *plasmin* (81). Unlike the enzyme thrombin, which has a relatively narrow substrate specificity, the serine protease plasmin has a much broader spectrum of activity, with a number of substrates. Indeed, it hydrolyzes both fibrinogen and fibrin into degradation products (FDPs) and degrades factors V, VIII, IX, and XI, adrenocorticotropic hormone (ACTH), growth hormone, insulin, components of the complement system, and many other proteins

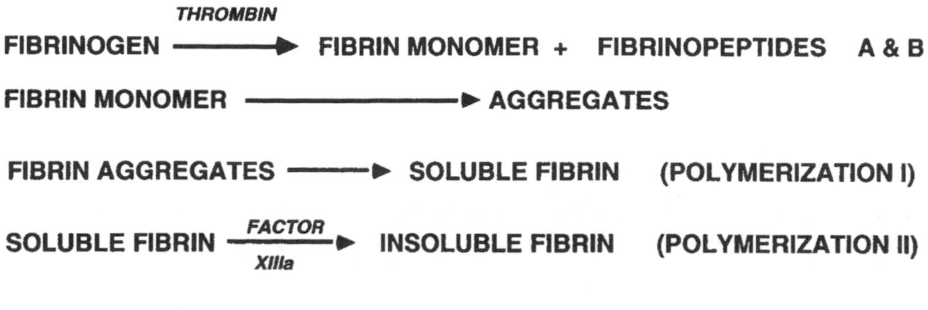

FIGURE 9.6. The conversion of fibrinogen to fibrin.

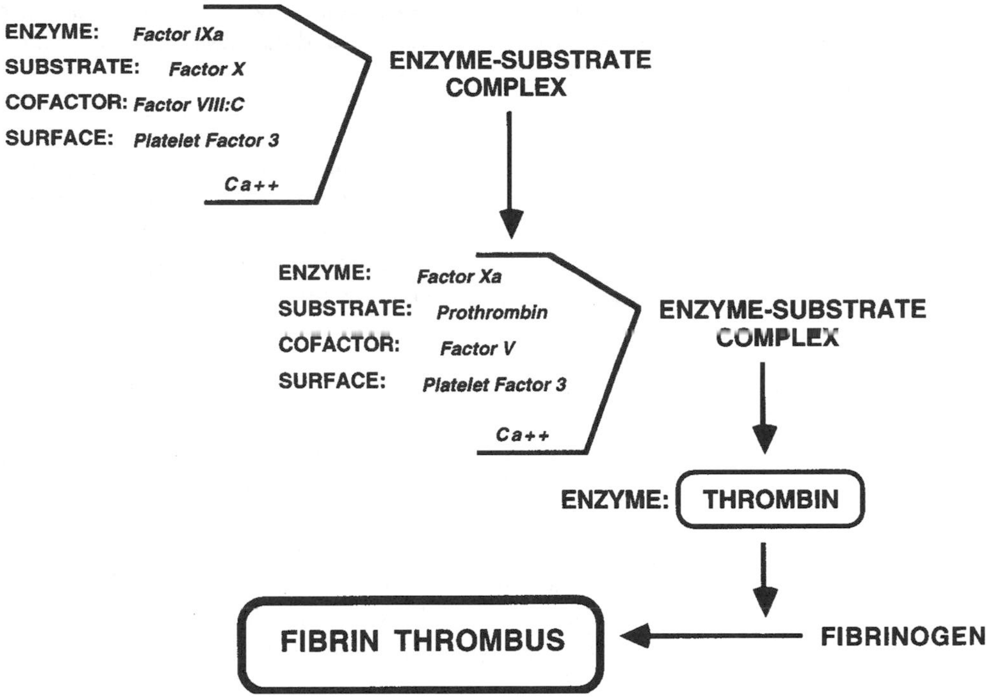

FIGURE 9.7. Summary of the key reactions in final fibrin formation.

(82–84). There are two recognized and well-characterized physiologic activation pathways of the fibrinolytic system. A primary one involves endothelial cell–derived plasminogen activator (t-PA), which converts plasminogen to plasmin directly (85). Another, probably of less physiologic significance, involves factor XIIa (generated by many triggers), which converts a proactivator (prekallikrein) into an activator (kallikrein), which, in turn, converts plasminogen into plasmin (86–88).

The fibrinolytic system is modulated by many inhibitors. α_2-Antiplasmin is an extraordinarily rapid inhibitor of plasmin activity (1,79,89). Although present in

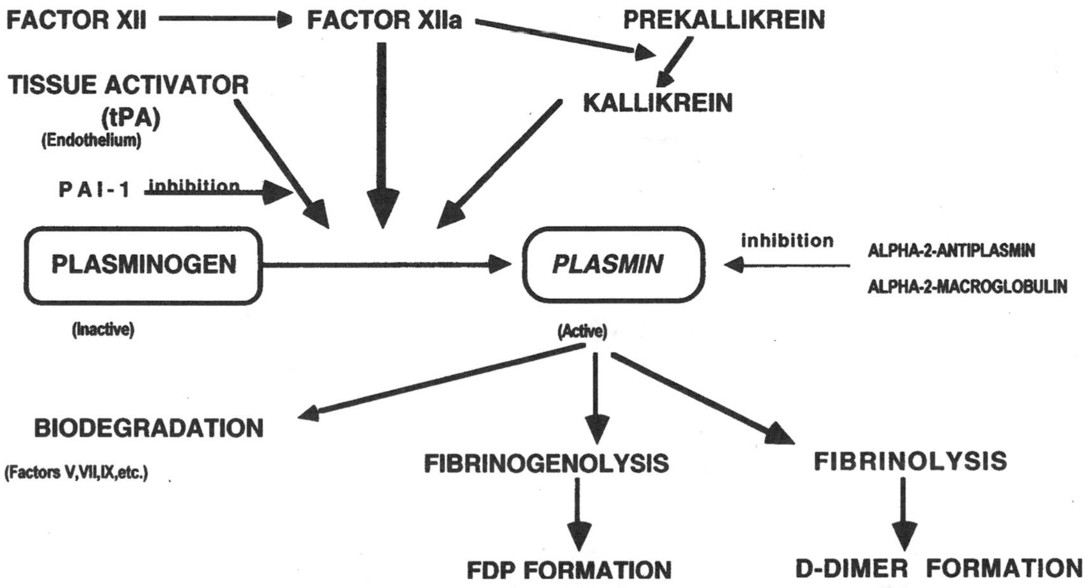

FIGURE 9.8. Physiology of the fibrinolytic system. *PAI-1*, plasminogen activator inhibitor type 1; *FDP*, fibrinogen degradation product.

very low concentration in plasma, α_2-antiplasmin, with its extraordinary affinity for plasmin (resulting in an irreversible covalent complex), is the primary candidate for the major regulator of fibrinolysis in vivo. There are several inhibitors of t-PA (90,91), including plasminogen activator inhibitors types 1 and 2 (PAI-1 and PAI-2). PAI-1 is the primary modulator (1). A number of cells produce this protein, including platelets, supporting the hypothesis that at sites of injury, platelet aggregation facilitates the survival of the fibrin and thus the integrity of the hemostatic plug (1,92). Aprotinin is a potent exogenous (pharmacologic) inhibitor of plasmin (93).

In contrast to thrombin, which cleaves fibrinopeptides A and B from the amino terminus of fibrinogen, creating fibrin monomer, plasmin begins to degrade fibrin(ogen) at the carboxy terminus of the A-α chain and continues to further hydrolyze the matrix in various other loci, yielding soluble degradation products. Figure 9.9 depicts the characterized FDPs (1). These are illustrated in descending order of molecular size, with fibrinogen having a molecular weight of approximately 340,000; fragment X, approximately 265,000; fragment Y, approximately 155,000; fragment D, approximately 95,000; and fragment E, about 50,000. The presence of FDPs in the circulation may seriously compromise hemostasis by interference with fibrin monomer polymerization and platelet function (1,92,94,95).

Complement Activation

Whereas complement activation is generally not considered an integral part of the hemostatic system, its role in the pathophysiology of thrombohemorrhagic disorders is of considerable importance (1). It is a multimolecular self-assembling system constituting the primary humoral mediator of inflammation and tissue damage (1,96,97). It involves a series of sequential reactions similar to the coagulation system and is depicted in Fig. 9.10 (1). A primary "classic" activation pathway involves the activation of C1 by antigen–antibody complexes, and an "alternate" (properdin) activation pathway involves the direct activation of C3. The activation of C1 through C5 is called the "activation phase," and the activation of C5 through C9 is called the "attack phase," leading to cell lysis, or the destruction of pathogens by phagocytes (opsonization) (1). This includes osmotic lysis of red cells and platelets, releasing procoagulant material in the form of membrane lipoprotein, as well as ADP, both serving to accelerate the coagulation process (98–100). It is of interest to note that, although it is diffi-

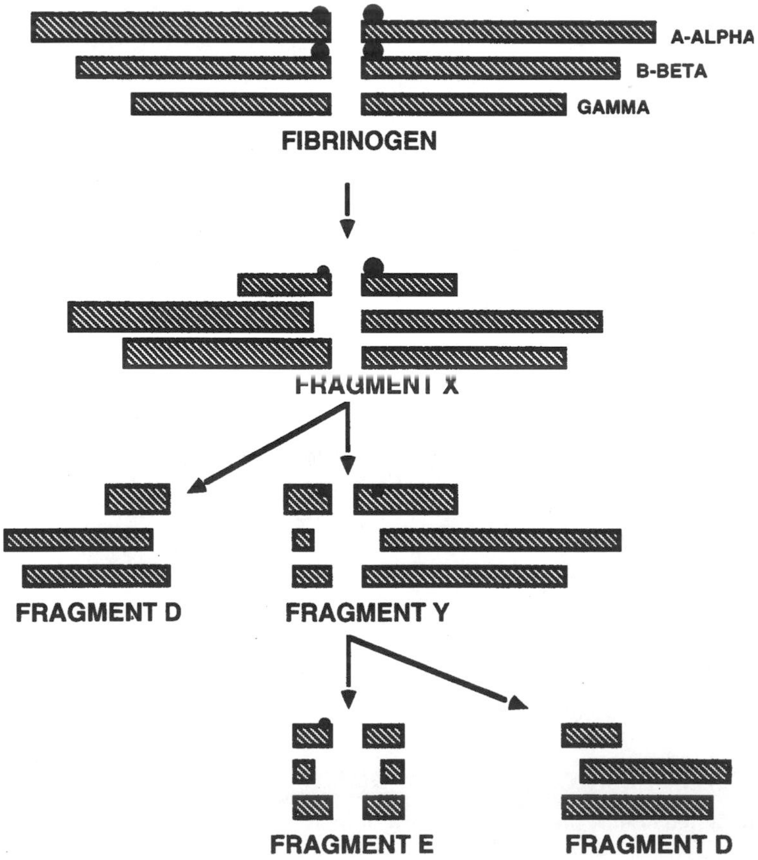

FIGURE 9.9. Formation of fibrin(ogen) degradation products.

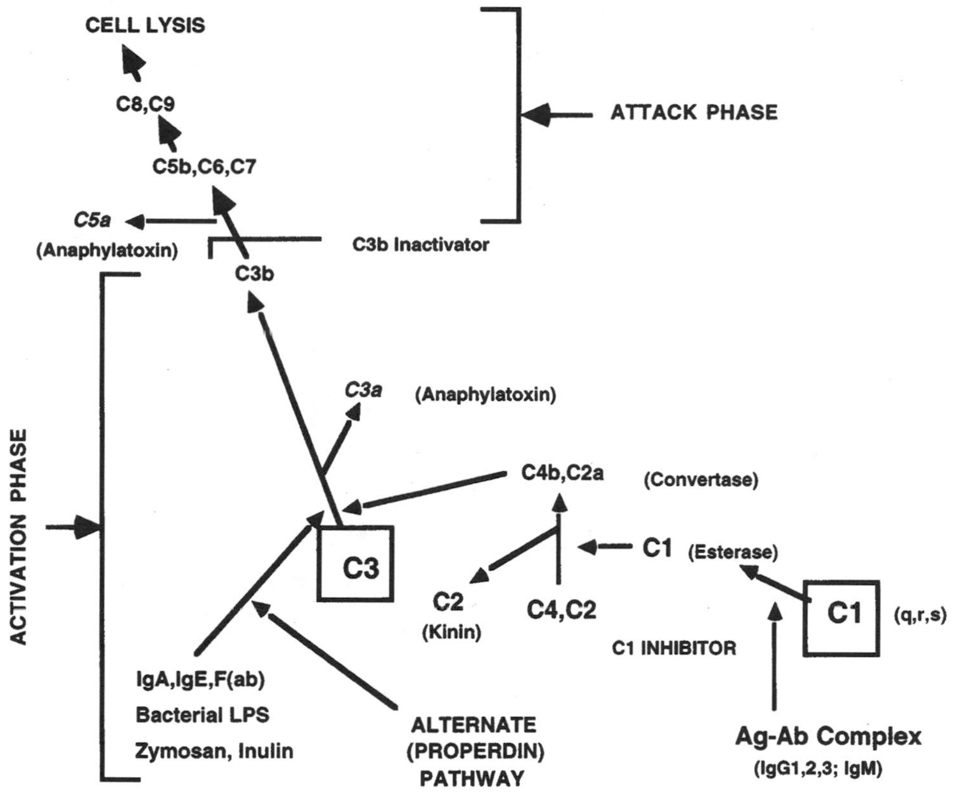

FIGURE 9.10. The complement system.

cult to assess its pathophysiologic relevance, plasmin generated either by t-PA or through the Hageman factor pathway can directly activate C1 or C3 independent of antigen–antibody complexes (1). Aprotinin is capable of the inhibition of kallikrein–C1-inhibitor complexes and C1–C1-inhibitor complexes (101). In many instances of pronounced activation of the fibrinolytic system, one might envision significant plasmin-induced activation of the complement system, leading to serious clinical consequences (1,60,102).

Kinin Generation

The importance of kinin generation during thrombohemorrhagic disorders has been appreciated only recently. Kinins increase vascular permeability and induce vascular dilation leading to hypotension, shock, and potential end-organ damage, common occurrences in syndromes of DIC (60,103–105). Like complement activation, generation of kinins centers around Hageman factor (factor XII) activation (1). As noted earlier, factor XIIa, in addition to activating factor XI to factor XIa, converts prekallikrein (Fletcher factor) into kallikrein, which converts kininogens to kinins (1). Factor XIIa also is further digested into factor XIIa fragments by plasmin; these fragments, although void of procoagulant activity, can further activate prekallikrein to kallikrein, with ensuing generation of kinins. Aprotinin is a potent inhibitor of kallikrein (106).

Figure 9.11 illustrates the important interrelations between the coagulation system, the fibrinolytic system, the complement system, and the kinin system. Factor XII is converted to active factor XIIa by various compounds ("surfaces"), including collagen and phospholipids; factor XIIa converts prekallikrein to kallikrein, which converts plasminogen to plasmin. Plasmin activates C1 and/or C3 of the complement system. Plasmin-induced factor XIIa fragments also convert prekallikrein to kallikrein, which, in addition to generating more plasmin, converts kininogens to kinins. These activation pathways, although difficult to assess quantitatively, based on a multitude of clinical observations, likely play important roles in the pathophysiology of disseminated intravascular coagulation, often leading to catastrophic clinical consequences (1,60,101).

Inhibitor Systems

Like other biologic processes, the blood coagulation system is governed by many inhibitory mechanisms designed to limit the extent of the various biochemical reactions and possible dissemination of the coagulation process. To this extent, the regulation of coagulation is effected by a number of negative-feedback loops, the involvement of specific inhibitors, and the compartmentalization of function, all of which serve to restrict clotting to a localized process. Table 9.6 summarizes inhibitory systems in hemostasis (107,108).

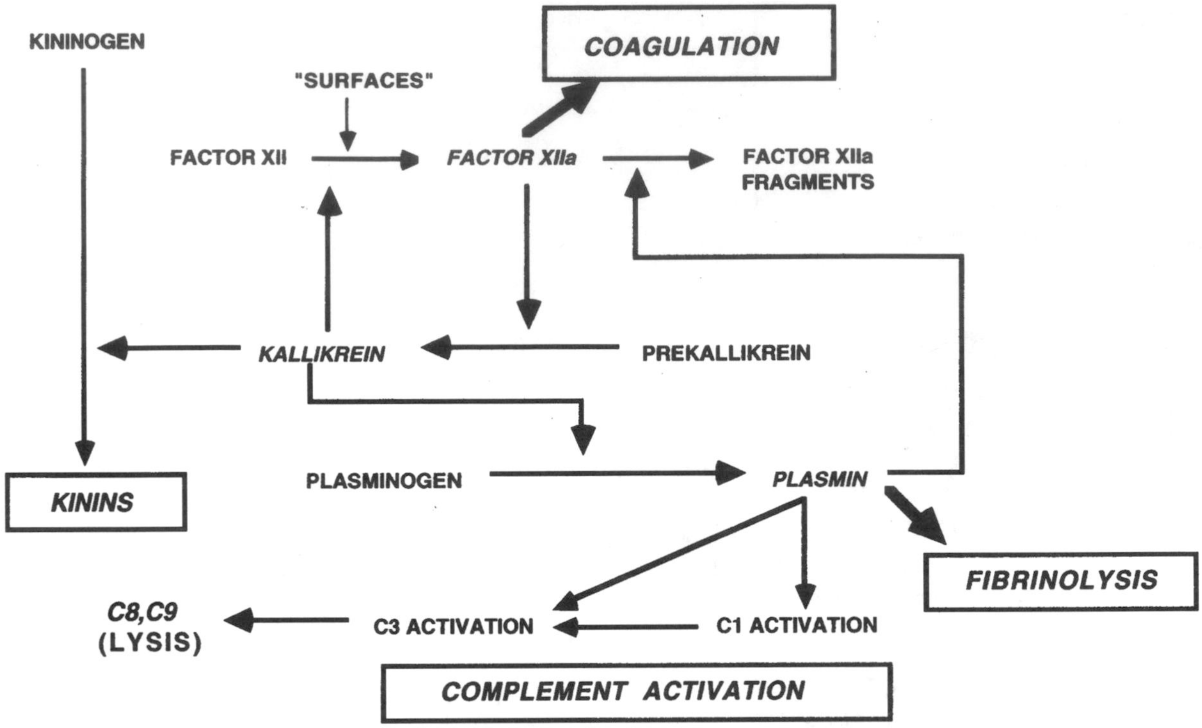

FIGURE 9.11. Interaction of coagulation, fibrinolysis, complement, and kinins.

Many of these mechanisms assume major importance in pathophysiology. First, there is the inactivation of factors V and VIII:c by the activated protein C and protein S systems (1,109). This mechanism involves the interaction of the enzyme thrombin with an endothelial cell component thrombomodulin, resulting in an *in situ* complex incapable of converting fibrinogen to fibrin but fully active in converting protein C (a proenzyme) to protein Ca (an enzyme). This enzyme (protein Ca) in turn, and in the presence of another protein (protein S), inactivates (by proteolysis) factors V and VIII:c, essentially halting further fibrin deposition (Fig. 9.12). Dahlback et al. (110) identified an "activated protein C cofactor/resistance," a molecular defect in factor V (factor V Leiden), which leads to familial thrombosis. In concert with procoagulant inhibitor activity is the observation that protein Ca enhances fibrinolysis, perhaps by depressing the activity of naturally occurring fibrinolytic inhibitors and/or by enhancing the activity of plasminogen activators (1). Aprotinin also is a potent inhibitor of activated protein C (111). The inhibitory activity of active protein C is itself modulated by another endothelial cell–derived inhibitor.

Another mechanism identified as playing a primary role in modulating hemostasis is the inhibition of the serine proteases thrombin, factor Xa, factor IXa, factor XIIa, and kallikrein by antithrombin (AT) (1). The inhibitory activity of AT is markedly enhanced by heparin (112–116). Figure 9.13 depicts a model illustrating the interaction of AT with serine proteases (1). Arginine-rich centers in AT react irreversibly with the serine center of serine proteases. In Fig. 9.13, thrombin serves as an example. Heparin, when used in therapy, reacts with lysine sites in antithrombin, making the arginine-rich center more available, thereby enhancing AT inhibitory activity. This ternary complex then dissociates to yield an inactive thrombin–AT complex and free heparin. The complex is then cleared from the circulation.

TABLE 9.6. MAJOR INHIBITORY MECHANISMS IN HEMOSTASIS

A. Inactivation of factors V and VIII by thrombin and activated protein C and protein S
B. Inhibition of prothrombin activation and fibrin formation by prothrombin fragments
C. Inhibition of factor Xa by activated protein C
D. Inhibition of thrombin or factor Xa formation by suboptimal "complex" components
E. Inhibition of thrombin factors Xa, IXa, XIa, XIIa, and kallikrein by antithrombin
F. Inhibition of thrombin activity by absorbing to fibrin
G. Inhibition of fibrin monomer polymerization and platelet function by fibrinolytic degradation products
H. Tissue factor pathway inhibitor (TFPI) in neutralizing tissue factor and tissue factor VIIa Xa and other complexes

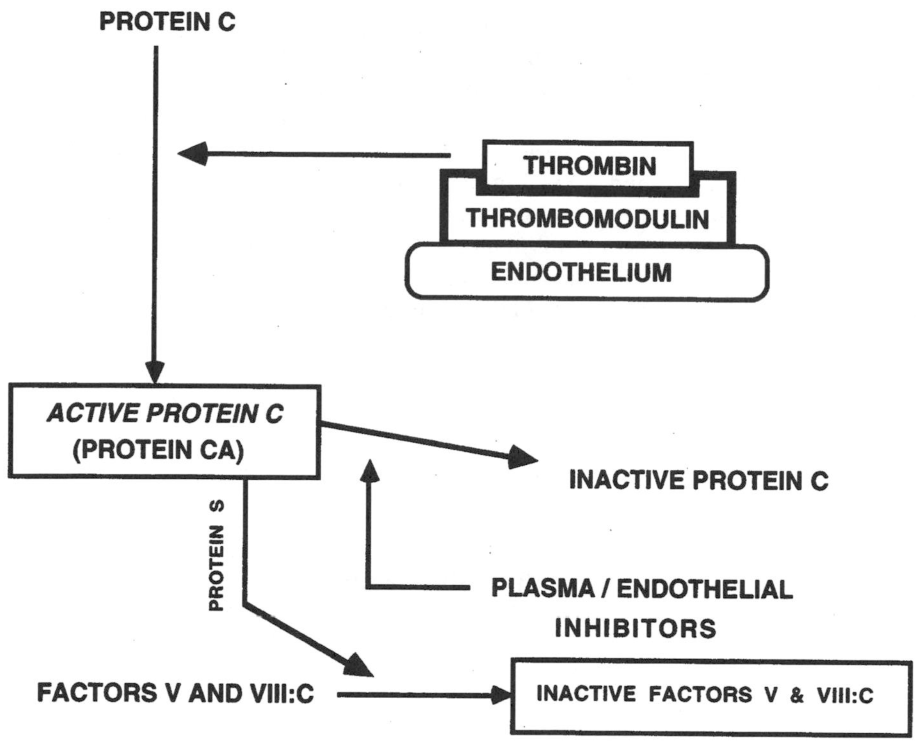

FIGURE 9.12. Protein C and S activity.

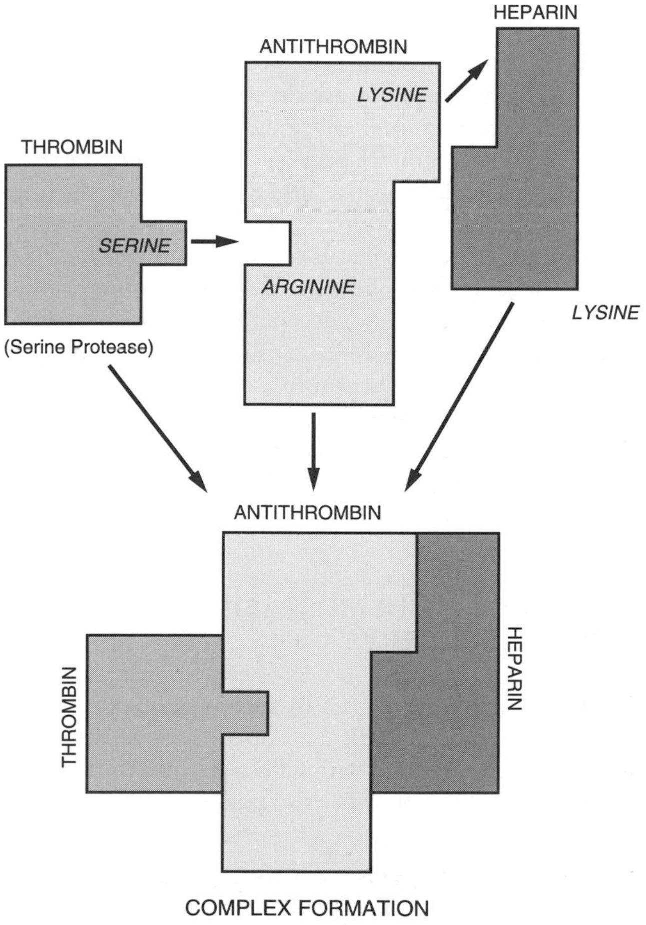

FIGURE 9.13. Antithrombin–heparin inhibitory activity.

The elucidation of this mechanism has served as a fundamental premise rationalizing heparin/miniheparin therapy (1).

Although the vast majority of evidence shows that these two systems (protein C and AT) likely are the most important modulators of coagulation, the contribution by other mechanisms listed in Table 9.6 is probably not trivial. For instance, prothrombin fragments produced when thrombin is generated are known to interfere with further prothrombin conversion and with fibrin polymerization. As fibrin is formed, it absorbs thrombin, thus decreasing thrombin availability. Inhibition of fibrin monomer polymerization and platelet function by FDPs also may occur. If FDPs complex with fibrin monomer, it becomes "solubilized" and unavailable for polymerization. Late degradation products, especially fragments D and E, have a high affinity for platelet membranes and render platelets markedly dysfunctional. Sometimes this activity can lead to significant clinical hemorrhage (117).

Other Interactive Components

Evidence is mounting that many other interactive components including vascular proteoglycans, fibronectin, complement derivatives, neutrophils/monocytes, cytokines, and other thus far uncharacterized agents may play important roles in modulating hemostasis (1).

Fibronectin is a high-molecular-weight glycoprotein that is soluble in plasma (118). An insoluble form is found in connective tissue and basement membranes (119). It binds to collagen, fibrin, fibrinogen, and intact cells, especially fibroblasts (1,119–121). It is synthesized by vascular endothelium and also is found in the α granules of platelets (1,30). It is cleaved by thrombin and trypsin, coprecipitates with fibrin, and is covalently cross-linked to fibrin by factor XIIIa (122–124). Fibronectin is needed to support cell growth, to enhance cellular migration into a fibrin clot, and to provide an extracellular matrix that eventually replaces a fibrin clot (1). As clot formation occurs, approximately 50% of plasma fibronectin is lost (123). This loss is because of cross-linking of fibronectin to the α chain of fibrin (by factor XIIIa), thus accounting for approximately 5% of the total protein of a fibrin clot (1). Fibronectin is necessary for cryoprecipitation of fibrinogen–fibrin complexes and accounts for the laboratory "cryoprecipitation" seen in DIC (1). Fibronectin is commonly decreased not only in DIC, but also in postoperative states, in patients sustaining major trauma (especially burns), and in patients with solid tumor metastases (124).

Other activities associated with this molecule relate to the potentiation of plasminogen activators, thus mediating clot lysis and matrix turnover, the mediation of activation of platelets by damaged tissue, opsonization of bacteria by neutrophils, attachment of bacteria to damaged tissues, and inhibition of the endothelial uptake of low-density lipoprotein. The fibronectin associated with α granules of platelets is released during collagen- or thrombin-induced platelet aggregation; after release, it binds to the platelet surface, further enhancing collagen–platelet adhesion and further stimulating collagen-induced platelet aggregation and release. The interaction with collagen (122) and probably other vascular proteoglycans (heparan sulfate, hyaluronic acid, and chondroitin sulfate) is mediated by cross-linking by factor XIIIa. Heparin may accelerate the binding of fibronectin to both fibrinogen and collagen; however, the binding of heparin to fibronectin does not appear to change the "anticoagulant" nature of the bound heparin (124).

Vascular proteoglycans are a heterogeneous group of high-molecular-weight protein polysaccharides consisting of carbohydrate polymers (glycosaminoglycans) covalently linked to a protein core (125). The common vascular proteoglycans are hyaluronic acid, chondroitin-4-sulfate, chondroitin-6-sulfate, dermatan sulfate, keratin sulfate, heparin sulfate, heparan sulfate, and heparin (126). Heparan sulfate is a low-sulfated D-glucuronic acid–rich polysaccharide, whereas heparin is a highly sulfated, L-iduronic acid–rich polysaccharide. The amount of each particular type of proteoglycan differs in various regions of the vasculature. Most are concentrated in the intimal layer. The concentration of dermatan and heparan sulfate correlates closely with antithrombotic activity. Selected proteoglycans inhibit collagen- and thrombin-induced platelet aggregation, accelerate AT inhibitory activity, and induce the release of platelet factor 4. Their concentrations change with the development of atherosclerotic plaques. Physiologically, vascular proteoglycans support vascular integrity, maintain the viscoelastic properties of vessels, regulate permeability of macromolecules, and regulate arterial lipid deposition. All these properties encompass modulating functions in the interaction of blood proteins with the vascular wall. Several complement derivatives, especially C3a and C5a, may play key roles in hemostasis. These components not only regulate vascular tone but also may induce a neutrophil/monocyte release of enzymes like elastases and collagenases, important in the degradation of fibrinogen, fibrin, and FDPs. Complement derivatives also modulate release of granulocyte/monocyte procoagulant activity, may modulate platelet reactivity, and influence the neutrophil/monocyte interaction with fibronectin (127). Granulocytes and monocytes contain procoagulant activity that may be released under pathologic conditions, such as in acute leukemia (1,128,129).

Concluding Remarks

The consequences of acute insults to the hemostatic system, whether congenital or acquired, often present a considerable challenge in diagnosis and therapy. Logical and effective management depends on (a) the proper identification of the hemostatic compartments involved; (b) an appreciation for the considerably complex, delicately modulated interplays of various enzyme–inhibitor systems; and (c) knowledge of the mechanism by which a variety of apparently unrelated disease processes precipitate sometimes catastrophic events: thrombosis/embolism/hemorrhage. The section on plasma proteins pays particular attention to biocybernetic principles (positive/negative-feedback loops) and to the interrelation of enzyme systems involved in coagulation, fibrinolysis, kinin generation, and complement activation, as these systems are often disrupted during cardiac surgery. A working knowledge of basic mechanisms not only provides advantages in diagnostic/therapeutic management, but also serves as a firm foundation for the development of novel diagnostic and therapeutic modalities, particularly as relates to prevention, diagnosis, and management of hemorrhage or thrombosis associated with cardiac surgery and cardiovascular medicine (1).

PATHOLOGY OF HEMOSTASIS DURING CARDIAC SURGERY

Cardiopulmonary bypass (CPB) surgery has become conventional in clinical medicine, and the severe defects in hemostasis that can occur with CPB may dramatically compromise morbidity or mortality of patients.

Prevention of Cardiac Surgical Bleeding

Hemorrhage associated with cardiac surgery may be devastating and life threatening; overcautiousness regarding prevention, differential diagnosis, and rapid effective therapy are essential. Attention must be paid to preventing surgical hemorrhage by uncovering hereditary, acquired, or drug-induced bleeding tendencies before CPB. A preexisting bleeding diathesis, although mild, when coupled with the changes of hemostasis induced by cardiac surgery, may lead to calamitous results (130). Recently there has been great interest in aprotinin and other drugs as agents to decrease blood loss during cardiac surgery (131–135).

TABLE 9.7. PRESURGICAL HEMOSTASIS SCREEN

Complete blood and platelet count (CBC)
Prothrombin time
Partial thromboplastin time
Template bleeding time or PFA-100
Thrombin time (CPB surgery) (observe clot for 5 min)
Cryoglobulins and cold agglutinins (hypothermic cardiopulmonary bypass)

PFA-100, platelet/vascular function screen; CPB, cardiopulmonary bypass.

Laboratory Screening

Any preoperative laboratory and hemostasis screen should generally be simple and incur a minimum of expense to the patient while providing adequate information; however, presurgical or precardiac bypass hemostasis screens are often insufficient (136–138). As with an adequate history and physical examination, one must be knowledgeable in screening for defects in hemostasis when a surgical procedure is planned. When preexisting hemostatic defects are combined with the defects in hemostasis created by CPB, the resultant hemorrhage is often catastrophic but often can be averted by wise screening of patients. The usually ordered biochemical screening survey, electrolytes, and complete blood and platelet count will detect the common acquired disorders often associated with a bleeding tendency, such as chronic liver disease, renal disease, and instances of "hypersplenism" or bone marrow failure. Most commonly, a presurgical screen consists only of a prothrombin time, activated partial thromboplastin time, and a platelet count. Although these simple tests will detect most coagulation protein problems and thrombocytopenia, they provide absolutely no information about vascular or platelet function and ignore the possibility of pathologic fibrinolysis.

Most nontechnical hemorrhage associated with cardiac surgery is caused by platelet-function defects, and less commonly, coagulation protein or vascular defects; it is important to realize that platelet defects are a more common cause of surgical bleeding than are coagulation protein problems! Therefore, one simple procedure is often added to the routine preoperative surgical screen. This test is the standardized template bleeding time, as described by Mielke et al. (139), and is performed before a cardiac surgical procedure; this provides a screen for adequate vascular and platelet function, but is not always reliable (140). The template bleeding time should not be done until adequate platelet numbers (greater than 100×10^9/L) are documented by count or smear evaluation. For CPB patients, a thrombin time may be added to the preoperative screen (141,142). If performed, the resultant clot should be observed for 5 minutes after the test is done. A normal thrombin time assures the absence of significant hypofibrinogenemia, dysfibrinogenemia, fibrinolysis, or FDP elevation. The use of these tests in the presurgical screen adds only minimal cost and laboratory time while providing valuable information not given by a simple prothrombin time, activated partial thromboplastin time, or platelet count. If hypothermic perfusion is to be done, cryoglobulins and cold agglutinins also should be assessed before bypass (143–148). The preoperative surgical and bypass hemostasis screen is summarized in Table 9.7 (139,149–152).

Hemostasis in Cardiac Surgery

Hemorrhage during or after bypass is of more than fleeting significance, as it may lead to substantial morbidity and mortality from an elective procedure, places formidable demands on blood bank facilities, and can lead to prolonged, costly hospitalizations (142,153–156). The actual incidence of life-threatening hemorrhage associated with CPB varies from 5% to 25% and may be higher in pediatric heart surgery, approaching 35% (142,153–160).

Formerly, the pathophysiology of altered hemostasis created by CPB was poorly understood. Various investigators attributed the hemorrhagic syndrome of CPB surgery to an assorted spectrum of defects; each investigator, moreover, ranked each defect by diverse degrees of importance, depending on which particular hemostatic parameters were monitored. Indeed, the basic pathophysiology of altered hemostasis during CPB remains bewildering to many. Clearly, basic mechanisms of altered hemostasis associated with CPB should be completely understood and appreciated before a useful approach to rapid diagnosis and effective therapy can be effectively designed.

Thrombocytopenia

Early studies of hemostasis during CPB noted significant thrombocytopenia, about 50×10^9/L, in patients undergoing bypass surgery; many authors thought this responsible for bypass hemorrhage. Kevy (161) also noted that thrombocytopenia was related to time on bypass, and was more pronounced with perfusions lasting longer than 60 minutes. A relation between thrombocytopenia and time on bypass also was reported by Signore et al. (162). Later studies noted similar findings (163,164); Porter and Silver (163) observed that in most patients undergoing CPB, the platelet count decreased to one third of the preoperative level; it also was found that thrombocytopenia did not abate until several days after CPB. Earlier studies by Wright et al. (165) and von Kaulla and Swan (166) also recognized thrombocytopenia in association with CPB, but these investigators decided that thrombocytopenia bore little, if any, relation to actual bypass hemorrhage. Some studies finding thrombocytopenia during CPB concluded that this represented thrombocytopenia of DIC (167–170). Bick et al. (138,142,154,171–174) and others (175–177) failed to find significant thrombocytopenia during CPB. This wide variability in experience probably represents different surgical and pumping techniques, such as flow rates, normothermic or hypothermic perfusion, the oxygenation system used, time on bypass, and the priming solution. Figure 9.14 shows changes in platelet number during CPB. The solid diamonds represent the mean platelet counts in membrane oxygenation–pumped patients, and the dotted squares represent bubble-oxygenation patients (138,154,178). A total of 300 consecutive patients is depicted. In our experience, the type of oxygenation mechanism used appears to play little role, if any, in causing clinically significant thrombocytopenia (138,154,178). Thrombocytopenia with bubble oxygenators is slightly greater than that seen with membrane oxygenators, but this does not often reach clinical significance. The most commonly cited mechanisms for the development of CPB thrombocytopenia are (a) hemodilution, (b) formation of intravascular platelet thrombi, (c) platelet utilization in the pump or oxygenation system, and (d) peripheral use because of DIC. We have failed to find a correlation between CPB hematocrit and platelet count, suggesting that hemodilution is not a major factor (137,174,179). The role, if any, of these mechanisms in producing CPB thrombocytopenia is unclear. An additional problem in cardiac surgery, during which heparin is always used, is that of heparin-induced thrombocytopenia (HIT) (180). Although in non–cardiac surgery patients, HIT is based on clinical criteria and the noting of a platelet count of less than 150×10^9/L or a decrease in the platelet count to 30% to 50% from baseline (before heparin platelet count), postoperative cardiac surgery patients have a particular problem, because many patients have a platelet count between 100×10^9/L

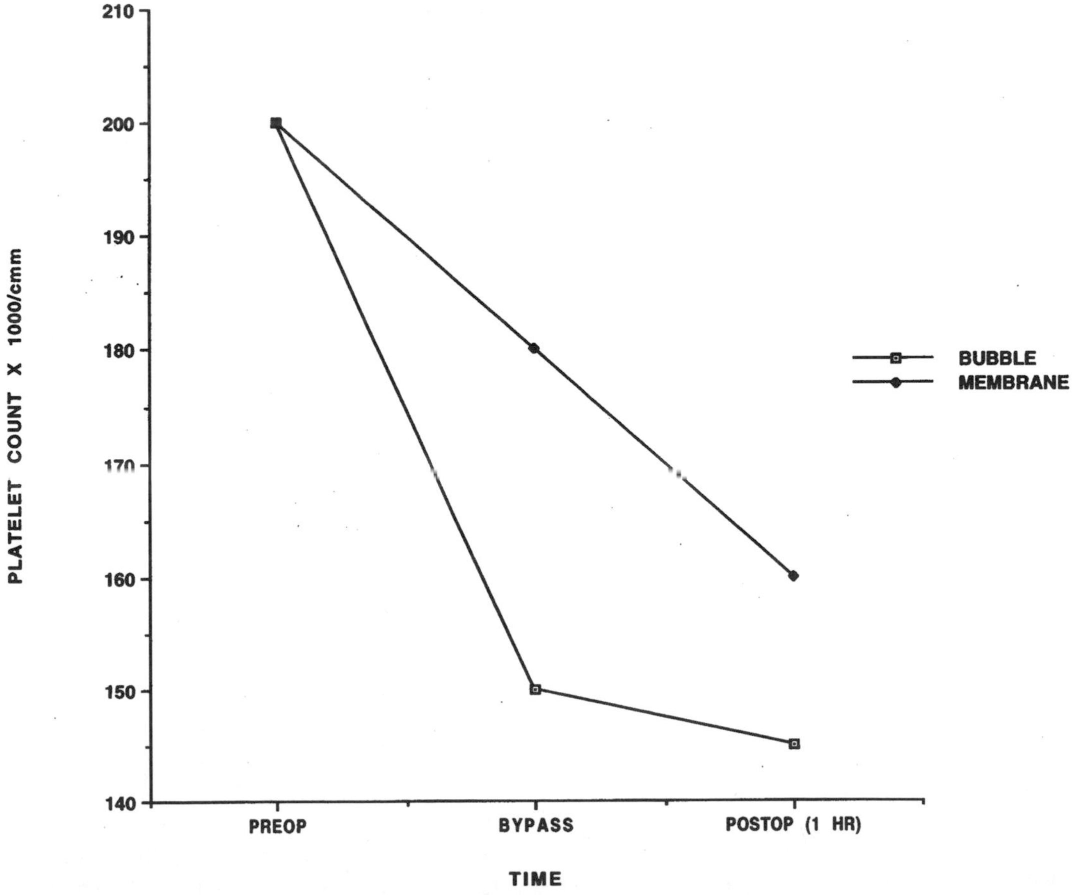

FIGURE 9.14. Platelet counts during cardiopulmonary bypass, membrane versus bubble oxygenation, in 300 consecutive patients.

and 150×10^9/L on postoperative day 1 (181,182). In these patients, therefore, a diagnosis of HIT should be suspected when there is a 20% to 30% reduction in the platelet count, using the postoperative day 1 platelets count as a baseline. If there is a 50% reduction with the postoperative day 1 baseline count, HIT is highly likely (180–183).

Platelet-function Defects

In contrast to the prolific investigations regarding platelet number during CPB, there has been a surprising lack of interest in assessing platelet function during this procedure. Early investigators suspected that abnormalities of platelet function might happen, as faulty clot retraction was noted (162). These results were of unclear significance, however, because other changes known to affect clot retraction, such as hypofibrinogenemia and thrombocytopenia, also were present. Another early study assessed platelet function before placing patients on CPB but did not examine platelet function during or after bypass (184). In this study, abnormal preoperative platelet adhesion in glass-bead columns was associated with increased postoperative bleeding. Salzman (185) studied platelet adhesion before, during, and after bypass and noted decreased adhesion to glass-bead columns in patients during bypass; however, the significance of this defect was difficult to evaluate because all patients had marked thrombocytopenia, which is definitely known to alter adhesion studies (186–188). However, adhesion studies are now generally thought to be without any particular clinical significance (140,189,190). Further information from this study was that heparin, in doses used during CPB, did not alter platelet adhesion. This study concluded that a circulating anticoagulant might be responsible for the platelet-function defect noted, as plasma from CPB patients altered adhesion when added to normal platelets. This circulating anticoagulant probably represented FDPs (142). Salzman's (185) study also noted that perfusion temperature and the type of priming solution did not correlate with the development of abnormal platelet function. Platelet-adhesion studies also have been performed in patients undergoing CPB without significant thrombocytopenia (171,173,174,179). In these studies, platelet function, as measured by adhesion, decreased profoundly in all patients at the initiation of bypass; most patients showed adhesion, which decreased to 17% of preoperative levels. In one study, little correlation was noted between hematocrit, fibrinogen level, or FDP titer and abnormal adhesion (173). Poor correlation also was noted between chest-tube blood loss and abnormal platelet function, as assessed by adhesion. It must again be stressed that recent studies have questioned the clinical importance of platelet adhesion by the glass-bead column technique (140,189,190). However, this degree of abnormal platelet function would surely be expected to compromise hemostasis severely. The platelet-function defect is slightly more severe and tends to correct more slowly when a membrane oxygenator is used, as compared with a bubble oxygenator. Platelet function as assessed by template bleeding times or platelet aggregation or lumi-aggregation is abnormal in patients with platelet-function defects (140,188), von Willebrand syndrome (ristocetin aggregation only) (187), and myeloproliferative disorders (191). Many factors, some possibly altered by CPB, may affect platelet function; these include (a) pH, (b) absolute platelet count, (c) hematocrit, (d) drugs, (e) the presence of FDPs, (f) the type of pump prime, and (g) the type of oxygenation system used (142,192–198). Although most studies do not clearly define the reasons for abnormal platelet function during CPB, they do suggest that several of these mechanisms are probably not involved. The finding of platelet counts greater than 100×10^9/L and hematocrits greater than 30% in most patients with marked platelet dysfunction 1 hour after CPB suggests that the absolute platelet count and the hematocrit do not account for altered platelet function. Most patients have a normal or near-normal pH 1 hour after bypass surgery, so a change in pH is unlikely to account for abnormal platelet function during bypass surgery. Heparin, at levels higher than those attained in patients undergoing CPB, has been shown not to alter platelet function (153,185,188). Circulating FDPs are known to interfere with platelet function, and these are present in about 85% of patients undergoing CPB (142,193,197). However, there is poor correlation between levels of circulating FDP and abnormal platelet function during bypass surgery (173,179). In addition, defective platelet function occurs in 100% of patients undergoing CPB; thus circulating FDP cannot account for altered platelet function in many instances (137,142,154, 173,179).

Other possible mechanisms of altered platelet function during CPB include platelet membrane damage by shearing force or contact with foreign material, resulting in a partial release of platelet contents; platelet membrane coating with nonspecific proteins or protein degradation products; or incomplete release reaction or nonspecific platelet damage induced by flow rates. More recent studies have shown selective platelet degranulation to occur during bypass surgery (199). However, no studies reported yet allow conclusions to be drawn regarding the contribution of any of these mechanisms to altered platelet function during CPB. One preliminary study has reported platelet-aggregation studies during CPB. In this series of 29 patients, only 20% developed aggregation abnormalities during CPB; however, after heparin reversal with protamine sulfate, aggregation abnormalities developed in 90% of patients. These authors attributed this finding to a protamine/platelet interaction and not to the bypass itself (200). We have evaluated platelets by lumi-aggregation in patients undergoing CPB surgery, and in all patients, platelet aggregation and platelet release were markedly altered (153,154,201). Typical midbypass and postbypass lumi-aggregation patterns seen in cardiac surgery patients are depicted in Figs. 9.15 and 9.16. In all patients

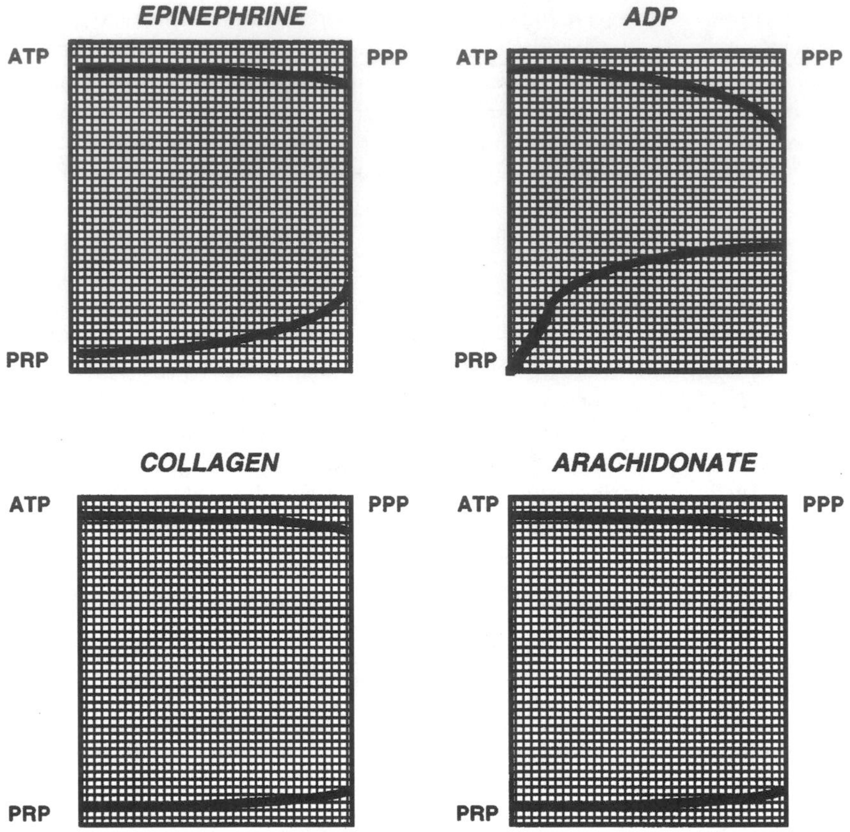

FIGURE 9.15. Cardiopulmonary bypass surgery: platelet lumi-aggregation patterns, mid-bypass. *PRP*, platelet-rich plasma; *PPP*, platelet-poor plasma; *ATP*, adenosine triphosphate release.

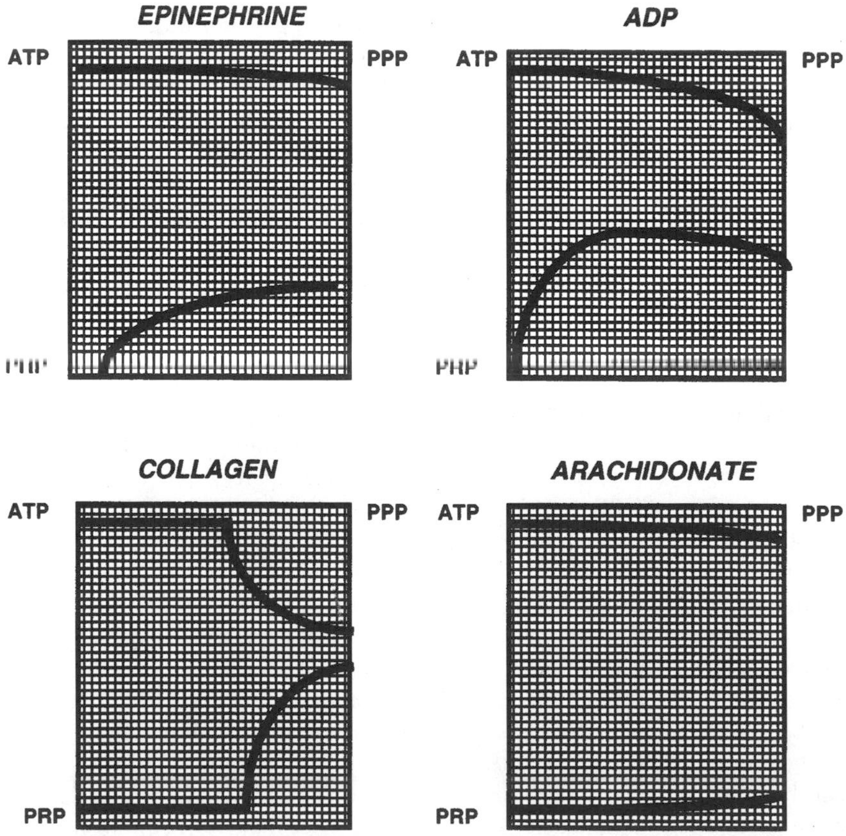

FIGURE 9.16. Cardiopulmonary bypass surgery platelet lumi-aggregation patterns, after bypass. *PRP*, platelet-rich plasma; *PPP*, platelet-poor plasma; *ATP*, adenosine triphosphate release.

assessed, the aggregation and release reaction defects happened within 10 to 15 minutes of starting bypass. We also have noted that in all patients, platelet factor 4 levels increase rapidly with the initiation of bypass. The aggregation defects appear to be similar with both membrane- and bubble-type oxygenators; however, the type of priming solution, albumin versus hydroxyethyl starch, does seem to change the types of defects seen (201). A new concern during bypass surgery is the noting of infrequent cases of graft-versus-host disease from transfusions, thus prompting many to use irradiated blood and blood products. It has recently been noted that platelet function remains intact after radiation of whole blood; thus this will not contribute to platelet dysfunction in the cardiac patient (202).

Despite the mechanism(s) involved, studies to date clearly disclose a significant platelet-function defect that is induced in all patients undergoing CPB surgery. The magnitude of this defect would certainly be expected to have potential serious consequences for hemostasis during and after bypass. In addition, patients who have ingested drugs known to interfere with platelet function would be expected to have more blood loss than would those not ingesting such agents. In such patients, this would be expected to compound the defects already induced by CPB and to potentiate the chance for hemorrhage. One small study has supplied evidence for this conclusion (196). Although diagnosis and management of hemorrhage associated with CPB are discussed later, it should be pointed out that this platelet-function defect is of major importance in post-CPB hemorrhage. The use of platelet concentrates in those with a normal platelet count will usually promptly correct or significantly reduce most episodes of CPB or post-CPB hemorrhage. DDAVP (1-deamino-8-D-arginine vasopressin; desmopressin acetate) was initially thought to decrease bleeding after open-heart surgery; because of this finding, many surgeons began the empiric, and sometimes irrational use of DDAVP during and after open-heart surgery. However, more recent blinded randomized trials have failed to show any significant differences in post-CPB blood loss between DDAVP and placebo (203–205). DDAVP also releases t-PA (endothelial), potentially activating the fibrinolytic system and enhancing or inducing hemorrhage, so many using this agent recommend the concomitant use of aminocaproic acid to abort any possible hemorrhage (206–209). Because of current evidence, there appears to be little, if any, rationale for the empiric use of DDAVP during CPB; those using this agent should be aware of the potential for enhancing hemorrhage and for increased risk of coronary artery and cerebrovascular thrombosis.

Isolated Coagulation Factor Defects

Many studies have examined and reported coagulation factor deficiencies during CPB. A wide variety of findings have been observed and, like the finding of thrombocytopenia, may reflect only differences in surgical or pumping techniques, such as flow rate, priming solution, etc. Most studies have noted significant hypofibrinogenemia, which does not seem to be correlated with perfusion time (157, 163–165,173,174). We (173,174,193) and others (157, 164) have found fibrinogen levels to be closely correlated with CPB fibrinolysis; however, other investigators reported little correlation between hypofibrinogenemia and degree of CPB fibrinolysis (168,210). Figure 9.17 depicts correlations noted between fibrinogen, plasminogen, circulating plasmin, and FDPs during CPB. The dashed lines represent membrane-pumped patients, and the solid lines represent bubble oxygenator–pumped patients (137,154,178). Some studies have concluded that hypofibrinogenemia happens primarily because of DIC during pump surgery (167,169,170); however, others did not find hypofibrinogenemia during CPB (211,212). It seems reasonable to conclude from the studies reported that hypofibrinogenemia secondary to hyperfibrinolysis may be a frequent event during CPB. Fibrinolysis occurs in about 85% of patients undergoing bypass surgery. Most studies also have noted other coagulation deficiencies in association with CPB; those most commonly decreased and reported to play a role in CPB hemorrhage are factor II, factor V, and factor VIII:c (157,161,165,167,170). It has been noted that some patients undergoing CPB for valvular heart disease have low factor VIII:vW high-molecular-weight monomers; these monomers also may increase during the CPB procedure (204). Some concluded that these changes are secondary to DIC (167,177), whereas others ascribed these decreases to a primary fibrinolytic syndrome and plasmin-induced degradation of coagulation proteins (137,142,157,173, 174,193). Still others did not find a significant decrease in most coagulation factors during bypass surgery (161,211, 212), and two authors (211,213) reported increased factor VIII:c levels during perfusion.

Disseminated Intravascular Coagulation

The question of DIC developing during bypass surgery has caused much confusion regarding altered hemostasis both during and after bypass. Many early studies of hemostasis during CPB concluded that DIC occurred (167,169,170, 214,215). However, many such studies monitored only isolated coagulation factors; the measured decreases were empirically ascribed to presumed DIC, as no other clear explanation was evident. Specifically, the findings of isolated fibrinogen, factor VIII:c (165,169), or prothrombin complex factor deficiencies (176) were often assumed, usually erroneously, to be secondary to DIC, without proper confirmatory laboratory testing. Two more recent reports also concluded that DIC accounts for altered hemostasis during CPB (177,216). In these reports of nine patients, it was concluded that DIC was present, after noting that several parameters of hemostasis worsened after heparin reversal with protamine. Specifically, FDPs elevation, hypofib-

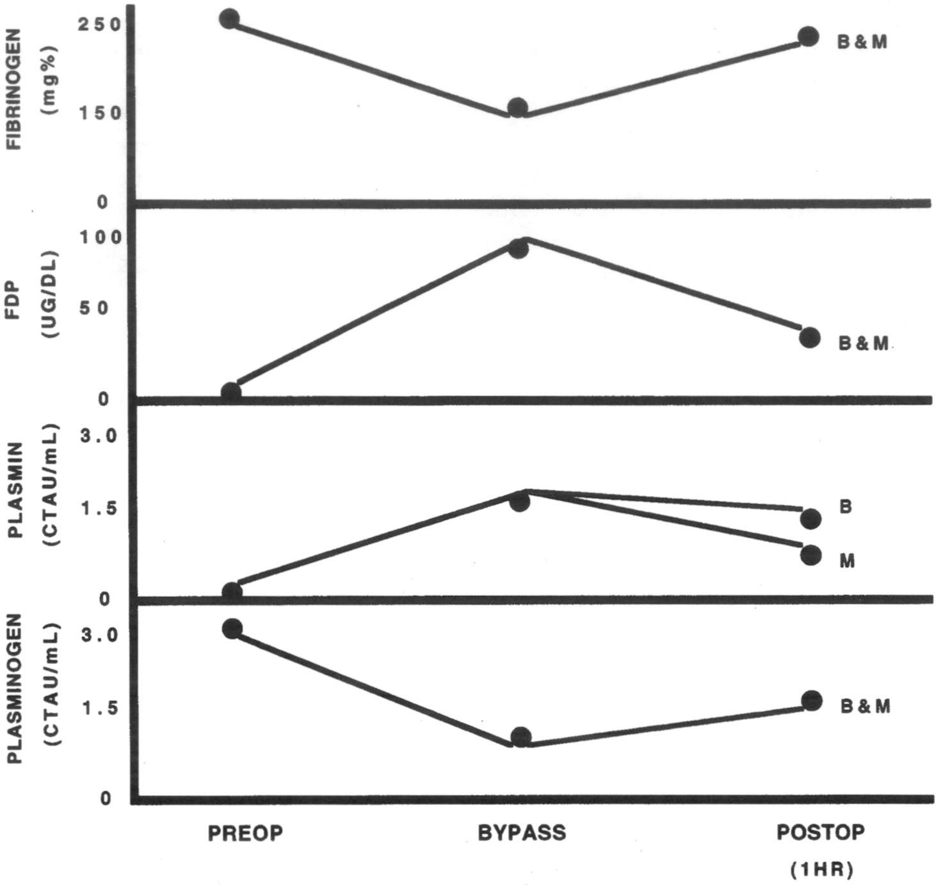

FIGURE 9.17. Fibrinolytic activity during cardiopulmonary bypass. *B*, bubble oxygenator; *M*, membrane oxygenator.

rinogenemia, and hypoplasminogenemia appeared to become accentuated after the infusion of protamine. However, our experience (137,138,142,153,173,174) and that of others (157,162,163,166,212,217) has been the opposite; hypofibrinogenemia, hypoplasminogenemia, and FDPs elevation are usually noted to correct rapidly and uniformly after the administration of protamine sulfate.

These findings would suggest that DIC is not generally associated with CPB surgery. DIC during cardiac surgery also seems unlikely, in view of massive heparinization and the absence of significant or uniform thrombocytopenia reported in many studies in which hemostasis appeared to be markedly abnormal. Another finding that would surely suggest that DIC is not present during CPB is the presence of normal or near-normal AT levels during CPB (137,153, 157,179); evidence suggests that decreased AT levels are a good indicator of the development of acute or chronic DIC (218–221). Only one study has shown decreased AT during CPB (179); however, in the nine patients described, all had low levels of AT III before bypass was started. The method used was quite old, and possibly influenced by the presence of FDPs or heparin, making interpretation of these results unclear. Another consideration negating the probability that DIC occurs during CPB is that if DIC were present in patients undergoing CPB, the infusion of intravenous protamine sulfate would be expected to cause a massive precipitation of soluble fibrin monomer, with resultant extensive micro- or macrovascular occlusion. In my experience, only two of several thousand patients have had true DIC in association with CPB (137,142,154). In both patients, DIC developed before CPB, one from cardiac arrest and the other from septicemia. In these two instances, bypass surgery was finished without incidents; however, when protamine sulfate was infused, massive vascular occlusion, including carotid and renal artery thrombosis, occurred.

To summarize, although most early and several recent studies have detected primary fibrinolysis in association with CPB, a few have concluded that DIC might occur. These conclusions probably emanate from the marked superficial similarities between primary fibrinolysis and DIC and the usual secondary fibrinolytic response and from the difficulty in making a clear-cut differential diagnosis between these two states without sophisticated and complete coagulation studies.

Primary Fibrinolysis

Fibrinolytic activity is generally decreased or inhibited during and after most general surgical procedures (222–225). However, most studies using a variety of laboratory modalities have found increased fibrinolysis during and after CPB surgery (137,142,154,157,173–175,193–195,201,210,217, 226). Many earlier studies of hemostasis during CPB assessed fibrinolysis with the euglobulin lysis time, and the finding of fibrinolysis was of unclear significance for a long time (227,228). More recent studies of CPB hemostasis (137,153,154,163,173,174,179), which have used more specific methods for assessing fibrinolysis, primarily synthetic substrate assays (220,229–233), have confirmed earlier reports of a primary fibrino(geno)lytic syndrome in most patients undergoing CPB surgery. Figure 9.17 depicts changes in the fibrinolytic system in patients undergoing CPB. Because of early reports detecting primary fibrinolysis during CPB, the empiric use of antifibrinolytics, usually ε-aminocaproic acid (EACA) has become commonplace. Despite the attendant hazards of this agent, which include hypokalemia, hypotension, ventricular arrhythmias, local or disseminated thromboses, and DIC syndromes (234,235), many cardiovascular surgeons have often used this drug. Controlled studies with and without antifibrinolytics have failed to show any clear-cut differences in CPB hemorrhage (157,164,210,236,237), and Gomes and McGoon (217) and Tsuji et al. (212) demonstrated an increase in post-CPB hemorrhage with the empiric use of antifibrinolytics. The need to use EACA to control CPB hemorrhage is extremely rare (137,138,142,154); this agent should generally be used only when clear laboratory evidence of primary fibrinolysis is noted in the severely hemorrhaging CPB patient who did not respond to adequate platelet transfusions. Two recent randomized studies, however, demonstrated significant reductions in intraoperative and postoperative blood loss with the empiric use of tranexamic acid (Cyklokapron); the doses used were 160 mg/kg as one intravenous (i.v.) dose after induction of anesthesia in one study, and in the other study, the dose was 20 mg/kg i.v. at time of skin incision, followed by an i.v. infusion of 2 mg/kg per hour during the duration of surgery (238,239). Despite studies showing no benefit of empiric use of EACA, one recent small study (30 randomized patients) study demonstrated a significant reduction in blood loss, but at the expense of thrombosis in the EACA group (240).

Several investigators finding primary fibrinolysis during CPB have concluded this to be inconsequential as a cause of postperfusion hemorrhage (162,164), whereas others have thought that this syndrome is triggered only by specific events, such as pyrogenicity of equipment, the use of dextran 10 (Rheomacrodex), or induction of anesthesia (166,241,242). Because primary fibrinolysis happens in most patients subjected to CPB surgery, it seems likelier that activation of the fibrinolytic system may be happening in the oxygenation mechanism, or alternatively, that pump-induced accelerated flow rates may activate the plasminogen–plasmin system or may alter endothelial plasminogen activator, or inhibitor, activity. There is marked activation of factor XII in patients undergoing CPB surgery with about 70% of factor XII being converted to factor XIIa, possibly a consequence of complement system activation (243). This is another potential activation pathway for the initiation of a primary fibrinolytic syndrome. However, the exact pathogenesis of fibrinolytic activation during CPB remains unclear. Although many investigators have noted enhanced fibrinolysis during CPB, a few studies have found only elevated fibrinolytic activator activity, with no systemically circulating plasmin (161,210,214). A few studies also failed to find any evidence of primary fibrinolysis in association with CPB (164,165,214,236).

Other Defects in Cardiac Surgery

Heparin "rebound" has received significant attention as a potential cause of CPB hemorrhage (242,244–247). This was observed more often in earlier studies. With today's generally accepted doses of both heparin and protamine, both heparin rebound and inadequate heparinization are rarely, if ever, seen (137,142,153,168,174,177,179). Neither heparin rebound nor inadequate heparin neutralization has ever been documented as an actual cause of CPB hemorrhage (137,138,153,168,169). Similarly, protamine excess has occasionally been incriminated as a cause of CPB hemorrhage; however, several studies have failed to note this phenomenon in a single patient undergoing CPB (142,159, 173–175,245,248). Although protamine sulfate is a well-known in vitro anticoagulant, it is unlikely that this agent is the cause of clinical hemorrhage (249).

Several authors have reported that both coagulation defects and significant CPB hemorrhage may be associated with hypothermic perfusion (164,166,236,242); our experience in comparing normothermic with hypothermic perfusions has led to the same conclusion (226). Gomes and McGoon (217) and Porter and Silver (163) found no increased incidence of CPB hemorrhage resulting from hypothermic perfusion. Many patients undergoing coronary artery bypass grafting (CABG) for coronary occlusive disease have been taking warfarin-type drugs. Verska et al. (236) noted that although the prothrombin time returns to normal before CPB, patients previously receiving warfarin therapy show more hemorrhage than do those not earlier taking these agents. This observation applies to general surgery patients as well. One study (152) noted that increased hemorrhage was associated with a repeated bypass procedure; others, however, noted no increased hemorrhage in association with a second procedure (170,217). Patients undergoing CPB for correction of cyanotic heart disease also appear to have more severe derangements in hemostasis during perfusion and a propensity to hemorrhage than do those operated on for noncyanotic heart disease (162,217). Increased hemorrhagic risk during and after CPB surgery is associated with (a) the prior use of warfarin drugs, (b) hypothermic perfusion, (c) surgery for correction of cyanotic heart disease, (d) repeated bypass procedure, (e) long perfusion/aortic cross-clamp times, and (f) preoperative ingestion of drugs interfering with platelet function (137,138,153,154). Advancing age does not appear to be associated with increased risk of hemorrhage with CPB (250,251).

Summary of Cardiopulmonary Bypass Hemostasis Pathophysiology

Many conclusions regarding altered hemostasis and resultant hemorrhage during CPB surgery are of questionable significance; for example, it appears that overheparinization, heparin rebound, inadequate protamine neutralization, and protamine excess, although receiving at least theoretic attention as potential sources of CPB hemorrhage, have not been documented as causes of bleeding associated with bypass surgery. Similarly, thrombocytopenia, almost surely a potential source of hemorrhage, is an inconsistent finding during cardiac bypass surgery. The finding of isolated coagulation defects during CPB has added little to an understanding of altered hemostasis during bypass surgery; probably these isolated findings simply represent isolated measurements of the results of fibrinolysis and systemically circulating plasmin.

Although DIC has been thought by some to occur during CPB, most carefully done studies have not documented this. The significant doses of heparin used during CPB, the absence of consistent thrombocytopenia, and the general correction of hypofibrinogenemia, hypoplasminogenemia, and elevated FDPs after heparin neutralization all suggest that the presence of DIC during cardiac surgery is a very rare event. DIC may be associated with cardiac surgery when another triggering event is provided, such as sepsis, shock, massive transfusions, or a frank hemolytic transfusion reaction.

Predisposing factors associated with enhanced cardiac surgery hemorrhage are (a) long perfusion times, (b) prior ingestion of warfarin-type drugs, (c) cyanotic heart disease, (d) hypothermic perfusions, (e) the preoperative ingestion of drugs known to interfere with platelet function, and (f) prolonged perfusion/aortic cross-clamp times. These predisposing risk factors are summarized in Table 9.8. Prevailing evidence suggests that in most patients undergoing CPB surgery, a primary fibrinolytic syndrome develops, although the exact triggering mechanisms are unclear, but may result from factor XII activation. However, the resultant secondary derangements in hemostasis will certainly create a potential for CPB hemorrhage. In most patients undergoing CPB procedures, severe platelet dysfunction develops. It is unclear whether this defect results from coating of platelet surfaces by FDP, membrane damage from the oxygenation mechanism, platelet damage from fast flow rates, or other unrecognized mechanisms. Whatever the triggering mechanism(s), it is quite clear that the most important alterations in hemostasis associated with CPB surgery are defective platelet function and primary fibrinolysis. These two defects alone or in combination certainly account for most nonsurgical and nontechnical hemorrhage in patients undergoing CPB; platelet-function defects account for far more hemorrhagic episodes than does primary fibrinolysis.

TABLE 9.8. FACTORS PREDISPOSING TO HEMORRHAGE DURING CARDIOPULMONARY BYPASS

1. Long perfusion times
2. Prior use of warfarins
3. Cyanotic heart disease
4. Hypothermic perfusion
5. Preop ingestion of antiplatelet drugs
6. Repeated bypass procedure

Diagnosis of Cardiopulmonary Bypass Hemorrhage

When bleeding happens during or after bypass, it is obviously extremely important to define the defect as quickly as possible; only in this manner can specific and effective therapy be delivered (138,142,154,159,252). As earlier mentioned, many instances of CPB hemorrhage are clearly the result of inadequate surgical technique, but alterations of hemostasis also may be responsible for accentuating CPB hemorrhage. This discussion is limited to nontechnical causes of CPB hemorrhage. The types of hemorrhage that occur during CPB are somewhat limited and are depicted in Table 9.9 in descending order of probability.

The primary distinction to be made is between strictly surgical bleeding, defects in hemostasis, and a combination of the two. This distinction becomes more difficult and more important after the patient has left the operating room; during this period, a decision must be made regarding reexploration and the adequacy of hemostasis for reexploration. In distinguishing between surgical and nonsurgical bleeding, many physical findings are helpful: is the bleeding localized or systemic? If the patient is already in the recovery room, the recognition of hematuria in association with petechiae and purpura, and oozing from i.v. sites

TABLE 9.9. HEMORRHAGIC SYNDROMES SEEN WITH CARDIOPULMONARY BYPASS SURGERY: DESCENDING ORDER OF PROBABILITY

Severe platelet dysfunction
  CPB induced
  Drug induced
Primary fibrinolytic syndrome
Thrombocytopenia
Hyperheparinemia or rebound ??
Disseminated intravascular coagulation (exceedingly rare)

CPB, cardiopulmonary bypass.

in conjunction with increased chest tube blood loss and oozing from surgical sites, including the sternotomy wound and saphenous vein harvest site, means a defect in hemostasis. Increased chest tube blood loss alone often signifies a technical bleeding problem. When the patient is in the operating room, these same findings hold true, and the surgeon will usually note bleeding or oozing throughout the surgical field in nontechnical bleeding. It is important, therefore, that communication between the surgeon and the hematologist or internist occurs. Clinical suggestions of a systemic instead of local cause of CPB hemorrhage are depicted in Table 9.10.

When CPB hemorrhage is seen or suspected, the following laboratory tests are ordered: prothrombin time, activated partial thromboplastin time, CBC and platelet count, examination of a peripheral smear, FDPs and D-dimer or prothrombin fragment 1+2 (PF 1+2) levels, heparin assay by synthetic substrate (anti-Xa), thrombin time, and plasminogen/plasmin levels by synthetic substrate methods (139,153,154,159). Evaluation of the heparin level will provide rapid information regarding the status of heparin and its potential effects on other tests of hemostasis. The resultant clot from the thrombin time is always observed for 5 minutes for evidence of lysis, supplying rapid additional information regarding the presence or absence of a clinically significant primary fibrino(geno)lytic syndrome. More evidence for or against primary lysis is obtained by noting the FDP and D-dimer/PF 1+2 levels (219,253–255). A peripheral blood smear and platelet count are invaluable for rapid evaluation of the potential for thrombocytopenic bleeding. Plasminogen and plasmin levels obtained by synthetic substrate technique are not time consuming but are not used for an immediate diagnosis; however, they are invaluable in making decisions regarding antifibrinolytic therapy later (139,153,154,159). If significant primary fibrinolysis is present, FDPs will be significantly elevated, the D-dimer/PF 1+2 level normal or near normal, and hypoplasminogenemia and circulating plasmin will be detected. If available, fibrinopeptide A levels will not be elevated, but B-β 15-42–related peptides will be elevated. If, on the other hand, excess heparin is a potential problem, this is noted by the heparin assay, and in addition, the thrombin time will be markedly prolonged. If no significant clot lysis is observed in the clot formed during measurement of the thrombin time, and significant FDP elevation is not present, primary fibrinolysis should not be dwelled on. All patients undergoing CPB have a platelet-function defect; when bleeding occurs, it is prudent to assume this defect is always present, and although it might not be the primary reason for hemorrhage, platelet dysfunction can be assumed to be additive to any other defect, whether surgical or resulting from altered hemostasis. No tests of platelet function need to be routinely done, therefore, but platelet levels are immediately ordered for any patient who demonstrates intrabypass or postbypass hemorrhage (137,138,154). The time period when hemorrhage occurs (that is, intraoperatively, after heparin neutralization, or in the recovery room) appears to bare little relation to the etiology of the primary hemostatic defect responsible for hemorrhage. Exceptions to this are thrombocytopenic bleeding, which usually happens after the patient is in the recovery room, and a significant drug-induced platelet-function defect, which is usually manifest as significant oozing immediately after the operative procedure is started. Tests ordered for the differential diagnosis of the etiology of hemorrhage during CPB surgery are listed in Table 9.11.

During the past decade, more and more cardiac surgeons are using several methods to graft and bypass coronary arteries on the beating heart, thus without need for bypass pumps. The experience with this technique has demonstrated much less thrombocytopenia and blood loss. The significant decrease in blood loss certainly implies fewer or perhaps minimal to no defects in hemostasis in the absence of the CPB pump, although no actual hemostasis studies have as yet been published. This is an exiting new area, as morbidity, mortality, and overall outcome results thus far equal those of patients undergoing CABG with a bypass pump (256–261).

TABLE 9.10. CLINICAL EVALUATION OF HEMORRHAGE IN THE CBP PATIENT

Chest tube blood loss only? or associated with
Petechiae, purpura, or ecchymoses
Hematuria
Oozing from intraarterial line sites
Oozing from intravenous sites
Oozing from venipunctures
Oozing from sternotomy wound
Oozing from saphenous vein graft site
Other systemic bleeding sites
Clots forming in chest tube?

CPB, cardiopulmonary bypass.

TABLE 9.11. LABORATORY EVALUATION OF CARDIAC BYPASS HEMORRHAGE (ORDERED "STAT")

Platelet count and CBC
Peripheral blood smear evaluation
Prothrombin time
Partial thromboplastin time
FDP titer
D-dimer assay
Heparin assay[a]
Thrombin time[b]
Plasminogen assay[c]
Plasmin assay[c]

CBC, complete blood count; FDP, fibrin degradation product.
[a]Anti-Xa level.
[b]Observe for clot lysis × 5 min.
[c]Synthetic substrate methods.

Management of Cardiopulmonary Bypass Hemorrhage

When first encountering a patient with intraoperative or postoperative CPB hemorrhage, it is of prime importance (a) to note the type of bleeding (systemic vs. local), (b) to order a stat laboratory screen as outlined earlier, and (c) to administer 6 to 8 units of platelet concentrates as quickly as possible. Although the use of platelet concentrates is somewhat empiric at this point, it is done for several sound reasons: (a) all patients have a significant platelet-function defect that may be the primary reason for hemorrhage, and usually it is a nontechnical bleed; or (b) this defect is likely to accentuate bleeding from other causes, whether it be a surgical defect or defective hemostasis. The quick administration of platelet concentrates while awaiting the earlier-mentioned laboratory evaluation will often stop or significantly reduce most instances of nontechnical CPB hemorrhage (137,138,154). Recently a fibrin "glue" in paste or spray form has been applied with reasonable success to bleeding sites in patients undergoing CPB hemorrhage; the source for this fibrin glue may be autologous or allogeneic (262–265).

When bleeding begins immediately on initiation of surgery, a platelet-function defect, usually drug induced, can be assumed to be present until further laboratory investigation can be done. In this instance, the patient should be given 6 to 8 units of platelet concentrates as quickly as possible, and the surgical wound should be closed if feasible. If a platelet-function defect is responsible for the hemorrhage (no laboratory evidence of significant fibrinolysis or hyperheparinemia), 6 to 8 units of platelet concentrates should be repeated the evening after surgery and for two postoperative mornings. Thrombocytopenic CPB hemorrhage should be controlled in the same manner, although greater numbers of platelet concentrates may be needed, as dictated by the initial platelet count, the site and severity of hemorrhage, and the response to platelet transfusions. Hyperheparinemia and heparin rebound, if thought to be a real clinical problem as documented by synthetic substrate assays, are managed by delivering 25% of the original calculated protamine sulfate dose; this is repeated every 30 to 60 minutes until bleeding stops. It should again be stressed that hyperheparinemia and heparin rebound are unlikely to be responsible for bleeding and should not be dwelled on unless concrete laboratory proof of hyperheparinemia is present, and evidence of primary fibrinolysis is clearly absent. I have seen many instances of excessive heparinization resulting from mistakes in calculations and solution preparation; none of these instances was associated with significant cardiac surgical hemorrhage. Similarly, protamine excess is rarely, if ever, a clinical problem. This situation should never call for therapy and should not be dwelled on at the risk of ignoring other potential defects in hemostasis.

Primary fibrinolysis is commonly present and may or may not be responsible for hemorrhage. This syndrome should not be treated empirically; antifibrinolytic therapy should be considered if the patient has failed to respond to platelet concentrates, and there is documented laboratory evidence for this syndrome, as noted by the presence of hypoplasminogenemia, circulating plasmin, and elevated FDPs. For those having appropriate testing systems available, the absence of elevated fibrinopeptide A, the absence of elevated D-dimer, and the presence of elevated B-β 15-42–related peptides offer further evidence for primary lysis. Primary fibrino(geno)lytic bleeding is generally treated with EACA given as an initial dose of 5 to10 g slow intravenous push followed by 1 to 2 g per hour until bleeding stops or slows to a non–life-threatening level. It should be recalled that EACA may be associated with ventricular arrhythmias (tachycardia or fibrillation), hypotension, hypokalemia, localized or diffuse thrombosis, and frank DIC. This agent should be injected slowly, and patients should be monitored carefully for cardiac status, renal output, blood pressure, and electrolytes. Another antifibrinolytic agent now available is tranexamic acid (266).

THROMBOHEMORRHAGIC COMPLICATIONS OF PROSTHETIC DEVICES AND OTHER EXTRACORPOREAL CIRCUITS

Exposure of the blood to foreign surfaces is often linked with thrombosis, which provides a major clinical obstacle to the use of prosthetic devices. The use of prosthetic devices and extracorporeal circuits has become commonplace in the management of patients with cardiovascular disease and for common angiographic studies or therapeutic angioplasty (153,267,268). The hemostatic complications after the insertion of prosthetic devices include consumption of coagulation factors, other plasma proteins, or platelets; the generation of microthrombi of little clinical consequence; and thrombosis or thromboembolism that may give rise to serious, life-threatening, or terminal vasoocclusion. Under normal circumstances, the blood remains fluid because of numerous obvious factors including a nonthrombogenic endothelial surface, endogenous fibrinolytic activity, natural protease inhibitors such as AT III, protein C, and protein S, and the dilution and dispersion of procoagulant components of the blood (112,269,270). All of these protective mechanisms are lost, to some degree, with the use of prosthetic devices (138,153,268).

In general, slow flow rates are associated with local thrombotic events; however, fast flow rates are more commonly associated with a high shear force and embolization (254). In addition, smooth prosthetic surfaces tend to favor little adhesiveness of a formed thrombus, and thus embolization is more likely to occur than with a rough surface, which tends to favor firm fibrin clot formation and eventual neovascularization (271). When blood is exposed to prosthetic devices or any foreign surface, including extracorporeal circuits, plasma proteins are immediately absorbed, primarily fibrinogen, albumin, α- and β-globulins, γ-globulin, factor VIII:c, factor XII, factor XI, and thrombin (272,273). Factors XII and XI may simply be absorbed or, alternatively, may become activated. Fibrinogen appears to be the major plasma protein absorbed and promotes subsequent platelet adhesion, with platelets adhering as a monolayer and then aggregating. Platelet adhesion will be enhanced/induced not only by fibrinogen but also by γ-globulin, thrombin, and subsequent factor XII and factor XI activation (274). In addition, the activation of factors XII and/or XI may induce intrinsic coagulation, with further fibrin formation generating a platelet–fibrin thrombus. As thrombotic surfaces form and embolize in the aforementioned manner, they may eventually overwhelm the ability of the reticuloendothelial system to clear them; subsequent thromboembolization with vascular occlusion and subsequent end-organ infarction may occur (275).

The most common defects that may generally occur with prosthetic devices are as follows: (a) there may be a frank coagulation factor and platelet consumption with subsequent thrombocytopenia and resultant hemorrhage; (b) devices may cause partial platelet degranulation, with subsequent defective platelet function and resultant hemorrhage; (c) in cases of oxygenation/dialysis membranes, fibrin–platelet deposition will render the exchange ineffective and provide a focus for thromboembolus; and (d) micro- or macrothromboemboli of platelets and/or fibrin may give rise to serious clinical vasoocclusive problems (138,153). The use of anticoagulants, including warfarin-type drugs, heparin, and platelet-suppressive agents, tends to normalize thrombotic and thromboembolic complications with prosthetic devices (138,153). However, the problem still remains clinically significant, especially during CPB surgery, hemodialysis, angiographic studies, prosthetic heart valve placement, long-term i.v. catheterization, and the use of LeVeen shunts (138,153).

Arterial and Venous Catheters

Intraarterial or intravenous catheters are coated with fibrin and/or platelet aggregates when used for angiographic studies, therapeutic angioplasty, long-term chemotherapy, infusions of fluids, and long-term parenteral hyperalimentation (138,153,267,276). Thromboembolism occurs in approximately 2% of individuals catheterized for angiographic studies (138,153,267,276,277). An additional complication is that an existing atherosclerotic plaque may be disrupted and embolize. The thromboembolic complications of short-term or long-term catheterization are usually minimized by the use of subcutaneous low-molecular-weight (LMW) heparin or unfractionated (UF) heparin. In addition to the aforementioned intraarterial catheters, i.v. catheters also can be associated with thrombotic events, but are most usually associated with localized phlebitis around the introduction site. This complication can occur in up to 20% to 30% of patients, and only 10% of these are diagnosed before the i.v. catheter is removed (278). The diagnosis of phlebitis may be made between 60 and 80 hours after starting the i.v. and appears to occur later in diabetics and earlier in patients with intravenous catheters for peripheral hyperalimentation (153,267,278). In addition, there is an inordinately increased incidence of local phlebitis in those patients who are undergoing i.v. therapy and have an associated infectious process (279).

Intraaortic Balloon Pump

Intraaortic balloon pumping (IABP) has been in clinical use since 1968 and is commonly used for the control of cardiogenic shock or low-output failure after CPB (280–282). Common current indications also include (a) acute myocardial infarction with cardiogenic shock, remaining unresponsive to immediate medical management; (b) unstable cardiac status after cardiac catheterization, coronary angiography, or coronary angioplasty; (c) impaired left ventricular function; (d) refractory low cardiac output after CPB procedures; and (e) occasionally for arrhythmias (280–283).

These devices are usually constructed of polyurethane and are inserted surgically or percutaneously into the left common femoral artery (280). The most common complications of intraaortic balloon pumping are (a) leg ischemia of several causes; (b) local or distal arterial injury/thrombosis; (c) aortic dissection; (d) destruction or activation of numerous blood elements including red cells, platelets, and coagulation proteins; and (e) infections, which are, of course, more common when the percutaneous insertion route is used (153,284,285). Despite the high frequency of thrombus and thromboembolus formation, there is no uniform anticoagulation regimen used with these devices. Some clinicians advocate the routine use of heparin to be delivered before, during, and until the point of removal of these balloons (286); however, others use heparin only in medical patients and use aspirin and/or LMW dextrans in surgical patients (153,267,283), and even other clinicians use no anticoagulants at all unless there is another underlying indication besides balloon assist (287). Another approach has been to use dextran plus heparin (282). Although it has been suggested that the routine use of anticoagulants may decrease the incidence of thrombus or thromboembolus (161,164), there are no clear guidelines.

Several mechanisms are operative to induce thrombus, thromboembolus, and resultant end-organ infarction in patients undergoing IABP. Thrombi adherent to the aortic intima along the path of the balloon often develop, and emboli may easily develop (285). These mural thrombi may detach fragments of existing thrombus, denuded endothelium, and/or platelet macroaggregates that may embolize downstream (during systole) or upstream (during diastole), and may infarct essentially any end organ or any other site, including the upper or lower extremities, depending on the direction of embolization and the size of the embolus (285,288). It has been noted that after 3 days of balloon assist, there is marked denuding of aortic endothelium adjacent to the balloon. After this, there is the usual expected platelet hyperactivity with subsequent platelet activation and release of procoagulant and vasoactive materials, leading to more platelet activation, activation of the coagulation system, more thrombi, emboli, thromboembolic showers, and vasoconstriction (136). Embolization is frequently to upper extremities, lower extremities, central nervous system, kidneys, spleen, superior mesenteric artery, or small bowel (284,285,288,289). Embolization is noted to occur most frequently in debilitated patients or in patients with severe cardiac failure.

Leg ischemia can develop from local thrombus formation in the aortic or iliofemoral vessels, or from emboli (283–285). Local thrombosis is especially common if the insertion is inadvertently made into the superficial femoral artery (284). Leg ischemia due to thrombus or thromboembolus is the most frequent early complication of intraaortic balloon assist devices (284). It has been suggested that the use of heparin/LMW heparin may decrease the incidence of this serious complication (153,156,267, 284). Leg ischemia due to local thrombosis or thromboembolus may be severe enough to give rise to an anterior compartment syndrome, necessitating fasciotomy or even amputation in severe cases (283). The incidence of leg ischemia secondary to thrombosis or thromboembolus is thought to be related to the time on balloon assist (284). In addition, the presence of atherosclerosis in the iliofemoral system is another important predisposing factor for vasoocclusion and the development of leg ischemia; the use of heparin will obviously not be preventive with this mechanism (284). The type of balloon also may influence the incidence of thrombus or thromboembolus (283). Even bilateral renal artery thrombi have been noted in association with IABP (289). Limb ischemia due to thrombosis or thromboembolus associated with IABP is common, occurring in up to 36% of patients (153,267,282,283). Because this complication can lead to obviously serious morbidity or even mortality, careful monitoring and the use of anticoagulants, preferably heparin in nonsurgical patients, is mandatory. Evaluation of the dorsalis pedis and posterior tibial pulses coupled with Doppler ultrasonography of the thigh vessels should be performed every 4 hours in these patients (283,284); digits should be inspected to assess capillary filling every 4 hours (284). The development of leg ischemia dictates immediate removal of the balloon if medically possible.

Hemorrhage is another potentially serious complication of IABP. Wound hemorrhage is the most common bleeding seen; however, retroperitoneal hemorrhage, gastrointestinal bleeding, genitourinary bleeding, central nervous system bleeding, and frank DIC also may occur (138,153,267,282, 283). The most common etiologic mechanism for hemorrhage associated with IABP is thrombocytopenia (138, 282,283); the degree of thrombocytopenia is clearly related to time on the device and may be of multiple etiologies including consumption in an aortic mural thrombus or consumption secondary to DIC. The development of DIC also appears to be related to time on the device, and these authors have noted DIC to develop only in patients undergoing at least 5 days of IABP; however, DIC may occur at only 1 day of balloon assist (288). There are multiple mechanisms by which DIC may develop in patients undergoing IABP. One such mechanism is simply activation of the hemostasis system by massive platelet release; another is "consumption" due to massive aortic intramural thrombus formation. Intravascular hemolysis may commonly develop, especially if a patient is on the device for more than 2 days (284); this also may trigger DIC (102,290). In this regard, balloon-induced hemolytic anemia and thrombocytopenia may be so severe that support with washed packed red cells and platelet concentrates is required (284). An additional triggering event for DIC is the high incidence of bacteremia, which is most commonly seen in patients receiving the balloon by percutaneous insertion (102,284).

In summary, IABP has now become a common therapeutic modality for patients with selected indications including cardiogenic shock and "weaning" from CPB with unstable hemodynamics or left ventricular dysfunction. These devices can be associated with very severe thrombotic, thromboembolic, and hemorrhagic problems of multifaceted etiology. In general, the careful monitoring of patients, in association with the judicious use of anticoagulants and a familiarity with the types of thrombotic or hemorrhagic disorders that may develop, are important to ward off these serious complications.

Vascular Shunts

Access shunts in the form of surgically created arteriovenous (AV) shunts or prosthetic AV shunts are necessary for hemodialysis patients, frequently transfused patients, patients undergoing long-term parenteral hyperalimentation, patients undergoing long-term chemotherapy, and patients committed to a long-term apheresis program (291,292). Surgically created AV shunts tend to have fewer thrombotic complications than prosthetic shunts. Although thrombosis of the shunt remains the major significant problem with these devices, infection also is of concern. Prosthetic shunts and surgically created shunts are usually "declotted" by the use of surgery or medical thrombolysis with reasonably good success (138,293,294). Anticoagulant therapy has not become commonplace for patients with AV shunts; however, it has been shown that dipyridamole will correct decreased platelet survival and increased platelet consumption in patients with these devices (295). Aspirin alone will not decrease the incidence of shunt thrombosis. Prosthetic vascular grafts are primarily constructed of Dacron, with sufficient porosity to allow for neovascularization, thrombus organization, and nutrient blood flow. Thrombotic occlusion of prosthetic grafts is not well controlled with heparin- or warfarin-type drugs and is now most commonly treated with platelet suppressive therapy (138,153,267).

Peritoneovenous shunting using a LeVeen valve or Denver valve has become a palliative procedure for the treatment of intractable ascites associated with severe liver disease and malignant ascites (296,297). A generalized hemorrhagic diathesis is frequently seen with the use of LeVeen shunts and appears to represent a straightforward DIC-type syndrome associated with accelerated fibrinogen and platelet destruction (60,138,267,298–302). The removal of ascitic fluid at the time of valve implantation, as well as the use of anticoagulants, has been advocated to abort DIC in patients receiving LeVeen shunts (60,138). Sitting the patient upright will often totally abort, or significantly blunt, the DIC process, and should be used as a short-term palliative measure in patients developing DIC with LeVeen shunts (60).

Prosthetic Heart Valves

The use of prosthetic heart valves has become common and has greatly reduced morbidity and mortality in patients with valvular heart disease. However, complications of these devices, which include thromboembolism, infection, hemolysis, and detachment, also may significantly alter morbidity and mortality (303). Of these complications, thromboembolism is the most common and can be the most serious; the most likely sites of embolism are the central nervous system, coronary arteries, retinae, and extremities (304). Early in the history of cardiac valve placement, it was discovered that warfarin could decrease, but not alleviate, the thromboembolic events occurring with mitral and aortic valves (305). Thromboembolism is much more common with mitral valves than with aortic valves, especially if atrial fibrillation or left atrial enlargement is present (303,305–307). Initial valves, which had metal exposed to blood, were associated with a 50% incidence of thromboembolism, which could be reduced to 13% with the use of warfarin (308). Original aortic valves were associated with a 35% incidence of thromboembolism, which was reduced to 8% with the use of warfarin (309). Valvular thromboemboli arise from platelets; after valve replacement, platelets adhere to the foreign surface by adhesion and aggregation (138,153,267,303,310,311). An additional impetus for platelet aggregation may come from ADP liberated during red cell hemolysis (267). Because of this platelet consumption on valvular surfaces, many patients with prosthetic valves demonstrate decreased platelet survival and increased platelet turnover; the decreased survival appears to correlate reasonably well with the incidence of thromboemboli (312–314). However, patients with rheumatic valve disease without prosthetic valves also demonstrate decreased platelet survival and increased platelet consumption and, in addition, an increased incidence of thromboembolism (315). Valvular platelet consumption has decreased progressively with new valve design, but still has not been totally alleviated. Platelet deposits and thromboemboli were most pronounced with the early metal valves, and decreased in incidence with second-generation cloth-bound valves, which would induce neoendothelialization of the valve surface and, it was hoped, an inert valve. Newer xenograft (porcine) valves are associated with an even greater reduction in thromboembolic complications. In spite of this improvement, however, there is still a significant incidence of serious thromboembolism in patients with prosthetic aortic or mitral valves, and most are committed to long-term or life-long anticoagulation of some type.

It has been noted that both dipyridamole and sulfinpyrazone will normalize decreased platelet survival in patients with prosthetic valves, but aspirin alone does not demonstrate this effect (312,316). However, aspirin will potentiate the effect of dipyridamole in normalizing platelet survival in patients (312). The mechanisms for this are unclear, as the doses of dipyridamole and sulfinpyrazone that will normalize platelet survival are lower than doses required to alter platelet aggregation in vitro. It also has been noted that sulfinpyrazone will normalize decreased platelet survival in patients with rheumatic mitral valvular disease who do not have prosthetic valves (315). These observations led to interest in antiplatelet drugs for the control of thromboembolism associated with prosthetic heart valves, and numerous clinical trials have proven the efficacy of several agents, including aspirin and dipyridamole (317–321). One early trial demonstrated a reduction from 14% to a 1.3% incidence of thromboemboli by adding dipyridamole to a warfarin regimen (317). Another early trial revealed that the addition of aspirin to the warfarin regimen decreased the incidence of thromboembolism by 80% (318). The efficacy of antiplatelet agents alone remains unclear; one trial found aspirin plus dipyridamole alone (no warfarin) to be effective (322), but another trial found this regimen to be ineffective (323).

Thus even though the role of antiplatelet agents alone remains unclear, it is clear that an antiplatelet agent might be considered in conjunction with warfarin in some patients with prosthetic valves. There is now generally little uniformity in anticoagulant regimens for patients with prosthetic cardiac valves. One suggestion has been that the incidence of thromboembolism decreases with time, and after a given period, an anticoagulant is no longer needed in selected patients (324–326). Another recommendation is to use adequate doses of warfarin (2.5 × the control time) plus aspirin or dipyridamole (311). Yet another recommended regimen is to use warfarin in patients with mitral or double valve replacement but antiplatelet agents alone in patients with aortic valves (307). Another author (313) suggested combination antiplatelet agents alone in prosthetic valve patients; the aspirin dose suggested is 330 mg, t.i.d., and the dipyridamole dose recommended is 75 mg, t.i.d. (313). Another recommendation is that of Frankl (303), who recommended that patients with aortic valves receive adequate doses of aspirin plus dipyridamole, and patients with mitral valve replacement or double valve replacement should be treated with aspirin (ASA) plus dipyridamole plus warfarin. In 1998, specific antithrombotic recommendations for patients with mechanical or bioprosthetic heart valves were offered by the American College of Chest Physicians (ACCP) (327). These recommendations are generally summarized as follows: all patients with mechanical heart valves should receive oral anticoagulants; an international normalized ratio (INR) of 2.5 is recommended for patients with an aortic bileaflet mechanical valve, provided the left atrium is of normal size and the patient exhibits normal sinus rhythm and a normal ejection fraction. An INR of 3.0 (2.5 to 3.5) is recommended for patients with tilting disk valves and bileaflet mechanical valves in the mitral region; an alternative for this scenario is an INR of 2.5 (2.0 to 3.0) in conjunction with ASA at 80 to 100 mg per day. In patients with caged ball or caged disk valves, an INR of 3.0 (2.5 to 3.5) plus ASA at 80 to 100 mg per day is recommended. It is recommended that patients with mechanical valves plus an additional risk factor receive oral anticoagulant at an intensity of 3.0 (2.5 to 3.0) in conjunction with ASA at 81 mg per day. Patients with mechanical heart valves who have systemic embolization despite adequate antithrombotic therapy with oral anticoagulants should have ASA at 81 mg per day added to the antithrombotic regimen. For patients with bioprosthetic valves, the following general recommendations are provided by the ACCP: those with bioprosthetic valves in the mitral or aortic position should receive oral anticoagulant therapy, with the INR 2 to 3, for 3 months after placement. If patients with aortic or mitral position bioprosthetic valves have accompanying atrial fibrillation, therapy with oral anticoagulants, at INR of 2 to 3 should be over the long term. If patients with bioprosthetic valves have an atrial thrombus, a permanent pacemaker, or systemic embolization, oral anticoagulants with an INR of 2 to 3 should be used over the long term. If patients with bioprosthetic heart valves are in sinus rhythm, the ACCP recommends ASA at 162 mg per day.

SUMMARY

This discussion has provided a review of altered hemostasis associated with CPB surgery and selected cardiovascular devices. The key to prevention of CPB hemorrhage is to obtain an adequate preoperative evaluation. An adequate history for bleeding tendencies and thrombotic tendencies in both the patient and the family are of importance, as is a careful history regarding the use of drugs affecting hemostasis, especially drugs known to interfere with platelet function, should be obtained. A careful physical examination, searching for clues of a real or potential bleeding diathesis, also may prevent catastrophic cases of hemorrhage. An adequate presurgical screen must be done in CPB candidates. Besides the usual prothrombin time, partial thromboplastin time, and platelet count, a standardized template bleeding time and thrombin time should be done. The use of these simple testing modalities will guard against significant defects in vascular and platelet function. Most instances of nontechnical cardiovascular surgical hemorrhage are because of several well-defined defects in hemostasis, which should be easily controlled if approached in a logical manner as a team effort among cardiac surgeons, pathologists, and hematologists.

REFERENCES

1. Bick RL, Murano G. Physiology of hemostasis. *Clin Lab Med* 1994;14:677.
2. Muller-Berghaus G. Pathophysiologic and biochemical events in disseminated intravascular coagulation: dysregulation of procoagulant and anticoagulant pathways. *Semin Thromb Hemost* 1989;15:58.
3. Ryan TJ. The investigation of vasculitis. In: *Microvascular injury*. Philadelphia: WB Saunders, 1976:333.
4. Sheppard B, French JE. Platelet adhesion in the rabbit abdominal aorta following the removal of endothelium: a scanning and transmission electron microscopic study. *Proc R Soc Lond* 1971; 176:427.
5. Wessler S, Yin ET. On the mechanism of thrombosis. *Prog Hematol* 1969;4:201.
6. Friedman RJ, Burns ER. Role of platelets in the proliferative response of the injured artery. *Prog Hemost Thromb* 1978;4: 2498.
7. Harker LA, Schwartz SM, Ross R. Endothelium and arteriosclerosis. *Thromb Clin Haematol* 1981;10:283.
8. Roberts WC, Ferrans VJ. The role of thrombosis in the etiology of atherosclerosis (a positive one) and in precipitating fatal ischemic heart disease (a negative one). *Semin Thromb Hemost* 1976;2:123.
9. Sinzinger H. Role of platelets in atherosclerosis. *Semin Thromb Hemost* 1986;12:124.
10. Henry RL. Platelet function in hemostasis. In: Murano G, Bick RL, eds. *Basic concepts of hemostasis and thrombosis.* Boca Raton, Fla: CRC Press, 1980:17.
11. Triplett DA. The platelet: a review. In: Triplett DA, ed. *Platelet function.* Chicago: ASCP Press, 1978:1.
12. Astrup T. Fibrinolysis: an overview. In: Davidson JF, Rowan RM, Samama MM, et al., eds. *Progress in chemical fibrinolysis.* Vol 3. New York: Raven Press, 1978:1.
13. Kwaan HC. The role of fibrinolysis in disease states. *Semin Thromb Hemost* 1984;10:71.
14. Mammen EF. Inhibitor abnormalities. *Semin Thromb Hemost* 1983;9:42.

15. Ruggeri ZM, Zimmerman TS. von Willebrand factor and von Willebrand disease. *Blood* 1987;70:895.
16. White GC, Shoemaker CB. Factor VIII gene and hemophilia. *Blood* 1989;73:1.
17. Walsh P. The effect of collagen and kaolin on the intrinsic coagulation activity of platelets: evidence for an alternative pathway in intrinsic coagulation not requiring factor XII. *Br J Haematol* 1972;22:393.
18. Wilner GD, Nossel HL, LeRoy EL. Activation of Hageman factor by collagen. *J Clin Invest* 1968;47:2608.
19. Ginbrane MA. *Vascular endothelium in hemostasis and thrombosis.* London: Churchill Livingston, 1986:250.
20. Leonard EF, Turitto VT, Vroman L, eds. Blood in contact with natural and artifical surfaces. *Ann N Y Acad Sci* 1987;516:688.
21. Ruggeri ZM, Fulcher CA, Ware J. Progress in vascular biology, hemostasis and thrombosis. *Ann N Y Acad Sci* 1991;614:311.
22. Stern DM, Nawroth PP, eds. Vessel wall. *Semin Thromb Hemost* 1987;13:39-536.
23. Ulutin ON, et al., eds. Modulation of endothelium and control of vascular and thrombotic disorders. *Semin Thromb Hemost Suppl* 1988;14:114.
24. Droller MJ. Ultrastructure of the platelet release reaction in response to various aggregating agents and their inhibitors. *Lab Invest* 1973;29:595.
25. Stuart MJ. Inherited defects of platelet function. *Semin Hematol* 1975;12:233.
26. White JG. Identification of platelet secretion in the electron microscope. *Ser Haematol* 1973;6:429.
27. Nachman RL. Platelet proteins. *Semin Hematol* 1968;5:18.
28. Day NJ, Stormorken, Holmsen H. Subcellular localization of platelet factor 3 and platelet factor 4. *Proc 12th Congr Int Soc Hematol* Mexico City, 1968:172.
29. Packham MA, Mustard JF. Platelet reactions. *Semin Hematol* 1971;8:30.
30. Thomas DP, Niewiarowski S, Ream VJ. Release of adenosine nucleotides and platelet factor 4 from platelets of man and four other species. *J Lab Clin Med* 1970;75:607.
31. Born GVR, Cross MJ. The aggregation of blood platelets. *J Physiol* 1963;168:178.
32. Zucker MB, Peterson J. Serotonin, platelet factor 3 activity and platelet aggregating agent released by adenosine diphosphate. *Blood* 1967;30:556.
33. Davis RB, Mecker WR, Bailey WL. Serotonin release after injection of *E. coli* endotoxin in the rabbit. *Fed Proc* 1961;20:261.
34. Des Prez RM, Horowitz HI, Hoo EW. Effects of bacterial endotoxin on rabbit platelets, I: platelet aggregation and release of platelet factors in vitro. *J Exp Med* 1961;114:857.
35. Mueller-Eckhardt C, Luscher EF. Immune reactions of human blood platelets, I: a comparative study on the effects on platelets of heterologous antiplatelet antiserum, antigen-antibody complexes, aggregation gamma-globulin, and thrombin. *Thromb Diath Haemorrh* 1968;20:155.
36. Pfueller SL, Luscher F. The effects of immune complexes on blood and their relationship to complement activation. *Immunochemistry* 1972;9:1151.
37. Haslam RJ. Interactions of the pharmacological receptors of blood platelets with adenylate cyclase. *Ser Haematol* 1973;6:333.
38. Salzman EW. Cyclic AMP and platelet function. *N Engl J Med* 1972;286:358.
39. Cole B, Robison GA, Hartman RC. Effects of prostaglandin E and theophylline on aggregation and cyclic AMP levels of human blood platelets. *Fed Proc* 1970;29:316.
40. Horlington M, Watson PA. Inhibition of 3′-5′-cyclic-AMP, phosphodiesterase by some platelet aggregation inhibitors. *Biochem Pharmacol* 1970;19:955.
41. Gerrard JM, White JG. Prostaglandins and thromboxanes: "middlemen" modulating platelet function in hemostasis and thrombosis. *Prog Hemost Thromb* 1978;4:87.
42. Gryglewski RJ, Bunting S, Moncada S, et al. Arterial walls are protected against deposition of platelet thrombi by a substance (prostaglandin X) which they make from prostaglandin endoperoxides. *Prostaglandins* 1976;12:685.
43. Moncada S, Gryglewski R, Bunting S, et al. A lipid peroxide inhibits the enzyme in blood vessel microsomes that generate from prostaglandin endoperoxides the substance (prostaglandin X) which prevents platelet aggregation. *Prostaglandins* 1976;12:715.
44. Turpie AGG. Antiplatelet therapy. *Thromb Clin Haematol* 1981;10:497.
45. Berndt MC, Caen JP. Platelet glycoproteins. *Prog Hemost Thromb* 1984;7:111.
46. Davies GE, Palek J. Platelet protein organization: analysis by treatment with membrane-permeable cross-linking reagents. *Blood* 1982;59:502.
47. Lusher JM, et al., eds. Factor VIII/vWF and platelet formation and function in health and disease. *Ann N Y Acad Sci* 1987;509:223.
48. Berndt MC, Gregory C, Chong BH. Additional glycoprotein defects in Bernard-Soulier syndrome: confirmation of genetic basis of parental analysis. *Blood* 1983;62:800.
49. Clemetson KJ, McGregor JL, James E. Characterization of the platelet membrane glycoprotein abnormalities in Bernard-Soulier syndrome and comparison with normal by surface-labeled techniques and high-resolution two-dimensional gel electrophoresis. *J Clin Invest* 1982;70:304.
50. Meyer D, Baumgartner HR. Role of von Willebrand factor in platelet adhesion to the subendothelium. *Br J Haematol* 1983;54:1.
51. Bick RL. Platelet function defects: a clinical review. *Semin Thromb Hemost* 1992;18:167.
52. Kunicki TJ, Russell N, Nurden AT. Further studies of the human platelet receptor for quinine and quinidine-dependent antibodies. *J Immunol* 1981;126:398.
53. Berendt MC, Phillips DR. Interaction of thrombin with platelets: purification of the thrombin substrate. *Ann N Y Acad Sci* 1981;370:87.
54. Gogstad GO, Hagen J, Korsmo R. Characterization of the proteins of isolated human platelet alpha granules, evidence for a separate alpha granule pool of the glycoproteins IIb and IIIa. *Biochim Biophys Acta* 1981;670:150.
55. Fujimura K, Phillips DR. Binding of Ca++ to glycoprotein IIb from human platelet plasma membranes. *Thromb Haemost* 1983;50:251.
56. McMillan R, Mason D, Tani P. Evaluation of platelet surface antigens: localization of the pla-1 alloantigen. *Br J Haematol* 1981;51:297.
57. White JG. Inherited disorders of the platelet membrane and secretory granules. *Hum Pathol* 1987;18:123.
58. Lawler J, Hynes RO. Structural organization of the thrombospondin molecule. *Semin Thromb Hemost* 1987;13:245.
59. Santoro SA. Thrombospondin and the adhesive behavior of platelets. *Semin Thromb Hemost* 1987;13:290.
60. Bick RL. Disseminated intravascular coagulation and related syndromes: a clinical review. *Semin Thromb Hemost* 1988;14:299.
61. McKusick VA. *Mendelian inheritance in man: catalogs of autosomal dominant, autosomal recessive and X-linked phenotypes.* 9th ed. Baltimore: Johns Hopkins University Press, 1990.
62. Kaplan AP. Initiation of the intrinsic coagulation and fibrinolytic pathways of man: the role of surfaces, Hageman factor, prekallikrein, high molecular weight kininogen, and factor XI. *Prog Hemost Thromb* 1978;4:127.

63. Kaplan AJ, Meier HL, Mandle R. The Hageman factor dependent pathways of coagulation, fibrinolysis, and kinin generation. *Semin Thromb Hemost* 1976;3:1.
64. Griffin JH, Cochrane CG. Recent advances in the understanding of contact activation reactions. *Semin Thromb Hemost* 1979; 5:254.
65. Manuhalter CH, ed. Contact phase coagulation disorders. *Semin Thromb Hemost* 1987;13:130.
66. Irwin JF, Seegers WH, Andary JTJ, et al. Blood coagulation as a cybernetic system: control of autoprothrombin C (Xa) formation. *Thromb Res* 1975;6:431.
67. Jesty J, Maynard JR, Radcliffe RD, et al. Initiation and control of the extrinsic pathway of coagulation. In: Reich E, Rifkin DB, Shaw E, eds. *Proteases and biological control.* Cold Springs Harbor, NY: Cold Springs Harbor Labs, 1975:171.
68. Silverberg AS, Nemerson Y, Zur M. Kinetics of the activation of bovine factor XII by components of the extrinsic pathway. *J Biol Chem* 1977;252:8481.
69. Chabbat J, Porte P, Tellier M, et al. Aprotinin is a competitive inhibitor of the factor VIIa-tissue factor complex. *Thromb Res* 1993;71:205.
70. Seegers WH. Prothrombin complex. *Semin Thromb Hemost* 1981;7:291.
71. Stenflo J. Vitamin K, prothrombin, and gamma-carboxy-glutamic acid. *N Engl J Med* 1977;296:624.
72. Denson KWE. The levels of factor II, VII, IX, and X by antibody neutralization techniques in the plasma of patients receiving phenindione therapy. *Br J Haematol* 1971;20:643.
73. Mackie MJ, Douglas AS. Drug induced disorders of coagulation. In: Ratnoff OD, Forbes CD, eds. *Disorders of hemostasis.* Philadelphia: WB Saunders, 1991:493.
74. Walz DA, Fenton JW, Shuman MA, eds. Bioregulatory functions of thrombin. *Ann N Y Acad Sci* 1986;485:1–450.
75. Fenton JW, ed. Thrombin and hemostasis. *Semin Thromb Hemost* 1993;19:321–424.
76. Mosesson MW, Doolittle RF, eds. Molecular biology of fibrinogen and fibrin. *Ann N Y Acad Sci* 1983;408:1–672.
77. Alami SY, Hampton JW, Race GH, et al. Fibrin stabilizing factor (factor XIII). *Am J Med*1968;44:1.
78. Ratnoff OD. The molecular basis of hereditary clotting disorders. *Prog Hemost Thromb* 1972;1:39.
79. Aoki N, Harpel PC. Inhibitors of the fibrinolytic enzyme system. *Semin Thromb Hemost* 1984;10:24.
80. Wiman B, Hamsten A. The fibrinolytic enzyme system and its role in the etiology of thromboembolic disease. *Semin Thromb Hemost* 1990;16:207.
81. Castellino FJ. Biochemistry of human plasminogen. *Semin Thromb Hemost* 1984;10:18.
82. Aoki N, ed. Fibrinolysis. *Semin Thromb Hemost* 1984;10:107.
83. Ratnoff OD, Naff GB. The conversion of C′1s to C′1 esterase by plasmin and trypsin. *J Exp Med* 1967;125:337.
84. Robbins KM. Present status of the fibrinolytic system. In: Fareed J, Messmore HL, Fenton J, et al., eds. *Perspectives in hemostasis.* New York: Pergamon Press, 1980:53.
85. Bachmann F, Kruithof KO. Tissue plasminogen activator: chemical and physiological aspects. *Semin Thromb Hemost* 1984;10:6.
86. Goldsmith GN, Saito H, Ratnoff OD. The activation of plasminogen by Hageman factor (factor XII) and Hageman factor fragments. *J Clin Invest* 1978;21:54.
87. Kaplan AP, Austin F. The fibrinolytic pathway of human plasma: isolation and characterization of the plasminogen proactivator. *J Exp Med* 1972;135:1378.
88. Stump DC, Taylor FB, Neshein ME. Pathologic fibrinolysis as a cause of clinical bleeding. *Semin Thromb Hemost* 1990;16: 260.
89. Schreiber AD. Plasma inhibitors of the Hageman factor dependent pathways. *Semin Thromb Hemost* 1976;3:43.
90. Astedt B, Lecander I, Ny T. The placental type plasminogen activator inhibitor: PAI-2. *Fibrinolysis* 1987;1:203.
91. Loskutoff DJ, Sawdey M, Mimuro J. Type 1 plasminogen activator inhibitor. *Prog Hemost Thromb* 1989;9:87.
92. Emeis JJ, Brommer EJP, Kluft C. Progress in fibrinolysis. In: Poller L, ed. *Recent advances in blood coagulation.* Edinburgh: Churchill Livingstone, 1985:11.
93. Yee JA, Yan L, Dominguez JC, et al. Plasminogen-dependent activation of latent transforming growth factor beta (TGF-beta) by growing cultures of osteoblast-like cells. *J Cell Physiol* 1993; 157:528.
94. Marder VJ. Molecular aspects of fibrin formation and dissolution. *Semin Thromb Hemost* 1982;8:74.
95. Marder VJ, Shulman NR. High molecular weight derivatives of human fibrinogen produced by plasmin: mechanism of their anticoagulant activity. *J Biol Chem* 1969;244:2120.
96. Rosse WF. Complement. In: Williams WJ, Beutler E, Erslev AJ, et al., eds. *Hematology.* New York: McGraw-Hill, 1977:87.
97. Ruddy S, Gigli I, Austen KF. The complement system in man, I: activation, control, and products of the reaction sequences. *N Engl J Med* 1972;278:489.
98. Gotze O. Proteases of the properdin system. In: Reich E, Rifkin DB, Shaw E, eds. *Proteases and biological control.* Cold Springs Harbor, NY: Cold Spring Harbor Symposium, 1975:255.
99. Muller-Eberhard HJ. Complement. *Annu Rev Biochem* 1975; 44:667.
100. Pillomer L, Blum L, Lepow IH. The properdin system and immunity, I: demonstration and isolation of a new serum protein, properdin, and its role in immune phenomena. *Science* 1954;120:279.
101. Wachtfogel YT, Kucich U, Hack CE, et al. Aprotinin inhibits the contact, neutrophil, and platelet activation systems during simulated extracorporeal circulation. *J Thorac Cardiovasc Surg* 1993;106:1.
102. Bick RL. Disseminated intravascular coagulation: pathophysiological mechanisms and manifestations. *Semin Thromb Hemost* 1998;24:3.
103. Bennett B, Ogston D. Role of complement, coagulation, fibrinolysis, and kinins in normal haemostasis and disease. In: Bloom AL, Thomas DP, eds. *Haemostasis and thrombosis.* London: Churchill Livingston, 1981:236.
104. Ryan JW, Ryan US. Biochemical and morphological aspects of the actions and metabolism of kinins. In: Pisano JJ, Austen KF, eds. *Chemistry and biology of the kallikrein-kinin system in health and disease.* Bethesda, Md: DHEW Pub 76-791, U.S. Department of Health, Education, and Welfare, 1974:315.
105. Van Arman CG, Bohidar HR. Role of the kallikrein-kinin system in inflammation. In: Pisano JJ, Austin KF, eds. *Chemistry and biology of the kallekrein-kinin system in health and disease.* Bethesda, Md: DHEW Publ 76-791, U.S. Department of Health, Education and Welfare, 1974:471.
106. Swies J, Chopicki S, Gryglewski RJ. Kinins and thrombolysis. *J Physiol Pharmacol* 1993;44:171.
107. Comp PC. Hereditary disorders predisposing to thrombosis. *Prog Hemost Thromb* 1986;8:71.
108. Joist JH. Hypercoagulability: introduction and perspective. *Semin Thromb Hemost* 1990;16:151.
109. Esmon CT, ed. Protein C. *Semin Thromb Hemost* 1984;10: 109–172.
110. Dalbach B, Carlsson M, Svensson PJ. Familial thrombophilia due to a previously unrecognized mechanism characterized by poor anticoagulant response to activated protein C: prediction of a cofactor to activated protein C. *Proc Natl Acad Sci U S A* 1994;90:1004.

111. Taby O, Chabbat J, Steinbuch M. Inhibition of activated protein C by aprotinin and the use of the insolubilized inhibitor for its purification. *Thromb Res* 1990;59:27.
112. Bick RL. Clinical relevance of antithrombin III. *Semin Thromb Hemost* 1982;8:276.
113. Jaques LB, McDuffie NM. The chemical and anticoagulant nature of heparin. *Semin Thromb Hemost* 1978;4:277.
114. Rosenberg RD. The effect of heparin on factor XIa and plasmin. *Thromb Diath Haemorrh* 1975;33:51.
115. Rosenberg RD, Damus P. The purification and mechanism of action of human antithrombin-heparin cofactor. *J Biol Chem* 1973;248:6490.
116. Seegers WH. Antithrombin III. *Semin Thromb Hemost* 1981;7:263.
117. Bick RL. The clinical significance of fibrinogen degradation products. *Semin Thromb Hemost* 1982;8:302.
118. Moseson MW. Cold-insoluble globulin: a circulating cell surface protein. *Thromb Haemost* 1977;38:742.
119. Pearlstein E, Gold LI, Garcia-Pardo A. Fibronectin: a review of its structure and biological activity. *Mol Cell Biochem* 1980;29:103.
120. Couchman JR, Austria MR, Woods A. Fibronectin-cell interactions. *J Invest Dermatol* 1990;94:7.
121. Moser DF. Fibronectin. *Prog Hemost Thromb* 1980;5:111.
122. Moser DF, Schad PE, Kleinman HK. Cross-linking of fibronectin to collagen by blood coagulation factor XIIIa. *J Clin Invest* 1979;64:781.
123. Moseson MW, Umfleet RA. The cold-insoluble globulin of plasma. *J Biol Chem* 1970;254:5728.
124. Wagner DD, Hynes RO. Domain structure of fibronectin and its relationship to function. *J Biol Chem* 1979;254:6746.
125. Wight TN. Vessel proteoglycans and thrombogenesis. *Prog Hemost Thromb* 1980;5:1.
126. Ofusu FA, Danishefsky I, Hirsh J, eds. Heparin and related polysaccharides. *Ann N Y Acad Sci* 1989;556:1–501.
127. Goldstein IM, Perez HD. Biologically active peptides derived from the fifth component of complement. *Prog Hemost Thromb* 1980;5:41.
128. Galloway MJ, Mackie MJ, McVerry BA. Combinations of increased thrombin, plasmin, and non-specific protease activity in patients with acute leukemia. *Haemostasis* 1983;13:322.
129. Lisiewicz J. Disseminated intravascular coagulation in acute leukemia. *Semin Thromb Hemost* 1988;14:339.
130. Bick RL. Assessment of patients with hemorrhage. In: *Disorders of thrombosis and hemostasis: clinical and laboratory practice.* Chicago: ASCP Press, 1992:27.
131. Teylor KM. Effect of aprotinin on blood loss and blood use after cardiopulmonary bypass. In: Pifarre R, ed. *Anticoagulation, hemostasis, and blood conservation in cardiovascular surgery.* St. Louis: Hanley, Belfus/Mosby, 1993:129.
132. Orchard MA, Goodchield CS, Prentice CR, et al. Aprotinin reduces cardiopulmonary bypass-induced blood loss and inhibits fibrinolysis without influencing platelets. *Br J Haematol* 1993;85:533.
133. Schonberger JP, Bredee JJ, van Oeveren W, et al. Preoperative therapy of low-dose aspirin in internal mammary bypass operations with and without aprotinin. *J Thorac Cardiovasc Surg* 1993;106:262.
134. Hardy JF, Desroches J, Belisle S, et al. Low-dose aprotinin infusion is not clinically useful to reduce bleeding and transfusion of homologous blood products in high-risk cardiac surgical patients. *Can J Anaesth* 1993;40:625.
135. Royston D. Controversies in the practical use of aprotinin In: Bifarre R, ed. *Anticoagulation, hemostasis, and blood conservation in cardiovascular surgery.* St. Louis: Hanley and Belfus, Mosby, 1993:147.
136. Bick RL, Tse N. Hemostasis abnormalities associated with prosthetic devices and organ transplantation. *Lab Med* 1992;23:462–486.
137. Bick RL. Hemostasis defects with cardiac surgery, general surgery, and prosthetic devices. In: *Disorders of thrombosis and hemostasis: clinical and laboratory practice.* Chicago: ASCP Press, 1992:195.
138. Bick RL, Fareed J. Hemostasis processes during cardiovascular bypass and intravascular cardiovascular devices. In: Pifarre R, ed. *New anticoagulants for the cardiovascular patient.* Philadelphia: Hanley & Belfus, 1997:551.
139. Mielke CHMM, Kaneshiro LA, Maher J, et al. The standardized normal Ivy bleeding time and its prolongation by aspirin. *Blood* 1969;34:204.
140. Bick RL. Platelet defects. In: *Disorders of hemostasis and thrombosis: principles of clinical practice.* New York: Thieme, 1985:65.
141. Bick RL, Murano G. Primary hyperfibrino(geno)lytic syndromes. In: Murano G, Bick RL, eds. *Basic concepts of hemostasis and thrombosis.* Boca Raton, Fla: CRC Press, 1980:181.
142. Bick RL. Syndromes associated with hyperfibrino(geno)lysis. In: *Disseminated intravascular coagulation.* Boca Raton, Fla: CRC Press, 1983:105.
143. Shahian DM, Wallach SR, Bern MM. Open heart surgery in patients with cold-reactive proteins. *Surg Clin North Am* 1985;65:315.
144. Landymore R, Isom W, Barlam B. Management of patients with cold agglutinins who require open-heart surgery. *Can J Surg* 1983;26:79.
145. Guena L, Kwabena KA, Addei A. Intraoperative hypothermia in a patient with cold agglutinin disease. *JAMA* 1982;74:691.
146. Klein HG, Faltz LL, McIntosh CL, et al. Surgical hypothermia in a patient with a cold agglutinin. *Transfusion* 1980;20:354.
147. Leach AB, Van Hasselt GL, Edwards JC. Cold agglutinins and deep hypothermia. *Anaesthesia* 1983;38:140.
148. Moore RA, Geller EA, Mathews ES, et al. The effect of hypothermic cardiopulmonary bypass on patients with low-titer, non-specific cold agglutinins. *Ann Thorac Surg* 1984;37:233.
149. Brecker G, Cronkite EP. Morphology and enumeration of human blood platelets. *J Appl Physiol* 1950;3:365.
150. Hougie C. *Fundamentals of blood coagulation in clinical medicine.* New York: McGraw-Hill, 1963:241.
151. Proctor RR, Rapaport SI. The partial thromboplastin time with kaolin: a simple screening test for first stage plasma clotting factor deficiencies. *Am J Clin Pathol* 1961;36:212.
152. Quick AJ, Stanley-Brown M, Bancroft FW. A study of the coagulation defect in hemophilia and in jaundice. *Am J Med Sci* 1935;190:501.
153. Bick RL. Alterations of hemostasis associated with surgery, cardiopulmonary bypass surgery, prosthetic devices and transplantation. In: Ratnoff OD, Forbes CD, eds. *Disorders of hemostasis.* 2nd ed. Philadelphia: WB Saunders, 1991:382.
154. Bick RL. Hemostasis defects associated with cardiac surgery, prosthetic devices, and other extracorporeal circuits. *Semin Thromb Hemost* 1985;11:249.
155. Beall C, Yow EM, Blodwell RD, et al. Open heart surgery without blood transfusion. *Arch Surg* 1967;94:567.
156. Cordell AR. Hematological complications of extracorporeal circulation. In: Cordell AR, Ellison RG, eds. *Complications of intrathoracic surgery.* Boston: Little, Brown, 1979:27.
157. Mammen EF. Natural proteinase inhibitors in extracorporeal circulation. *Ann N Y Acad Sci* 1968;146:754.
158. Koets MH, Washington BC, Wolk LW, et al. Hemostasis changes during cardiovascular bypass surgery. *Semin Thromb Hemost* 1985;11:281.
159. Bick RL. Pathophysiology of hemostasis and thrombosis. In:

Sodeman's pathologic physiology, mechanisms of disease. 7th ed. Philadelphia: WB Saunders, 1985:705.

160. Silveira FM, Lourenco DM, Maluf M, et al. Hemostatic changes in children treated with open heart surgery with cardiopulmonary bypass. *Arq Brasil Cardiol* 1998;70:29.
161. Kevy SV, Glickman RM, Bernhard WF, et al. The pathogenesis and control of the hemorrhagic defect in open-heart surgery. *Surg Gynecol Obstet* 1966;123:313.
162. Signori EE, Penner JA, Kahn DR. Coagulation defects and bleeding in open heart surgery. *Ann Thorac Surg* 1969;8:521.
163. Porter JM, Silver D. Alterations in fibrinolysis and coagulation associated with cardiopulmonary bypass. *J Thorac Cardiovasc Surg* 1968;56:869.
164. Tice DA, Worth MH. Recognition and treatment of postoperative bleeding associated with open heart surgery. *Ann N Y Acad Sci* 1968;146:745.
165. Wright TA, Darte J, Mustard WT. Postoperative bleeding after extracorporeal circulation. *Can J Surg* 1959;2:142.
166. von Kaulla KN, Swan H. Clotting deviations in man during cardiac bypass: fibrinolysis and circulating anticoagulants. *J Thorac Surg* 1958;36:519.
167. Blomback M, Noren I, Senning A. Coagulation disturbances during extracorporeal circulation and the postoperative period. *Acta Chir Scand* 1964;127:433.
168. Deiter RA, Neville WE, Piffare R, et al. Preoperative coagulation profiles and posthemodilution cardiopulmonary bypass hemorrhage. *Am J Surg* 1971;121:689.
169. Penick GD, Averette HE, Peters RM, et al. The hemorrhagic syndrome complicating extracorporeal shunting of blood: an experimental study of its pathogenesis. *Thromb Diath Haemorrh* 1958;2:218.
170. Trimble AS, Herst R, Grady M, et al. Blood loss in open heart surgery. *Arch Surg* 1966;93:323.
171. Bick RL, Arbegast NR, Holtermann N, et al. Platelet function abnormalities in cardiopulmonary bypass. *Circulation* 1974;50(suppl):301.
172. Bick RL, Schmalhorst WR, Crawford L, et al. The hemorrhagic diathesis created by cardiopulmonary bypass. *Am J Clin Pathol* 1975;63:588.
173. Bick RL, Arbegast NR, Crawford L, et al. Hemostatic defects induced by cardiopulmonary bypass. *Vasc Surg* 1975;9:228.
174. Bick RL, Schmalhorst WR, Arbegast NR. Alterations of hemostasis associated with cardiopulmonary bypass. *Am J Clin Pathol* 1975;63:588.
175. Casteneda AR. Must heparin be neutralized following open heart operations? *J Thorac Cardiovasc Surg* 1966.52:716.
176. deVries SI, von Creveld S, Green P, et al. Studies on the coagulation of the blood in patients treated with extracorporeal circulation. *Thromb Diath Haemorrh* 1961;5:426.
177. Muller N, Popov-Cenic S, Buttner W, et al. Studies of fibrinolytic and coagulation factors during open-heart surgery, II: postoperative bleeding tendencies and changes in the coagulation system. *Thromb Res* 1975;7:589.
178. Bick RL. Alterations of hemostasis during cardiopulmonary bypass: a comparison between membrane and bubble oxygenators. *Am J Clin Pathol* 1980;73:300.
179. Bick RL, Schmalhorst SW, Arbegast NR. Alterations of hemostasis associated with cardiopulmonary bypass. *Thromb Res* 1976;8:285.
180. Bick RL. Heparin therapy and monitoring: guidelines and practice parameters for clinical and laboratory approaches. *J Clin Appl Thromb Hemost* 1996;2(suppl 1):12.
181. Walenga JM, Bick RL. Heparin-induced thrombocytopenia, paradoxical thromboembolism, and other side effects of heparin therapy. *Cardiol Clin Ann Drug Ther* 1998;2:123.
182. Walenga JM, Bick RL. Heparin-induced thrombocytopenia, paradoxical thromboembolism, and other side effects of heparin therapy. *Med Clin North Am* 1998;82:635.
183. Lewis BE, Walenga JM, Wallis DE. Anticoagulation with Novostan (argatroban) in patients with heparin-induced thrombocytopenia and heparin-induced thrombocytopenia and thrombosis syndrome. *Semin Thromb Hemost* 1997;23:197.
184. Holswade GR, Nachman RL, Killip T. Thrombocytopathies in patients with open-heart surgery: preoperative treatment with corticosteroids. *Arch Surg* 1967;94:365.
185. Salzman WE. Blood platelets and extracorporeal circulation. *Transfusion* 1963;3:274.
186. Bick RL, Adams T, Schmalhorst WR. Bleeding times, platelet adhesion, and aspirin. *Am J Clin Pathol* 1976;65:69.
187. Bowie EJW, Owen CA, Thompson JH. Platelet adhesiveness in von Willebrand's disease. *Am J Clin Pathol* 1969;52:69.
188. Bowie EJW, Owen CA. The value of measuring platelet adhesiveness in the diagnosis of bleeding diseases. *Am J Clin Pathol* 1973;60:302.
189. Hirsh J. Laboratory diagnosis of thrombosis. In: Coleman RW, Hirsh J, Marder VJ, et al., eds. *Basic principles and clinical practice.* Philadelphia: JB Lippincott, 1982:789.
190. Zimmerman TS, Meyer D. Factor VIII-von Willebrand factor and the molecular basis of von Willebrand's disease. In: Coleman RW, Hirsch J, Marder VM, eds. *Hemostasis and thrombosis: basic principles and clinical practice.* Philadelphia: JB Lippincott, 1982:54.
191. Adams T, Schutz L, Goldberg L. Platelet function abnormalities in the myeloproliferative disorders. *Scand J Haematol* 1975;13:215.
192. Mustard JF, Packham MA. Factors influencing platelet function: adhesion, release, and aggregation. *Pharmacol Rev* 1970;23 97.
193. Bick RL. The clinical significance of fibrinogen degradation products. *Semin Thromb Hemost* 1982;8:302.
194. Sarin CL, Yalav Y, Clement AJ, et al. Thrombo-embolism after Starr valve replacement. *Br Heart J* 1971;33:111.
195. Hellem AJ. The advances of human blood platelets in vitro. *Scand J Clin Lab Invest Suppl* 1960;51:1.
196. Bick RL, Fekete LF. Cardiopulmonary bypass hemorrhage: aggravation by pre-op ingestion of antiplatelet agents. *Vasc Surg* 1979;13:277.
197. Kowalski E, Kopec M, Wegrzynowicz Z. Influence of fibrinogen degradation products (FDP) on platelet aggregation, adhesiveness, and viscous metamorphosis. *Thromb Diath Haemorrh* 1963;10:406.
198. Kowalski E. Fibrinogen derivatives and their biologic activities. *Semin Hematol* 1968;5:45.
199. Harker LA, Malpass TW, Branson HE, et al. Mechanisms of abnormal bleeding in patients undergoing cardiopulmonary bypass: acquired transient platelet dysfunction associated with selective alpha-granule release. *Blood* 1980;56:824.
200. Stass S, Bishop C, Fosberg R, et al. Platelets as affected by cardiopulmonary bypass. *Trans Am Soc Clin Pathol* 1976:35[abst].
201. Saunders CR, Carlisle L Bick RL. Hydroxyethyl starch versus albumin in cardiopulmonary bypass prime solutions. *Ann Thorac Surg* 1982;36:532.
202. Lavee J, Shinfeld A, Savion N, et al. Irradiation of fresh whole blood for prevention of transfusion-associated graft-versus-host disease does not impair platelet function and clinical hemostasis after open heart surgery. *Vox Sang* 1995;69:104.
203. Salzman EW, Weinstein MJ, Weintraub RM, et al. Treatment with desmopressin acetate to reduce blood loss after cardiac surgery. *N Engl J Med* 1986;314:1402.
204. Weinstein M, Ware JA, Troll J, et al. Changes in von Willebrand factor during cardiac surgery: effect of desmopressin acetate. *Blood* 1988;71:1648.

205. Rocha E, Llorens R, Paramo JA, et al. Does desmopressin acetate reduce blood loss after surgery in patients on cardiopulmonary bypass? *Circulation* 1988;77:1319.
206. Mannucci PM. Desmopressin (DDAVP) for treatment of disorders of hemostasis. *Prog Hemost Thromb* 1986;8:19.
207. Warrier I, Lusher JM. DDAVP: a useful alternative to blood components in moderate hemophilia A and von Willebrand's disease. *J Pediatr* 1983;102:228.
208. Mariani G, Ciavarella N, Mazzucconi MG. Evaluation of the effectiveness of DDAVP in surgery and in bleeding episodes in hemophilia and von Willebrand's disease: a study of 43 patients. *Clin Lab Haematol* 1984;6:229.
209. De La Fuente B, Kasper CK, Rickles FR. Response of patients with mild hemophilia A and von Willebrand's disease to treatment with desmopressin. *Ann Intern Med* 1985;103:6.
210. Derman UM, Rand PW, Barker N. Fibrinolysis after cardiopulmonary bypass and its relationship to fibrinogen. *J Thorac Cardiovasc Surg* 1966;51:223.
211. Bachmann F, McKenna R, Cole ER, et al. The hemostatic mechanisms after open-heart surgery, I: studies on plasma coagulation factors and fibrinolysis in 512 patients after extracorporeal circulation. *J Thorac Cardiovasc Surg* 1975;70:76.
212. Tsuji HK, Redington JV, Kay JH, et al. The study of fibrinolytic and coagulation factors during open heart surgery. *Ann N Y Acad Sci* 1968;146:763.
213. Woods JE, Kirklin JW, Owen CA, et al. The effect of bypass surgery on coagulation sensitive clotting factors. *Mayo Clin Proc* 1967;42:724.
214. Gans H, Subramanian V, John S, et al. Theoretical and practical (clinical) considerations concerning proteolytic enzymes and their inhibitors with particular reference to changes in the plasminogen-plasmin system during assisted circulation in man. *Ann N Y Acad Sci* 1968;146:721.
215. Palester-Chlebowzyk M, Strzyzewska E, Sitowski W, et al. Detection of the intravascular coagulation of blood clotting, II: Results of the paracoagulation test in patients under-going open-heart surgery, with extracorporeal circulation. *Pol Med J* 1972;11:59.
216. Kladetsky RG, Popov-Cenic S, Buttner W, et al. Studies of fibrinolytic and coagulation factors during open-heart surgery with ECC. *Thromb Res* 1975;7:579.
217. Gomes MM, McGoon D. Bleeding patterns after open heart surgery. *J Thorac Cardiovasc Surg* 1970;60:87.
218. Bick RL. Disseminated intravascular coagulation. In: *Disorders of thrombosis and hemostasis: clinical and laboratory practice.* Chicago: ASCP Press, 1992:37.
219. Bick RL. Disseminated intravascular coagulation and related syndromes: a clinical review. *Semin Thromb Hemost* 1988;14:299.
220. Bick RL. Clinical hemostasis practice: the major impact of laboratory automation. *Semin Thromb Hemost* 1983;9:139.
221. Bick RL, Kovacs I, Fekete LF. A new two stage functional assay for antithrombin III (heparin cofactor): clinical and laboratory evaluation. *Thromb Res* 1976;8:745.
222. Lackner H, Javid JP. The clinical significance of the plasminogen level. *Am J Clin Pathol* 1973;60:175.
223. Tsitouris G, Bellet S, Eilberg R, et al. Effects of major surgery on plasmin-plasminogen systems. *Arch Intern Med* 1961;108:98.
224. Wuelfing D, Brandau KP. Fibrinolytic activity after surgery. *Minn Med* 1968;51:1503.
225. Ygge J. Changes in blood coagulation and fibrinolysis during the postoperative period. *Am J Surg* 1970;119:225.
226. Bick RL, Bishop RC, Warren M, et al. Changes in fibrinolysis and fibrinolytic enzymes during extra-corporeal circulation. *Trans Am Soc Hematol* 1971;109.
227. Graeff H, Beller FK. Fibrinolytic activity in whole blood, dilute blood, and euglobulin lysis time tests. In: Bang N, Beller FK, Deutsch E, eds. *Thrombosis and bleeding disorders, theory and methods.* New York: Academic Press, 1970:328.
228. Menon IS. A study of the possible correlation of euglobulin lysis time and dilute blood clot lysis time in the determination of fibrinolytic activity. *Lab Pract* 1968;17:334.
229. Bick RL, Bishop RC, Shanbrom ES. Fibrinolytic activity in acute myocardial infarction. *Am J Clin Pathol* 1972;57:359.
230. Bishop RC, Ekert H, Gilchrist G, et al. The preparation and evaluation of a standardized fibrin plate for the assessment of fibrinolytic activity. *Thromb Diath Haemorrh* 1970;23:202.
231. Fareed J. New methods in hemostatic testing. In: Fareed J, Messmore H, Fenton J, eds. *Perspectives in hemostasis.* New York: Pergamon Press, 1981:310.
232. Fareed J, Messmore HL, Bermes EW. New perspectives in coagulation testing. *Clin Chem* 1980;26:1380.
233. Huseby RM, Smith RE. Synthetic oligopeptide substrates: their diagnostic application in blood coagulation, fibrinolysis, and other pathologic states. *Semin Thromb Hemost* 1980;6:173.
234. Naeye RL. Thrombotic state after a hemorrhagic diathesis: a possible complication of therapy with epsilon amino-caproic acid. *Blood* 1962;19:694.
235. Ratnoff OD. Epsilon aminocaproic acid: a dangerous weapon. *N Engl J Med* 1969;280:1124.
236. Verska JJ, Lonser ER, Brewer LA. Predisposing factors and management of hemorrhage following open-heart surgery. *J Cardiovasc Surg (Torino)* 1972;13:361.
237. Verska J. Letter to the editor. *Ann Thorac Surg* 1972;13:87.
238. Okuyama K, Matsukawa T, Abe F, et al. Comparative effect of tranexamic acid on the reduction of bleeding during and after cardiac surgery. *Jpn J Anesth* 1998;47:861.
239. Shore-Lesserson L, Reich DL, Vela-Cantos F, et al. Tranexamic acid reduces transfusions and mediastinal drainage in repeat cardiac surgery. *Anesth Analg* 1996;83:18.
240. Aprile AE, Palmer TJ. The intraoperative use of Amicar to reduce bleeding associated with open heart surgery. *AANA J* 1995;63:325.
241. Brooks DH, Bahnson HT. An outbreak of hemorrhage following cardiopulmonary bypass. *J Thorac Cardiovasc Surg* 1972;63:449.
242. O'Neill JA, Ende N, Collins IS, et al. A quantitative determination of perfusion fibrinolysis. *Surgery*1966;60:809.
243. Bick RL, Frazier BL, Saunders CL, et al. Alterations of hemostasis during cardiopulmonary bypass: the potential role of factor XII activation in inducing primary fibrino(geno)lysis. *Blood* 1984;64:926.
244. Akkerman JW, Runne WC, Sixma JJ, et al. Improved survival rates in dogs after extracorporeal circulation by improved control of heparin levels. *J Thorac Cardiovasc Surg* 1974;68:59.
245. Ellison N, Betty CP, Blake DR, et al. Heparin rebound: studies in patients and volunteers. *J Thorac Cardiovasc Surg* 1974;67:723.
246. Gollub S. Heparin rebound in open-heart surgery. *Surg Gynecol Obstet* 1967;124:337.
247. Jaberi M, Bell WR, Benson DW. Control of heparin therapy in open-heart surgery. *J Thorac Cardiovasc Surg* 1974;67:133.
248. Ellison N, Ominsky AJ, Wollman H. Is protamine a clinically important anticoagulant? A negative answer. *Anesthesiology* 1971;35:621.
249. Ollendorff P. The nature of the anticoagulant effect of heparin, protamine, Polybrene, and toluidine blue. *Scand J Clin Lab Invest* 1962;14:267.
250. Tsai TP, Matloff JM, Gray RJ, et al. Cardiac surgery in the octagenarian. *J Thorac Surg* 1986;91:924.
251. Horneffer PJ, Gardner TJ, Manolio TA, et al. The effects of age

on outcome after coronary bypass surgery. *Circulation* 1987; 76:v–6.
252. Soloway HB, Cornett BM, Donahoo V, et al. Differentiation of bleeding diathesis which occurs following protamine correction of heparin anticoagulation. *Am J Clin Pathol* 1973;60:188.
253. Lewis JH, Wilson HJ, Brandon JM. Counterelectrophoresis test for molecules immunologically similar to fibrinogen. *Am J Clin Pathol* 1972;58:400.
254. Salzman EW. The events that lead to thrombosis. *Bull N Y Acad Med* 1972;48:225.
255. Bick RL, Baker WF. Diagnostic efficacy of the D-dimer assay in DIC and related disorders. *Blood* 1968;68:329.
256. Nader ND, Khadra WZ, Reich NT, et al. Blood product use in cardiac revascularization: comparison of on- and off-pump techniques. *Ann Thorac Surg* 1999;68:1640.
257. Gundry SR, Romano MA, Shattuck OH, et al. Seven year follow-up of coronary artery bypass performed with and without cardiopulmonary bypass. *J Thorac Cardiovasc Surg* 1998;115:1273.
258. Puskas JD, Wright CE, Ronson RS, et al. Off-pump multivessel coronary bypass via sternotomy is safe and effective. *Ann Thorac Surg* 1998;66:1068.
259. Cartier R, Brann S, Dagenais F, et al. Systematic off-pump coronary artery revascularization in multivessel disease: experience of three hundred cases. *J Thorac Cardiovasc Surg* 2000; 119:221.
260. Cartier R. Systematic off-pump coronary artery revascularization: experience of 275 cases. *Ann Thorac Surg* 1999;68:1494.
261. Turner WF. "Off- pump" coronary artery bypass grafting: the first one hundred cases of the Rose City experience. *Ann Thorac Surg* 1999;68:1482.
262. Rousou JA, Engelman RM, Breyer RH. Fibrin glue: an effective hemostatic agent for nonsuturable intraoperative bleeding. *Ann Thorac Surg* 1984;38:409.
263. Rousou J. Randomized clinical trial of fibrin glue sealant in patients undergoing resternotomy or reoperation after cardiac operations: a multicenter study. *J Thorac Surg* 1989;97:194.
264. Garcia-Rinaldi R, Simmons P, Salcedo V, et al. A technique for spot application of fibrin glue during open heart operations. *Ann Thorac Surg* 1989;47:59.
265. Dresdale A, Bowman FO, Malm JR, et al. Hemostatic effectiveness of fibrin glue derived from single-donor fresh frozen plasma. *Ann Thorac Surg* 1985;40:385.
266. Verstraete M. Clinical application of inhibitors of fibrinolysis. *Drugs* 1985;29:236.
267. Bick RL. Thrombotic and hemorrhagic problems during cardiopulmonary bypass surgery and cardiovascular procedures. In: Pifarre R, ed. *Management of bleeding in cardiovascular surgery.* Philadelphia: Hanley & Belfus, 2000:9.
268. Forbes CD. Thrombosis and artificial surfaces. *Thromb Clin Haematol* 1981;10:653.
269. Bick RL. Basic mechanisms of hemostasis pertaining to DIC. In: *Disseminated intravascular coagulation.* Boca Raton, Fla: CRC Press, 1983:1.
270. Esmon CT. Protein C: biochemistry, physiology, and clinical implications. *Blood* 1983;62:1155.
271. Braunwald NS, Bonchek L. Prevention of thrombus formation on rigid prosthetic heart valves by the ingrowth of autogenous tissue. *J Thorac Cardiovasc Surg* 1967;54:630.
272. Bagnall RD. Absorption of plasma proteins on hydrophobic surfaces, II: fibrinogen and fibrinogen-containing protein mixtures. *Biomed Biomater Res* 1978;12:203.
273. Hubbard D, Lucas GL. Ionic charges of glass surfaces and other materials and their possible role in the coagulation of blood. *J Appl Physiol* 1960;15:265.
274. Mason RG. The interaction of blood hemostatic elements with artificial surfaces. In: Spaet TH, ed. *Progress in hemostasis and thrombosis.* New York: Grune & Stratton, 1941:141.
275. Knieriem HJ, Chandler AB. The effect of warfarin sodium on the duration of platelet aggregation. *Thromb Diath Haemorrh* 1967;18:766.
276. Lessin LS, Jensen WH, Kelser GA. Scanning electron microscopy of thrombogenesis on vascular catheter surfaces. *N Engl J Med* 1972;286:139.
277. Moore CH, Wolma FJ, Brown RW, et al. Complications of cardiovascular radiology: a review of 1204 cases. *Am J Surg* 1970; 120:591.
278. Hershey CO, Tomford JW, McLaren CE, et al. The natural history of intravenous catheter-associated phlebitis. *Arch Intern Med* 1984;144:1373.
279. Tomford JW, Hershey CO. The effect of an intravenous therapy team on peripheral venous catheter associated phlebitis. *Clin Res* 1982;30:770A.
280. Bolooki H. Indications for use of IABP. In: *Clinical application of intra-aortic balloon pump.* Mt. Kisco, NY: Futura, 1984:293.
281. Okada M, Shiozawa T, Iizuka M, et al. Experimental and clinical studies on the effect of intra-aortic balloon pumping for cardiogenic shock following acute myocardial infarction. *Artif Organs* 1979;3:271.
282. McEnany MT, Kay HR, Buckley J, et al. Clinical experience with intra-aortic balloon pump support in 728 patients. *Circulation* 1978;58:124.
283. Alpert J, Bhaktan EK, Gielchinsky I, et al. Vascular complications of intra-aortic balloon pumping. *Arch Surg* 1976;111: 1190.
284. Balooki H. Complications of balloon pumping: diagnosis, prevention, and treatment. In: *Clinical application of intra-aortic balloon pump.* Mt. Kisco, NY: Futura, 1984:133.
285. Isner JM, Cohen SR, Virmani R, et al. Complications of the intra-aortic balloon counter-pulsation device: clinical and morphologic observations in 45 necropsy patients. *Am J Cardiol* 1980;45:260.
286. Karlson K. Discussion: vascular complications of intra-aortic balloon pumping. *Arch Surg* 1976;111:1190.
287. Curtis JJ, Barnhorst DA, Pluth JR, et al. Intra-aortic balloon assist: initial. Mayo Clinic experience and current concepts. *Mayo Clin Proc* 1977;52:723.
288. Schneider MD, Kaye MP, Blatt SJ, et al. Safety of intraaortic balloon pumping, II: physical injury to aortic endothelium due to mechanical pump action. *Thromb Res* 1974;4:399.
289. Baciewicz FA, Kaplan BM, Murphy TE, et al. Bilateral renal artery thrombotic occlusion: a unique complication following removal of a transthoracic intra-aortic balloon. *Ann Thorac Surg* 1982;33:631.
290. Bick RL. Disseminated intravascular coagulation: objective criteria for clinical laboratory diagnosis and assessment of therapeutic response. *Clin Appl Thromb Hemost* 1995;1:3–23.
291. Bick RL, Strauss JF, Frenkel EP. Thrombosis and hemorrhage in oncology patients. *Hematol Oncol Clin North Am* 1996;10:875.
292. Gajewski JL, Champlin RE. Vascular access. In: Haskell CM, ed. *Cancer treatment.* Philadelphia: WB Saunders, 1990:866.
293. Murano G, Bick RL. Thrombolytic therapy. In: Murano G, Bick RL, eds. *Basic concepts of hemostasis and thrombosis.* Boca Raton, Fla: CRC Press, 1980:259.
294. Bick RL. Thrombolytic therapy. In: *Disorders of hemostasis and thrombosis.* New York: Thieme, 1985:352.
295. Harker LA, Slichter SJ. Platelet and fibrinogen survival in man. *N Engl J Med* 1972;287:999.
296. LeVeen HH, Christoudias G, Ip M, et al. Peritoneovenous shunting for ascites. *Ann Surg* 1974;180:580.
297. Reinhardt GF, Stanley MM. Peritoneovenous shunting for ascites. *Surg Gynecol Obstet* 1977;145:419.

298. Bick RL. Disseminated intravascular coagulation: objective laboratory diagnostic criteria and guidelines for management. *Clin Lab Med* 1994;14:729.
299. Lerner RG, Nelson JC, Corines P, et al. Disseminated intravascular coagulation: complication of LeVeen peritoneovenous shunts. *JAMA* 1978;240:2064.
300. Harmon DC, Demirjian Z, Ellman Z, et al. Disseminated intravascular coagulation with the peritoneovenous shunt. *Ann Intern Med* 1979;90:774.
301. Strin SF, Fulenwider JT, Ansley JD, et al. Accelerated fibrinogen and platelet destruction after peritoneovenous shunting. *Arch Intern Med* 1981;141:1149.
302. Baker WF. Clinical aspects of disseminated intravascular coagulation. *Semin Thromb Hemost* 1989;15:1.
303. Frankl WS. Indications for anticoagulants in cardiovascular disease. In: Jepson JH, Frankl WS, eds. *Hematological complications in cardiac practice.* Philadelphia: WB Saunders, 1975:182.
304. Kaltman AJ. Late complications of heart valve replacement. *Annu Rev Med* 1971;2:343.
305. Fraser RS, Waddell J. Systemic embolization after aortic valve replacement. *J Thorac Cardiovasc Surg* 1967;54:81.
306. Effler DB, Favaloro R, Groves LK. Heart valve replacement: clinical experience. *Ann Thorac Surg* 1965;1:4.
307. Mason RG, Chuang HYK, Mohammad SF, et al. Thrombosis and artificial surfaces. In: van de Loo J, Prentice CRM, Beller FK, eds. *The thromboembolic disorders.* Stuttgart: Schattauer Verlag, 1983:533.
308. Akbarian M, Austen WG, Yurchak PM, et al. Thromboembolic complications of prosthetic cardiac valves. *Circulation* 1968;37:826.
309. Duvoisin GE, Brandenburg RO, McGoon DC. Factors affecting thromboembolism associated with prosthetic heart valves. *Circulation* 1967;35:70.
310. Berger S, Salzman EW. Thromboembolic complications of prosthetic devices. *Prog Hemost Thromb* 1974;2:273.
311. Weiss HJ. Antiplatelet drugs in clinical medicine. In: *Platelets: pathophysiology and antiplatelet drug therapy.* New York: Alan R. Liss, 1982:75.
312. Harker LA, Slichter SJ. Studies of platelet and fibrinogen kinetics in patients with prosthetic heart valves. *N Engl J Med* 1970; 283:1302.
313. Harker LA, Hirsh J, Gent M, et al. Critical evaluation of platelet-inhibiting drugs in thrombotic disease. *Prog Hematol* 1975;9:229.
314. Weily HS, Steele PP, Davies H, et al. Platelet survival in patients with substitute heart valves. *N Engl J Med* 1974;290:534.
315. Steele PP, Weily NS, Davies H, et al. Platelet survival in patients with rheumatic heart disease. *N Engl J Med* 1974;290:537.
316. Weily HW, Genton E. Altered platelet function in patients with prosthetic mitral valves: effects of sulfinpyrazone therapy. *Circulation* 1970;42:967.
317. Sullivan JM, Harken DE, Gorlin R. Pharmacologic control of thromboembolic complications of cardiac-valve replacement. *N Engl J Med* 1971;284:1391.
318. Dale J, Myhre E, Storstein A, et al. Prevention of arterial thromboembolism with acetylsalicylic acid. *Am Heart J* 1977;94:101.
319. Dale J, Myhre E, Lowe D. Bleeding during acetylsalicylic acid and anticoagulant therapy in patients with reduced platelet reactivity after aortic valve replacement. *Am Heart J* 1980;99:746.
320. Altman R, Boullon F, Rouvier J, et al. Aspirin and prophylaxis of thromboembolic complications in patients with substitute heart valves. *J Thorac Cardiovasc Surg* 1976;72:127.
321. Arrants JE, Hairston E. Use of persantine in preventing thromboembolism following valve replacement. *Ann Surg* 1972;38: 432.
322. Taguchi K, Matsumura H, Washizu T, et al. Effect of atherombogenic therapy, especially high dose therapy of dipyridamole, after prosthetic valve replacement. *J Cardiovasc Surg* 1975;16:8.
323. Bjork VO, Henz A. Management of thrombo-embolism after aortic valve replacement with the Bjork-Shiley tilting disc valve. *Scand J Thorac Cardiovasc Surg* 1975;9:183.
324. Sarin CL, Yalav E, Clement AJ, et al. Thrombo-embolism after Starr valve replacement. *Br Heart J* 1971;33:111.
325. Gadboys HL, Litwak RS, Niemetz J, et al. Role of anticoagulants in preventing embolization from prosthetic heart valves. *JAMA* 1967;202:282.
326. Friedli B, Aerichide N, Grondin P, et al. Thrombo-embolic complications of heart valve prostheses. *Am Heart J* 1971;81: 702.
327. Stein PD, Alpert JS, Copeland JG, et al. Antithrombotic therapy in patients with mechanical and biological prosthetic heart valves. *Chest* 1998;114(suppl):602.

Disorders of Thrombosis and Hemostasis: Clinical and Laboratory Practice, Third Edition, edited by Rodger L. Bick.
Lippincott Williams & Wilkins, Philadelphia © 2002

10

ACQUIRED BLOOD COAGULATION INHIBITORS

YALE S. ARKEL
DE-HUI W. KU

Inhibitors of the blood coagulation system are well known to be associated with the inherited clotting factor deficiencies such as in hemophilia A and B. However, acquired inhibitors, also known as circulating anticoagulants, occur with coagulation factors in patients with no inherited deficiency and may be associated with severe hemorrhage. In addition, there is evidence that antibodies may affect components of the coagulation system and be associated with an increased risk for thrombosis. In this chapter, we review the acquired coagulation inhibitors that may be associated with hemorrhage and, in some instances, the inhibitors that may be associated with thrombosis. The antiphospholipid antibody and the lupus inhibitor, also called lupus anticoagulant (LA), and inhibitors associated with the congenital factor deficiencies (hemophilia A and B) are addressed in greater detail in another section of this volume.

In their review in 1961, Margolus et al. (1) defined inhibitors as " abnormal endogenous components of blood, which inhibit the coagulation of normal blood." For the most part, this definition is still appropriate. Their review of 40 cases and the then existing literature provides an excellent early resource on the subject of inhibitors to coagulation factors. The review by Shapiro and Hultin (2) on coagulation inhibitors remains very current.

With the exception of natural anticoagulant substances that have heparin-like properties and exogenous heparin that is administered therapeutically or the new synthetically derived antithrombins, inhibitors are for the most part immunoglobulins. These antibodies may bind to the factor and cause a deficiency by increasing the clearance of the factor, or they may affect the active site(s) of the factor, resulting in dysfunction with resultant loss of coagulation activity. Inhibitors are a significant problem in many of the patients in which they appear. They cause bleeding and/or thrombosis, complicate the management of the underlying disease, and prevent needed surgical procedures or increase the morbidity and mortality that is associated with needed invasive procedures. In many of the patients with autoinhibitors, the bleeding diathesis is the main determinant for morbidity and mortality.

The presence of an inhibitor should be suspected when a patient with no prior bleeding history develops unprovoked or spontaneous bleeding manifestations such as excessive bruising, hematomas, or mucosal bleeding. It also should be considered when patients who have had surgery, invasive procedures, or trauma have unexplained excessive or prolonged bleeding that is unusual for the situation. The diagnosis is made when coagulation testing reveals that the patient's plasma causes abnormal clotting in the normal control plasma. In practical application, the diagnosis of blood coagulation inhibitors is often a difficult and perplexing challenge. Global screening tests such as the activated partial thromboplastin time (aPTT) or the prothrombin time (PT) are usually the tests first noted to be affected. When the aPTT is the only prolonged or abnormal test, the major categories that come into consideration in the patient with bleeding issues are (a) the hemophilia patient who is resistant to replacement therapy with factor concentrates, or (b) in the nonhemophilia patient, the acquired inhibitor. Inhibitors may more rarely affect other coagulation systems or factors with prolongation of the prothrombin time (i.e., factor V) or the thrombin time due to heparin-like inhibitors or antithrombin inhibitors such as seen after bovine thrombin use in surgery. The screening test for an inhibitor is based on the results of the affected global tests of clotting time when the patient's plasma is mixed in a 50:50 mixture with normal plasma. This will correct a pure factor deficiency, whereas an inhibitor will prolong the normal plasma clotting time. To define an inhibitor to a specific factor, one would test the effect of the patient's plasma on known quantities of the individual factors. The measurement of inhibitors was standardized by the work of Kasper

Y. S. Arkel and D-H. W. Ku: Departments of Obstetrics/Gynecology, Maternal/Fetal Medicine, Thrombophilia Research Program, New York University School of Medicine, New York, New York

et al. (3,4). In 1995 the Bethesda assay method was modified, and the specificity and reliability of the assay was improved, particularly for the low-titer inhibitors (5). Based on these methods, the inhibitor is expressed in Bethesda units (BU). One BU is defined as the amount of anti–factor VIII necessary to neutralize 50% of factor VIII in 1 mL of pooled normal plasma after incubation for 2 hours at 37°C. The Bethesda assay can be adapted for the determination of the titer of inhibitor to other coagulation factors such as factors IX, XI, and V. Sahud (6) reviewed the subject of the laboratory evaluation for an inhibitor, and the reader is referred to his article for details. In the evaluation of a prolonged aPTT, it is important to differentiate a lupus-type inhibitor (lupus anticoagulant; LA) from a true factor inhibitor. This can be differentiated by the correction of the factor levels by serial dilution of the test plasma and shortening of the clotting time with the addition of platelets or phospholipid to the test mixture. Several tests are commonly used in the detection and confirmation of the lupus inhibitor. These include the dilute Russell viper venom time (DRVVT), hexagonal phase assay, and the platelet neutralizing procedure (PNP), among others. The confirmatory tests for lupus inhibitors are generally based on the finding that the prolonged clotting times are corrected by the addition of platelet material or phospholipid to the test system (7). A potent single factor inhibitor, such as to factor VIII, may appear to have multiple factor deficiencies. This is due to the effect of the inhibitor on the normal test substrate. Specifically this is noted when performing factor IX or XI assays in plasma with factor VIII inhibitor. The factor VIII inhibitor will decrease the factor VIII in the normal substrate used in the assay system. Serial dilution of the test sample will correct for the nondeficient factors, and by adding a high concentration of factor VIII, in the case of a factor VIII inhibitor, will tend to correct the assays for the factor XI and IX assays. Unlike the true factor inhibitors, such as those to factor VIII, the lupus inhibitor is very rarely associated with hemorrhage. However, there are reports of patients with factor inhibitors in addition to the lupus-type inhibitor (17). In rare cases, bleeding has been reported as a complication of the lupus inhibitor. This may be due to a prothrombin deficiency, possibly related to true prothrombin antibodies and/or thrombocytopenia that occurs in a number of patients with the LA/anticardiolipin syndrome (9–11). We reported a patient with an acquired von Willebrand syndrome in association with the anticardiolipin syndrome and LA (12). The acquired von Willebrand disease (vWD) responded to treatment with high-dose intravenous immuno(γ)globulin (IVIG). The anticardiolipin antibody syndrome is discussed in detail elsewhere in this volume.

In the following pages, we review in some detail the autoimmune factor inhibitors. Although we will touch on the inhibitors associated with the congenital factor deficiencies, the detailed in-depth discussion will be left to other sections.

FACTOR VIII INHIBITORS

Factor VIII inhibitors (13–24,60) occur in patients with an inherited deficiency of factor VIII (hemophilia A), with an estimated incidence of 15% to 35% or, in nondeficient patients on an autoimmune basis, one to four per million (acquired factor VIII inhibitors also called spontaneous inhibitors or acquired hemophilia). Acquired auto–factor VIII inhibitors, although a rarer clinical condition, have been discussed in the medical literature for many years. Its fascination may be due to its rather unexpected occurrence in otherwise healthy individuals or as a sudden complication of an unrelated underlying disease or treatment. As we noted earlier, there have been several excellent reviews over the years, and the reader is referred to these for further detail.

General Approach to Detection of Factor VIII Inhibitor

1. Usually the presenting laboratory finding is a prolonged aPTT, with normal prothrombin time.
2. The aPTT, using mixtures of patient's plasma and normal plasma, reveals that the patient's plasma prolongs the time of normal plasma. This is the key laboratory finding to indicate the presence of an inhibitor.
3. Tests are performed to exclude a lupus-like inhibitor (see earlier).
4. Factor assay(s) are performed to determine specificity of the inhibitor.
5. Bethesda assay may be used to measure the titer of the inhibitor.
6. Tests are done for antibody cross-reactivity to porcine factor VIII.

The domains of the factor VIII molecule and their interaction with anti–factor VIII antibodies in hemophilia A patients have been determined. Factor VIII is a 265-kDa protein procoagulant molecule that functions as a cofactor for factor IX, in the proteolytic activation of factor X (25–27). It is a phospholipid-binding protein that complexes with factors IX and X and binds to the surface of activated platelets (28,29). In patients with inherited severe deficiency of factor VIII, hemophilia A, there is an expected incidence of greater than 30% for the development of inhibitors, whereas there is only a 3% to 5% incidence in those with severe hemophilia B (30). In one study, as many as 50% of the severe group will develop demonstrable antibodies when exposed to factor VIII concentrates (31). It is the severe deficiency group of hemophilia patients that have the great majority of inhibitors. An interchromosomal inversion due to the mutation in the intron 22 region of the factor VIII gene is present in some 45% of patients with severe hemophilia A (less than 1% factor activity). In these patients, there is an absence of the factor VIII protein. This may make them more susceptible to the development of antibodies (32,33). In a large retrospective study of previously untreated patients with hemophilia A, the mutation type and inhibitor incidence were assessed (34). Mutations were determined in 28 patients with inhibitors and 67 patients without inhibitors. The data confirm the previously reported data that inhibitor formation occurred mainly in patients with intron 22 inversions with a relative risk (RR) of 1.5; nonsense mutations, RR 2.1; and large deletions, RR 4.6. The patients with missense mutations and small deletions had relatively low risks of 0.1 and 0.6, respectively. Scandella (35) reviewed the properties of anti–factor VIII inhibitor antibodies in hemophilia A patients. She stated that the major epitopes for inhibitor specificity are contained within the A2, C2, and A3–C1 domains. Hemophilia patients treated with plasma-derived or recombinant factor VIII were identified with inhibitors to the A2 domain or the light chain. In a subgroup of the patients with the light chain–specific antibodies, there was a relation to the C2 domain. Antibodies to two or more domains are noted in a significant number of the patients. In the congenital hemophilia patients, the antibodies are usually immunoglobulin G (IgG_4), less often IgG_1, nonprecipitating immunoglobulins and non–complement fixing directed to the functional epitopes of the factor VIII molecule (36). Most usually the antibodies bind to the 44-kDa of the factor VIII heavy chain (A2 domain) or to the light chain in the area of the C2 domain on the 72-kDa portion (37–39). Inhibitors may arise in hemophilia patients with mild or moderate-severity disease. The latter usually appear under unusual circumstances associated with acute-phase reactivity or inflammation. This may cause stimulation of the immune system, as does the use of additional factor concentrate (40–42). In the analysis of the immune responses to factor VIII in mild to moderate hemophilia A patients, it was noted that the carboxy-terminal part of the C1 domain is an important source of the antigenic determinants (43). The data indicate that the C1 domain contains antigenic determinants for both T and B lymphocytes and that the mutation of the an arginine residue (Arg2150) eliminates certain T- and B-cell epitopes that are likely to favor the development of an immune response to normal factor VIII. Hodge and Han (44) reported on the effect of factor VIII concentrate on antigen-presenting cell/ T-cell interactions in vitro and the relevance to inhibitor formation and tolerance induction. Inhibitor formation is dependent on effective T-cell/B-cell interactions, especially B cell CD40 with T cell CD40L (45). In a review of their work, at the Scientific Program at the American Society of Hematology in San Francisco, December 2000, Conti-Fine et al. (46) discussed the use of a mouse model to explain inhibitor development. Synthesis of factor VIII inhibitors requires $CD4^+$ T-helper cells. There is a lower frequency and intensity of the $CD4^+$ T-cell responses to factor VIII in healthy subjects as compared with patients with hemophilia. There is inadequate toleration of $CD4^+$ cells to factor VIII, due to the lack of endogenous factor VIII, in hemophilia. This may be clinically important in the devlopment of anti–factor VIII antibodies. In patients with severe hemophilia, inhibitors usually develop at a young age relatively shortly after factor exposure. Usually an increase in the inhibitor levels is detected 2 to 4 days after factor administration; they may reach their high point at 1 to 3 weeks. High-titer inhibitors tend to persist for longer periods even without factor treatment, and the low-titer inhibitors can disappear. The low titer inhibitors may not reappear with further factor VIII treatment. Those patients in whom the inhibitor levels do not increase after treatment with factor are considered *low responders*. These patients usually have inhibitor titers less than 5 BU and less than 10 BU after factor VIII infusion. The patients in whom the titer increases after factor infusion are classified as *high responders*. This classification is important in the treatment of hemophilia patients with factor replacement, as will be discussed. Patients with acquired auto–factor VIII inhibitors are rarely high responders. In the severe hemophilia patients, approximately 50% of the inhibitors are high titer, and the frequency in racial and ethnic backgrounds seem to support a genetic basis for vulnerability to inhibitor development. Black and Hispanic hemophilia A patients are more vulnerable to develop inhibitors. The epitopes noted with the inhibitors from the mild-to-moderate cases were noted in one case to be the same for the severe hemophilia group (47), whereas in other such patients studied, there were variable characteristics to the binding of the inhibitor to regions of factor VIII and their interactions with endogenous versus exogenous factor VIII. Alterations have been reported in the factor VIII molecule due to the heating and pasteurization process as a cause of transient inhibitor formation. It was noted that a series of cases of inhibitors occurred in the patients treated with a new factor VIII concentrate that had been heat/pasteurized treated. The antibodies were directed to the C2 domain, possibly due to alterations in this region by the processing of the factor concentrate (48,49). The inhibitors disappeared when the product was no longer used.

Acquired Factor VIII Inhibitor (Acquired Hemophilia A)

The reviews noted earlier contain most of the information in this section. In contrast to inhibitors in the patients with inherited hemophilia A, acquired hemophilia due to an autoantibody to factor VIII is rare (50–58,422) and is estimated to occur in one to four per million population, with more recent data that would suggest a higher frequency. The cumulative experience indicates that the autoimmune inhibitors have bleeding that is severe in 87% of the cases and may be life threatening in the period of the early presentation or diagnosis. Mortality due to bleeding from acquired hemophilia is reported as between 7.9% and 22% of the patients (59–61). Lechner (62), in 1974, reviewed the occurrence of inhibitors in nonhemophilic patients. He grouped the patients with factor VIII inhibitors into five categories, *postpartum, autoimmune diseases,* or *allergic diseases, paraproteinemias, drug hypersensitivity,* and *without a definite underlying illness.* For the most part, this grouping still is valid today. He included in the *autoimmune or allergic group* patients with *rheumatoid arthritis (RA), systemic lupus erythematosus (SLE), bullous dermatitis, pemphigus, ulcerative colitis, temporal arteritis, rheumatoid spondylitis, bronchial asthma, hypersensitivity angiitis,* and *rheumatoid heart disease.* One of the common features of these patients, with the exception of the pregnancy-related inhibitors, is the older age, and the appearance of the inhibitor at a later stage in the patient's illness. In the RA patients, the average time from the onset of the underlying disease to the appearance of the inhibitor was 16 years, whereas the time lags for patients with skin diseases such as bullous dermatitis and pemphigus was 5.7 years. Patients with drug sensitivity had an onset of the inhibitor in a matter of days (4 to 90). In the pregnancy (postpartum) group, which included 22 cases, the time of onset varied from 2 days to 12 months, with an average of 91 days. The ages of the patient groups were older but with quite a range. The RA patients were aged a mean of 61 years; range, 56 to 73; SLE, an average of 42 years, with a range of 21 to 71 years; and dermatologic disorders, 69 years, with a range of 57 to 82 years. The drug-hypersensitivity patients varied from age 25 to 83 years. Apart from the patients with drug hypersensitivity and the pregnancy-related inhibitors, spontaneous remissions were rare. There was no evidence that the inhibitor paralleled the exacerbation or remission of the underlying disease. The patients without an underlying disease formed the greatest number, and had a mean age of 58 years, with a range of 13 to 82 years. In their review of the clinical overview of factor VIII inhibitors, White et al. (63) noted that 10% of spontaneous inhibitors will regress or disappear without treatment, and an additional 45% will disappear in association with corticosteroid and other therapy.

As noted earlier, auto–factor VIII inhibitors have been described in a wide variety of clinical situations (64–69). In approximately 50% of the cases, the inhibitors are idiopathic, and half of the cases occurred in patients older than 50 years. The clinical features of acquired hemophilia are most commonly bruising, and bleeding into soft tissues, muscle, gastrointestinal tract, and the urogenital system. Bleeding into the joint spaces is much less common than in congenital hemophilia. In general the patients have no history of bleeding problems and have not used blood products. The course of the inhibitor in relation to the underlying disorder is variable. There is a report of a remission of the inhibitor with resection of the affected bowel with enteritis (70). In other reports, such as in a patient with lymphoma, immunosuppressive treatment resulted in disappearance of the inhibitor and persistence of the lymphoma (428). Green and Lechner (14) noted in their survey of 215 nonhemophilic patients with inhibitors to factor VIII that 53% were male and 47% female patients (14). In addition to the overall group who tended to be older than 50 years, there was the postpartum group with an age peak between 21 and 30 years. Forty-six percent had no underlying disorder, but the list of disorders in the other patients was quite extensive. Most autoantibodies appear to be directed to a single domain of factor VIII. They are more likely to be anti-C2 than anti-A2 (71). Antibodies in hemophilia appear to be directed to both domains (72). Antibodies with inhibitor activity, described as directed to C2, inhibit binding of factor VIII to vWF and phospholipid (73,74). Antibodies to the A3–C1 domains have been demonstrated to prevent the interaction between factor VIII and factor IXa (75). Other immunoglobulins can function as inhibitors, as is seen in patients with dysproteinemias due to plasma cell and lymphoproliferative disorders, which can have IgA and IgM factor VIII inhibitors (76). A patient with a factor VIII inhibitor, 700 BU, with a monoclonal IgM disorder, Waldenström macroglobulinemia, was described. The inhibitor, however, was actually due to a polyclonal IgG. The inhibitor had type II kinetics and was directed to the A2 domain of the factor VIII heavy chain. This indicates that although paraproteins can have inhibitor properties and be responsible for the bleeding, it also is possible for other causative antibodies to be present in these patients (77).

Auto–factor VIII inhibitors, unlike the majority of inhibitors in hemophilia A, are type II[1] in their kinetics and therefore do not completely inactivate factor VIII at high concentrations (78). Less commonly, autoantibodies can follow type I[2] kinetics, which is the usual form noted in hemophilia, with total inactivation of factor VIII activity (79). Nogami et al. (80) studied three patients with type II factor VIII autoantibodies who had normal levels of factor VIII antigen and low levels of factor VIII activity. The antibodies were ascribed to the A3–C1 domains, which was unusual. Heavy and light chains of factor VIII were detected in plasma-derived immune complexes that were extracted. The three autoantibodies blocked the factor VIII binding to activated protein C (APC) and therefore inhibited the proteolytic inactivation of factor VIII. It was suggested that this might explain the persistence of factor VIII immune complexes in the type II inhibitors.

The auto–factor VIII antibodies inhibit factor VIII activity by several hypothesized mechanisms (81–85).

---

[1]Type II inhibitors: More commonly in autoantibodies, with incomplete neutralization of factor VIII activity.

[2]Type I inhibitors: More commonly seen in alloantibodies, with complete neutralization of factor VIII activity.

1. Affect the A2 domain and therefore the coagulant activity.
2. Affect the FVIII–phospholipid interaction by their anti-C2 properties.
3. Impair thrombin cleavage of factor VIII.
4. Decrease the ability of FVIII to activate factor X.
5. Inhibit the FVIII–vWF interaction.

The disappearance of auto–factor VIII inhibitors is unpredictable, as demonstrated by the case report of a patient with a very high titer inhibitor (86). In their patient, the factor VIII inhibitor was 3,600 BU at its maximal level, with specificity to the A2 and C2 domains. The inhibitor decreased and could no longer be detected over several years. This was followed shortly by autoimmune hemolytic anemia. Antiidiotypic antibodies to the anti–factor VIII antibodies were not found to explain the decreasing titer. The disappearance of the inhibitor was postulated to be due to "clonal exhaustion" of antigen-specific memory B lymphocyte cells. Sultan et al. (85) reported that recovery from anti–factor VIII autoimune antibodies is dependent on antiidiotypes against anti–factor VIII autoantibodies. They found a higher frequency of neutralizing antibodies against anti–factor VIII autoantibodies in the IgG from aged donors and multiparous women compared with random donors. Using pooled donors for their IgG resulted in greater expression of antiidiotypic activity to auto–factor VIII antibodies. Approximately 20% of randomly screened healthy blood donors have natural IgG anti–factor VIII antibodies. The autoantibodies that are affected by the anti-iodiotypic antibodies in IVIG are based on the paratope-related idiotypes, which are different from those expressed by natural anti–factor VIII antibodies. The response to IVIG in the suppression of factor VIII inhibitors has been postulated to be due to antiidiotypic expression of the IVIG to auto–factor VIII inhibitors (88). Therefore it is possible that the immune system may alter to produce antiidiotypic antibodies to factor VIII inhibitors that decrease the level of the inhibitor or cause its disappearance (Table 10.1).

In a retrospective study reported by Sallah et al. (89), the characteristics of the inhibitors were assessed in patients with acquired hemophilia and solid and hematologic tumors, older than 25 years. A total of 41 patients was evaluable and compared with 116 patients with factor VIII inhibitors without malignancy. They found that 59% of the patients had solid tumors, and adenocarcinoma was 67% of this group. Hematologic malignancies represented 41% of the entire group, with chronic lymphocytic leukemia forming 35% of the hematologic malignancy group. There was no statistical difference in the mean factor VIII level in the malignancy group versus the nonmalignancy group (3.7% to 4.5% mean factor VIII levels). Neither was there a significant difference in the inhibitor levels in these groups (mean, 66 to 81 BU/mL). The time to disappearance of the inhibitor was 20

TABLE 10.1. LIST OF DISORDERS NOTED TO BE ASSOCIATED WITH INHIBITORS TO FACTOR VIII

No disorder detected	46%
Autoimmune disease (419–426)	
Rheumatoid arthritis	7.9%
Systemic lupus erythematosus	5.6%
Other autoimmune diseases	4.5%
(Temporal arteritis, ulcerative colitis, *inflammatory bowel disease* (427), dermatomyositis, myasthenia gravis, polymyositis, Sjøgren syndrome)	
Postpartum	7.3%
Malignancy	6.7%
Lymphocytic leukemia and lymphoma (428), solid tumors [carcinoma of lung, colon, kidney, *hepatocellular carcinoma* (429) *prostate, cervical carcinoma, myeloma* (430), *gastric malignancy, testicular tumor, astrocytoma, and lymphoproliferative diseases*] (17, 430–436)	
Dermatologic disorders	4.5%
Psoriasis, pemphigus, exfoliative dermatitis, erythema annularis centrifugum, *dermatitis herpetiformis* (437–442)	
Respiratory disorders	3.9%
Asthma (443), sarcoid, respiratory failure	
Other disorders	5.1%
Diabetes, hyperglobulinemia, glomerulonephritis, polycythemia, *lung abscess* (444), *liver disease, hepatitis* (445, 446), *cytomegalovirus infection* (22), *chronic graft-versus-host disease* (447), *after electric shock therapy* (448)	
Drug related	5.6%
Penicillin, ampicillin, phenytoin, chloramphenicol, *sulfa drugs, nitrofurazone, phenylbutazone, dilantin, depot thioanthene* (2, 13, 14, 449, 450)	
Multiple transfusions	2.8%
When all the autoimmune conditions are combined, they represent the largest group of 18%; the other large groups are the pregnancy, postpartum, followed by the patients with malignancy	

Modified from Green D, Lechner K. A survey of 215 nonhemophilic patients with inhibitors to factor VIII. *Thromb Haemost* 1981;45:200. Additional disorders from other reports in italics with the percentages for the underlying disorders, as noted by Green and Lechner).

weeks for the malignancy patients compared with 95 weeks for the other patients ($p = 0.02$). This was thought to reflect the response of therapy for malignancy. The incidences of the major groups of disorders and patients without underlying disorders are fairly consistent for the several reviews of factor VIII inhibitors, as listed in Table 10.1. Several medications have been associated with the occurrence of inhibitors. In addition to these, there are isolated reports of other agents that have been implicated in possibly causing auto-factor inhibitors. One such report includes a patient with hemophilia A who was treated with interferon-α for chronic hepatitis C and in whom a factor VIII inhibitor developed (90). Although it is possible that the inhibitor was related to the underlying disorders, the patient had clinical evidence for the inhibitor several months after the completion of interferon therapy. There had been no evidence for an inhibitor on previous evaluations. The patient had been treated for hemophilia with factor concentrates. The authors made the point that interferon is associated with autoimmune complications. Regina et al. (91) reported a patient with Hodgkin disease and acquired factor VIII inhibitor who was treated with interferon-α. The patient had been treated with chemotherapy, radiotherapy, and surgery. She also had an autologous bone marrow transplantation and subsequently received interferon treatment. Hypothyroidism and a factor VIII inhibitor with bleeding complicated the course. At the time of the diagnosis of the inhibitor, the Hodgkin disease was in remission. The inhibitor responded to treatment with corticosteroids, and the patient remained in complete remission from the Hodgkin disease and inhibitor for 2 years at the time of last assessment. In another report, interferon-γ2a was used successfully in the treatment of a patient with postpartum factor VIII inhibitor (92). However, generalization from a single postpartum patient is problematic.

As already noted, there are patients (*de novo*) with no obvious disorder who have an acquired factor VIII inhibitor. Although the patients with *de novo* inhibitors to factor VIII are generally elderly, they may well appear in younger patients with an equal distribution in male and female patients (93).

In their review of 16 patients with acquired factor VIII, Lottenberg et al. (94) found that the hemorrhagic diathesis was distinct from the inherited hemophilias. They found fewer hemarthroses compared with the hemophilia patients, with frequent skin and soft tissue hematomas. Hematuria was a significant problem. In their study, two patients had a fatal hemorrhage, and five patients had a spontaneous remission. They found that long-term survival is not incompatible with the diagnosis. They suggest that attempts to treat all patients with immunosuppression therapy may not be required. Söhngen et al. (95) reported on their experience from 1980 to 1995 with 10 nonhemophilia patients with factor VIII inhibitors. Their experience was very much similar to that in other reported reviews. Of their 10 patients, four had asthma, three had rheumatic disease, and two had early cytomegalovirus (CMV) infection. The association with asthma and CMV infection seemed to be unusually high. Most of the cases in their review had bleeding shortly after an injury or surgery. The range of the inhibitor titer, as in other studies, was wide, from 2 to 128 BU. The correlation between factor VIII level, titer of the inhibitor, the aPTT, and bleeding complications was very low. In some of the patients, the infused factor VIII was rapidly cleared, even though there was no detectable inhibitor by the Bethesda assay. Antibodies undetected by the Bethesda assay may be demonstrated by immunoblot analysis. This would support the management approach of treating according to the clinical findings and the bleeding manifestations instead of the inhibitor level. In seven of the 10 patients, treatment with immunosuppression with azathioprine or cyclophosphamide in combination with methylprednisolone led to complete disappearance of the inhibitor within 6 weeks (95).

In the Green and Lechner (66) survey study, major bleeding complications that required transfusions occurred in 87% of the patients, and 22% died directly or indirectly of the bleeding. The bleeding episodes included melena, hematuria, and intracranial or retroperitoneal hemorrhage. In 11 (38%) patients, the inhibitor spontaneously disappeared, after having been present for an average of 14 months (1 to 48 months). These patients were either postpartum or those without underlying diseases who had low-titer inhibitors. It was more likely for patients without chronic diseases to have a greater chance for the inhibitor to disappear. In one of the postpartum patients, the inhibitor reappeared in a subsequent pregnancy. This is discussed in the pregnancy section later. In about 50% of the patients treated with varying doses of corticosteroids, or with cyclophosphamide and in 19 (68%) of 28 treated with azathioprine, there was disappearance of or decline in the inhibitor. The responders included patients with chronic diseases. There were a large number of patients with no underlying disorder in the responders. In analysis of the responses, based on the underlying diagnosis of RA and postpartum inhibitors, it was noted that with the diagnosis of RA, there was, with one exception, no incidence of the inhibitor disappearing or declining without therapy. The use of an alkylating agent was associated with a disappearance of the inhibitor in eight of 10 cases. In the postpartum patients, the inhibitor disappeared in eight of 13 spontaneously or with corticosteroids alone. The data from this study reveal a variable natural history and response to treatment. It would appear the patients with high titer and autoimmune disorders and possibly malignancy have a greater need for treatment to decrease the inhibitor titer. The study indicated that inhibitors disappear relatively infrequently in untreated patients and usually in those with low titers. Coots and Glueck (96) described a patient with an acquired inhibitor to factor VIII who was observed for 20 years. They performed analysis of the inhibitor over the last 8 years of the patient's life by using preparative isofocusing, affinity chromatography, and immunoglobulin subtyping. They were able to detect that the antibody consisted of mixtures of IgG1 and IgG4 with both κ and λ light chains. They concluded that the inhibitor was polyclonal and that the changes in the inhibitor were a dynamic process, with some inhibitors persisting, and others with different characteristics being formed. A definitive underlying disorder was not diagnosed, but an autoimmune hemolytic anemia developed just before his death at age 83 years. The authors concluded that several different groups of cells were responsible for the inhibitors during the 8-year interval, and that only three persisted. Therefore in this case, the anti–factor VIII inhibitor was in a changing or evolving process. A review of 17 new cases of acquired hemophilia in two Italian Centers in 1977 by DiBona et al. (17) revealed that, as in other studies, the mean age of the patients was 50 years; 59% of the patients had underlying disorders; and 29% were postpartum. They used DDAVP (desmopressin; 1-deamino-8-D-arginine vasopressin) successfully in five cases for minor bleeding. They had two of 15 patients with fatal hemorrhage within 2 days of diagnosis; 52% of the patients achieved complete remission (four postpartum). In three patients with SLE, a lupus-like anticoagulant was noted by tissue thromboplastin inhibition test, platelet neutralizing test, and positive antiphospholipid antibodies. The postpartum inhibitors, as is discussed later, occurred in five previously healthy primiparas, 1 to 7 months after delivery. All five patients were treated with corticosteroids, and four had a complete remission. One patient required immunosuppression treatment. These authors concluded that acquired hemophilia is a severe bleeding disorder and there is a tendency to treat patients with either corticosteroids or immunosuppression. Corticosteroids are generally found to be associated with a remission or decrease in the inhibitor titer in about 40% of the cases (97). In a randomized trial, corticosteroids alone were effective in five of 13 patients (98). Lian et al. (99) reported that 11 of 12 nonhemophilic patients with a factor VIII inhibitor treated with corticosteroids, cyclophosphamide, and vincristine had a remission. DiBona et al. (17) suggested that aggressive chemotherapy for immunosuppression should be used only in those patients with high-titer inhibitors. They noted that cyclosporine is a safe and effective drug that may have a role in the treatment of factor VIII inhibitors. The experience of the DiBona group with IVIG was reported as poor. They did have a good experience with DDAVP, and they noted that they increased factor VIII in three patients to more than 2%, 30 minutes after infusion. The treatment with DDAVP showed fair results with subcutaneous hematomas, with poorer results with deeper bleeds or open hemorrhage. Repeated daily doses were complicated by the well-known phenomenon of tachyphylaxis (102,103). The authors thought that porcine factor VIII was the most useful therapy, particularly for patients with high-titer inhibitors and those with severe bleeding.

Factor VIII Inhibitors Associated with Pregnancy

Postpartum inhibitors to factor VIII (104–109) are serious and can be a life-threatening complication that tends to occur in otherwise uncomplicated pregnancies. It usually occurs with or after the first pregnancy, with the bleeding noted in the postpartum period. As listed earlier, there have been several reviews and case studies of patients with pregnancy-related factor VIII inhibitor. Rosenthal et al. (110) in 1937 and Madison and Quick (111) in 1945 reported this entity, and Fantl and Nance (112) in 1946 reported the actual defect. They described the finding that the patient's plasma had a defect that induced a hemophilia-like state in normal plasma. Further work by Chargaff and West (113) in 1946, Dreskin and Rosenthal (114) in 1950, and Frick (115) in 1953 studied postpartum inhibitors and showed that they were directed to factor VIII. The immunoglobulin nature of the abnormality was described in the 1960s (116–118). It was noted that the responsible immunoglobulins in postpartum acquired hemophilia were the same as noted in congenital hemophilia with inhibitors. Most usually a factor VIII inhibitor is noted in the postpartum period, with excessive or prolonged vaginal bleeding as the most common finding, although the bleeding picture can be similar to that of other patients with factor VIII inhibitors. In an early review of this entity in some 30 cases, it was noted that there was a wide time frame as to when the inhibitor might appear in relation to the pregnancy and delivery. They noted that this might be from 1 week to 1 year. Case reports of the inhibitor appearing during the later stages of the pregnancy are noted. We reported on an aspect of the hypercoagulability related to treatment with activated prothrombin complex concentrate (aPCC) in a patient who had severe postsurgical bleeding during early pregnancy and whose pregnancy was undiagnosed until the complications of the bleeding and the inhibitor were noted (119). In reviewing the early literature of postpartum factor VIII inhibitors, it is very possible that some of the reports are due to other forms of inhibitors or coagulation disorders. A patient is reported in whom there was postpartum bleeding after her first delivery. She had another pregnancy some 10 weeks after the first. This was associated with normalization of her bleeding symptoms after the second month and through the pregnancy and postpartum period. A definite inhibitor was not identified (120). The occurrence of an inhibitor is reported to be more common in the first pregnancy, and most usually the pregnancy and delivery are otherwise very normal. The inhibitors can be noted after spontaneous abortion, and most of the pregnant women with factor VIII inhibitors do not have underlying disorders. The clinical presentation is usually that of a mild to severe bleeding diathesis, and the duration of the disorder can vary from 3 months to 11 years or longer, as noted in other studies. It is most usual for women in whom the inhibitor has disappeared to have uneventful subsequent pregnancies. In a review of acquired hemophilia A in 215 patients, an underlying disorder was detectable in 47% of the patients; however, in 7% of the postpartum women, an underlying disorder was noted (121). The occurrence of postpartum factor VIII inhibitors is rare. Michiels (122) described their first case in 1978 and reviewed 27 cases in the literature at that time. They noted that there were 12 documented cases since then. In their review of the literature, only one patient had a hemorrhagic diathesis during pregnancy. We noted earlier that our reported patient with the factor VIII inhibitor diagnosed during pregnancy had bleeding provoked by abdominal surgery. The time of the onset of bleeding varied, with one study revealing a distribution from right after an abortion (one), immediately after delivery (eight), in a few weeks (four), 1 to 4 months (18), and 4 to 12 months in nine patients. The inhibitor has developed in primi- and multiparae with male and female babies. The prevailing theory is that the mother is sensitized by the fetal factor VIII (123). Most studies have indicated a low rate of recurrence of the inhibitor in subsequent pregnancies (124). Spontaneous disappearance of the inhibitor during a subsequent pregnancy is reported (125). However, in a small number of patients, the inhibitor persisted during the pregnancy and a subsequent pregnancy and was detected in the child (126,127). In the Michiels review of the literature, from 1943 to 1978, there were three deaths in 28 patients (128). In the more current review, year 2000, there was one death. They followed up a total of 11 patients who did not enter a remission, and this ranged up to 24 years. In those followed up who entered a remission, a total of 25 of 40, this occurred up to 96 months with a mean, in the earlier study, of 33 months and 14 months in the more recent study. The patients who died had reported respiratory obstruction from a sublingual hematoma, massive retroperitoneal hemorrhage, and one died from uncontrollable hemorrhage after delivery. The type and titer of the inhibitor noted in the postpartum were important determinants of the bleeding and response to treatment (129). The majority of postpartum factor VIII inhibitors are type II, and the titer is relatively low (130). Therefore the inhibitor will show incomplete inactivation of infused factor VIII. In the type II inhibitors, the use of intravenous γ-globulin can be effective in decreasing the inhibitor titer and providing an increase in the factor level (131). Hauser et al. (132) addressed the effect of treatment on the disappearance of the inhibitor in 51 patients. In this retrospective review, 77% of the 51 patients achieved complete remission during the observation period. Three patients died of bleeding at 1, 5, and 36 months after the onset of symptoms. In nine patients, the inhibitor was still detectable at the last visit, which was from 2 to 29 months after onset of symptoms. A Kaplan–Meier analysis of all the patients independent of treatment revealed a probability of complete remission (CR) of almost 100%. The median time to CR was 11 months. Although one patient died of bleeding 36 months after diagnosis, the calculated probability of survival at 2 years was 97%. The use of corticosteroids did not appear to be superior to no treatment, whereas the patients treated with immunosuppressive (with or without steroids) drugs such as cyclophosphamide, azathioprine, and 6-mercaptopurine had a shorter time to complete remission compared with steroids alone ($p = 0.05$). They found that in 18 patients treated with immunosuppressives, the mean time for the loss of the inhibitor was 8 months; in 23 patients, 12 months treated with corticosteroids; in 10 patients treated with neither steroids nor immunosuppressives, 16 months. However, there was no significant difference in the final outcomes in the untreated patients, the corticosteroid group, and the immunosuppressive-treated group.

In summary, the postpartum factor VIII inhibitor is usually type II of moderate titer and enters spontaneous remission. At present there is no universally agreed-on treatment for bleeding in the postpartum inhibitor patients, based on prospective randomized trials. The immediate goal is to control the active bleeding, which may be achieved with factor VIII concentrates (133). This may be in the form of human, recombinant factor VIII or with porcine factor VIII (134). If there is a high titer, and there is a high titer of cross-reactivity to porcine factor VIII, the use of activated coagulation preparations such as aPCCs or recombinant factor VIIa (rFVIIa) may be necessary. The use of porcine factor VIII for type I or type II inhibitors in patients who do not have cross-reactive antibodies to the porcine factor is probably now the treatment of choice. IVIG in the type II inhibitors may reduce the inhibitor titer and increase the factor level for several days to weeks and enhance hemostasis and reduce the amount of factor replacement required to control bleeding (135–140). As noted in the review by Hauser et al. (132), there seems to be an advantage in treating the postpartum inhibitor patients with immunosuppressive drugs to shorten the time to remission from the inhibitor. This must be considered on an individual case-by-case basis, weighing the risks associated with immunosuppressive therapy versus a more prolonged time for the patient to have an elevated inhibitor titer. (For greater detail on treatment recommendations, see the following.)

Treatment of Patients with Factor VIII Inhibitors

Listed are agents used to control or prevent hemorrhage in addition to human factor VIII concentrates or recombinant factor VIII. The responses to the several treatments for inhibitors to factor VIII are not universally effective and individual assessment must be made in each case.

Prothrombin Complex Concentrates[3]

Activated Prothrombin Complex Concentrates[4]

The prothrombin complex concentrates (PCCs) were reported to be effective in the treatment of hemarthrosis in hemophilia patients, in 50% of the episodes (141). The

[3]PCCs: Proplex-T, Baxter Healthcare; Konyne, Bayer Biological; Profilnine, Alpha Therapeutic; Bebulin, Baxter Healthcare.

[4]aPCCs: FEIBA-VH, Baxter Healthcare; and Autoplex-T, Nabi.

aPCCs such as in the commercial products Factor VIII Inhibitor Bypassing Activity (FEIBA)-VH and Autoplex, have been generally been found to have a higher degree of effectiveness than the nonactivated PCCs, 64% versus 52% in one study (142). Although in another study, there was no advantage demonstrated for the aPCC, Autoplex compared with PCC (143). Several other studies have reported response rates with FEIBA from 75% to 95% (144,145). The aPCCs have the disadvantage of being human blood products that can transmit viral disorders. PCCs and aPCCs have been associated with thrombotic events including venous thrombosis, pulmonary embolism, disseminated intravascular coagulation, and acute myocardial infarctions (146–153). Turecek et al. (154) studied the mechanism of action of FEIBA. They were able to characterize the inhibitor-bypassing activity and potency of the components of FEIBA as being due to factor Xa, and prothrombin. The Xa/prothrombin complex associates with factor V (FVa) with the formation of the prothrombinase complex on activated platelets. This leads to thrombin formation at the site of injury. There also is stimulation of the intrinsic pathway with prothrombin facilitating factor XI binding to platelets. In the hemophilia A inhibitor patients with previous anamnestic responses to factor VIII concentrates, the use of FEIBA may be associated with anamnesis in 32% to 36% of patients (155,156). With Autoplex, the incidence of anamnesis has been reported to be variably lower. Abildgaard et al. (157–159) found no incidence, whereas others reported 6% to 20% incidence of anamnesis. White (160) reviewed 17 years of experience with Autoplex in patients with severe hemophilia and inhibitors. He reported on the treatment of 23 hemophilia A patients with high titer (more than 10 BU) and noted that there was effective or partially effective hemostatic control in 72 hours in 94% of the cases (85% effective and 9% partial). There were no thrombotic complications, and there was little tendency for Autoplex to cause an anamnestic response, noted in one of the 19 bleeding episodes. There was no postoperative bleeding in the three patients who required invasive procedures. Kantrowitz et al. (159) reported satisfactory responses with Autoplex in 87% of bleeding episodes. They did not report the occurrence of thrombotic complications.

Although there appears to be no significant reported incidence of thrombosis with Autoplex, caution is recommended in the use of PCCs and aPCCs with repeated doses or high-dose regimens (see rFVIIa later).

1. Porcine factor VIII (Hyate:C, Speywood, U.K.) represented a major advance in the treatment of factor VIII inhibitors. In one retrospective study, antibody cross-reactivity to porcine factor VIII was noted in 15% of the patients with inhibitors. The Bethesda assay did not reveal the inhibitor in 27% of these patients (161). In three studies, porcine factor VIII was shown to be effective in controlling bleeding in up to 90% of the episodes (162–164). Anamnesis in hemophilia A patients with porcine factor VIII can occur in up to 35% of the infusions.

2. Porcine factor VIII has been shown to provide clinical benefit in patients who have high titers of inhibitors to human and porcine factor VIII (165). Brettler et al. (166) and Lozier et al. (167) reported using porcine factor VIII in 12 bleeding episodes in hemophilia A patients with inhibitors greater than 12 BU (14 to 1,000 BU). They administered porcine factor VIII, 50 to 150 U/kg, Lozier at a higher dose schedule, averaging 148 U/kg per bleeding episode. In eight evaluable treatments, there was good to excellent hemostasis with no measurable factor VIII activity. In two of five instances in which the postinfusion factor VIII was less than 1%, there was excellent hemostasis. The mechanism(s) is unclear by which porcine factor VIII continues to provide good hemostasis in spite of little to no increase in the factor VIII level in some patients. It may be due to differences in the reaction kinetics between human factor VIII antibodies and porcine factor VIII, with dissociation of the factor VIII from the antibody. Other postulates are that porcine factor VIII may have hemostatic activity, even when not detected by standard factor VIII assays. There may be greater factor VIII activity on a weight basis in porcine versus human factor VIII. Porcine factor VIII may stimulate or activate platelets. There may be a hemostatic effect due to residual porcine vWF in the preparation. (165).

3. A major advantage in the use of porcine factor VIII is the lack of transmission of viruses such as human immunodeficiency virus (HIV) and the hepatitis viruses B and C.

4. Problems with use of porcine factor VIII, in hemophilia A, are anamnesis, thrombocytopenia, and reactions with infusions.

- Thrombocytopenia is commonly transiently noted and has little clinical significance. Platelet agglutination is associated with the intensive treatment with porcine factor VIII and may be due to the porcine vWF in the concentrate (168). It has been postulated that the control of bleeding without an increase in the factor VIII level may be related to the platelet agglutination and the porcine vWF effect (169).
- The reactions to porcine factor VIII are usually mild and may occur in up to 5% of the infusions.
- The use of continuous intravenous infusion of porcine factor VIII may decrease the risk for reactions and thrombocytopenia (170).

Activated Recombinant Factor VII

The use of a new form of an activated coagulation preparation, recombinant activated factor VII (rFVIIa; NovoSeven)5 has been described in several studies (171–174). rFVIIa is a genetic product of hamster kidney cells that have been trans-

[5]rFVIIa, NovoSeven, Novo Nordisk Pharmaceuticals, Inc., Princeton, NJ, U.S.A.

fected with the human factor VII gene. The factor VII is converted to the active form, FVIIa. The rFVIIa has activation properties similar to those of the naturally derived factor VIIa. There is no evidence that it produces an anamnestic response. Data so far indicate that thrombogenecity is not a significant issue. One case of myocardial infarction related to the use of rFVIIa has been reported in a 72-year-old man with severe hemophilia A and a high-titer inhibitor. He was treated with bolus and continuous infusion of rFVIIa and with tranexamic acid. The patient who had high risk factors for atherogenic disease had a coronary thrombosis and, on angiography, had atheromatous disease. It was postulated that the tissue factor in the atherosclerotic lesions had interacted with the rFVIIa (175). NovoSeven has been reported to control bleeding successfully in two patients, one with hemophilia A and inhibitor and one with acquired hemophilia, who had been treated with aPCCs and had related myocardial infarction. The use of NovoSeven was not associated with recurrent myocardial or thrombotic complications (176). It is suggested that the advantage to rFVIIa is that it functions through tissue factor and therefore at the sites of vascular injury. However, if increased tissue factor is being generated in arterial atheromatous lesions, there may be a risk for arterial or coronary thrombosis. rFVIIa has the advantage of not being a blood-derived product. Patients hypersensitive to mouse, hamster, and bovine proteins may have a problem with rFVIIa.

rFVIIa (NovoSeven) is now commercially available and should be the agent of choice when an activated coagulation agent is required and the future chance of exposure to blood products is less likely. There is mounting evidence that rFVIIa is an effective and safe agent in the management of several forms of inhibitors with bleeding, in addition to a wide variety of serious bleeding disorders (177).

rFVIIa has been reported in 38 patients with 74 bleeding episodes. These were severe bleeds in patients who failed to respond to other treatment. There was a good response in 75% of the bleeding episodes, with an additional partial response in 17%. All responses occurred in 8 to 24 hours; therefore alternative therapy is to be considered if hemostasis has not occurred within this time frame (178). Liebman et al. (179) reported on the successful use of rFVIIa in the treatment of abdominal hemorrhage in six of seven patients with acquired or hemophilia inhibitors. One patient had a partial response. Makris et al. (180) reported a patient with continued bleeding after a nephrectomy and an acquired factor VIII inhibitor, with 532 BU. The patient received 20 doses of rFVIIa with continued bleeding. The bleeding was eventually controlled by the use of porcine factor VIII. This case serves as pointer that no single treatment for bleeding with factor VIII inhibitors is universally successful and that adjustment in management must be made in the patient who is not adequately responding.

In a 1998 review, rFVIIa was reported to be effective in controlling bleeding in 81% of major surgical procedures, in 86% of minor procedures, and in 92% of dental procedures. It was further reported to be effective in 62% to 88% of various forms of 518 bleeding episodes. These ranged from muscle, oral and nasal mucosal, central nervous system, joint and retroperitoneal hemorrhage (181).

It would be appropriate to exert caution in the use of rFVIIa in patients with atheromatous disease. It was suggested by some that when aPCC treatment is needed, minimal doses be used, and if higher doses or more prolonged

TABLE 10.2. OUTLINE FOR THE MANAGEMENT OF ACUTE BLEEDING IN HEMOPHILIA A PATIENTS WITH INHIBITORS

Type of Inhibitor Response	Minor Bleed	Severe Bleed
Low responder	r-human FVIII[a] Porcine FVIII[b] FEIBA[b] rFVIIa[b]	r-human FVIII[a] Porcine FVIII[a] FEIBA[b] rFVIIa[b]
High responder with baseline <5 BU	rFVIIa[ad] Porcine FVIII[b]	Porcine FVIII[ae] or rFVIIa[a]
High responder with >5 BU	rFVIIa[ad] FEIBA[a] Porcine FVIII[b]	Porcine FVIII[ae] rFVIIa[b] FEIBA[b] Plasmapheresis or immunoadsorption[c]

BU, Bethesda unit.
[a]Primary choice of treatment.
[b]Next choice if poor response to initial choice of treatment.
[c]Option in selected patients and situations.
[d]Use agents that give the least chance for anamnesis.
[e]If there is no evidence for a high-titer anti–porcine factor VIII antibody.
Modified from Hay CRM, Baglin TP, Collins PW, et al. Guideline: the diagnosis and management of factor VIII and IV inhibitors: a guideline from the Haemophilia Centre Doctor's Organization. *Br J Haematol 2000;111:78–90,* and Canadian Directors of Hemophilia Center Subcommittee on Inhibitors. Suggestions for the management of factor VIII inhibitors. *Haemophilia 2000; 6(suppl 1):52–59.*

use is needed to control bleeding, that rFVIIa be used. They suggested that antifibrinolytics be avoided in this setting and that myocardial status should be monitored.

Because of its short half-life ($T_{½}$), frequent dosing may be necessary. No specific available clinically laboratory method measures the effect of rFVIIa. There is a shortening of the aPTT after infusion in inhibitor patients. This does not correlate with the clinical response, and the use of the aPTT in determining the response to rFVIIa is not indicated.

The dose schedule for rFVIIa has been assessed in several reports, but serious bleeding with factor VIII or factor IX inhibitors may best be treated with 90 mg/kg, when this dose was compared with a schedule of 35 mg/kg (171). The most effective dose schedule for rFVIIa by bolus or continuous infusion has not been conclusively established, although dose schedules from 30 mg/kg to 90 mg/kg as a bolus have been reported. Schedules for the successful use of continuous administration of rFVIIa also are reported.

- The use of transexamic acid and fibrin glue with the rFVIIa have been reported to provide more effective hemostasis, with a decreased amount of rFVIIa required (182,183). See factor V inhibitor section later on the complications with fibrin glue and topical thrombin (Table 10.2).

Caution should be exercised in the use of antifibrinolytic agents, as mentioned earlier, in relation to patients who might be at risk becausee of the complications of atheromatous disease.

MANAGEMENT OF ACQUIRED FACTOR VIII INHIBITORS (TABLE 10.3)

The following is based in part on the guidelines report of the United Kingdom Haemophilia Center Directors Organization (UKHCDO) Inhibitor Working Party and the Canadian Hemophilia Center Directors Subcommittee on Inhibitors (184–186).

General Initial Approach in Bleeding Patient

1. Make an accurate diagnosis and exclude other possible causes of prolonged aPTT.
2. Determine factor VIII level and the inhibitor titer by using Bethesda assay (BU).
3. Determine if there is a positive anti porcine factor VIII antibody and its titer.
4. Porcine factor VIII is usually more successful than human factor VIII, particularly when the inhibitor has little to no cross-reactivity to porcine factor VIII.
5. Investigate patient for possible underlying condition or drugs and institute appropriate treatment.
6. The inhibitor titer as per the BU has poor correlation with the clinical bleeding pattern in the acquired hemophilia patients.
7. If factor VIII inhibitor–bypassing agent is indicated, the treatment of choice is rFVIIa (NovoSeven) over the standard aPCCs. This is particularly true for patients who have not previously received blood products and may not receive such in the future.

General Suggested Approach for Immunosuppressive Treatment of Acquired Factor VIII Inhibitor

1. Initiate immunosuppressive therapy as soon as diagnosis of acquired hemophilia is noted.
2. Start with corticosteroids in the bleeding patient (not threatening life or limb), prednisone, 1 mg/kg/day, for 3 weeks or until the elimination of the inhibitor or whatever comes first.

TABLE 10.3. TREATMENT OF ACQUIRED HEMOPHILIA

Agent	Source
Prednisolone, 1 mg/kg/day Inhibitor disappears 30%	Green and Lechner 1981 (14) Spero et al. 1981 (451) Green 1968 (424)
Prednisolone + cyclophosphamide, 50–100 mg/day 60–70% response	Green and Lechner 1981 (14) Green et al. 1993 (98)
Other options Prednisolone + azathioprine or cyclophosphamide and vincristine	Green and Lechner 1981 (14) Lian et al. 1989 (452)
or IVIG, 2 g/kg × 2–5 days 30% partial to complete responses	Sultan et al. 1984 (453) Green and Kwaan 1987 (454) Struillou et al. 1993 (455) Schwartz et al. 1995 (456)
Cyclosporine. 10–15 mg/kg/day Serum levels of 150–350 ng/mL	Hart et al. 1988 (100) Pfliegler et al. 1989 (457) Schulman et al. 1996 (458)

IVIG, intravenous immunoglobulin.

3. If more serious bleeding occurs, begin corticosteroids and IVIG simultaneously.

4. Immunoglobulins (IVIGs) may be tried in a dose of 0.4 g/kg/day for 5 days. The response is variable. High-dose IVIG, 2 g/kg over 2 to 5 days, is successful in 30% to 50% of patients. (Response to IVIG usually noted within 5 days because of an antiidiotype effect) (87,88).

5. Alternatively can treat with prednisolone, 1 mg/kg/day, with oral cyclophosphamide, 50 to 100 mg/day (larger doses by i.v. pulse), particularly if response is not adequate.

6. Based on uncontrolled trials, corticosteroids and cyclophosphamide may be effective when used individually or in combination.

- It may take weeks or months to reduce the titer significantly.
- The use of cyclophosphamide or azathioprine can be considered for a period of 8 to 12 weeks to eradicate the inhibitor.
- Immunosuppressive drugs are contraindicated in pregnancy and during lactation. They should be used with caution in children.
- Treat with prednisolone alone or possibly with azathioprine in women of reproductive age.

7. With no or poor response, use multiple immunosuppressive agent therapy and possibly cyclosporine.

8. In patients with very low titers or in patients with postpartum inhibitors, the inhibitors may be transient, and aggressive therapy may not be needed.

See Table 10.3 for an outline of the guidelines for inhibitor suppression.

Treatment of Bleeding Episodes in Acquired Hemophilia A[6]

Patients with Low-titer and Residual Factor VIII Activity (Bleeding Not Threatening Life or Limb)

DDAVP (0.3 μg/kg, i.v. or subcutaneously or intranasally, and can be repeated in 24 hours; response to repeated doses is diminished) can be tried for minor bleeds involving superficial sites and is not recommended for open bleeding lesions or when there is no plasma factor VIII response (187,188).

1. DDAVP should not be used with severe bleeding or with very low to nondetectable factor levels. If bleeding persists or response is not adequate to DDAVP or for more serious bleeding, give porcine factor VIII (50 to 100 IU/kg). Porcine factor VIII is indicated based on the relatively low incidence of cross-reactive antibodies to the porcine product and unusual occurrence of anamnesis (189–193). The response in the control of bleeding may not be associated with immediate increase in the factor VIII level after porcine factor VIII infusion. Repeated doses on an intermittent basis at 12- to 24-hour intervals or by continuous intravenous infusion (5 to 10 U/kg/h).

- The Bethesda Units are less predictive of response to factor replacement in the acquired inhibitors.
- Actual measurements of factor VIII levels in response to factor infusions are more informative.
- Porcine factor VIII infusion is reported to have good to excellent responses in 78% of bleeds (194).
- Monitor FVIII levels with porcine treatment. If FVIII level is increased with porcine infusion in spite of increased antiporcine inhibitor levels, can continue with treatment if bleeding is controlled (see porcine factor VIII earlier).
- Anamnesis is reported in a small number of patients with single treatment episodes (4%).

2. If porcine FVIII fails or there is evidence of antibody cross-reactivity or there is refractoriness to porcine factor VIII, can treat with bypassing agents such as aPCC[7] or rFVIIa[8] (195–205).

Patients with More Serious Bleeding That May Threaten Life or Limb

The use of corticosteroids and IVIG, as noted earlier, should be initiated.

- To control the bleeding, the choice is between porcine factor VIII and rFVIIa. If there is a high titer and the patient has recently received porcine factor VIII, would start with rFVIIa.
- Patients with serious bleeding should receive 75 to 100 IU/kg of porcine factor VIII.
- If the factor VIII responses are adequate to greater than 0.5 IU/mL, the doses should be followed at 8- to 12-hour intervals or with continuous intravenous infusion at 5 to 10 IU/kg/h.
- If the response is less than desired, repeat bolus dose, 100 to 200 IU/kg, and test for factor level response.
- If inadequate, change to rFVIIa or aPCC.
- The dose of rFVIIa is currently recommended at 70 to 90 μg/kg every 2 hours, as needed.
- aPCCs should be given at 50 to 100 IU/kg every 6 to 12 hours for four to six doses.

[6]Abstracted from Guideline: the diagnosis and management of factor VIII and IX inhibitors: a guideline from the Haemophilia Centre Doctor's Organization. Hay CRM, Baglin TP, Collins PW, et al. *Br J Haematol* 2000;111:78–90 and Canadian Hemophilia Center Directors Subcommittee on Inhibitors. *Hemophilia* 2000;6 (suppl 1):52–59.

[7]FEIBA Factor VIII Inhibitor Bypassing Activity (Baxter-Immuno) and Autoplex T (Nabi).

[8]rFVIIa, NovoSeven.

- The use of antifibrinolytics should be avoided with aPCCs but can be used with rFVIIa and porcine factor VIII.
- (a) Failure of the above can be followed by the use of plasmapheresis or extracorporeal immunoadsorption with porcine factor VIII or rFVIIa after the procedure;
- (b) Failure to irradicate the inhibitor can be followed by repeated doses of corticosteroids, IVIG; or
- (c) Cyclosporine (4 mg/kg/day in two divided doses to maintain plasma cyclosporine levels at 125 to 225 mg/mL).

FACTOR XI INHIBITORS

The literature on factor XI inhibitors is relatively sparse compared with that on factor VIII. This reflects its infrequent occurrence. *Factor XI (plasma thromboplastin antecedent, PTA)* is a glycoprotein (GP) homodimer of 607 amino acids that is activated to become a serine protease. The activation is accomplished by cleavage by factor XIIa or thrombin. Factor XIa converts factor IX to factor IXa. In 1991 it was reported that thrombin has the capacity to activate factor XI, and this was an alternative route for the activation of factor XI (206–208). In the new revised model of the activation of blood coagulation, the contact factors have little to no role in the physiologic process of blood coagulation. The new schema would have the extrinsic system being stimulated with the resultant generation of thrombin. The activation of factor Xa leads to a downregulation of the extrinsic system by the stimulation of the tissue factor pathway inhibitor (TFPI). The continued formation of thrombin would then depend on a feedback system due to the thrombin-induced activation of factors V, VIII, and XI. It would appear that factor XI increases the rate of thrombin formation and is important in the coagulation phase of low tissue factor concentrations. It also is now known that factor XI plays an important role in regulating the fibrinolytic process by its stimulation of thrombin activatable fibrinolysis inhibitor (TAFI) (209,210). This may explain the predilection for bleeding to occur in factor XI–deficient patients at sites with greater fibrinolytic activity, such as the oral mucosa. Inherited factor XI deficiency, first reported by Rosenthal in 1953, is inherited as an autosomal recessive disorder with variable expression in heterozygotes. Homozygotes have up to 20% levels of factor XI antigen, and heterozygotes may have 30% to 70% levels. Factor XI deficiency is found predominantly in Ashkenazi Jews but occurs in all other groups (211,212). Usually little or no bleeding is associated with the defect (213). The incidence of bleeding in homozygotes is reported at about 50%. Although patients with severe deficiency will bleed more frequently than will those with the milder deficiencies, patients with milder heterozygous deficiency states, with nearly normal levels of factor, may bleed after surgery or other invasive procedures (214). Because of the benign behavior of the deficiency, most patients with congenital factor XI deficiency will not receive blood products or plasma infusions. However, a small minority of factor XI–deficient patients have mild to moderated bleeding histories, particularly with invasive procedures that involve mucous membranes. Factor XI inhibitors in this group of patients can form after infusion of blood components (215,216,229). In addition, there are reports of patients with inherited factor XI deficiency developing inhibitors without documented exposure to blood products. Chediak et al. reported a patient with congenital factor XI deficiency, with no known exposure to blood products and carcinoma of the prostate, in whom a factor XI inhibitor developed (217). There is not an abundance of literature on the development and management of factor XI antibodies (218). The low incidence of inhibitors in congenital factor XI deficiency is ascribed to the infrequent use of plasma or blood component treatment, immune tolerance due to the presence of plasma factor, and that factor XI may not be so immunogenic as is factor VIII (219). However, there are reports of the inhibitor being associated with severe hemorrhage, thrombosis, and increased platelet aggregation. The inhibitor may be associated with autoimmune disease such as systemic lupus; with drugs such as procainamide or chlopromazine; or with other disorders such as Waldenström macroglobulinemia, bronchial carcinoma, acute myeloid leukemia, and psoriasis (220–232,240). Goodrick et al. (233) reported a 71-year-old man with acquired factor XI inhibitor, who had chronic lymphocytic leukemia. He had excessive bleeding after a resection of the prostate and had a factor XI level of 18% and 0.8 BU. The inhibitor activity was abolished by 2-mercaptoethanol, which suggested that the inhibitor was an IgM antibody. There was no evidence of a paraprotein. The factor level increased to 30%, with loss of measurable inhibitor after treatment with corticosteroids and chlorambucil. Factor XI inhibitors have generally been characterized as IgG4 and transient IgM antibodies (76). De la Cadena et al. (234) described antibody in two cases as binding to the heavy chain of factor XI. The antibodies inhibited different functions, with one binding to high-molecular-weight (HMW) kininogen, and the other, to the site for substrate factor IX (234). Shapiro and Hultin (2) noted in their review of acquired inhibitors that only seven cases in 1975 had been reported of inhibitors to factor XI or factor XIa. All were female patients, and only one was congenitally deficient in factor XI; the others had systemic lupus. The association with SLE probably explains the increased female incidence for the inhibitor. Only one of the six patients had bleeding, and none of the acquired inhibitor cases had been previously transfused. As also has been noted by other investigators, three of the six acquired factor XI patients had decreased factor XII. Patients with autoimmune diseases such as SLE may have antibodies that affect the components of the contact system and may therefore appear to be inhibitors of factor XI. Inhibitors of the contact coagulation factors may be associated with prolongation of the aPTT. Schnall et al. (229) reported four patients with factor XI deficiency. In three, the inhibitors were noted after plasma infusions. In one case with a milder factor XI deficiency of 25%, no infusions were involved. This patient had a transient inhibitor. They noted that transient inhibitors to factor XI had been previously reported, and these are usually related to other intercurrent illnesses. The patients with acquired factor XI inhibitors have a rather heterogeneous clinical picture, with most having few to no bleeding manifestations. In their report, Goldsmith and Silverman (232) examined IgG inhibitors from four patients and assessed the effect of the inhibitors on specific functions of factor XI. They noted that the inhibitors from patients with inherited factor XI deficiency and the acquired variety exhibit similar patterns of factor XI inhibition. They tended to interfere more often with the surface-bound factor XI than with the coagulant properties of factor XIa. They concluded that the principal binding sites for the acquired inhibitors of factor XI are the domains involved with surface binding, and the conversion of factor XI to factor XIa had less effect on the factor XIa enzymatic activity. In their study, there were two patients with hereditary deficiency but in whom there was no explanation for the inhibitor, such as use of blood products, and two patients with newly diagnosed adenocarcinoma. The inhibitors were polyclonal IgG. They commented that their patients, like most with this type of inhibitor, had no evidence of abnormal bleeding. One of their patients, with a high titer of inhibitor, underwent surgery without significant bleeding. Overall the studies of factor XI inhibitors revealed that inhibitors from different patients possess widely varying mechanisms of factor XI inhibition. It is not apparent whether the absence of inhibitor-associated bleeding in these patients is reflective of alternative pathways for factor IX activation or whether the function of factor XI is somehow protected from these inhibitors. The diagnosis of factor XI inhibitors must include a diligent examination for the possibility of a lupus-like inhibitor that may well appear to be a specific factor XI inhibitor. It is possible that some of the previously reported factor XI inhibitors without bleeding complications and possibly some of those associated with thrombosis were due to lupus-like inhibitors. The recommended treatment of severe bleeding, in the factor XI inhibitor patients, is to attempt to bypass the inhibitor effect with the aPCCs or with the use of the rFVIIa concentrate (235–237). In a report of two patients with factor XI inhibitors who required cardiac intervention, the successful use of treatment with immunosuppressive therapy and plasma exchange was described (238). These two cases demonstrated that patients can be prepared for surgery by immunosuppression and/or plasma exchange. However, a larger number of carefully studied cases would be required before definitive management recommendations can be established. The case reports and literature on factor XI inhibitors tend to classify those patients with congenital factor XI deficiency who receive blood components such as fresh frozen plasma or factor XI concentrates with subsequent inhibitors as *acquired.* The inhibitors that occur in association with other conditions are classified as *spontaneous.*

The relation of factor XI to fibrinolysis is put forth to explain the increased tendency for bleeding, in factor XI–deficient patients, from mucous membrane sites. It is postulated that the production of fibrin in factor XI–deficient patients is less resistant to fibrinolytic enzymes that are prevalent in the secretions of the mucous membranes. In animal experiments, it was noted that in the presence of anti–factor XI antibody in a rabbit model, there was increased lysis of fibrin clots. It was indicated by the data that thrombin generation continues in a factor XI–dependent manner after clot formation has occurred. The thrombin increases the formation of TAFI (239). One can then postulate that in some patients with factor XI inhibitors, there is an inhibition of the factor XI function of promoting TAFI activation. There is now evidence that increased levels of factor XI can be associated with an increased incidence of venous thrombosis. This is postulated to be mediated through the TAFI system. It is not a major jump to postulate that, in some patients with factor XI inhibitors, there is an inhibition of the stimulation of TAFI that may contribute to a bleeding problem. Further studies are necessary to look at the relation of the factor XI inhibitors and TAFI and their effect on bleeding.

Reece et al. (240) reported on seven cases and review of the literature of spontaneous factor XI inhibitors. Their study covered a period of 10 years, and 12 cases were identified. The factor XI levels ranged from 2% to 27%. As was noted in other reports, there was a marked reduction in factor XII in one patient and slight reduction in two others. It was thought that the reduced factor XII noted was a cross-reactivity of the inhibitor in the factor XII assays. In four cases that were studied previously, two were found to have antibodies to factor XI and two against factor XIa. In the cases they collected, 55% had no hemorrhagic manifestations, 33% had mucous membrane bleeding, 27% had ecchymosis, and 11% had easy bruising. There was a subgroup of patients, 16% with thrombocytopenia, 11% with spontaneous abortion, and 11% with thrombosis. This might suggest the possibility of the lupus inhibitor, anticardiolipin syndrome, or autoimmune disease. In 55% of the patients, the inhibitor disappeared spontaneously with no treatment. Compatible with other reports, 72% of the patients had autoimmune disease, and the hemorrhagic problems were mild, with most bleeding episodes related to mucosal surfaces. Only one patient with another major coagulopathy had a serious hemorrhage in the central nervous system.

It would seem, therefore, from the accumulated data that factor XI inhibitor patients have a clinical picture of mild to no bleeding, with occasional cases of severe hemorrhage. There are reports of increased thrombosis in patients with factor XI inhibitors. This has been associated with a deficiency of factor XII or an associated inhibitor to factor XII. However, it is quite possible that these patients represented forms of lupus-like inhibitors that are well known to be related to thrombosis. SLE is associated with an increased incidence of thrombosis, and many of the patients with factor XI inhibitors are noted to have SLE. Circulating anticoagulants against factor XI and factor XII have been reported in association with spontaneous platelet aggregation. In other reports, the inhibitors have been associated with recurrent thrombosis (241,242). Vercellotti and Mosher (243) described a patient with factor XI deficiency and SLE in 1982. They were not able to demonstrate an actual inhibitor to factor XI, but the factor XI was less than 2% and improved to 33% and then to 56% after treatment with corticosteroids. Chromatography studies revealed the presence of a substance in the patient's plasma that bound factor XI into large aggregates. Although an inhibitor was not demonstrated in coagulation assays, there was evidence that there was a substance in the patient's plasma that most likely was an immunoglobulin. A pseudo-factor XI deficiency that was thought to be due to plasma activity that inhibited the adsorption of factor XI to glass surfaces was described by Schiffman et al. (244). The patient was a 16-year-old boy of non-Jewish origin in whom findings of ulcerative colitis developed. He had no prior bleeding history, and there was no family history of a bleeding tendency. He was noted to have a prolonged aPTT and a factor XI of 18%. No other coagulation defect was noted. The patient had bleeding postoperatively in spite of plasma administration. The aPTT did not shorten significantly after infusion. The evaluation revealed an inhibitor to reactions involving factor XI. There were no positive confirmatory tests for the lupus-like inhibitor, and infusion of normal plasma led to less than expected recovery of factor XI. This suggested that there was a plasma substance that was neutralizing exogenous factor XI. Although they did not identify the specific type of inhibitor, this was an early case that demonstrated the rather wide variety of inhibitory activities that can affect factor XI. It also demonstrates an inhibitor that was associated with bleeding after one surgery, but was managed satisfactorily in a subsequent surgery with fresh frozen plasma. That this was associated with an autoimmune disorder increased the probability that it was due to an antibody-mediated mechanism. Circulating anticoagulants to factor XIa have been described in SLE patients (245,246). Chiu Poon et al. (247) in 1984 reported an acquired inhibitor to factor XI in a patient with SLE; it was a precipitating IgG-λ autoantibody. The inhibitor interfered with the binding of factor XI onto reactive surfaces. It also inhibited surface-mediated proteolytic cleavage of factor XI. The authors excluded a lupus-like inhibitor by a negative dilute PT test. Other confirmatory tests for lupus inhibitor were not done. The patient of Poon et al. had no symptoms of a spontaneous bleeding diathesis. Ginsberg et al. (248) described the delivery of a patient with congenital factor XI deficiency (4%) and an inhibitor, who had a bleeding history including epistaxis, easy bruising, and bleeding after dental extraction. Preparatory to surgery for a bone tumor, she was treated with fresh frozen plasma with no shortening of the PTT. A factor XI inhibitor was noted with BU of 50 units. aPCC in the form of Autoplex was administered and halted the bleeding. The inhibitor titer increased to 300 units, with the level remaining at 4%. Autoplex was again given with control of bleeding for further surgery. The inhibitor decreased over time, and the factor XI was 6% when the BU was 1.2. The inhibitor was an IgG. The patient became pregnant and had an elective cesarean section at 37 weeks with the administration of the aPCC, FEIBA, just before the surgery. There was no excessive bleeding. The cesarean was elected because of the possibility for the inhibitor to affect the fetus and the danger of serious bleeding during the delivery.

In summary, acquired factor XI inhibitors are rarer forms of autofactor antibodies. For the most part, they do not cause serious bleeding and are most commonly associated with autoimmune diseases. However, they can be responsible for serious bleeding with invasive procedures. It also is important to differentiate true factor XI inhibitors from lupus-like inhibitors that can be associated with thrombotic disease and pregnancy complications. In addition, true factor XI inhibitors should be differentiated from inhibition of the contact phase factors that can prolong the aPTT and appear to be factor XI inhibitors. Treatment of bleeding or the prevention of bleeding with invasive procedures consists of the use of rFVIIa or aPCC. As described earlier, the use of plasma exchange with apheresis techniques and replacement with fresh frozen plasma has been reported to manage patients successfully during surgery.

FACTOR IX INHIBITORS IN HEMOPHILIA B AND ACQUIRED ANTI–FACTOR IX ANTIBODIES

Inhibitors are noted in about 3% of patients with hemophilia B, with a distribution similar to that seen in hemophilia A patients (249,250). The alloantibodies in hemophilia B are associated with deletions of the factor IX gene and are more common in sibling pairs and within families (251). In a report of previously untreated hemophilia B patients who were being followed up in the recombinant factor IX study, 62 were assessed for factor IX inhibitors by the Bethesda Inhibitor Assay method (BU) and an enzyme-linked immunosorbent assay (ELISA) (252). The latter was thought to be more sensitive to inhibitors. Two patients had high-titer inhibitors by both BU and ELISA. Another patient had a transient inhibitor detected only by ELISA. All these three had the same factor IX gene mutation with a single base pair change at nucleotide 6,460 in the factor IX gene. Another patient had this gene mutation without (as yet) evidence for inhibitor formation. The 6,460 C-to-T mutation has been previously reported in high association for inhibitor and anaphylactoid reactions after plasma-derived factor IX infusions. The 1999 Hemophilia DataBase of point mutations and short additions and deletions revealed that of the 21 inhibitor patients, 33% had this mutation. The presence of this mutation represents a high risk for inhibitor development. The antibodies, unlike hemophilia A, are not temperature or time dependent and, as in hemophilia A, are predominantly IgG4, either monoclonal or polyclonal (253–256). Lechner (254) described a patient with a factor IX inhibitor that was present in IgG-poor components of the patient's serum. These inhibitors can exhibit an anamnestic response after treatment with plasma or factor IX concentrate. Inhibitors to factor IX in nonhemophilic patients are rare but have been reported in patients with SLE, other autoimmune disorders, hepatitis, multiple sclerosis, after surgery, and in the postpartum (257–259). In a review of the Italian registry for acquired factor VIII/IX inhibitors, Baudo and Mostarda. (260) reported an overall frequency of 0.2 to 1 per million population per year. In the 90 inhibitor patients observed over a 19-year period, only one patient had a factor IX inhibitor. A 7-year-old black patient without hemophilia B is described with an inhibitor to factor IX and bleeding after dental extraction. The BU was 5.5 units, and the baseline factor IX was 5%. The bleeding and inhibitor responded to treatment with rFVIIa, IVIG, and corticiosteroids. It was thought that the inhibitor was related to previous viral infection or to the treatment with amoxicillin (261). An acquired deficiency of factor IX was reported with Gaucher disease (262). Ten patients with Gaucher disease were studied, and a low level of factor IX was found in eight. Other factor levels were decreased in fewer patients. It is postulated that the accumulation of cerebroside may influence the activity of factor IX. The patient studied did not exhibit bleeding tendencies, and the infused factor IX had a shortened half-life, suggesting that this was related to the Gaucher disease. Other investigators reported on the decrease in factor IX plasma levels with nephrotic syndrome, with a return to normal with remission of the proteinuria (263). These forms of acquired factor IX deficiency are not thought to be due to a circulating inhibitor. The treatment for the bleeding associated with severe factor IX deficiency with an inhibitor is through the use of high-purity factor IX concentrates and aPCCs. The successful use of rFVIIa has been described (264), as has immunosuppressive therapy and plasma exchange with plasmapheresis. In general, the approach to the patient with a factor IX inhibitor is much the same as that outlined for the factor VIII inhibitor.

ACQUIRED VON WILLEBRAND DISEASE

vWF (265–273) is a large adhesive GP that is synthesized in endothelial cells and megakaryocytes and has a major role in primary hemostasis. It has two major physiologic functions in the regulation of hemostasis (274). It aids the formation of the platelet plug at sites of vascular injury by mediating, through the binding of vWF to the platelet GPIb and GPIIa/IIIb, platelet-to-platelet interaction and the adhesion of platelets to the vessel surface (275–277). vWF mediates the adhesion and aggregation of platelets to the subendothelium in high-shear-rate environments when there is vessel perturbation. The other function relates to serving as the carrier and stabilizer for the antihemophilia coagulant activity (antihemophilic factor; AHF) protein. The platelet-associated activities of vWF are related to the HMW forms of the multimeric components. An inherited or acquired deficiency or functional abnormality of vWF can result in a bleeding disorder. Classic vWD is an inherited disorder in which there may be mild to severe quantitative deficiency or qualitative functional defect of the von Willebrand factor (vWF). The majority of the patients with the less severe deficiencies (type 1) have mild to inconsequential bleeding histories. Inhibitors are noted in the patients with the inherited severe (type 3) form of vWD when there have been multiple transfusions. Shelton-Inloes et al. (278) reported in 1987 gene deletions that correlated with the development of alloantibodies. In their study of 19 patients with severe type 3 vWD, two patients were noted to have large deletions within the vWF gene. They were the only ones noted to have inhibitory alloantibodies to vWF. Their study included in addition to the 19 type 3 patients, 19 with autosomal dominant type 1. In a survey including Western Europe and Israel, eight of 106 patients with severe vWD were noted to have alloantibodies, for a prevalence of 7.6% (279). In further work, it was demonstrated that there are striking differences in the inhibitor specificity (280). The inhibitors may block the vWF ristocetin cofactor function (vWF:RCoF) and have been described as polyclonal heterologous antibodies with variable targets on the vWF (281). The inhibitors can recognize the vWF domain involved in the platelet GPIb–vWF interaction (282–288). A patient was described with severe anaphylactic reactions to infusions of FVIII/vWF concentrates. This was related to the formation of vWF–IgG complexes and the subsequent activation of complement. The use of recombinant factor VIII concentrates without vWF secured hemostasis and was not associated with reactions; therefore the antibody was directed to the vWF component of the complex. This study indicated a cause–effect relation between the formation of IgG–vWF complexes and complement activation in posttransfusion non–IgE-mediated anaphylactic reactions. They also demonstrated that the use of recombinant factor VIII concentrates is an effective alternative manner of increasing the factor VIII level in patients with severe vWD and a history of anaphylactic reactions to factor VIII–vWF concentrates (289). The occurrence of inhibitors in vWD is not as severe a life-threatening problem as in hemophilia, but it makes the treatment and management more difficult.

Acquired vWD (AvWD) has been reported in the literature since 1968 with the case study by Simone et al. (290) of a 12-year-old boy with SLE who had a bleeding problem. Van Genderen and Michiels (293) noted in their review in 1998 that an 200 additional cases of AvWD had appeared in the English language literature, and Tefferi and Nichols (267,272) in their review noted only 100 well-documentated cases. The clinical picture of the disorder is very similar to that of the inherited form, with abnormal bleeding time, decreased levels of factor VIII coagulant activity, and vWF. AvWD is associated with a moderate-to-severe bleeding tendency from mucosal surfaces, as demonstrated by epistaxis, gingival and gastrointestinal bleeding, and bleeding after surgery and invasive procedures. The bleeding is usually a new occurrence in the patient's history and occurs rapidly after a surgical procedure. There is usually no history of a bleeding tendency in the family. AvWD occurs in all ages and can affect both sexes equally. The disorders that have been associated with AvWD have a spectrum similar to that of acquired factor VIII inhibitors, which include the lymphoproliferative disease, autoimmune diseases, malignancies, and dysproteinemias (see the following list of associated disorders). Although AvWD is noted most frequently in the lymphocyte–plasma cell disorders, it has a somewhat wider spectrum that includes metabolic and vascular disorders.

Causes of Acquired von Willebrand Disease

Tefferi and Nichols (267) reviewed the mechanisms for AvWD and noted that the most frequently involved process is immune mediated, with the resultant inhibition of vWF. Approximately 50% to 60% of the cases of AvWD are associated with a lymphoproliferative disease and/or a monoclonal gammopathy, and a minority will have a demonstrable inhibitor to vWF (273,293). As noted for factor VIII inhibitors, most of the identified vWF inhibitors in AvWD are IgG and occasionally IgM or IgA. The inhibition of vWF is generally related to a generalized autoimmune process or caused by antibodies directed specifically to vWF (291–300). The disorders in which these mechanisms have been determined are the lymphoproliferative diseases, autoimmune disorders such as the antiphosholipid syndrome, and the monoclonal gammopathies. The immune mechanism also has been described in other disorders such as angiodysplasia and polycythemia vera (PV) (301,302). The inhibitors have been demonstrated in the IgG fraction of the patients' sera or in the monoclonal globulin (292,295–297, 301,302). The formation of immune complexes of vWF with immunoglobulins can lead to the accelerated clearance of vWF and the HMW multimeric forms (303). Other mechanisms for AvWD have been described, as in the decreased synthesis in hypothyroidism, proteolysis of the large multimers in a drug-related case, and absorption/adsorption of vWF by tumor cells. The adsorption mechanism has been described in cases of monoclonal gammopathy (monoclonal gammopathies of undetermined significance; MGUS), myeloma, and Waldenström macroglobulinemia and adrenal carcinoma (267). Richard et al. (304) in 1990 described the selective absorption of vWF by plasma cells. There had been a previous report of selective immunoadsorption to lymphocytes in a patient with Waldenström macroglobulinemia (305). In the former report, the authors described AvWD in a patient with IgA-λ myeloma, and through the use of indirect immunofluorescence with anti-vWF antibodies, they were able to demonstrate selective adsorption of vWF to myeloma cells. This was associated with a low level of plasma vWF. Tefferi et al. (306) described a patient with lymphoma, serious bleeding and AvWD, in whom there was demonstrated platelet GPIb on the lymphoma cells. There was no evidence of circulating vWF inhibitor, as per the effect of the patient's plasma on normal plasma in the vWF:RCoF assay. The bleeding improved after splenectomy, with further improvement after chemotherapy. The patient was noted to have a biclonal gammopathy. The gammopathy, lymphoma, and AvWD had remained in remission for 2 years at the time of last follow-up evaluation.

AvWD has been described in at least nine patients, all girls, in whom the diagnosis of hypothyroidism was made after symptoms of bleeding triggered an evaluation of thyroid function. All of the patients were younger than 18 years, and four had findings to suggest a juvenile form of hypothyroidism. In their report, Aylesworth et al. (307) described a postpartum patient with hypothyroidism with AvWD. The findings were resolved by replacement treatment with thyroxine. The authors related that hypothyroidism is common after delivery. It is possible that the AvWD and bleeding in the postpartum period may relate to the hypothyroidism.

A retrospective review of 10 patients with AvWS, which were diagnosed over a period of 17 years, revealed that the bleeding tendency varied from mild to severe (268). In eight of the 10 patients, the abnormality had a type 1 pattern with normal multimers with type 2A, and with type 3 in the others. Actual autoantibodies against vWF were detected in only two cases. In three cases, resolution of the underlying disease led to remission of the coagulopathy. The median age, as noted in other reviews, at the time of diagnosis was 51 years, with a range of 22 to 67 years; six were female and four male patients. The clinical features were similar to those of congenital vWD, with mostly mucosal bleeding. The bleeding manifestations in the 10 patients were epistaxis (three), easy bruising (three), gastrointestinal bleeding (one), and postdental bleeding (one). Two patients had more serious postoperative bleeding. The laboratory evaluation revealed a prolonged aPTT in all 10, with evidence for vWD in all. The vWF ranged between 3 and 55 U/dL, with a median of 18 U/dL (normal range, 50 to 150 U/dL). The normal multimeric analysis in eight of 10 patients varied from the experience in the literature, in which type 2A patterns are reported to be more common. The template bleeding times were prolonged in six of eight patients studied. No inhibitors, as by the Bethesda assay, to factor VIII were detected in the 10 patients. The screening for inhibitor to vWF by using ristocetin-induced platelet aggregation (RIPA) revealed a reduction in aggregation by 25% in normal plasma by patients' plasma in two patients. In the other four patients studied, no evidence of inhibitor or reduction in RIPA in normal plasma was effected by the patients' plasma. An underlying condition was determined in eight of 10 patients, and the disorders were as noted by other reviews and are included in the overall listing later. The management was based on the treatment of the underlying disorders and included treatment for hypothyroidism, chemotherapy for malignancy, plasmapheresis for macroglobulinemia; two patients received immunosuppression for the inhibitor. A patient with myeloma and the inhibitor went into remission after stem cell–transplantation treatment. In a study of seven patients with AvWD associated with lymphoproliferative disorders or benign monoclonal gammopathies, Mannucci et al. (308) found that the platelet vWF values (antigen and vWF:RCoF) were normal. In addition, they found that the multimers of the vWF in plasma and platelets were normal. The vWF and bleeding time responded to DDAVP, indicating that the endothelial cell production and release of vWF were normal. However, the duration of the response to DDAVP was shorter than corresponding levels of deficiencies seen in congenital vWD (308). AvWD can be due to antibodies directed to the HMW multimers of the vWF, with clearance of the immune complex with the vWF by the reticuloendothelial system. Another mechanism is the binding of vWF to tumor cells by direct binding to GPIb receptors or the binding through Fc receptors of the vWF–antibody complex.

Antibody-Induced Acquired von Willebrand Disease

Type of Antibody

- Specific antibodies to vWF can be IgG more than IgM or IgA (309).
- Paraproteins with anti-vWF activity
- *Neutralizing antibodies* inhibit the function of active sites and diminish the activity of the functional site by steric hindrance.
- *Nonneutralizing antibodies* that do not impair the function of vWF but can form immune complexes with vWF and may cause rapid clearance of vWF from the circulation.

Non–Antibody-Induced Acquired von Willebrand Disease

1. Decreased synthesis of vWF is associated with reported cases of the following.

- Hypothyroidism, which responded to treatment with thyroxine, response possibly due to increased protein production (310–312).
- Angiodysplasia, postulated to be due to decreased endothelial cell production of vWF. Paraproteins have been reported in some cases with angiodysplasia (313–315).
- Associated with medications such as valproic acid (316).

2. Adsorption/absorption of vWF to malignant cells (304,305,306,317,318).

- Absortion is demonstrated by immunochemical staining of vWF in malignant cells.
- Flow cytometric analysis of cells demonstrated vWF on cells such as monocytes.
- Expression of platelet GPIb on tumor cells has been demonstrated.

3. Proteolysis of plasma vWF has been reported.

- Decreased vWF noted in myeloproliferative disorders (MPDs), related to the platelet count (calpain-like vWF fragments associated with high platelet counts. Reduction of platelet count associated with return of normal vWF and vWF multimers.) (319–321)

- Treatment with ciprofloxacin, thrombolytic agents (322, 323)
- Blood flow at high shear rates (i.e., cardiac valvular disorders) (324)
- Diabetes with poor glucose control (325,326)
- Idiopathic hyperfibrinoloysis (327)

4. Precipitation of vWF

- Hydroxyethyl starch (HES) used in large volumes causes precipitation of factor VIII/vWF (328).

Specific Issues Related to Acquired von Willebrand Disease in Malignancy

The mechanisms noted (319,320,337) are as described earlier and can be summarized as

1. Antibodies produced by the malignant clones of cells that attack circulating factor VIII /vWF subunits.
2. Adsorption of factor VIII/vWF on malignant cells.
3. Monoclonal antibody forms immune complex with the vWF and is removed by the reticuloendothelial system.
4. In patients with MGUS, the most likely mechanism causing AvWD is accelerated clearance of vWF, probably by formation of immune complexes with antibody and vWF interaction. It would appear that there is a satisfactory response with an increase in the HMW multimers (HMWMs) after DDAVP infusion. DDAVP should be considered for the treatment of bleeding in MGUS patients with AvWD.
5. Patients with nephroblastoma are reported with AvWD, which may well be due to vWF adsorption to tumor cells or to hyaluronic acid interference with the functions of vWF and affecting the assays for vWF.
6. AvWD in the MPDs is most commonly seen with essential thrombocythemia (ET) and less frequently with PV and chronic granulocytic leukemia (CGL). The syndrome in the MPDs is characterized by very high platelet counts, variable bleeding time, normal factor VIII and vWF antigen, but a decreased vWF:RCoF, decreased collagen-binding activity, and a decrease in the HMWMs with a type 2 pattern of vWF deficiency (320). In a review of 110 and 128 ET and PV patients, respectively, there was an inverse relation between the platelet count and the ratio of vWF:RCoF to vWF:Ag. The vWF changes did not correlate to the WBC. The absence of the HMWM correlated with the higher platelet counts. The authors noted that patients with reactive thrombocytosis also had a decrease in the HMWMs. It is postulated that there is increased proteolysis of the vWF. However, the possibility of an immune mechanism in MPD cannot be totally excluded. Platelets may remove vWF from the circulation. The treatment of AvWD with MPDs, particularly ET, should be centered about the reduction in the platelet counts. This can be achieved by plateletpheresis in the acute setting or by cytoreduction agents such as hydroxyurea, anagrelide, or interferon-α (319).
7. In patients with lymphoproliferative diseases and monoclonal gammopathies, the use of IVIG has proved to be efficacious. Treatment of the bleeding problems includes these and the use of the following:

- DDAVP, 0.3 μg/kg i.v., or 3 μg/kg intranasal.
- There may be no shortening of the bleeding time with DDAVP, but there is usually an increase in the vWF. This form of treatment is adequate for non–life-threatening bleeding or as a prophylactic to prevent bleeding with invasive procedures.
- With severe bleeding, the use of concentrates of factor VIII/vWF cryoprecipitates in addition to DDAVP is recommended.
- Extracorporeal immunoadsorption combined with the administration of factor VIII/vWF concentrates can be tried in those patients refractory to these who are thought to have a vWF inhibitor and in whom bleeding remains a serious issue. Table 10.4 lists disorders associated with AvWD.

Diagnosis

The diagnosis of AvWD should be considered particularly in patients with new onset of bleeding problems and in whom there is no previous history of bleeding or history of a congenital bleeding diathesis having been denoted in the family. The index of suspicion should be increased in those patients with monoclonal gammopathies, lymphoproliferative diseases, MPDs, other malignancies, and autoimmune diseases. The laboratory testing should be directed to the components of vWF and factor VIII. The aPTT is commonly prolonged because of the decrease in factor VIII. The aPTT can also be prolonged because of other inhibitors. This might be a true anti–factor VIII inhibitor or a lupus inhibitor, as in the patient we reported with a lupus inhibitor and AvWD (294). The evaluation of the prolonged aPTT should follow the format described in the previous sections. The assays for factor VIII:c, ristocetin cofactor activity (vWF:RCoF), and vWF antigen (vWF:Ag) should be performed when the possibility of AvWD is considered. The vWF:RCoF assay is most informative. The measurement of another functional aspect of vWF, the collagen-binding activity, may reveal additional cases. Multimeric analysis of the vWF may be informative if there is discordance in the vWF:RCoF and vWF:Ag. Most reviews indicate that a type 2A multimeric pattern is commonly seen in AvWD. A minority of patients in the literature have been demonstrated with a circulating inhibitor to vWF. Other studies that are appropriate are protein electrophoresis and immunoelectrophoresis to screen for a dysproteinemia, because of the common occurrence of monoclonal

TABLE 10.4. ASSOCIATED DISORDERS WITH AVWD

Lymphoproliferative disorders and dysproteinemias	Monoclonal gammopathy of unknown significance (MGUS)
	Multiple myeloma
	Waldenström macroglobulinemia
	Chronic lymphocytic leukemia
	Hairy cell leukemia
	Non-Hodgkin lymphoma
Myeloproliferative disorders	Chronic granulocytic leukemia
	Essential thrombocythemia
	Polycythemia vera
	Myelofibrosis
Malignancy and tumors	Wilm tumor
	Adenocarcinomas
	Prostate hyperplasia
	Astrocytoma
	Lung carcinoma
Autoimmune diseases	Systemic lupus erythematosus
	Scleroderma
	Mixed connective tissue disease
	Anticardiolipin syndrome
	Sjögren disease
	Graft-versus-host disease
Metabolic Endocrine disorders	Hypothyroidism
	Diabetes mellitus
	Glycogen storage disorders
Other conditions	Hemoglobinopathies (i.e., thalassemia, sickle cell disease)
	Hemolytic anemia
	Secondary amyloid
	Fibrinolysis
	Allogeneic bone marrow transplantation
	Acquired and congenital heart disease
	Hydatid disease of the spleen
	HIV
	Epstein–Barr virus infection
	Uremia
Medications and other agents	Ciprofloxacin
	Valproic acid
	Hydroxyethyl starch (HES)
	Recombinant factor VIII
	Griseofulvin
	Tetracycline
	Pesticide
	Thrombolytic treatment
	Use of recombinant FVIII
Vascular disorders	Angiodysplasia
	Telangiectasia
	Ehlers–Danlos syndrome
	Congenital heart valve defects
	Vascular shear stress

HIV, human immunodeficiency virus; AvWD, acquired von Willebrand disease.
Data from Jakway (265), Tefferi and Nichols (267), Nitu-Whalley and Lee (268), Van Genderen and Michiels (272), and Rinder et al. (273).

gammopathies in this syndrome. As noted earlier, detection by flow cytometry of vWF:Ag or platelet GPIb on suspected malignant cells and lymphocytes might indicate absorption or adsorption of vWF to explain a deficiency of vWF in the plasma.

Outline of Evaluation for Acquired von Willebrand Disease

Hemostatic Screening Tests

1. The *aPTT* may be prolonged *if there is a deficiency of factor VIII* due to the decreased or inhibited vWF. The aPTT can be prolonged if there are other forms of inhibitor activity such as *lupus inhibitor or a true anti–factor VIII inhibitor* (272).

2. The *template bleeding time* is usually prolonged *because of the decrease in vWF.*

3. The *vWF,* as assessed by the functional assay for the *RCoF,* is usually diminished.

4. A discordant decrease in the RCoF compared with the vWF antigen usually indicates a *loss of the HMWMs* with a *type 2 pattern.*

5. The other standard hemostasis tests are usually normal, including the PT, platelet count, and other factor assays.

Detection of Anti–von Willebrand Factor Antibody

Standard mixing studies of patient plasma with normal plasma frequently does not reveal the presence of the inhibitor (272).

Suggested modifications of the mixing study test technique have been described to improve the sensitivity of the test.

- Preheating of the patient's plasma to 56°C to dissociate complexes of vWF with inhibitor (329)
- Mixing studies often will not detect antibodies because they are limited to those inhibitors that affect the RCoF function (330).
- These methods usually fail to detect nonneutralizing antibodies.
- Use of *Staphylococcus* protein A has been proposed to remove antigen–antibody complexes.
- Testing for other functions of vWF such as collagen binding, which is due to the inhibition of the A1 and A3 domains (309)

Therefore it is suggested that *several functional assays should be included in the evaluation.*

1. Other techniques are based on the detection of binding of the antibody to vWF by *ELISA-type techniques.*

2. The principle is based on the use of *immobilized vWF on ELISA plates or on immunobeads.*

- Labeled anti–IgM, IgG, and IgA are used to detect the presence of antibody on the vWF (331,330).

3. Alternatively, *immunoprecipitation methods* with radiolabeled vWF fragments have been described to detect the presence of anti-vWF inhibitor (309).

4. The use of *vW antigen II (vWF:Ag II),* the propeptide of vWF, is thought to be useful in differentiating

congenital vWF type 1 from 2 and in assessing endothelial activation. In a study of eight patients with AvWD, there was increased clearance of vWF. The vWF:Ag II was higher in all the AvWD cases. This was thought to be due either to a compensatory mechanism or to perturbation of the endothelium by immune complexes. These data would suggest that the use of vWF:Ag II may be of benefit in discriminating the patients with decreased vWF production from those with increased rates of clearance (332–335).

Management of Acquired von Willebrand Disease

The treatment of AvWD (265,267,268,272,273) depends very much on the underlying disorder and the mechanism responsible for the effect on vWF. The basic approach to the bleeding issues evolved through the general experience with the treatment of congenital vWD. Therefore initially the use of cryoprecipitates and later on DDAVP were the mainstays of treatment for active bleeding or to prevent bleeding in patients undergoing surgery or invasive procedures. Commercial factor VIII concentrates, with high levels of vWF, have been successfully used in congenital vWD and AvWD. The overall management has been modified by the demonstrated utility of IVIG in suppressing the inhibitor with monoclonal gammopathies and lymphoproliferative disorders. The use of DDAVP has the distinct advantage over plasma-derived products of not having the risk of blood-transmitted diseases. The commercial factor VIII:vWF concentrates that are heat treated or chemically treated are safer overall than are cryoprecipitates in respect to the hepatitis viruses and HIV. However, all human blood–derived products must be used with the knowledge that unsuspected viruses or other infectious agents may subsequently be noted.

Principles of Management Based on Reports in the Literature of Successful Responses

1. Because of the high incidence of an underlying disease or condition associated with AvWD, an extensive search for an underlying condition should be conducted.

2. Spontaneous regression of the inhibitor is infrequently noted and may occur in the setting of a transient viral infection, as noted with other inhibitors in children (336).

3. Treatment of the underlying malignancy with reported successes with all the standard approaches appropriate to the specific malignancy including surgery, chemotherapy, and radiation (267,337). Patients with lymphoplasma cell disorders usually respond to chemotherapy. Patients with MGUS could be treated with intermittent high-dose dexamethasone to reduce the level of pathogenic immunoglobulin (338). AvWD associated with an IgM monoclonal gammopathy 2-chlorodeoxyadenosine has been suggested (273).

4. Therapy for other underlying diseases such as hypothyroidism.

5. Responses have been reported in patients who underwent the following procedures and treatments.

- Surgical resection of solid tumor (317,339–440)
- Chemotherapy (341)
- Radiotherapy (342)
- Surgical repair of defective heart valves (343)
- Hormone-replacement therapy (310)
- Discontinuation of offending drugs (322,344)
- Cytoreduction of high platelet count in MPD (321)

6. Treatment of the inhibitor with corticosteroids, high-dose intravenous γ-globulin, plasma exchange, DDAVP, and concentrates containing vWF (Humate-P) (267,269, 294,337).

The use of von Willebrand Factor Replacement Therapy.

1. Use of DDAVP has been described to stimulate endothelial cell release of vWF. In many cases, this form of treatment is limited because of the short-lived increase in the level of vWF.

2. The use of plasma component therapy rich in vWF [cryoprecipitates or commercial factor VIII concentrates (i.e., Humate-P)]. The treatment goal is to increase the vWF:RCoF, which tends to correlate with effectiveness. The increase in vWF activity in most cases has duration of about 2 to 3 hours.

Treatment to Reduce the Anti–von Willebrand Factor Inhibitor

1. The use of high-dose IVIG has been reported in several articles to induce a remission effectively with a disappearance of the inhibitor. We reported on a patient with a lupus inhibitor and anticardiolipin syndrome who had AvWD. He was treated with IVIG with complete remission of the AvWD, allowing the successful completion of orthopedic surgery (294). Several articles described the successful use of IVIG and are listed in the review by Rinder et al. (273).

2. IVIG, given at 0.5 to 2 g/kg over a period of 1 to 2 days, has been noted generally to produce a desirable lasting effect. Patients so treated can very often have surgery or other procedures in 1 to 2 days after the IVIG infusion. The bleeding manifestations due to AvWD usually respond very rapidly to IVIG. The good responses to IVIG are noted in those patients with lymphoproliferative disorders due to monoclonal gammopathies. There is little experience in the use of IVIG for patients with other malignancies, MPDs, or drug-induced AvWD. The duration of response to IVIG is reported to be from 5 days to more than 21 days.

3. IVIG is thought to exert its effect through two mechanisms: (a) by blocking Fc receptors on the monocyte phagocytic cells, thereby decreasing the clearance of inhibitor–vWF complexes from the circulation; and (b) as an antiidiotype antibody effect.

4. The use of immunosuppressive therapy to treat an underlying lymphoproliferative disease is reported to have success, whereas the use of immunosuppressive therapy for the inhibitor *per se* has been reported to have disappointing results (345).

5. Other treatments that have been described are plasma exchange and extracorporeal immunoadsorption. These would be considered in patients not responding to IVIG when bleeding is not controlled or invasive procedures are planned (346,347). In one case, the response was short lived, and the patient was treated with Humate-P to increase the vWF level after immnunoadsorption (348).

ACQUIRED FACTOR V INHIBITORS

Factor V is a plasma GP with a molecular mass of 330 kDa. There are three type A domains and two type C domains that are similar to factor VIII (349–356,363–368). The connecting region, the B domain, is proteolytically removed by thrombin activation. The B domain of factor V is not homologous to factor VIII. There is approximately 84% to 86% identity for human and bovine factor V in the C domains, with approximately 59% for the B domain. The activated factor V molecule is a cofactor for factor Xa in the presence of calcium ions and phospholipid membrane surface. This is called the prothrombinase complex. Antibodies that affect the prothrombinase activity of factor V tend to be associated with the bleeding tendencies. These antibodies tend to bind to the C2 domain of the factor V (356). Most factor V inhibitors are characterized as IgG, but IgM has been reported (357). The antibodies in patients with spontaneous factor V inhibitors, seven autoantibodies and five with cross-reacting bovine thrombin-induced antibodies, were characterized (372). All had antibody binding to the light chain of factor Va. The patients, consisting of both of the auto- and cross-reacting groups who had bleeding, were noted to have antibody that bound to the amino-terminal region of the C2 domain of the light chain. In four of the asymptomatic patients, one had binding to the entire C2 domain, and one to the C1, with two that could not be defined. The inhibitor exhibits immediate inhibition of normal plasma without incubation. There may be additional inhibition on incubation for 1 hour. The presence of the inhibitor is suspected when there is prolongation of the PT and aPTT, with findings to suggest an inhibitor on mixing studies with the PT and aPTT systems. Severe bleeding has been reported with factor V inhibitors (358–361). Factor V is found in platelets, and this may be a significant source of factor V when released from the platelet at the site of vascular injury. Bleeding due to an acquired inhibitor of platelet-associated factor V has been reported (362).

The first reports of inhibitors to factor V (labile factor) were in the mid-1950s (363). Knobl and Lechner, in 1998 (364), reviewed the published experience with inhibitors to factor V and noted that only 105 cases had been published between 1955 and 1997. They grouped the inhibitors in five general categories.

1. Patients exposed to bovine thrombin,
2. Postsurgical patients without bovine thrombin exposure,
3. Those with other associated conditions,
4. Those with idiopathic inhibitors (365), and
5. Patients with congenital factor V deficiency.

Laboratory manifestations (372) include the following.

1. Prolonged prothrombin time,
2. Prolonged aPTT,
3. Decreased factor V levels,
4. Demonstration of inhibitor by mixing studies,
5. Quantitative measurement by the Bethesda assay method,
6. Normal thrombin clotting time in the spontaneous autoantibodies,
7. Prolonged thrombin clotting time in patients with bovine thrombin–related antibodies (when bovine thrombin is used for thrombin clotting time),
8. Use of human thrombin in the thrombin clotting time may correct the prolongation,
9. Antibodies to bovine prothrombin may be detected by ELISA with bovine thrombin antibodies,
10. Some patients will have positive tests for lupus inhibitor (366,367), and
11. About 50% of patients with anti–factor V antibodies after bovine thrombin have increased levels of anticardiolipin antibodies.

Ortel (368) described the mechanisms for the development of factor V antibodies as three groups.

1. Spontaneous autoantibodies
   - In patients who are otherwise hemostatically normal, who develop the inhibitor after treatment with antibiotics, blood transfusions, recent surgery, or with malignancy and autoimmune disorders.
   - The findings are those of an isolated factor V inhibitor with normal thrombin clotting time, and prolonged PT and aPTT.
2. Alloantibodies in patients with congenital factor V deficiency.
   - This is rare, usually after treatment with plasma, and there is a prolonged PT, aPTT, and normal thrombin clotting time.
3. Cross-reacting anti–bovine factor V antibodies due to the use of bovine thrombin preparations in surgery.
   - Develop after exposure to topical bovine thrombin used in surgery.
   - Topical thrombin preparations have been used as hemostatic agents during cardiovascular surgery and

are applied in a spray form, a paste, or as fibrin glue. The thrombin preparations used in the United States are prepared from bovine plasma. Patients exposed to these bovine preparations can develop cross-reacting antibodies to human coagulation proteins, particularly factor V, and may be associated with hemorrhage. In addition, antibodies to other human coagulation proteins can occur after use of bovine thrombin (387).

- The standard coagulation tests that are affected by antibodies formed to coagulation proteins after the use of bovine thrombin are, if there is an anti–factor V cross-reacting to human factor V, prolonged PT and aPTT. The thrombin clotting time (TT) may be prolonged if there is anti–bovine thrombin inhibitor and bovine thrombin is used in the testing. A relatively small number of patients with prolonged TT have antithrombin antibodies (see later).

Although spontaneous anti–factor V antibodies are considered to be rare and usually asymptomatic, it would appear that antibodies to factor V related to the use of bovine thrombin may be much more common. These antibodies have been reported to be associated with either hemorrhagic or thrombotic complications (368).

The increase in the incidence of factor V inhibitors since the 1980s is most likely due to the common use of bovine thrombin in cardiovascular surgical procedures.

General Features of Factor V Inhibitors

The median age at diagnosis in the reported 105 cases was 65 years, with a greater incidence in men: 1:0.79. The most commonly noted conditions were surgery, with cardiovascular surgery being the most frequent. Other common associations were transfusion of blood components and use of β-lactam antibiotics. The exposure to bovine proteins is noted in a large subgroup. Other conditions, such as malignant diseases and autoimmune diseases, occur in 16% and 7%, respectively. There is a 6% incidence in patients who received streptomycin, with very infrequent occurrence noted in congenital factor V deficiency (homozygous) (1.9%). The cases considered idiopathic with no underlying condition determined were noted in 18%. Factor V inhibitors were reported with pregnancy in 1% of the inhibitor cases (364,369–371). Other drugs and medications reported to be associated with factor V inhibitors are the aminoglycosides, cephalosporins (cephradine), penicillin, and derivatives (372–374). The clinical manifestations of factor V inhibitors are wide ranging, from severe bleeding to purely a laboratory abnormality in the coagulation tests to the other end of the spectrum of thromboembolic disease.

The occurrence of thrombotic complications with spontaneous anti–factor V antibodies has been described (375–377). The anti–factor V antibody of one of the patients with thrombosis was found to bind to the light chain of factor Va, inhibited the procoagulant activity of factor Va, and did not seem to inhibit APC (377). In three of the reported cases, there was evidence for an LA in two of the patients. One patient had increased levels of antocardiolipin antibodies. The case without the LA or anticardiolipin antibodies was complicated by recurrent strokes. Additional patients have been reported with thrombosis occurring as the factor V inhibitor was improving (378,379). Obviously it is important to exclude the LA or anticardiolipin antibodies in the evaluation of a patient with suspected factor V inhibitor. The occurrence of coumarin skin necrosis associated with a factor V inhibitor with lupus-like inhibitor features was reported by Kamphuisen et al. (380). The patient was being treated for a deep vein thrombosis (DVT) after major cancer surgery. A factor V inhibitor was noted without bleeding symptoms. The evaluation revealed positive DRVVT and anticardiolipin antibodies. There was no exposure to topical bovine thrombin during surgery. On day 4 of heparin and coumarin treatment, a hemorrhagic bullous skin necrosis on the leg developed, which progressed to necrosis. It is suggested that the LA may be a significant finding in the causation of the coumarin necrosis, in addition to the factor V inhibitor.

Postoperative Factor V Inhibitors and Those Related to the Use of Bovine Thrombin

The most common surgical procedures associated with the occurrence of factor V inhibitors were cardiovascular and abdominal. However, many of the patients in this category also had been given blood transfusions or treated with β-lactam antibiotics. The antibodies in this group react specifically to human factor V.

Several groups have reported the development of inhibitors to bovine thrombin and human factor V, as related to the use of fibrin glue and bovine thrombin in surgery. Banninger et al. (381) prospectively studied 34 patients who had received fibrin glue as part of cardiac and neurosurgery. Eleven of 24 patients with cardiac surgery and two of 10 after neurosurgery had prolongation of the thrombin clotting time, and two had greater prolongation of the thrombin time after reexposure to the fibrin glue. In all 13 patients with an acquired thrombin inhibitor, there was a decreased factor V level. The factor V level was within the normal range in the 21 patients without evidence of a thrombin inhibitor. Their data indicated that the formation of a factor V inhibitor is frequent when fibrin glue is used. This was related to the type of surgery, with cardiovascular procedures particularly prominent. The quantity of the fibrin glue applied during the surgical procedure correlated with the occurrence of the inhibitors. None of the patients in this study who developed factor V inhibitors had a bleeding problem. Other reports that have demonstrated the development of anti–bovine thrombin antibodies after surgical procedures have noted their occurrence in neurosurgery and cardiac surgery with the placement of prosthetic cardiac valves (382,383). Rapaport et al. (384) addressed the significance of the development of antibodies to bovine and human thrombin and factor V after the use of bovine thrombin in surgery (384). They noted that the use of substrates that contain bovine factor V in the coagulation testing may cause what appear to be several factor defects with anti–bovine factor V antibodies. They set three criteria for the diagnosis of bovine thrombin–related factor V inhibitor: (a) documentation of the use of bovine thrombin in the surgery; (b) evidence that there are coexisting antibodies to bovine thrombin as manifest by a prolonged thrombin clotting time; and (c) demonstration that the factor V antibodies have higher neutralizing titer against factor V in bovine plasma than against the factor V in human plasma. It is possible for cross-reacting antibodies to human factor V to form, and this might happen without the formation of antithrombin antibodies, and therefore the thrombin clotting time would be normal. In a study reported by Dorion et al. (385), 12 of 120 patients, when exposed to bovine thrombin, developed antibodies to thrombin and other coagulation factors. Patients with multiple exposures were 8 times more likely to develop antibodies than were those with a single exposure. Antibody development was unrelated to age or gender. The antibody-positive group had longer hospital stays than the antibody-negative patients. This probably indicates that the antibody-positive patients had more complicated and serious illnesses. Other antibodies were noted in the group, with three for human factor II, five for bovine factor II, eight for bovine factor IX, and eight had antibodies for bovine factor X by Western blot analysis. One patient had a decreased factor V level. Two patients were found to have significant bleeding problems. The occurrence of solely antithrombin antibodies is probably not associated with bleeding problems, and the simultaneous occurrence of other factor inhibitors is responsible for bleeding. All the positive patients were those with cardiovascular procedures. Zehnder and Leung (386) reported the association of recurrent bleeding in a patient exposed to topical bovine thrombin who developed antibodies to thrombin and factor V. Ortel et al. (387) studied in a prospective manner the immunologic response to exposure to bovine thrombin with cardiac surgical procedures and assessed the patients for adverse clinical events. They studied 151 patients undergoing cardiac surgical procedures before and after exposure to surgery and bovine thrombin for bovine and human antibodies to coagulation proteins. They noted that a small but not insignificant number of patients had elevated levels of antibodies without a known prior exposure to bovine thrombin. The adverse outcome after surgery correlated with the patients having elevated levels of antibodies to multiple factors. Tests for changes in the coagulation system also were performed. They found that patients who had an exposure to bovine thrombin had antibodies to one or more bovine coagulation proteins (95% were antibody seropositive to bovine proteins, and 51% had elevated antibody levels to the corresponding human coagulation proteins). In 80.7% and 90.7%, IgG antibodies developed to factor V and Va, respectively, after exposure to bovine thrombin. Fifty-one percent of the patients had elevated antibody levels to human coagulation proteins after surgery, predominantly against factor V, thrombin, or both. The occurrence of human antibodies was not related to the amount of topical thrombin used or having had a prior surgical procedure. In four of 11 patients with human thrombin antibodies, there were no increases in bovine prothrombin or thrombin antibodies. In only eight patients was a prolonged thrombin clotting time noted, and all eight of these patients had elevated antibody levels to the topical thrombin used in the surgery. Hemorrhagic complications also correlated with the development of antibodies to multiple factors. Only a small number of patients (7%) developed a prolonged bovine thrombin clotting time, which reveals its ineffectiveness as a screen for bovine thrombin–induced antibodies. Most patients with bovine thrombin–induced anti–factor V antibodies are asymptomatic, with a few having serious life-threatening bleeding (388–390). In one study, the duration of the antibody as assessed by a prolonged PT was as long as 3.5 months (387).

Other Conditions with Factor V Inhibitors

1. In this group (387), the malignant diseases represent a large block, with monoclonal gammopathies noted in a small number, contrary to the vWF inhibitors. The autoimmune group consisted of Sjögren syndrome, celiac disease, and pemphigoid. Autoantibodies to factor V have been observed in association with pregnancy, tuberculosis, malignancy, and after liver transplantation (362,373,374, 391–395).

2. The association with streptomycin was noted in earlier reports, and isolated reports of the inhibitor in HIV patients have been noted (396). These patients had other complicating conditions, such as lymphoma and problems requiring extensive blood-product administration.

3. Homozygous congenital factor V deficiency is rare, with even rarer reports of inhibitors after treatment with blood products (397,398).

Treatment of Patients with Factor V Inhibitors

1. In the asymptomatic patient with only laboratory evidence of an inhibitor to factor V, no specific therapy is most likely needed (368).

2. In the patients with bleeding due to antifactor V antibodies
   - Platelet transfusions have been tried with some success (361) (platelets are rich in factor V).
   - Fresh frozen plasma is often nonproductive in controlling the bleeding (368).
   - aPCCs have been used with some success (399).
3. Attempts to reduce the inhibitor with
   - Steroids (358)
   - Cytotoxic therapy (361)
   - IVIG (400)
   - Plasmapheresis (360)
4. Inhibitors due to bovine thrombin exposure
   - Limit number of exposures; multiple exposures are more likely to be associated with complications.
   - Try to use the most pure thrombin product, one that has the least contaminants with other factors.

In the case report of Tarantino et al. (400), they treated a 9-year-old girl in whom a factor V inhibitor developed after cardiovascular surgery and exposure to bovine thrombin. The bleeding continued in spite of treatment with blood-product transfusions. She was then treated with IVIG, 400 mg/kg daily for 9 days. There was almost an immediate improvement in the coagulation tests, and bleeding stopped by the fifth IVIG treatment. The human anti–factor V and antithrombin antibodies did not return, but the bovine antibodies persisted after the IVIG treatment. This would indicate that the IVIG can be effective in suppressing the cross-reacting human antibodies that are thought to be responsible for the bleeding and possibly thrombotic complications associated with the use of bovine thrombin. Larger studies are necessary to make definitive statements. The use of IVIG in the other forms of spontaneous factor V inhibitors should be explored.

Israels and Leaker (401) reported on the use of LMW heparin (LMWH) in a patient with inhibitors to factors V and X after the exposure to topical thrombin. In a 4-year-old patient who had extensive cardiac valvular surgeries and who required continued anticoagulation, fibrin glue and topical bovine thrombin were used during the surgery. Markedly prolonged PT and aPTT were noted several days after the surgery when treatment with oral anticoaguation was to be initiated. The factor V was 2%, and an inhibitor to factor V was demonstrated. The patient was treated with LMWH because of the difficulty in monitoring the oral anticoagulation with the PT. The dose of the LMWH was decreased because of the high anti-Xa levels, but the levels did not respond to the lower doses. A bovine factor X inhibitor was noted. As the factor V inhibitor decreased, the dose of LMWH could be increased with proportionate responses in the anti-Xa levels. This patient did not experience thrombotic or bleeding complications. The commercial assay kit for the anti-Xa proved the Xa bovine in origin, and therefore the anti–bovine X inhibitor was interfering with the heparin assay. The authors alerted us to the problems in monitoring anticoagulation treatment when anti–bovine factor inhibitors are present and when bovine factors are used in the assay systems.

The occurrence of other antibodies with exposure to bovine thrombin and bleeding complications was described in a patient who had coronary bypass surgery 3 years previously (402). The presence of a factor V inhibitor was demonstrated. The patient's IgG was shown to bind to thrombin (bovine greater than human), fibrinogen, and to factor V. The antibody was shown to inhibit several functions of thrombin, including its procoagulant and anticoagulant activities and its cellular interactions. This was the first instance of an antibody binding to fibrinogen in this syndrome.

CIRCULATING HEPARAN–HEPARIN-LIKE ANTICOAGULANTS

A heparan sulfate anticoagulant was identified in a patient with multiple myeloma, and an IgG4λ monoclonal gammopathy was reported by Palmer et al. (403). The inhibitor had cofactor activity with antithrombin III that was abolished by protamine sulfate or platelet factor 4 (PF-4). A previous case of heparin-like anticoagulant was reported in a patient with IgAκ myeloma (404). Bussel et al. (405) reported a heparin-like anticoagulant in a child with acute monoblastic leukemia. The coagulation data in this case revealed that all coagulation factors were decreased, particularly factor V. The PT, aPTT, and TT all were prolonged. The reptilase was normal, and the fibrinogen was only slightly reduced. Protamine and PF-4 corrected the thrombin time. Preincubation with heparinase eliminated all heparin-like activity found in the urine. The possibility that the factor V was binding to the leukemia cells was considered, based on a previously reported case (406). These cases have in common an underlying hematologic malignancy, with a heparin-like anticoagulant associated with severe life-threatening bleeding.

ANTIBODIES AND INHIBITORS FOR PROTHROMBIN

Antibodies to prothrombin have been reported not infrequently with the lupus inhibitor and the anticardiolipin syndrome. Lee et al. (407) reported a transient hemorrhagic diathesis associated with an inhibitor of prothrombin in a young girl with the lupus anticoagulant. It is postulated that the hypoprothrombinemia noted in patients with the lupus inhibitor is due to the binding of nonneutralizing antibodies to prothrombin that result in the rapid clearance of prothrombin–immune complexes from the circulation (408). However, antibody to prothrombin is noted in a substantial number of patients with lupus inhibitor without hypoprothrombinemia. This is due to the presence of polyreactive antibodies in the lupus-inhibitor patients (409). Vivaldi et al. (410) reported severe bleeding due to acquired hypoprothrombimemia–lupus anticoagulant syndrome. The patient responded with disappearance of the inhibitor and improvement in the factor II level after corticosteroid and IVIG treatment. Erkan et al. (411) reported on two patients with SLE who had hemorrrhagic episodes and were found to have the lupus anticoagulant and decreased factor II activity. They found nonneutralizing antibodies directed against factor II. The bleeding stopped promptly after treatment with high-dose corticosteroids. They emphasized that although the occurrence of hypoprothrombinemia in the anticardiolipin antibody–positive patients is rare, it should be assessed in the patient with a bleeding diathesis.

Antibodies to prothrombin have been implicated as a risk factor for thrombosis. Paluso et al. (412) reported the correlation of high levels of prothrombin antibodies in deep venous thrombosis (DVT) and pulmonary embolism in middle-aged men. They examined the sera of 265 cases of DVT or pulmonary embolism with no previous thrombotic events. This was compared with 265 matched controls. The risk for thrombotic events was significantly increased only in relation to high levels of antiprothrombin antibodies. The same group studied the relation of antiprothrombin antibodies to the risk for myocardial infarction in middle-aged men (413). A high level of antiprothrombin antibodies predicted a 2.5-fold increase in the risk of myocardial infarction or cardiac death. The combination of antiprothrombin antibodies with increased triglyceride level, lipoprotein (a), and smoking increased the risk. The authors suggested that antiprothrombin antibodies are a newly recognized risk factor for myocardial infarction. Antiprothrombin antibodies and anti-beta$_2$-glycoprotein I (anti-β_2-GPI) antibodies were assessed by Galli et al. (414). They noted that the kaolin clotting time (KCT) was affected by the antiprothrombin antibodies, and the anti-β_2-GPI antibodies affected the DRVVT. The presence of antiphospholipid antibodies was frequently associated with acquired resistance to APC. The authors studied 42 patients, 24 with abnormal DRVVT and 18 with abnormal KCT. Fifteen of the patients had venous thrombosis, with 73% of these with evidence of delayed inactivation of activated factor Va, compared with 56% of the patients without thrombosis. The anti-β_2-GPI antibodies, but not the antiprothrombin antibodies, hampered the inactivation of factor Va. This suggested that the anti-β_2-GPI antibodies found in the anticardiolipin syndrome might be prothrombotic, through their effect on APC. However, Galli and Barbui (415) emphasized that antiprothrombin antibodies are found in 50% to 90% of patients with antiphospholipid antibodies, and their role in thrombosis, when determined by immunoassays, remains to be determined.

ANTIBODIES AND INHIBITORS OF ACTIVATED PROTEIN C

Zivelin et al. (416) reported a patient with recurrent major venous and arterial thrombosis with resistance to APC (APCR). There was no evidence for a mutation in the gene for factor V. The IgG from the patient's plasma decreased the APCR ratio, suggesting induced resistance. The patient's IgG affected the ability to inactivate factor Va. The authors suggested that acquired APCR be considered as a cause for severe venous and arterial thrombosis. Skin necrosis developed in this patient while she was receiving warfarin treatment for venous thrombosis. She was treated with LMWH and high-dose corticosteroids. The necrosis improved. Cavernous sinus thrombosis developed while she was receiving a lower dose of the LMWH, once daily. This was increased to an every-12-hour dose schedule, but the dose had to be doubled when she had multiple brain infarcts. She continued to do well on this dose and daily acetylsalicylic acid (ASA). Acquired APCR, as mentioned earlier, has been associated with lupus anticoagulants and thrombotic events. Male et al. (417) demonstrated the association of APCR and the lupus inhibitor and thrombosis in pediatric patients with SLE. They found in 59 patients with SLE that 17% had thrombotic events. Acquired APCR was found in 31% of the 58 patients. The APCR was found in association more with the lupus inhibitor than with the anticardiolipin antibodies. The APCR was significantly associated with the thromotic events, and an association was found between APCR and the lupus inhibitors in the patients with thrombotic events. The authors suggest that the lupus inhibitors were associated with inhibitors of the protein C pathway. Although a specific antibody to APC was not identified in this study, the association of APCR with the lupus inhibitor suggests an immune-based dysfunction of APC. Acquired APCR with the lupus inhibitor appears to be a significant indicator for the risk for thrombosis.

INHIBITORS TO FACTOR XIII

Acquired inhibitors to factor XIII are very rare, and the few that have been reported have been mostly related to drug treatment (418). The most common offender is isoniazid, but penicillin, procainamide, and the phenytoin group are included. The antibodies are usually IgG. The development of an inhibitor has been reported in rare patients with congenital deficiency of factor XIII with, in one case, the patient having had multiple transfusions. The antibodies have been described as directed to a variety of functions and sites in the factor XIII molecule or activities. The diagnosis of a factor XIII inhibitor is more difficult because of the usually normal global screening coagulation tests, such as the PT and the aPTT. The diagnosis is suspect in the patient with sudden onset of a bleeding diathesis during or after prolonged treatment with medications, particularly those mentioned earlier. In congenital factor XIII deficiency, the incidence of inhibitors is approximately 1%. The diagnosis is established when the patient's plasma inhibits normal plasma factor XIII activity. The patients may have a serious bleeding diathesis, and a variety of treatments have been used, including plasmapheresis and platelet concentrates.

In the previous pages, we surveyed some of the important inhibitors of coagulation associated with bleeding and some of the less-well-recognized antibodies and inhibitors of components of the coagulation system that may be implicated in thrombosis. The reader is referred to the many source articles and reviews listed in each section for more detailed information on specific issues.

REFERENCES

1. Margolius A, Jackson DP, Ratnoff OD. Circulating anticoagulants: a study of 40 cases and a review of the literature. *Medicine* 1961;40:145.
2. Shapiro SS, Hultin M. Acquired inhibitors to blood coagulation factors. *Semin Thromb Hemost* 1975;1:336–385.
3. Kasper CK, Aledort LM, Counts RB, et al. A more uniform measurement of factor VIII inhibitors. *Thromb Diath Haemorrh* 1975;34:875–876.
4. Kasper CK. Laboratory tests for factor VIII inhibitors; their variation, significance and interpretation. *Blood Coagul Fibrinolysis* 1991;2:(suppl 1):7–10.
5. Verbruggen B, Novakova I, Wessels H, et al. The Nijmegan modification of the Bethesda assay for factor VIII:C inhibitors: improved specificity and reliability. *Thromb Haemost* 1995;73: 247–251.
6. Sahud MA. Laboratory diagnosis of inhibitors. *Semin Thromb Hemost* 2000;26:195–203.
7. Goldsmith JC. Diagnosis of factor VIII versus nonspecific inhibitors. *Semin Hematol* 1993;30(suppl 1):3–6.
8. Reference deleted.
9. Lee MT, Nardi MA, Hu G, et al. Transient hemorrhagic diathesis associated with an inhibitor of prothrombin with lupus anticoagulant in a 1 1/2-year old girl: report of a case and review of the literature. *Am J Hematol* 1996;51:307–314.
10. Vivaldi P, Rossetti G, Galli M, et al. Severe bleeding due to acquired hypoprothrombinemia-lupus anticoagulant syndrome: case report and review of the literature. *Haematologica* 1997;82: 345–347.
11. Italian Registry of APA. Thrombosis and thrombocytopenia in the APA syndrome: first report from the Italian Registry. *Haematologica* 1993;78:313–318.
12. Hanley D, Arkel YS, Lynch J, et al. Acquired vonWillebrand's syndrome in association with lupus-like anticoagulant corrected by intravenous gammaglobulin. *Am J Hematol* 1994;46: 141–146.
13. Lechner K. Acquired inhibitor in nonhemophilic patients. *Hemostasis* 1974;3:65.
14. Green D, Lechner K. A survey of 215 nonhemophilic patients with inhibitors to factor VIII. *Thromb Haemost* 1981;45:200.
15. Saxena R, Mishra DK, Kashyap R, et al. Acquired haemophilia: a study of ten cases. *Haemophilia* 2000;6:78–83.
16. Lottenberg R, Kentro TB, Kitchens CS. Acquired hemophilia. *Arch Intern Med* 1987;147:1077–1081.
17. Di Bona E, Schiavoni M, Castaman G, et al. Acquired haemophilia: experience of two Italian centers with 17 new cases. *Haemophilia* 1977;3:183–188.
18. Shapiro SS. The immunologic character of acquired inhibitors of antihemophilic globulin (factor VIII) and the kinetics of their interaction. *J Clin Invest* 1967;46:147.
19. Kasper CK. Incidence and course of inhibitors among patients with classic hemophilia. *Thromb Diath Haemorrh* 1973;30:264.
20. McMillan CW, Shapiro SS, Whitehurst D, et al. The natural history of factor VIII inhibitors in patients with hemophilia A: a national cooperative study, II: observations on the initial development of factor VIII inhibitors. *Blood* 1988;71:344.
21. Hoyer LW. The incidence of factor VIII inhibitors in patients with severe hemophilia A. In: Aledort LM, Hoyer LW, Lusher JM, et al., eds. *Inhibitors to coagulation factors.* Chapel Hill: Plenum, 1995:46.
22. Sohngen D, Specker C, Bach D, et al Acquired factor VIII inhibitors in nonhemophilic patients. *Ann Hematol* 1997;74: 89–93.
23. Brettler DB. Inhibitors of factor VIII and IX. *Haemophilia* 1995;(suppl 1):35–39.
24. Lusher JM. Considerations for the current and future management of haemophilia and its complications. *Haemophilia* 1995; 1:2–10.
25. Scandella D. Properties of anti-factor VIII inhibitor antibodies in hemophilia A patients. *Semin Thromb Hemost* 2000;26: 137–142.
26. Kane WH, Davie EW. Blood coagulation factors V and VIII: structural and functional similarities and their relationship to hemorrhagic and thrombotic disorders. *Blood* 1988;71:539–555.
27. Vehar GA, Keyt B, Eaton D, et al. Structure of human factor VIII. *Nature* 1984;312:342–347.
28. Muntean W, Leschnik B. Factor VIII influences binding of factor IX and factor X to intact human platelets. *Thromb Res* 1989;55:537–548.
29. Gilbert GE, Drinkwater D. Specific membrane binding of factor VIII is mediated by *O*-phospho-L-serine, a moiety of phosphatidylserine. *Biochemistry* 1993;32:9577–9585.
30. Katz J. Prevalence of factor IX inhibitors among patients with hemophilia B: results of a large-scale North American study. *Haemophilia* 1996;2:28–31.
31. McMillan CW, Shapiro SS, Whitehurst D, et al. The natural history of factor VIII inhibitors in patients with hemophilia A: a national cooperative study, II: observations on the development of factor VIII C inhibitors. *Blood* 1988;71:344–348.
32. Lakich D, Kazazian HH, Antonarakis SE, et al. Inversions disrupting the factor VIII gene are a common cause of severe hemophilia A. *Nat Genet* 1993;5:236–241.
33. Antonarakis SE, Kazzazian HH, Tuddenham EGD. Molecular etiology of factor VIII deficiency in hemophilia A. *Hum Mutat* 1995;5:1–22.
34. Oldenburg J, Brackmann HH, Effenberger W, et al. Mutation type and inhibitor incidence in a large retrospective study of previously untreated patients with hemophilia A. *Haemophilia* 2000;6:283(abst).
35. Scandella DH. Properties of anti-factor VIII inhibitor antibodies in hemophilia A patients. *Semin Thromb Hemost* 2000;26: 137–142.

36. Hoyer LW, Scandella D. Factor VIII inhibitors: structure and function in autoantibody and hemophilia A patients. *Semin Hematol* 1994;31(suppl 4):1–5.
37. Fulcher CA, Mahoney SDG, Roberts JR, et al. Localization of human factor VIII inhibitor epitopes to two polypeptide fragments. *Proc Natl Acad Sci U S A* 1985;82:7728–7732.
38. Scandella D, Mattingly M, de Graaf S, et al. Colocalization of epitopes for human factor VIII inhibitor antibodies by immunoblotting and antibody neutralization. *Blood* 1989;74: 1618–1628.
39. Prescott R, Nakai H, Saendo EL, et al. The inhibitor antibody response is more complex in hemophilia A patients than in most nonhemophilics with factor VIII autoantibodies: Recombinant and Kogenate Study Groups. *Blood* 1997;89: 3663–3671.
40. McMillan CW, Shapiro SS, Whitehurst D, et al. The natural history of factor VIII inhibitors in patients with hemophilia A: a national cooperative study, II: observations on the initial development of factor VIII inhibitors. *Blood* 1988;71:344–348.
41. Beck P, Giddings JC, Blood AL. Inhibitor of factor VIII in mild hemophilia. *Br J Haematol* 1969;17:283.
42. Lechner K, Ludwig E, Niessner H, et al. Factor VIII inhibitor in a patient with mild haemophilia A. *Haemostasis* 1972;73: 261.
43. Jacquemin M, Burny W, Vantomme V, et al. Clonal analysis of the immune responses towards factor VIII in mild/moderate hemophilia A patients: the carboxy-terminal part of the C1 domain is an important source of antigenic determinants. *Haemophilia* 2000;6:283(abst).
44. Hodge G, Han P. Effect of factor VIII concentrate on antigen-presenting cell (APC) T-cell interactions in vitro: relevance to inhibitor formation and tolerance induction. *Br J Haematol* 2000;109:195–200.
45. Foy TM, Laman JD, Ledbetter JA, et al. gp39-CD40 interactions are essential for germinal center formation and the development of B cell memory. *J Exp Med* 1994;180:157–163.
46. Conti-Fine BM, Wu H, Okita DK, et al. 2000 Scientific program, American Society of Hematology, 58–59.
47. Duplicate of ref. 35.
48. Rosendaal FR, Nieuwenhuis HK, van der Berg HM, et al. A sudden increase in factor VIII inhibitor development in multitransfused hemophilia A patients in the Netherlands. *Blood* 1993;81:2180–2184.
49. Peerlink K, Arnout J, Gilles JG, et al. A higher than expected incidence of factor VIII inhibitors in multitransfused hemophilia A patients treated with an intermediate purity pasteurized factor VIII concentrate. *Thromb Haemost* 1993;69:115–118.
50. Biggs R, Denson KWE, Nossel HL. A patient with an unusual circulating anticoagulant. *Thromb Diath Haemorrh* 1964;12:1–11.
51. Deutsch E. Acquired inhibitors in coagulation. In: Schmer G, ed. *Symposium on current topics in coagulation.* New York: Academic Press, 1972:135–163.
52. Green D. Circulating anticoagulants. *Med Clin North Am* 1972;56:145–151.
53. Hocking DR. Acquired coagulation-factor deficiencies. *Med J Aust* 1970;1:657–659.
54. Horowitz HI, Fujinmoto MM. Acquired hemophilia due to a circulating anticoagulant. *Am J Med* 1962;33:501–509.
55. Hougie C. Studies on an acquired anticoagulant directed against factor VIII. *J Lab Clin Med* 1967;70:384–392.
56. Pinkerton PH, Dagg JH, Taylor F. A circulating anticoagulant inhibiting antihemophilic globulin. *J Clin Pathol* 1965;18: 334–338.
57. Poon MC, Wine AC, Ratnoff OD, et al. Heterogeneity of human circulating anticoagulants against antihemophilic factor (factor VIII). *Blood* 1975;46:409–416.
58. Ross SA. Naturally occurring anticoagulants. *N Z Med J* 1968; 67:411–413.
59. Hay CRM, Colvin BT, Ludlam CA, et al. Recommendations for the treatment of factor VIII inhibitors: from the UK Haemophilia Centre Directors' Organization Inhibitor Working Party. *Blood Coagul Fibrinolysis* 1996;7:134–138.
60. Hay CRM, Baglin TP, Collins PW, et al. Guideline: the diagnosis and management of factor VIII and IX inhibitors: a guideline from the UK Haemophilia Centre Doctors' Organization (UKHCDO). *Br J Haematol* 2000;111:78–90.
61. Morrison AE, Ludlam CA, Kessler C, et al. Porcine factor VIII in the treatment of patients with acquired hemophilia. *Blood* 1993;81:1513–1520.
62. Duplicate of ref. 13.
63. White GC, Mcmillan CW, Blatt PM, et al. Factor VIII inhibitors: a clinical overview. *Am J Hematol* 1982;13:335–342.
64. Margolius A, Jackson DP, Ratnoff OD. Circulating anticoagulants: a study of 40 cases and review of the literature. *Medicine* 1961;40:145–202.
65. Lottenberg R, Kentro TB, Kitchens CS. Acquired hemophilia. *Arch Intern Med* 1987;147:1077–1081.
66. Green D, Lechner K. A survey of 215 non-hemophilic patients with inhibitors to factor VIII. *Thromb Haemost* 1981;45: 200–203.
67. Kessler CM, Ludlam CA. International Acquired Hemophilia Study Group: the treatment of acquired factor VIII inhibitors: worldwide experience with porcine factor VIII concentrate. *Semin Hematol* 1993;30:22–27.
68. Soriano RM, Mathews JM, Guerdo-Parra E. Acquired hemophilia and rheumatoid arthritis. *Br J Rheumtol* 1987;26: 381–383.
69. Struillou L, Fiks-Sigaud M, Barrier JH, et al. Acquired hemophilia and rheumatoid arthritis: success of immunoglobulin therapy. *J Intern Med* 1993;233:304–305.
70. Ellis H, Handley DA, Taylor KB. Surgery in a patient with an acquired circulating anticoagulant. *Lancet* 1959;1:1167–1170.
71. Prescott R, Nakai H, Saenko EL, for the Recombinant and Kogenate Study Groups. The inhibitor antibody response is more complex in hemophilia A than in most nonhemophiliacs with factor VIII autoantibodies. *Blood* 1997;89:3663–3671.
72. Scandella D, de Graaf Mahoney S, Mattingly M, et al. Epitopes mapping of human factor VIII inhibitor antibodies by deletion analysis of factor VIII fragments expressed in *E. coli. Proc Natl Acad Sci U S A* 1988;85:6152–6156.
73. Shima M, Nakai H, Scandella D, et al. Common inhibitory effects of human anti-C2 domain inhibitor alloantibodies on factor VIII binding to vWF. *Br J Haematol* 1995;91:714–721.
74. Scandella D, Gilbert GE, Shima M, et al. Some factor VIII inhibitor antibodies recognize a common epitope corresponding to C2 domain amino acids 2248-2312, which overlap a phospholipid-binding site. *Blood* 1995;86:1811–1819.
75. Zhong D, Saenko EL, Shima M, et al. Some human inhibitor antibodies interfere with factor VIII binding to factor IX. *Blood.* 1998;92:136–142.
76. Cohen AJ, Kessler CM. Acquired inhibitors. *Baillierres Clin Haematol* 1996;9:331–354.
77. Endo T, Yatomi Y, Amemiya N, et al. Antibody studies of factor VIII inhibitor in a case with Waldenström's macroglobulimenia. *Am J Hematol* 2000;63:145–148.
78. Biggs R, Austen DEG, Denson KWE, et al. The mode of action of antibodies which destroy factor VIII: antibodies which give complex concentration graphs. *Br J Haematol* 1923;23: 137–155.
79. Kessler CM. New products for managing inhibitors to coagulation factors: a focus on recombinant factor VIIa concentrate. *Curr Opin Hematol* 2000;7:408–413.

80. Nogami K, Shima M, Giddings JC, et al. Circulating factor VIII immune complexes in patients with type 2 acquired hemophilia A and protection from activated protein C-mediated proteolysis. *Blood* 2001;97:669–677.
81. Cohen AJ, Kessler CM. Acquired inhibitors. *Baillierres Clin Haematol* 1996;9:331–354.
82. Scandella D, Mattingly M, Prescott R. A recombinant factor VIII A2 domain polypeptide quantitatively neutralizes human inhibitor antibodies that bind to A2. *Blood* 1993;82:1767–1775.
83. Foster PA, Fulcher CA, Houghten RA, et al. Synthetic factor VIII peptides with amino acid sequences contained within the C2 domain of factor VIII inhibit factor VIII binding by phosphatidylserine. *Blood* 1990;75:1999–2004.
84. Lazarchick J, Ashby MA, Lazarchick JJ, et al. Mechanism of actor VIII inactivation by human antibodies, IV: antibody binding prevents factor VIII proteolysis by thrombin. *Ann Clin Lab Sci* 1986;16:497–501.
85. Foster PA, Fulcher CA, Houghten RA, et al. An immunogenic region within residues of the factor VIII light chain induces antibodies which inhibit binding of factor VIII to vWF. *J Biol Chem* 1988;263:5230–5234.
86. Van Den Brink EN, Turenhout EAM, Wijn-Maas ECM, et al. Disappearance of factor VIII autoantibodies preceding autoimmune haemolytic anemia. *Haemophilia* 2000;6:698–701.
88. Sultan Y, Rossi F, Kazatchkine MD. Recovery from anti-factor VIII autoimmune disease is dependent on the generation of anti-idiotypes against anti-factor VIII autoantibodies. *Proc Natl Acad Sci U S A* 1987;84:828–831.
88. Sultan Y, Kazatchkine MD, Maisonneuve P, et al. Anti-idiotypic suppression of autoantibodies to factor VIII by high dose-dose intravenous gammaglobulin. *Lancet* 1984;8406:765–768.
89. Sallah S, Dugdalel M, Chesney C, et al. Inhibitors against factor VIII in patients with underlying malignancy: a clinicopathologic study. *Haemophilia* 2000;6:279(abst).
90. Castenkiold EC, Colvin BT, Kelsey SM. Acquired factor VIII inhibitor associated with chronic interferon-alpha therapy in a patient with hemophilia A. *Br J Haematol* 1994;87:434–436.
91. Regina S, Colombat P, Fimbel B, et al. Acquired inhibitor to factor VIII following interferon alpha therapy in a patient with Hodgkin's disease. *Haemophilia* 2000;6:279–280(abst).
92. Schwertfeger R, Hintz G, Huhn D. Successful treatment of a patient with postpartum factor VIII inhibitor with recombinant human interferon alpha 2a. *Am J Hematol* 1991;37:190–193.
93. Margolius A, Jackson DP, Ratnoff OD. Circulating anticoagulants: a study of 40 cases and review of the literature. *Medicine (Baltimore)* 1961;40:145–202.
94. Lottenberg R, Kentro T, Kitchens CS. Acquired hemophilia: a natural history study of 16 patients with factor VIII inhibitors receiving little or no therapy. *Arch Intern Med* 1987;147:1077–1081.
95. Sohngen D, Specker C, Bach D, et al. Acquired factor VIII inhibitors in nonhemophilic patients. *Ann Hematol* 1997;74:89–93.
96. Coots MC, Glueck HI. An acquired inhibitor to factor VIII in a non-hemophiliac: twenty years of observation and characterization. *Am J Hematol* 1987;24:415–424.
97. Green D. Cytotoxic suppression of acquired factor VIII inhibitors. *Am J Med* 1991;91:14s–9s.
98. Green D, Rademaker AW, Briet E. A prospective randomized trial of prednisone and cyclophosphamide in the treatment of patients with factor VIII autoantibodies. *Thromb Haemost* 1993;70:753–757.
99. Lian ECY, Larcada A, Chiu AYZ. Combination immunosuppressive therapy after factor VIII infusion for acquired factor VIII inhibitor. *Ann Intern Med* 1989;110:774–778.
100. Hart HC, Kraaijenhagen RJ, Kerkhaert JAM, et al. A patient with a spontaneous factor VIII autoantibody: successful treatment with cyclosporine. *Transplant Proc* 1988;20(3 suppl 4):323–328.
101. Pfliegler G, Boda Z, Harsfalvi J, et al. Cyclosporin treatment of a woman with acquired hemophilia due to factor VIII inhibitor. *Postgrad Med J* 1989;65:400–402.
102. Bond LR, Chitolie A, Bevan DH. Desmopressin therapy in patients with acquired factor VIII inhibitors. *Lancet* 1988;1:366.
103. Mudad R, Kane WH. DDAVP in acquired hemophilia: a case report and review of the literature. *Am J Hematol* 1993;43:295–299.
104. Hauser I, Schneider B, Lechner K. Post-partum factor VIII inhibitors: a review of the literature with special reference to the value of steroid and immunosuppressive treatment. *Thromb Haemost* 1995;73:1–5.
105. Voke J, Letsky E. Pregnancy and antibody to factor VIII. *J Clin Pathol* 1977;30:928–932.
106. Shitamoto BS, Leslie KO, Galloway WB. Postpartum hemophilia. *Am J Clin Pathol* 1982;78:789–791.
107. Reece AE, Fox HE, Rapoport F. Factor VIII inhibitor: a cause of severe postpartum hemorrhage. *Am J Obstet Gynecol* 1982;144:985–987.
108. Marengo-Rowe AJ, Muriff G, Leveson JE, et al. Hemophilia-like disease associated with pregnancy. *Obstet Gynecol* 1972;40:56–64.
109. Michiels JJ. Acquired hemophilia A in women postpartum: clinical manifestations, diagnosis, and treatment. *Clin Appl Thromb Hemost* 2000;6:82–86.
110. Rosenthal N, Vogel P, Beres D. Acquired hemophilia in a female. In: Geist SJ, et al., eds. *Anniversary volume for Robert Tilden Frank by his colleagues, collaborators, associates and friends.* St. Louis: CV Mosby, 1937.
111. Madison FW, Quick AJ. Hemophilia-like disease in the female. *Am J Med Sci* 1945;209:443–447.
112. Fantl P, Nance MH. An acquired haemorrhagic disease in a female due to an inhibitor of blood coagulation. *Med J Aust* 1946;2:125–128.
113. Chargaff E, West R. The biological significance of the thromboplastic proein of blood. *J Biol Chem* 1946;166:189–197.
114. Dreskin OH, Rosenthal N. A hemophilia-like disease with prolonged coagulation time and a circulating anticoagulant: report of a case in a female. *Blood* 1950;5:46–60.
115. Frick PG. Hemophilia-like disease following pregnancy, with transplacental transfer of an acquired circulating anticoagulant. *Blood* 1953;8:598–608.
116. Shapiro SS. The immunologic character of acquired inhibitors of antihaemophilic globulin (factor VIII) and the kinetics of their interaction with factor VIII. *J Clin Invest* 1967;46:147–156.
117. Robboy SJ, Lewis EJ, Schur PH, et al. Circulating anticoagulants to factor VIII: immunological studies and clinical response to factor VIII concentratres. *Am J Med* 1970;49:742–752.
118. Leitner A, Bidwell E, Dike GWR. An antihaemophilic globulin inhibitor: purification, characterization and reaction kinetics. *Br J Haematol* 1963;9:245–258.
119. Arkel YS, Bodner R, Ku DHW, et al. Thrombus precursor protein as a measure of prothrombotic activity in a patient with factor VIII inhibitor treated with activated prothrombin complex concentrates. *Thromb Haemost* 1999;82:152–153.
120. Voke J, Letsky E. Pregnancy and antibody to factor VIII. *J Clin Pathol* 1977;30:928–932.
121. Green D, Lechner K. A survey of 215 nonhemophilic patients with inhibitors to factor VIII. *Thromb Haemost* 1981;45:200.
122. Duplicate of ref. 109.
123. Coller BS, Hultin MB, Hoyer LW, et al. Normal pregnancy in a

patient with prior postpartum factor VIII inhibitor: with observations on the pathogenesis and prognosis. *Blood* 1981;58:619.
124. Michiels JJ, Bosch LJ, van der Plas PM, et al. Factor VIII inhibitor postpartum. Scand J Haematol 1978;20:97.
125. Voke J, Letssky E. Pregnancy and antibody to factor VIII. *J Clin Pathol* 1997;30:928.
126. Vicente V, Alberca I, Gonzalez R, et al. Normal pregnancy in a patient with a postpartum factor VIII inhibitor. *Am J Hematol* 1987;24:107.
127. Frick PG. Hemophilia-like disease following pregnancy. *Blood* 1953;8:598.
128. Duplicate of ref. 109.
129. Gawryl MS, Hoyer LW. Inactivation of factor VIII coagulant activity by two different types of human antibodies. *Blood* 1982;60:1103.
130. Hauser I, Schneider B, Lechner K. Postpartum factor VIII inhibitors. *Thromb Haemost* 1995;73:1.
131. Michiels JJ, Hamulyak K, Nieuwenhuis HK, et al. Acquired haemophilia A in women postpartum: natural history of the factor VIII inhibitor and management of bleeding episodes. *Eur J Haematol* 1997;59:105.
132. Hauser I, Schneider B, Lechner K. Postpartum factor VIII inhibitors. *Thromb Haemost* 1995;73:1.
133. Kasper CK. Treatment of factor VIII inhibitors. *Prog Hemost Thromb* 1989;9:57–86.
134. Morrison AE, Ludlam CA, Kessler C. Use of porcine factor VIII in the treatment of patients with acquired hemophilia. *Blood* 1993;81:1513–1520.
135. Morrison AE, Ludham CA, Kessler C. Use of porcine factor VIII in the treatment of patients with acquired hemophilia. *Blood* 1993;81:1513.
136. Morrison AE, Ludham CA. Acquired haemophilia and its management. *Br J Haematol* 1995;89:231.
137. Green D, Rademaker AW, Briet E. A prospective randomized trial of prednisone and cyclophosphamide in the treatment of patients with factor VIII autoantibodies. *Thromb Haemost* 1993;70:753.
138. Hay CRM. Acquired hemophilia. *Baillieres Clin Haematol* 1998;11:287.
139. Kessler CM, Ludlam CA. International Acquired Hemophilia Study Group: the treatment of acquired factor VIII inhibitors: worldwide experience with porcine factor VIII concentrate. *Semin Hematol* 1993;30:22–27.
140. Meili EO, Dazzi H, von Felten A. Recombinant activated factor VII (Novoseven(tm) Novo Nordisk) for hemostasis in a patient with an acquired factor VIII inhibitor. *Schweiz Med Wochenschr* 1995;125:405–411.
141. Lusher JM, Shapiro SS, Palascak JE, et al. Efficacy of prothrombin complex concentrates in hemophiliacs with antibodies to factor VIII: a multicenter therapeutic trial. *N Engl J Med* 1980;303:421–425.
142. Sjamsoedin LJ, Heijnen L, Mauser-Bunschoten EP, et al. The effect of activated prothrombin-complex concentrate (FIEBA) on joint and muscle bleeding in patients with hemophilia and antibodies to factor VIII: a double-blind clinical trial. *N Engl J Med* 1981;305:717–721.
143. Lusher JM, Blatt PM, Penner JA, et al. Autoplex versus proplex, a controlled, double -blind study of effectiveness in acute hemarthroses in hemophiliacs with inhibitors to factor VIII. *Blood* 1983;62:1135–1138.
144. Hilgartner MW, Knatterud GL, the FEIBA Study Group. The use of FEIBA for the treatment of bleeding epsiodes in hemophiliacs with inhibitors. *Blood.*1983;61:36–40.
145. Negrier C, Goudemand J, Sultan Y, et al. Multicenter retrospective study on the utilization of FEIBA in France in patients with factor VIII and factor IX inhibitors. *Thromb Haemost* 1997;77:1113–1119.
146. Lusher JM Myocardial necrosis after therapy with PCC [Letter]. *N Engl J Med* 1984;310:464.
147. Lusher JM Thrombogenicity associated with factor IX complex concentrates. *Semin Hematol* 1991;28:3–5.
148. Lusher JM. Prediction and management of adverse events associated with the use of factor IX complex concentrates. *Semin Hematol 1*993;30:36–40.
149. Duplicate of ref. 141.
150. Green D, Snapper H, Abu-Jawdeh G, et al. Acute myocardial infarction, non-bacterial thrombotic endocarditis, and disseminated intravascular coagulation in a severe hemophiliac. *Am J Hematol* 1990;35:210–212.
151. Chavin SI, Siegel DM, Rocco TA. Acute myocardial infarction during treatment with activated PCC in a patient with factor VIII deficiency and factor VIII inhibitor. *Am J Med* 1988; 85:244–249.
152. Mizon P, Goudemand J, Jude B, et al. Myocardial infarction after FEIBA therapy in a hemophilia-B patient with a factor IX inhibitor. *Ann Haematol* 1992;64:309–311.
153. Lusher JM. Use of PCC in management of bleeding in hemophiliacs with inhibitors: benefits and limitations. *Semin Haematol* 1994;31:49–52.
154. Turecek PL, Varadi K, Gritsch H, et al. Factor Xa and prothrombin: mechanism of action of FEIBA. *Vox Sang* 1999; 77(suppl 1):72–79.
155. Negrier C, Goudemand J, Sultan Y, et al. Multicenter retrospective study on the utilization of FEIBA in France in patients with factor VIII and factor IX inhibitors. *Thromb Haemost* 1997;77:1113–1119.
156. Kasper CK. Effect of prothrombin complex concentrates of factor VIII inhibitor levels. *Blood* 1979;54:1358–1368.
157. Laurian Y, Girma JP, Lambert T, et al. Incidence of immune response following 102 infusions of autoplex in 18 hemophilic patients with antibody to factor VIII. *Blood* 1984; 63:457–462.
158. Abilgaard CF, Penner JA, Watson Williams EJ. Anti-inhibitor complex (Autoplex)for the treatment of factor VIII inhibitors in hemophilia. *Blood* 1980;56:978–984.
159. Kantrowitz JL, Lee ML, McLure DA, et al. Early experience with the use of anti-inhibitor coagulation complex to treat bleeding in hemophiliacs with inhibitors to factor VIII. *Clin Ther* 1987;9:405–419.
160. White GC. Seventeen years' experience with Autoplex/Autoplex T: evaluation of inpatients with severe hemophilia A and factor VIII inhibitors at a major hemophilia center. *Haemophilia* 2000;6:508–512.
161. Duplicate of ref. 59.
162. Gatti L, Mannucci PM. Use of porcine factor VIII in the management of 17 patients with factor VIII antibodies. *Thromb Haemost* 1984;51:379–384.
163. Kernoff PBA, Thomas ND, Lilley PA, et al. Clinical experience with polyelectrolyte-fractionated porcine factor VIII concentrate in the treatment of haemophiliacs with antibodies to factor VIII. *Blood* 1984;63:31–41.
164. Brettler DB, Forsberg A, Levine PH. The use of porcine factor VIII in the treatment of patients with inhibitor antibodies to factor VIII: a multicenter US trial. *Arch Intern Med* 1989;149: 1381–1385.
165. Gribble J, Garvey MB. Porcine factor VIII provides clinical benefit to patients with high levels of inhibitors to human and porcine factor VIII: review article. *Haemophilia* 2000;6: 482–486.
166. Brettler DB, Forsberg AD, Levine PH, et al. The use of porcine factor VIII concentrate (HYALTE:C) in the treatment of patients with inhibitor antibodies to factor VIII. *Arch Intern Med* 1989;149:1381–1385.
167. Lozier JN, Santagostino E, Kasper CK, et al. Use of porcine fac-

tor VIII for surgical procedures in hemophilia A patients with inhibitors. *Semin Hematol* 1993;30(suppl 1):10–21.
168. Altieri DC, Capitanio AM, Mannucci PM. Von Willebrand factor containing porcine factor VIII concentrate causes platelet aggregation. *Br J Haematol* 1986;63:703–711.
169. Chang H, Mody M, Lazarus AH, et al. Platelet activation induced by porcine factor VIII. *Am J Haematol* 1998;57: 200–205.
170. Bona RD, Riberio M, Klatsky AU, et al. continuous infusion of porcine factor VIII in the treatment of patients with factor VIII inhibitors. *Semin Haematol* 1993;30:32–35.
171. Shapiro AD, Gilchrist GS, Hoots WK, et al. Prospective, randomized trial of two doses of rFVIIa (Novoseven) in hemophilia patients with inhibitors undergoing surgery. *Thromb Haemost* 1998;80:773–778.
172. Hedner U, Glazer S, Falch J. Recombinant activated factor VII in the treatment of bleeding episodes in patients with inherited and acquired bleeding disorders. *Transfus Med Rev* 1993;7: 78–83.
173. Macik BG, Lindley CM, Lusher J, et al. Safety and initial efficacy of three dose levels of recombinant activated factor VII (rFVIIa): results of a phase 1 study. *Blood Coagul Fibrinolysis* 1993;4:521–527.
174. Doughty HA, Northeast A, Sklaire L, et al. The use of rFVIIa in a patient with acquired haemophilia A undergoing surgery. *Blood Coagul Fibrinolysis* 1995;6:125–128.
175. Peerlinck K, Vermylen J. Acute myocardial infarction following administration of recombinant activated factor VII (Novo seven) in a patient with haemophilia A and inhibitor [Letter]. *Thromb Haemost* 1999;82:1775–1776.
176. Hough RE, Hampton KK, Preston FE, et al. Recombinant VIIa concentrate in the management of bleeding following prothrombin complex concentrate-related myocardial infarction in patients with hemophilia and inhibitors. *Br J Haematol* 2000; 111:974–979.
177. Roberts H, ed. Fifth Novo Nordisk Symposium of the treatment of bleeding and thrombotic disorders: proceedings of the Copenhagen Meeting, May 7-8, 1999. *Blood Coagul Fibrinolysis* 2000;11(suppl 1).
178. Hay CRM, Negrier C, Ludlam CA. The treatment of bleeding in acquired hemophilia with recombinant factor VIIa. *Thromb Haemost* 1997;78:1463–1467.
179. Liebman HA, Chediak J, Fink KI, et al. Activated recombinant human coagulation factor VII (rFVIIa) therapy for abdominal bleeding in patients with inhibitors to factor VIII. *Am J Hematol* 2000;63:109.
180. Makris M, Hampton KK, Preston EE. Failure of recombinant factor VIIa as treatment for abdominal bleeding in acquired hemophilia [Letter]. *Am J Hematol* 2001;66:67–71.
181. Lusher JM, Ingerslev J, Roberts H, et al. Clinical experience with recombinant factor VIIa. *Blood Coagul Fibrinolysis* 1998; 9:119–128.
182. Mauser- Bunschoten EP, de Goede-Bolder, et al. Continuous infusion of recombinant factor VIIa in patients with hemophilia and inhibitors: experience in the Netherlands and Belgium. *Neth J Med* 1998;53:249–255.
183. Schulman S, Bech Jensen M, Varon D, et al. Feasibility of using recombinant factor VIIa in a continuous infusion. *Thromb Haemost* 1996;75:432–436.
184. Duplicate of ref. 59.
185. Duplicate of ref. 60.
186. Inhibitor Subcommittee of the Association of Hemophilia Clinic Directors of Canada. Suggestions for the management of factor VIII inhibitors. *Haemophilia* 2000;6(suppl 1):52–59.
187. Chistolini A, Ghirardini A, Tirindeli MC. Inhibitor to factor VIII in a non-hemophilic patient: evaluation of the response to DDAVP and the in vitro kinetics of factor VIII. *Neuve Rev Fr Haematol* 1987;29:221–224.
188. Mudad R, Kane WH. DDAVP in acquired hemophilia A: case report and review of the literature. *Am J Hematol* 1993;43: 295–299.
189. Bona RD, Riberio M, Klatsky AU, et al. Continuous infusion of porcine factor VIII for the treatment of patients with factor VIII inhibitors. *Semin Haematol* 1993;30:32–35.
190. Hay CRM, Lozier JN, Lee CA. Porcine factor VIII therapy in patients with congenital hemophilia and inhibitors: efficacy, patient selection, and side effects. *Semin Hematol* 1994;31:20–25.
191. Morrison AE, Ludlum CA, Kessler C. Use of porcine facor VIII in the treatment of patients with acquired hemophilia. *Blood* 1993;81:1513–1520.
192. Rubinger M, Houston DS, Schwetz N, et al. Continuous infusion of porcine factor VIII in patients with acquired haemophilia. *Am J Hematol* 1997;56:112–118.
193. Kessler CM. New products for managing inhibitors to coagulation factors: a focus on recombinaant factor VIIa concentrate. *Curr Opin Hematol* 2000;7:408–413.
194. Morrison AE, Ludlam CA, Kessler C. Use of porcine factor VIII in the treatment of patients with acquired hemophilia. *Blood* 1993;81:1513–1520.
195. Duplicate of ref. 141.
196. Lusher JM. Use of prothrombin complex concentrates in the management of bleeding in hemophiliacs with inhibitors: benefits and linitations. *Semin Haematol* 1994;31:49–52.
197. Hedner U, Glazer S, Falch J. Recombinant activated factor VII in the treatment of bleeding episodes in patients with inherited and acquired bleeding disorders. *Transfus Med Rev* 1993;7: 78–83.
198. Macik BG, Lindley CM, Lusher J, et al. Safety and initial efficacy of three dose levels of recombinant activted factor VII (rFVIIa): results of a phase 1 study. *Blood Coagul Fibrinolysis* 1993;4:521–527.
199. Doughty HA, Northeast A, Sklaire L, et al. The use of rFVIIa in a patient with acquired haemophilia A undergoing surgery. *Blood Coagul Fibrinolysis* 1995;6:125–128.
200. White GC, Roberts HR, Kingdon HS, et al.: Prothrombin complex concentrates: potentially thrombogenic materials and clues to the mechanism of thrombosis in vivo. *Blood* 1997;49:159–170.
201. Kessler CM. New products for managing inhibitors to coagulation factors: a focus on recombinant factor VIIa concentrate. *Curr Opin Hematol* 2000;7:408–413.
202. Key NS, Aledort LM, Beardsley D, et al. Home treatment of mild to moderate bleeding episodes using recombinant factor VIIa in haemophiliacs with inhibitors. *Thromb Haemost* 1998; 80:912–918.
203. Negrier C, Lienhart A. Overall experience with Novoseven. *Blood Coagul Fibrinolysis* 2000;11(suppl 1):19–24.
204. Ingerslev J, Christiansen K, Calatzis A, et al: Management and monitoring of recombinant activated factor VII. *Blood Coagul Fibrinolysis* 2000;11(suppl 1):25–30.
205. Lusher JM, for the Novoseven Compassionate Use investigators. Recombinant factor VIIa (NovoSeven) in the treatment of internal bleeding in patients with factor VIII and IX inhibitors. *Haemostasis* 1996;26(suppl 1):124–130.
206. Naito K, Fuijikawa K. Activation of human blood coagulation factor XI independent of factor XII. *J Biol Chem* 1991;266: 7353–7358
207. Gailani D, Broze GJ. Factor XI activation in a revised model of blood coagulation. *Science* 1991;253:909–911.
208. Minnema MC, Ten Cate H, Hack EC. The role of factor XI in coagulation: a matter of revision. *Semin Thromb Hemost* 1999; 25:419–428.

209. Von dem Borne PA, Bajzar L, Meijers JC, et al. Thrombin-mediated activation of factor XI results in a thrombin-activatable fibrinolysis inhibitor-dependent inhibition of fibrinolysis. *J Clin Invest* 1997;99:2323–2327.
210. Bajzar L. Thrombin activatable fibrinolysis inhibitor and antifibrinolytic pathway. *Arteroscler Thromb Vasc Biol* 2000;20: 2511–2518.
211. Seligsohn U. High frequency of factor XI (PTA) deficiency in Ashkenazi Jews. *Blood* 1978;51:1223–1228.
212. Bolton-Maggs PHB. Factor XI deficiency and its management. *Haemophilia* 2000;6(suppl 1):100–109.
213. Ragni MV, Sinha D, Seaman F, et al. Comparison of bleeding tendency, factor XI coagulant activity and factor XI antigen in 25 factor XI deficient kindreds. *Blood* 1985;65:719–724.
214. Ragni MV, Sinha D, Seaman F, et al. Comparison of the bleeding tendency, factor XI activity and FXI antigen in 25 factor XI-deficient kindreds. *Blood* 1985;65:719.
215. Stern DM, Nossel HL, Owen J. Acquired antibody to factor XI in a patient with congenital factor XI deficiency. *J Clin Invest* 1982;69:1270.
216. Josephson AM, Lisker R. Demonstration of a circulating anticoagulant in plasma thromboplastin antecedent deficiency. *J Clin Invest* 1958;37:148.
217. Chediak J, Madej-Zevin P, Ratnoff OD, et al. Studies on a circulating anticoagulant inhibiting factor XI in a patient with congenital deficiency and carcinoma of the prostate. *Br J Haematol* 1986;63:123–133.
218. Schnall SF, Duffy TP, Clyne LP. Acquired factor XI inhibitors in congenitally deficient patients. *Am J Hematol* 1987;26: 323–328.
219. Lawler P, White B, Rajan S, et al. Inhibitor formation in a patient with inherited factor XI deficiency. *Haemophilia* 2000;6:280(abst).
220. Aberg H, Nilsson IM. Recurrent thrombosis in a young woman with a circulating inhibitor directed against factors XI and XII. *Acta Med Scand* 1972;192:419–425.
221. Cronberg S, Nilsson IM. Circulating anticoagulant against factor XI and XII together with massive spontaneous platelet aggregation. *Scand J Haematol* 1973;10:309–314
222. Leone G, Accorra F, Boni P. Circulating anticoagulant against factor XI and thrombocytopenia with platelet aggregation inhibition in systemic lupus erythematosus. *Acta Haematol* 1977; 58:240–245.
223. Bell WR, Boxx GR, Wolfson JS. Circulating anticoagulants in procainamide-induced lupus syndrome. *Arch Intern Med* 1977; 137:1471–1473.
224. Zucker S, Zarrabi MH, Romano G, et al. IgM inhibitors of the contact activation phase of coagulation in chlorpromazine treated patients. *Br J Haematol* 1978;406:447–457.
225. DiSabatino CA, Clyne LP, Malawista SE. A circulating anticoagulant directed against factor XIa in systemic lupus erythematosus. *Arthritis Rheum* 1979;22:1135–1138.
226. Vercellotti GM, Mosher DF. Acquired factor XI deficiency in systemic lupus erythematosus. *Thromb Haemost* 1982;48: 250–252.
227. Rustgi RN, LaDuca FM, Tourbaf KD. Circulating anticoagulant against factor XI in psoriasis. *J Med* 1982;13:289–301.
228. Reese EA, Clyne LP, Romero R, et al. Spntaneous factor XI inhibitor: seven additional cases and a review of the literature. *Arch Intern Med* 1984;144:525–529.
229. Schnall SF, Duffy TP, Clyne LP. Acquired factor XI inhibitors in congenitally deficient patients. *Am J Hematol* 1987;26: 323–328.
230. Castro D, Farber LR, Clyne LP. Circulating anticoagulants against factors IX and XI in systemic lupus erythematosus. *Ann Intern Med* 1972;77:543–548.
231. Krieger H, Leddy JP, Breckenbridge RT. Studies on circulating anticoagulant in systemic lupus erythematosus: evidence for inhibition of the function of activated plasma thromboplastin antecedent (factor XIa). *Blood* 1975;46:189–197.
232. Goldsmith GH, Silverman P. Inhibitors of plasma thromboplastin antecendent (factor XI): studies on the mechanism of inhibition. *J Lab Clin Med* 1985;106:279–285.
233. Goodrick MJ, Prentice AG, Copplestone JA, et al. Acquired factor XI inhibitor in chronic lymphocytic leukemia. *J Clin Pathol* 1992;45:352–353.
234. De la Cadena RA, Baglia FA, Johnson CA, et al. Naturally occurring human antibodies against two distinct functional domains in the heaavy chain of FXI/FXIa. *Blood* 1988;72:1748.
235. Rolovic Z, Elezovic I, Obrenovic B, et al. Life threatening bleeding due to an acquired inhibitor to factor XI/XII successfully treated with activated prothrombin complex concentrate. *Br J Haematol* 1982;51:659.
236. Connelly NR, Brull SJ. Anesthetic management of a patient with factor XI deficiency and factor XI inhibitor undergoing a cesarean section. *Anesth Analg* 1993;51:659.
237. Morgan K, Schiffman S, Feinstein D. Acquired factor XI inhibitors in two patients with hereditary factor XI deficiency. *Thromb Haemost* 1984;51:371–375.
238. Teruya J, Styler M. Management of factor XI inhibitor for cardiac intervention: successful treatment with immunosuppressive therapy and plasma exchange. *Haemophilia* 2000;6:158–161.
239. Von dem Borne PAK, Bajzar L, Meijers JCM, et al. Thrombin-mediated activation of factor XI results in a TAFI dependent inhibition of fibrinolysis. *J Clin Invest* 1997;99:2323–2327.
240. Reece EA, Clyne LP, Romero R, et al. Spontaneous factor XI inhibitors. *Arch Intern Med* 1984;144:525–529.
241. Duplicate of ref. 221.
242. Aberg H, Nilsson IM. Recurrent thrombosis in a young women with a circulating anticoagulant directed against factors XI and XII. *Acta Med Scand* 1972;192:419–425.
243. Vercellotti GM, Mosher DF. Acquired factor XI deficiency in systemic lupus erythematosus. *Thromb Haemost* 1982;48:250–252.
244. Schiffman S, Margalit R, Rosove M, et al. Factor-XI deficiency: effect of an inhibitor of factor XI adsorption to surface. *Blood* 1981;57:437–443.
245. DiSabatino CA, Clyne LP, Malawista SE. A circulating anticoagulant against factor XIa in patients with systemic lupus erythematosus. *Arthritis Rheum* 1979;22:1135.
246. Krieger H, Leddy JP, Breckenridge RT. Studies on a circulating anticoagulant in systemic lupus erythematosus: evidence for inhibition of the function of activated plasma thromboplastin antecedent (factor XIa). *Blood* 1975;46:189.
247. Chiu [illegible] M, [illegible] H, [illegible] WJ. A unique precipitating autoantibody against plasma thromboplastin antecedent associated with multiple apparent plasma clotting factor deficiencies in a patient with systemic lupus erythematosus. *Blood* 1984:63: 1309–1317.
248. Ginsberg SS, Clyne LP, McPhedran P, et al. Successful childbirth by a patient with congenital factor XI deficiency and acquired inhibitor. *Br J Haematol* 1993;84:172–174.
249. Eherenforth S, Kreuz W, Scharrer I, et al. Incidence of the development of factor VIII and factor IX inhibitors in hemophiliacs. *Lancet* 1992;339:594–598.
250. Nilsson IM, Hedner U, Bjorlin B. Suppression of factor IX by cyclophosphamide. *Ann Intern Med* 1973;78:91–95
251. Ljung RC. Gene mutations and inhibitor formation in patients with haemophilia B. *Acta Haematol* 1995;94(suppl 1):49–52.
252. Rup BJ, Gill J, Pollman H, et al. Factor IX gene mutation and anti-factor IX antibodies formation in hemophilia B previously untreated patients (PUPs) treated with recombinant factor IX (rFIX). *Haemophilia* 2000;6:286(abst).

253. Reisner HM, Roberts HR, Krumholz S, et al. Immunochemical characterization of a polyclonal human antibody to factor IX. *Blood* 1977;50:11.
254. Lechner K. Factor IX inhibitors: report of 2 cases and a study of the biological, chemical and immunological properties of the inhibitors. *Thromb Diath Haemorrh* 1971;25:447.
255. Orstavik KH. Alloantibodies to factor IX in hemophilia B characterized by cross immunoelectrophoresis and enzyme-conjugated antisera to human immunoglobulins. *Br J Haematol* 1981;48:15.
256. Pike IM, Yount WJ, Puritz EM, et al. Immunochemical characterization of a monoclonal IgG4 lambda human antibody to factor IX. *Blood* 1972;40:1.
257. Sanchez-Medal I, Liker R, Lopez ET. Unusual circulating anticoagulants in a patient with systemic lupus erythematosus. *Acta Haematol* 1963;29:117–122.
258. Largo R, von Felton A, Strauh PW. Acquired factor IX inhibitor in a nonhemophiliac patient with autoimmune disease. *Br J Haematol* 1974;26:129–140.
259. Ozsoylu S, Ozer FL. Acquired factor IX deficiency. *Acta Haematol* 1973;50:38–44.
260. Baudo F, Mostrada G, on behalf of the Italian Association of Hemophilia Centers. Factor VIII/IX acquired inhibitors: report from the Italian register. *Haemophilia* 2000;6:280(abst).
261. Stein DT, Farley DM, Ohler SA, et al. Acquired factor IX inhibitor in a patient without haemophilia. *Haemophilia* 2000; 6:284(abst).
262. Boklan BF, Sawitsky A. Factor IX deficiency in Gaucher disease. *Arch Intern Med* 1976;136:489–492
263. Handley DA, Lawrence JR. Factor IX deficiency in the nephrotic syndrome. *Lancet* 1967;1:1079–1081.
264. Scharrer I. Recombinant factor VIIa for patients with inhibitors to factor VIII or factor IX of factor VII deficiency. *Haemophilia* 1999;5:253–259.
265. Jakway J. Acquired von Willebrand's disease. *Hematol Oncol Clin North Am* 1992;6:1409–1419.
266. Phillips MD, Santhouse A. von Willebrand disease: recent advances in pathophysiology and treatment. *Am J Med Sci* 1998;316:77–86.
267. Tefferi A, Nichols WL. Acquired von Willebrand disease: concise review of occurrence, diagnosis, pathogenesis, and treatment. *Am J Med* 1997;103:536–540.
268. Nitu-Whalley IC, Lee CA. Acquired von Willebrand syndrome: report of 10 cases and review of the literature. *Haemophilia* 1999;5:318–326.
269. Jakway JL. Acquired von Willebrand's disease in malignancy. *Semin Thromb Hemost* 1992;18:434–439.
270. Van Genderen PJJ, Paptsonis DNM, Michiels JJ, et al. High-dose intravenous gammaglobulin therapy for acquired von Willebrand disease. *Postgrad Med J* 1994;70:916–920.
271. Mannuccio PM. Platelet von Willebrand factor in inherited and acquired bleeding disorders. *Proc Natl Acad Sci U S A* 1995;92: 2428–2432.
272. Van Genderen PJ, Michiels JJ. Acquired von Willebrand disease. *Baillieres Clin Hematol* 1998;11:319–330.
273. Rinder MR, Richard RE, Rinder H. Acquired von Willebrand's disease: a concise review. *Am J Hematol* 1997;54:139–145.
274. Ruggeri ZM, Ware J. The structure and function of von Willebrand's factor. *Thromb Haemost* 1992;67:594–599.
275. Fujimura Y, Ruggeri ZM, Zimmerman TS. Structure and function of human von Willebrand factor. In: Zimmerman T, Ruggeri Z, eds. *Coagulation and bleeding disorders: the role of factor VIII and vWF.* New York: Marcel Dekker, 1989:77.
276. Girma JD, Meyer CL, Verweij H, et al. Structure function relationship of human vWF. *Blood* 1987;70:605.
277. Weiss HJ, Sussman II, Hoyer L. Stabilization of factor VIII in plasma by the vWF: studies on the post-transfusion and dissociated factor VIII and in patients with vWF. *J Clin Invest* 1977; 60:390.
278. Shelton-Inloes BB, Chehab FF, Mannucci PM, et al. Gene deletions correlate with the development of alloantibodies in vWD. *J Clin Invest* 1987:79:1459–1465
279. Mannucci PM, Mari D. Antibodies to factor VIII-vWF in congenital and acquired vWD. In: Hoyer LW, ed. *Factor VIII inhibitors.* New York: Alan R Liss, 1984:109–122.
280. Lopez-Fernandez MF, Martin R, Lopez-Berges C, et al. Further specificity characterization of vWF inhibitors developed in 2 patients with severe vWD. *Blood* 1988;72:116–120.
281. Fernandez MF, Ginsberg MH, Ruggeri ZM, et al. Multimeric structure of platelet factor VIII/von Willebrand factor: the presence of larger multimers and their reassociation with thrombin-stimulated platelets. *Blood* 1982;60:1132–1138.
282. Sarji KE, Stratton RD, Wagner RH, et al. Nature of vWF: a new assay and a specific inhibitor. *Proc Natl Acad Sci U S A* 1974;71:2937.
283. Stratton RD, Wagner RH, Webster WP, et al. Antibody nature of circulating inhibitor of plasma vWF. *Proc Natl Acad Sci U S A* 1975;72:4167.
284. Mannucci PM, Meyer D, Kouts J, et al. Precipitating antibodies in vWD. *Nature* 1976;262:141.
285. Egberg N, Blomback M. On the characterization of acquired inhibitors to ristocetin-induced platelet aggregation found in patients with vWD. *Thromb Res* 1976;9:957.
286. Maragall S, Castillo R, Ordinas FL, et al. Inhibition of vWF in vWD. *Thromb Res* 1979;14:495.
287. Mannucci PM, Ruggeri ZM, Ciavarella N, et al. Preccipitating antibodies to factor VIII/vWF in vWD: effects on replacement therapy. *Blood* 1981;57:25.
288. Ruggeri ZM, Ciavarella N, Mannucci PM, et al. Familial incidence of precipitating antibodies in vWD: a study of four cases. *J Lab Clin Med* 1979;94:60.
289. Bergamaschini L, Mannucci PM, Federici AB, et al. Posttransfusion anaphylactic reactions in a patient with severe vWD: role of complement and alloantibodies to vWF. *J Lab Clin Med* 1995;125:348–355.
290. Simone JV, Comet JA, Abildgaard CF. Acquired von Willebrand's syndrome in systemic lupus erythematosus. *Blood* 1968; 31:806–812.
291. Igarashi N, Miura M, Kato E, et al. Acquired von Willebrand's syndrome with lupus-like serology. *Am J Pediatr Hematol Oncol* 1989;11:32–35.
292. Handin RI, Martin V, Moloney WC. Antibody-induced vWD: a newly defined inhibitor syndrome. *Blood* 1976;48:393–405.
293. Van Genderen PJ, Vink T, Michiels JJ, et al. Acquired vWD caused by an autoantibody selectively inhibiting the binding of VWF to collagen. *Blood.* 1994;84:3378–3384.
294. Hanley D, Arkel Y, Lynch J, et al. Acquired von Willebrand's syndrome in association with a lupus-like inhibitor corrected by intravenous immunoglobulin. *Am J Hematol* 1994;46:141–146.
295. Sampson BM, Greaves M, Malia RG, et al. Acquired vWD: demonstration of a circulating inhibitor to the factor VIII complex in four cases. *Br J Haematol* 1983;54:233–244.
296. Fricke WA, Brinkhous KM, Garris JB, et al. Comparison of inhibitory and binding characteristics of an antibody causing acquired vWS: an assay for vWF binding by antibody. *Blood* 1985;66:562–569.
297. Bovill EG, Ershler WB, Golden EA, et al. A human myeloma-produced monoclonal protein directed against the active subpopulation of vWF. *Am J Clin Pathol* 1986;85:115–123.
298. Mohri H, Noguchi T, Kodama F, et al. Acquired vWD due to inhibitor of human myeloma protein specific for vWF. *Am J Clin Pathol* 1987;87:663–668.

299. Mazurier C, Parquet-Gernez A, Descamps J, et al. Acquired vWS in the course of Waldenström's disease. *Thromb Haemost* 1980;44:115–118.
300. Goudemand J, Samor B, Caron C, et al. Acquired type II vWD: demonstration of a complexed inhibitor of the vWF-plaelet interaction and response to treatment. *Br J Haematol* 1988;68: 227–233.
301. McGrath KM, Johnson CA, Stuart JJ. Acquired vWD associated with an inhibitor to factor VIII antigen and gastrointestinal telangiectasia. *Am J Med* 1979;67:693–696.
302. Lazarchick J, Pappas AA, Kizer J, et al. Acquired vWS due to an inhibitor specific for vWF antigens. *Am J Hematol* 1986;21: 305–314.
303. Gan TE, Sawers RJ, Koutts J. Pathogenesis of antibody-induced acquired vWS. *Am J Hematol* 1980;9:363–371.
304. Richard C, Cuadrado MA, Prieto M, et al. Acquired von Willebrand's disease in multiple myeloma secondary to absorption of von Willebrand's factor by plasma cells. *Am J Hematol* 1990; 35:114–117.
305. Brody JI, Haidar ME, Rossman RE. A hemorrhagic syndrome in Waldenström's macroglobulinemia secondary to immunoadsorptionof factor VIII. *N Engl J Med* 1979;300:408.
306. Tefferi A, Hanson CA, Kurtin PJ, et al. Acquired vWD due to aberrant expression of platelet glycoprotein Ib by marginal zone lymphoma cells. *Br J Haematol* 1997;96:850–853.
307. Aylesworth CA, Smallridge RC, Rick ME, et al. Acquired vWD: a rare manifestation of postpartum thyroiditis. *Am J Hematol* 1995;50:217–219.
308. Mannucci PM, Lombardi R, Bader R, et al. Studies of the pathophysiology of acquired von Willebrand's disease in seven patients with lymphoproliferative disorders or benign monoclonal gammopathies. *Blood* 1984;64:614–621.
309. Duplicate of ref. 293.
310. Dalton RG, Dewar MS, Savidge GF, et al. Hypothyroidism as a cause of AvWD. *Lancet* 1987;i:1007–1009.
311. Bruggers CS, McElliogott K, Rallison ML. AvWD in twins with autoimmune hypothyroidism: response to DDAVP and L-thyroxine therapy. *J Pediatr* 1994;125:911.
312. Coccia MR, Barnes HV. Hypothyroidism and AvWD. *J Adolesc Health* 1991;12:152.
313. Cass AJ, Bliss BP, Bolton RP, et al. Gastrointestinal bleeding, angiodysplasia of the colon and AvWD. *Br J Surg* 1980;67: 639–641.
314. Wautier JL, Caen JP, Rymer R. Angiodysplasia in AvWD. *Lancet* 1976;ii:973.
315. Foutch PG. Angiodysplasia of the gastrointestinal tract. *Am J Gastroenterol* 1993;88:807–818.
316. Kreuz W, Linde R, Funk M, et al. Induction of von Willebrand's disease type I by valproic acid. *Lancet* 1990;i: 1350–1351.
317. Facon T, Caron C, Courtin P, et al. Acquired type 2 vWD associated with adrenal cortical carcinoma. *Br J Haematol* 1992;80: 488–494.
318. Scrobohaci ML, Daniel MT, Levy et al. Expression of GPIb on plasma cells in a patient with monoclonal IgG and acquired vWD. *Br J Haematol* 1993;84:471–475.
319. Michiels JJ Acquired vWD due to increasing platelet count can readily explain in the paradox of thrombosis and bleeding in thrombocythemia. *Clin Appl Thromb Hemost* 1999;5:147–151.
320. Van Genderen PJJ, Leenknegt H, Michiels JJ, et al. Acquired vWD in myeloproliferative disorders. *Leukemia Lymphoma* 1996;22(suppl 1):79–82.
321. Budde U, van Genderen PJJ. Acquired vWD in patients with high platelet counts. *Semin Thromb Hemost* 1997;23:425–431.
322. Castaman G, Lattuada A, Mannucci PM, et al. Characterization of two cases of acquired transitory vWD with ciprofloxacin: evidence for heightened proteolysis of vWF. *Am J Hematol* 1995;49:83–86
323. Federici AB, Berkowitz SD, Zimmerman TS, et al. Proteolysis of vWF after thrombolytic therapy in patients with acute myocardial infarction. *Blood* 1992;79:38–44.
324. Tsai HM, Sussman II, Nagel RL. Shear stress enhances the proteolysis of vWF in normal plasma. *Blood* 1994;83: 2171–2179.
325. Pasi KJ, Enayat MS, Horrocks PM, et al. Qualitative and quantitative abnormalities of vW antigen in patients with diabetes mellitus. *Thromb Res* 1990;59:581–591.
326. Federici AB, Elder JH, DeMarco L, et al. Carbohydrate moiety of vWF is not necessary for maintaining multimeric structure and ristocetin cofactor activity but protects from proteolytic degradation. *J Clin Invest* 1984;74:2049–2055.
327. Eikenboom JCJ, van der Meer FJM, Briet E. Acquired vWD due to excessive fibrinoloysis. *Br J Haematol* 1993;81:618–620.
328. Trieb J, Haass A, Pindur G, Coagulation disorders caused by hydroxyethyl starch. *Thromb Haemost* 1997;78:974–983.
329. Goudemand J, Samor B, Caron C, et al. Acquired type II vWD: demonstration of a complexed inhibitor of the vWF-platelet interaction and response to treatment. *Br J Haematol* 1988; 68:227–233.
330. Soff GA, Geen D. Autoantibody to vWF in systemic lupus erythematosus. *J Lab Clin Med* 1993;121:424–430.
331. Stewart AK, Etches WS, Shaw ARE, et al. vWF inhibitor detection by competitive ELISA. *J Immunol Methods* 1997;200: 113–119.
332. Fay PJ, Kawai Y, Wagner DD, et al. Propolypeptide of vWF circulates in blood and is identical to vW antigen II. *Science* 1986;232:995–999.
333. McCarroll DR, Ruggeri ZM, Montgomery RR. Correlation between circulating levels of vW:Ag II and vWF: discrimination between type I and II vWD. *J Lab Clin Med* 1984;103:704–711.
334. Borchiellini A, Fijnvandraat K, ten Cate JW, et al. Quantitative analysis of vWF propetide release in vivo: effect of experimental endotoxemia and administration of DDAVP in humans. *Blood* 1996;88:2951–2958.
335. van Genderen PJJJ, Boertjes R, van Mourik JA. Quantitative analysis of vWF and its propeptide in plasma in acquired vWD. *Thromb Haemost* 1998;80:495–498.
336. Kinoshita S, Yoshioka K, Kasahara M, et al. AvWD after Epstein-Barr virus infection. *J Pediatr* 1991;119:595–598.
337. Jakway J. Acquired vWD in malignancy. *Semin Thromb Hemost.* 1992;18:434–439.
338. Alexanian R, Dimoupoulos MA, Delasaille K, et al. Primary dexamethasone treatment of multiple myeloma. *Blood* 1992; 80:887.
339. Scott JP, Montgomery RR, Tubergen DG, et al. AvWD in association with Wilm's tumor: regression following treatment. *Blood* 1961;58:665–669.
340. Richard C, Sedano MC, Cuadrado MA, et al. AvWD associated with hydatid disease of the spleen: disappearance after splenectomy. *Thromb Haemost* 1984;52:90–93.
341. Duran-Saurez JR, Pico M, Zuazu J, et al. Acquired vWD caused by chronic granulocytic leukemia. *Br J Haematol* 1981;48: 173–175.
342. Joist JH, Cowan JF, Zimmerman TS. AvWD evidence for a quantitative and qualitative factor VIII disorder. *N Engl J Med* 1978;298:988–991.
343. Gill JC, Wilson AD, Endres-Brooks J, et al. Loss of largest vWF multimers from the plasma of patients with congenital cardiac defects. *Blood* 1966;67:758–761.
344. Dalrymple-Hay M, Aitchison R, Collins P, et al. HES induced acquired vWD. *Clin Lab Haematol* 1992;14:209–211.
345. Stewart AK, Glynn MFX. AvWD associated with free lambda

light chain monoclonal gammopathy, normal bleeding time and response to prednisone. *Postgrad Med J* 1990;66:560–562.
346. Silberstein LE, Abraham J, Shattil SJ. The efficacy of intensive plasma exchange in AvWD. *Transfusion* 1987;27:234–237.
347. Uelinger J, Rose E, Aledort LM, et al. Successful treatment of an acquired vWF antibody by extracorporeal immunoadsorption. *N Engl J Med* 1991;320:254–255..
348. Jehlinger J, Rose E, Aledort LM. Successful treatment of an acquired vWF antibody to extracorporeal immunoadsorption. *N Engl J Med* 1989;320:254.
349. Israels SJ, Leaker MT. Acquired inhibitors to factor V and X after exposure to topical thrombin: interference with monitoring of low molecular weight heparin and warfarin *J Pediatr* 1997;131:480–483.
350. Rapaport SI, Zivelin A, Minow RA, et al. Clinical significance of antibodies to bovine and human thrombin and factor V after surgical use of bovine thrombin. *Am J Clin Pathol* 1992;97:84–91.
351. Banninger H, Hardegger T, Tobler A, et al. Fibrin glue in surgery: frequent development of inhibitors of bovine thrombin and human factor V. *Br J Haematol* 1993;85:528–532.
352. Dorion P, Hamati HF, Landis B, et al. Risk and clinical significance of developing antibodies induced by topical thrombin preparations. *Arch Pathol Lab Med* 1998;122:887–894.
353. Zehnder JL, Leung LLK. Development of antibodies to thrombin and factor V with recurrent bleeding in a patient exposed to topical bovine thrombin. *Blood* 1990;76:2011–2016.
354. Lawson JH, Pennell BJ, Olson JD, et al. Isolation and characterization of an acquired antithrombin antibody. *Blood* 1990; 76:2249–2257.
355. Chouhan VD, De La Cadena, Nagaswami C, et al. Simultaneous occurrence of human antibodies directed against fibrinogen, thrombin, and factor V following exposure to bovine thrombin: effects on blood coagulation, protein C activation and platelet function. *Thromb Haemost* 1997;77:343–349.
356. Ortel TL, Moore KD, Quinn-Allen MA, et al. Inhibitory anti-factor V antibodies bind to the factor V C2 domain and are associated with hemorrhagic manifestations. *Blood* 1998;91: 4188–4196.
357. Crowell EB. Observations on a factor V inhibitor. *Br J Haematol* 1975;29:397.
358. Smid WM, de Wolf JTM, Nijland JH, et al. Severe bleeding caused by an inhibitor to coagulation factor V: a case report. *Blood Coagul Fibrinolysis* 1994;5:133.
359. Shastri KA, Ho C, Logue G. An acquired factor V inhibitor: clinical and laboratory features. *J Med* 1999;30:357–366.
360. Coots MC, Muhleman AF, Glueck HI. Hemorrhagic death with high titer factor V inhibitor. *Am J Hematol* 1978;4:193.
361. Chediak J, Ashenhurst JB, Garlick I, et al. Successful management of bleeding in a patient with factor V inhibitor by platelet transfusions. *Blood* 1980;56:835.
362. Grigg AP, Dauer R, Thurlow PJ. Bleeding due to an acquired inhibitor of platelet associated factor V. *Aust N Z J Med* 1989; 19:310–314.
363. Ferguson JH, Johnston CL, Howell DA. Anti-AcG: a specific circulating inhibitor of the labile clotting factor. *Proc Soc Exp Biol Med* 1957;95:567–568.
364. Knobl P, Lechner K. Acquired factor V inhibitors. *Baillieres Clin Haematol* 1998;11:305–318.
365. Chong LL, Wong YC. A case of factor V inhibitor. *Am J Hematol* 1985;19:395–399.
366. Kapur A, Kelsey PR, Isaacs PET. Factor V inhibitor in thrombosis . *Am J Hematol* 1993;42:384–388.
367. Kamphuisen PW, Haan J, Rosekrans PCM, et al. Deep-vein thrombosis and coumarin skin necrosis associated with a factor V inhibitor with lupus-like features. *Am J Hematol* 1998;57: 176–178.
368. Ortel TL. Clinical and laboratory manifestation of anti-factor V antibodies. *J Lab Clin Med* 1999;133:326–334.
369. Feinstein DI. Acquired inhibitors of factor V. *Thromb Haemost* 1978;39:663–674.
370. Feinstein DI, Rapaport SI, Chong MMY. Factor V inhibitor: report of a case, with comments on a possible effect of streptomycin. *Ann Intern Med* 1973;78:385–388.
371. Feinstein DI, Rapaport SI, McGehee WG, et al. Factor V anticoagulants: clinical, biochemical and immunological observations. *J Clin Invest* 1970;49:1578–1588.
372. Duplicate of ref. 356.
373. Duplicate of ref. 371.
374. Nesheim ME, Nichols WL, Cole TL, et al. Isolation and study of an acquired inhibitor of human factor V. *J Clin Invest* 1986; 77:405.
375. Kapur A, Kelsey PR, Isaacs PET. Factor V inhibitor in thrombosis. *Am J Hematol* 1993;42:384–388.
376. Duplicate of ref. 367.
377. Koyama T, Saito T, Kusano T, et al. Factor V inhibitor associated with Sjögren syndrome. *Br J Haematol* 1995;89:893–896.
378. Berruyer M, Amiral J, French P, et al. Immunization by bovine thrombin used with fibrin glue during cardiovascular operations: development of thrombin and factor V inhibitors. *J Thorac Cardiovasc Surg* 1993;105:892–897.
379. George S, Nagabhushana MS, Cyran EM. Coagulopathy due to an acquired factor V inhibitor and subsequently thrombosis. *Am J Hematol* 1995;49:98–100.
380. Duplicate of ref. 367.
381. Banninger H, Hardegger T, Tobler A, et al. Fibrin glue in surgery: frequent development of inhibitors of bovine thrombin and human factor V. *Br J Haematol* 1993;85:528–532.
382. Martin JD, Sikkink RA, Gilchrist GS, et al. Development of anti-bovine thrombin antibodies following neurosurgical procedures. *Br J Haematol* 1990;74:369–370.
383. Sticker RB, Lane PK, Leffert JD, et al. Development of antithrombin antibodies following surgery in patients with prosthetic cardiac valves. *Blood* 1988;72:1375–1380.
384. Rapaport SI, Zivelin A, Minow RA, et al. Clinical significance of antibodies to bovine and human thrombin and factor V after surgical use of bovine thrombin. *Am J Clin Pathol* 1992;97:84–91.
385. Dorion RP, Hamati HF, Landis B, et al. Risk and clinical significance of developing antibodies induced by topical thrombin preparations. *Arch Pathol Lab Med* 1998;122:887–894.
386. Zehnder JL, Leung LLK. Development of antibodies to thrombin and factor V with recurrent bleeding in a patient exposed to topical bovine thrombin. *Blood* 1990;76:2011–2016.
387. Ortel TL, Mercer MC, Thames EH, et al. Immunologic impact and clinical outcomes after surgical exposure to bovine thrombin. *Ann Surg* 2001;233:88–96.
388. Zehnder JL, Leung LLK. Development of antibodies to thrombin and factor V with recurrent bleeding in a patient exposed to topical bovine thrombin. *Blood* 1990;76:2011–2016.
389. Cmolik BL, Spero JA, Magovern GL, et al. Redo cardiac surgery: late bleeding complications from topical thrombin-induced factor V deficiency. *J Thorac Cardiovasc Surg* 1993;105: 222–228.
390. Muntean W, Zenz W, Edlinger G, et al. Severe bleeding due to factor V inhibitor after repeated operations using fibrin sealant containing bovine thrombin. *Thromb Haemost* 1997;77:1223.
391. Taillan B, Fuzibet J-G, Vinti H, et al. Factor V inhibitor in celiac disease. *Am J Med* 1989;87:360.
392. Gordon B, Haire W, Duggan M, et al. Factor V inhibitor developing after liver transplantation in a 3 year old. *Pediatrics* 1991; 88:156–159.
393. Raman BKS, Batchev C, Shurafa M. Acquired factor V inhibitors showing positive platelet neutralizing test and

responding to platelet transfusions: report of 4 cases. *Thromb Haemost* 1995;73:1426(abst).

394. Bryning K, Leslie J. Factor V inhibitor and bullous pemphigoid. *Br Med J* 1977;2:677–678.
395. Suehisa E, Toku M, Akita N, et al. Study on an antibody against F1F2 fragment of human factor V in a patient with Hashimoto's disease and bullous pemphigoid. *Thromb Res* 1995;77:63–68.
396. Brickner LA, Scannell KA, Sahud MA. Acquired factor V inhibitor in a patient with acquired human immunodeficiency syndrome. *Am J Hematol* 1996;52:332–333.
397. Fratantoni JC, Hilgartner M, Nachman RL. Nature of the defect in congenital factor V deficiency: study in a patient with an acquired circulating anticoagulant. *Blood* 1972;39:751–758.
398. Mazzucconi MG, Solinas S, Chistolini A, et al. Inhibitor to factor V in severe factor V congenital deficiency: a case report. *Nouv Rev Fr Hematol* 1985;27:303–305.
399. Vickars LM, Coupland RW, Naiman SC. The response of acquired factor V inhibitor to activated factor IX concentrate. *Tranfusion* 1985;25:51–53.
400. Tarantino MD, Ross MP, Danielos TM, et al. Modulation of an acquired coagulation factor V inhibitor with IVIG. *J Pediatr Hematol Oncol* 1997;19:226–231.
401. Israels SJ, Leaker MT. Acquired inhibitors to factors V and X after exposure to topical thrombin: interference with monitoring of low molecular weight heparin and warfarin. *J Pediatr* 1997;131:480–483.
402. Chouhan VD, De La Cadena RA, Nagaswami C, et al. Simultaneous occurrence of human antibodies directed against fibrinogen, thrombin, and factor V following exposure to bovine thrombin: effects on blood coagulation, protein C activation and platelet function. *Thromb Haemost* 1997;77:343–349.
403. Palmer RN, Rick ME, Rick PD, et al. Circulating heparan sulfate anticoagulant in a patient with a fatal bleeding disorder. *N Engl J Med* 1984;310:1696–1699.
404. Khoory MS, Nesheim ME, Bowie EJW, et al. Circulating heparan sulfate proteoglycan anticoagulant from a patient with a plasma cell disorder. *J Clin Invest* 1980;65:666–674.
405. Bussel JB, Steinherz PG, Miller DR, et al. A heparin-like anticoagulant in an 8-month-old boy with acute monoblastic leukemia. *Am J Hematol* 1984;16:83–90.
406. Hasegawa DK, Bennet AJ, Coccia PF, et al. Factor V deficiency in Philadelphia-positive chronic myelogenous leukemia. *Blood* 1980;56:585–595.
407. Duplicate of ref. 9.
408. Bajaj SP, Rapaport SI, Fierer DS. A mechanism for the hypoprothrombinemia of the acquired hypoprothrombinemia-lupus anticoagulant syndrome. *Blood* 1983;61:684.
409. Fleck R, Rapaport SI, Rao LVM. Anti-prothrombin antibodies and the lupus anticoagulant. *Blood* 1988;72:512.
410. Vivaldi P, Rossetti G, Galli M, et al. Severe bleeding due to acquired hypoprothrombinemia-lupus anticoagulant syndrome: case report and review of the literature. *Haematologica* 1997;82:345–347.
411. Erkan D, Bateman H, Lockshin MD. Lupus anticoagulant-hypoprothrombinemia syndrome associated with systemic lupus erythematosus: report of 2 cases and review of the literature. *Lupus* 1999;8:560–564.
412. Palossuo T, Virtamo J, Haukka J, et al. High antibody levels to prothrombin imply a risk of deep venous thrombosis and pulmonary embolism in middle-aged men. *Thromb Haemost* 1997;78:1178–1182.
413. Vaarala O, Puurunen M, Manttari M, et al. Antibodies to prothrombin imply a risk of myocardial infarction in middle-aged men. *Thromb Haemost* 1996;75:456–459.
414. Galli M, Ruggeri L, Barbui T. Differential effects of anti-beta2 GPI and antiprothrombin antibodies on the anticoagulant activity of activated protein C. *Blood* 1998;91:1999–2004.
415. Galli M, Barbui T. Prothrombin as a cofactor for antiphospholipids. *Lupus* 1998;7(suppl 2):S37–S40.
416. Zivelin A, Gitel S, Griffin JH, et al. Extensive venous and arterial thrombosis associated with an inhibitor to activated protein C. *Blood* 1999;94:895–901.
417. Male C, Mitchell L, Julian J, et al. Acquired activated protein C resistance is associated with lupus anticoagulants and thrombotic events in pediatric patients with systemic lupus erythematosus. *Blood* 2001;97:844–849.
418. McDonaugh J. Structure and function of factor XIII. In: Coleman R, Hirsch J, Marder V, et al., eds. *Hemostasis thrombosis: basic principles and clinical practice.* 3rd ed. Philadelphia: JB Lippincott, 1994:309–310.
419. Payne RW, Harris MC. Factor VIII inhibitor: acquired haemostatic defect in a non-haemophilic patient with rheumatoid arthritis. *Scott Med J* 1972;17:310–313.
420. Sise HS, Gauthier J, Desforges J, et al. Spontaneous circulating anticoagulant (antiVIII). *Am J Med* 1962;32:964–975.
421. Gobbi F, Stefanini M. Circulating anti-AHG anticoagulant in a patient with lupus erythematosus disseminatus. *Acta Haematol (Basel)* 1962;28:155–162.
422. Robboy SJ, Lewis EJ, Schur PH, et al. Circulating anticoagulants to factor VIII. *Am J Med* 1970;49:742–752.
423. Whitfield AGW, Meynell MJ, Fessey BM, et al. A circulating anticoagulant occurring after temporal arteritis and controlled by corticosteroids therapy. *J Clin Pathol* 1962;15:357–360.
424. Green D. Spontaneous inhibitors of factor VIII. *Br J Haematol* 1968;15:57–75.
425. Rizza CR, Adgcumbe JOP, Pitney WR, et al. The treatment of patients having spontaneously occurring antibodies to antihaemophilic factor VIII. *Thromb Diath Haemorrh* 1972;28:120–128.
426. DeHoratius RJ. Treatment of acquired factor VIII inhibitor using IVIG in two patients with systemic lupus erythematosis. *Arthritis Rheum* 1997;40:775–778.
427. Shapiro SS. The immunologic character of acquired inhibitors of antihemophilic globulin (factor VIII) and the kinetics of their interaction with factor VIII. *J Clin Invest* 1967;46:147–156.
428. Wenz B, Friedman G. Acquired factor VIII inhibitor in a patient with malignant lymphoma. *Am J Med Sci* 1974;268:295–299.
429. Neilson RF, Walker ID, Robertson M. Factor VIII inhibitor associated with hepatocellular carcinoma. *Clin Lab Haematol* 1993;15:145–148.
430. Glueck HI, Hong R. A circulating anticoagulant in gamma1A-multiple myeloma: its modification by penicillin. *J Clin Invest* 1965;44:1866–1881.
431. Castaldi PA, Penny R. A macroglobulin with inhibitory activity against factor VIII. *Blood* 1970;35:370–376.
432. Nilsson IM, Hedner U, Holmberg L. Suppression of factor VIII antibody by combined factor VIII and cyclophosphamide. *Acta Med Scand* 1972;195:65–72.
433. Neilson RF, Walker ID, Robertson M. Factor VIII inhibitor associated with hepatocellular carcinoma. *Clin Lab Haematol* 1993;15:145–148.
434. Heyd R, Kirchner J, Kollath J, et al. Acquired factor VIII inhibitor in advanced cervical carcinoma. *Tumor Diagn Ther* 1995;16:242–245.
435. Moccia F, Tognoni E, Boccaccio P. Acquired factor VIII inhibitor associated with prostatic cancer: successful treatment with steroid and immunosuppressive therapy. *Ann Ital Med Int* 2000;15:172–176.
436. Harada Y, Iwai M, Ueda Y, et al. Life threatening hemorrhage

in a patient with gastric cancer and acquired hemophilia. *Am J Gastroenterol* 1998;93:1372–1373.

437. Lechner K. Immunologisch bedingte Koaglopathein. *Thromb Diath Haemorrh* 1969;(suppl 34):33–47.
438. Nussey AM, Dawson DW. Haemophilia-like disease due to an autoantibody. *Br Med J* 1957;2:1077–1079.
439. Sherman LA, Goldstein MA, Sise HS. Circulating anticoagulant (antifactor VIII) treated with immunosuppressive drugs. *Thromb Diath Haemorrh* 1969;21:249–258.
440. Andersen BR, Troup SB. gammaG-antibody to human antihemophilic globulin (factor VIII). *J Immunol* 1968;100: 175–186.
441. Green D. Suppression of an antibody to factor VIII by a combination of factor VIII and cyclophosphamide. *Blood* 1971;37: 381–387.
442. Fisher M, Lechner K, Raith W. Hemmkorperhaemophilie bei bullosem Pemphigoid (Lever). *Hautarzt* 1968;l10:459–462.
443. Goudemand M, Hutin A. Maladie hemorrhagique acquise par anticoagulant circulant inhabant la thromboplastinoformation. *Sang* 1959;30:395–405.
444. Ganly PS, Issacs JD, Laffan MA, et al. Acquired factor VIII inhibitor associated with lung abscess. *Br Med J* 1987;295:811.
445. Usohima N, Ootuki R, Hiramori N, et al. A case of liver cirrhosis with acquired factor VIII inhibitor. *Kyoto Daini Seki-Juji Byoin Igaku Zasshi* 1993;10:187–193(abst).
446. Sugishta K, Nagase H, Takahashi T, et al. Acquired factor VIII inhibitor in a non-hemophilic patient with chronic C viral infection. *Intern Med* 1999;38:283–286.
447. Seidler CW, Mills LE, Flowers MED, et al. Spontaneous factor VIII inhibitor occurring in association with chronic graft-versus-host disease. *Am J Hematol* 1994;45:240–243.
448. Ollendorf P, Amris CJ. A case of factor VIII inhibitor developed after electric shock therapy. *Scand J Haematol* 1967;4:401–410.
449. Green D. Spontaneous inhibitors of factor VIII. *Br J Haematol* 1968;15:57–75.
450. Stewart AJ, Manson LM, Dasani H, et al. Acquired haemophilia in recipients of depot thioxanthenes. *Haemophilia* 2000;6:709–712.
451. Spero JA, Lewis JH, Hasiba U. Corticosteroid therapy for acquired factor VIII inhibitors. *Br J Haematol* 1981;48:635–642.
452. Lian ECY, Larcada AF, Chiu AYZ. Combination immunosuppressive therapy after factor VIII infusion for acquired factor VIII inhibitor. *Ann Intern Med* 1989;110:774–778.
453. Sultan Y, Kazatchkine MD, Caisonneuve P, et al. Anti-idiotype suppression of autoantibodies to factor VIII by high-dose intravenous immunoglobulin. *Lancet* 1984;ii:765–768.
454. Green D, Kwaan CH. An acquired factor VIII inhibitor responsive to high-dose gamma globulin. *Thromb Haemost* 1987;57: 521–522.
455. Struillou L, Fiks-Sigaud M, Barrier JH, et al. Acquired haemophilia and rheumatoid arthritis: success of immunoglobulin therapy. *J Intern Med* 1993;233:304–305.
456. Schwartz RS, Gabriel DA, Aledort LM, et al. A prospective study of the treatment of acquired factor VIII inhibitors with high dose intravenous gammaglobulin. *Blood* 1995;86: 797–804.
457. Pfliegler G, Boda Z, Harsfalvi H, et al. Cyclosporin treatment of a women with acquired hemophilia due to factor VIII inhibitor. *Postgrad Med J* 1989;65:400–402.
458. Schulman S, Langevitz P, Livneh A, et al. Cyclosporin therapy for acquired factor VIII inhibitor in a patient with systemic lupus erythematosus. *Thromb Haemost* 1996;76:344–346.

11

CLINICAL APPROACH TO THE PATIENT WITH THROMBOSIS, THROMBOEMBOLUS, AND PULMONARY EMBOLUS

RODGER L. BICK
WILLIAM F. BAKER, JR.

Thrombosis, thromboembolus, and pulmonary embolus (PE) are common clinical problems seen throughout a broad spectrum of clinical practices. PE is a prominent cause of death in the United States, and thus it is important to diagnose promptly those individuals who are predisposed to thrombosis and thromboembolus and to diagnose and treat immediately those who are already afflicted with thromboembolic disease. As in all practice of medicine, a comprehensive clinical assessment of the patient is the mainstay of diagnosis, and only after a rigorous clinical evaluation should adjunct studies including laboratory assessment, radiographic examination, nuclear imaging, and invasive procedures (including angiography) be accomplished. Only in the appropriate clinical circumstance can the results of these ancillary investigations be appropriately interpreted and a clear diagnosis made, thus resulting in precise, effective, and expeditious therapy.

The diagnostic evaluation of the patient with suspected deep vein thrombosis (DVT) and PE is rapidly changing as the result of clinical studies that clarify the relation between clinical features and the results of laboratory and imaging studies. The history and physical examination determine a clinical probability, which guides test selection and interpretation. Newly available diagnostic modalities allow greater diagnostic accuracy, lower cost, and greater convenience. New algorithms combine clinical features with ancillary measures such as the rapid enzyme-linked immunosorbent assay (ELISA) (VIDAS) D-dimer assay, compression ultrasonography, the ventilation/perfusion (V/Q) scan, and spiral computed tomographic imaging.

Morbidity and mortality studies indicate that 73% of PE cases diagnosed at autopsy were not detected clinically (1) and that PE has a mortality rate of 18% to 30% without treatment (2). More than 90% of PE cases arise from DVT, and as many as 50% of patients with leg symptoms are proven to have a diagnosis other than DVT (Table 11.1) (3–6). Classic symptoms for PE, such as pleuritic chest pain and hemoptysis, are not particularly useful in establishing the diagnosis of PE (2). Thus clinical features alone are inadequate for a firm diagnosis.

Although often viewed as distinct clinical entities, DVT and PE represent manifestations of a continuum of disease. More than 50% of cases (7) of PE may not have recognized sources of DVT. Many patients with proximal DVT have clinically silent PE. Symptomatic thrombi are usually found in proximal veins (8,9); however, at least 50% of PE occur in asymptomatic patients (10). Whereas the majority of DVT occurs in infrapopliteal veins, the primary source of PE is proximal DVT (3,11,12). Calf DVT propagates proximally in at least 20% to 30% of cases (12).

Predisposition to venous thromboembolic disease results from specific clinical conditions, and hereditary and acquired blood defects (13–17). High clinical probability occurs in malignancy, stasis, the postoperative state (especially orthopedic), sepsis, trauma, cardiac disease, burns, hematologic malignancy, immobility, pregnancy, and the use of estrogen-containing compounds. Hereditary and acquired blood protein defects include protein C and S deficiency, antithrombin (AT) deficiency, hyperhomocyst(e)inemia, factor V Leiden mutation (18–20), factor V Cambridge mutation (21), prothrombin G20210A mutation (22–24), antiphospholipid syndrome, lupus anticoagulant, heparin cofactor II deficiency, plasminogen defects,

R. L. Bick: Department of Medicine and Pathology, University of Texas Southwestern Medical Center; Dallas Thrombosis/Hemostasis Clinical Center; ThromboCare Laboratories, Dallas, Texas.

W. F. Baker, JR.: Department of Medicine, Center for Health Sciences, University of California at Los Angeles, Los Angeles, California; Department of Medicine, Kern Medical Center, Bakersfield, California; and California Clinical Thrombosis Center, Bakersfield, California.

TABLE 11.1. ALTERNATIVE DIAGNOSES IN PATIENTS WITH SUSPECTED LOWER EXTREMITY DEEP VEIN THROMBOSIS

Postphlebitic syndrome, varices
Congestive heart failure
Trauma
Direct twisting injury to the leg
Muscle strain with unaccustomed exercise
Muscle tear
Weber fracture of the ankle
Surgery
Blunt trauma with subfascial hematoma
Hematoma
Internal derangement of the knee
Venous reflux
Baker cyst
Cellulitis
Lymphangitis
Inguinal abcess
Malignancy with venous or lymphatic obstruction
Exacerbation of rheumatoid arthritis
Contact dermatitis
Gout
Erythema nodosum
Pregnancy
Paralysis
Superficial phlebitis

tissue plasminogen activator defects, plasminogen activator inhibitor defects, sticky platelet syndrome, dysfibrinogenemia, and factor XII defects (25–27). Successful diagnosis, treatment, and secondary prevention require definition and management of not only the thrombotic process but also the underlying risk factors.

THE HISTORY

A history and a physical examination that identify patients at risk are essential to diagnosis because the presenting signs and symptoms of DVT may be minimal, misleading, or absent. Wells et al. (28) demonstrated that [illegible]% of patients with high clinical probability are proven to have DVT, compared with only 5% with low pretest probability. Classically, the chief complaint in a patient with DVT is a painful, swollen leg. The location of the thrombus determines the location of swelling. In complete iliofemoral thrombosis, the entire leg is usually swollen distal to the site of thrombosis. In calf vein or partial occlusion, swelling may be more localized. Bilateral iliofemoral or vena caval thrombosis results in bilateral leg swelling. Unfortunately, other edema-forming states may cause a similar presentation. Pain resulting from focal inflammation at the site of thrombosis may suggest DVT; however, pain and tenderness also may occur with superficial venous thrombosis and other conditions, making the complaint of leg pain generally unreliable. Upper extremity swelling has fewer causes and may be more reliable as a symptom of thrombosis of the axillary–subclavian system, associated with mechanical impingement or cannulation of the subclavian vein.

The first presentation of DVT may be cardiovascular collapse, cardiorespiratory arrest, or sudden death due to PE (1,3). Particularly observed in the high-risk patient, this catastrophic presentation may occur without prodromal signs or symptoms. Symptoms of PE typically include the sudden onset of chest pain (especially pleuritic), shortness of breath, diaphoresis, and anxiety. The character of chest pain is particularly significant, as patients with constant pain have a much lower pretest probability of a positive V/Q scan (29). Paradoxic embolization through an atrial septal defect appears as a cerebrovascular accident. Uncommon presentations include fever of undetermined origin, unexplained dyspnea in the absence of other typical symptoms or signs, unexplained pelvic or abdominal pain, and upper extremity pain associated with shoulder abduction. PE without prodromal symptoms or signs usually results from DVT of the pelvic veins. Because interpretation of the V/Q scan is partly dependent on the identification of underlying chronic or acute lung disorders, symptoms of chronic lung disease and acute respiratory infections may be particularly relevant (30).

The medical history may indicate underlying risk factors or prior thrombotic events. The family history may identify hereditary blood defects or other medical illnesses predisposing to DVT. A family history of specific inherited coagulation defects may be unknown, because the laboratory-testing capabilities for many disorders have only recently been developed.

When evaluating the patient with a predisposition to thrombus formation or a suspected thrombotic event, one must first solicit a chief complaint including a detailed description of symptoms and how long the symptoms have been present. Subsequently, the patient should be questioned about other disease conditions, with emphasis on conditions and situations known to be associated with a predisposition to venous or arterial thrombotic events. The patient should be asked about oral contraceptive/hormone-replacement use; obesity; a history of malignancy; a history of abdominal, thoracic, obstetrical, or orthopedic surgery; pregnancy; heart disease; a history of venous thrombosis; and a history of chronic venous insufficiency or varicosities; and clinical suggestions of rare predisposing disorders such as Behçet syndrome and cystathionine β-synthetase deficiency, and so on. If a predisposition to arterial thrombotic events is suspected, the patient should be carefully questioned about the presence or absence of ischemic heart disease, hypertension, hypercholesterolemia, hyperlipidemia, obesity, tobacco smoking, hyperglycemia, peripheral vascular occlusive disease, a history of myocardial infarction, history of angina, history of high dietary fat intake, lack of exercise, and a history of the use of oral contraceptives, both estrogenic and progestational. The presence or absence of obesity and the gender of the patient also may be relevant.

After this, inquiry about associated disease conditions known to be associated with an enhanced predisposition to venous or arterial thrombotic events should be instituted; the patient should be questioned about regular drug intake, with particular attention to the use of contraceptive agents, estrogens, or progestational agents. A history regarding the use of aspirin, aspirin-containing compounds, antihypertensives, cough medications, digitalis, hormones, cortisone, insulin, diabetic medications, thyroid medications, analgesics, weight-reducing pills, anticoagulants (including antiplatelet agents), dilantin, diuretics, antibiotics, barbiturates, tranquilizers, or antidepressants also must be elicited.

The presence or absence of a medical history of angina, coronary artery disease, heart disease, diabetes, emphysema, recurrent bronchitis, recurrent pneumonia, asthma, tuberculosis, herpes zoster, measles, mumps, chicken pox, rheumatic fever, scarlet fever, hepatitis, peptic ulcer disease, liver disease, jaundice, renal disease, hives, venereal disease, anemia, seizures, or mental disease, including a history of chronic venous insufficiency, a history of any type of arterial or venous thrombotic event, or a history of varicosities should be noted. A rigorous surgical history should be obtained, particularly an immediate past surgical history for abdominal, thoracic, gynecologic, or orthopedic surgery. The patient should be questioned about any recent injuries or accidents, especially those involving the extremities or chest. The patient should be asked about any known allergy to medications or any other agents.

After this, a review of systems should include a personal history of generalized weakness, fevers, chills, skin rashes, poorly healing sores, enlarging moles, chills, drenching night sweats, weight loss, loss of appetite, recurrent localized headaches, dizzy spells, or any unexplored loss of consciousness. A careful history of blurred vision, double vision, persistent scotomata, tinnitus, hearing loss, lateralization of hearing, or sore tongue should be noted. The patient also must be queried about gingival bleeding with tooth brushing, the presence of dentures, frequent upper respiratory infections, difficulty swallowing, unexplained hoarseness, cervical pain, or the noting of supraclavicular, cervical, submental, axillary, epitrochlear, inguinal, or deep iliac adenopathy. The patient should be questioned about productive cough, hemoptysis, blood-tinged sputum, coughing episodes, dyspnea at rest or exertion, angina or other types of chest pain, a history of heart disease, hypertension, or the presence of tachycardia, palpitations, or ankle edema. The patient also should be questioned concerning frequent preprandial or postprandial epigastric distress, epigastric pain, nausea, emesis, hematemesis, melena, hematochezia, or deviations in bowel habits within the last 6 months. A genitourinary history must encompass a history of burning or stinging on urination, nocturia, hematuria, port wine– or root beer–colored urine, and a history of renal stones or renal disease. A history of joint pain, back pain, or bone pain also should be noted.

In the female patient, the age at onset of menses and the age at first pregnancy should be recorded. The presence or absence of continued menses also should be noted, including the date of the last menstrual period and the year menses stopped, whether naturally or by surgical means. The patient must be painstakingly questioned about ingesting any type of oral contraceptives, and the exact nature of these contraceptives and when they were stopped, if discontinued, should be documented. The female patient also should be questioned about excessive vaginal discharge, recurrent vaginal infections, intramenstrual bleeding, or the noting of lumps, discharge, or irritation of her breasts. The date of the last Pap smear and pelvic examination should be obtained. After this a pregnancy history should be taken, including number of pregnancies, number of miscarriages, number of premature births, number of children born alive, number and nature of cesarean sections, number of stillborns, number of abortions, and any potential complications of pregnancy including any suspicion of preeclampsia or eclampsia, the blood pressure during these episodes, and any thrombotic problems. Male patients should be questioned about difficulty in starting the urinary stream, a history of prostatic disease, and type of prostatic disease if present.

After this, a personal history should be accomplished, including a detailed smoking history incorporating the amount smoked per day, and whether the patient smokes cigarettes, pipe, cigars, or uses snuff or chewing tobacco. An ethanol history including the amount ingested per day and the type of ethanol consumed should be noted. A diligent dietary history should be obtained including any special diets or food faddism. A detailed occupational history should be obtained including careful inquiry into the potential exposure to radiation, carbon tetrachloride, benzene, industrial toxins, lead, asbestos, and pesticides. In addition, any potential injuries, particularly to the extremities and chest, should be recorded.

A family history should include the presence or absence of any venous or arterial thrombotic events, PE, or the presence of hypertension, cerebrovascular thrombotic or ischemic events, renal disease, the presence or absence of myocardial infarction or any other situations known to be associated with increased family risk. The patient also should be asked about the general health of the spouse and children. A family history of cerebrovascular thrombosis, hypertension, tuberculosis, diabetes mellitus, thyroid disease including goiter, gout, arthritis, any type of bleeding or thrombotic trends, coronary artery disease, pulmonary disease including PE, the existence of gastrointestinal disease including gastric or duodenal ulcer, ulcerative colitis, renal disease, anemia, or other hematologic disease is noted.

PHYSICAL EXAMINATION

As often as 50% of the time, the physical examination of patients with DVT and PE is misleading (4–6,31). The classic signs of leg edema, erythema, increased warmth, a palpable cord, positive Homan sign, and tenderness occur relatively infrequently. There may be evidence of unilateral edema or tenderness without other signs. Hull et al. (32) noted that in symptomatic patients, DVT is confirmed in only 59% of those with leg pain, tenderness, and swelling; 22% with pain and tenderness; and 11% of patients with isolated leg swelling.

Chronic lower extremity edema, stasis dermatitis, and stasis ulcers may result from recurrent lower extremity or pelvic DVT. Acute DVT may be mimicked by the postphlebitic syndrome, which results in dependent swelling and calf fullness made worse by prolonged standing and walking but relieved by rest and leg elevation (33,34). Unfortunately, PE may occur without signs of DVT in the lower extremities (1,10,12,35).

PE typically occurs with apprehension, diaphoresis, tachycardia, and a rapid respiratory rate. A vast array of physical signs may be observed in patients with illnesses predisposing to DVT and PE. Establishing the diagnosis of an underlying disease may be as important as confirming the presence of thrombosis.

Landefeld et al. (36,37), Wells et al. (38), and Michiels (39) have quantified the risk associated with selected clinical findings and have ranked these according to the clinical probability of a positive venographic study for DVT. Michielis designed a scoring system for clinical features, which may assist the clinician in assigning clinical probability. One point each is assigned to (a) active cancer treatment (current, within 6 months, palliative); (b) paralysis, paresis, or immobilization of the lower extremities; (c) generalized immobilization for longer than 3 days or major surgery within 4 days; (d) focal tenderness and/or pain corresponding to the distribution of deep veins; (e) generalized leg edema, calf swelling (measured 10 cm below the tibial tuberosity), with the symptomatic leg more than 2 cm larger than the asymptomatic leg; (f) pitting edema more prominent in the symptomatic leg; or (g) the presence of collateral superficial veins. Low pretest clinical probability (PCP) is a score of 0; moderate, a score of 1 to 2; and high is greater than 3 (39). Diagnostic evaluation can be specifically designed for the degree of clinical probability.

The physical examination should begin with an evaluation of body habitus and general health, with the noting of obesity, muscle wasting, skin complexion, skin turgor, and general hygiene. After this, the vital signs are recorded including the height; weight; temperature; sitting, standing, and supine blood pressure; and the pulse, including character and regularity. Next, the head is examined for subcutaneous nodules in the scalp, followed by search of occipital, periauricular, cervical, submental, or supraclavicular lymphadenopathy. The pupils are assessed for reactivity to light and accommodation, and the palpebral and bulbar conjunctivae are evaluated. The equality of the pupils should be noted. A funduscopic examination follows; if a PE is suspected, the detection of retinal venous dilation is indicative of a pulmonary artery pressure greater than 30 mm Hg. Hearing should be appraised and both Weber and Rinne testing performed. Weber testing may lateralize in the presence of transient ischemic attacks (TIAs), small stroke syndromes, or a frank cerebrovascular thrombotic event. The oral mucosa is explored, including the sublingual area, for vascular anomalies. The carotid pulses should be evaluated and auscultated for bruits. The noting of jugular venous distention suggests a pulmonary artery pressure of more than 30 to 35 mm Hg and may indicate a sizable PE in the appropriate clinical setting. The patient should be assessed for sternal tenderness, rib tenderness, cervical tenderness, thoracic tenderness, lumbosacral spine tenderness, and costovertebral angle tenderness. The chest should be auscultated and percussed, and diaphragmatic excursion should be noted. The prevalent physical findings of a patient with a PE may be unremarkable, or one may note findings compatible with pleural effusion; there may be tachypnea, localized inspiratory wheezing, rhonchi, or rales. A pleural friction rub, findings of consolidation, or as mentioned, findings harmonious with pleural effusion may be found; there may be increased tactile fremitus, dullness to percussion, or tubular breath sounds. An evaluation of the heart must be accomplished, with noting of heart sounds, murmurs, and findings suggestive of acute cor pulmonale, including a right ventricular heave, a right-sided gallop, accentuated second heart sound, or a murmur of tricuspid insufficiency. Distended jugular veins and a positive hepatojugular reflex should be recorded when conjecturing a PE. These findings are suggestive of increased pulmonary artery pressure. After evaluation of the heart, the peripheral pulses including the brachial pulse, radial pulse, ulnar pulse, and femoral, popliteal, dorsalis pedis, and posterior tibial pulses are noted. Both the femoral arteries and the aorta should be auscultated for the presence or absence of murmurs. The popliteal pulse, posterior tibial pulse, and dorsalis pedis pulses are customarily evaluated with assessment of the extremities.

After the cardiorespiratory evaluation, the abdomen is evaluated for tenderness, bowel sounds, the presence of hepatomegaly, hepatic tenderness, splenomegaly, splenic tenderness, costovertebral angle tenderness or bruits, and the presence of abdominal masses. A rectal examination is performed unless there is a contraindication. In male patients, prostatic enlargement and localized tenderness are noted, and analysis of the stool for occult blood should be done in all patients undergoing rectal examination. After the rectal examination, the genitalia are examined, including noting of testicular swelling or tenderness in men, and a pelvic in women is done, unless recently performed by the primary care physician. Evaluation of the extremities is important in a patient with suspected venous thrombosis, because the physical findings of DVT are unreliable; however, reliability is increased by careful evaluation. The presence of chronic venous insufficiency including varicosities, ankle edema, and chronic hemosiderin deposits should be carefully searched for and noted. Popliteal pulses, dorsalis pedis pulses, and posterior tibial pulses are assessed for presence and intensity. The toes and toenails should be sufficiently examined for evidence of pallor, cyanosis, chronic ulcerative changes, or chronic atrophic changes suggestive of chronic vascular insufficiency. Capillary refill should be recorded. The inguinal areas, anterior medial thighs, popliteal fossae, and calves should be carefully evaluated for evidence of erythema, tenderness, swelling, hyperpyrexia, or a frank venous cord. In this regard, the palpation of a distinct cord is the most dependable physical finding of a venous thrombus; however, detection of a demonstrable increase in diameter of the calf, popliteal area, or thigh, and associated edema also is a reliable finding. Alternatively, the presence or absence of Homan sign is less reliable. It must be recollected that in the presence of substantial venous thrombosis, there may be a compartmental compression syndrome, either anterior tibial, posterior tibial, or a compartmental compression syndrome of the thigh (extensor or flexor compartment), and with this, there may be arterial and neurologic (neurovascular bundle impairment) compromise with not only extreme pain, cyanosis, redness, swelling, and tenderness in the area of a cord noted in association with venous disease, but also interference with arterial vascular flow, leading to more cyanosis, pallor, intensified swelling, and a dull persistent ache in conjunction with decreased or absent pulses by palpation; the pulses however, are usually demonstrable by Doppler.

Subsequent to a careful evaluation of the extremities for the physical findings of venous thrombosis or arterial disease, an inspection of the integument should be performed, looking for the presence of petechiae, purpura, ecchymoses, or any unexplained cyanosis, edema, clubbing, discoloration, or unexplained rash. A careful neurologic examination should be performed and not only should the cerebrum and cerebellum be assessed but also the cranial nerves, the biceps, triceps, and ulnar reflexes and the patellar and Achilles reflexes. In addition, pinpoint sensation, two-point sensation, and vibratory sensation should be appraised.

Ancillary studies are customarily required when assessing patients who are hypercoagulable or are suspected of having venous or arterial thrombotic or thromboembolic events or PE. With respect to PE, ancillary diagnostic aids are readily available; however, they must be interpreted in the appropriate clinical setting. Usually one will note elevated enzymes including lactate dehydrogenase (LDH), aspartate aminotransferase (SGOT), and creatine phosphokinase (CPK); however, these are nonspecific findings. Close to 90% of patients with a PE will have a PO_2 of less than 80 mm Hg. Further laboratory tests often found positive are elevated fibrin(ogen) degradation products and D-dimer, circulating soluble fibrin monomer by ELISA (so-called thrombin precursor protein), and depressed AT-III, protein C and protein S. Moreover, elevated fibrinopeptide A and B levels and elevated platelet factor 4 and β-thromboglobulin levels are frequently observed in patients with PE or extensive DVT. A baseline electrocardiogram (ECG) should always be done in a patient with venous thrombosis or suspected PE. The ECG may be normal in PE; more typically, the ECG will exhibit findings of acute cor pulmonale and right ventricular failure. Usually a sinus tachycardia will be present; however, transient atrial premature systoles, atrial flutter, or atrial fibrillation also may be present in the presence of a PE. The extremity leads commonly show an S_1Q_3 pattern, having a deep S wave in lead 1, a prominent Q wave, an inverted T wave in lead 3, and depression of ST segments in leads 2 and 1. The precordial leads will often show T-wave inversions in right precordial leads, a complete or incomplete right bundle branch block, and a QR pattern in leads V_3, V_1, and V_2, in association with negative T waves. Because of widespread myocardial ischemia, the precordial leads also may show ST-segment depressions or T-wave inversions. The following patterns are strongly suggestive of an acute PE and acute right heart failure: $S_1Q_3T_3$ pattern associated with T-wave inversion in the right precordial leads, and S_1T_3 pattern or T-wave inversion in lead 3 and the right precordial leads, and an $S_1Q_3T_3$ pattern in association with a complete or incomplete right bundle branch block.

A baseline chest radiograph must always be obtained in patients with suspected thrombus or PE. Most individuals with a PE will have an abnormal chest radiograph, albeit in numerous findings, these are not diagnostic. The most common defect found is that of a patchy infiltrate; however, characteristic humped-shaped infarcts at the lung base or in other areas of the pulmonary parenchyma also may be found. Less commonly, a pleural effusion will be noted; there may be local constriction of pulmonary vessels and fullness of pulmonary arteries at the hilus. There may be an area of oligemia (Westermark sign). These findings must be correlated with V/Q lung scans. Customarily one will note perfusion defects in the same areas as pulmonary infiltrates; if the pulmonary infiltrate is smaller than the perfusion defect, a PE is probable. Alternatively, if the infiltrative anomaly on the chest radiograph is larger than the perfusion defect, the probability of PE is doubtful. Ventilation scans of low probability for a PE are those showing single or multiple defects less than 3 to 4 cm in diameter or, as mentioned, a perfusion defect that is smaller than a radiographic infiltrate. However, the presence of a perfusion defect that is larger than a radiographic infiltrate or a perfusion defect that is larger than a segment in size may be considered positive. Perfusion defects equal to or smaller than chest radiograph infiltrates fall into an intermediate probability category, and in this instance, the patient should be treated as having a PE or should be subjected to pulmonary angiography (PA) if the findings will modify the therapy being proposed for the patient. The noting of a normal V/Q lung scan is strong evidence that the patient has not sustained a PE. However, the finding of a normal chest radiograph is not evidence for the absence of a PE, and when appropriate clinical suspicion is aroused, a V/Q scan must always be performed.

About 95% of PEs arise from DVTs of the lower extremities; these venous thrombi are most commonly proximal to the popliteal vein and are less commonly noted to be present in the calf veins. However, a PE arising from calf veins is much more common than often appreciated. When a patient has a documented PE, a search for presence or absence of venous thrombi should be done. PEs may sporadically arise from thrombi in the subclavian, basilic, or ovarian veins and the inferior vena cava. Alternatively, in the patient without a PE but with only clinically suspected DVT, confirmatory procedures must be performed. There are associated difficulties with some invasive procedures; the radioactive fibrinogen scan is associated with a high incidence of false negatives and false positives and is insensitive to thrombi above the lower thigh because of increased radioactive background activity in the pelvic vessels and bladder. Positive results also will emanate from perivascular hemorrhage or inflammation. Furthermore, radioactive fibrinogen scanning cannot discriminate between old and new thrombi. Doppler ultrasonography is of high reliability, except for lesions below the knee; however, the results may be influenced by collateral circulation and venous recanalization. Doppler techniques are discussed subsequently. Contrast venography is a time-tested technique to prove venous thrombi of the lower extremities; however, the method is exceedingly painful and time consuming, is associated with allergic reactions, and Doppler appears just as reliable. An associated 10% incidence of postvenogram venous thrombosis may occur.

SUPPORTIVE DIAGNOSTIC MODALITIES

Clinical criteria alone are not adequate to establish the diagnosis of DVT or PE. The Prospective Investigation of Pulmonary Embolism Diagnosis (PIOPED) study of patients with suspected PE determined that if the pretest clinical probability of PE was 80% to 100% (10% of patients), the diagnosis was correctly predicted in only 68%. When the clinical probability was none to 19% (26% of patients), PE was excluded in 91%. Unfortunately, in the majority of patients (64%), the clinical diagnosis was noncommittal (20% to 79% probability of PE) (40,41). The PIOPED study clearly demonstrates that pretest probability correlates primarily with negative diagnostic studies. The recent development of the highly sensitive, automated, rapid ELISA (VIDAS) D-dimer assay, however, with a negative predictive value of 99.5% to 100%, may profoundly affect the approach to suspected venous thromboembolism (39, 42–45). The reference standards for diagnosis are ascending contrast venography and PA, respectively. Impedance plethysmography, Doppler flow analysis, and radiolabeled fibrinogen uptake have been replaced by compression ultrasound (US) and color flow Duplex imaging for DVT. Spiral computed tomographic imaging has been added to the diagnostic armamentarium for the diagnosis of PE.

Deep Vein Thrombosis

Real-time B-mode Compression Ultrasound

Real-time B-mode compression ultrasound (CUS) is the imaging modality of choice for the diagnosis of proximal DVT. The primary diagnostic finding is the presence (normal) or absence (thrombosis) of compressibility of the vein. Useful findings also include the lack of movement of the venous valves and walls with direct pressure and maneuvers such as respiration and Valsalva. The external iliac, common femoral, and popliteal veins are examined. The veins of the calf may be excluded from examination because of the low sensitivity to calf thrombi (9,46–49).

Numerous investigators have confirmed that CUS is nearly 100% sensitive and specific for the diagnosis of proximal DVT (47,49,50–52). CUS fails to identify calf thrombi adequately (less than 50% sensitivity) (49,53,54); however, only 20% to 30% of calf thrombi extend proximally, and these are rarely asymptomatic (12). Follow-up studies performed 7 days after an initially negative CUS have identified only 1% (51) to 1.4% (52) of patients with the subsequent development of DVT. The incidence of PE in the patients who were treated without anticoagulation based on the negative US was only 0.7% in the study by Cogo et al. (51) and 0.6% in the series of Birdwell et al. (52).

CUS is limited by the inaccuracy in detecting pelvic DVT and the relatively low sensitivity and specificity in asymptomatic patients. False-negative CUS may occur as the result of (a) thrombosis involving less than 3 cm of the distal popliteal vein; (b) a single-lumen thrombosis of a duplicate popliteal vein; (c) edema; (d) distortion of the venous anatomy due to malignancy or cellulitis; (e) common femoral vein involvement by a short tail of thrombus originating in the deep femoral vein; and (f) unknown reasons (50,55).

Repeated CUS, after an initially negative study, may be indicated in symptomatic hospitalized patients (39,50) and in symptomatic outpatients (55), particularly in the setting of high clinical probability and a positive D-dimer assay. In clinical situations in which the diagnosis of pelvic or calf vein thrombosis is critical, or if there is particularly poor laboratory-to-clinical correlation, contrast venography or magnetic resonance imaging (MRI) may be required. CUS also may be included in the diagnostic evaluation of patients with intermediate-probability V/Q lung scans.

Real-time B-mode Ultrasound with Color Doppler (Duplex Scanning)

Improvement in the diagnostic accuracy and specificity of standard CUS may result from enhancement of B-mode US with color Doppler (Duplex). US analysis augmented by color Doppler analysis with a 3- to 5-mHz Doppler transducer compares favorably with contrast venography (50). The Doppler component allows the examiner to determine areas of abnormality and focus on changes in blood-flow spontaneity, phasicity, and augmentation. Venous patency is confirmed by normal phasic flow signals and obliteration of the venous lumen by direct compression of the vein with the transducer. Thrombotic venous occlusion eliminates normal Doppler signals, and the lumen is rendered noncompressible with direct pressure. Nonocclusive clots result in partial obliteration of the lumen with pressure and continuous (rather than phasic) venous signals. Evaluation of calf veins requires foot compression and monitoring of signals from the posterior tibial vein. Very recent thrombi resemble flowing blood with Doppler and are compressible with CUS. Older clots are not compressible and are somewhat less echogenic (56).

As with CUS, Duplex is 97% to 100% sensitive and specific in symptomatic patients with proximal DVT (50). Numerous studies also have demonstrated that Duplex scanning is not cost effective for screening high-risk, asymptomatic patients and should primarily be applied in patients with symptoms (57,58).

Ascending Contrast Venography

The radiocontrast venogram remains the reference standard for the diagnosis of DVT (32,57). Although highly reliable, ascending contrast venography is limited by the difficulty encountered in venous cannulation and a patient history of allergy to iodine or radiocontrast media. As many as 20% of hospitalized patients may not be suitable candidates for study (59). In addition, thrombogenicity of iodinated radiocontrast results in a 2% to 4% risk of developing DVT from the procedure (60).

Magnetic Resonance Imaging

MRI is primarily used for the diagnosis of DVT in pregnant women. The diagnostic evaluation of lower extremity edema in this group is often difficult, and the risk of DVT in pregnancy is high. Spitzer et al. (61) applied MRI and determined a sensitivity for detecting thrombi of 87% in the calf and 97% to 100% above the knee. MRI also may be useful in the patient with suspected pelvic, iliac, or caval thrombosis, in spite of a negative venous Duplex scan of the lower extremities (62).

Pulmonary Embolism

Chest Radiograph

Chest radiography is usually of little or no value in confirming the diagnosis of PE. Approximately 40% of patients with PE have a normal chest radiograph. Classic abnormalities include the "cut-off" sign of central pulmonary artery occlusion with increased lucency of the lung field, atelectasis, small pleural effusions, and a pleural-based, wedge-shaped density of pulmonary infarction (63). In the majority of patients, the chest radiograph is primarily of value in suggesting alternative diagnoses and in clarifying the etiology of matching defects on the V/Q scan.

Electrocardiogram

The ECG of a patient with PE usually is normal or reveals sinus tachycardia. The classic findings of S_1T_3, T inversion in the right precordial leads, right axis deviation, and incomplete or complete bundle branch block due to right ventricular enlargement and strain may be observed but are not diagnostic (64). Most often, the ECG serves as an indicator of underlying illness and is infrequently of value in confirming the diagnosis of PE.

Arterial Blood Gas

Reliance on the arterial blood gas for useful diagnostic information is perhaps the most common mistake in evaluating the patient with suspected PE. Patients with acute PE may have both matching and nonmatching abnormalities of ventilation and perfusion, and many have underlying disease as a cause of an abnormal arterial blood gas. Characteristic findings include a decrease in the normal PO_2 and PCO_2, and thus a widening of the arterial–alveolar oxygen gradient accompanied by an alkalotic pH. Among PE patients with no prior cardiopulmonary disease, 30% or more will have a PO_2 greater than 80 mm Hg (63). A normal blood gas does not exclude PE, and an abnormal result does not confirm PE.

Ventilation/Perfusion Lung Scan

V/Q is the diagnostic procedure of choice to confirm a suspected PE. Perfusion scanning is performed by venous administration of isotopically labeled macroaggregates of human albumin. Ventilation scanning involves the inhalation of aerosols of either ^{127}Xe or technetium. A normal scan exhibits homogeneous and matching distribution of the aerosol and the macroaggregated albumin throughout both lungs.

The degree of V/Q match guides interpretation. Scans consistent with PE exhibit areas of V/Q mismatch characterized by absence of perfusion in the presence of normal ventilation. Matching defects are typical of lung disease. Peripherally based, large perfusion defects in areas of normal ventilation are strongly suggestive of PE, whereas matching, small, central or ill-defined defects are less likely to represent PE. The scans are interpreted as high probability, intermediate probability, low probability, very low probability, or normal, as defined by PIOPED criteria (40). Pretest clinical suspicion plays a major role in establishing the diagnosis. With a strong pretest suggestion of PE and a high probability scan, the V/Q is 96% accurate in identifying PE. A moderate clinical probability combined with a high-probability scan confirms PE in only 80% to 88% of cases (33,40,65). The primary challenge has been to develop management strategies for patients with intermediate-probability scans, because patients with high to moderately high clinical suspicion and high-probability scans represent only 12% to 32% of patients with abnormal scans. Among patients with a low clinical suspicion and high-probability scan, only 56% are confirmed to have PE. Fewer than 6% of patients with low clinical suspicion of PE and a low-probability scan will be determined to have a PE (40).

High pretest probability and a high-probability scan as well as low pretest probability and a low-probability scan reliably confirm the diagnosis and guide therapy. Remaining is the more than 50% of patients for whom the diagnosis is not clear, based on the clinical findings and V/Q result (30).

Pulmonary Angiography

PA is the primary reference standard for diagnosis of PE. Analysis of the PIOPED data has demonstrated that PA is about 98% accurate for the diagnosis of PE (40). Although the error rate is low, in the selected patient with ongoing clinical indications of thromboembolic disease, further evaluation may be indicated (41,62,63). As an invasive procedure, PA is not without risk of complications (66). Accepted morbidity and mortality rates (due to severe allergic reactions to radiocontrast, cardiac perforation, and serious cardiac arrhythmias) are 0.2% and 1.9%, respectively (67).

Clearly the risk of failure to diagnose PE is great, and the risk/benefit ratio of PA must be weighed in each patient. Oudkerk et al. (67) concluded that the inclusion of PA in a diagnostic algorithm was important and cost effective. PA was most useful when performed in patients with non–high-probability scans and normal leg US (67). The consensus of most proposals has been that PA should be performed whenever the V/Q is interpreted as intermediate or low probability, the leg US is normal, the clinical probability is intermediate or high, and the D-dimer assay is abnormal. PA also has been recommended whenever there is a strong clinical indication of PE, even in the absence of a positive V/Q or US (67–69).

Spiral Computed Tomographic Angiography

Spiral CT angiography (SCTA) is a noninvasive alternative to PA that provides three-dimensional visualization of pulmonary thromboemboli. Sensitivity for diagnosis of PE with SCTA is 95.5% (range, 64% to 100%), with a specificity of 97.6% (range, 89% to 100%) (70,71). When PEs are confined to subsegmental pulmonary arteries, sensitivity is lower (as low as 36%) (70,72). Subsegmental emboli have been demonstrated in as many as 30% of patients with intermediate-probability V/Q scans (70). Stein and Henry (73) resolved the concern regarding subsegmental emboli, noting that only 6% of PEs detected among all PIOPED patients were subsegmental and that these corresponded to low-probability V/Q scans.

Evaluation of a diagnostic algorithm for the diagnosis of PE, proposed by van Erkel et al. (70) in 1996, confirmed that SCTA could be an important component of the best approach to diagnosis. D-dimer was used to exclude DVT and PE, and SCTA was used to confirm PE in all patients with non–high-probability V/Q scans. Both clinical outcome and cost-effectiveness data were superior to those of other approaches (70). Subsequent studies have confirmed the superiority of SCTA over V/Q scanning for the diagnosis of PE. Mayo et al. (74) compared SCTA and V/Q scanning, determining sensitivity and specificity for CTA of 95% and 94% versus 87% and 65% for V/Q scanning (74). Garg et al. (75) compared the two modalities and clearly demonstrated the superiority of CTA over V/Q scanning. SCTA exhibited greater accuracy and specificity and was recommended as the primary screening technique for PE. Notably, SCTA provided significant, clinically useful information not available from V/Q scanning, as old clots were distinguishable from new, and an alternative diagnosis was established in 31% of patients (75). Cross et al. (76) performed a similar analysis and recommended that SCTA replace V/Q scanning as the initial diagnostic study in patients with suspected PE.

LABORATORY EVALUATION

Few laboratory studies are particularly useful in confirming suspected DVT or PE. The complete blood count and chemistry analysis are of little value in diagnosis of DVT and PE but may aid considerably in the identification of underlying illness predisposing to or initiating thrombosis. Only the D-dimer assay and AT level are useful in evaluating a patient for suspected DVT or PE.

The AT level [normal, 85% to 125% of normal human plasma (NHP)] is diminished to a degree corresponding to the severity of thrombosis, as AT binds to thrombin. The AT level should be obtained in patients suspected of having DVT as a diagnostic adjunct and to assess the suitability for heparin therapy (77).

The D-dimer assay of the end products of cross-linked fibrin degradation by plasmin has emerged as an important tool for the diagnosis of suspected DVT and PE (29). Numerous reports have indicated the considerable diagnostic value of the D-dimer assay as an indicator of active thrombosis (45,78,79). Wells et al. (44) reported a D-dimer sensitivity of 93% for proximal DVT, 70% for calf DVT, an overall specificity of 77%, and a negative predictive value of

98% for proximal DVT (44). Becker et al. (80) presented an analysis of 29 studies that evaluated the use of the D-dimer test for diagnosis of venous thromboembolism. These studies used the (SimpliRed) semiquantitative whole-blood agglutination assay.

Janssen et al. (41,43), Freyburger et al. (42), de Moerloose et al. (81), D'Angelo et al. (82), Reber et al. (83), and Perrier et al. (84,85) analyzed application of the automated rapid ELISA (VIDAS) D-dimer assay for the exclusion of venous thromboembolism. Remarkably, 99.5% to 100% negative predictive value was determined for the exclusion of DVT and PE. These results remain to be confirmed in a prospective multicenter United States trial of outpatients with suspected DVT and PE; however, it is clear that the significance of such a sensitive and readily available assay may dramatically change the approach to diagnosis of DVT and PE. As Michiels (39,69) noted, the algorithms proposed for diagnosis must be necessarily altered in light of the essentially 100% negative predictive value of the rapid ELISA (VIDAS) D-dimer assay. Regardless of the clinical probability, the diagnoses of DVT and PE are excluded in patients with a negative rapid ELISA (VIDAS) D-dimer (39,41–45,69). In the United States, the (VIDAS) ELISA assay, from BioMerieux Vitek, Inc., is not readily available. The SimpliRed latex assay is of considerable value, however, because the sensitivity is only 95%; confirmatory testing is still required, and anticoagulation cannot be withheld solely on the basis of the D-dimer result (86). Other D-dimer assays, such as Asserchrome and Fibrinostica, are not similarly useful. With the (VIDAS) ELISA D-dimer assay, it appears that many venous CUSs and V/Q scans may be avoided, anticoagulation withheld, and hospitalizations unnecessary, at remarkable cost savings.

RECOMMENDED DIAGNOSTIC STRATEGIES

The evaluation of the patient with suspected DVT or PE begins with a thorough history and physical examination. A clinical probability is then developed to guide the selection of diagnostic studies. Test results are interpreted with knowledge of the clinical context and the outcome of other studies. Figures 11.1 through 11.6 illustrate various approaches to suspected DVT and PE. The algorithms in Figs. 11.1 through 11.3 reflect use of the D-dimer assay most widely available in the United States and with the

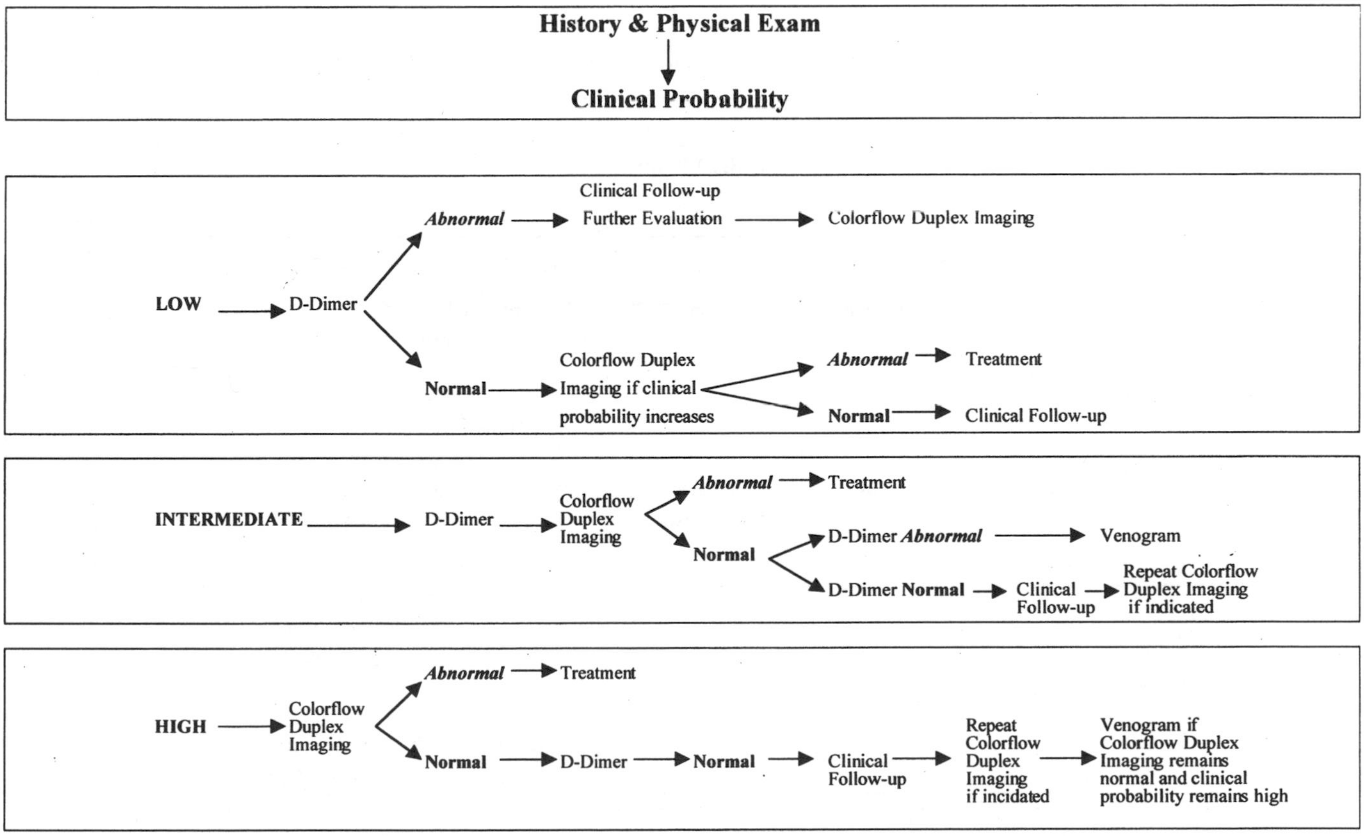

FIGURE 11.1. Diagnostic evaluation for suspected deep vein thrombosis.

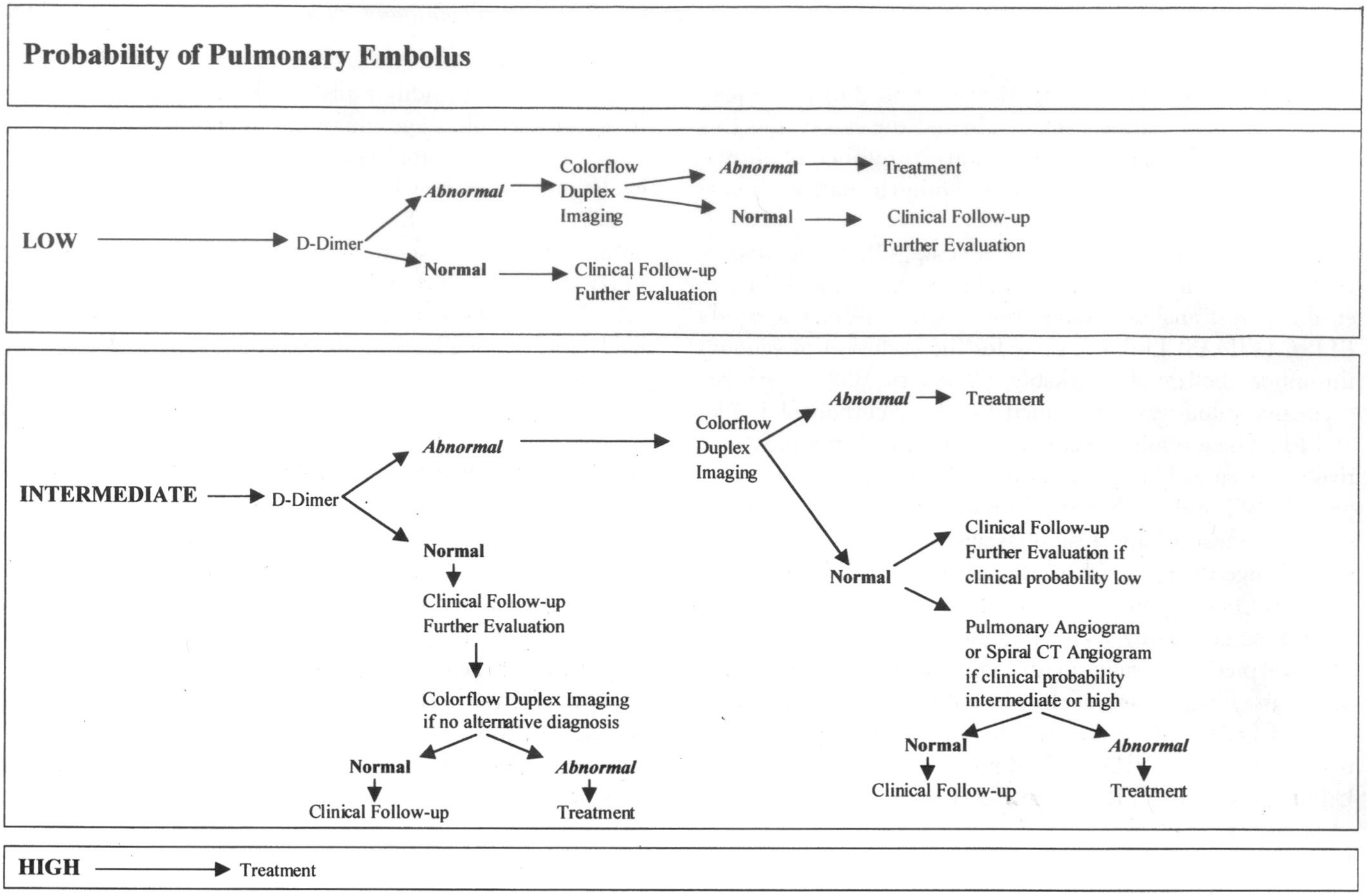

FIGURE 11.2. Ventilation/perfusion scan diagnosis of pulmonary embolus.

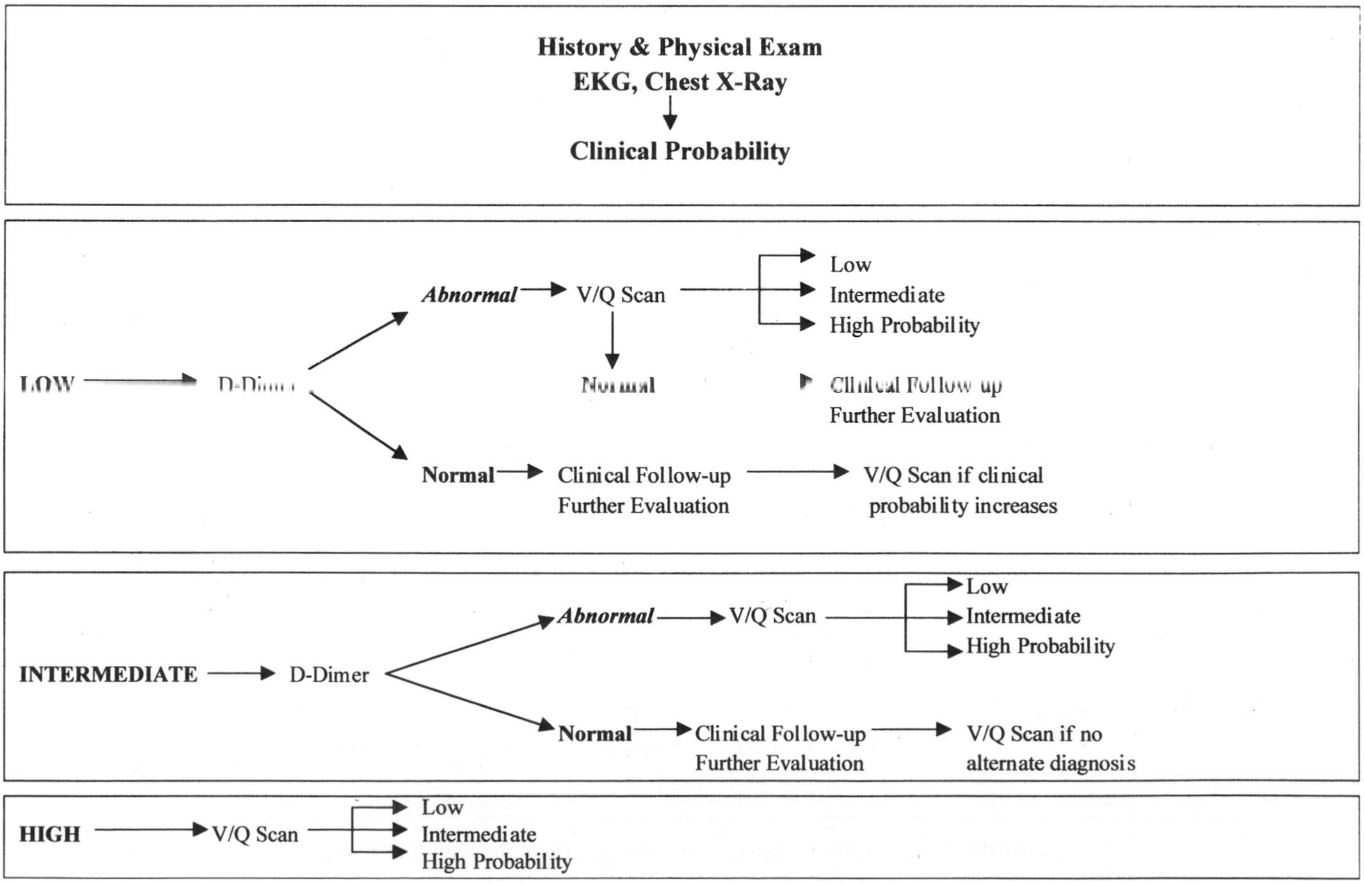

FIGURE 11.3. Diagnostic evaluation for suspected pulmonary embolus.

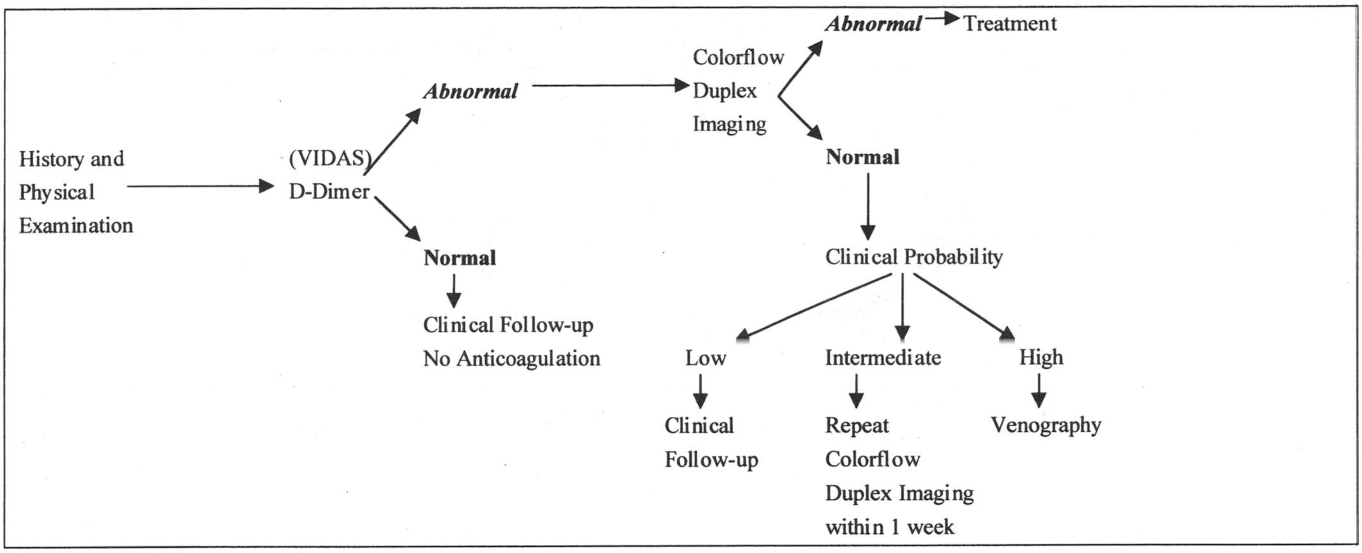

FIGURE 11.4. D-dimer–directed evaluation for suspected deep vein thrombosis.

highest negative predictive value (SimpliRed). Figures 11.4 and 11.5 incorporate the rapid ELISA (VIDAS) D-dimer assay as the primary screening instrument.

Clinical probability and the results of the D-dimer assay [normal rapid (VIDAS) ELISA D-dimer is less than 500 μg/L] direct the algorithm. The diagnosis must always be confirmed by clinical follow-up and may require serial testing. In the algorithms, CUS may be used interchangeably with Duplex. The indication for repeated imaging with Duplex has been extensively reviewed (39,51–54). Repeated imaging is indicated primarily in patients with high clinical probability, an initially negative Duplex, and continuing symptoms, even

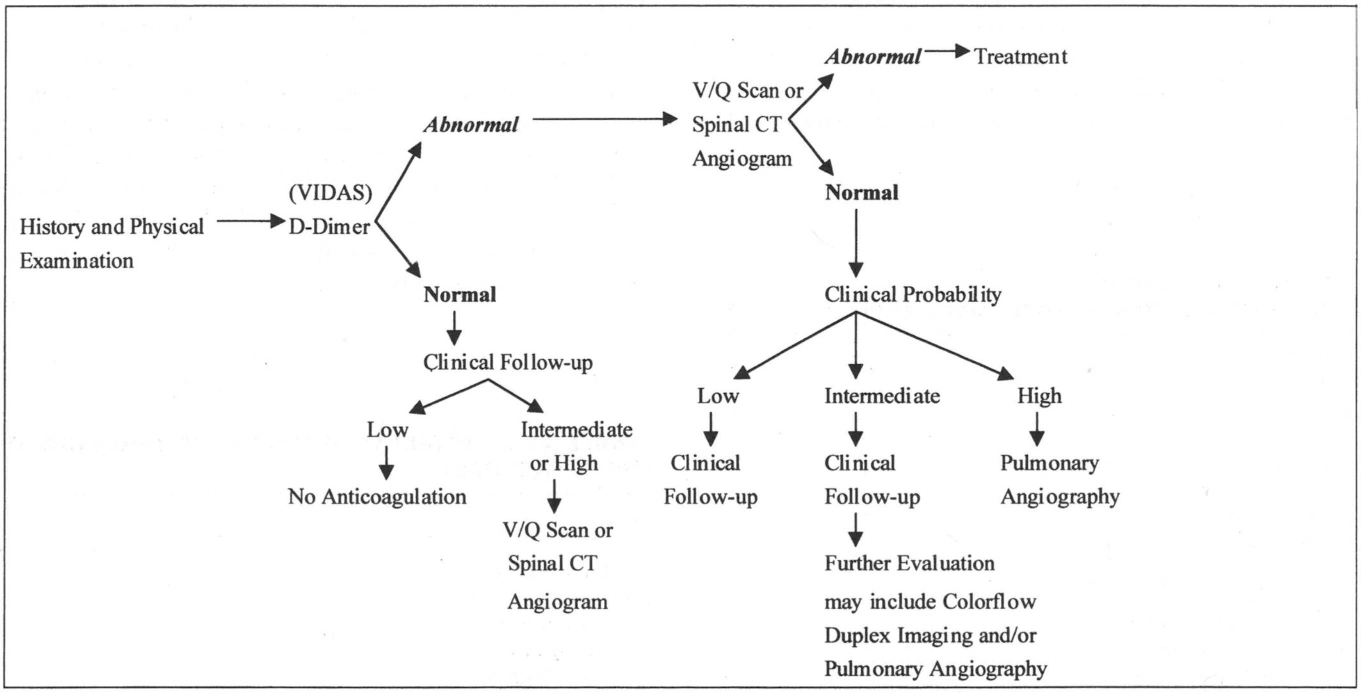

FIGURE 11.5. D-dimer evaluation for suspected pulmonary embolus.

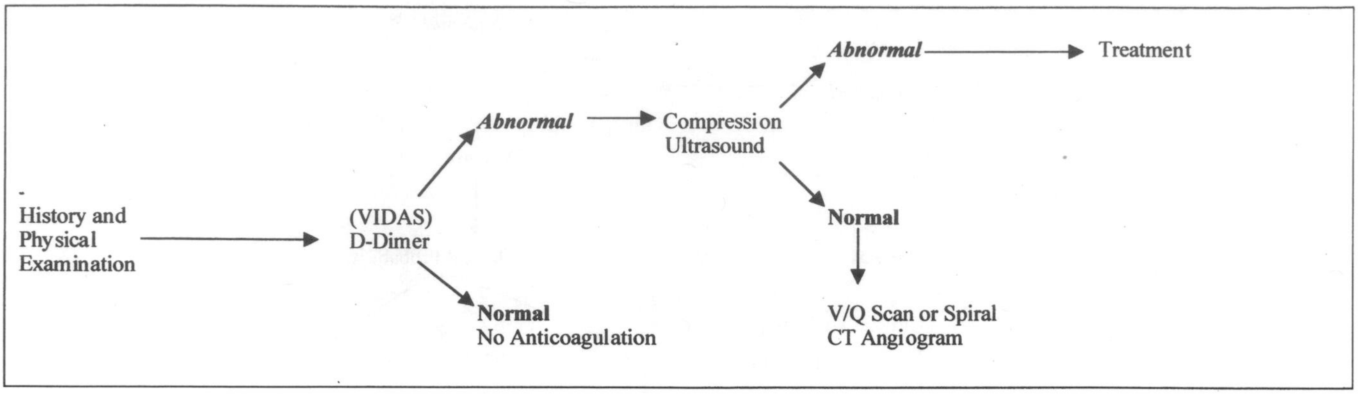

FIGURE 11.6. D-dimer and compression ultrasound for suspected pulmonary embolism.

if the D-dimer is normal. Venography or MRI is reserved for the 1% of cases for whom the clinical probability remains high and the diagnosis remains obscure.

The highest clinical probability of PE is present in patients with known risk factors who have new-onset pleuritic chest pain, shortness of breath, or acute cardiovascular collapse. The diagnostic procedure of first choice when PE is suspected and the D-dimer is abnormal is the V/Q scan or SCTA (depending on availability). The SCTA should now be preferred. Pulmonary radiocontrast angiography is indicated only when the basic studies are inadequate to establish a firm diagnosis and clinical probability is high. The algorithms presented in Figs. 11.2, 11.3, and 11.5 combine clinical probability, the V/Q scan, and other studies. Patients with intermediate-probability V/Q scans may require additional diagnostic studies, including CUS or Duplex and careful clinical follow-up. Figure 11.5 reflects the superiority of SCTA as the initial investigation for patients with suspected PE. Figure 11.6 is a proposed algorithm based on the data presented by Perrier et al. (85), in which approximately 50% of patients with suspected PE are successfully managed with neither V/Q scan nor SCTA.

TABLE 11.2. VENOUS THROMBOSIS/THROMBOEMBOLUS (RISK FACTORS)

Obesity
Oral contraceptives
Varicose veins
Infection
Trauma
Surgery
General anesthesia
Pregnancy
Malignancy
Immobility
Congestive heart failure
Nephrotic syndrome
Blood protein defects

SUMMARY

Because thrombotic or thromboembolic events are customary irreversible perils potentially leading to extraordinary morbidity and, indeed, mortality in patients, it is of obvious extreme gravity to assess these patients painstakingly from the clinical standpoint, including use of ancillary testing procedures. This principle applies to patients who are hypercoagulable as well as to patients who recently had a thrombotic event. Only in this manner can prophylactic therapy or therapy to treat the underlying event be instituted before the patient has sustained an unalterable and often catastrophic insult that will lead to prolonged morbidity or to mortality. The clinical situations affiliated with venous thrombosis are summarized in Table 11.2, and the clinical disorders related to either arterial or venous thrombosis are denoted in Table 11.3.

TABLE 11.3. ARTERIAL AND VENOUS THROMBOSIS (RISK FACTORS)

Age
Obesity
Blood group A
Oral contraceptives
Homocystinuria
Behçet syndrome
Thromboangiitis obliterans?

REFERENCES

1. Landefeld CS, Chren M-M, Myers A, et al. Diagnostic yield of the autopsy in a university hospital and a community hospital. *N Engl J Med* 1988;318:1249.
2. Kemp PM, Tarver D, Batty V, et al. Pulmonary embolism: is the clinical history a useful adjunct to aid interpretation of the equivocal lung scan? *Clin Nucl Med* 1996;21:203.
3. Kistwer RL, Ball JJ, Nordyke RA, et al. Incidence of pulmonary embolism in the course of thrombophlebitis of the lower extremities. *Am J Surg* 1972;124:169.
4. Johnson WC. Evaluation of newer techniques for the diagnosis of venous thrombosis. *J Surg Res* 1974;16:473.
5. Nicolaides AN, Kakar VV, Field ES, et al. The origin of venous thrombosis: a venographic study. *Br J Radiol* 1971;44:653.
6. Sigel B, Felix RJ, Popky GL, et al. Diagnosis of lower limb thrombosis by Doppler ultrasonic technique. *Arch Surg* 1972;104:174.
7. Eze AR, Comerota AJ, Kerr RP, et al. Is duplex imaging an appropriate initial screening test for patients with suspected pulmonary embolism. *Ann Vasc Surg* 1996;10:220.
8. Heijboer H, Brandjes DPM, Lensing AWA, et al. Efficacy of real-time B-mode ultrasonography in the diagnosis of deep vein thrombosis in symptomatic outpatients. *Thromb Haemost* 1991;65:804.
9. Heijboer H, Cogo A, Buller HR, et al. Detection of deep vein thrombosis with impedance plethysmography and real-time compression ultrasonography in hospitalized patients. *Arch Intern Med* 1992;152:1901.
10. Clagett GP, Salzman EW. Prevention of venous thromboembolism in surgical patients. *N Engl J Med* 1974;290:93.
11. Moser KM, Brach BB, Dolan GF. Clinically suspected deep venous thrombosis of the lower extremities. *JAMA* 1977;237:2195.
12. Philbrick JT, Becker DM. Calf deep vein thrombosis: a wolf in sheep's clothing? *Arch Intern Med* 1988;148:2131.
13. Bick RL, Baker WF. Frequency of disorders associated with deep vein thrombosis and pulmonary embolus. *Thromb Haemost* 1991; 65:1170.
14. Briet E, Engesser L, Brommer EJP. Thrombophilia: its causes and a rough estimate of its prevalence. *Thromb Haemost* 1987;58:39.
15. Meade T. Risk associations in the thrombotic disorders. *Clin Haematol* 1981;10:391.
16. Tabernero MD, Tomas JF, Alberca I. Incidence and clinical characteristics of hereditary disorders associated with venous thrombosis. *Am J Hematol* 1991;36:249.
17. Tripodi A, Mannucci PM. A survey of inherited thrombotic syndromes in Italy. *Res Clin Lab* 1989;19:67.
18. Manten B, Westendorp RG, Koster T, et al. Risk factor profiles in patients with different clinical manifestations of venous thromboembolism: a focus on the factor V Leiden mutation. *Thromb Haemost* 1996;76:520.
19. Melichart M, Kyrle PA, Eichinger S, et al. Thrombotic tendency in 75 symptomatic unrelated patients with APC resistance. *Wien Klin Wochenschr* 1996;108:607.
20. Simioni P, Prandoni P, Lensing AW, et al. The risk of recurrent venous thromboembolism in patients with an Arg506→Gln mutation in the gene for factor V (factor V Leiden). *N Engl J Med* 1997;336:399.
21. Williamson D, Brown K, Luddington R, et al. Factor V Cambridge: a new mutation (Arg306→Thr) associated with resistance to activated protein C. *Blood* 1998;91:1140.
22. Arruda VR, Annichino-Bizzacchi JM, Goncalves MS, et al. Prevalence of the prothrombin gene variant (nt20210A) in venous thrombosis and arterial disease. *Thromb Haemost* 1997;78:1430.
23. Makris M, Preston FE, Beuachamp NJ, et al. Co-inheritance of the 20210A allele of the prothrombin gene increases the risk of thrombosis in subjects with familial thrombophilia. *Thromb Haemost* 1997;78:1426–1429.
24. Martinelli I, Sacchi E, Landi G, et al. High risk of cerebral-vein thrombosis in carriers of a prothrombin-gene mutation and in users of oral contraceptives. *N Engl J Med* 1998;338:1793.
25. Bertina RM. Factor V Leiden and other coagulation factor mutations affecting thrombotic risk. *Clin Chem* 1997;43:1678.
26. Bick R. Hereditary coagulation protein defects. In: *Disorders of thrombosis and hemostasis: clinical and laboratory practice.* Chicago: ASCP Press, 1992:109–136.
27. Bick R. Syndromes of thrombosis and hypercoagulability. In: Cullen JH, ed. *Current concepts of thrombosis.* Vol 82. Philadelphia: WB Saunders, 1998:409–458.
28. Wells PS, Hirsh J, Anderson DR, et al. Accuracy of clinical assessment of deep-vein thrombosis. *Lancet* 1995;345:1326.
29. Perrier A, Bounameaux H, Morabia A, et al. Diagnosis of pulmonary embolism by a decision analysis-based strategy including clinical probability, D-dimer levels, and ultrasonography: a management study. *Arch Intern Med* 1996;156:531.
30. Stein PD, Henry JW, Gottschalk A. The addition of clinical assessment to stratification according to prior cardiopulmonary disease further optimizes the interpretation of ventilation/perfusion lung scans in pulmonary embolism. *Chest* 1993;104:1472.
31. Barnes RW, Wu KK, Hoak JC. Fallibility of the clinical diagnosis of venous thrombosis. *JAMA* 1975;234:605.
32. Hull RD, Hirsh J, Sackett DL, et al. Clinical validity of a negative venogram in patients with clinically suspected venous thrombosis. *Circulation* 1981;64:622.
33. Hirsch J, Hoak J. Management of deep vein thrombosis and pulmonary embolism: a statement for healthcare professionals. *Circulation* 1996;93:2212.
34. Leclerc JR, Jay RM, Hull RD, et al. Recurrent leg symptoms following deep vein thrombosis: a diagnostic challenge. *Arch Intern Med* 1985;145:1867.
35. Moser KM, LeMoine JR. Is embolic risk conditioned by location of deep venous thrombosis? *Ann Intern Med* 1981;94:439.
36. Landefeld CS, McGuire E, Cohen C. Clinical findings associated with acute proximal deep vein thrombosis: a basis for quantifying clinical judgment. *Am J Med* 1990;88:382.
37. Wells P, Hirsh J, Lensing A, et al. Accuracy of clinical assessment of deep-vein thrombosis. *Lancet* 1995;i:1326.
38. Wells P, Anderson D, Bormanis J, et al. Value of assessment of pretest probability of deep-vein thrombosis in clinical management. *Lancet* 1997;350:1795.
39. Michiels JJ. Rational diagnosis of deep vein thrombosis (RADIA DVT) in symptomatic outpatients with suspected DVT: simplification and improvement of decision rule analysis for the exclusion and diagnosis of DVT by the combined use of a simple clinical model, a rapid ELISA D-dimer test and compression ultrasonography (CUS). *Semin Thromb Hemost* 1998;24:401.
40. PIOPED Investigators. Value of the ventilation/perfusion scan in acute pulmonary embolism: results of the Prospective Investigation of Pulmonary Embolism Diagnosis (PIOPED). *JAMA* 1990;263:2753.
41. Janssen M, Heebels A, de Mertz M, et al. Reliability of five rapid D-dimer assays compared to ELISA in the exclusion of deep vein thrombosis. *Thromb Haemost* 1997;77:262.
42. Freyburger G, Trillaud H, Labrouche S, et al. D-dimer strategy in thrombosis exclusion: a gold standard study in 100 patients suspected of deep vein thrombosis or pulmonary embolism: 88 DD methods compared. *Thromb Haemost* 1998;79:31.
43. Janssen M, Wollersheim H, Verbruggen, Novakova R. Rapid D-dimer assays to exclude deep venous thrombosis and pulmonary embolism: current status and new developments. *Semin Thromb Hemost* 1998;23:393.

44. Wells P, Brill-Edwards P, Stevens P, et al. A novel and rapid whole-blood assay for D-dimer in patients with clinically suspected deep vein thrombosis. *Circulation* 1995;91:2184.
45. Pittet JL, de Moerloose P, Reber G, et al. VIDAS D-dimer: fast quantitative ELISA for measuring D-dimer in plasma. *Clin Chem* 1996;42:3.
46. Cronan JJ, Dorfman GS, Scola FH, et al. Deep venous thrombosis: US assessment using vein compression. *Radiology* 1887;162:191.
47. Appelman PT, Dejong TE, Lampmann LE. Deep vein thrombosis of the leg: US findings. *Radiology* 1987;163:743.
48. Lensing AWA, Prandoni P, Brandjes D, et al. Detection of deep-vein thrombosis by real-time B-mode ultrasonography. *N Engl Med* 1989;320:342.
49. Monreal M, Montserrat E, Salvador R, et al. Real-time ultrasound for diagnosis of symptomatic venous thrombosis and for screening of patients at risk: correlation with ascending conventional venography. *Angiology* 1989;40:527.
50. Pedersen OM, Aslaksen A, Vik-Mo H, et al. Compression ultrasonography in hospitalized patients with suspected deep vein thrombosis. *Arch Intern Med* 1991;151:2217.
51. Cogo A, Lensing A, Koopman M, et al. Compression ultrasonography with clinically suspected deep vein thrombosis: a cohort study. *Br Med J* 1998;316:17.
52. Birdwell B, Raskob G, Whitsett T, et al. The clinical validity of normal compression ultrasonography in outpatients suspected of having deep vein thrombosis. *Ann Intern Med* 1998;128:1.
53. Cogo A, Lensing A, Prandoni P, et al. Distribution of thrombosis in patients with symptomatic deep vein thrombosis. *Arch Intern Med* 1993;153:2777.
54. Kearon C, Julian J, Math M, et al. Noninvasive diagnosis of deep venous thrombosis. *Ann Intern Med* 1998;128:663.
55. Raghavendra BN, Rosen RJ, Lam S, et el. Deep vein thrombosis: detection by high resolution real-time ultrasonography. *Radiology* 1984;152:789.
56. Langsfeld M, Hershey FB, Thorpe L, et al. Duplex B-mode imaging for the diagnosis of deep venous thrombosis. *Arch Surg* 1987;122:587.
57. Davidson BL, Elliott CG, Lensing AWA. Low accuracy of color Doppler ultrasound in the detection of proximal leg vein thrombosis in asymptomatic high-risk patients. *Ann Intern Med* 1992; 117:735.
58. Barnes RW, Nix ML, Barnes CL, et al. Perioperative asymptomatic venous thrombosis: role of duplex scanning versus venography. *J Vasc Surg* 1989;9:251.
59. Heijboer H, Buller HR, Lensing AW, et al. A comparison of real-time compression ultrasonography with impedance plethysmography for diagnosis of deep vein thrombosis in symptomatic outpatients. *N Engl J Med* 1993;329:1365
60. Albrechtsson U, Olsson CG. Thrombotic side effects of lower-limb phlebography. *Lancet* 1976;1:723.
61. Spritzer CE, Evans AC, Kay JJ. Magnetic resonance imaging of deep venous thrombosis in pregnant women with lower extremity edema. *Obstet Gynecol* 1995;85:603.
62. Brown H, Hiett A. Deep vein thrombosis and pulmonary embolism. *Clin Obstet Gynecol* 1996;39:87.
63. Bergus GR, Barloon TS. An approach to diagnostic imaging of suspected pulmonary embolism. *Am Fam Physician* 1996;53:1259.
64. Georgopoulos DC. Diagnosis of pulmonary embolism. *Monaldi Arch Chest Dis* 1996;51:306.
65. Hull RD, Hirsh J, Carter C, et al. Diagnostic value of ventilation-perfusion lung scanning in patients with suspected pulmonary embolism. *Chest* 1985;8:8190.
66. Stein PD, Athanasoulis C, Alavi A, et al. Complications and validity of pulmonary angiography in acute pulmonary embolism. *Circulation* 1992;85:462.
67. Oudkerk M, van Beek EJ, van Putten WL, et al. Cost-effectiveness analysis of various strategies in the diagnostic management of pulmonary embolism. *Arch Intern Med* 1993;153:947.
68. Hull RD, Feldstein W, Stein PD, et al. Cost-effectiveness of pulmonary embolism diagnosis. *Arch Intern Med* 1996;156:68.
69. Michiels JJ. Rational diagnosis of pulmonary embolism (RADI-APE) in symptomatic outpatients with suspected PE: an improved strategy to exclude or diagnosis venous thromboembolism by the sequential use of a clinical model, rapid ELISA D-dimer test, perfusion lung scan, ultrasonography, spiral CT and pulmonary angiography. *Semin Thromb Hemost* 1998;24:413.
70. Van Erkel AR, van Rossum AB, Bloem J, et al. Spiral CT angiography for suspected pulmonary embolism: a cost-effectiveness analysis. *Radiology* 1996;201:29.
71. Van Rossum AB, Treurniet FE, Kieft G, et al. Role of spiral volumetric computed tomographic scanning in the assessment of patients with clinical suspicion of pulmonary embolism and an abnormal ventilation/perfusion lung scan. *Thorax* 1996;51:23.
72. Godman LR, Curtin JJ, Mewissen MW, et al. Detection of pulmonary embolism in patients with unresolved clinical and scintigraphic diagnosis: helical CT versus angiography. *Am J Radiol* 1995;164:1369.
73. Stein PD, Henry JW. Prevalence of acute pulmonary embolism in central and subsegmental pulmonary arteries and relation to probability interpretation of ventilation/perfusion lung scans. *Chest* 1997;111:1246.
74. Mayo JR, Remy-Jardin M, Muller NL, et al. Pulmonary embolism: prospective comparison of spiral CT with ventilation-perfusion scintigraphy. *Radiology* 1997;205:447.
75. Garg K, Welsh C, Feyerabend A, et al. Pulmonary embolism: diagnosis with spiral CT and ventilation-perfusion scanning: correlation with pulmonary angiographic results or clinical outcome. *Radiology* 1998;208:201.
76. Cross J, Kemp P, Walsh, et al. A randomized trial of spiral CT and ventilation perfusion scintigraphy for the diagnosis of pulmonary embolism. *Clin Radiol* 1998;53:17.
77. Bick RL. Clinical relevance of antithrombin III. *Semin Thromb Hemost* 1982;8:276.
78. Ginsberg JS, Brill-Edwards PA, Demers C. D-dimer in patients with clinically suspected pulmonary embolism. *Chest* 1993;104: 1679.
79. Bounameaux H, Cirafici P, De Moerloose P. Measurement of D-dimer in plasma as diagnostic aid in suspected pulmonary embolism. *Lancet* 1991;337:196.
80. Becker DM, Philbrick JT, Bachhuber TL, et al. D-dimer testing and acute venous thromboembolism. *Arch Intern Med* 1996;156: 939.
81. de Moerloose P, Desmarais S, Bounameaux H, et al. Contribution of a new, rapid, individual and quantitative automated D-dimer ELISA to exclude pulmonary embolism. *Thromb Haemost* 1996;75:11.
82. D'Angelo A, D'Alessandro G, Tomassini L, et al. Evaluation of a new rapid quantitative D-dimer assay in patients with clinically suspected deep vein thrombosis. *Thromb Haemost* 1996;75:412.
83. Reber G, de Moerloose P, Coquoz C, et al. Comparison of two rapid D-dimer assays for the exclusion of venous thromboembolism. *Blood Coagul Fibrinolysis* 1998;9:387.
84. Perrier A, Buswell L, Bounameaux H, et al. Keeping down diagnostic costs for pulmonary embolism. *Cardiol Rev* 1998;15:28.
85. Perrier A, Desmarais S, Miron MJ, et al. Non-invasive diagnosis of venous thromboembolism in outpatients. *Lancet* 1999;353:190.

Disorders of Thrombosis and Hemostasis: Clinical and Laboratory Practice, Third Edition, edited by Rodger L. Bick.
Lippincott Williams & Wilkins, Philadelphia © 2002

12

THROMBOHEMORRHAGIC DEFECTS ASSOCIATED WITH MALIGNANCY

EUGENE P. FRENKEL
RODGER L. BICK

Thrombohemorrhagic events commonly complicate the clinical status of patients with cancer. Hemorrhagic findings are commonly seen in leukemia and lymphoma and often can be further precipitated by cytoreductive chemotherapy that further suppresses the hematopoietic system. In general these events are clinically evident and have a rational basis. By contrast, thrombosis is more commonly seen than is hemorrhage. In some circumstances, its occurrence appears to be the expected result of a complication of recent surgery, prolonged immobility, or chemotherapy. A more complex situation is the development of spontaneous, often migratory, recurrent venous thrombosis, arterial emboli, or both, in patients with cancer, a syndrome so classically related to the presence of a neoplasm by Trousseau (1) that it continues to bear his name. This recognition of the thrombotic diathesis led to extensive attempts to define its clinical and pathophysiologic features and characterize therapeutic approaches (2–6). It is clear that the changes in hemostasis secondary to malignancy are multifaceted, and the development of hemorrhages or thrombotic events in the cancer patient are the result of a combination of factors (4,5).

HYPERCOAGULABILITY AND THROMBOSIS

Pathophysiology

The clinical and laboratory pattern in malignancy-associated thrombosis is that of chronic disseminated intravascular coagulation (DIC) (2–6). Extensive studies have pursued a unitary mechanism for the hypercoagulability (5–15). Elevated clotting factor levels have been seen, especially factors I, V, VII:c, IX, and XI (6,7,12,16). Shortened activated or nonactivated partial thromboplastin times, accelerated prothrombin times, and accelerated clotting times have been seen (5,12,16). Unfortunately, none of these findings correlates with the development of a clinical thrombotic episode in any individual patient (2–5).

Increased fibrinogen and platelet catabolism (increased turnover and decreased survival) occur in many patients with disseminated malignancy (17). Similarly, increased levels of fibrin(ogen) degradation products (FDPs), D-dimer, prothrombin fragment 1.2 (PF1.2), fibrinopeptide A and B, cryofibrinogens, fibrin monomer, B-β 15-42 and related peptides, platelet factor 4, β-thromboglobulin, and altered fibronectin and antithrombin levels also are seen in many patients with disseminated malignancy (7,17–27). These laboratory findings clearly demonstrate that many patients with cancer have an ongoing low-grade disseminated intravascular clotting (DIC) process (2,3,28,29). The shortened survival of fibrinogen and platelets often is followed by an overcompensatory increase in coagulation factors and fibrinolytic enzymes (30). These changes are frequently accompanied by significant decrease in major coagulation inhibitors including antithrombin, protein C, and protein S, although these decrease and may be the result of "consumption" (10,12,30,31). These changes may predispose the patient to localized intravascular coagulation (thrombosis/thromboembolism) or a classic DIC-type syndrome (28,29,32–34).

The mechanism(s) by which malignant tissues may initiate localized or DIC are highly complex. It has long been evident that malignant tissues could release procoagulant moieties and sometimes fibrinolytic materials into the systemic circulation (2–5). The nature of the procoagulant material has been difficult to define. Many malignant tissues can initiate fibrin formation without apparent later activation of the fibrinolytic system (35,36).

Mucinous adenocarcinomas have been the most commonly associated with thrombus formation (2,3,5,14,16).

E. P. Frenkel: Departments of Medicine and Radiology, University of Texas Southwestern Medical School; Simmons Cancer Center, Zale-Lipshy University Hospital, Dallas, Texas.

R. L. Bick: Department of Medicine and Pathology, University of Texas Southwestern Medical Center, Dallas, Texas.

Evidence that these malignancies have a sialic acid moiety of secreted mucin that can initiate coagulation by the nonenzymatic activation of factor X to factor Xa has had significant focus (5,8,16,37). For those associated with pancreatic carcinoma, it has been shown that the release of systemic trypsin, which has the potential to trigger intravascular coagulation events, can occur (5). In spite of the clinical correlate that mucin-producing tumors are more commonly associated with thrombosis than are non–mucin-type malignancies, it has been difficult to implicate the mucin as the procoagulant moiety. Careful histologic studies in pancreatic carcinoma have failed to define a relation between the mucin production and the presence of multiple thrombi (3,38). Virtually all of the recent data support the procoagulant activity in mucin to be tissue factor; that exposure of the blood to tumor cell tissue factor is the basis for the hypercoagulability and chronic DIC that produces the thrombotic diathesis (3). It is now evident that the cancer cell expresses tissue factor on its surface.

Because not all cancers are associated with thrombosis, a second feature is now known to be an intrinsic requirement for the thrombotic diathesis. It is that the cancer cells are so situated that cell membranes or shed material is exposed to the blood or the lymphatic system (3). With the recent recognition of tumor-associated angiogenesis, it is no longer difficult to visualize such circumstances.

That this construct has some simplicity to it is emphasized by prostate cancer. DIC certainly represents the true "coagulopathy" of adenocarcinoma of the prostate (39,40). Nevertheless, malignant prostatic tissue not only activates the procoagulant system but also independently activates the fibrinolytic system. Thus both DIC and secondary fibrinolysis in association with inordinately excessive fibrino(geno)lysis from both primary activation and activation secondary to DIC can occur. In this circumstance, the clinical presentation is one of hemorrhage rather than thrombosis, thereby emphasizing the wide variability of clinical expression in DIC, depending on the balance between activation of the procoagulant system and activation of the fibrino(geno)lytic system. Therapy for prostatic carcinoma is often followed by an alleviation of general hemostatic abnormalities, including changes of the procoagulant and fibrinolytic systems. This is particularly true with administration of estrogens, whereas testosterone has been noted to enhance the coagulation abnormalities (19,41,42).

Hypercoagulability in cancer patients also may arise from platelet abnormalities. The role of platelets in contributing to thrombosis in malignancy was suspected many years ago, and the first large study of this phenomenon, initiated by Moolten in 1949 (43), showed abnormal increases in platelet numbers and abnormal morphology, platelet lysis, and defective adhesion to glass wool. In addition, a correlation was noted between increased platelet adhesiveness and the development of thrombosis (44); the increased platelet adhesion was better correlated with thrombosis in malignancy than was thrombocytosis (45, 46). It is unclear whether the platelet changes are primary disturbances caused by the malignancy, or whether they are the result of the earlier changes in the coagulation system that "activate" platelets and make them "hyperaggregable" (4). Although thrombocytosis is a well-recognized accompaniment of malignancy, it and increased platelet aggregability generally correlate poorly with the actual development of a clinical thrombotic event in any individual patient, making the significance of the platelet changes unclear.

TABLE 12.1. MALIGNANCIES OFTEN ASSOCIATED WITH THROMBOSIS

Colon
Gallbladder
Gastric
Lung (any cell type)
Myeloproliferative syndromes
Ovary
Pancreas
Paraprotein disorders

In spite of viewing the thrombotic diathesis in generic terms, some malignancies have a higher incidence than others. The malignancies most commonly associated with thrombosis are depicted in Table 12.1. The general incidence of thrombosis in malignancy is about 15%, but may be higher in specific tumors such as pancreatic carcinoma, in which it may occur in more than 50% of patients (3–5,10,14). Comorbid states importantly affect the occurrence and frequency of thrombotic events. Thus surgery appears to be an added comorbidity in the development of thrombosis. Patients with malignancy are more likely to develop postoperative deep venous thrombosis (DVT) than are patients without cancer. For cancer of the gastrointestinal tract, the chance of postoperative thrombosis and thromboembolus approaches 40% (5,8,16,37,47).

Management of Thrombosis and Thromboembolus in Patients with Malignancy

Antineoplastic therapy is associated with some correction of abnormal hemostasis, and this is especially evident in prostatic cancer. Treated patients are less susceptible to thrombosis and thromboembolus; when thrombotic episodes develop in untreated patients, consideration should be given to antineoplastic therapy. Cancer patients are notoriously resistant to anticoagulant therapy, and thrombotic events commonly continue after initiation of antithrombotic therapy (3,5,48).

Warfarin not only is often ineffective, but it may also be associated with significant bleeding problems in patients with malignancy. Presently the treatment of choice is heparin and, in most circumstances, low-molecular-weight heparin. It merits emphasis that patients with central nervous system tumors, either primary or metastatic, are at particular risk for hemorrhage with any form of anticoagulation and should be treated with such agents only with great caution and then only when no other therapy is applicable or available. A serious consideration is the duration of therapy once it has been instituted. In those patients in whom a comorbid state was present and then treated or removed, it is often possible to discontinue the therapy after such event and at a time when the cancer has been effectively controlled. Significantly more difficult is the patient with ongoing DIC of the "Trousseau-type," because these patients require heparin therapy for very long durations, commonly for life, because of the malignant nature of their prothrombotic diathesis. This latter circumstance is the common clinical pattern in most patients.

HEMORRHAGE

Leukemias

Hemorrhage may precede the overt clinical diagnosis of leukemia by several months; this is especially noted in acute leukemias (49–52). Petechiae, purpura, and ecchymoses are the most common prediagnostic manifestations, and these are present in 40% to 70% of patients with acute leukemia at the time of diagnosis (5,53–55). The most prevalent sites of hemorrhage in patients with acute leukemia are the skin, eye, and mucosal membranes, including epistaxis, gingival bleeding, and gastrointestinal bleeding (5,50,51); however, retinal bleeding can be found in about 15% of patients at presentation and in 50% of patients with acute leukemia as the disease progresses (5,52,53,56). In acute leukemia, hemorrhage is a common cause of death and is the mechanism of death in nearly 40% of patients (52,53,57). During the past three decades, infection has surpassed hemorrhage as the most common cause of death in patients with acute leukemia, resulting from more intensive chemotherapy and attendant immunosuppression. A major impact on the risk of bleeding has been the availability of platelet concentrates to control thrombocytopenia, the most common cause of fatal hemorrhage in acute leukemia (5,50–52,58).

Hemorrhage is less commonly a problem in chronic myeloid or lymphoid leukemias (5,50–52,59). However, in both, local or diffuse thromboses or thromboembolism are not uncommon (4,48,60). Many patients with chronic leukemia have bothersome bleeding, usually manifest as petechiae, purpura, ecchymoses, or oozing from mucosal membranes (5,61). Only rarely do these patients have retinal bleeding or serious life-threatening bleeding unless severe thrombocytopenia develops (5).

Hemorrhage may occur in any of the leukemias, but is most common in acute promyelocytic (FAB-M3) leukemia, acute myelomonocytic (FAB-M4) leukemia, and acute granulocytic (FAB-M2 and M2) leukemia and to a lesser extent in acute monocytic leukemia (4,5,50–52,62–64).

The most common single cause of serious or life-threatening hemorrhage in the leukemias is thrombocytopenia (4,50,51). Thrombocytopenia is usually due to chemotherapy or marrow infiltration. However, less common causes of thrombocytopenia in patients with leukemia are the development of DIC with consumption of platelets, infection-induced immune or nonimmune thrombocytopenia, or the development of splenomegaly and associated hypersplenism with increased platelet sequestration. In clinical practice when severe thrombocytopenia in patients with leukemia occurs, these mechanisms must be recalled because, although the most common cause of thrombocytopenia is drug induced or secondary to marrow infiltration, any combination(s) of several or many of the mentioned earlier mechanisms may be present and must be corrected if life-threatening hemorrhage is to be treated successfully. Mechanisms of thrombocytopenia in leukemia are summarized in Table 12.2.

In patients with acute myelogenous leukemia, the platelet count commonly decreases to less than 10,000/μL, and at levels less than 5,000/μL, hemorrhage represents a potential clinical event. Currently prophylactic platelet concentrate therapy is given when the platelet count is less than 5,000/μL and is continued until the platelet count is consistently higher than 10,000/μL and any significant bleeding is controlled (65,66).

These same management approaches are applicable to bleeding in the other leukemias or lymphomas. The availability of interleukin 2 (IL-2; Neumega) and thrombopoietin have now afforded alternate therapeutic approaches in chemotherapy-induced thrombocytopenia (14).

An additional factor in the thrombocytopenia can be the presence of significant platelet dysfunction. This is particularly true in chronic myelogenous leukemia, essential thrombocythemia, and other myeloproliferative syndromes, even with normal platelet numbers (3–5,45,50,52). These platelet-function defects can contribute to significant hemorrhage. Although many types of defects are seen, the most common is impaired aggregation to adenosine diphosphate

TABLE 12.2. MECHANISMS OF THROMBOCYTOPENIA IN LEUKEMIA

Bone marrow infiltration (myelophthisis)
Chemotherapy
Radiation therapy
Bacteremia
Disseminated intravascular coagulation
Infection-induced (immune and nonimmune)
Splenomegaly and hypersplenism
Immune thrombocytopenia purpura
Myelofibrosis
Richter syndrome (CLL)

CLL, chronic lymphocytic leukemia.

(ADP) and epinephrine and defective PF-3 release (67–69). A deficiency or absence of α granules also can be seen in patients with myeloproliferative syndromes (70). Although platelet-function defects in chronic myelogenous leukemia and other of the myeloproliferative disorders are known to contribute to significant hemorrhage, the role of abnormal platelet function as a dominant cause of hemorrhage is unclear (70–75).

Another factor contributing to hemorrhage in malignancy is the presence of coagulation protein abnormalities. Liver infiltration with ensuing defective or decreased synthesis of the vitamin K–dependent factors is common in acute leukemias, and impaired synthesis of other factors also may occur (50,52,76). Therefore if, in a patient with acute leukemia, significant liver infiltration develops, there may be defective or decreased synthesis of any combination of not only factors II, VII, IX, and X, but also fibrinogen, factor V, factor VIII:c, factor XI, factor XII, factor XIII, prekallikrein, and high-molecular-weight kininogen, plasminogen, or antithrombin, protein S, and protein C (3–5, 30,50–52). In addition, cholestasis occurs in some patients with acute leukemia and may lead to defective synthesis of the vitamin K–dependent clotting factors; at times, cholestasis may lead to overt DIC (50,51,77). Chronic lymphocytic leukemia may be associated with substantial liver infiltration, especially as the disease progresses and approaches terminal states (5,50,52,76,78), and lead to impaired or decreased synthesis of the vitamin K–dependent factors. However, defective hepatic synthesis of coagulation factors resulting from hepatic infiltration in chronic lymphocytic leukemia is an uncommon cause of life-threatening hemorrhage. Chronic myelogenous leukemias also may be associated with hepatic infiltration; however, this is much less common than even in leukemias or chronic lymphocytic leukemia (50,62).

Finally, acquired von Willebrand syndrome can occur in association with many hematologic malignancies, including chronic lymphocytic leukemia, hairy cell leukemia, myelodysplastic syndromes, multiple myeloma, chronic myelogenous leukemia, polycythemia vera, primary (essential) thrombocythemia, and myelofibrosis (79–86). In most cases examined, the variant has been type II. The two mechanisms defined have been the development of a circulating inhibitor to von Willebrand factor or proteolysis of von Willebrand factor. Treatment of the underlying malignant disorder sometimes has been accompanied by partial or complete correction of bleeding. The use of 1-deamino-8-D-arginine vasopressin (DDAVP) has alleviated bleeding in some patients with malignancy-associated von Willebrand syndrome. Malignancies associated with acquired von Willebrand syndrome are summarized in Table 12.3.

Changes in the fibrinolytic system of patients with cancer, particularly with acute leukemia, have been reported. However, the findings have been inconsistent, with increased fibrinolytic activity reported by some (74) and decreased fibrinolytic activity noted by others (87,88). These findings did not correlate with findings suggestive of procoagulant activity or findings of DIC, and these fibrinolytic changes appear to be independent of intravascular procoagulant activity or findings of DIC (88–91). As mentioned, in prostate cancer, and perhaps in pancreatic cancer, activated fibrinolysis may contribute to a symptomatic coagulopathy.

TABLE 12.3. MALIGNANCIES ASOCIATED WITH ACQUIRED VON WILLEBRAND DISEASE

Wilm tumor
Renal cell carcinoma
Malignant lymphoma
Waldenström disease
Multiple myeloma
Chronic lymphocytic leukemia
Hairy cell leukemia
Chronic myelogenous leukemia
Polycythemia vera
Primary essential thrombocythemia
Myelodysplastic syndromes

DISSEMINATED INTRAVASCULAR COAGULATION IN LEUKEMIA

DIC is a common occurrence in leukemia and is a major factor in morbidity. Myeloblasts, promyelocytes, monocytes, and lymphoblasts all contain and can release procoagulant materials or enzymes in patients with acute leukemia (3–5,50–52,64,92–97). DIC may complicate the course of acute leukemia in as many as 50% of patients (98,99). Blasts may have fibrinolytic activity or fibrinolytic system activator activity (3–5,50,51,88,94,100–103). Granulocytes in chronic granulocytic leukemia also are capable of releasing procoagulant enzymes, procoagulant activity, and antithrombin-type materials (52,62). These can release an antiheparin-like activity that is derived from myeloperoxidase (50,104). Mature lymphocytes in chronic lymphocytic leukemia also release procoagulant materials that are phospholipoprotein- or "thromboplastin-like" in composition (5,50,52,60,78), although this uncommonly results in clinical problems. Because of this ability to release procoagulant materials into the systemic circulation and potentially activate the coagulation system, essentially any leukemia may be associated with low-grade or even fulminant DIC (3,4,28,29,105–107). The most common leukemia associated with DIC is acute promyelocytic leukemia (FAB-M3), followed by acute myelomonocytic leukemia (FAB-M4), acute myeloblastic leukemia (FAB-M1 and 2), and acute lymphoblastic leukemia (FAB-L1-3) in descending order of probability (5,28,29,105,106). Fulminant DIC is uncommon in the chronic leukemias, and if present, is seen in chronic myelogenous leukemia. The

TABLE 12.4. DEFECTIVE HEMOSTASIS IN LEUKEMIA PATIENTS (DESCENDING ORDER OF PROBABILITY)

Thrombocytopenia
Platelet dysfunction
Disseminated intravascular coagulation
Leukemia cell procoagulant activity
Bacteremia
Massive transfusions
Shock
Coagulation protein defects
Liver infiltration
Cholestasis
Drug induced
Primary fibrinolysis
Leukemia cell proteolytic activity
Drug induced
Vascular defects
Infiltration
Hyperviscosity/leukostasis
Extramedullary hematopoiesis

development of DIC influences survival in acute leukemias; and in acute promyelocytic leukemia (FAB-M3), it is a common and serious event. The survival of patients with acute progranulocytic leukemia can be dramatically improved by suppressing the development of DIC or by attenuating an existing DIC with heparin and the addition of retinoic acid–differentiating agents, thereby delimiting the presence and availability of the procoagulant granules (5,28,29,105,106,108,109).

Vascular defects also are recognized in patients with acute leukemia, and these may be responsible for or contribute to significant hemorrhage (5,50,51). Patients with acute leukemias commonly display increased vascular permeability because of (a) infiltration of the vasculature by leukemic cells, (b) hyperviscosity or leukostasis of the vasa vasorum, or (c) altered structural stability due to foci of extramedullary hematopoiesis in the vessel wall (4, 110–112).

Thus a variety of defects of hemostasis may occur in leukemia. When significant hemorrhage occurs, the defects may be multifactorial and require careful clinical and laboratory evaluation to define rational and effective therapy. Coagulation alterations associated with leukemia are summarized in Table 12.4.

Hemorrhage and Solid Tumors

Although thrombosis is the usual hemostatic defect in solid tumors, hemorrhage also may be a significant clinical problem in patients with solid tumors (4,5). Intravascular coagulation is present in many patients with malignancy and can have varying clinical expressions, the most extreme form being acute fulminant DIC with catastrophic hemorrhage and thrombosis. DIC in cancer patients may be low grade or fulminant (4,5,28,32,48,105–107). The low-grade form is slightly more common and is manifest by mild to moderate bleeding, usually of the skin or mucous membranes (4,5,29,32,105). Easy and spontaneous bruising, petechiae and purpura, ecchymoses, gingival bleeding, and minor gastrointestinal bleeding, coupled with thrombosis are the usual manifestations. In contrast, fulminant DIC is characterized by an explosive catastrophic hemorrhage, with bleeding usually from at least three unrelated sites simultaneously (29,32). In addition, most patients with fulminant DIC will manifest oozing from an intravenous site or site of other invasive procedures, such as intraarterial lines, central lines, subclavian catheters, and hepatic artery catheters (4,5,28,29,32,105–107). Although these are the most common bleeding manifestations, life-threatening bleeding with intracranial or intrapulmonary hemorrhage also may occur. Fulminant DIC has been noted in association with almost all types of solid tumors, but is most common in carcinoma of the lung, gallbladder, stomach, colon, breast, ovary, malignant melanoma (5,12,16,37,113–116), and is especially common in carcinoma of the prostate (19, 39,40,117). Table 12.5 lists the malignancies most commonly associated with DIC. It is of interest that initiation of chemotherapy has occasionally been associated with the "triggering" or acceleration of DIC (7,92,105,115,118), presumably related to the release of tissue factor or other clot-promoting materials or enzymes from necrotic tumor cells. In acute promyelocytic leukemia, low-dose heparin therapy given before starting cytotoxic drugs may protect against this development (105,108,109,119). Most patients with disseminated cancer have some laboratory or clinical evidence of DIC, although no clinical effect is seen. The patient with extensive disseminated cancer is a special problem, because the DIC may be manifest as thrombosis or hemorrhage or both (4,105–107).

There are many potential mechanisms by which cancer provides triggers for DIC. The hemorrhagic syndrome associated with prostatic carcinoma was long confusing because

TABLE 12.5. MALIGNANCIES COMMONLY ASSOCIATED WITH DISSEMINATED INTRAVASCULAR COAGULATION

Acute promyelocytic leukemia
Acute myelomonocytic leukemia
Acute myeloblastic leukemia
Lymphomas (immunoblastic)
Hodgkin disease
Biliary cancer
Breast cancer
Colon cancer
Gastric cancer
Lung cancer
Malignant melanoma
Ovarian cancer
Prostate cancer

it appeared to be DIC with secondary fibrinolysis, although a primary (hyper)fibrinolytic syndrome appeared evident (40,116,120). It is now recognized that both processes may occur in malignant prostatic disease and may even occur in benign prostatic disease. Malignant prostatic tissue contains procoagulant materials that may be released into the circulation, triggering a disseminated intravascular clotting process with the usual secondary fibrinolytic response (4,5). In addition, malignant prostatic tissue may independently activate the fibrinolytic system, leading to a primary fibrino(geno)lytic syndrome (4). Prostatic carcinoma is commonly associated with DIC and the usual secondary fibrinolytic response plus a primary fibrino(geno)lytic syndrome. This helps explain why patients with prostatic carcinoma often appear to have an overwhelming fibrino(geno)lytic syndrome with only a minimal procoagulant problem, and the clinical manifestation is hemorrhage rather than diffuse thrombosis (1). Indeed, evidence of DIC, as defined by elevated FDPs and soluble fibrin monomer, is noted in many patients before surgery for prostatic cancer (121). After transurethral resection of the prostate (TURP), blood loss appears to be correlated with preoperative evidence of DIC (105,121).

DIC also is commonly associated with pancreatic carcinoma. The DIC is more commonly manifest as diffuse thrombosis instead of diffuse hemorrhage, as the procoagulant activity dominates, and secondary fibrinolysis is minimal. DIC, manifest as acute disseminated thrombosis, is more commonly seen in carcinoma of the body and tail of the pancreas, probably because these are often associated with some limited ductal obstruction, resulting in release of trypsin into the circulation, where the trypsin has thrombin-like activity. In carcinoma of the head of the pancreas, there is more ductal obstruction and less trypsin released in the systemic circulation, and it less commonly has associated DIC or thrombotic syndrome (5,28).

In patients with adenocarcinomas at a variety of other primary sites, the mechanism for DIC may be multifaceted. However, the sialic acid moiety of secreted mucin from adenocarcinomatous tissue can invoke the nonenzymatic activation of factor X to factor Xa (16,37). This can easily provide a trigger for systemic thrombin generation and subsequent fulminant or subacute DIC (105,122). This sequence may lead to thrombosis (5,105–107). Other less well-defined mechanisms exist for initiating DIC in malignancy and include systemic release of necrotic tumor tissue and/or enzymes with procoagulant or phospholipoprotein-like activity. Many such tumors undergo neovascularization; this process could potentially produce abnormal endothelial cell lining, which may cause either a platelet release or generation of factors VIIa and Via with subsequent procoagulant activation and the development of DIC (105–107,123,124). Table 12.6 lists the usual laboratory features found in most patients with disseminated malignancy and disrupted hemostasis (5,28,29,46).

TABLE 12.6. COMMON LABORATORY MANIFESTATIONS OF DISSEMINATED INTRAVASCULAR COAGULATION IN PATIENTS WITH METASTATIC MALIGNANCY

Microangiopathic hemolytic anemia
Schistocytosis
Reticulocytosis leukocytosis
Elevated fibrin(ogen) degradation products
Circulating soluble fibrin monomer
Decreased antithrombin III
Decreased protein C
Elevated fibrinopeptide A
Elevated B-β 15–42–related peptides
Decreased fibronectin
Clotting factors: normal, up, or down
Hypoplasminogenemia
Circulating plasmin
Decreased antiplasmin
Thrombocytopenia
Decreased platelet survival
Large "young" platelets
Elevated platelet factor 4
Elevated β-thromboglobulin
Elevated prothrombin fragment 1.2

Another potential precipitating mechanism for DIC in the patient with malignancy is the use of LeVeen or Denver shunts for the treatment of malignant ascites. Patients with malignant ascites must be carefully chosen for this procedure; if ascitic fluid is positive for malignant cells, the placement of a LeVeen shunt is usually not successful (125), does not lead to significant improved quality of life, and is commonly associated with the development of DIC (28,29,32, 126–129). DIC may be blunted or aborted by removal of ascitic fluid at the time of shunt placement (130). Another potential complication of LeVeen shunting in the patient with malignant ascites is that of thromboembolism (125).

DIAGNOSIS OF DISSEMINATED INTRAVASCULAR COAGULATION IN MALIGNANCY

Clinical Assessment

The clinical diagnosis of DIC need not be difficult; the key is a high index of suspicion and the recognition of the type of bleeding and/or thrombosis in the patient with malignancy (2,3,5,105). The type of bleeding manifest by most patients with DIC suggests multiple hemostatic compartment defects. For example, most patients with fulminant DIC will bleed from at least three unrelated sites simultaneously (3,4,28,29,105–107). When bleeding from multiple hemostatic compartment is seen in patients with cancer, DIC is an almost certain diagnosis. With fulminant DIC shock, end-organ hypoxia and ischemia may be seen (5, 105). As a result of occlusive vascular changes, renal or lung failure may occur, as well as a central nervous system syndrome. Because interplay between coagulation proteins and other protein systems may occur, kinin generation and complement activation may result in pain and shock. Finally, when the patient with malignancy has diffuse thrombosis, DIC should be strongly considered, the patient appropriately studied for confirmatory proof, and proper therapy started if the diagnosis is confirmed (1–5,48, 105–107,131).

Laboratory Diagnosis

The laboratory diagnosis of DIC is complex. Although noting the expected type of bleeding in the appropriate clinical setting can essentially assure a diagnosis of DIC, laboratory confirmation is appropriate, if not mandatory, before committing a cancer patient to heparin or other antiprocoagulant therapy. Understanding the pathophysiology of DIC makes it clear that these patients have numerous abnormal laboratory tests of hemostasis. Most laboratory tests that might be expected to be abnormal in DIC are abnormal in only the fulminant form of DIC. In subacute or low-grade DIC associated with malignancy, many laboratory parameters of hemostasis may be difficult to interpret or are within normal limits (5,105–107,131). In addition, other comorbid complications occurring in cancer patients may induce DIC; they include sepsis, initiation of radiation therapy, microangiopathic hemolytic anemia, hemolysis of any etiology, hemolytic transfusion reactions, and transfusions of large amounts of banked whole blood (28,29,32,105,106).

Therapy for Disseminated Intravascular Coagulation in Malignancy

Therapy for DIC in the cancer patient is a major clinical challenge: one approach is outlined in Table 12.7. Effective therapy is multiphasic and is best approached in a sequential and logical manner (28,29,32,105,132). The first and essential modality is to treat the malignancy, because this is supplying the procoagulant material stimulating intravascular coagulation. Therapy may be surgical, radiotherapy, chemotherapy, or endocrine manipulation, or a combination as the clinical situation warrants. Treatment of the tumor is often associated with cessation or significant improvement of DIC. Until attempts at antineoplastic therapy are introduced, therapy for bleeding or thrombosis often is unsuccessful. This is especially true if the manifestation is well controlled; cancer patients are notoriously resistant to anticoagulant therapy (4,5,48,105). Therapy also must be highly individualized, depending on the overall medical condition of the patient, sites and severity of hemorrhage and thrombosis, sites of metastases, hemodynamic status, and age of the patient. If significant bleeding continues after reasonable attempts to control the malignancy, anticoagulant therapy must be considered. For the patient with malignancy and fulminant DIC, antithrombin concentrates or low-dose heparin therapy can be given, as the site and severity of hemorrhage or thrombosis dictate (5,29,105). Patients with low-grade DIC and bothersome but not life-threatening hemorrhage may be started on such antiplatelet agents as acetylsalicylic acid (ASA) and dipyridamole (5). These are usually successful at stopping a low-grade intravascular clotting process. The use of antiplatelet agents in chronic DIC will usually need 24 to 36 hours for an effect on the intravascular clotting process, whereas the use of low-dose heparin will usually stop the process within 4 to 8 hours (4,29).

TABLE 12.7. SEQUENTIAL TREATMENT OF DIC IN MALIGNANCY

1. Treat the malignancy
   Surgery as indicated
   Radiation as indicated
   Chemo/hormonal therapy as indicated
2. Stop intravascular clotting process
   Antiplatelet drug therapy
   Subcutaneous heparin[a]
   Intravenous heparin[a]
3. Component therapy as indicated
   Platelet concentrates
   Packed red cells (washed)
   Fresh frozen pasma
   AT III concentrates
4. Component therapy as indicated
   Rarely, if ever, indicated
   Tranexamic acid
   Aminocaproic acid
5. Individualize therapy
   Type of malignancy
   Site(s) of bleeding and thrombosis
   Age
   Hemodynamic and medical status

[a]Contraindicated with CNS metastases.
AT, antithrombin.

OTHER DEFECTS IN MALIGNANCY

Cancer patients also may develop bleeding from other coagulation factor abnormalities. These are less common and are usually associated with less serious hemorrhage than is seen with DIC. Patients with malignancy, especially those with liver metastases, may acquire deficiencies of the vitamin K–dependent factors (12,117). When this results in significant or life-threatening bleeding, vitamin K is usually ineffective, and the hemorrhage must be controlled with fresh frozen plasma or prothrombin complex concentrates (133). However, before using such therapy, DIC must be excluded. In addition, cancers of the extra- or intrahepatic biliary tree and obstruction and cholestasis often have malabsorption of vitamin K and defective synthesis of the vitamin K–dependent factors (4,5).

Factor XIII deficiency or dysfunction is common in malignancy and is most pronounced in patients with liver metastases (116,134). This may result from decreased factor XIII activators or impaired removal of factor XIII inhibitors by the invaded liver (4). Because factor XIII is associated with albumin, cancer patients with hypoalbuminemia may be factor XIII deficient. Acquired factor XIII deficiency may cause hemorrhage, although more commonly, impaired clot formation and poor wound healing are noted. When factor XIII deficiency is thought to cause or contribute to hemorrhage in cancer patients, it is managed with transfusions with fresh frozen plasma given at a dose of 5 mL/kg every 7 to 10 days (135).

Patients with liver metastases often have low levels of other clotting factors synthesized in the liver, including fibrinogen, factor V, factor VIII:c, factor XI, factor XII, prekallikrein, high-molecular-weight kininogen, plasminogen, antithrombin, protein C, protein S, and fibronectin (4). However, the decreased synthesis of these is of unclear clinical significance. Of particular concern in malignancy is the development of a dysfibrinogenemia with either primary hepatoma or liver metastases. Abnormalities in fibrin monomer polymerization are manifestations of this dysfibrinogenemia and may lead to hemorrhage in patients with disseminated malignancy and liver metastases or in patients with primary hepatoma (4).

Acquired circulating anticoagulants may develop in a wide variety of tumors; however, these have been isolated findings in cancer patients and often have an unclear relation to actual hemorrhage. Many are heparinoid and are found in association with carcinoma of the lung and in myeloma (4,48,136–140). Some appear to inhibit the activation phase of coagulation or act as antithrombins, and these have been most commonly noted in association with carcinoma of the breast (134). Of significance, circulating anticoagulant in the form of FDPs may assume paramount clinical importance in a cancer patient with low-grade covert intravascular coagulation (4,141).

PRIMARY FIBRINO(GENO)LYSIS IN SOLID TUMORS

Primary fibrino(geno)lysis has been seen in patients with metastatic malignancy (4,5,19,32,42,116). In this disorder, hemorrhage is caused by plasmin-induced biodegradation of many clotting factors including fibrinogen, factor V, factor VII:c, and the impairment of hemostasis by circulating FDPs, which interfere with fibrin monomer polymerization, thrombin generation, and platelet function (141,142). Although primary fibrinolysis occurs in malignancy, DIC is a far more common cause of hemorrhage in cancer patients. Many malignant tissues are capable of spontaneous fibrinolytic activity and activation of the fibrinolytic system (143). This has been noted in patients with carcinoma of the breast, thyroid, colon, and stomach; however, the greatest activity is seen in patients with disseminated sarcoma (4,5,33). If patients with carcinoma develop a systemic hemorrhagic syndrome, the cause is usually DIC, and only rarely is it because of primary activation of the fibrinolytic system and a primary fibrino(geno)lytic syndrome (4). The opposite is true in patients with disseminated sarcoma (4). If a systemic hemorrhage syndrome develops in these patients, the most common cause is primary fibrino(geno)-lysis, and only rarely is it from DIC (4,33). Kwaan (144) noted a decrease in tumor fibrinolytic activity in patients with liver metastases and ascribed this phenomena to increased levels of fibrinolytic inhibitors that appear with liver involvement. Primary fibrino(geno)lytic hemorrhage is treated with agents that inhibit the fibrinolytic system. One approach is to give ε-aminocaproic acid or tranexamic acid. The use of antifibrinolytics is contraindicated in patients with DIC (105).

PLATELETS AND BLEEDING

Thrombocytopenia

Thrombocytopenia is clearly the most common cause of hemorrhage in patients with both solid tumors and hematologic malignancies (5,17). Thrombocytopenia is commonly the result of bone marrow suppression by radiation therapy or chemotherapy (145–147). It also may result from bone marrow invasion by tumor, and in that circumstance, the degree of thrombocytopenia correlates well with the degree of marrow involvement (4,7,12,17). Marrow metastases should be suspected and searched for when unexplained thrombocytopenia develops in patients with malignancy, particularly when leukoerythroblastosis is evident in the peripheral blood. This is best done by examination of the bone marrow (4,5,148–152).

Aside from bone marrow–suppressive therapy and marrow metastases, other types of thrombocytopenia may develop in cancer patients. When splenomegaly develops as a part of the malignant process, hypersplenism and later thrombocytopenia may follow (4,5,147,153). Development of splenic metastases also is more common than generally recognized, especially in carcinoma of the lung, breast, prostate, colon, and stomach (4,5,154,155), and this may lead to reactive hypersplenism with thrombocytopenia (4,5,17,147). It is rare for congestive splenomegaly to result in a significant platelet reduction to levels associated with bleeding. Thus it rarely requires any therapeutic interdiction. By contrast, thrombocytopenia and bleeding can result from decreased bone marrow production. In that circumstance, platelet concentrates have generally been the treatment of choice (147). Presently, IL-2 (Neumega) and recombinant thrombopoietin provide alternatives in selected circumstances (see Chapter 5). In general, platelet counts less than 10,000/μL are commonly associated with spontaneous and serious hemorrhage, whereas platelet counts greater than 30,000/μL are usually not associated with bleeding unless the patient is challenged with trauma or surgical stress (147,156). Immune thrombocytopenic purpura (ITP) occasionally occurs in patients with solid tumors, but is more commonly noted in patients with lymphoid malignancies (147,157,158). When ITP occurs in association with malignancy, the approach to management should be that generally used for this disorder: in general, steroids and possibly splenectomy if indicated (159,160). Another type of increased platelet destruction that may sometimes be associated with malignancy is thrombotic thrombocytopenia purpura (TTP) (5,147,161,162). This rare syndrome is commonly fatal when it develops in the cancer patient but may respond to vigorous plasma exchange.

Platelet-function Defects

Abnormalities of platelet function are commonly found in both solid and hematologic malignancies. Because of frequent episodes of intravascular coagulation and the resultant elevated fibrin degradation products (FDPs) noted in cancer patients, the coating of platelet surfaces by these fragments probably is the most common cause of platelet dysfunction in oncology patients (3,4,141). However, other platelet-function abnormalities also are noted in cancer patients. PF-3 is commonly decreased in patients with cancer (163). Other platelet-function defects also have been consistently noted in cancer patients. These include defective platelet aggregation to ADP and other presumptive evidence of platelet dysfunction, as manifest by a prolonged thromboplastin generation test, prolonged template bleeding times, positive tourniquet tests, and poor clot retraction (7,163–165). It is unclear whether these defects develop secondary to the malignancy itself, whether they develop from partial release of platelet contents after contact with malignant tissue, or whether they develop in response to circulating activated clotting factors. The malignant paraprotein disorders are frequently associated with platelet-function abnormalities, which develop from coating of platelet surfaces by circulating immunoglobulin (Ig) (4,5, 166,167). Consistent platelet-aggregation abnormalities are found in the myeloproliferative and myelodysplastic syndromes (4,5,45,163). The significance of platelet-function defects in contributing to hemorrhage in patients with solid tumors is unclear. However, these defects may correlate better with the development of hemorrhage in cancer patients than does the platelet count (4,5,163,164). At the very least, these defects must be presumed to be active in aggravating bleeding in cancer patients who already have severely compromised hemostasis systems or attendant thrombocytopenia (4,5).

Clinical clues to platelet dysfunction include easy or spontaneous bruising, gingival bleeding, petechiae and purpura, and other minor forms of mucosal membrane bleeding with a normal platelet count. Serious bleeding is uncommon but can be approached as for thrombocytopenia with platelet concentrates. The patient with malignancy and a documented associated platelet-function defect should be cautioned regarding use of drugs known to interfere with platelet function.

HEMOSTASIS IN MALIGNANT PARAPROTEIN DISORDERS

Defects in hemostasis associated with malignant paraprotein disorders are in a special category because these commonly lead to significant clinical hemorrhage. Alterations of hemostasis in malignant paraprotein disorders are expressed as either hemorrhage or thrombosis, or a combination of the two; however, hemorrhage is more common than thrombosis (3,166).

The actual incidence of hemorrhage in malignant paraprotein disorders varies somewhat depending on the particular disease present. About 15% of patients with IgG myeloma experience hemorrhage, whereas those with IgA myeloma have a 40% chance of hemorrhage (4,166). Patients with Waldenström macroglobulinemia or IgM myeloma have a greater than 60% chance of significant hemorrhage (6,166,168,169).

There are many reasons for hemorrhage in patients with malignant paraprotein disorders, and some of these are not simply because of changes of the hemostatic system. The most common bases for hemorrhage are abnormalities in hemostasis, which are manifestations of circulating paraprotein. Uremia and attendant abnormal platelet function account for significant hemorrhage in many of these patients. Liver failure or hypersplenism also may be associated with defects in hemostasis in patients with malignant paraprotein disorders (4,48,166). Hypersplenism is a frequent accompaniment of malignant paraprotein disorders, and significant thrombocytopenia resulting from splenic sequestration of platelets may develop, although this rarely results in bleeding unless through associated amyloidosis. In many patients with malignant paraprotein disorders, liver disease develops, with resultant decreased synthesis of the vitamin K–dependent factors, abnormal fibrinogen (dysfibrinogenemia), abnormal fibrinolytic activity, and other coagulation protein defects associated with diffuse myelomatous involvement of the liver. DIC has been reported in myeloma and may account for hemorrhage in some patients.

Thrombocytopenia resulting from chemotherapy or radiation therapy also may lead to hemorrhage in patients with malignant paraprotein disorders. Significant thrombocytopenia obviously may result from bone marrow replacement in multiple myeloma, light-chain disease, or Waldenström macroglobulinemia. In general, thrombocytopenia is not severe and is not a significant cause of bleeding, although it may be additive to other hemostatic alterations.

Platelet-function defects are more common causes of hemorrhage in malignant paraprotein disorders than is thrombocytopenia (4,166). Many patients with multiple myeloma have a prolonged template bleeding time, which correlates poorly with clinical bleeding; however, many patients have normal or shortened bleeding times even with marked defects in platelet function. Platelet aggregation or lumi-aggregation studies are usually markedly abnormal in most patients with circulating paraprotein, and these studies correlate better with predisposition to clinical hemorrhage (4,5,166). Abnormalities of platelet function in multiple myeloma have not been clearly defined, but usually result from coating of platelet membrane surfaces by paraprotein (4,5,166). Platelet-aggregation abnormalities are seen in about 80% of patients with myeloma. There appears to be poor correlation with the type of paraprotein present (4,166). However, there appears to be some correlation with the quantity of paraprotein circulating. It is thought that platelet membrane coating by paraprotein is not an antigen–antibody reaction but simply a chemical paraprotein–protein interaction with platelet membrane receptor sites. There is poor correlation between platelet-aggregation abnormalities and template bleeding times in multiple myeloma or other malignant paraprotein disorders. Up to 80% of patients with malignant paraprotein disorders have markedly abnormal aggregation and release; epinephrine-induced aggregation is abnormal in about 90% of patients, ADP-induced aggregation and release is abnormal in about 60% of patients, and collagen-induced aggregation is abnormal in about 60% of patients with malignant paraprotein disorders (170). The most sensitive indicator of abnormal platelet aggregation in multiple myeloma is epinephrine-induced platelet aggregation (4,166). It is of interest that some individuals show markedly abnormal platelet lumi-aggregation but have normal template bleeding times and the absence of clinical bleeding.

Other mechanisms for abnormal platelet function occur in patients with multiple myeloma; the most important and prominent of which include uremia, the development of liver disease, and the occurrence of circulating FDPs. In addition, the malignant paraproteins may coat the vasculature, interfere with normal endothelial function, or may precipitate in the vasa vasorum, interfering with vascular function.

The malignant paraprotein itself may interfere with coagulation proteins. Probably the most noted change of the coagulation system in malignant paraprotein disorders is inhibition of a single specific clotting factor, such as factor VIII:c. However, in reality, this phenomenon is rare and the least common cause of hemorrhage by paraprotein–coagulation protein interactions. When specific inhibition of blood coagulation factors by paraprotein does happen, it is usually somewhat selective; for example, IgG paraprotein is commonly directed against factors II, VII X, or thrombin; alternatively, IgA and IgM paraprotein is more commonly directed against the larger coagulation proteins, usually factor V and factor VIII:c activity. The most common coagulation protein interaction is inhibition of fibrin monomer polymerization. Paraprotein selectively attacks fibrin monomer and hampers polymerization into a stable fibrin clot. It is unclear whether paraprotein coats the intact fibrinogen molecule and hinders the generation of fibrin monomer after exposure to thrombin, or alternatively, paraprotein attacks fibrin monomer only after its generation from fibrinogen (166,167). It has been proposed, but not proven, that the Fab segment is the primary site of attachment to fibrin monomer by paraprotein. An abnormal thrombin time or reptilase time is a good indication of inhibition of fibrin monomer polymerization in paraprotein disorders and correlates well with clinical hemorrhage resulting from this phenomenon (4,166). An abnormal thrombin time or reptilase time has been noted in more than 50% of patients with malignant paraprotein disorders (4,166). However, there is not good correlation between abnormal prolonged thrombin times and reptilase times and the quantity or type of paraprotein present. Rarely, acquired von Willebrand syndrome may be noted in association with malignant paraprotein diseases; in myeloma, this has been noted to be because of an inhibition, by paraprotein, of von Willebrand factor (171–173)

The treatment of hemorrhage in patients with malignant or benign paraprotein disorders presents difficult management problems. The exact alterations of hemostasis associated with hypersplenism, uremia, liver infiltration, and bone marrow infiltration are usually best controlled by proper management of the paraprotein disorder itself. This applies also to paraprotein inhibition of platelet function, coagulation protein defects, or interference by paraprotein of fibrin monomer polymerization. Often these defects will correct partly, and sometimes completely, with decreases in the myeloma cell population induced by chemotherapy or radiation therapy. When bleeding becomes severe and rapid control of hemorrhage is called for, vigorous plasmapheresis is usually effective for rapidly lowering the paraprotein concentration and restoring normal or near-normal hemostasis (174). DDAVP has been useful in aborting bleeding associated with acquired von Willebrand syndrome in myeloma.

EFFECTS OF CHEMOTHERAPY ON HEMOSTASIS

Chemotherapeutic agents may alter hemostasis by a variety of mechanisms (4,5). The most common and significant of these include the thrombocytopenia associated with bone marrow–suppressive cytotoxic drugs or the initiation or enhancement of DIC by cytotoxic drugs or hormones in both solid tumors and acute promyelocytic or myelomonocytic leukemia.

L-Asparaginase therapy often is accompanied by substantial hypofibrinogenemia, a common complication of this drug. Although earlier investigators attributed this phenomenon to decreased fibrinogen synthesis (175), others have shown this to result from the synthesis of functionally abnormal fibrinogen. This arises from reactions between L-asparaginase and asparagine residues of the fibrinogen molecule (176). In addition, L-asparaginase may induce a DIC-type syndrome. Actinomycin D also is associated with hemorrhage; actinomycin D is a potent vitamin K antagonist and causes defective synthesis of factors II, VII, IX, and X (177,178). Mitomycin is associated with the development of a microangiopathic hemolytic anemia (179–182). Doxorubicin (Adriamycin) (183) and daunomycin (184) cause primary activation of the fibrinolytic system and later clinical hemorrhage. Melphalan, cytosine arabinoside, vincristine, and vinblastine induce platelet dysfunction that may contribute to bleeding in patients receiving these anticancer drugs (4,185). Thrombosis resulting from single- or multiple-agent chemotherapy or hormonal therapy has been repeatedly reported (5,186–190).

HEMOSTASIS AND BONE MARROW TRANSPLANTATION

The most common defect in hemostasis associated with bone marrow transplantation is hepatic venoocclusive disease. This syndrome occurs 10 to 20 days after transplantation, is probably related to aggressive preconditioning radiochemotherapy, and is characterized by sudden weight gain, hepatomegaly, ascites, hyperbilirubinemia, and hepatic encephalopathy. This syndrome is commonly preceded by 3 to 4 days of thrombocytopenia, usually refractory to platelet transfusions. It was first thought that hepatic venoocclusive disease after transplantation might be related to graft-versus-host disease (GVH); however, there is probably no such relation. The early symptoms of hepatic venoocclusive disease can be confused with GVH disease. The incidence in major transplantation centers is about 40%, with the highest incidence being noted in aggressively preconditioned patients with acute leukemia or in patients who have pretransplantation transaminasemia. The mortality reaches 30% to 40% (191,192). The pathophysiology of this devastating complication of transplantation has been thoroughly studied by Shulman (193), who found an overall incidence of 21% among transplant patients, with a mortality of 33%. This study evaluated the molecular and cellular events associated with venoocclusive disease by use of immunofluorescent staining with anti–factor VIII, antifibrinogen, and antibody to platelet glycoprotein Ib. In the 11 patients studied, eight had widespread hepatic changes, and three had patchy lesions. The lesions were associated with marked widening of the subendothelial zone of terminal hepatic venules and sublobular veins by fragmented red cells within an edematous background. The central lobar area had severe congestion with hemorrhagic necrosis of hepatocytes. Five of eight patients with late venoocclusive disease had diffuse fibrous obliteration of most central venules, associated with atrophy of central lobar hepatocytes, sinusoidal widening, and fibrosis. The remaining three patients with late venoocclusive disease had only focal fibrotic obliterative changes of the central venules. Immunohistochemical stains revealed that nine of the 11 patients with early venoocclusive disease demonstrated intense immunostaining of the adventitial portion of the central vein walls (intima) with anti–factor VIII, and some patients had additional immunostaining for anti–factor VIII in the subendothelial zone. It also was noted that a significant number of patients with early venoocclusive disease had antifibrinogen staining on both the central venules and in the central lobar areas. However, none of the patients had evident immunostaining for antibody to platelet glycoprotein Ib. This study indicates that in the early stages of venoocclusive disease, the coagulation system is activated around and within the walls of the central venules. Venoocclusive disease and its sequelae, the deposition of interstitial collagens, can be considered a form of localized wound healing confined to the central lobar area of the liver acinus. The liver immunohistochemical studies suggest that coagulation proteins are first deposited within the adventitial zone of the affected terminal hepatic venules before involving the subendothelial zone. Shulman et al. (193) could not explain the lack of antiplatelet glycoprotein Ib, but suggested that this may have resulted from either postmortem autolysis or from lysis of platelet thrombi after aggregation. Another complication that has, on occasion, been associated with bone marrow transplantation is nonbacterial thrombotic endocarditis. Jerman and Fick (194) reported two patients treated with bone marrow transplantation who later developed fatal nonbacterial thrombotic endocarditis. These patients developed typical findings of DIC, soft systolic cardiac murmurs, hematuria, and signs of cerebral embolic events. The overall incidence of nonbacterial thrombotic endocarditis in bone marrow transplant recipients may approximate 10% (195).

Because of the high risk of venoocclusive disease and its potential mortality, prevention efforts have focused on alterations of doses of the conditioning regimens and continuous-infusion heparin during the pretransplantation conditioning. For actual cases of venoocclusive disease, recombinant human tissue plasminogen activator (t-PA) and heparin have been used.

CATHETER-RELATED THROMBOSIS IN PATIENTS WITH MALIGNANCY

The use of indwelling central venous catheters and ports has become a standard adjunctive measure in the practice of oncology. With increased use of vascular-access devices, it has become evident that two complications result from their presence: infection and thrombosis (196), and the clinician who uses these must be able to recognize these events and appropriately manage them. The placement of an intravascular catheter is followed by fibrin deposition on the surface of the catheter and potentially initiates a complex series of events related to the presence of the foreign body and the endothelium. It is now evident that four types of catheter thrombotic lesions can occur (197). These include an intraluminal thrombus, a mural thrombus, a fibrin sheath thrombosis, and a fibrin tail thrombosis. As expected, the intraluminal thrombus develops within the lumen of the catheter. A mural thrombus is believed to occur when the fibrin generated from the stimulus of the initial "injury" to the vessel wall binds to the fibrin on the catheter surface. The fibrin sheath thrombus also has been termed the fibrin sleeve thrombus; it occurs when fibrin that is generated adheres to the external portion of the catheter. Finally, the fibrin tail thrombosis, sometimes termed the fibrin flap thrombosis, occurs when the fibrin adheres to the end of the catheter (197,198).

Catheter-associated thrombosis has been documented in approximately one third of patients studied prospectively with extremity venography (199,200). An autopsy study of patients with malignancy demonstrated mural thrombus in 38% of catheters placed in veins, compared with 1.4% incidence of thrombus in the corresponding contralateral vessel (196). Because infection is the other major complication of catheters, it is very impressive that all of the episodes of catheter-associated sepsis in the patients studied were in patients who also had thrombosis. It is very important to emphasize that many of the thromboses are asymptomatic when diagnosed in prospective studies. The clinical diagnosis is often first manifest by impaired function of the catheter "withdrawal occlusion" (201) or by pain in the upper chest or neck, or by swelling in the shoulder, upper chest, arm, or the face.

Patients suspected of having catheter-associated thrombosis require an evaluation to assess both the catheter and the vein. The evaluation should include imaging to confirm the appropriate position of the catheter and to determine whether it is patent. The possibility of flow constrained by a fibrin sheath should be sought because it presents the risk for extravasation of infused chemotherapy drugs (202). Possible thrombosis of the axillary, innominate, or subclavian vein, and/or the superior vena cava should be evaluated with extremity venography or Doppler ultrasound. It has been suggested that most obstructing thrombi are not in the catheter lumen, but are instead in the vessel at or near the catheter end (198,203–205).

In the absence of mural thrombus, patency of the catheter can often be restored with instillation of a thrombolytic agent. In the past urokinase became a favored agent, but purity problems led to its removal from the market. A randomized trial of treatment for catheters proven radiographically to have occluding thrombus found a bolus injection of 2 mg recombinant t-PA more effective than urokinase (206). As a result, t-PA (Alteplase) has become the therapeutic agent of choice (198). A recent consensus conference provided excellent guidelines for the use of t-PA for the management of a partial thrombotic occlusion of a catheter, as shown in Fig. 12.1, and for the approach to a complete occlusion, as shown in Fig. 12.2 (198).

Venous thrombosis associated with vascular-access devices is increasingly being treated in a manner similar to DVT in other sites. Although the risk associated with venous thrombosis of the upper extremities was previously considered low, there have been a number of reports of pulmonary emboli in these circumstances (207,208). Effective treatment has been reported with intravenous heparin followed by warfarin (201) and with thrombolytic therapy with catheter-directed thrombolytic infusion (209). Safe and effective treatment with low-molecular-weight heparin also has been shown to be effective (210).

Finally, it merits stress that the high risk of thrombosis has led to interest in a variety of prophylactic approaches. In one randomized trial of patients studied prospectively with venography, it was demonstrated that a significant reduction in the occurrence of catheter-associated thrombosis was achieved with the use of 1 mg warfarin daily (200).

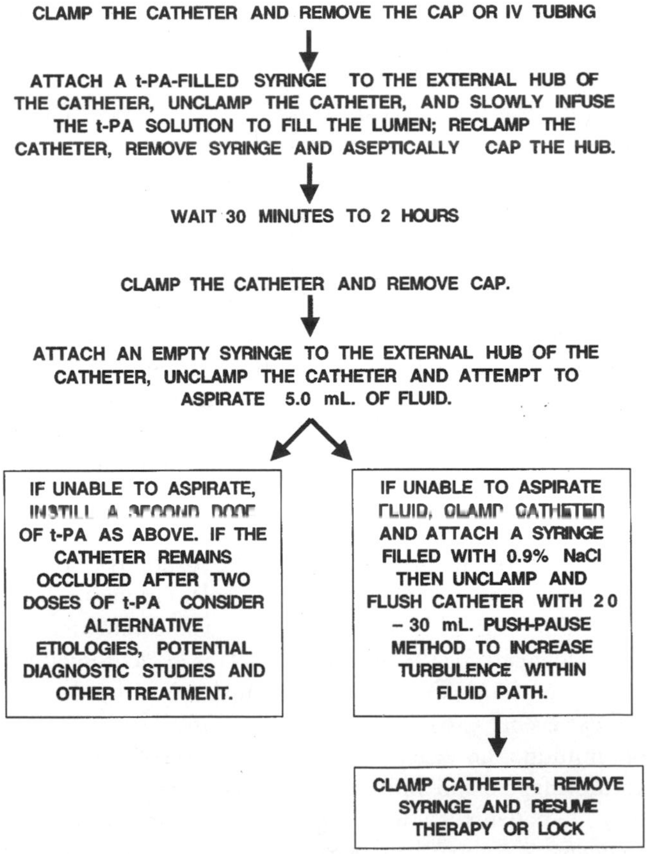
CLAMP THE CATHETER AND REMOVE THE CAP OR IV TUBING
ATTACH A t-PA-FILLED SYRINGE TO THE EXTERNAL HUB OF THE CATHETER, UNCLAMP THE CATHETER, AND SLOWLY INFUSE THE t-PA SOLUTION TO FILL THE LUMEN; RECLAMP THE CATHETER, REMOVE SYRINGE AND ASEPTICALLY CAP THE HUB.
WAIT 30 MINUTES TO 2 HOURS
CLAMP THE CATHETER AND REMOVE CAP.
ATTACH AN EMPTY SYRINGE TO THE EXTERNAL HUB OF THE CATHETER, UNCLAMP THE CATHETER AND ATTEMPT TO ASPIRATE 5.0 mL. OF FLUID.
IF UNABLE TO ASPIRATE, INSTILL A SECOND DOSE OF t-PA AS ABOVE. IF THE CATHETER REMAINS OCCLUDED AFTER TWO DOSES OF t-PA CONSIDER ALTERNATIVE ETIOLOGIES, POTENTIAL DIAGNOSTIC STUDIES AND OTHER TREATMENT.
IF UNABLE TO ASPIRATE FLUID, CLAMP CATHETER AND ATTACH A SYRINGE FILLED WITH 0.9% NaCl THEN UNCLAMP AND FLUSH CATHETER WITH 20 – 30 mL. PUSH-PAUSE METHOD TO INCREASE TURBULENCE WITHIN FLUID PATH.
CLAMP CATHETER, REMOVE SYRINGE AND RESUME THERAPY OR LOCK

FIGURE 12.1. Suggested tissue plasminogen activator (t-PA; alteplase) treatment for partial thrombotic occlusion of a central venous catheter. (Modified from Haire WD, Herbst SL. The use of alteplase (t-PA) for the management of thrombotic catheter dysfunction. *Clinician* 2000; 18:1, with permission.)

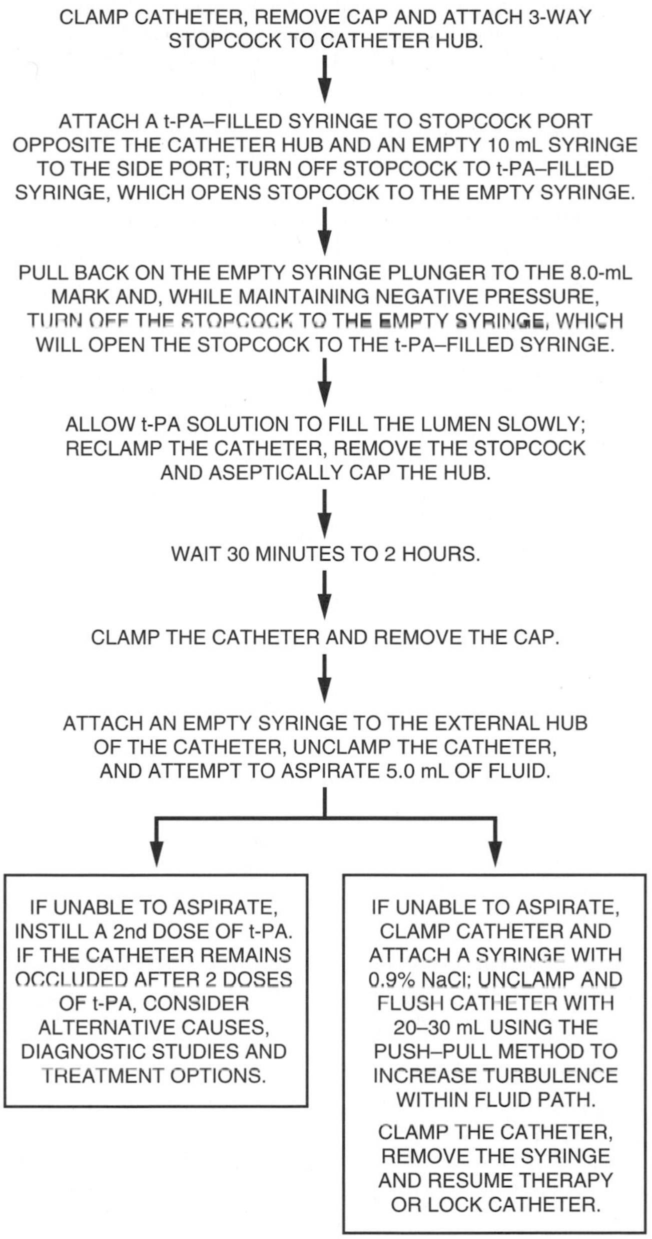
CLAMP CATHETER, REMOVE CAP AND ATTACH 3-WAY STOPCOCK TO CATHETER HUB.
ATTACH A t-PA–FILLED SYRINGE TO STOPCOCK PORT OPPOSITE THE CATHETER HUB AND AN EMPTY 10 mL SYRINGE TO THE SIDE PORT; TURN OFF STOPCOCK TO t-PA–FILLED SYRINGE, WHICH OPENS STOPCOCK TO THE EMPTY SYRINGE.
PULL BACK ON THE EMPTY SYRINGE PLUNGER TO THE 8.0-mL MARK AND, WHILE MAINTAINING NEGATIVE PRESSURE, TURN OFF THE STOPCOCK TO THE EMPTY SYRINGE, WHICH WILL OPEN THE STOPCOCK TO THE t-PA–FILLED SYRINGE.
ALLOW t-PA SOLUTION TO FILL THE LUMEN SLOWLY; RECLAMP THE CATHETER, REMOVE THE STOPCOCK AND ASEPTICALLY CAP THE HUB.
WAIT 30 MINUTES TO 2 HOURS.
CLAMP THE CATHETER AND REMOVE THE CAP.
ATTACH AN EMPTY SYRINGE TO THE EXTERNAL HUB OF THE CATHETER, UNCLAMP THE CATHETER, AND ATTEMPT TO ASPIRATE 5.0 mL OF FLUID.
IF UNABLE TO ASPIRATE, INSTILL A 2nd DOSE OF t-PA. IF THE CATHETER REMAINS OCCLUDED AFTER 2 DOSES OF t-PA, CONSIDER ALTERNATIVE CAUSES, DIAGNOSTIC STUDIES AND TREATMENT OPTIONS.
IF UNABLE TO ASPIRATE, CLAMP CATHETER AND ATTACH A SYRINGE WITH 0.9% NaCl; UNCLAMP AND FLUSH CATHETER WITH 20–30 mL USING THE PUSH–PULL METHOD TO INCREASE TURBULENCE WITHIN FLUID PATH.
CLAMP THE CATHETER, REMOVE THE SYRINGE AND RESUME THERAPY OR LOCK CATHETER.

FIGURE 12.2. Suggested tissue plasminogen activator (t-PA; alteplase) treatment for total thrombotic occlusion of a central venous catheter. (Modified from Haire WD, Herbst SL. The use of alteplase (t-PA) for the management of thrombotic catheter dysfunction. *Clinician* 2000;18:1, with permission.)

THE SEARCH FOR UNDERLYING MALIGNANCY IN *DE NOVO* THROMBOTIC DISEASE

The recognition that thrombotic–thromboembolic disease has a variety of definable pathogenetic mechanisms (e.g., thrombophilia, founder coagulation defects, thrombocythemia) that can affect therapy and future management of the patient has led to consideration of underlying cancer as an important predisposing factor. The correlate questions then are which patients should be screened and how should they be screened for the presence of an underlying malignancy when a patient has a new thrombosis (9).

Several large studies have focused on the recognition of cancer in patients seen with a thrombotic event (2,3,211–230). Gore et al. (222) identified a statistically significant incidence of cancer in a group of 610 patients studied over the 2-year period after an episode of angiographically documented pulmonary embolization. Similarly, by using impedance plethysmography to define peripheral venous thrombotic disease in 1,546 patients, they noted a 2.7 relative risk for the development of cancer when such patients were followed up over a 5-year period (223). A similar study of 660 patients by the Mayo Clinic group followed up for 4 years, however, failed to identify an increased incidence of cancer in these patients with a documented thromboembolic event (224). In another study (226), cancer was the final diagnosis in 25% of patients with unexplained DVT. Similarly, Cornuz et al. (226) noted that 12% of patients with unexplained DVT were rendered a diagnosis of cancer by 34 months of median follow-up.

Thus all of the current reports have identified an increased incidence of cancer in patients with a thrombotic event when the period of evaluation extends through the first 6 to 12 months after that incident (227–230). Although the statistical definition has varied, the odds ratios have been in the range of 3 (227,228), and a meta-type analysis was 3.2 (229). A recent remarkable report from the Danish Epidemiology Science Center examined registry data from 1977 through 1992 of 15,348 patients with DVT and 11, 305 patients with pulmonary embolism (230). The risk of underlying cancer was approximately 3 times the expected for each cohort examined. It is noteworthy that this increased risk existed for the first 6 months and then declined to 2.2 at 1 year, and then was only marginal (1.1) thereafter (230). Because these studies covered a long temporal era during which there was a significant evolution of technology applicable to the diagnosis and definition of thrombotic disease, their final numbers may have (slightly) underestimated the true risk (231).

A very important subset of patients is those with recurrent thrombotic episodes. When such subsets have been examined, the odds ratios have been significantly increased over those of a primary episode. These range up to 45.3 (as compared with 2.3) (228) or 3.2 (as compared with 2.3) (230) in representative studies. One study suggested that patients with recurrent idiopathic DVT have a 10-fold increased risk of occult malignancy (227).

In summary, one can expect an underlying neoplasm to be recognized in 5% to 10% of patients who have an idiopathic thrombotic episode, and the higher number reasonably can be expected in those with recurrent thrombotic events. The incidence may be higher if DVT is recurrent,

TABLE 12.8. CLINICAL CHARACTERISTICS OF THROMBOTIC EVENTS THAT SUGGEST THE PRESENCE OF AN UNDERLYING CANCER

Idiopathic thrombosis after age 50 yr
Recurrent recent thrombosis
Thrombosis involving both superficial and deep veins
Thrombosis at multiple or unusual sites
Idiopathic arterial thrombosis
Refractoriness of the thrombosis to coumadin therapy

the patient is older than 50 years, the patient experiences both superficial and deep venous thrombosis, the DVT involves multiple or unusual sites, arterial thrombosis or thromboembolism is present, or if the DVT is refractory to coumadin therapy (218,232); these features are shown in Table 12.8. It must, however, be appreciated that the incidence of occult malignancy in patients with idiopathic DVT will be highly dependent on the vigor of the workup. This caveat has often been exploited to demand an extensive evaluation of all patients with DVT in the absence of a precipitating factor. It is suggested that, unless otherwise dictated by clinical examination, routine laboratory tests (that include a complete blood count and biochemical profile) and chest radiograph are cost effective, whereas empiric extensive additional evaluation may not be. Unfortunately, no simple algorithm exists to provide the clinician with an easy template. Clinical judgment is absolutely critical to define the extent of the search for an underlying malignancy. Recent data from the Danish National Registry provided evidence that cancer identified at the same time as or within 1 year of an episode of venous thromboembolism is associated with an advanced stage of the cancer and a poor prognosis (233). These observations help provide perspective for appropriate clinical judgment in the pursuit of such underlying etiologic mechanisms.

REFERENCES

1. Trousseau A. Phlegmasia alba dolens. In: *Clinique medicale de L'Hotel Dieu de Paris.* 2nd ed. Paris: Balliere, 1865:3.
2. Sack JRGH, Levin J, Bell WR. Trousseau's syndrome and other manifestations of chronic disseminated coagulopathy in patients with neoplasms: clinical, pathophysiologic, and therapeutic features. *Medicine* 1977;56:1.
3. Callander N, Rappaport SI. Trousseau's syndrome. *West J Med* 1993;158:364.
4. Bick RL. Alterations of hemostasis in malignancy. In: Bick RL, Bennett JM, Byrnes RK, eds. *Hematology: clinical and laboratory practice.* St. Louis: CV Mosby, 1993:83.
5. Bick RL, Strauss JF, Frenkel EP. Thrombosis and hemorrhage in oncology patients. *Hematol Oncol Clin North Am* 1996;10:875.
6. Arkel YS. Thrombosis and cancer. *Semin Oncol* 2000;27:362.
7. Davis RB, Theologides A, Kennedy BJ. Comparative studies of blood coagulation and platelet aggregation in patients with cancer and non-malignant disease. *Ann Intern Med* 1969;71:67.
8. Edwards EA. Migrating thrombophlebitis associated with carcinoma. *N Engl J Med* 1949;240:1031.
9. Frenkel EP, Bick RL. Issues of thrombosis and hemorrhagic events in patients with cancer. *In Vivo* 1998;12:625.
10. Innerfield I, Anrist A, Benjamin JW. Plasma antithrombin patterns in disturbances of the pancreas. *Gastroenterology* 1951;19:843.
11. Goldsmith GH. Hemostatic disorders associated with malignancy. In: Ratnoff OD, Forbes CD, eds. *Disorders of hemostasis.* Philadelphia: WB Saunders, 1991:352.
12. Miller SP, Sanchez-Avalos J, Stefanski T. Coagulation disorders in cancer, I: clinical and laboratory studies. *Cancer* 1967;20:1452.
13. Scates SM. Diagnosis and treatment of cancer-related thrombosis. *Hematol Oncol Clin North Am* 1992;6:1329.
14. Sproul EF. Carcinoma and venous thrombosis: the frequency of association of carcinoma in the body or tail of the pancreas with multiple venous thrombosis. *Am J Cancer* 1938;34:566.
15. Rosen PJ. Bleeding problems in the cancer patient. *Hematol Oncol Clin North Am* 1992;6:1315.
16. Pineo GF, Brain MC, Gallus AS. Tumors, mucus production, and hypercoagulability. *Ann N Y Acad Sci* 1974;230:262.
17. Slickter SJ, Harker LA. Hemostasis in malignancy. *Ann N Y Acad Sci* 1974;230:252.
18. Astedt B, Svanberg L, Nilsson IM. Cancer, FDP, and radiotherapy. *Br Med J* 1972;2:47.
19. Phillips LL, Skrodelis V, Furey CA. The fibrinolytic enzyme system in prostatic cancer. *Cancer* 1959;12:721.
20. Yip ML, Lee S, Sacks HJ. Nonspecificity of the protamine sulfate test for intravascular coagulation. *Am J Clin Pathol* 1972;57:487.
21. Boughton BJ, Simpson A. Plasma fibronectin in acute leukemia. *Br J Haematol* 1982;51:487.
22. Rickles FR, Edwards RL, Barb C. Abnormalities of blood coagulation in patients with cancer: fibrinopeptide A generation and tumor growth. *Cancer* 1983;51:301.
23. Douglas JT, Lowe GDO, Forbes CD. Beta-thromboglobulin and platelet counts: effect of malignancy, infection, age, and obesity. *Thromb Res* 1982;25:459.
24. Yodo Y, Abe T. Fibrinopeptide A (FPA) level and fibrinogen kinetics in patients with malignant disease. *Thromb Haemost* 1981;46:706.
25. Choate JJ, Mosher DF. Fibronectin concentration in plasma of patients with breast cancer, colon cancer, and acute leukemia. *Cancer* 1983;51:1142.
26. Walenga JM, Fareed J, Mariani G. Diagnostic efficacy of a simple radioimmunoassay test for fibrinogen/fibrin fragments containing the B-beta 15-42 sequence. *Semin Thromb Hemost* 1984;10:252.
27. Fareed J, Walenga JM, Bick RL. Impact of automation on the quantitation of low molecular weight markers of hemostatic defects. *Semin Thromb Hemost* 1983;9:355.
28. Bick RL. Disseminated intravascular coagulation and related syndromes. In: *Disorders of thrombosis and hemostasis: clinical and laboratory practice.* Chicago: ASCP Press, 1992:137.
29. Bick RL. Disseminated intravascular coagulation: objective criteria for diagnosis and management. *Med Clin North Am* 1994;78:511.
30. Bick RL, Adams T. Fibrinolytic activity in myeloproliferative disorders. *Clin Res* 1973;21:264.
31. Bick RL. Disseminated intravascular coagulation: objective laboratory diagnostic criteria and guidelines for management. *Clin Lab Med* 1994;14:729.
32. Bick RL, Kunkel L. Disseminated intravascular coagulation. *Int J Hematol* 1992;55:1.
33. Cliffton EE, Grossi CE. Fibrinolytic activity of human tumors as measured by the fibrinplate method. *Cancer* 1955;8:1146.
34. Enck RE, Rios CN. Tamoxifen treatment of metastatic breast cancer and antithrombin III levels. *Cancer* 1984;53:2607.

35. Boggust WA, O'Brien DJ, O'Meara RA. The coagulative factors of normal human and human cancer tissue. *Ir J Med Sci* 1963;6:131.
36. O'Meara R. Coagulation properties of cancers. *Ir J Med Sci* 1958;394:474.
37. Pineo GF, Regorczi F, Hatton MWC. The activation of coagulation by extracts of mucin: a possible pathway of intravascular coagulation accompanying adenocarcinomas. *J Lab Clin Med* 1973;82:255.
38. Lafler CJ, Hinerman DL. A morphologic study of pancreatic carcinoma with reference to multiple thrombi. *Cancer* 1961; 944:14.
39. Owen CA, Oels HC, Bowie EJW. Chronic intravascular coagulation syndrome. *Thromb Diath Haemorrh* 1969;136:197.
40. Rapaport SI, Chapman CG. Coexistent hypercoagulability and acute hypofibrinogenemia in a patient with prostatic carcinoma. *Am J Med* 1959;27:144.
41. Brown RC, Campbell DC, Thompson JH. Increased fibrinolysin with malignant disease. *Arch Intern Med* 1962;109:29.
42. Omar JB, Saxena HS, Mitel HS. Fibrinolytic activity in malignant diseases. *J Assoc Physicians India* 1971;19:293.
43. Moolton SE, Vroman L, Broman GMS. Role of blood platelets in thromboembolism. *Arch Intern Med* 1949;84:667.
44. Levin J, Conley CL. Thrombocytosis associated with malignant disease. *Arch Intern Med* 1964;114:487.
45. Adams T, Shultz L, Goldberg L. Platelet function abnormalities in the myeloproliferative disorders. *Scand J Haematol* 1974; 13:215.
46. Bick RL. Hypercoagulability and thrombosis. In: *Disorders of thrombosis and hemostasis: clinical and laboratory practice.* Chicago: ASCP Press, 1992:261.
47. Patterson WP, Ringenberg QS. The pathophysiology of thrombosis in cancer. *Semin Oncol* 1990;17:140.
48. Bick RL. Treatment of bleeding and thrombosis in the patient with cancer. In: Nealon T, ed. *Management of the patient with cancer.* Philadelphia: Saunders, 1976:48.
49. Kumar S, Monorama B. Pre-leukemic acute myelogenous leukemia. *Acta Haematol* 1970;3:21.
50. Lisiewicz J. Mechanisms of hemorrhage in leukemias. *Semin Thromb Hemost* 1978;4:241.
51. Coleman RW, Rubin RN. Disseminated intravascular coagulation due to malignancy. *Semin Oncol* 1990;17:172.
52. Lisiewicz J. Disseminated intravascular coagulation in acute leukemia. *Semin Thromb Hemost* 1988;14:339.
53. Boggs DR, Wintrobe MM, Cartwright CE. Acute leukemias: analysis of 322 cases and review of the literature. *Medicine* 1962;41:163.
54. Evans HE, Wolman IJ. Problems in the diagnosis and management of acute leukemia in childhood. *Clin Pediatr* 1971; 10:571.
55. Moszczynski P, Lisiewicz J. The liver function in leukemic patients in the light of enzymatic studies. *Pol Tyg Leg* 1974; 29:1925.
56. Holt JM, Gordon-Smith EG. Retinal abnormalities in diseases of the blood. *Br J Ophthalmol* 1969;53:145.
57. Hersh EM, Bodey GP, Nies BA. Causes of death in acute leukemia: a ten year study of 414 patients from 1954-1963. *JAMA* 1965;193:105.
58. Han T, Stutzman L, Cohen E. Effect of platelet transfusion on hemorrhage in patients with acute leukemia. *Cancer* 1966;19: 1937.
59. Moszczynski P, Lisiewicz J. Early symptoms of acute and chronic leukemias in 300 patients. *Med Wiejska* 1973;8:249.
60. Kuznik BI, Kuzmiehco EL, Alnikov GP. On the role of leukocytes in the process of blood coagulation in chronic lymphocytic leukemia. *Probl Gematol Pereliv Krovi* 1969;14:3.
61. Seifter EJ, Bell WR. Platelet disorders In: Bell, WR, ed. *Coagulation disorders in the cancer patient.* Mt Kisco, NY: Futura Publishing, 1984:15.
62. Lisiewicz J. Chronic granulocytic leukemia. In: *Hemorrhage in leukemias.* Warsaw: Polish Medical Publishing, 1976:82.
63. Brakman P, Synder J, Henderson ES. Blood coagulation and fibrinolysis in acute leukemia. *Br J Haematol* 1970;18:135.
64. Ventura GJ, Hester JP, Dixon DO. Analysis of risk factors for fatal hemorrhage during induction therapy of patients with acute promyelocytic leukemia. *Hematol Pathol* 1989;3:23.
65. Foon KA, Champlin RE, Gale RP. Acute myelogenous leukemia and the myelodysplastic syndromes. In: Haskell CM, ed. *Cancer treatment.* Philadelphia: WB Saunders, 1990:589.
66. Rosove MH, Schwartz GE. Hematologic complications of cancer and its treatment. In: Haskell CM, ed). *Cancer treatment.* Philadelphia: WB Saunders, 1990:850.
67. Caen J, Sinakoz Z, Sultan V. Les troubles du functionnement des plaquettes dans les leukemies myeloides chroniques. *Nouv Rev Fr Hematol* 1966;6:719.
68. Cardamone JM, Edson J, McArthur JK. Abnormalities of platelet function in the myeloproliferative disorders. *JAMA* 1972;221:270.
69. Sultan Y, Delobel J, Caen J. Anomalies de l'hemostase primaire au cours des leucemies myeloides chroniques et des autres syndromes myeloproliferatifs. *Actual Hematol (Paris)* 1969;3:95.
70. Miyagawa K, Kawakita Y. Ultrastructure of blood platelets in various hematologic disorders. *Acta Haematol (Japan)* 1969; 32:64.
71. Bick RL, Wilson WL. Essential (hemorrhagic) thrombocythemia: a clinical and laboratory study of 14 patients. *Am J Clin Pathol* 1984;81:799.
72. Bick RL. Essential (primary) thrombocythemia: hematology check sample #H-86-4. *Am Soc Clin Pathol Hematol* 1989;31:4.
73. Wehmeier A, Scharf RE, Fricke S. Bleeding and thrombosis in chronic myeloproliferative disorders: relation of platelet disorders to clinical aspects of the disease. *Haemostasis* 1989;19:251.
74. Rosner F, Dobbs JV, Ritz DN. Disturbances of hemostasis in acute myeloblastic leukemia. *Acta Haematol* 1970;43:65.
75. Cowan DM, Haut MJ. Platelet function in acute leukemia. *J Lab Clin Med* 1972;79:893.
76. Lisiewicz J, Moszczynski P. Disturbances of hemostasis in patients with various leukemia types in the light of results of basic tests of blood coagulation and fibrinolysis. *Przegl Lek* 1972;29:389.
77. Diebold J, Camilieri TP, Delarue J. Les lesions hepatiques au cours des leucoses: etude histopathologique. *Ann Anat Pathol (Paris)* 1969;14:41.
78. Lisiewicz J. Chronic lymphocytic leukemia. In: *Hemorrhage in leukemias.* Warsaw: Polish Medical Publishers, 1976:104.
79. Lazarachick J, Pappas AA, Kizer J. Acquired von Willebrand's syndrome due to an inhibitor specific for von Willebrand factor antigens. *Am J Hematol* 1986;21:305.
80. Mohri H. Acquired von Willebrand's disease and storage pool disease in chronic myelocytic leukemia. *Am J Hematol* 1986;22: 391.
81. Budde U, Dent JA, Berkowitz SD. Subunit composition of plasma von Willebrand factor in patients with the myeloproliferative syndrome. *Blood* 1986;68:1213.
82. Fabris F, Casonato A, Del Ben MG. Abnormalities of von Willebrand factor in myeloproliferative disease: a relationship with bleeding diathesis. *Br J Haematol* 1986;63:75.
83. Goudemand J, Samor B, Caron C. Acquired type II von Willebrand's disease: demonstration of a complexed inhibitor of the von Willebrand factor-platelet interaction and response to treatment. *Br J Haematol* 1988;68:227.
84. Meschengieser S, Blanco A, Maugeri N. Platelet and intraplate-

let von Willebrand factor antigen and fibrinogen in myelodysplastic syndromes. *Thromb Res* 1987;46:601.

85. Mohri H, Noguchi T, Kodama F. Acquired von Willebrand disease due to inhibitor of human myeloma protein specific for von Willebrand factor. *Am J Clin Pathol* 1987;87:663.
86. Tatewaki W, Takahashi H, Wada K. Plasma von Willebrand factor proteolysis in patients with chronic myeloproliferative disorders: no possibility of ex vivo degradation by calcium-dependent proteolysis. *Thromb Res* 1989;56:191.
87. Takahashi H, Nagayama R, Tanabe Y. DDAVP in acquired von Willebrand syndrome associated with multiple myeloma. *Am J Hematol* 1986;22:421.
88. Lisiewicz J, Moszcynski P. Leukocytosis and fibrinolytic activity of the blood in the leukemic patients. *Rev Med Intern* 1975;1:37.
89. Tatarsky J, Sinakos Z, Larrieu MJ. Leukocytes et fibrinolyse, II: etudes des leukocytes pathologiques. *Nouv Rev Fr Hematol* 1967;7:95.
90. Kirchmayer S, Stalowa I, Biernacka B. Measurements of proteolytic activity of leukoblasts: a new diagnostic method. *Pol Arch Med Wesn* 1970;44:365.
91. Wado H, Nagano T, Tomeoku M. Coagulant and fibrinolytic activities in the leukemic cell lysates. *Thromb Res* 1982;30:315.
92. Gralnick HR, Tan HK. Acute promyelocytic leukemia: a model for understanding the role of the malignant cells in hemostasis. *Hum Pathol* 1974;5:661.
93. Gordon SG. Cancer cell procoagulants and their implications. *Hematol Oncol Clin North Am* 1992;6:1359.
94. Girolami A, Cliffton EE. Fibrinolytic and proteolytic activity in acute and chronic leukemia. *Am J Med Sci* 1966;51:638.
95. Polliack A. Acute promyelocytic leukemia with disseminated intravascular coagulation. *Am J Clin Pathol* 1971;56:155.
96. Galloway MJ, Mackie MJ, McVerry BA. Combinations of increased thrombin, plasmin, and non-specific protease activity in patients with acute leukemia. *Haemostasis* 1983;13:322.
97. Matsuoka M, Onishi Y. Pathologic cells as procoagulant substances of disseminated intravascular coagulation syndrome in acute promyelocytic leukemia. *Thromb Res* 1976;8:263.
98. Sultan C, Gounault M, Varet B. Relationship between the cell morphology of acute myeloblastic leukemia and occurrence of a syndrome of disseminated intravascular coagulation. XIV International Congress of Hematology, Sao Paulo, 1972: Abstract 603.
99. Huth K, Loffler H, Lechlemayer U. Verbrauchskoagulopathie bei unreifzelligen keukosen. *Verh Dtsch Ges Inn Med* 1968;74:147.
100. van Creveld J, Mochtar JA. Fibrinolysis in acute leukemia. *Pediatr Ann* 1960;194:65.
101. Fisher S, Ramot B, Kreisler B. Fibrinolysis in acute leukemia. *Isr Med J* 1960;19:195.
102. Cooperberg AA, Neiman GMA. Fibrinogenopenia and fibrinolysis in acute myelogenous leukemia. *Ann Intern Med* 1955;42:706.
103. Pisciotta AV, Schulz EJ. Fibrinolytic purpura in acute leukemia. *Am J Med* 1955;19:824.
104. Sznajd J, Naskalski J, Liciewicz J. Antiheparin activity of myeloperoxidase and ribonuclease of chronic granulocytic leukemia leukocytes. *Pol Arch Med Wewn* 1969;42:207.
105. Bick RL, Scates S. Disseminated intravascular coagulation. *Lab Med* 1992;23:161.
106. Bick RL, Baker WF. Disseminated intravascular coagulation syndromes. *Hematol Pathol* 1992;6:1.
107. Bick RL. Disseminated intravascular coagulation and related syndromes: a review. *Am J Hematol* 1978;5:265.
108. Gralnick HR, Bagley J, Abrell E. Heparin treatment for the hemorrhagic diathesis of acute promyelocytic leukemia. *Am J Med* 1974;52:167.
109. Bennett RM. Acute leukemia. In: Rappaport H, ed. Tutorial in hematopathology. Chicago: University of Chicago Press, 1980:42–70.
110. Shustrova NM. On the permeability of vascular walls in some disorders of the blood system. Doctoral dissertation. Alma-Ata, 1965.
111. Trunova LE. The pathogenesis of the hemorrhagic system in acute leukemia. *Vrach Delo* 1965;11:41.
112. Valkov J. Histologic studies of extramedullary hemopoiesis in leukemias and its relationship to the blood vessels. *Med Fizkult* 1963;42:35.
113. Luzzatto G, Schaffer AI. The prethrombotic state in cancer. *Semin Oncol* 1990;17:147.
114. Didisheim P, Bowie EJW, Owen CA. Intravascular coagulation fibrinolysis (ICF) syndrome and malignancy: historical review and report of two cases with metastatic carcinoid and with acute myelomonocytic leukemia. *Thromb Diath Haemorrh* 1969;36:215.
115. Goodnight SH. Bleeding and intravascular clotting in malignancy: a review. *Ann N Y Acad Sci* 1974;230:271.
116. Soong BCF, Miller SP. Coagulation disorders in cancer: fibrinolysis and inhibitors. *Cancer* 1970;25:867.
117. Frick PG. Acute hemorrhagic syndrome with hypofibrinogenemia in metastatic cancer. *Acta Haematol (Basel)* 1956;16:11.
118. Leavy RA, Kahn SB, Brodsky I. Disseminated intravascular coagulation: a complication of chemotherapy in acute promyelocytic leukemia. *Cancer* 1970;26:142.
119. Henderson ES. Acute myelogenous leukemia. In: Williams WJ, Beutler E, Erslev AL, et al., eds. *Hematology.* New York: McGraw-Hill, 1977:830.
120. Brassinne C, Coone A, Jijs M. Characterization of two direct fibrinogenolytic activities and one proteolytic inhibitor activity in the human prostate. *Thromb Res* 1976;8:803.
121. Mertins BF, Green LF, Bowie EJW. Fibrinolytic split products and ethanol gelation test in pre-operative evaluation of patients with prostatic disease. *Mayo Clin Proc* 1974;49:642.
122. Bick RL. Basic mechanisms of hemostasis pertaining to DIC. In: Bick RL, ed. *Disseminated intravascular coagulation and related syndromes.* Boca Raton, Fla: CRC Press, 1983:1.
123. Bull B, Rubenberg M, Dacie J. Microangiopathic hemolytic anemia: mechanisms of red-cell fragmentation. *Br J Haematol* 1968;14:643.
124. Folkman J. Tumor angiogenesis: therapeutic implications. *N Engl J Med* 1971;285:1182.
125. Cheung DK, Raaf JH. Selection of patients with malignant ascites for a peritoneovenous shunt. *Cancer* 1982;50:1204.
126. Bick RL. Alterations of hemostasis associated with surgery, cardiopulmonary bypass surgery, and prosthetic devices. In: Ratnoff OD, Forbes CD, eds. *Disorders of hemostasis.* Philadelphia: WB Saunders, 1991:382.
127. Lerner RG, Nelson JC, Corines P, et al. Disseminated intravascular coagulation: complication of LeVeen peritoneovenous shunts. *JAMA* 1984;240:2064.
128. Harmon DC, Demirjian Z, Ellman L. Disseminated intravascular coagulation with the peritoneovenous shunt. *Ann Intern Med* 1979;90:714.
129. Stein SF, Fulenwider JT, Ansley JD. Accelerated fibrinogen and platelet destruction after peritoneovenous shunting. *Arch Intern Med* 1981;141:1149.
130. Qazi R, Savlov ED. Peritoneovenous shunt for palliation of malignant ascites. *Cancer* 1982;49:600.
131. Bick RL. Disseminated intravascular coagulation: a clinical/laboratory study of 48 patients. In: Walz DA, McCoy LE, eds. *Contributions to hemostasis. Ann N Y Acad Sci* 1981;370:843.
132. Feinstein DI. Treatment of disseminated intravascular coagulation. *Semin Thromb Hemost* 1988;14:351.
133. Bick RL, Schmalhorst WR, Shanbrom E. Prothrombin complex concentrates: use in controlling the hemorrhagic diathesis of chronic liver disease. *Am J Dig Dis* 1975;20:741.
134. Marguliusa A, Jackson DP, Ratnoff OD. Circulating anticoagu-

lants: a study of 40 cases and review of the literature. *Medicine (Baltimore)* 1961;40:145.

135. Ikkala E. Transfusion therapy in congenital deficiencies of plasma factor XIII. *Ann N Y Acad Sci* 1972;202:200.
136. Bick RL. Circulating heparin activity in multiple myeloma. *Blood* 1984;64:924.
137. Palmer RN, Rick ME, Rick PD. Circulating heparan sulfate anticoagulant in a patient with a fatal bleeding disorder. *N Engl J Med* 1984;310:1696.
138. Khoory MS, Nesheim ME, Bowie EJW. Circulating heparan sulfate proteoglycan anticoagulant from a patient with a plasma cell disorder. *J Clin Invest* 1980;65:666.
139. Bussel JB, Steinherz PG, Miller DR. A heparin-like anticoagulant in an 8-month-old boy with acute monoblastic leukemia. *Am J Hematol* 1984;16:83.
140. Kunkel LA. Acquired circulating anticoagulants. *Hematol Oncol Clin North Am* 1992;6:1359.
141. Bick RL. The clinical significance of fibrinogen degradation products. *Semin Thromb Hemost* 1982;8:302.
142. Bick RL. Congenital and acquired coagulation protein defects associated with hemorrhage or thrombosis. In: Powers J, ed. *Diagnostic hematology: clinical and technical aspects.* St. Louis: CV Mosby, 1989:375.
143. Bick RL. Syndromes associated with hyperfibrino(geno)lysis. In: Bick RL, ed. *Disseminated intravascular coagulation and related syndromes.* Boca Raton, Fla: CRC Press, 1983:105.
144. Kwaan HC, Lo R, McFadzean AJS. Antifibrinolytic activity in primary carcinoma of the liver. *Clin Sci* 1959;18:251.
145. Livingston RB, Carter SK. *Single agents in cancer chemotherapy.* New York: Plenum Press, 1970.
146. Rubin P, Casareh GW. *Clinical radiation pathology.* Philadelphia: WB Saunders, 1968:778.
147. Bick RL. Qualitative (functional) platelet defects. In: *Disorders of thrombosis and hemostasis: clinical and laboratory practice.* Chicago: ASCP Press, 1992:49.
148. Berkheiser SW. The incidence of malignant cells in routine bone marrow examination. *Cancer* 1955;8:958.
149. Hansen HH, Muggia FM, Selawry OS. Bone marrow examination in 100 consecutive patients with bronchogenic carcinoma. *Lancet* 1971;1:443.
150. Jamshidi K, Swaim WR. Bone marrow biopsy with unaltered architecture: a new biopsy device. *J Lab Clin Med* 1971;77:335.
151. Jonsson U, Rundles RW. Tumor metastases in bone marrow. *Blood* 1951;6:16.
152. Lanier PF. Sternal marrow in patients with metastatic cancer. *Arch Intern Med* 1949;84:891.
153. Harker LA, Finch CA. Thrombokinetics in man. *J Clin Invest* 1969;48:963.
154. Marymount JH, Gross S. Patterns of metastatic cancer in the spleen. *Am J Clin Pathol* 1963;40:58.
155. Miale JB. *Laboratory medicine hematology.* St. Louis: CV Mosby, 1972:53.
156. Gardner GF. Platelet transfusion. In: Baldini MG, Elbe S, eds. *Platelets: production, function and storage.* New York: Grune & Stratton, 1974:393.
157. Heustis DW, Bove JR, Busch S. *Practical blood transfusion.* Boston: Little, Brown, 1969.
158. Ey FS, Goodnight SH. Bleeding disorders in cancer. *Semin Oncol* 1990;17:187.
159. Ahn YS, Harrington WJ, Seelman RC. Vincristine therapy of idiopathic and secondary thrombocytopenias. *N Engl J Med* 1974;291:376.
160. Marmont AM, Damasio EE, Gori E. Vinblastine sulfate in idiopathic thrombocytopenic purpura. *Lancet* 1971;2:94.
161. Nalbandian RM, Henry RL, Bick RL. Thrombotic thrombocytopenic purpura. *Semin Thromb Hemost* 1979;5:216.
162. Brook J, Konwaler BE. Thrombotic thrombocytopenic purpura: association with metastatic gastric carcinoma and a possible auto-immune disorder. *Calif Med* 1965;102:222.
163. Friedman IA, Schwartz SO, Leifhold SL. Platelet function defects with bleeding. *Arch Intern Med* 1964;113:177.
164. Perry S. Coagulation defects in leukemia. *J Lab Clin Med* 1957; 50:229.
165. Sanchez-Avalos J, Soong BCF, Miller SP. Coagulation disorders in cancer, II: multiple myeloma. *Cancer* 1969;23:1388.
166. Bick RL. Acquired circulating anticoagulants and defective hemostasis in malignant paraprotein disorders. In: Murano G, Bick RL, eds. *Basic concepts of hemostasis and thrombosis.* Boca Raton, Fla: CRC Press, 1980:205.
167. Glaspy JA. Hemostatic defects in multiple myeloma and related disorders. *Hematol Oncol Clin North Am* 1992;6:1301.
168. Patterson WP, Caldwell CW, Doll DC. Hyperviscosity syndromes and coagulopathies. *Semin Oncol* 1990;17:210.
169. Bick RL, Adams T, Schmalhorst RS. Bleeding times, platelet adhesion, and aspirin. *Am J Clin Pathol* 1976;65:69.
170. Bick RL, Klein CA, Fekete LF. Alterations of hemostasis associated with malignant paraprotein disorders. *Trans Am Soc Hematol* 1976:163.
171. Silberstein, LE, Abrahm J, Shattil SJ. The efficacy of intensive plasma exchange in acquired von Willebrand's disease. *Transfusion* 1987;27:234.
172. Bovill EG, Ershler WB, Golden EA. A human myeloma-produced monoclonal protein directed against the active subpopulation of von Willebrand factor. *Am J Clin Pathol* 1986;85:115.
173. Horellou MH, Baumelou E, Sitbon N. Four cases of acquired Willebrand factor deficiency associated with monoclonal dysglobulinemia. *Ann Med Intern (Paris)* 1983;134:707.
174. Schwab PJ, Fahey JL. Treatment of Waldenströms macroglobulinemia by plasmapheresis. *N Engl J Med* 1960;263:574.
175. Bettigole RF, Himelstein ES, Oettgen HF. Hypofibrinogenemia due to L-asparaginase: studies of fibrinogen survival using autologous ^{131}I-fibrinogen. *Blood* 1970;35:195.
176. Brodsky I, Conroy JF. The effects of chemotherapy on hemostasis. *Cancer Chemother* 1972;2:85.
177. Monto RW, Talley RW, Caldwell MJ. Observation on the mechanisms of hemorrhagic toxicity in mithramycin therapy. *Cancer Res* 1969;29:697.
178. Olson RE. Vitamin K-induced prothrombin formation antagonism by actinomycin-D. *Science* 1964;145:926.
179. Hayano K, Fukui H, Otsuka Y. Three cases of renal failure associated with microangiopathic hemolytic anemia after mitomycin C therapy. *Nippon Jinzo Gakki Shi* 1988;30:835.
180. Jain S, Seymour AE. Mitomycin C associated hemolytic uremic syndrome. *Pathology* 1987;19:58.
181. Sheldon R, Slaughter D. A syndrome of microangiopathic hemolytic anemia, renal impairment, and pulmonary edema in chemotherapy-treated patients with adenocarcinoma. *Cancer* 1986;58:1428.
182. McCarthy JT, Staats BA. Pulmonary hypertension, hemolytic anemia, and renal failure: a mitomycin-associated syndrome. *Chest* 1986;89:608.
183. Bick RL, Fekete LF, Wilson WL. Adriamycin and fibrinolysis. *Thromb Res* 1976;8:467.
184. Bick RL, Fekete L, Murano G. Daunomycin and fibrinolysis. *Thromb Res* 1976;9:201.
185. Klener P, Kubisz P, Suranova J. Influence of cytotoxic drugs on platelet functions and coagulation. *Thromb Hemost* 1977;37:53.
186. Feffer SE, Carmosino LS, Fox RL. Acquired protein C deficiency in patients with breast cancer receiving cyclophosphamide, methotrexate, and 5-fluorouracil. *Cancer* 1989;63: 1303.
187. Milne A, Talbot S, Bevan D. Thrombosis during cytotoxic chemotherapy. *Br Med J* 1988;297:624.
188. Levin MN, Gent M, Hirsh J. The thrombogenic effect of anti-

cancer drug therapy in women with stage II breast cancer. *N Engl J Med* 1988;318:404.

189. Goodnough CT, Saito H, Manni A. Increased incidence of thromboembolism in stage IV breast cancer patients treated with a five drug chemotherapy regimen. *Cancer* 1984;54:1264.
190. Weiss RB, Tormey DC, Holland JF. Venous thrombosis during multimodal treatment of primary breast carcinoma. *Cancer Treat Rep* 1981;65:677.
191. Farbstein MJ, Blume KG. Acute leukemia. In: Blume KG, Petz LD, eds. *Clinical bone marrow transplantation.* New York: Churchill Livingstone, 1983:271.
192. Sullivan KM. Graft-versus-host disease. In: Blume KG, Petz LD, eds. *Clinical bone marrow transplantation.* New York: Churchill Livingstone, 1983:91.
193. Shulman HM, Gown AM, Nugent DJ. Hepatic veno-occlusive disease after bone marrow transplantation. *Am J Pathol* 1987; 127:549.
194. Jerman MR, Fick RB. Nonbacterial thrombotic endocarditis associated with bone marrow transplantation. *Chest* 1986; 90:919.
195. Kuramoto K, Matsushita S, Yamanouchi H. Nonbacterial thrombotic endocarditis as a cause of cerebral and myocardial infarction. *Jpn Circ J* 1984;48:1000.
196. Raad II, Luna M, Khalil SA, et al. The relationship between the thrombotic and infectious complications of central venous catheters. *JAMA* 1994;271:1014–1016.
197. Kaplan LK, McKinnon BT. Vascular access devices: managing occlusions and related complications in home infusion. *Infusion* 1998;4:SI.
198. Haire WD, Herbst SL. The use of alteplase (t-PA) for the management of thrombotic catheter dysfunction. *Clinician* 2000;18:1.
199. Horne MK III, May DJ, Alexander HR, et al. Venographic surveillance of tunneled venous access devices in adult oncology patients. *Ann Surg Oncol* 1995;2:174–178.
200. Bern MM, Lokich JJ, Wallach SR, et al. Very low doses of warfarin can prevent thrombosis in central venous catheters: a randomized prospective trial. *Ann Intern Med* 1990;112:423–428.
201. Gould JR, Carloss HW, Skinner WL. Groshong catheter-associated subclavian venous thrombosis. *Am J Med* 1993;95: 419–423.
202. Mayo DJ, Pearson DC. Chemotherapy extravasation: a consequence of fibrin sheath formation around vascular access devices. *Oncol Nurs Forum* 1995;22:675–680.
203. Stephens LC, Haire WD, Kotuclak GD. Are clinical signs accurate indicators of the cause of central venous catheter occlusion. *J Parent Enter Nutr* 1995;19:75.
204. Tolar B, Gould JR. The timing and sequence of multiple device related complications in patients with long term in dwelling Groshong catheters. *Cancer* 1996;78:1308.
205. Young C, Gould JR. The timing and sequence of multiple device related complications in patients with indwelling subcutaneous ports. *Am J Surg* 1997;174;417.
206. Haire WD, Atkinson JB, Stephens LC, et al. Urokinase versus recombinant tissue plasminogen activator in thrombosed central venous catheters: a double-blinded, randomized trial. *Thromb Haemost* 1994;72:543–547.
207. Leiby JM, Purcell H, DeMaria JJ, et al. Pulmonary embolism as a result of Hickman catheter-related thrombosis. *Am J Med* 1989;86:228–231.
208. Monreal M, Raventos A, Lerma R, et al. Pulmonary embolism in patients with upper extremity DVT associated with venous central lines: a prospective study. *Thromb Haemost* 1994;72:548–550.
209. Seigel EL, Jew AC, Delcore R, et al. Thrombolytic therapy for catheter-related thrombosis. *Am J Surg* 1993;166:716–718; discussion 718–719.
210. Drakos PE, Nagler A, Or R, et al. Low molecular weight heparin for Hickman catheter-induced thrombosis in thrombocytopenic patients undergoing bone marrow transplantation. *Cancer* 1992;70:1895–1898.
211. Hoerr SO, Harper JR. On peripheral thrombophlebitis: its occurrence as a presenting symptom of malignant disease of pancreas, biliary tract or duodenum. *JAMA* 1957;164:233.
212. Lieberman JS, Borrero J, Urdanetta E, et al. Thrombophlebitis and cancer. *JAMA* 1961;177:542.
213. Klastersky J, Daneau D, Verhest A. Causes of death in patients with cancer. *Eur J Cancer* 1972;8:149.
214. Inagaki J, Rodriguez V, Bodey GP. Causes of death in cancer patients. *Cancer* 1974;33:568.
215. Ambrus JL, Ambrus CM, Mink IB, et al. Causes of death in cancer patients: *J Med* 1975;6:61.
216. Thompson CM, Rodgers RL. Analysis of autopsy records of 157 cases of carcinoma of the pancreas with particular reference to the incidence of thromboembolism. *Am J Med Sci* 1952; 223:469.
217. Rahr HB, Sorenson JV. Venous thromboembolism and cancer. *Blood Coagul Fibrinolysis* 1992;3:451.
218. Francis JL, Biggerstaff J, Amirkhosravi A. Hemostasis and malignancy. *Semin Thromb Hemost* 1998;24:93.
219. Luzatto G, Schafer AI. The prethrombotic state in cancer. *Semin Oncol* 1990;17:147.
220. Dvorak HF. Thrombosis and cancer. *Hum Pathol* 1987;18:275.
221. Wooling KR, Schick RM. Thrombophlebitis: a possible clue to cryptic malignant lesion. *Proc Staff Meet Mayo Clin* 1956;31: 227.
222. Gore JM, Appelbaum JS, Greene HL, et al. Occult cancer in patients with acute pulmonary embolism. *Ann Intern Med* 1982;96:556.
223. Goldberg RJ, Seneff M, Gore JM, et al. Occult malignant neoplasm in patients with deep venous thrombosis. *Arch Intern Med* 1987;147:251.
224. Griffen MR, Stanton AW, Brown ML, et al. Deep venous thrombosis and pulmonary embolism: risk of subsequent malignant neoplasms. *Arch Intern Med* 1987;147:1907.
225. Bastounis EA, Karayiannakis AJ, Makri GG, et al. The incidence of occult cancer in patients with deep venous thrombosis: a prospective study. *J Intern Med* 1996;239:153.
226. Cornuz J, Pearon SD, Creager MA, et al. Importance of findings of the initial evaluation for cancer in patients with symptomatic idiopathic deep venous thrombosis. *Ann Intern Med* 1996;125:785.
227. Pradoni P, Lensinq AWA, Buler HR, et al. Deep vein thrombosis and the incidence of subsequent cancer. *N Engl J Med* 1992; 327:1128.
228. Nordstrom M, Lindblad G, Anderson H, et al. Deep vein thrombosis and occult malignancy: an epidemiological study. *BMJ* 1994;308:891.
229. Prins MH, Hettiarachchi RJ, Lensin AW, et al. Newly diagnosed malignancy in patients with venous thromboembolism: search or wait and see? *Thromb Haemost* 1997;25:185.
230. Sorensen HT, Mellemkjaer L, Steffensen FH, et al. The risk of a diagnosis of cancer after primary deep venous thrombosis or pulmonary embolism. *N Engl J Med* 1998;338:1169.
231. Buller H, Wouter ten Cate JW. Primary thromboembolism and cancer screening. *N Engl J Med* 1998;338:1221.
232. Adamson DJA, Currie JM. Occult malignancy is associated with venous thrombosis unresponsive to adequate anticoagulation. *Br J Clin Pract* 1993;47:190.
233. Sorensen HT, Mellemkjaer L, Olsen JH, et al. Prognosis of cancers associated with venous thromboembolism. *N Engl J Med* 2000;343:1846.

13

HEREDITARY THROMBOPHILIC DISORDERS

RODGER L. BICK
WILLIAM F. BAKER, JR.

Thrombosis is clearly the most common cause of death in the United States. About 2 million individuals die each year of an arterial or venous thrombosis or the consequences thereof (1). About 80% to 90% of all causes of thrombosis can now be defined. Of these, in more than 50% of all patients, a congenital or acquired blood coagulation protein or platelet defect caused the thrombotic event. It is obviously of major importance to define those individuals with such a defect, as this allows (a) appropriate antithrombotic therapy to decrease risks of recurrence, (b) determination of the length of time the patient must receive therapy for secondary prevention, and (c) testing of family members of those with a hereditary blood coagulation protein or platelet defect (about 50% of all coagulation and platelet defects mentioned earlier). These and common clinical defects leading to thrombosis are discussed later and are found in Table 13.1. Aside from mortality, significant additional morbidity occurs from both arterial or venous thrombotic events, including, but not limited to, paralysis (nonfatal thrombotic stroke), cardiac disability (repeated coronary events), loss of vision (retinal vascular thrombosis), and fetal wastage syndrome (placental vascular thrombosis), stasis ulcers, and other manifestations of postphlebitic syndrome [recurrent deep vein thrombosis (DVT)], and so on.

THROMBOTIC EVENTS

Specific examples are as follows:

R. L. Bick: Department of Medicine and Pathology, University of Texas Southwestern Medical Center; Dallas Thrombosis/Hemostasis Clinical Center; ThromboCare Laboratories, Dallas, Texas.

W. F. Baker, JR.: Department of Medicine, Center for Health Sciences, University of California at Los Angeles, Los Angeles, California; Department of Medicine, Kern Medical Center, Bakersfield, California; and California Clinical Thrombosis Center, Bakersfield, California.

Deep Vein Thrombosis

The incidence of DVT in the United States is about 159 per 100,000 or about 398,000 per year (1,2). A definable etiology can be found in 80% to 90% of these patients; this allows effective therapy to be delivered and allows the other advantages of defining the blood coagulation protein or platelet defects, mentioned earlier. For example, about 28% of these patients will have antiphospholipid syndrome, and oral anticoagulants will fail (rethrombosis will occur) in about 65% (2). About 30% to 50% of these patients will have congenital coagulation protein or platelet defects; thus family members should be assessed and, obviously, antithrombotic therapy for the afflicted patient should be prolonged, not 6 weeks to 3 months.

Pulmonary Embolus

The overall incidence of pulmonary embolus (PE) in the United States is about 139 per 100,000 or about 347,000 cases per year (clinical data); the incidence of fatal PE in the United States is 94 per 100,000 or about 235,000 deaths (autopsy data) (1–3). The same scenario as that for DVT prevails for PE. If the PE is not fatal, every attempt should be made to define the blood coagulation protein or platelet defect responsible.

Coronary Artery Thrombosis (Acute Myocardial Infarction)

Approximately 1,500,000 individuals in the United States will have an acute myocardial infarction (AMI) per year; 50% will be fatal, and 50% will be a premature/precocious event (1,4). Thus there are about 750,000 deaths of coronary artery thrombosis per year. Of these coronary thrombotic events, 67% of patients have a coagulation blood protein or platelet defect leading to thrombosis. Fifty percent of these coagulation protein or platelet defects will be hereditary, thus emphasizing the importance of defining the

TABLE 13.1. CAUSES OF THROMBOSIS

Clinical Conditions: Arterial	Clinical Conditions: Venous	Blood Protein and Platelet Defects
Atherosclerosis	General surgery	Antiphospholipid syndrome
Cigarette smoking	Orthopedic surgery	APC resistance
Hypertension	Arthroscopy	Factor V Leiden
Diabetes mellitus	Trauma	Sticky platelet syndrome
LDL Cholesterol	Malignancy	Prothrombin G 20210A
Hypertriglyceridemia	Immobility	Protein S defects
Family history	Sepsis	Protein C defects
Left ventricular failure	Congestive heart failure	Antithrombin defects
Oral contraceptives	Nephrotic syndrome	Heparin cofactor II defects
Estrogens	Obesity	Plasminogen defects
Lipoprotein (a)	Varicose veins	TPA defects
Polycythemia	Postphlebitic syndrome	PAI-1 defects
Hyperviscosity syndromes	Oral contraceptives	Factor XII defects
Leukostasis syndromes	Estrogens	Dysfibrinogenemia
Inflammation/sepsis	Inflammation/sepsis	Homocystinemia
		MTHFR mutations
		Factor V Cambridge
		Factor V Hong Kong
		Factor V HR2 mutation
		Immune vasculitis

MTHFR, 5,10-methylene tetrahydrofolate reductase; LDL, low-density lipoprotein; APC, activated protein C; t-PA, tissue plasminogen activator; PAI, plasminogen activator inhibitor.

presence and type of defect in survivors of AMI. Defining the defect also will allow one to optimize antithrombotic therapy for secondary prevention.

Cerebrovascular Thrombosis

Cerebrovascular thrombosis (CVT) occurs in more than 1,500,000 individuals yearly in the United States; of these, 66% die or have severe permanent paralysis. In those with CVT, including transient cerebral ischemic attacks (TIAs), small stroke syndrome (SSS), and frank thrombotic stroke, at least 30% have a blood coagulation protein or platelet defect causing thrombosis. Like the disorders discussed earlier, the need for defining the presence or absence and type of defect is of obvious importance.

Although the incidence of retinal arterial or venous thrombosis is unclear, and death does not occur, significant visual morbidity is a major problem. Like those with CVT, about 30% of individuals sustaining retinal vascular thrombosis have a blood coagulation protein or platelet defect; reasons for defining these are as obvious as for the other disorders discussed.

Recurrent Miscarriage Syndrome

Many women have miscarriages. Although there are anatomic, hormonal, and genetic/chromosomal causes, defects in blood coagulation proteins or platelets, leading to early placental vascular thrombosis and nonviability of the fetus, account for about 30% to 50% of all cases of fetal wastage syndrome (FWS) (5). Clearly defining the coagulation defect almost always allows antithrombotic therapy, which will lead to normal term pregnancy.

ETIOLOGIES OF THROMBOSIS

Comparative incidence rates for thrombotic deaths compared with cancer deaths in the United States are found in Table 13.2; note that only the most common thrombotic problems leading to significant morbidity or mortality are included (6). Table 13.1 summarizes the etiologic factors known to be responsible for many of these events; this table illustrates the types of defects and prevalence, which should be considered, thus allowing appropriate therapy to be instituted when such defects are found.

The etiologies of hypercoagulability and overt thrombosis are becoming more clear and often definitive with enhanced knowledge of hemostasis and the development and extended use of testing systems for evaluating patients with thrombotic and thromboembolic disorders. With these test systems, in conjunction with careful clinical assessment of patients, about 80% to 90% of patients with thrombosis will have a defined etiology. Many of these will have an obvious clinical condition leading to thrombosis, and at least 50% to 80% will have an underlying hereditary or acquired blood protein/platelet defect causing thrombosis. Many clinical conditions are associated with an increased risk of arterial or venous thrombosis and thromboembolism; the more common of these are summarized in Table 13.1.

TABLE 13.2. INCIDENCE OF THROMBOSIS IN THE UNITED STATES

Disease	U.S.A. Incidence100,000	Total in U.S.A.Year (Cases)	Definable Reason
Deep vein thrombosis (DVT)	159	398,000	90%
Pulmonary embolus (PE)	139	347,000	90%
Fatal pulmonary embolus	94	235,000	90%
Acute myocardial infarction (AMI)	600	1,500,000	67%
Fatal myocardial infarction	300	750,000	67%
Cerebrovascular thrombosis (CVT)	600	1,500,000	30%
Fatal cerebrovascular thrombosis	396	990,000	30%
Total serious thromboses in U.S.A.	1498	3,742,000	50%
Total deaths from above thromboses	790	1,990,000	50%
All cancer in U.S.A, 1996	544	1,359,150	
Cancer deaths in U.S.A, 1996	222	554,740	

It must be remembered and emphasized that a diagnosis of thrombosis is similar to and as generic as a diagnosis of "anemia"; one must, in all instances, as in anemia, ask next, WHAT IS THE ETIOLOGY OF THE THROMBOSIS? As for anemia, the specific and appropriate therapy is highly dependent on defining the etiology. Thrombosis, be it arterial or venous, can no longer be viewed as a generic diagnosis; approaching thrombosis in this manner probably accounts not only for many treatment failures, but also for often confusing and conflicting results of clinical trials. Most clinicians and most trialists approaching thrombosis as a generic diagnosis fail to note that a very heterogeneous population is likely to be present, and outcomes will depend on designing therapy specific for a given etiology. As a simple example, it would not make sense to treat patients with thrombosis and sticky platelet syndrome (SPS) with heparin or coumadin when they actually need aspirin, nor would it make sense to treat a patient with antiphospholipid syndrome and thrombosis with aspirin (no response) or warfarin (65% failure rate), when they respond most ideally to heparin.

This chapter is limited to hereditary changes in circulating blood associated with thrombotic and thromboembolic disease. These disorders are best classified as hereditary versus acquired and more common versus less common. The acquired thrombophilias are discussed in Chapter 14.

In the rapidly changing field of thrombosis and hemostasis, diagnosis has become increasingly challenging as new disorders are discovered and an array of new laboratory studies are developed. Therapy is no less complex, as clinical studies continue to identify more effective treatment regimens. This chapter summarizes currently accepted approaches to the diagnosis and treatment of inherited disorders of hemostasis predisposing to thrombosis. Immediate therapeutic intervention as well as prophylaxis is addressed. Whereas issues surrounding diagnosis are essential to proper therapy, only attention to diagnosis will relate to the laboratory and clinical tools necessary to guide and properly direct treatment. The clinical course of thrombophilic patients is highly dynamic. When the response to therapy is not as expected, it must be remembered that more than one cause of thrombophilia may be present in any patient. Treatment must address the primary coagulopathy as well as any precipitating factors. Furthermore, over the course of time, the nature of the problem may change. As summarized in Table 13.3, thrombophilic disorders may be inherited, both inherited and acquired, and only acquired.

The decision to treat, in patients with both inherited and acquired thrombophilia, will depend on several factors. As van den Belt et al. (7) pointed out, the critical information for each disorder will include (a) the incidence of thrombo-

TABLE 13.3. HEREDITARY AND ACQUIRED THROMBOPHILIC DISORDERS

- Inherited Disorders
  - APC resistance
    - Factor V Leiden mutation
    - Factor V Cambridge mutation
    - Factor V Hong Kong
    - Factor V HR2 mutation
    - Prothrombin 20210A mutation
  - Factor XII deficiency (Hageman trait)
  - Dysfibrinogenemia
  - Hyperhomocyst(e)inemia
  - Platelet defects
    - Wein–Penzing defect
    - Sticky platelet syndrome
- Disorders both inherited and acquired
  - Antithrombin deficiency
  - Heparin cofactor II deficiency
  - Protein C deficiency
  - Protein S deficiency
  - Plasminogen deficiency
  - APC resistance
- Acquired disorders
  - Antiphospholipid antibodies
    - Anticardiolipin antibodies
    - Lupus anticoagulant
  - Myeloproliferative syndromes
  - Trousseau syndrome

APC, activated protein C.

sis, (b) the proportion of idiopathic to secondary thrombotic events, and (c) the probability of a fatal outcome. The risk of pharmacologic intervention must be balanced against the likelihood of real benefit. If the incidence of thrombosis in a given disorder is low and if the mortality rate for these events is similarly low, therapy with an agent known to be associated with a high risk of complications, such as warfarin, would not be indicated. If thrombotic events are seen primarily after surgery or in other high-risk situations, therapy might be limited to a fixed period. Conversely, if the ongoing risk of idiopathic thrombosis remains high or if a history of recurrent thrombotic events dictates, life-long therapy might be indicated. Unfortunately, for the disorders of inherited thrombophilia, randomized, blinded, controlled studies are rarely available. Some studies are controlled, but many are uncontrolled trials. The recommendations that follow are based on the available studies for each. As blinded, controlled trials are published, the indications for therapy and the therapeutic agent of choice will undoubtedly evolve.

PHARMACOLOGIC INTERVENTION

The choice of therapeutic agent must be guided by the clinical setting. The pharmacologic agents in general use at present are summarized in Table 13.4. Antithrombotic therapy currently understood to be of the greatest overall efficacy with the lowest risk, and in the setting of acute venous and arterial thrombosis is low-molecular-weight heparin (LMWH) (8–12). Outpatient or short-stay inpatient management of DVT/PE with LMWH also is much more cost effective than a traditional course of 7 to 10 days of intravenous unfractionated heparin (UFH) (11–16). Likewise, when long-term management requires a form of heparin, LMWH is preferred over UFH because of greater efficacy and fewer complications (16,17). The increased cost of LMWH over UFH is more than offset by the savings that result from treatment in the outpatient setting and reduced need for laboratory monitoring (16). Anticoagulation with warfarin has been recommended in a variety of settings. Warfarin therapy is generally recommended after antithrombotic therapy with UFH or LMWH for acute DVT (18,19). Frequent failures and an incidence of major hemorrhage of up to 3% to 12% per year and fatal bleeding of 0.4% per year complicate management of warfarin therapy (20–24). For long-term therapy, LMWH has been demonstrated to be of equal or greater efficacy and with lower risk than warfarin (16,17,25).

The action of all forms of heparin is primarily to induce a conformational change in antithrombin (AT), accelerating the action of AT in binding and inactivating thrombin, factor Xa, and a variety of serine proteases (26). With lower-molecular-weight preparations, the inactivation of factor Xa increases, and the degree of inactivation of factor IIA (thrombin) decreases. Bleeding risk correlates with the degree of inactivation of factor IIa, whereas therapeutic anticoagulation correlates with the degree of inactivation of factor Xa (27,28). UFH therapy is guided by the activated partial thromboplastin time (aPTT). In patients with acute DVT/PE treated with full-dose anticoagulation, the target aPTT is about 1.5 to 3 times normal, provided new recommendations for calibrating the aPTT to heparin levels is performed; this is discussed in Chapter 17 (18). Usually, low-dose UFH therapy is administered as a fixed dose of 5,000 units subcutaneously every 8 to 12 hours. LMWH dosing will vary according to the preparation chosen. Dalteparin is administered at a dose of 200 units/kg once daily for full-dose anticoagulation and 2,500 to 5,000 units once daily for prophylaxis. Dalteparin is available as 2,500 units/0.2 mL or 5,000 units/mL in fixed-dose syringes or as a multidose vial containing 95,000 units/9.5 mL. Enoxaparin should be given at 1 mg/kg every 12 hours for full-dose anticoagulation and 0.5 mg/kg every 12 hours, or 30 to 40 mg once a day for subsequent prophylaxis. Risks of all forms of heparin are similar; however, the risk of heparin-induced thrombocytopenia (HIT) (29–31) is lower with LMWH than with UFH. The other major risk of long-term therapy with heparin is osteoporosis (32).

Warfarin has the primary advantages over UFH and LMWH of oral administration and lower drug-related cost.

TABLE 13.4. ANTICOAGULATION THERAPY

Drug	Indication	Dose
Unfractionated heparin	Acute arterial and venous thrombosis	Bolus: 5,000 U i.v. Maintenance: i.v. infusion adjust dose to PTT, 1.5 to 2.0 × control. Heparin level: anti-Xa –0.3 to 0.7 U/mL
	Prophylaxis	5,000 U s.c. every 8 to 12 h
Low-molecular-weight heparin	Acute arterial and venous thrombosis	Dalteparin: 200 U/kg s.c. every 24 h Enoxaparin: 1 mg/kg s.c. every 12 h
	Prophylaxis	Dalteparin: 2,500–5,000 U s.c. every 24 h Enoxaparin: 30–40 mg/kg s.c. every 24 h
Warfarin	Arterial and venous thromboprophylaxis	5 mg by mouth daily for 3 days and then adjust dose per PT to achieve INR of 2.0 to 3.0

PTT, partial thromboplastin time; PT, prothrombin time; INR, international normalized ratio.

The primary action of warfarin is as a vitamin K antagonist. Vitamin K–dependent synthesis of coagulation factors II, VII, IX and X, as well as protein C and protein S is inhibited (33–35). The onset of action of warfarin is about 8 to 12 hours, with anticoagulation effect usually reached within 36 hours. The duration of action of warfarin is about 72 hours (36). Factor VII level decreases rapidly on initiation of warfarin and correlates best with the prothrombin time (PT). Decreases in factors II (half-life, 72 hours) and X best correlate with clinical anticoagulant effect and hemorrhagic risk. Patients with protein C and protein S deficiency who are started on warfarin experience an early, rapid decrease in protein C and S levels (half-life, 6 hours), resulting in a transient hypercoagulable state (29). This may further explain the need for an overlap in heparin therapy with warfarin in the treatment of acute venous thromboembolism. Loading doses of warfarin are no longer recommended, because this approach simply serves to increase the risk of hemorrhage (37). A dose of 5 mg per day monitored with a daily PT usually produces a therapeutic international normalized ratio (INR) within 36 to 72 hours. The target INR for patients with acute DVT/PE is 2.0 to 3.0 (18,38). Excessive anticoagulation with warfarin, without evidence of hemorrhage and with an INR less than 10.0, may be effectively treated by withholding one or two doses of warfarin and administering 1.0 (39) to 2.5 mg (40) of vitamin K orally.

Antiplatelet therapy is evolving with the availability of newer agents. Aspirin remains the primary choice in most settings (41–43). Clopidogrel, a selective inhibitor of the adenosine diphosphate (ADP)-induced activation of the platelet glycoprotein IIb/IIIa receptor [inhibiting platelet binding of fibrinogen (44–46)] replaces ticlopidine as the agent of choice when another drug is required by aspirin allergy, intolerance, or failure (47). An enhanced awareness of the risk of pancytopenia (48,49) and thrombotic thrombocytopenic purpura (TTP) associated with ticlopidine (50–52) suggests that clopidogrel is the preferred agent in situations previously indicated for ticlopidine therapy, as these complications are extremely rare with clopidogrel (47,53–55). The phosphodiesterase inhibitor dipyridamole is a less potent agent than clopidogrel or ticlopidine and should probably only be used as an adjunct to aspirin or other agents (56,57). The platelet glycoprotein IIb/IIIa inhibitors abciximab, tirofiban, and eptifibatide also have been demonstrated to be particularly effective in the treatment of patients with acute myocardial ischemia. Abciximab has proven safe and cost effective when used after percutaneous transluminal coronary angioplasty (PTCA) to enhance patency (58–61). Tirofiban has been demonstrated to be efficacious in patients with unstable angina, non–Q-wave myocardial infarction, and those undergoing PTCA (62,63). Eptifibatide also appears to decrease mortality when used in patients with unstable angina, AMI, and those treated with PTCA (64). Antiplatelet agents are summarized in Table 13.5.

Monitoring of drug therapy varies with the agent chosen (Table 13.6). In general clinical practice, the aPTT remains the measurement of choice for adjusting the dose of unfractionated heparin. Full anticoagulation for continuous intravenous infusion targets an aPTT of 1.5 to 3.0 times normal control (depending on the commercial aPTT reagent used and calibration of the aPTT with heparin levels) (18). A weight-adjusted nomogram also may be used, consisting of an 80-U/kg intravenous bolus followed by an infusion at 18 U/kg/hour (65). The target aPTT should provide a target anti-Xa heparin level of 0.3 to 0.75 to 1.0 U/mL (18). Although it is recognized that the aPTT is not closely correlated with heparin levels or clinical efficacy, it continues to be the primary tool for laboratory monitoring, provided that the aPTT has been calibrated according to recent guidelines, as discussed in Chapter 17 (66). Heparin therapy, whether UFH or LMWH, also requires monitoring for HIT (30,31,67), with a platelet count at least every 2 days for the first 14 days of therapy and then periodically thereafter. Because the most frequent serious complication of all forms of anticoagulation remains hemorrhage, a measurement of the hemoglobin is indicated at least weekly for the first few weeks and later at least every 1 to 2 months, or as clinically indicated.

The PT provides the guide to therapy with warfarin. The use of the INR has many limitations but remains the accepted laboratory standard for dose adjustment (68). Most instances of DVT and PE, treated with warfarin after

TABLE 13.5. ANTIPLATELET AGENTS

Drug	Site of Action	Indication
Aspirin	Cyclooxygenase	Arterial and venous thrombosis: acute intervention and prophylaxis
Dipyridamole	Phosphodiesterase	Arterial and venous thrombosis; prophylaxis
Ticlopidine	Inhibits ADP-induced platelet activation	Arterial and venous thrombosis
Clopidogrel	Inhibits ADP-induced platelet activation and endothelial procoagulants	Transient ischemic attack including acute coronary syndromes, after PTCA and to maintain patency after coronary and peripheral vascular surgery
Abciximab	Glycoprotein IIb/IIIa	Acute coronary syndromes refractory to standard therapy, PTCA

PTCA, percutaneous transluminal coronary angioplasty; ADP, adenosine diphosphate.

TABLE 13.6. RECOMMENDED MONITORING OF LONG-TERM PHARMACOLOGIC THERAPY

Drug	Monitoring
Heparin	CBC baseline and every 2 days for the first 14 days (UFH or LMWH) of therapy, then weekly for the first month, then monthly. Heparin levels (anti-Xa) weekly for the first month and then monthly. Bone density analysis baseline and every 6–12 months. Liver-function tests every 3 months
Warfarin	CBC and PT/INR baseline, then PT/INR monthly to every 2 months in the most stable patients. Dose adjustments require repeated PT/INR weekly or more often. CBC every 1 to 3 months. Periodic UA and stool occult blood in selected patients
Aspirin	CBC baseline and then if any symptoms or signs of bleeding or GI side effects, do CBC. May take with liquid antacid. GI studies if indicated
Clopidogrel	CBC ADP aggregation and baseline; repeated CBC q week × 4 weeks and repeated ADP aggregation in 4 weeks to note blunted effect, and then CBC if any symptoms or signs of bleeding or GI side effects. GI studies if indicated

CBC, complete blood count; LMWH, low-molecular-weight heparin; UA, urinalysis; PT, prothrombin time; GI, gastrointestinal; ADP, adenosine diphosphate; UFH, unfractionated heparin; INR, international normalized ratio.

heparin therapy, target an INR of 2.0 to 3.0 (18,69). Patients who are treated with warfarin anticoagulation may require a change in therapy at the time of interventional vascular procedures, dental work, or minor or major surgery. Rather than an abrupt discontinuation of anticoagulation, a transition from warfarin to heparin is required (70). The objective is to minimize the period during which the patient is vulnerable to thrombosis. Intravenous UFH or LMWH may be used for high-risk patients undergoing a major surgical procedure, whereas simply discontinuation of warfarin, without introducing another agent, may be appropriate for dental work and minor procedures (71).

The monitoring of antiplatelet therapy generally does not require routine laboratory studies, except for the monitoring of patients taking ticlopidine for pancytopenia. Ticlopidine-treated patients require a complete blood count every 2 weeks for the first 3 months of therapy. The recognition of ticlopidine-induced TTP further emphasizes the importance of following these guidelines (50). In patients with significant thrombotic problems, we routinely obtain aggregation to ADP after several weeks of clopidogrel therapy to assure an effect.

INHERITED DISORDERS

Factor V Leiden

As many as 5% of whites (72) and 20% to 50% of unselected patients with DVT (73,74) are demonstrated to have a single point mutation (at point 1691) in the gene responsible for the production of factor V. As a result, the factor V produced is abnormal, with a glutamine (Q) for arginine (R) substitution at position 506 (FV:R506Q, factor V Leiden). Inactivation of factor Va by activated protein C (APC) is impaired, resulting in a life-long hypercoagulable state (73–80). APC resistance also may be acquired, as occurs with the use of oral contraceptives or in the presence of elevated factor VIII:c (81). Regardless of the source of the APC abnormality, the clinical manifestations are similar. Because a hypercoagulable state is present, patients have either venous or arterial thrombosis (82,83) or recurrent miscarriage syndrome (RMS) (84).

At issue is the question of primary and secondary prophylaxis. Although there is a 5 to 10 times increased risk of thrombosis in heterozygous carriers of FV:R506Q, there is no major effect on life expectancy. Additionally, because there may be long intervals between episodes of thrombosis, it appears clear that life-long primary prophylactic anticoagulation may not be indicated (85,86). For the same reasons, screening of family members of patients with the mutation also is not recommended until they are of an age at which other risks, such as contact sports, surgery, trauma, oral contraceptives, or hormone-replacement therapy is contemplated (87). Proper management becomes more critical in homozygous individuals, who may be at 50 to 100 times greater risk of thrombosis than are the general population (88). One recent study of 355 FV:R506Q patients with an initial episode of symptomatic DVT detected a recurrence rate of 30.3% after 8 years (89). Patients with factor V Leiden mutation, in another study, were demonstrated to be four times more likely to have a recurrent event than were first DVT patients without the mutation. Recurrences often follow discontinuation of anticoagulation (90). A prospective trial of 251 patients after first DVT detected a FV:R506Q rate of 16.3%. Over an 8-year follow-up period, patients with factor V Leiden mutation had a recurrence rate of 39.7%, compared with 18.3% for those without the mutation (91). An additional study comparing homozygous and heterozygous individuals determined that the rate of recurrence was 9.5% per patient per year for homozygotes and 4.8% for heterozygotes. The rate for heterozygotes compared with that for individuals without the mutation was 5% per patient per year (92).

Life-long anticoagulation with warfarin or heparin may be considered in selected heterozygous individuals with recurrent thrombotic events but is not, therefore, widely recommended. Homozygotes with an initial episode of DVT may be considered for long-term anticoagulation on a case-by-case basis. Treatment of acute episodes of thrombosis should follow accepted recommendations, which include 6 weeks of anticoagulation after DVT, associated with a reversible risk factor and 3 to 6 months of anticoagulation in idiopathic disease (18). Patients with inherited or acquired thrombophilia who have recurrent, unprovoked venous thromboembolism should be considered for long-term anticoagulation (93).

The risk of thrombosis in individuals with FV:R506Q is compounded by the presence of other thrombophilic conditions. The risk associated with the use of oral contraceptives is increased from fourfold in genetically unaffected persons to 30-fold in FV:R506Q patients (94–96). In symptomatic patients with protein C deficiency, the prevalence of factor V Leiden was 14% (97). Analysis of families with the concomitant presence of factor V Leiden mutation and protein S deficiency detected a history of thrombosis in 72% of individuals with both abnormalities and 19% with either defect alone (98). Patients with both hyperhomocyst(e)inemia and FV:R506Q are at 20 times increased risk of idiopathic venous thrombosis compared with those with neither defect. The likelihood of thrombosis was significantly greater in the presence of both abnormalities than with either in isolation (99). Management of patients with more than one thrombophilic disorder must consider the enhanced risk and be adapted accordingly. Furthermore, therapy should target both disorders.

Patients with FV:R506Q who also experience RMS have been effectively treated with UFH or LMWH, when therapy begins from first diagnosis and is continued to delivery (84). Homozygous patients in high-risk settings, particularly in the presence of additional risk factors such as oral contraceptive use, should be treated with a prophylactic dose of LMWH. During pregnancy and the puerperium, the risk of venous thromboembolism also is substantially increased (87). Individuals with the factor V Leiden mutation experience additional risk. One small study of pregnant women with acute thromboembolism detected a 40% to 59% incidence of APC resistance or FV:R506Q. An important role is suggested for heparin prophylaxis (100). Controlled follow-up studies are, however, lacking.

Monitoring of patients with factor V Leiden mutation or with other forms of APC resistance focuses primarily on the form of therapy used. Antiplatelet therapy with aspirin or clopidogrel requires no monitoring. Anticoagulation with warfarin should achieve a target INR of 2.0 to 3.0 (19). Antithrombotic therapy with LMWH requires no monitoring except for a platelet count at least every 3 days during the first 2 weeks of treatment to assist in the early detection of HIT/heparin-induced thrombocytopenia and thrombosis (HITT) (101,102). The primary objective and clinical goals of treatment are avoidance of additional thrombotic events and, in the case of pregnancy, delivery of a healthy newborn to a healthy mother.

Factor V Cambridge

The recent characterization of another genetic mutation in factor V as a cause of APC resistance emphasizes the notion that a variety of genetic mutations are responsible for a propensity to both venous and arterial thrombosis. In this mutation, the arginine (AGG) at position 306 was changed to threonine (ACG). This was found to result in removal of the recognition site for the restriction enzyme *Bst*NI. Factor V Cambridge increases the risk for thrombosis in a similar manner as does factor V Leiden. Both mutations exhibit the same clinical manifestations and the same degree of APC resistance in the laboratory (103,104).

Treatment of patients with the factor V Cambridge mutation is the same as with FV:R506Q. Intervention in acute thrombosis with antithrombotic therapy followed by anticoagulation with warfarin is indicated. Long-term secondary prophylaxis with warfarin or heparin may be appropriate in selected patients. The pharmacologic agent chosen guides monitoring.

Factor V HR2 Haplotype

The HR2 haplotype represents a defect of six base substitutions in exons 13 and 16, with two amino acid changes. This mutation is associated with APC resistance in both carriers and noncarriers of factor V Leiden. The mutation, when found in association with factor V Leiden, imparts an additional three- to fourfold increase of venous thrombosis over that of carriers of factor V Leiden alone (105). Patients with the factor V haplotype also are prone to thrombosis in individuals without factor V Leiden. Unlike factor V Leiden, which is predominantly found in white populations, the factor V HR2 haplotype has been found in with about equal frequency in white, Italian, Indian, and Somalian individuals (106).

Factor V Hong Kong

This phenotype, thus far only found in Hong Kong Chinese, actually represents two different genotypes, referred to as factor V Hong Kong 1 and 2. The first mutation is an Arg485 to Lys mutation at exon 10; this is the result of a G1691A mutation. The second genotype (factor V Hong Kong 2) is a Arg306 to Gly substitution, resulting from an A1090G mutation. Both appear to lead to thrombosis. The first mutation is associated with a high tendency for thrombosis, but the second has not been assessed long enough to know the prevalence of thrombosis (107,108).

Prothrombin G20210A Mutation

Presence of a replacement of guanidine with adenine at position 20210 in the sequence of the 3′-untranslated region of the prothrombin gene (20210 G/A or 20210A) has been identified as a common genetic defect predisposing to thrombosis. The risk of venous thrombosis is nearly three times that of a control population (109). Clinical manifestations include both venous thromboembolism and, possibly, arterial thrombosis. The risk of arterial disease in patients with the prothrombin 20210A mutation is debated. A Brazilian study of 116 patients with venous disease and 71 with arterial disease (compared with 295 controls) demonstrated an allele frequency of 4.3% in DVT patients, 5.7% in arterial disease patients, and 0.33% among controls. Arterial disease patients were those with a history of MI, cerebral arterial occlusive disease, or occlusive peripheral arterial disease, in the absence of the accepted risk factors of hyperlipoproteinemia, hypertension, and diabetes mellitus (110). In an Italian study, 132 patients with venous thrombosis and 195 patients with cerebrovascular or coronary artery disease were compared with 161 controls. Whereas 16% of patients with venous thrombosis were found to have the GA genotype (4% of controls), the GA allele frequency was not increased in arterial disease patients (111). It is clear from several studies that the risk of venous thrombosis increases significantly in patients with other concomitant thrombophilic defects. Makris et al. (112) demonstrated that, in the presence of protein C or S deficiency, AT deficiency, or factor V Leiden, the likelihood of thrombosis greatly increases. Double heterozygotes have a much greater frequency of events and younger age at onset. Synergism appears to exist between increased prothrombin levels as the result of the 20210A mutation and the delayed activation of factor V Leiden substrate and cofactor in the prothrombinase complex (111). Oral contraceptive use in patients with prothrombin 20210A appears to increase greatly the risk of thrombosis, including of the cerebral venous system (113,114) and the coeliac artery (115).

Management includes the discontinuation of oral contraceptives and appropriate intervention for acute thrombosis. Because, in as many as 40% of patients, factor V Leiden also is present (109), therapy must consider the enhanced thrombophilia associated with the concomitant presence of both disorders. Treatment with antithrombotic agents for acute venous thrombosis, as well as for acute cerebrovascular or coronary arterial thrombosis, should follow accepted protocols (18,56). Because the risk for recurrent thrombosis is high, patients heterozygous for factor V Leiden or other mutations and 20210A must be considered for long-term therapy with warfarin or heparin. No long-term, controlled trials are available to confirm this approach; however, Ferraresi et al. (111) noted that 70% of their study population with more than one genetic defect experienced recurrent thrombosis.

Although the prothrombin level is significantly increased in patients with the prothrombin mutation, measurement of the PT and other global clotting tests are not useful for diagnosis or surveillance of the disorder (111,112,115, 116). Monitoring with clinical and laboratory testing is guided by the therapy chosen. Measurement of the PT is required to follow warfarin therapy (target INR, 2.0 to 3.0) and serial platelet counts to monitor the heparin therapy, as previously discussed.

Factor XII (Hageman Trait)

Deficiency of factor XII (Hageman trait) (117) may result from either autosomal recessive or dominant inheritance (118). Whereas heterozygous individuals possess approximately 50% of normal factor XII levels, homozygous patients have very low levels (119). Clinical manifestations vary from mild hemorrhage (rarely serious or fatal) to fatal venous thromboembolism or MI (120–123).

Because patients rarely bleed, factor replacement is not generally required. If major hemorrhage does occur, hemostasis can be readily achieved with the infusion of fresh frozen plasma. In view of the defect in surface-mediated activation of fibrinolysis that is associated with the Hageman trait, there is some question as to whether treatment with a medication such as stanozolol to enhance fibrinolysis is indicated prophylactically. Clearly, in the setting of increased thrombotic risk associated with a variety of medical and surgical disorders, LMWH or other prophylaxis is indicated. When thrombosis occurs, treatment should proceed according to accepted guidelines (18,19). No specific monitoring is usually required for the management of Hageman patients. Although a diagnosis is made by determination of a markedly prolonged aPTT with a normal PT and a low factor XII, none of these determinations is generally useful for guiding therapy.

Fibrinogen

Congenital dysfibrinogenemia (124) is identified in more than 100 specific molecular variants (125,126). The usual consequence of dysfibrinogenemia is mild to moderate hemorrhage. Only about 10% of patients have thrombosis (124), mostly venous, but also arterial (127). Although most of the dysfibrinogenemias associated with thrombosis have not been fully characterized, some defects appear to involve abnormal fibrin monomer polymerization, impaired activation of fibrinolysis, or resistance to fibrinolysis (128,129). Treatment of patients who exhibit thrombosis consists of antithrombotic therapy with UFH or LMWH followed by warfarin, as clinically appropriate. The propensity for hemorrhage requires careful monitoring of treatment.

Homocyst(e)inemia

Homocyst(e)inemia refers to the combined pool of homocysteine, homocystine, mixed disulfides involving homocysteine, and homocysteine thiolactone (130). Homocystinuria is a rare, autosomal recessive disorder in which the activity of cystathionine β-synthetase is decreased, resulting in disordered methionine metabolism. The result is homocystinemia, methioninemia, and homocystinuria. Patients with congenital deficiency exhibit typical features of ectopia lentis, mental retardation, and skeletal deformities (131–133). As described by McCully in 1969 (134), severe atherosclerosis develops at a young age. Venous and arterial thrombosis also are common (135). High total levels of homocyst(e)ine have recently been identified as the result of a mutation in the methylenetetrahydrofolate reductase (MTHFR) gene(C-to-T mutation at nucleotide 677) (136,137), rendering the enzyme thermolabile (137–140).

Severe hyperhomocyst(e)inemia is rare, but mild elevations of homocyst(e)ine are present in 5% to 7% of adults (141,142). A study of 212 North American coronary disease patients detected 17% with decreased activity of MTHFR, compared with 5% of 202 controls (143). Estimates of incidence in arterial vascular disease have varied from 13% to 47% of patients (141,144–147). The manifestations of recurrent venous and arterial thrombosis and precocious coronary and peripheral vascular disease develop in the third and fourth decade of life. Although the pathophysiologic influence of homocyst(e)ine on hemostasis is poorly characterized, it is clear that hyperhomosyct(e)inemia is associated with both arterial (130,148) and venous (149–151) thrombosis (152). Accelerated and severe atherosclerosis involves coronary (143,153–157), cerebral (158–160), and peripheral arteries (161,162). Marchant et al. (163) determined coagulation profiles as well as homocyst(e)ine levels in patients with a history of thrombosis. An elevated homocyst(e)ine level was confirmed as an independent risk factor for thrombosis (163). Presentation is with DVT, angina, or an acute coronary syndrome, stroke, or claudication.

Hyperhomocyst(e)inemia is managed primarily by the administration of folic acid with or without pyridoxine (vitamin B_6) (144,145,153,157,164–172). Boushey et al. (145) estimated that an increased intake of 350 μg per day in men and 280 μg per day in women could prevent as many as 56,000 deaths from cardiovascular disease per year in the United States. The recommended dietary supplement of 400 μg per day is sufficient to decrease the total homocyst(e)ine levels by about 5-μ*M*/L (145). The recent study of Malinow (172) demonstrated the lack of efficacy of vitamin B_6 and vitamin B_{12} supplementation alone in reducing homocyst(e)ine levels. They showed, however, that supplementation with cereals containing 499 μg and 665 μg of folic acid decreased homocyst(e)ine levels by 11.0% and 14.0%, respectively. Whether subsequent reductions of homocyst(e)ine correlate with a reduction in the incidence of atherosclerosis or venous or arterial thrombosis, and whether the addition of supplementation with vitamin B_6 has additional value, has not been determined by blinded controlled studies (130,153,157,172). Immediate intervention for thrombosis follows accepted an protocol for arterial or venous events. In addition to folic acid, prophylaxis requires antiplatelet therapy. Monitoring consists of clinical and radiologic follow-up of sites of vascular occlusion and measurement of homocyst(e)ine levels.

Antithrombin

AT deficiency may be both inherited and acquired. AT is an essential inhibitor of thrombin (173), factors Xa, IXa, XIa, and XIIa, plasmin, and kallikrein and has activity against protein C and protein S (174–181). Although the etiologies of AT deficiency may differ, the clinical and laboratory consequences are similar. Likewise, therapy is the same for both inherited and acquired forms.

Hereditary deficiency of AT is an autosomal dominant disorder characterized by either absence of AT or the presence of a dysfunctional form. The majority of affected individuals are heterozygotes (182). Whereas a functional AT level of more than 50% to 70% of normal human plasma appears to be required to avoid thrombosis, some patients with lower levels may be unaffected (183–187). Venous thrombosis is the primary presentation, usually begins in adolescence, and is frequently accompanied by PE (188). High-risk events such as surgery, trauma, pregnancy, and oral contraceptive use may initiate the first thrombotic event (189). Patients with acquired deficiency, in whom recurrent thrombotic events develop, require life-long anticoagulation.

The management of patients with both inherited and acquired AT deficiency has advanced considerably with the wide availability of AT concentrates (190). Because patients with AT deficiency lack the available site of action for heparin, anticoagulation of patients with congenital deficiency who have acute venous thrombosis or PE, with heparin alone, is ineffective. Administration of AT concentrates must accompany anticoagulation with heparin. Antithrombin concentrates also may be efficacious in patients with inherited deficiency, even without heparin (191). Prophylaxis with AT for congenitally deficient patients in high-risk settings may be indicated; however, controlled studies are not available to confirm this. Pregnancy represents a special risk for deficient patients. Subcutaneous heparin or LMWH is recommended throughout pregnancy. Warfarin is contraindicated because of teratogenicity. AT concentrates may be indicated at the time of greatest risk, during the puerperium, and for obstetric emergencies (192).

Vinazzer et al. (193) demonstrated the efficacy of AT concentrates. The formula for administration of therapeutic AT concentrates is as follows:

Units required Baseline AT level is expressed as a percentage of normal level based on functional AT assay. Dosing frequency is generally every 12 hours, guided by repeated AT assays (194).

Generally a dose of 50 U/kg is recommended for a patient with a baseline functional level of 50%. Repeated administration of 60% of the loading dose every 24 hours will usually maintain adequate levels in patients with congenital deficiency (194). The dose requirement may be much higher in patients with DIC and similar conditions that actively deplete AT.

Monitoring of patients with AT deficiency varies considerably between those with inherited and those with acquired states. Patients with the inherited disorder who experience recurrent thrombosis require life-long anticoagulation, usually with warfarin and the determination of the PT at regular intervals (goal is to maintain INR, 2.0 to 3.0). As the clinical circumstance changes, the intervals of follow-up and monitoring may change. For clinical purposes, the assay of choice is the functional AT assay, reported as percentage of normal human plasma. Immunologic assays of AT are of no clinical value. In the acutely ill patient receiving AT concentrates, repeated AT levels may be required at intervals of 6 to 12 hours.

Heparin Cofactor II

Heparin cofactor II (HC II) directly inactivates the activity of thrombin on fibrinogen (195) and inhibits thrombin-induced platelet activation (196). Congenital deficiency of HC II appears to be very rare and is associated with an increased risk of both arterial and venous thrombosis (197–202). Heterozygous individuals have 50% of normal levels, and thrombotic risk appears to increase when levels decrease to less than 60% (198,199). Treatment is based on the clinical circumstances. Treatment with anticoagulation should proceed according to accepted guidelines for the clinical condition (18). Heparin will be effective in the presence of HC II deficiency. Long-term anticoagulation and prophylaxis for high-risk situations should be considered for individuals with a history of recurrent thrombosis. Because the populations studied are small, firm recommendations are not available.

Protein C

Protein C is a vitamin K–dependent protein that inhibits the coagulation system primarily through inactivation of factors V and VIII:c, the cofactors required for activation of thrombin and factor Xa (203). This serine protease is inhibited by AT (204) and enhanced by protein S (205). The presence of protein C is essential to maintain hemostatic balance. Deficiencies of protein C may be either congenital or acquired (206).

Congenital deficiency is autosomal dominant and is characterized by recurrent venous thrombosis and thromboembolism beginning in adolescence (207–209). Most homozygous patients die of thromboembolic disease in infancy (210,211). Both absence and dysfunctional forms of the disorder are observed. Type I disease is characterized by reduction in both antigenic and functional levels, and type II, in which functional levels are decreased much more than antigenic levels (212—217).

Homozygous patients have been successfully managed with infusions of fresh frozen plasma or certain factor IX concentrates (containing large amounts of protein C and S), together with heparin (207,210,218). Maintenance of an INR of 3.5 or higher may be necessary to prevent recurrence of severe skin necrosis (219). Considering the need for life-long anticoagulation, the need for high-dose warfarin, the difficulties attendant on maintenance of a consistent level of anticoagulation, and the risks of major hemorrhage, LMWH appears to be preferred for long-term management (220).

Anticoagulation is the treatment of choice in patients with heterozygous protein C deficiency. Heparin or LMWH are used according to accepted guidelines for acute thrombotic events (18,19). Long-term anticoagulation with warfarin is indicated after an acute event and as prophylaxis. Warfarin-induced skin necrosis is a major therapeutic problem (221—223). With the institution of warfarin, the reduction of protein C (half-life, 6 hours) occurs at a faster rate than the reduction in the other vitamin K–dependent factors II (half-life, 72 hours), VII, and X. This results in a transient hypercoagulable state, predisposing to thrombosis, including skin necrosis (18,29). Recent studies have demonstrated that this problem can be controlled by maintaining full anticoagulation with heparin until the PT is well into the therapeutic range (target INR, 3.0 to 3.5). Maintaining a therapeutic PT is, subsequently, essential to avoiding recurrent thrombosis. Despite therapeutic anticoagulation with warfarin, there are treatment failures. Long-term therapy with heparin/LMWH may be required. Protein C concentrates are now available for treatment failures (224).

Therapy is monitored with the appropriate laboratory test, depending on the pharmacologic agent selected. The target INR for warfarin therapy is 3.0 to 3.5. Therapy with LMWH is weight adjusted and does not require monitoring, except for a platelet count every 2 to 3 days for the first 2 weeks of treatment. Although the measurement of the biologic and immunologic activity of protein C is required for diagnosis (225), follow-up analysis is not required. When evaluating a patient with unexplained thrombosis, however, it is essential to obtain the laboratory tests for protein C deficiency before therapy is initiated, because warfarin immediately reduces the vitamin K–dependent hepatic production of protein C. The levels of both protein C and S decrease to 40% to 60% of normal immediately and return to about 70% of normal after several weeks of therapy. Measurement of the protein C and S levels should wait for several weeks after initiation of warfarin therapy. On repeated evaluation of protein C and S, if levels greater than 60% are not detected, congenital deficiency should be considered (224).

Protein S

Protein S is a cofactor for the protein C–induced inactivation of factor V (226) and the protein C–induced inactivation of factor VIII:c (226). Protein S is also a cofactor in the protein C acceleration of fibrinolysis (227) and appears to have anticoagulant functions independent of protein C by direct inhibition of procoagulant enzyme complexes (228,229). Congenital protein S deficiency is autosomal dominant and is fairly common, identified in as many as 10% of patients younger than 45 years presenting with DVT (230). Incidence in other selected groups has varied from to 1.5% to 7% (231,232). Simmonds et al. (233) have recently reported analysis of a 122-member family in which 44 members were identified with the protein S gene mutation substitution, Gly295 to Val. The probability of remaining thrombosis free was 0.97 for unaffected family members, and 0.5 for those with the mutation (233). Homozygotes have a severe propensity to thrombosis and may present with purpura fulminans soon after birth (234). Heterozygous patients are at high risk for thrombosis throughout life. An asymptomatic variant also may exist (235,236).

Management of patients with protein S deficiency is similar to that of those with protein C deficiency. Acute thrombosis is managed with heparin anticoagulation according to accepted guidelines dependent on the site and severity of disease. Long-term anticoagulation with warfarin is indicated after heparin therapy for an acute event and for prophylaxis (18,19). Follow-up of patients involves repeated clinical evaluation in the immediate setting, and monitoring is dependent on the form of anticoagulation selected. LMWH requires only periodic evaluation of the platelet count. Warfarin is monitored with the PT to maintain a target INR of 2.0 to 3.0. Repeated analysis of the protein S level is usually not required if evaluation is performed before initiation of warfarin therapy. Subsequent measurement should wait for several weeks, as discussed with protein C (224). In warfarin failures, long-term therapy with UFH or LMWH may be required. As with other thrombophilic disorders, the patient and family members should be counseled regarding the need for diagnostic screening and the need to intervene in high-risk circumstances. These include but are not limited to the avoidance of oral contraceptives, the control of obesity, and prophylactic anticoagulation at the time of surgery, prolonged immobility, pregnancy, and the puerperium.

Fibrinolytic Defects and Thrombosis

A variety of abnormalities of the fibrinolytic system predispose to thrombosis. Plasminogen may be decreased because of impaired synthesis. Tissue plasminogen activator (t-PA) may be decreased, or there may be abnormal factor XII activation. t-PA inhibitor type I (PAI-1) may be present in increased amounts, or there may be an increase in fibrinolytic inhibitors, α_2-antiplasmin, α_2-macroglobulin, and α_1-antitrypsin. A variety of clinical conditions are associated with elevated levels of fibrinolytic inhibitors, including diabetes mellitus (237), TTP (238), MI (239,240), malignancy, DVT and PE, (241), scleroderma, pulmonary fibrosis, pregnancy, oral contraceptive use (242), serious infections, and surgery (243,244). Patients with generalized atherosclerosis may exhibit decreased plasminogen activity because of damage to the vascular intima (245,246). Treatment of impaired fibrinolysis must include treatment of the underlying disease with the appropriate modalities, as well as anticoagulation. Caution must be exercised in the application of thrombolytic agents because, in the absence of adequate levels of plasminogen, t-PA, streptokinase, and urokinase may be less effective than expected.

Patients with congenital plasminogen deficiency have clinical features similar to those of patients with congenital protein C, protein S, and AT deficiency. Symptomatic patients generally have DVT or PE (247). The disorder is of autosomal recessive inheritance and is characterized by the onset of DVT and PE in adolescence (248). As many as 2% to 3% of young patients with idiopathic DVT may be so affected (249). Both the absence form and dysfunctional form exist, with the dysfunctional form the more common (247,248,250). Although the significance of congenital plasminogen deficiency has been disputed as a risk factor for thrombosis (1), both forms have been correlated with some increased risk, particularly when associated with other thrombophilic abnormalities or circumstantial risk factors (251,252). Thrombosis is primarily venous and usually is correlated with a plasminogen level less than 40% of normal (250).

Treatment in patients with acute thrombosis should follow accepted guidelines for DVT and PE (18,19). Warfarin therapy should target an INR of 2.0 to 3.0. Immediate intervention may include urokinase, when clinically indicated in the setting of massive PE and severe or recurrent iliofemoral thrombosis (250,253). Antiplatelet therapy also may play a role in management (250,253).

Monitoring must rely on clinical parameters and evaluation of the plasminogen level. In patients with the dysfunctional form rather than the absence form of the disorder, the biologic functional assay will be abnormal, whereas the immunologic quantitative assay will be normal (254).

Patients with congenital t-PA deficiency and with congenitally elevated levels of PAI are rare, and are characterized by the same increased risk of thrombosis as seen with congenital deficiency of plasminogen (255–257). Three polymorphic alterations in the human PAI-1 gene have been associated with elevated plasma PAI-1 levels; these are (a) a *Hin*dIII restriction fragment length polymorphism; (b) a (C-A)n dinucleotide repeat polymorphism; and (c) a single nucleotide insertion/deletion polymorphism (4G/5G). The *Hin*dIII polymorphism develops because of a base change in the 3′-untranslated region; the 1/1 genotype exhibits higher PAI-1 levels than do 1/2 or 2/2 genotypes. The smaller alleles of an eight-allele dinucleotide repeat polymorphism also are noted to be associated with increased PAI-1 activity (258,259). Regarding the sequence length polymorphism, which occurs in the promoter region of the PAI-1 gene, the (4G/4G) genotype correlates with higher PAI-1 activity compared with genotypes possessing a 5G allele. Both the 4G and 5G alleles bind a transcriptional activator, but only the 5G allele binds a repressor protein; as a result, the 4G/4G genotype has a higher basal PAI-1 transcription rate and higher plasma PAI-1 levels. The association of the 4G/4G PAI-1 polymorphism with thrombosis has given conflicting results. In an evaluation of 94 men with AMI before age 45 years, an increased prevalence of the 4G allele compared with a healthy control population was noted (260). However, although another study confirmed an association between PAI-1 elevation and 4G/4G genotype, there were not differences in 4G allele prevalence between patients with MI and controls (261). The Physicians Health Study did not find an increased prevalence of the 4G allele in those with MI or venous thrombosis (262). Thus although suggestive, more studies are needed to define clearly the association between these polymorphisms and thrombosis. This topic is extensively reviewed by Hong and Kwaan (263).

Treatment is the same, and monitoring requires assay of t-PA or PAI-1. Treatment is based on therapy for the primary disease. Awareness of the underlying decrease in fibrinolytic activity associated with decreased plasminogen activity should prompt greater attention to appropriate antithrombotic therapy, both in the setting of acute thrombosis and as prophylaxis in high-risk circumstances.

HEREDITARY PLATELET DEFECTS LEADING TO THROMBOPHILIA

Wein–Penzing Defect

The Wein–Penzing defect is extremely rare. A deficiency is present in the lipooxygenase metabolic pathway with resulting increases in cyclooxygenase pathway products, including thromboxane, prostaglandin E_2, and prostaglandin D_2. The two reported patients experienced AMI at an early age (264). Management is with aspirin.

Sticky Platelet Syndrome

However, another platelet defect that (a) appears quite common, (b) accounts for many episodes of arterial and venous thrombosis and significant morbidity and mortality, (c) is easy to diagnose, and (d) is easy to treat is SPS. SPS was first described by Mammen et al. (265) in 1983 at the Ninth International Joint Conference on Stroke and Cerebral Circulation. Subsequently Mammen et al. (266,267) described 41 patients with coronary artery disease and SPS; this was followed by a report in 1986 delineating this syndrome in a number of individuals with cerebrovascular disease; the inheritance was noted to be autosomal dominant. Finally in 1995, more than 200 families were described with a wide variety of arterial and venous thrombotic events due to SPS (268,269). Although these publications have clearly delineated SPS as a common inherited and easily diagnosed and treated syndrome leading to significant, and often preventable, arterial and venous thrombosis, most clinicians and laboratory scientists are still unfamiliar with the prevalence of SPS and fail to consider this diagnosis in appropriate patient populations. In addition, the actual prevalence remains unclear, especially as relates to venous versus arterial events. A more recent study (270) assessed the prevalence of SPS in a wide variety of patients with various types of arterial and venous events. One-hundred fifty patients were referred for evaluation to determine the etiology, if possible, for unexplained arterial or venous events; 78 had had venous events consisting of DVT with or without PE. Seventy-five patients were referred for evaluation of arterial events; these patients had coronary artery thrombosis (21%), cerebrovascular thrombosis (50.6%), TIAs (13.3%), retinal vascular thrombosis (6.6%), or peripheral arterial thrombosis (8%). Peripheral arterial thrombotic events consisted of unexplained thrombosis of renal (two), radial (one), popliteal (one), and mesenteric (one) arteries. All patients referred for determining the etiology of an unexplained thrombotic event were subjected to a complete history and physical examination and then were studied for hypercoagulability syndromes, including SPS.

Based on these studies, it appears that SPS is a common cause of both arterial and venous events. A similar study was performed by Anderson et al. (271); this also was a prospective study wherein 195 patients with arterial, venous, or arterial plus venous thrombosis were assessed for hypercoagulability. SPS was the singular most common defect found, being detected in 28% of the entire population. The authors also concluded, as in the previous study, that SPS is a common inherited prothrombotic disorder leading to arterial and venous thrombosis. The association of SPS as a cause of young-age cerebrovascular thrombosis also recently was noted by German investigators (272). It appears that SPS accounts for about 14% of unexplained venous thrombotic events and between 12% (peripheral arterial thrombosis) and 33% (TIAs) of arterial events, so this hereditary platelet-function defect should be strongly suspected, and searched for, in any individual with an otherwise unexplained arterial or venous event. If one assumes, based on prevalence studies, that the congenital blood coagulation protein defects, including AT defects, protein S, protein C, and other rare defects account for about 20% of all venous events, and APC resistance (factor V Leiden) accounts for another 20% of unexplained venous events, then, when adding SPS (at 14%), it may be concluded that

TABLE 13.7. RECOMMENDED LONG-TERM PHARMACOLOGIC THERAPY FOR SYMPTOMATIC THROMBOPHILIA

Disorder	Therapy
APC resistance	Warfarin (INR 2.0–3.0); fixed, low-dose s.c. UFH or LMWH
FV Leiden	
FV Cambridge	
Prothrombin 20210A	
Factor XII deficiency (Hageman trait)	Fixed, low-dose s.c. UFH or LMWH
Dysfibrinogenemia	Fixed, low-dose s.c. UFH or LMWH, or warfarin (INR 2.3–3.0)
Hyperhomocyst(e)inemia	Folic acid, 5 mg/day Consider additional vitamin B_6 (50 mg/day) ASA prophylaxis for atherosclerosis
Antithrombin deficiency	Warfarin (INR 2.3–3.0) Antithrombin concentrates for acute intervention or LMWH
Heparin cofactor II deficiency	Warfarin (INR 2.0–3.0), fixed, low-dose s.c. UFH or LMWH
Protein C deficiency	Warfarin (INR 2.0–3.0), fixed, low-dose s.c. UFH or LMWH
Protein S	Warfarin (INR 2.0–3.0), fixed, low-dose s.c. UFH or LMWH
Plasminogen deficiency/inhibition	Warfarin (INR 2.0–3.0), fixed, low-dose s.c. UFH or LMWH
Antiphospholipid antibodies	Dependent on syndrome type (see Table 3)
Platelet defects	
Wein–Penzing defect	ASA (81–325 mg/day)
Sticky platelet syndrome	
Myeloproliferative disorders	Phlebotomy, ASA (81–325 mg/day), anagrelide, hydroxyurea
Trousseau syndrome	PTT adjusted dose UFH i.v. or s.c. or LMWH (full dose)

INR, international normalized ratio; PTT, partial thromboplastin time; LMWH, low-molecular-weight heparin; ASA, acetylsalicylic acid; UFH, unfractionated heparin; APC, activated protein C.

congenital defects account for about 50% to 60% of unexplained venous events. If it is then considered that antiphospholipid syndrome, based on prevalence studies, accounts for another 25% of venous events, then it may be reasonably concluded that about 80% to 90% of venous events and a somewhat lesser number of arterial events can be defined as to cause. Because the treatment(s) for these disorders may differ and because about half are hereditary, it is important to define the presence of hereditary and acquired coagulation protein or platelet defects whenever possible. This leads to the inescapable conclusion that a diagnosis of thrombosis, like a diagnosis of anemia, is only a partial diagnosis, and the precise nature and cause must next be defined. In the case of SPS, warfarin or heparin therapy would not generally be indicated, and aspirin appears to be the treatment of choice.

CONCLUSION

In all patients with thrombophilia, management is determined not solely by the presence of the laboratory abnormality but also by the clinical consequences. Prophylaxis in asymptomatic patients is reserved for those disorders with the highest risk of idiopathic thrombosis. The choice of pharmacologic agent will necessarily vary with the likelihood of serious or life-threatening thrombosis. Intervention includes a spectrum from no treatment to full-dose anticoagulation. Blinded, controlled studies to validate many of these recommendations are frequently lacking. Understanding of the pathophysiology of the disorder, review of the available studies and reports, and clinical experience must guide management decisions. Our recommendations for treatment of the thrombophilic disorders are presented in Table 13.7.

REFERENCES

1. Bick RL, Fareed J. Current status of thrombosis: a multidisciplinary medical issue and major American health problem: beyond the year 2000. *Clin Appl Thromb Hemost* 1997;3(suppl 1):1.
2. Bergqvist D, Lundblad B. Incidence of venous thromboembolism in medical and surgical patients. In: Bergqvist D, Comerota A, Nicolaides A, et al., eds. *Prevention of venous thromboembolism.* London: Med-Orion Press, 1994:3.
3. Ramaswami G, Nicolaides AN. The natural history of deep vein thrombosis In: Bergqvist D, Comerota A, Nicolaides A, et al., eds. *Prevention of venous thromboembolism.* London: Med-Orion Press, 1994:409.
4. American Heart Association. *Heart and stroke: 1997.* Dallas, Tex: American Heart Association National Headquarters, 1996.
5. Bick RL. Recurrent miscarriage syndrome and infertility caused by blood coagulation protein or platelet defects. *Hematol Oncol Clin North Am* 2000;14:1117.
6. American Cancer Society. *Cancer: facts and figures: 1996.* Atlanta: American Cancer Society, 1996.

7. Van den Belt AGM, Prins M, Huisman MH, et al. Familial thrombophilia: a review analysis. *Clin Appl Thromb Hemost* 1996;2:227–236.
8. Buckley M, Sorkin E. Enoxaparin: a review of its pharmacology and clinical applications in the prevention and treatment of thromboembolic disorders. *Drugs* 1992;44:465.
9. Ewenstein BM. Antithrombotic agents and thromboembolic disease. *N Engl J Med* 1997;337:1383–1384.
10. Armstrong PW. Heparin in acute coronary disease: requiem for a heavyweight? *N Engl J Med* 1997;337:492–494.
11. Hull RD, Raskob GE, Pineo GF, et al. The treatment of proximal vein thrombosis with subcutaneous low-molecular-weight heparin compared with intravenous heparin. *Clin Appl Thromb Hemost* 1995;1:151–159.
12. Harenburg J, Schmitz-Huebner U, Breddin K, et al. Treatment of deep vein thrombosis with low-molecular-weight heparins: a consensus statement of the Gesellschaft fur Thrombose-und Hamostaseforschung (GTH). *Semin Thromb Hemost* 1997;23:91–96.
13. Buller HRMG, Gallus AS, Ginsberg J, et al. Low-molecular-weight heparin in the treatment of patients with venous thromboembolism. *N Engl J Med* 1997;337:657–662.
14. Van den Belt AG, Bossuyt PM, Prins MH, et al. Replacing inpatient care by outpatient care in the treatment of deep venous thrombosis: an economic evaluation. *Thromb Haemost* 1998;79:259.
15. Bick RL. Proficient and cost-effective approaches for the prevention and treatment of venous thrombosis and thromboembolism. *Drugs* 2000;60:575.
16. Crowther M, Hirsh J. Low-molecular-weight heparin for the out-of-hospital treatment of venous thrombosis: rationale and clinical results. *Semin Thromb Hemost* 1997;23:77–81.
17. Hirsch J, Raschke R, Warkentin TE, et al. Heparin: mechanism of action, pharmacokinetics, dosing considerations, monitoring, efficacy, and safety. *Chest* 1995;108(4 suppl):258S—275S.
18. Hirsh J, Hoak J. Management of deep vein thrombosis and pulmonary embolism: a statement for healthcare professionals. *Circulation* 1996;93:2212–2245.
19. Baker WF Jr, Bick RL. Deep vein thrombosis: diagnosis and management. *Med Clin North Am* 1994;82:685.
20. Hirsh J, Dalen J, Deykin D, et al. Oral anticoagulants: mechanism of action, clinical effectiveness and optimal therapeutic range. *Chest* 1992;102:312S.
21. Landefeld CS, Goldman L. Major bleeding in outpatients treated with warfarin: incidence and prediction by factors known at the start of outpatient therapy. *Am J Med* 1989;87:144.
22. Landefeld CS, Rosenblatt MW, Goldman L. Bleeding in outpatients treated with warfarin: relation to the prothrombin time and important remediable lesions. *Am J Med* 1989;87:153.
23. Levine MN, Raskob G, Hirsh J. Hemorrhagic complications of long-term anticoagulant treatment. *Chest* 1986;89:16.
24. Finn SD, McDonnell M, Martin D, et al. Risk factors for complications of chronic anticoagulation: a multicenter study: Warfarin Optimized Outpatient Follow-up Study Group. *Ann Intern Med* 1993;118:511–520.
25. Monreal M. Heparin in patients with venous thromboembolism and contraindications to oral anticoagulant therapy. *Semin Thromb Hemost* 1997;23:69–75.
26. Bick RL, Kunkel L. Hypercoagulability and thrombosis. *Lab Med* 1992;23:233.
27. Barrowcliffe TW, Johnson EA, Eggleton CA. Anticoagulant activities of lung and mucous heparins. *Thromb Res* 1977;12:27.
28. Losito R, Losito C. Molecular weight of heparin versus biologic activity. *Semin Thromb Hemost* 1985;11:29.
29. Warkentin TE, Elavathil LJ, Hayward CP, et al. The pathogenesis of venous limb gangrene associated with heparin-induced thrombocytopenia. *Ann Intern Med* 1997;127:804–812.
30. Warkentin TE, Levine MN, Hirsh J, et al. Heparin-induced thrombocytopenia in patients treated with low-molecular-weight heparin or unfractionated heparin. *N Engl J Med* 1995;332:1330–1335.
31. Walenga J, Bick RL. Heparin associated thrombocytopenia and other adverse effects of heparin therapy. *Med Clin North Am* 1998;82:635–658.
32. Hirsh J, Levine M. Low molecular weight heparin. *Blood* 1992;79:1.
33. Raskob GE, Carter CJ, Hull RD. Anticoagulant therapy for venous thromboembolism. *Prog Hemost Thromb* 1989;9:1.
34. Mackie MJ, Douglas AS. Drug-induced disorders of coagulation. In: Ratnoff OD, Forbes CD, eds. *Disorders of hemostasis.* Philadelphia: WB Saunders, 1991:493.
35. Stenflo J. Vitamin K, prothrombin, and gamma-carboxyglutamic acid. *N Engl J Med* 1977;296:624.
36. Loeliger EA, von der Esch B, Matten MJ. Behaviour of factors II, VII, IX, and X during long-term treatment with coumarin. *Thromb Diath Haemorrh* 1963;9:74.
37. Deykin D. Warfarin therapy. *N Engl J Med* 1970;287:691.
38. Hyers TM, Hull RD, Weg JG. Antithrombotic therapy for venous thromboembolic disease. *Chest* 1995;108:335S–351S.
39. Weibert RT, Le DT, Kayser SR, et al. Correction of excessive anticoagulation with low-dose oral vitamin K_1. *Ann Intern Med* 1997;126:959–962.
40. Crowther MA, Donovan D, Harrison L, et al. Low-dose oral vitamin K reliably reverses over-anticoagulation due to warfarin. *Thromb Haemost* 1998;79:116–118.
41. Folts JD, Cromwell EB, Rowe GG. Platelet agreggation in partially obstructed vessels and their elimination with aspirin. *Circulation* 1976;4:356.
42. Coller BS. Platelets in cardiovascular thrombosis and thrombolysis. In: Fossard HA, Haber E, Jennings RB, et al., eds. *The heart and cardiovascular system: scientific foundations.* New York: Raven Press, 1991:216.
43. Pantrano C. Aspirin as an antiplatelet drug. *Acta Obstet Gynecol Scand* 1994;330:1287.
44. Savi P, Heilman E, Nurden P, et al. Clopidogrel: an antithrombotic drug acting on the ADP-dependent activation pathway of human platelets. *Clin Appl Thromb Hemost* 1996;2:35–42.
45. Mills D, Puri R, Hu C-J, et al. Clopidogrel inhibits the binding of ADP analogues to the receptor mediating inhibition of platelet adenylate cyclase. *Arterioscler Thromb* 1992;12:430–436.
46. Roald HE, Barstad RM, Kierulf P, et al. Clopidogrel: a platelet inhibitor which inhibits thrombogenesis in non-anticoagulated human blood independently of the blood flow conditions. *Thromb Haemost* 1994;71:655–662.
47. Committee CS. A randomized blinded trial of clopidogrel versus aspirin in patients at risk of ischemic events. *Lancet* 1996;34:1129.
48. Wysowski DK, Bacsayani J. Blood dyscrasias and hematologic reactions in ticlopidine users [Letter]. *JAMA* 1996;276:952.
49. Defreyn G, Bernat A, Delebasse D, et al. Pharmacology of ticlopidine: review. *Semin Thromb Hemost* 1989;15:159–166.
50. Kovacs M, Soong PG, Chin-Yee IH. Thrombotic thrombocytopenic purpura associated with ticlopidine. *Ann Pharmacother* 1993;27:1060.
51. Becquemin J-P. Effect of ticlopidine on the long-term patency of saphenous-vein bypass grafts in the legs. *N Engl J Med* 1997;337:1726–1731.
52. Bennett CL, Weinberg PD, Rozenberg-Ben-Dror K, et al. Thrombotic thrombocytopenic purpura associated with ticlopidine: a review of 60 cases. *Ann Intern Med* 1998;128:541–544.

53. Berqvist D, Almgren B, Dickenson JP. Reduction of requirement for leg vascular surgery during long-term treatment of claudicant patients with ticlopidine: results from the Swedish Ticlopidine Multicentre Study (STIMS). *Eur J Endovasc Surg* 1995;10:69.
54. Hass WK, Easton JD, Adams HPJ, et al. A randomized trial comparing ticlopidine hydrochloride with aspirin for the prevention of stroke in high-risk patients. *N Engl J Med* 1989; 321:501–507.
55. Gent M, Blakely JA, Easton JD. The Canadian American Ticlopidine Study (CATS) in thromboembolic stroke. *Lancet* 1989; 1:1215–1220.
56. Baker WF Jr. Thrombosis and hemostasis in cardiology, part I. *Clin Appl Thromb Hemost* 1998;4:51–75.
57. Stein B, Fuster V, Israel DH, et al. Platelet inhibitor agents in cardiovascular disease: an update. *J Am Coll Cardiol* 1989;14: 813.
58. Coller BS, Anderson KM, Weisman HF. The anti-GPIIb/IIIa agents: fundamental and clinical aspects. *Hemostasis* 1996;26 (suppl 4):285.
59. Anderson HV, Jordan RE, Weisman HF. Concept and clinical application of platelet glycoprotein IIb/IIIa with abciximab (c7E3 Fab; ReoPro) for the prevention of acute ischemic syndromes. *Clin Appl Thromb Hemost* 1997;3:256–266.
60. The EPIC Investigators. Use of a monoclonal antibody directed against the platelet glycoprotein IIb/IIIa receptor in high-risk coronary angioplasty. *N Engl J Med* 1994;330:956–961.
61. The EPILOG Investigators. Platelet glycoprotein IIb/IIIa receptor blockade and low-dose heparin during percutaneous coronary revascularization. *N Engl J Med* 1997;336:1689–1696.
62. The Platelet Receptor Inhibition in Ischemic Syndrome Management (PRISM) Study Investigators. A comparison of aspirin plus tirofiban with aspirin plus heparin for unstable angina. *N Engl J Med* 1998;338:1498–1505.
63. The Platelet Receptor Inhibition in Ischemic Syndrome Management in Patients Limited by Unstable Signs and Symptoms (PRISM-PLUS) Study Investigators. Inhibition of the platelet glycoprotein IIb/IIIa receptor with tirofiban in unstable angina and non-Q wave myocardial infarction. *N Engl J Med* 1998; 338:1488–1497.
64. The Impact-II Investigators. Randomized placebo-controlled trial of effect of eptifibatide on complications of percutaneous coronary intervention: IMPACT-II. *Lancet* 1997;349: 1422–1428.
65. Raschke RA, Reilly BM, Guidry JR, et al. The weight-based heparin dosing nomogram compared with a standard care nomogram: a randomized controlled trial. *Ann Intern Med* 1993;119:8740–8881.
66. Hull RD, Raskob GE, Rosenbloom D, et al. Optimal therapeutic level of heparin therapy in patients with venous thrombosis. *Arch Intern Med* 1992;152:1589–1595.
67. Babcock RB, Dumper CW, Scharfman WB. Heparin-induced immune thrombocytopenia. *N Engl J Med* 1976;295:237–241.
68. Schmitz LL, Olson SL, Shapiro RS, et al. Failure to generate comparable international normalized ratio values using five different thromboplastin reagents in parallel studies of patients receiving warfarin. *Clin Appl Thromb Hemost* 1995;1:142–150.
69. Raskob GE, George JN. Thrombotic complications of antithrombotic therapy: a paradox with implications for clinical practice. *Ann Intern Med* 1997;127:839–840.
70. Nicolaides AN. Prevention of venous thromboembolism: international consensus statement, guidelines compiled in accordance with scientific evidence. *Int Angiol* 2001;20:1.
71. Haas S. Prevention of venous thromboembolism: recommendations based on the international consensus and the American College of Chest Physicians sixth consensus conference on antithrombotic therapy. *J Clin Appl Thromb Hemost* 2001;7: 171.
72. Rees DS, Cox M, Clegg JB. World distribution of factor V Leiden. *Lancet* 1995;346:1133–1134.
73. Svensson P, Dahlback B. Resistance to activated protein C as a basis for venous thrombosis. *N Engl J Med* 1994;330:517.
74. Koster T, Rosendaal FR, de Ronde H, et al. Venous thrombosis due to poor anticoagulant response to activated protein C: Leiden Thrombophilia Study. *Lancet* 1993;342:1503–1506.
75. Dahlback B, Carlsson M, Svensson PJ. Familial thrombophilia due to a previously unrecognized mechanism characterized by poor anticoagulant response to activated protein C: prediction of a cofactor to activated protein C. *Proc Natl Acad Sci U S A* 1993;90:1004–1008.
76. Bertina RM. Factor V Leiden and other coagulation factor mutations affecting thrombotic risk. *Clin Chem* 1997;43: 1678–1683.
77. Bertina RM, Reitsma PH, Rosendaal FR, et al. Resistance to activated protein C and factor V Leiden as risk factors for venous thrombosis. *Thromb Haemost* 1995;74:449–453.
78. Greengard JS, Fisher CL, Villoutreix B, et al. Structural basis for type I and type II deficiencies of antithrombotic plasma protein C: patterns revealed by three-dimensional molecular modeling of mutations of the protease domain. *Proteins* 1994;18:367–380.
79. Voorberg J, Roelse J, Koopman R, et al. Association of idiopathic venous thromboembolism with single-point mutation at Arg506 of factor V. *Lancet* 1994;343:1535.
80. Zoller B, Hillarp A, Berntorp E, et al. Activated protein C resistance due to a common factor V gene mutation is a major risk factor for venous thrombosis. *Annu Rev Med* 1997;48:45–58.
81. Laffan MA, Manning T. The influence of factor VIII on measurement of activated protein C resistance. *Blood Coagul Fibrinolysis*1996;7:761.
82. Bontempo FA. The factor V Leiden mutation: spectrum of thrombotic events and laboratory evaluation. *J Vasc Surg* 1997; 2:271–276.
83. Simioni P, Scalia D, Tormene D. Intra-arterial thrombosis and homozygous factor V Leiden mutation. *Clin Appl Thromb Hemost* 1997;3:215.
84. Bick RL, Laughlin HR, Cohen B. Fetal wastage syndrome due to blood protein/platelet defects: results of prevalence studies and treatment outcome with low-dose heparin and low-dose aspirin. *Clin Appl Thromb Hemost* 1995;1:286.
85. Hile ET, Westendorp RG, Vandenbroucke JP, et al. Mortality and causes of death in families with the factor V Leiden mutation (resistance to activated protein C). *Blood* 1997;89:1963.
86. Samama MM, Simon D, Horellou MH, et al. Diagnosis and clinical characteristics of inherited activated protein C resistance. *Haemostasis* 1996;26(suppl 4):315–330.
87. Middeldorp S, Henkens CM, Koopman MM, et al. The incidence of venous thrombembolism in family members of patients with factor V Leiden mutation and venous thrombosis. *Ann Intern Med* 1998;128:15–20.
88. Bick RL. Syndromes of thrombosis and hypercoagulability. In: Bick RL, ed. *Current concepts of thrombosis, medical clinics North America.* Philadelphia: WB Saunders, 1998:82–409.
89. Prandoni P, Lensing AW, Cogo A, et al. The long-term clinical course of acute deep venous thrombosis. *Ann Intern Med* 1996; 125:1–7.
90. Ridker PM, Miletich JP, Stampfer MJ, et al. Factor V Leiden and recurrent idiopathic venous thromboembolism. *Circulation* 1995;92:2800–2802.
91. Simioni P, Prandoni P, Lensing AW, et al. The risk of recurrent venous thromboembolism in patients with an Arg506 → Gln mutation in the gene for factor V (factor V Leiden). *N Engl J Med* 1997;336:399–403.

92. Rintelen C, Pabinger I, Knobl P, et al. Probability of recurrence of thrombosis in patients with and without factor V Leiden. *Thromb Haemost* 1996;75:229–232.
93. Levine MN, Hirsh J, Gent M, et al. Optimal duration of oral anticoagulant therapy: a randomized trial comparing four weeks with three months of warfarin in patients with proximal deep vein thrombosis. *Thromb Haemost* 1995;74:606–611.
94. Vandenbroucke JP, Koster T, Briet E, et al. Increased risk of venous thrombosis in oral-contraceptive users who are carriers of factor V Leiden mutation. *Lancet* 1994;344: 1453–1457.
95. Bloemenkamp KW, Rosendaal FR, Helmerhorst FM, et al. Enhancement by factor V Leiden mutation of risk of deep-vein thrombosis associated with oral contraceptives containing a third-generation progestagen. *Lancet* 1995;346:1593–1596.
96. Rintelen C, Mannhalter C, Ireland H, et al. Oral contraceptives enhance the risk of clinical manifestation of venous thrombosis at a young age in females homozygous for factor V Leiden. *Br J Haematol* 1996;93:487–490.
97. Gandrille S, Greengard JS, Alhenc-Gelac M, et al. Incidence of activated protein C resistance caused by the Arg 506 Gln mutation in factor V in 113 unrelated symptomatic protein C-deficient patients: the French network on the behalf of INSERM. *Blood* 1995;86:219–224.
98. Zoller B, Berntsdotter A, Garcia de Frutos P, et al. Resistance to activated protein C as an additional genetic risk factor in hereditary deficiency of protein S. *Blood* 1955;85:3518–3523.
99. Ridker PM, Hennekens CH, Selhub J, et al. Interrelation of hyperhomocyst(e)inemia, factor V Leiden, and risks of future venous thromboembolism. *Circulation* 1997;95:1777–1782.
100. Bokarewa MI, Bremme K, Blomback M. Arg506-Gln mutation in factor V and risk of thrombosis during pregnancy. *Br J Haematol* 1996;92:473–478.
101. Kibbe MR, Rhee RY. Heparin-induced thrombocytopenia: pathophysiology. *Semin Vasc Surg* 1996;9:284–291.
102. Wallis DE, Lewis BE, Messmore H, et al. Heparin-induced thrombocytopenia and thrombosis syndrome. *Clin Appl Thromb Hemost* 1998;4:160–163.
103. Williamson D, Brown K, Luddington R, et al. Factor V Cambridge: a new mutation (Arg306→Thr) associated with resistance to activated protein C. *Blood* 1998;91:1140–1144.
104. Santacroce R, Bossone A, Brancaccio V, et al. In the presence of other inherited or acquired high-risk situations, the FV Cambridge mutation may be an additional thrombophilic risk factor, through its effect on APC sensitivity. *Thromb Haemost* 2000;83:963.
105. Faioni EM, Franchi F, Bucciarelli P, et al. Coinheritance of the HR2 haplotype in the factor V gene confers an increased risk of venous thromboembolism in carriers of factor V R506Q (factor V Leiden). *Blood* 1999;94:3062.
106. Bernardi F, Faioni EM, Castoldi E, et al. A factor V genetic component differing from factor V R506Q contributes to the activated protein C resistance phenotype. *Blood* 1997;90:1552.
107. Chan WP, Lee CK, Kwong YL, et al. A novel mutation of Arg306 of factor V gene in Hong Kong Chinese. *Blood* 1998; 91:1135–1139.
108. Sugahara Y, Miura O, Aoki N. Protein C deficiency Hong Kong 1 and 2: hereditary protein C deficiency caused by two mutant alleles, a 5-nucleotide deletion and a missense mutation. *Blood* 1992;80:126.
109. Poort SR, Rosendaal FR, Reitsma PH, et al. A common genetic variation in the 3′-untranslated region of the prothrombin gene is associated with elevated plasma prothrombin levels and an increase in venous thrombosis. *Blood* 1996;88:3698–3703.
110. Arruda VR, Annichino-Bizacchi JM, Goncalves MS, et al. Prevalence of the prothrombin gene variant (nt20201A) in venous thrombosis and arterial disease. *Thromb Haemost* 1997; 78:1430–1433.
111. Ferraresi P, Marchetti G, Legnani C, et al. The heterozygous 20210 G/A prothrombin genotype is associated with early venous thrombosis in inherited thrombophilias and is not increased in frequency in artery disease. *Arterioscler Thromb Vasc Biol* 1997;17:2418–2422.
112. Makris M, Preston FE, Beauchamp NJ, et al. Co-inheritance of the 20210A allele of the prothrombin gene increases the risk of thrombosis in subjects with familial thrombophilia. *Thromb Haemost* 1997;78:1426–1429.
113. Bloem BR, van Putten MJ, van der Meer JM, et al. Superior sagittal sinus thrombosis in a patient heterozygous for the novel 20210A allele of the prothrombin gene. *Thromb Haemost* 1997; 79:235.
114. Martinelli I, Sacchi E, Landi G, et al. High risk of cerebral-vein thrombosis in carriers of a prothrombin-gene mutation and in users of oral contraceptives. *N Engl J Med* 1998;338: 1793–1797.
115. Gould J, Deam S, Dolan G. Prothrombin 20210A polymorphism and third generation oral contraceptives: a case report of coeliac axis thrombosis and splenic infarction. *Thromb Haemost* 1998;79:1214–1215.
116. Poort SR, Rosendaal FR, Reitsma PH, et al. A common genetic variation in the 3′-untranslated region of the prothrombin gene is associated with elevated plasma prothrombin levels and an increase in venous thrombosis. *Blood* 1996;88:3698–3703.
117. Ratnoff OD, Colopy JE. A familial hemorrhagic trait associated with a deficiency of clot-promoting fraction of plasma. *J Clin Invest* 1955;34:602.
118. Seegers WH. Factor X (autoprothrombin III). *Semin Thromb Hemost* 1981;7:233.
119. Bick RL. Hereditary coagulation protein defects. In: *Disorders of thrombosis and hemostasis: clinical and laboratory practice.* Chicago: ASCP Press, 1992:109–136.
120. McPherson RA. Thromboembolism in Hageman trait. *Am J Clin Pathol* 1977;68:240.
121. Hoak JC, Swanson LW, Warner ED, et al. Myocardial infarction associated with severe factor XI deficiency. *Lancet* 1966;2:884.
122. Ratnoff OD, Busse RJ, Sheon RP. The demise of John Hageman. *N Engl J Med* 1968;279:760.
123. Goodnough LT, Saito H, Ratnoff O. Thrombosis or myocardial infarction in congenital clotting factor abnormalities and chronic thrombocytopenias: a report of 21 patients and a review of 50 previously reported cases. *Medicine* 1983;62:248.
124. Di Imperato D, Dettori AG. Ipofibrinogenemia congenita con fibrinoastenia. *Helv Pediatr Acta* 1958;13:380.
125. Mosesson MW. Dysfibrinogenemia and thrombosis. *Semin Thromb Hemost* 1999;25:311.
126. Mammen EF. Fibrinogen abnormalities. *Semin Hemost Thromb* 1983;9:1.
127. Al Mondhiry H, Galanakis D. Dysfibrinogenemia and lupus anticoagulant in a patient with recurrent thrombosis. *J Lab Clin Med* 1987;110:726.
128. Lijnen HR, Soria J, Soria C. Dysfibrinogenemia (fibrinogen Dusard) associated with impaired fibrin-enhanced plasminogen activation. *Thromb Haemost* 1984;51:108.
129. Reber P, Furlan M, Henschen A. Three abnormal fibrinogen variants with the same amino acid substitution (gamma-275 Arg-His): fibrinogens Bergamo II, Essen and Perugia. *Thromb Haemost* 1986;56:401.
130. Welch GN, Loscalzo J. Homocysteine and atherothrombosis. *N Engl J Med* 1998;338:1042–1050.
131. Carson NAJ, Neill DW. Metabolic abnormalities detected in a survey of mentally backward individuals in Northern Ireland. *Arch Dis Child* 1962;37:505–513.

132. Mudd SH, Finkelstein JD, Irreverre F, et al. Homocystinuria: an enzymatic defect. *Science* 1964;143:1443–1445.
133. Valle D, Pai GS, Thomas GH, et al. Homocystinuria due to cystathione beta-synthetase deficiency: clinical manifestations and therapy. *Johns Hopkins Med J* 1980;146:110.
134. McCully KS. Vascular pathology of homocysteinemia: implications for the pathogenesis of arteriosclerosis. *Am J Pathol* 1969; 56:111–128.
135. Carey MC, Donovan DE, Fitzgerald O, et al. Homocystinuria, I: a clinical and pathologic study of nine subjects in six families. *Am J Med* 1968;45:17.
136. Goyette P, Sumner JS, Milos R, et al. Human methylenetetrahydrofolate reductase: isolation of cDNA, mapping and mutation identification. *Nat Genet* 1994;7:195–200.
137. Frosst P, Blom HJ, Milos R. A candidate genetic risk factor for vascular disease: a common mutation in methylenetetrahyrofolate reductase. *Nat Genet* 1995;10:111–113.
138. Van der Put NMJ, Steegers-Theunissen RPM, Frosst P. Mutated methylenetetrahydrofolate reductase as a risk factor for spina bifida. *Lancet* 1995;346:1070–1071.
139. Jacques PF, Bostom AG, Williams RR, et al. Relation between folate status, a common mutation in methylenetetrahydrofolate reductase, and plasma homocysteine concentrations. *Circulation* 1996;93:7–9.
140. Rozen R. Molecular genetic aspects of hyperhomocysteinemia and its relation to folic acid. *Clin Invest Med* 1996;19:171–178.
141. Guba SC, Fonseca V, Fink LM. Hyperhomocysteinemia and thrombosis. *Semin Thromb Hemost* 1999;25:291.
142. Stampfer MJ, Malinow MR, Wilett WC, et al. A prospective study of plasma homocyst(e)ine and risk of myocardial infarction and risk of myocardial infarction in US physicians. *JAMA* 1992;268:877–881.
143. Kang SS, Wong PWK, Susmano A, et al. Thermolabile methylenetetrahydrofolate reductase: an inherited risk factor for coronary artery disease. *Am J Hum Genet* 1991;48:536–545.
144. Malinow MR. Hyperhomocyst(e)inemia: a common and easily reversible risk factor for occlusive atherosclerosis. *Circulation* 1990;81:2004–2006.
145. Boushey CJ, Beresford AA, Omenn GS, et al. A quantitative assessment of plasma homocysteine as a risk factor for vascular disease: probable benefits of increasing folic acid intake. *JAMA* 1995;274:1049–1057.
146. Duell PB, Malinow MR. Plasma homocyst(e)ine: an important risk factor for atherosclerotic vascular disease. *Curr Opin Lipidol* 1997;8:28–34.
147. Mayer EL, Jacobsen DW, Robinson K. Homocysteine and coronary atherosclerosis. *J Am Coll Cardiol* 1996;27:517–527.
148. Nygard O, Nordrehaug JE, Refsum H, et al. Plasma homocysteine levels and mortality in patients with coronary artery disease. *N Engl J Med* 1997;337:230–236.
149. Cattaneo M, Martinelli I, Manucci PM. Hyperhomocysteinemia as a risk factor for deep-vein thrombosis. *N Engl J Med* 1997;336:1399.
150. Falcon CR, Cattaneo M, Panzeri D, et al. High prevalence of hyperhomocyst(e)inemia in patients with juvenile venous thrombosis. *Arterioscler Thromb* 1994;14:1080–1083.
151. Den Heijer M, Koster T, Blom HU. Hyperhomocysteinemia as a risk factor for deep- vein thrombosis. *N Engl J Med* 1996;334: 759–762.
152. Fermo I, Vigano D'Angelo S, et al. Prevalence of moderate hyperhomocysteinemia in patients with early-onset venous and arterial occlusive disease. *Ann Intern Med* 1995;123:747–753.
153. Moghadasian MH, McManus BM, Frohlich JJ. Homocyst(e)ine and coronary artery disease: clinical evidence and genetic and metabolic background. *Arch Intern Med* 1997;157: 2299–2308.
154. Robinson K, Mayer EL, Miller DP, et al. Hyperhomocystinemia and low pyridoxal phosphate: common and independent reversible risk factors for coronary artery disease. *Circulation* 1995;92:2825–2830.
155. Israelsson B, Brattstorm LE, Hultberg BL. Homocysteine and myocardial infarction. *Atherosclerosis* 1988;71:227–233.
156. Wu LL, Wu J, Hunt SC, et al. Plasma homocyst(e)ine as a risk factor for early familial coronary artery disease. *Clin Chem* 1994;40:552–561.
157. Wald NJ, Watt HC, Law MR, et al. Homocysteine and ischemic heart disease: results of a prospective study with implications regarding prevention. *Arch Intern Med* 1998;158: 862–867.
158. Araki A, Sako Y, Fukushima Y, et al. Plasma sulfhydryl-containing amino acids in patients with cerebral infarction and in hypertensive subjects. *Atherosclerosis* 1989;79:139–136.
159. Brattstrom L, Lindgren A, Israelsson B, et al. Hyperhomocysteinemia in stroke: prevalence, cause and relationship to type of stroke and stroke risk factors. *Eur J Clin Invest* 1992;22: 214–221.
160. Coull BM, Malinow MR, Beamer N, et al. Elevated plasma homocyst(e)ine concentration as a possible independent risk factor for stroke. *Stroke* 1990;21:572–576.
161. Molgaard J, Malinow MR, Lassvik C, et al. Hyperhomocyst(e)inaemia: an independent risk factor for intermittent claudication. *J Intern Med* 1992;231:273–279.
162. Van den Berg M, Stehouwer DA, Biedrager E, et al. Plasma homocysteine and severity of atherosclerosis in young patients with lower-limb atherosclerotic disease. *Arterioscler Thromb Vasc Biol* 1996;16:165–171.
163. Kottke-Marchant K, Green R, Jacobsen DW, et al. High plasma homocysteine: a risk factor for arterial and venous thrombosis in patients with normal coagulation profiles. *Clin Appl Thromb Hemost* 1997;3:239–244.
164. Franken DG, Boers GH, Blom HJ, et al. Treatment of mild hyperhomocysteinemia in vascular disease patients. *Arterioscler Thromb* 1994;14:465–470.
165. Brattstrom L, Israelsson B, Norving B, et al. Impaired homocysteine metabolism in early onset cerebral and peripheral occlusive arterial disease: effect of pyridoxine and folic acid treatment. *Atherosclerosis* 1990;81:51–60.
166. Brattsrom LE, Israelsson B, Jeppsson JO, et al. Folic acid: an innocuous means to reduce plasma homocysteine. *Scand J Clin Lab Invest* 1988;48:215–221.
167. Ubbink JB, Hayward Vermaak WJ, van der Merwe A, et al. Vitamin requirements for the treatment of hypercysteinemia in humans. *J Nutr* 1994;124:1927–1933.
168. Naurath HJ, Joosten E, Riezler R, et al. Effects of vitamin B12, folate, and vitamin B6 supplements in elderly people with normal serum vitamin concentrations. *Lancet* 1995;346:85–89.
169. Landgren P, Israelsson B, Lindgren A, et al. Plasma homocysteine in acute myocardial infarction: homocysteine lowering effect of folic acid. *J Intern Med* 1995;237:381–388.
170. Ward M, McNulty H, McPartlin J, et al. Plasma homocysteine, a risk factor for cardiovascular disease, is lowered by physiological doses of folic acid. *Q J Med* 1997;909:519–524.
171. Cuskelly GJ, McNulty H, McPartlin JM, et al. Plasma homocysteine response to folate intervention in young women. *Ir J Med Sci* 1995;164:3.
172. Malinow MR, Duell PB, Hess DL, et al. Reduction of plasma homocyst(e)ine levels by breakfast cereal fortified with folic acid in patients with coronary heart disease. *N Engl J Med* 1998; 338:1009–1015.
173. Abidgaard U. Purification of two progressive antithrombins of human plasma. *Scand J Clin Lab Invest* 1967;19:190.
174. Kurachi K, Schmer G, Hermodson M. Inhibition of bovine fac-

tor IXa and factor Xa by anti-thrombin-III. *Biochemistry* 1976; 15:368.
175. Lahiri K, Rosenberg RD, Talamo RC. Antithrombin-III: an inhibitor of human plasma kallikrein. *Fed Proc* 1974;33:642.
176. Seegers WH, Cole ER, Harmison CR. Neutralization of autoprothrombin-C activity with antithrombin. *Can J Biochem* 1964;42:359.
177. Walker F, Esmon C. The molecular mechanism of heparin action, II: separation of functionally different heparins by affinity chromatography. *Thromb Res* 1979;14:219.
178. Abildgaard U. Binding of thrombin to antithrombin III. *Scand J Clin Lab Invest* 1969;24:23.
179. Seegers WH, Schroer H, Kagami M. Interactivation of purified autoprothrombin I with antithrombin. *Can J Biochem* 1964;42: 1425.
180. Stead N, Kaplan AP, Rosenberg RD. Inhibition of activated factor XII by antithrombin-heparin cofactor. *J Biol Chem* 1976; 251:6481.
181. Vennerod AM, Laake K, Soleberg AK. Inactivation and binding of human plasma kallikrein by antithrombin III and heparin. *Thromb Res* 1976;9:457.
182. Fischer AM, Cornu P, Sternberg C. Antithrombin III Alger: a new homozygous ATIII variant. *Thromb Haemost* 1986;55:218.
183. Fagerhol M, Abildgaard U. Immunologic studies in human antithrombin III: influence of age, sex, and use of oral contraceptives on serum concentration. *Scand J Haematol* 1970;7:10.
184. Howie P, Mallinson A, Prentice C. Effect of combined oestrogen-progesterone contraceptives, oestrogen, and progesterone on antiplasmin and antithrombin activity. *Lancet* 1990;II:1329.
185. McKay E. Immunochemical analysis of active and inactive antithrombin III. *Br J Haematol* 1980;46:277.
186. Peterson C, Kelley R, Minard B. Antithrombin III: comparison of functional and immunologic assays. *Am J Clin Pathol* 1978; 69:500.
187. Sveger T. Antithrombin III in adolescents. *Thromb Res* 1979;15: 885.
188. Bick RL. Clinical relevance of antithrombin III. *Semin Hemost Thromb* 1982;8:276.
189. Candrina R, Goppini A. Antithrombin III deficiency. *Blood Rev* 1988;2:239.
190. Menache D, O'Malley JP, Schorr JB, et al. Evaluation of the safety, recovery, half-life, and clinical efficacy of antithrombin III (human) in patients with hereditary antithrombin III deficiency. *Blood* 1990;75:33.
191. Menache D. Replacement therapy in patients with hereditary antithrombin III deficiency. *Semin Hematol* 1991;28:31
192. Owen J. Antithrombin III replacement therapy in pregnancy. *Semin Hematol* 1991;28:46
193. Vinnazer H. Antithrombin III in shock and disseminated intravascular coagulation. *Clin Appl Thromb Hemost* 1995;1:62.
194. Vinazzer H. Hereditary and acquired antithrombin deficiency. *Semin Thromb Hemost* 1999;25:257.
195. Tollefson DM, Majerus DW, Blank MK. Heparin cofactor II: purification and properties of a heparin-dependent inhibitor of thrombin in human plasma. *J Biol Chem* 1982;257:2162.
196. Sie P, Fernandez F, Caranobe C. Inhibition of thrombin-induced platelet aggregation and serotonin release by antithrombin III and heparin cofactor II in the presence of standard heparin, dermatan sulfate and pentosan polysulfate. *Thromb Res* 1984;35:231.
197. Sie P, Dupouy D, Pichon J. Constitutional heparin cofactor II deficiency associated with recurrent thrombosis. *Lancet* 1985;II: 414.
198. Anderson T, Larsen M, Abildgaard U. Low heparin cofactor II associated with abnormal crossed immunoelectrophoresis pattern in two Norwegian families. *Thromb Res* 1987;47:243.
199. Bertina RM, Van der Linden IK, Engesser L, et al. Hereditary cofactor-II deficiency and the risk of development of thrombosis. *Thromb Haemost* 1987;57:196.
200. Frenkel EP, Bick RL. Prothrombin G202010A gene mutation: heparin cofactor II defects, primary (essential) thrombocythemia and thrombohemorrhagic manifestations. *Semin Thromb Hemost* 1999;25:375–386.
201. Toulin P, Vitoux JF, Capron L. Heparin cofactor II in patients with deep venous thrombosis under heparin and oral anticoagulant therapy. *Thromb Res* 1988;49:479.
202. Grau E, Oliver A, Felez J. Plasma and urinary heparin cofactor II levels in patients with nephrotic syndrome. *Thromb Haemost* 1988;60:137.
203. Stenflo J. Structure and function of protein C. *Semin Thromb Hemost* 1984;10:109.
204. Esmon CT, Esmon NL. Protein C activation. *Semin Thromb Hemost* 1984;10:122.
205. Walker FJ. Protein S and the regulation of activated protein C. *Semin Thromb Hemost* 1984;10:131.
206. Dahlback B. The protein C anticoagulant system: inherited defects as basis for venous thrombosis. *Thromb Res* 1995;77: 1–43.
207. Griffin JH. Clinical studies on protein C. *Semin Thromb Hemost* 1984;10:162.
208. Marlar RA, Endres-Brooks J. Recurrent thromboembolic disease due to heterozygous protein C deficiency. *Thromb Haemost* 1983;50:351.
209. Broekmans AW. Hereditary protein C deficiency. *Haemostasis* 1985;15:233.
210. Seligsohn U, Berger A, Abend M. Homozygous protein C deficiency manifested by massive venous thrombosis in the newborn. *N Engl J Med* 1984;310:559.
211. Marciniak E, Wilson HO, Marlar RA. Neonatal purpura fulminans: a genetic disorder related to the absence of protein C in blood. *Blood* 198;65:15.
212. Mammen EF. Inhibitor abnormalities. *Semin Thromb Hemost* 1983;9:42.
213. Reitsma PH, Poort SR, Allaart CF, et al. The spectrum of genetic defects in a panel of 40 Dutch families with symptomatic protein C deficiency type I: heterogeneity and founder effects. *Blood* 1991;78:890.
214. Comp PC, Nixon R, Esmon CT. Determination of functional levels of protein C, an antithrombotic protein, using thrombin/thrombomodulin complex. *Blood* 1984;63:15.
215. Griffin JH, Bezeaud A, Evatt B. Functional and immunologic studies of protein C in thromboembolic disease. *Blood* 1983;62: 301a.
216. Bick RL. Hypercoagulability and thrombosis. In: Bick RL, Bennett JM, Byrnes RK, eds. *Hematology: clinical and laboratory practice.* St. Louis: CV Mosby, 1993:155.
217. Nizzi FA, Kaplan HS. Protein C and S deficiency. *Semin Thromb Hemost* 1999;25:265.
218. Marlar RA, Sills RH, Montgomery RR. Protein C in commercial factor IX (F IX) concentrations (CONC) and its use in the treatment of "homozygous" protein C deficiency. *Blood* 1998; 62:303.
219. Pescatore P, Horellou H, Conard J, et al. Problems of oral anticoagulation in an adult with homozygous protein C deficiency and late onset of thrombosis. *Thromb Haemost* 1993;69:311–314.
220. Monagle P, Andrew M, Halton J, et al. Homozygous protein C deficiency: description of a new mutation and successful treatment with low molecular weight heparin. *Thromb Haemost* 1998;79:756–761.
221. Broekmans AW, Bertina RM, Loeliger EA, et al. Protein C and the development of skin necrosis during anticoagulant therapy. *Thromb Haemost* 1983;49:251.

222. Zauber NP, Stark MW. Successful warfarin anticoagulation despite protein C deficiency and a history of warfarin necrosis. *Ann Intern Med* 1986;104:659–660.
223. Samama M, Horellou MH, Soria J, et al. Successful progressive anticoagulation in a severe protein C deficiency and previous skin necrosis at the initiation of oral anticoagulation treatment [Letter]. *Thromb Haemost* 1984;51:132–133.
224. Bick RL, Kaplan H. Syndromes of thrombosis and hypercoagulability: congenital and acquired thrombophilias. *Clin Appl Thromb Hemost* 1998;4:25–50.
225. Miletich JP. Laboratory diagnosis of protein C. *Semin Thromb Hemost* 1990;16:169–176.
226. Gardiner JE, McGann MA, Berridge CW. Protein S as a cofactor for activated protein C in plasma and the inactivation of purified factor VIII:C. *Circulation* 1984;70:205.
227. De Fouw NJ, Haverkate F, Bertina RM. The cofactor role of protein S in the acceleration of whole blood clot lysis by activated protein C in vitro. *Blood* 1986;67:1189.
228. Hackeng TM, van't Veer C, Meijers JC, et al. Human protein S inhibits prothrombinase complex activity on endothelial cells and platelets via direct interactions with factors Va and Xa. *J Biol Chem* 1994;269:21051–21058.
229. Koppelman SJ, Hackeng TM, Sixma JJ, et al. Inhibition of the intrinsic factor X activating complex by protein S: evidence for specific binding of protein S to factor VIII. *Blood* 1995;86: 1062–1071.
230. Gladson KH, Griffin JH, Hach V. The incidence of protein C and protein S deficiency in 139 young thrombotic patients. *Thromb Hemost* 1988;59:18.
231. Heijboer H, Brandjes DP, Buller HR, et al. Deficiencies of coagulation-inhibiting and fibrinolytic proteins in outpatients with deep-vein thrombosis. *N Engl J Med* 1990;323: 1512–1516.
232. Tabernero MD, Tomas JF, Alberca I, et al. Incidence and clinical characteristics of hereditary disorders associated with venous thrombosis. *Am J Hematol* 1991;36:249–254.
233. Simmonds RE, Ireland H, Lane D, et al. Clarification of the risk for venous thrombosis associated with hereditary protein S deficiency by investigation of a large kindred with a characterized gene defect. *Ann Intern Med* 1998;128:8–14.
234. Mahasandana C, Suvatte V, Marlar RA, et al. Neonatal purpura fulminans associated with homozygous protein S deficiency. *Lancet* 1990;335:61–62.
235. Broekmans MA, Engesser L, Briet E. Clinical manifestations of hereditary protein S deficiency. *Thromb Haemost* 1985; 54:57.
236. Engesser L, Broekmans AW, Briet E, et al. Hereditary protein S deficiency: clinical manifestations. *Ann Intern Med* 1987;106: 677–682.
237. Juhan-Vague I, Roul C, Alessi MC, et al. Increased plasminogen activator inhibitor activity in non-insulin dependent diabetic patients: relationship with plasma insulin. *Thromb Haemost* 1989;61:370.
238. Nalbandian RM, Henry RL, Bick RL. Thrombotic thrombocytopenic purpura: an extended editorial. *Semin Thromb Hemost* 1979;5:216.
239. Bick RL, Bishop RC, Shanbrom E. Fibrinolytic activity in acute myocardial infarction. *Am J Clin Pathol* 1972;57:359.
240. Collen D, Juhan-Vague I. Fibrinolysis and atherosclerosis. *Semin Thromb Hemost* 1988;14:180.
241. Mansfield MO. Alterations in fibrinolysis associated with surgery and venous thrombosis. *Br J Surg* 1972;59:754.
242. Bick RL, Thompson WB. Fibrinolytic activity: changes induced with oral contraceptives. *Obstet Gynecol* 1972;39:213.
243. Marsh N. Fibrinolysis in disease. In: Marsh N, ed. *Fibrinolysis.* New York: John Wiley and Sons, 1981:125.
244. Hedner U, Nilsson IM. Urokinase inhibitors in serum in a clinical series. *Acta Med Scand* 1971;189:185–189.
245. Stemerman MB. Vascular intimal components: precursors of thrombosis. *Prog Hemost Thromb* 1974;2:1.
246. Wight T. Vessel proteoglycans and thrombogenesis. *Prog Hemost Thromb* 1980;5:1.
247. Mammen EF. Plasminogen abnormalities. *Semin Hemost Thromb* 1983;9:50.
248. Aoki N, Moroi M, Sakata Y. Abnormal plasminogen: a hereditary molecular abnormality found in a patient with recurrent thrombosis. *J Clin Invest* 1978;61:1186.
249. Blaisdell W. Acquired and congenital clotting syndromes. *World J Surg* 1990;14:664.
250. Hasegawa DK, Tyler BJ, Edson JR. Thrombotic disease in three families with inherited plasminogen deficiency. *Blood* 1982; 60:213.
251. Sartori MT, Patrassi GM, Girolami B, et al. Type I plasminogen deficiency should be included among familial thrombophilias [Letter]. *Clin Appl Thromb Hemost* 1997;3:218–219.
252. Biasutti FD, Sulzer I, Stucki B, et al. Is plasminogen deficiency a thrombotic risk factor? A study on 23 thrombophilic patients and their family members. *Thromb Haemost* 1998;80:167–170.
253. Kazama M, Tahara C, Suzki Z. Abnormal plasminogen: a case of recurrent thrombosis. *Thromb Res* 1981;21:517.
254. Bick RL. Clinical hemostasis practice: the major impact of laboratory automation. *Semin Thromb Hemost* 1983;9:139.
255. Nilsson IM, Tehgborn LA. A family with thrombosis associated with high level of tissue plasminogen activator inhibitor. *Haemostasis* 1984;14:24.
256. Petaja M, Rasi V, Myllyla G. Familial hypofibrinolysis and venous thrombosis. *Br J Haematol* 1989;71:393.
257. Brommer EJP, Engesser L, Briet E. Thrombophilia and hereditary increase in plasminogen activator inhibitor (PAI-1). *Fibrinolysis* 1988;2:83.
258. Dawson S, Hamsten A, Wiman B. Genetic variation at the plasminogen activator inhibitor-1 locus is associated with altered levels of plasma plasminogen activator inhibitor activity. *Ather oscler Thromb* 1991;11:183.
259. Li XN, Grenett HE, Benza RL. Genotype-specific transcriptional regulation of PAI-1 expression by hypertriglyceridemic VLDL and LP(a) in cultured human endothelial cells. *Atheroscler Thromb Vasc Biol* 1997;17:3215–3223.
260. Eriksson P, Kallin B, Van Hooft FM. Allele-specific increase in basal transcription of the plasminogen-activator inhibitor 1 gene is associated with myocardial infarction. *J Natl Acad Sci U S A* 1995;92:1851.
261. Ye S, Green FR, Scarabin PY. The 4G/5G genetic polymorphism in the promoter of the plasminogen activator inhibitor 1 (PAI-1) gene is associated with differences in plasma PAI-1 activity but not with the risk of myocardial infarction in the ECTIM study. *Thromb Haemost* 1995;74:837.
262. Ridker PM, Hennekens CH, Lindpaintner K. Arterial and venous thrombosis is not associated with the 4G/5G polymorphism in the promoter of the plasminogen activator inhibitor gene in a large cohort of US men. *Circulation* 1997; 95:59.
263. Hong JJ, Kwaan HC. Hereditary defects in fibrinolysis associated with thrombosis. *Semin Thromb Hemost* 1999;25:321.
264. Sinzinger H, Kaliman J, O'Grady J. Platelet lipoxygenase defect (Wein-Penzing defect). *Am J Hematol* 1991;36:202.
265. Mammen EF, Barnhart MI, Selik NR, et al. "Sticky platelet syndrome": a congenital platelet abnormality predisposing to thrombosis. *Folia Haematol* 1988;115:361.
266. Rubenfire M, Blevens RD, Barnhart MI, et al. Platelet hyperaggregability in patients with chest pain and angiographically normal coronary arteries. *Am J Cardiol* 1986;57:657.

267. Chittoor S, Elsehety AE, Roberts GF, et al. Sticky platelet syndrome: a case report and review of the literature. *J Clin Appl Thromb Hemost* 1998;4:280.
268. Mammen EF. Ten years' experience with the "sticky platelet syndrome." *J Clin Appl Thromb Hemost* 1995;1:66.
269. Mammen EF. Sticky platelet syndrome. *Semin Thromb Hemost* 1999;25:361.
270. Bick RL. Sticky platelet syndrome: a common cause of unexplained venous and arterial thrombosis: results of prevalence and treatment outcome. *J Clin Appl Thromb Hemost* 1998;4: 77–81.
271. Anderson JA, Bleeding and thrombosis in women. *Biomed Prog* 1999;12: 40.
272. Berg-Damer E, Henkes E, Trobisch H, et al. Sticky platelet syndrome: a cause of neurovascular thrombosis and thromboembolism. *Intervent Neuroradiol* 1997;3:145.

Disorders of Thrombosis and Hemostasis: Clinical and Laboratory Practice, Third Edition, edited by Rodger L. Bick.
Lippincott Williams & Wilkins, Philadelphia © 2002

14

ACQUIRED THROMBOPHILIA

RODGER L. BICK
WILLIAM F. BAKER, JR.

Patients recognized to be at increased risk for thrombosis have generally been referred to as having a "hypercoagulable" state, or "thrombophilia" (1). Many blood protein and platelet defects are now known to account for hypercoagulability and thrombosis; hereditary defects of blood proteins leading to thrombosis, such as antithrombin (AT), protein C and protein S, heparin cofactor II, and plasminogen deficiency, activated protein C resistance (APC resistance)/factor V Leiden, the prothrombin mutation G20210A, dysfibrinogenemia fibrinolytic system defects, and others, are generally termed the "hereditary thrombophilias." The hereditary thrombophilias are discussed in Chapter 13. Acquired blood protein and platelet-function defects also are associated with thrombosis, including acquired defects of protein C, protein S or AT, acquired APC resistance, and others. These are the "acquired thrombophilias," the topic of this chapter. Acquired blood protein defects leading to thrombosis are as common as the hereditary forms. The thrombophilias are depicted in Table 14.1.

ANTIPHOSPHOLIPID SYNDROME

Antiphospholipid thrombosis syndromes (APL-TS), which include not only the lupus anticoagulant (LA) and anticardiolipin antibodies (ACLAs), but also more recently recognized "subgroups" of antiphospholipid antibodies (antibodies against β_2-glycoprotein I (β_2-GpI), and antibodies to phosphatidylserine. phosphatidylethanolamine, phosphatidylglycerol, phosphatidylinositol, phosphatidylcholine, and antiannexin-V, all compose the APL-TSs. Antiphospholipid syndrome is the most common acquired blood protein defect(s) associated with either venous or arterial thrombosis or both (2). The thrombotic and thromboocclusive events associated with these antiphospholipid antibodies include thrombosis of the venous system, the arterial system, coronary artery thrombosis, cerebrovascular thrombosis, transient cerebral ischemic attacks (TIAs), retinal vascular thrombosis, and placental vascular thrombosis [leading to recurrent miscarriage syndrome (RMS)]; these antibodies also may be associated with related clinical syndromes, as discussed in this chapter (3).

The APL-TS consists of closely related but clearly distinct clinical syndromes that often are discordant with respect to types of antiphospholipid antibodies found: these are (a) the lupus anticoagulant thrombosis syndrome, (b) the ACLA thrombosis syndrome, and (c) thrombosis asso-

TABLE 14.1. HEREDITARY AND ACQUIRED THROMBOPHILIC DISORDERS

Inherited disorders
APC resistance
Factor V Leiden mutation
Factor V Cambridge mutation
Factor V Hong Kong
Factor V HR2 mutation
Prothrombin 20210A mutation
Factor XII deficiency (Hageman trait)
Dysfibrinogenemia
Hyperhomocyst(e)inemia
Platelet defects
Wein–Penzing defect
Sticky platelet syndrome
Disorders both inherited and acquired
Antithrombin deficiency
Heparin cofactor II deficiency
Protein C deficiency
Protein S deficiency
Plasminogen deficiency
Other fibrinolytic system defects
Acquired disorders
Antiphospholipid antibodies
Anticardiolipin antibodies
Lupus anticoagulant
Subgroup phospholipid antibodies
Myeloproliferative syndromes
Trousseau syndrome

APC, activated protein C.

R. L. Bick: Department of Medicine and Pathology, University of Texas Southwestern Medical Center; Dallas Thrombosis/Hemostasis Clinical Center; ThromboCare Laboratories, Dallas, Texas.

W. F. Baker, Jr.: Department of Medicine, Center for Health Sciences, University of California at Los Angeles, Los Angeles, California; Department of Medicine, Kern Medical Center, Bakersfield, California; and California Clinical Thrombosis Center, Bakersfield, California.

ciated with subgroups of antiphospholipid antibodies. There is poor correlation between thrombosis patients with ACLAs and those with LAs, and stronger, but still not concordant, correlation between thrombosis patients with anticardiolipin antibodies and those with antibodies to β_2-GpI, or antibodies to phosphatidylserine, phosphatidylethanolamine, phosphatidylglycerol, phosphatidylinositol, annexin-V, and phosphatidylcholine. Although there are similarities, there are, at times, clinical, laboratory, and biochemical differences, particularly regarding prevalence, etiology, possible mechanisms of thrombosis, clinical presentations, diagnosis, and, at times, management (4,5). The ACLA–thrombosis antiphospholipid syndrome is much more common than is the LA–thrombosis antiphospholipid syndrome, the ratio being about 5:1 (3,6,7). All of these syndromes may be associated with (a) arterial and venous thrombosis, (b) recurrent miscarriage, and (c) thrombocytopenia, in descending order of prevalence; however, the ACL syndrome is more commonly associated with both arterial and venous thrombosis, including typical deep vein thrombosis (DVT) and pulmonary embolus (PE), premature coronary artery disease, premature cerebrovascular disease (including TIAs, small stoke syndrome, and cerebrovascular thrombotic stroke), and retinal arterial and venous occlusive disease. The LA, although sometimes associated with arterial disease, is more commonly associated with venous thrombosis with or without PE. Patients with ACL–thrombosis syndrome also develop more predictable types of thrombosis than do those with the LA–thrombosis syndrome, and management of thrombotic problems can be quite different between the two syndromes. Thrombosis patients with antibodies to β_2-GpI, or antibodies to phosphatidylserine, phosphatidylethanolamine, phosphatidylglycerol, phosphatidylinositol, annexin-V, or phosphatidylcholine tend to resemble more closely patients with ACLAs than patients with isolated LA. Although all of these antiphospholipid antibody thrombosis syndromes may be seen in association with systemic lupus erythematosus (SLE), other connective tissue and autoimmune disorders, and other selected medical conditions such as lymphomas, the majority of individuals, about 90%, with any of the antiphospholipid thrombosis syndromes are otherwise healthy individuals, have no other underlying medical condition, and are classified as having *primary* rather than *secondary* antiphospholipid thrombosis syndrome (8). This distinction is of significance, as those with secondary antiphospholipid syndromes generally have heterogeneous antibodies that react with a variety of phospholipid moieties, including ACL, LA tests, or antibodies to β_2-GpI, phosphatidylserine, phosphatidylethanolamine, phosphatidylglycerol, phosphatidylinositol, annexin-V, or phosphatidylcholine, and render biologic false-positive tests for syphilis, whereas those with primary antiphospholipid thrombosis syndrome more commonly have homogeneous antibodies reacting with only one phospholipid moiety (8). Thus when evaluating published studies, one must carefully assess the population being studied for antiphospholipid antibodies. The findings and results of studies in patients with autoimmune disorders may not necessarily be extrapolated to studies or clinical and laboratory findings in patients with primary antiphospholipid thrombosis syndromes. These antiphospholipid thrombosis syndromes, including etiology, pathophysiology, clinical and laboratory diagnosis, and management principles, are herein discussed.

LUPUS ANTICOAGULANTS AND THROMBOSIS

In 1952, Conley and Hartmann (9) described a coagulation disorder in two patients with SLE; the patients exhibited anticoagulant activity by in vitro testing, which was manifested by a prolonged whole blood clotting time and prothrombin time (PT). It is now known that patients with SLE or other autoimmune diseases, an immunoglobulin may develop that has the ability to prolong phospholipid-dependent coagulation tests (10,11). About 10% of patients with SLE have an LA; however, the LA is commonly seen in other conditions as well, including malignancy, lymphoproliferative disorders, and viral infections, especially human immunodeficiency virus (HIV) infection (12–14). Most commonly, the LA develops in otherwise healthy individuals (primary LA–thrombosis syndrome). There also is an association with drug ingestion; commonly associated drugs include chlorpromazine, procainamide, quinidine, hydralazine, phenytoin (Dilantin), interferon, sulfoxidine and pyrimethamine (Fansidar), and cocaine (6,7,15–17). A common misconception is that patients with drug-induced LA, usually immunoglobulin M (IgM) idiotype, do not have thrombosis, but these patients also have an increased risk of thrombotic disease. The frequency of hemorrhage resulting from the LA is clearly less than 1%; however, it is important to recognize conditions that may predispose lupus patients with an LA to hemorrhage (18,19). Twenty-five percent of patients with SLE have concomitant prothrombin deficiency, and more than 40% may have thrombocytopenia; these accompanying defects are particularly noted in those with secondary LA–thrombosis syndromes (18,20).

Of greater clinical significance, patients with the LA are at increased risk for thromboembolic disease, most commonly DVT, PE, and thrombosis of other large vessels (21,22). Thromboembolism occurs in about 10% of patients with SLE; however, in patients with SLE and the LA, thromboembolism occurs in up to 50% of patients. In patients with a primary LA, the LA is estimated to account for about 6% to 8% of thrombosis in otherwise healthy individuals. There also have been associations with primary LA syndrome and recurrent miscarriage, neuropsychiatric disorders, renal vascular thrombosis, thrombosis of dermal vessels, and thrombocytopenia (17,20,23,24).

Primary LA–thrombosis syndrome is much more common than the secondary type and consists of patients with LA and thrombosis who have no other underlying disease; secondary LA–thrombosis syndrome consists of those patients with LA and thrombosis with an underlying disease, such as lupus or other autoimmune disorders, malignancy, infection, inflammation, or ingestion of drugs inducing the LA.

Patients with primary LA phospholipid syndrome primarily have venous thrombosis and PE. A wide variety of venous systems may become involved, including not only the extremities (most common presentation) but also mesenteric, renal, hepatic, portal, and superior and inferior vena cava (8,12). Although patients also may have arterial events, this is uncommon in primary LA–thrombosis syndrome, as opposed to primary ACLA–thrombosis syndrome, in which arterial events are almost as common as venous events. This is in contradistinction to patients with secondary LA–thrombosis syndrome, wherein patients, especially those with SLE and the LA, more commonly have arterial events than do those with primary LA–thrombosis syndrome. However, even in secondary LA–thrombosis syndrome, venous events are more common than arterial events. Arteries commonly involved include coronary, cerebral, carotid, aorta, mesenteric, renal, and those of the extremities (8,12,23,25–27).

Purified LA inhibits the Ca^{2+}-dependent binding of prothrombin and factor Xa to phospholipids, therefore inhibiting the activity of the phospholipid complex required for conversion of prothrombin to thrombin (11,18). Of interest, biologic false-positive tests for syphilis are seen in up to 40% of patients with SLE; the number increases to 90% in patients with SLE plus the LA (19,23,28). An abnormality often (theoretically) exists in the phospholipid-dependent coagulation reactions, including the PT, the activated partial thromboplastin time (aPTT), and the Russell's viper venom time (RVVT), as the LA is directed not against a specific factor, but against phospholipids. The inhibitor usually does not exert an increasing effect with prolonged incubation with normal plasma, and thus this simple screen can often be used to distinguish the lupus inhibitor from inhibitors that neutralize specific clotting factors. About 15% to 25% of LAs can, however, be time dependent, so this is not an absolute or definitive test. Incubation of the patients' plasma with normal plasma does not generally cause a sensitivity of the PTT to the inhibitor's effect, and one-stage assays for factors XII, XI, IX, and VII may yield low values when the standard dilutions of test plasma are used. Usually further dilution of the test plasma causes the measured level of these factors to approach the normal range; an exception occurs in rare patients with decreased concentration of prothrombin resulting from accelerated removal of prothrombin antigen–antibody complexes (29,30).

Multiple LA assays are currently in use (29). Sensitivity of the aPTT to the presence or absence of the LA is highly dependent on the reagents used. Many patients with thrombosis and the LA have normal aPTTs, even with the newer allegedly more "sensitive" reagents; thus the aPTT is *not* an appropriate screening test for LAs; when the presence of an LA is suspected, a more definitive test, preferably the dilute RVVT (dRVVT), should immediately be performed regardless of the PTT (6,7,31,32). The lupus inhibitor is identified by an ability to bind phospholipid and to inhibit phospholipid-dependent coagulant reactions. The assays are based on the use of limiting amounts of phospholipid, and therefore sensitized, in platelet-poor plasma. Initially, a PT was performed with dilute tissue thromboplastin and a reduced number of platelets in the mixture; however, IgM inhibitors were missed (19). A "modified" RVVT was developed in which the venom is diluted to give a "normal" time of 23 to 27 seconds, and the phospholipid is then diluted to a minimal level that continues to support this range. A prolongation of this system will not correct with a mixture of patient and normal plasma, and this system detects both IgG and IgM anticoagulants (33). This assay is known as the dRVVT and is the most sensitive of all assays purported to be useful in the screening or diagnosis of LAs (32). The kaolin clotting time (KCT) test has been modified to detect LAs. In this assay, platelet-poor plasma is mixed with varying proportions of test plasma and normal plasma. Kaolin is added, and the time required for clotting is determined (34). The KCT is then plotted against proportions of patients' plasma with normal plasma; an inhibitor is assumed to be present when a small portion of test plasma in comparison with normal plasma prolongs the assay system. A kaolin-activated aPTT, with rabbit brain phospholipid in a standard and fourfold increased "high" lipid concentration to normalize or "out-inhibit" the abnormal "standard" aPTT, also has been used in diagnosis of the lupus inhibitor (35). The best test at present is the dRVVT; if this test is prolonged, the confirmation of a lupus inhibitor, by noting correction of the prolonged dRVVT by adding phospholipid in some form (preferably void of platelet membrane material) is recommended, especially if the patient is receiving warfarin or heparin therapy. Both heparin and warfarin also are capable of prolonging the dRVVT. In our experience, the most sensitive and specific is the dRVVT available from American Diagnostics.

There is a correlation between elevated ACLAs and the LA in secondary antiphospholipid syndromes (those associated with other autoimmune diseases); however, the LA, ACLAs, and subgroups are separate entities, and most of the time ACLAs are found in the absence of the LA in the *primary* antiphospholipid thrombosis syndromes (18,36). The LA has a stronger association with binding phospholipids of a hexagonal composition such as phosphocholine, or after membrane damage by infection, interleukin-1 (IL-1), or other mechanisms leading to change from the lamellar to hexagonal form, whereas ACLAs usually have an affinity to lamellar phospholipids in a bilayer (lamellar) composition (11,37,38). IgG and IgM ACLAs are the most frequent idiotypes and can be detected by enzyme-linked immunosorbent assay (ELISA); IgA ACLAs occur slightly less frequently and also are detected by ELISA. Although the LA is associated with thrombosis, the mechanism(s) whereby thrombosis occurs remains unclear. It has been proposed that there might be an interaction with the vasculature, thereby altering prostaglandin release. There may be activation of platelets and changes in prostaglandin metabolism, or the antibodies block protein C, or the APC pathway, or alter phospholipid interactions with activated factor V (39). It also has been proposed that there may be hyperactivity of the fibrinolytic system and increased levels of plasminogen activation inhibitor (40). Despite many proposed mechanisms, there is no consensus on the precise mechanism(s) of action of LAs (6,7,41,42).

The clinical subclassification of types of thrombosis and LA and ACLA patients into groups may be important for choosing therapy (6,7,36). Patients can generally be divided into one of six clinical subgroups. Type I syndrome includes DVT of the upper and lower extremities; inferior vena cava; hepatic, portal, and renal veins; and PE. Type II syndrome includes patients with arterial thrombosis including the coronary arteries, peripheral (extremity) arteries, extracranial carotid arteries, and aorta. Type III syndrome includes patients with retinal or cerebral vascular thrombosis/ischemia, including those with TIAs. Several neurologic syndromes may be manifested including TIAs, migraine headaches, and optic neuritis (24). Type IV syndrome includes patients with combinations of the aforementioned types of thrombosis. Like ACLAs and other antiphospholipid subgroups, the LA has been associated with a RMS; this is type V. Abortion occurs frequently in the first, and less frequently in the second or third trimester. Placental vasculitis and vascular thrombosis may be apparent, and there may occasionally be an associated maternal thrombocytopenia (2,19,43). Type VI patients are those with LA with no apparent disease, including thrombosis.

Although patients with LA–thrombosis syndrome can be classified similar to those with ACL–thrombosis syndrome, most patients with *primary* LA–thrombosis syndrome will fit into type I. In secondary LA–thrombosis syndrome, however, more patients will belong in types II, III, and V than are seen in the primary syndrome.

The lupus inhibitor usually persists in patients with primary APL-TS, although it may sometimes disappear spontaneously. In the secondary LA–thrombosis APL syndrome, treatment of the underlying autoimmune disorder frequently results in reduction or disappearance of inhibitor activity. Corticosteroids may have a suppressive effect on the titer of the LA, and to a lesser degree on ACLAs, but they do not appear to decrease thrombotic risk. Thus there is no role for immunosuppressive therapy, including steroids, cyclophosphamide, or azathioprine, in patients with the primary LA–thrombosis syndrome. When steroids or other immunosuppressive therapy is warranted in the patient with an autoimmune disease and LA–thrombosis syndrome, the immunosuppression, although perhaps benefiting the underlying autoimmune disorder, will generally not alleviate propensity to thrombosis. Discovery of an LA, in the absence of underlying disease, and without evidence of thrombosis (type VI) does not necessarily require treatment, but current evidence suggests these individuals to have about a 40% chance of eventually having a thrombotic event over a 3-year follow-up period. Thus the decision to perform anticoagulation in an asymptomatic patient with the LA requires individualization and judgment, as no clear guidelines yet exist. However, patients with the LA or ACLAs and a history of thrombosis need to be taking long-term anticoagulant therapy. If they are untreated, there is a high incidence of thromboembolic recurrence (6,7,44,45). Patients with DVT or arterial thrombosis are generally best managed with long-term low-molecular-weight heparin (LMWH) therapy, as they are notoriously resistant to warfarin therapy (warfarin therapy eventually fails in about 50% to 65% of patients with APL-TS) (46,47). Over the past 24-month period, we have assessed 111 patients with thrombosis and APL syndrome (exclusive of recurrent miscarriage patients); of these, 59 patients were referred because of recurrent thrombosis on adequate doses of warfarin; on evaluation, they were found to have APLAs or were known APL-TS patients and gave a history of recurrence with adequate doses of warfarin. The failure rate with warfarin in this group was 59 (53%) of 111 patients. In contrast, in fewer than 2% of patients, fixed low-dose unfractionated porcine mucosal heparin will fail, and we have not yet seen a DVT failure with LMWH therapy (dalteparin) in patients with APL syndrome. After patients with DVT/PE are stable for a time with LMWH, consideration of changing to long-term clopidogrel may be entertained, as this agent has been effective in stable patients for whom LMWH has not failed. Patients with type II thrombosis (coronary artery, large peripheral arteries) are successfully treated with LMWH. Like those with type I, if the patient remains free of thrombotic events for a long period, clopidogrel may be successfully substituted, particularly if osteoporosis becomes a consideration. In patients with retinal or cerebral vascular thrombosis (type III), fixed-dose long-term LMWH plus clopidogrel for intracranial/cerebral vascular thrombosis is usually effective. If the patient remains symptom free for 6 to 12 months, consideration of stopping the LMWH and continuing with clopidogrel may be reasonable. Clopidogrel at 75 mg/day is usually effective for retinal vascular thrombosis, and if failure occurs, LMWH is added to the clopidogrel therapy. In those with mixtures of thrombotic sites (type IV), therapy is individualized, based on predominant sites and severity of thrombosis (6,7,43). The RMS (type V) is successfully treated, allowing term delivery, with initiation of low-dose ASA (81 mg/day) before conception and the addition of fixed low-dose unfractionated heparin (UFH) at 5,000 units every 12 hours, both used to term. With this regimen, our population of RMS patients with APL syndrome have experienced a 97% pregnancy success outcome (43,48). There is little or no role for prednisone in RMS because of the LA, if there is no underlying autoimmune disease.

ANTICARDIOLIPIN ANTIBODIES, "SUBGROUP" ANTIBODIES, AND THROMBOSIS

Interest in APLs began with discovery of the LA in about 10% of patients with SLE in 1952 (9), and shortly thereafter, it was recognized that presence of the LA was associated with thrombosis, instead of bleeding (49). It also was soon recognized that many patients without autoimmune disorders had LAs, and these APLAs have now been reported in many conditions including malignancy, immune thrombocytopenia purpura, leukemias, infections, in individuals ingesting chlorpromazine, phenytoin (Dilantin), sulfadoxine and pyrimethamine (Fansidar), hydralazine, quinidine, cocaine, interferon, or procainamide (secondary syndrome), and in many otherwise normal individuals (primary syndrome) (30,50–54). Because of a noted association between lupus, a biologic false-positive test for syphilis, and the presence of the LA, Harris et al. (55) in 1983 devised a new test for APLs using cardiolipin. This and subsequent modifications have now become known as the ACLA test; generally, IgG, IgA, and IgM ACL idiotypes are currently assessed (56). Shortly after development of the ACLA assay, it became apparent that these antibodies were not limited to the lupus patient population, but were found in patients without lupus as well. Of particular importance, these ACLAs are associated with (a) thrombosis and thromboembolus of both arterial and venous systems (8,41,57–59), (b) RMS (43,60,61), and (c) thrombocytopenia, in descending order of prevalence (62,63). More recently, it has become apparent that antibodies (all three idiotypes: IgG, IgA, and IgM) to β_2-GpI, phosphatidylserine, phosphatidylethanolamine, phosphatidylglycerol, phosphatidylinositol, annexin-V, or phosphatidylcholine are independent risk factors for thrombosis of all types (types I through V) (64). Although there is an association between the LA and ACLAs and an association between LAs and the aforementioned syndromes, it has become clear that LAs, ACLAs, and antibodies to β_2-GpI, phosphatidylserine, phosphatidylethanolamine, phosphatidylglycerol, phosphatidylinositol, phosphatidylcholine, or annexin-V are separate entities; most individuals with ACLAs do not have an LA, and most with the LA do not have ACLAs (65). However, many with subgroups have ACLAs, but 10% to 20% of patients demonstrate discordance (66), and subgroups are present in the absence of positive ELISA assays for ACLAs or LA. In our experience, discordance is noted in about the same percentages. In particular, in patients with type I, about 7% are discordant; in type II, 14% are discordant; in type III, 15% are discordant; and in type V, 22% are discordant (67). Thus when APL syndrome is suspected in a patient with thrombosis of any type and negative LA and negative ACL assays, the presence of isolated antibodies to β_2-GpI, phosphatidylserine, phosphatidylethanolamine, phosphatidylglycerol, phosphatidylinositol, annexin-V, or phosphatidylcholine should be suspected and tested for (64).

Regarding the primary APL-TS, the ACL-TS is at least fivefold more common than is the LA-TS (6,8). Other differences between LAs and ACLAs include not only (a) differing clinical presentations, but also (b) the noting that ACLs are usually, but not always, dependent on a cofactor, β_2-GpI (apolipoprotein H) in vitro, whereas in vitro LA activity appears independent of β_2-GpI, (c) ACLAs and LAs have different isoelectric points on chromatofocusing separation, (d) both appear to be directed against different combinations of phospholipid moieties and complexes, and (e) purified ACLAs do not generally prolong any of the phospholipid-dependent coagulation tests, such as the aPTT, dRVVT, PNP (platelet neutralization procedure), or KCT unless there is concomitant presence of an LA (68,69).

Initially it was assumed that only IgG ACLA was associated with thrombosis; however, it is now clear that IgA and IgM ACLAs also are associated with thrombosis (6,7). The presence of any one ACLA, a combination of two, or indeed, all three together may be associated with thrombosis and thromboembolus (70). Although different types of thrombosis occur, there also is no apparent association between the type of thrombotic event and the type or titer of ACLA present (6,7). The mechanism of action of ACLAs, or subgroups, in causing thrombosis is unknown, but several plausible theories have been proposed. ACLAs have an affinity for important phospholipids involved at many points in the hemostasis system; they are directed primarily against phosphatidylserine and phosphatidylinositol, but not phosphatidylcholine, another important phospholipid in hemostasis (71). The proposed mechanisms of action of ACLAs in interfering with hemostasis to induce thrombosis include (a) interference with endothelial release of prostacyclin (72); (b) interference with activation, via thrombomodulin, of protein C activation or interference with protein S activity as a cofactor for protein C (73); (c) interference with AT activity (74) (d) by interaction with platelet membrane phospholipids, leading to platelet activation (75), (e) by interference of prekallikrein activation to kallikrein (76), and (f) by interference with endothelial plasminogen activator release (77), or (g) by interference with the APC system (78). All these components of normal hemostasis are dependent on phospholipid, except possibly AT activity. These concepts are reviewed (6,8,41,42).

Anticardiolipins and Venous–Arterial Thrombosis

ACLAs are associated with many types of venous thrombotic problems including DVT of the upper and lower extremities, PE, intracranial veins, inferior and superior vena cava, hepatic vein (Budd–Chiari syndrome) (6,7,79), portal vein, renal vein, and retinal veins (80–82). Arterial thrombotic sites associated with ACLAs have included the coronary arteries, carotid arteries, cerebral arteries, retinal arteries, subclavian and/or axillary artery (aortic arch syndrome) (83), brachial arteries, mesenteric arteries (84), peripheral (extremity) arteries, and both proximal and distal aorta (85–87).

Anticardiolipins and Cardiac Disease

In an early study, it was found that 33% of coronary artery bypass graft (CABG) patients with late graft occlusion (as determined by coronary angiography 12 months after CABG surgery) had preoperative ACLA levels more than 2 standard deviations above control values, strongly suggesting an association between graft occlusion and APLAs. In 80% of patients, the ACLA levels increased to levels greater than the preoperative levels at some time. The observed increase in ACLA levels was greater in patients having had an acute myocardial infarction than in those who had not (88,89). Another study revealed more than 20% of young (younger than 45 years) survivors of acute myocardial infarction to have ACLAs; in those surviving, 61% having these antibodies experienced a later thromboembolic event (90). No association was found between the presence of ACLAs and antinuclear antibody or other clinical features that would have suggested the presence of SLE. ACLAs are suggested as an indicator of increased risk for thrombotic events after myocardial infarction and an indication for prophylactic anticoagulation or antiplatelet therapy (90). Despite continuous prophylactic treatment with ASA and warfarin, acute myocardial infarction has been documented in a patient with previously documented normal coronary arteries, treated successfully with tissue type plasminogen activator (t-PA) (91). In analyzing the relative frequency of acute myocardial infarction in patients with ACLAs, a study published in 1989 noted myocardial infarction in only five of 70 patients (significantly fewer than those experiencing cerebral arterial thromboses) (92). Another study revealed a very high percentage of young individuals (those younger 50 years) who have acute myocardial infarction, or who experience restenosis after percutaneous transluminal coronary angioplasty (PTCA) or CABG have ACLAs (93). Thus ACLAs appear to play a significant and probable major role in premature/precocious coronary artery disease; this may approach almost 70% of young patients with coronary artery disease (27,93).

ACLAs also are associated with cardiac valvular abnormalities. Cardiac disease in patients with SLE has been associated with valvular vegetations, regurgitation, and stenosis. Almost 8% to 9% of patients with SLE and valvular disease have been found to have APLAs, compared with only 44% of patients without valvular involvement. Although only 18% of all patients with lupus have valvular disease, cardiac valvular abnormalities are found in 36% of patients with the primary APL syndrome. The valvular abnormalities of the primary APL syndrome are characterized by significant, irregular thickening of the mitral and aortic valves, valvular regurgitation (but not stenosis), the potential for severe hemodynamic compromise, and surprisingly, an absence of valvular thrombi (94). Patients with concomitant SLE and APLAs have been found to have aortic and mitral valvulitis, including typical Libman–Sacks verrucous endocarditis (95,96). Additionally, in patients with SLE, the presence of APLAs is associated with isolated left ventricular dysfunction (97). An isolated instance has been reported of an intracardiac mass in the right ventricle, presumably resulting from the combined effects of abnormal intracardiac flow resulting from anomalous muscle bundles combined with enhanced thrombogenesis associated with APLAs. (98) In view of the high incidence of valvular abnormalities in patients with APLAs and arterial thromboembolism, Doppler echocardiography should routinely be considered (99).

Anticardiolipins and Cutaneous Manifestations

ACLAs are associated with livido reticularis, an unusual manifestation of cutaneous vascular stasis characterized by a distinctive pattern of cyanosis (57,100,101). This cutaneous finding has been associated with recurrent arterial and venous thromboses, valvular abnormalities, and cerebrovascular thromboses with concomitant essential hypertension (Sneddon syndrome) (57). Other cutaneous manifestations include a syndrome of recurrent DVT, necrotizing purpura, and stasis ulcers of the ankles (57,100,101). Skin lesions of Degos disease (a rare multisystem vasculopathy), characterized pathologically by cutaneous collagen necrosis, atrophy of the epidermis with an absence of inflammatory cells, have been linked to the other consequences of the disease such as cerebral and bowel infarction and ACLAs or an LA (102). Vascular thromboses may be manifest as ischemia or necrosis of entire extremities, as demonstrated in association with disseminated intravascular coagulation (DIC) (103) with resultant cutaneous necrosis or more patchy, widespread, demarcated areas of cutaneous necrosis, manifest by areas of painful purpura and necrosis with underlying dermal necrosis (104). Other common cutaneous manifestations include livido vasculitis/reticularis, nonfading acral microlivido, peripheral gangrene, necrotizing purpura, hemorrhage (ecchymosis and hematoma formation) (104), and crusted ulcers about the nail beds (105). See reference 101 for an excellent review of this topic.

Anticardiolipins and Neurologic Syndromes

The neurologic syndromes associated with ACLAs include TIAs, small stroke syndrome, arterial and venous retinal occlusive disease, cerebral arterial and venous thrombosis, migraine headaches, Degos disease, Sneddon syndrome, (106) Guillain–Barré syndrome (107), chorea, seizures, and optic neuritis (102,108,109). The central nervous system manifestations of SLE are commonly, but not always, associated with positive APLAs (110,111). Whereas it is clear that lupus patients with APLAs may experience cerebrovascular thromboses, cerebral ischemia, and infarction, these events occur more commonly in patients with the *primary* ACL-TS and absence of an underlying autoimmune disease. Multiple cerebral infarctions in patients with APLAs may result in dementia (112).

The primary phospholipid syndrome is often present in patients with a constellation of concomitant arterial occlusions, strokes, TIAs leading to multiple-infarct dementia, DVT associated with PE and resultant pulmonary hypertension, RMS, thrombocytopenia, positive Coomb test, and chorea (24,113). The primary distinction between patients with primary phospholipid syndrome and Sneddon syndrome is the involvement of large vessels in the former and exclusively medium-sized arteries in the latter (106,114,115). Patients with APLAs are more likely to experience cerebral ischemic or thrombotic events when also having primary hypertension or coronary disease, respectively (116). ACLAs and recurrent stroke also have been associated with thymoma (117). Recent studies have found that APLAs, including subgroups, particularly antiphosphatidylserine, are important etiologic factors. This is of major importance with respect to appropriate antithrombotic therapy, and these patients cannot be treated with simple antiplatelet therapy or warfarin therapy with success, as they require LMWH or UFH with or without an antiplatelet agent for adequate protection against recurrence. One recent study found that 46% of young individuals (age 50 or younger) with cerebral ischemic events had APLAs (118); another found 44% of young individuals (age 51 or younger) to have APLAs (119), but another study found only 18% of patients younger than 44 years to harbor APLAs (120). Subgroups only of APLAs have been noted in up to 23% of young patients with cerebral thrombotic events; thus it is of extreme importance to consider these (119). APLAs also are associated with cerebral venous events (121). Another recent study noted 65% of patients with cerebrovascular thrombosis younger than 60 years to have APLAs, and in the same study, 28% of patients with only TIAs had APLAs (122). Studies also have noted that those with APLAs tend to have the cerebrovascular occlusive/ischemic event about a decade earlier than those having cerebrovascular thrombotic or ischemic events in the absence of APLAs (123). Thus it is clear that APLAs are important in the etiology of cerebrovascular ischemic events (24,124). The primary importance of these findings is in making an appropriate diagnosis so that effective therapy may be instituted (LMWH or UFH) to afford effectual secondary prevention. The complicated topic of neurologic manifestations in APL-TSs has recently been reviewed (24,124).

Anticardiolipins and Autoimmune Collagen Disease

Although much of the initial research and many of the first descriptions of APLAs resulted from investigation of the LA in populations with SLE, it is now well established that APLAs occur in patients without SLE much more frequently than in those with lupus or other autoimmune disorders. In patients with lupus, the presence of livido reticularis may represent an important cutaneous marker for the presence, or the later development, of APLAs (100). APLAs may occur with increased frequency in individuals with other autoimmune disorders and have been reported in patients with mixed connective tissue disease, rheumatoid arthritis (104), Sjögren syndrome (96), Behçet syndrome (possible role in the pathogenesis of the multisystem manifestations of the syndrome) (125), and autoimmune thrombocytopenic purpura (62). Most patients with ACLA-TS, however, have a *primary* syndrome with no underlying autoimmune disorder. Fewer than 10% of patients with thrombosis and APLAs have, or will ever have, an autoimmune disease such as SLE, rheumatoid arthritis, mixed connective tissue disease, or a related syndrome. The clinical manifestations can be varied and substantial (23,115).

Anticardiolipins and Obstetric Syndromes

ACLAs are associated with a high incidence of RMS; the characteristics of this syndrome are (a) frequent abortion in the first trimester due to placental thrombosis/vasculitis; (b) recurrent fetal loss in the second and third trimesters, also due to placental thrombosis/vasculitis; and (c) maternal thrombocytopenia, in descending order of prevalence. This is especially likely in the presence of moderate or high IgG ACL levels (126). This syndrome has been successfully treated to normal term by institution of ASA, low-dose heparin, or plasma exchange (61,127–129). Women with ACLAs have about a 50% to 75% chance of fetal loss, and successful anticoagulant therapy can increase the chances of normal term delivery to about 97% (43,49).

Optimal therapy for the RMS has not yet been defined, but we have noted a 97% normal delivery outcome in 123 patients with RMS treated with preconception ASA at 81 mg/day, with the immediate postconception addition of UFH at 5,000 units q 12 hours, and both agents used to term (49). A variety of heparin doses have been used with significant success in carrying patients to term, and most of these have been in combination with ASA therapy. It is clear that in the primary APL syndrome (absence of an underlying autoimmune disorder such as SLE), the use of corticosteroids or other immunosuppressive therapy is not warranted and only enhances side effects. However, immunosuppressive therapy may be useful in those with ACL syndrome and lupus. A variety of vigorous antibody-removing/eradicating modes of therapy have been attempted with varying degrees of success, including plasmapheresis, plasma exchange, immunoadsorption column treatment, and intravenous immunoglobulin (IVIG). Based on available reports and our own experience, the use of low-dose ASA (about 81 mg/day) in combination with low-dose porcine mucosal heparin (5,000 units subcutaneously q 12 hours) appears now to be consistently the most effective therapy for term delivery. Our approach in treating the RMS is to start a patient on low-dose ASA (81 mg/day) at the time a diagnosis of RMS is made: the demonstration of ACLA, LA, or APL subgroups (seen in 22% of our patients with RMS and APLAs) and a history of recurrent abortion (130). Subgroup analysis, including anti–annexin-V antibodies, is particularly important in RMS (130). As soon as pregnancy is achieved, fixed low-dose porcine mucosal heparin (5,000 units q 12 hours) is added to the ASA and used to term. The low-dose heparin need not be stopped during delivery, as it is extremely unlikely to be associated with significant hemorrhage and affords peripartum and postpartum protection against thrombosis and thromboembolic disease. Thus far our success rate using this regimen has been 97% (43,49). LMWH also may be used, but in view of reported cases of perispinal/epidural bleeding with epidural anesthetics reported with enoxaparin, APLA patients receiving LMWH during pregnancy should be changed to UFH during the last trimester.

The incidence of APLAs in RMS has been studied by a number of groups. Most studies, however, have not used control pregnant populations. Lin (131) studied a population of 245 women with RMS and found 13.5% to have ACLAs. Parazzini et al. (132) studied 220 patients with two or more spontaneous abortions and found 19% to have ACLAs. Grandone et al. (133) assessed 32 patients with RMS and found 28% to have ACLAs, and Birdsall et al. (134) studied 81 patients with RMS, finding 41% to harbor ACLAs. Maclean et al. (135) assessed 243 patients with RMS (two or more spontaneous abortions) and found 17% to have ACLAs, 7% to have LAs, and 2% to have both. Howard et al. (136) assessed 29 patients without lupus but with RMS and found 48% to have LAs. Taylor et al. (137), in a study of 189 women with unexplained miscarriage, found LAs in 7% and ACLAs in 15%. The only two studies assessing matched controls were those of Parke et al. (138), who found 7% of pregnant women without RMS and 16% of those with RMS to have APLAs, and Parazzini et al. (132), who found an incidence of 3% ACLAs in control women. Thus it appears that a small population of normal pregnant females without symptoms of RMS also will have APLAs. This, of course, raises the question of treatment in the pregnant woman with APLAs but no history of spontaneous miscarriage; no data provide adequate direction for this dilemma.

ACLAs also are associated with a peculiar postpartum syndrome of spiking fevers, pleuritic chest pain, dyspnea and pleural effusion, patchy pulmonary infiltrates, cardiomyopathy, and ventricular arrhythmias. This syndrome characteristically occurs 2 to 10 days postpartum (139). Because the majority of patients with postpartum syndrome recover spontaneously, most require no therapy other than symptomatic treatment. It is unclear whether any type of antithrombotic therapy is warranted in this population, because recovery almost always occurs spontaneously.

Miscellaneous Disorders and Anticardiolipin Thrombosis Syndrome

ACLAs have recently been reported in patients with HIV infection, with or without immune thrombocytopenic purpura (140). Particularly elevated are IgG isotypes; however, there is no correlation between APLA level and disease progression or the incidence of thrombosis, despite a correlation with the titer and presence of thrombocytopenia (140–143). Elevations of one or more of the ACL isotypes has been observed after a number of acute infections, including ornithosis, *Mycoplasma* infection, adenovirus infection, rubella, varicella, mumps, malaria, and Lyme disease (144). Abnormalities of the aPTT in patients with hepatic cirrhosis have recently been attributed to the presence of APLAs (145). Drugs associated with the development of ACLAs include phenytoin (146), quinidine, sulfadoxine and pyrimethamine (Fansidar), hydralazine, procainamide, cocaine, interferon, and phenothiazines (with a predisposition to thrombosis, which does occur in drug-associated APL syndrome) (6,7,147). The ACL-TS can be divided into those that are primary and those that are secondary. Primary ACL-TS is much more common and consists of patients with ACLA and thrombosis who have no other underlying disease; secondary ACL-TS consists of those patients with ACLA and thrombosis with an underlying disease, such as lupus or other autoimmune disorder, malignancy, infection, inflammation, or ingestion of drugs inducing an ACLA.

ANTIPHOSPHOLIPID THROMBOSIS SYNDROMES

Classification of Antiphospholipid Syndromes

The finding of ACLAs, subgroups of APLAs, or LAs in association with thrombosis is referred to as the APL-TS. Patients with LA do not tend to have thromboses that are as predictable as those with ACLA or the subgroups of antibodies to β_2-GpI, phosphatidylserine, phosphatidylethanolamine, phosphatidylglycerol, phosphatidylinositol, phosphatidylcholine, or annexin-V; however, management principles, as far as is currently known, apply equally to all (64).

The APL-TS, associated with ACL or subgroup antibodies, can be divided into one of *six* subgroups: *type I* syndrome comprises patients with DVT and PE, *type II* syndrome comprises patients with coronary artery or peripheral arterial (including aorta and carotid artery) thrombosis, *type III* syndrome comprises patients with retinal or cerebrovascular (intracranial) thrombosis, and *type IV* patients are those with admixtures of the first three types. Type IV patients are uncommon, with most patients fitting into one of the first three types. *Type V* patients are those with RMS, and *type VI* patients are those with APL syndromes without any (as yet) clinical expression, including thrombosis. There is little overlap (about 10% or less) between these subtypes, and patients usually conveniently fit into only one of these clinical types. The types of APL-TS associated with ACLAs are summarized in Table 14.2 (3,5,67). Although there appears to be no correlation with the type, or titer, of ACLA and type of syndrome (I through VI), the subclassification of thrombosis and ACLA patients into these groups is important from the therapy standpoint (3,5,67). Type I patients are best managed by use of long-term fixed-dose LMWH or fixed-dose subcutaneous UFH therapy. If the patient remains thrombus free for 6 to 12 months or if osteoporosis becomes a consideration, long-term clopidogrel may eventually be substituted for the heparin. Type II patients also are best managed by long-term fixed-dose LMWH (about 5,000 units/24 hours) or fixed-dose subcutaneous UFH therapy (usually 5,000 units every 12 hours), and after long-term stability, clopidogrel may be an alternative. Type III patients, those with cerebrovascular disease or retinal vascular disease, should be treated with fixed-dose long-term LMWH plus clopidogrel for intracranial/cerebral vessel thrombosis/TIA; long-term stability can usually be achieved by stopping the heparin/LMWH and continuing clopidogrel. Clopidogrel (at 75 mg/day) is usually effective for retinal vascular thrombosis, and if failure occurs, LMWH is added to the clopidogrel therapy. Therapy for type IV depends on types and sites of thrombosis present (3,5,67). Patients with type V, RMS, are best treated with preconception initiation of low-dose ASA (81 mg/day) as soon as the diagnosis is made and then started on fixed low-dose porcine mucosal heparin (5,000 units, subcutaneously every 12 hours) immediately after conception, with both drugs being used to term delivery. Patients with type V syndrome are usually encouraged to stop the heparin after delivery (depending on the individual clinical situation), but to continue on long-term low-dose ASA indefinitely. The decision to continue ASA after delivery in these patients is empiric, but might ward off other minor thrombotic manifestations of APL syndrome. No guidelines demonstrate how to treat these patients after delivery, as most (fewer than 10%) will not develop a non-placental thrombosis.

Obviously, patients with thrombosis and ACLAs require long-term antithrombotic therapy, and treatment should be stopped only if the ACLA is persistently absent for at least 6 months before considering cessation of antithrombotic therapy (3,5,67). After persistent absence of the APLA for at least 6 months, we usually discuss the risks and benefits of continuing antithrombotic therapy and encourage patients to take one low-dose ASA (81 mg/day) or long-term clopidogrel [depending on the seriousness of the initial thrombotic event(s)], in hopes the antibody and thrombosis will not return. Obviously, patients with APL syndrome who are going to be taking long-term fixed low-dose UFH or LMWH therapy should have initial bone-density studies and should be cautioned about heparin-induced thrombocytopenia, mild alopecia, mild allergic reactions, osteoporosis, benign transaminasemia (seen in about 5% treated with UFH and in about 10% treated with LMWH), and the development of benign eosinophilia (148,149). Patients should be monitored with weekly heparin levels (anti-Xa method) and complete blood count (CBC)/platelet counts for the first month of therapy and monthly thereafter; this also applies to patients with type V syndrome. Table 14.3 outlines suggested antithrombotic therapy regimens, based on the type of ACL-TS. Because warfarin therapy fails for most patients with thrombosis and APLAs, the clinician should always suspect and search for APLAs when evaluating a patient for warfarin failure.

TABLE 14.2. SYNDROMES OF THROMBOSIS ASSOCIATED WITH ANTIPHOSPHOLIPID ANTIBODIES

Type I syndrome
Deep venous thrombosis with or without pulmonary embolus
Type II syndrome
Coronary artery thrombosis
Peripheral artery thrombosis
Aortic thrombosis
Carotid artery thrombosis
Type III syndrome
Retinal artery thrombosis
Retinal vein thrombosis
Cerebrovascular thrombosis
Transient cerebral ischemic attacks
Type IV syndrome
Mixtures of types I, II, and III
Type IV patients are rare
Type V (fetal wastage) syndrome
Placental vascular thrombosis
Fetal wastage common in first trimester
Fetal wastage can occur in second and third trimester
Maternal thrombocytopenia (uncommon)
Type VI syndrome
Antiphospholipid antibody
No apparent clinical manifestations

TABLE 14.3. RECOMMENDED ANTITHROMBOTIC REGIMEN FOR SYNDROMES OF THROMBOSIS ASSOCIATED WITH ANTIPHOSPHOLIPID ANTIBODIES

Type I syndrome
Short-term treatment with heparin/LMW heparin followed by long-term[a] self-administration of subcutaneous porcine heparin/LMW heparin
Clopidogrel long-term if stable
Type II syndrome
Short-term treatment with heparin/LMW heparin followed by long-term[a] self-administration of subcutaneous porcine heparin/LMW heparin
Clopidogrel long-term if stable
Type III syndrome
Cerebrovascular
Long-term clopidogrel plus long-term[a] self-administration of subcutaneous porcine heparin/LMW heparin
Retinal
Clopidogrel; if failure, add long-term[a] self-administration of subcutaneous porcine heparin/LMW heparin
Type IV syndrome
Therapy is dependent on type(s) and site(s) of thrombosis, as per above recommendations
Type V (fetal wastage) syndrome
Low-dose ASA (81 mg/day) before conception and add fixed low-dose porcine heparin at 5,000 Units every 12 h, immediately after conception
Type VI syndrome
No clear indications for antithrombotic therapy

ASA, acetylsalicylic acid.
[a]Antithrombotic therapy should not be stopped unless the anticardiolipin antibody has been absent for the preceding 4 to 6 months.

Clinical Presentations

It is becoming increasingly clear with increased experience in using the ACL assay in clinical practice, primary APL syndromes are much more common than suspected. Diagnostic evaluation of the patient to determine the etiology of a wide variety of thrombotic problems must now include assays for ACLAs, LAs, and when indicated, subgroups. Although it is appropriate to suspect APLAs in virtually any clinical problem complicated by thrombosis, certain presentations are stronger indicators than others.

In patients with type I disease, a strong index of suspicion is appropriate, particularly in individuals with DVT unaccompanied by another potential risk factor, such as exogenous estrogen administration, surgery, prolonged immobility, malignancy, or another hypercoagulable state. Likewise, patients may have recurrent DVT with or without a significant clinical risk factor. As is frequently observed in clinical practice, patients may be referred for evaluation only after a second episode of thrombosis. The initial thrombotic event may have appeared to result from a recognizable predisposing problem, only later proven to be present concomitant with ACLAs. Although the severity or location (iliofemoral, popliteal calf vein, or other sites) of thrombosis or the presence of PE does not correlate with the presence of ACLAs, recurrent thromboembolic events or multiple sites of thrombosis should strongly suggest an ACLA. Another very common presentation is a patient referred because of failure (rethrombosis) while receiving warfarin therapy. Failure with apparently adequate doses of warfarin should immediately alert the physician to consider strongly the APL-TS.

Patients with type II disease frequently have catastrophic illness. A history of myocardial infarction at a young age, recurrent myocardial infarction, early graft occlusion after CABG surgery, and early reocclusion after PTCA is typical. Aorta, subclavian, mesenteric, femoral, or other large vessel thrombosis may be seen with complete occlusion and acute symptoms of ischemia and threatened limb loss. Emergency diagnosis and appropriate therapy may decrease unnecessary morbidity and may be life saving.

Type III patients may be referred for a variety of problems. Acute loss or distortion of vision may lead to ophthalmologic confirmation of retinal arterial or venous thrombosis. Focal neurologic symptoms may suggest the presence of cerebrovascular thrombosis, resulting in symptoms of stroke or TIA. Alternatively, multiple-infarct dementia may occur more gradually, without clearly defined acute ischemic events. Early diagnosis is critical in type III patients, because failure to treat may result in irreversible cerebral or retinal injury.

Type IV patients, having a mixture of the aforementioned types, are extremely rare and compose only about 1% of patients with ACL-TS. A strong index of suspicion is required for the diagnosis, and therapy must be individualized depending on the particular combination of thromboses.

Type V patients are usually those with one or more spontaneous miscarriages and are most often referred by the obstetrician or high-risk reproductive experts. Most women relate a history of spontaneous miscarriage in the first trimester (most commonly weeks 6 to 12), but some also spontaneously miscarry in the second and third trimester.

Drugs associated with APL-TS are listed in Table 14.4.

TABLE 14.4. DRUGS ASSOCIATED WITH THE ANTIPHOSPHOLIPID THROMBOSIS SYNDROME

Phenytoin
Sulfadoxine and pyrimethamine (Fansidar)
Quinidine
Quinine
Hydralazine
Procainamide
Phenothiazines
Interferon α
Cocaine

Most are immunoglobulin M and are associated with thrombosis.

Prevalence of the Antiphospholipid Thrombosis Syndrome

Unfortunately, very little information is available on prevalence of APLAs, especially in asymptomatic individuals. Additionally, nothing is known about the potential propensity to develop thrombosis or other clinical manifestations when seemingly health individuals have these antibodies. Two recent studies have addressed this issue. The first was the Montpellier Antiphospholipid (MAP) study (150), wherein 1,014 patients (488 male and 526 female subjects) admitted to a general internal medicine department for a variety of reasons were assessed for IgG, IgA, and IgM ACLAs. LA assays were not performed. Of the patients tested, 72 (7.1%) were positive for at least one idiotype. Of these 72 patients, 20 (28%) were determined to have clinical manifestations of the APL-TS. Fifty-two patients, when questioned, had not yet demonstrated any manifestations of APL-TS, suggesting a false-positive incidence of 5.1%. However, long-term follow-up of the thus far asymptomatic patients has not occurred, and a follow-up report of the MAP study will be awaited with interest. In another recent study (151), 552 healthy blood donors were screened for study; IgG and IgM idiotypes and LA were assessed. It was found that 28 (6.5%) donors of the population had IgG, 38 (9.4%) donors of the population had IgM ACLAs, and five donors had both idiotypes. No donor was positive for LA. The donors were followed up for 12 months; during the follow-up time, no ACLA-positive patient had a thrombotic event. However, nine ACLA-positive donors had a family history of thrombosis, and three of the ACLA-positive donors had a history of unexplained miscarriage (151). In a recent survey of 100 consecutive patients with DVT or PE, 24% of patients were found to have ACLAs (46). It is suggested that ACLAs are common in patients with unexplained DVT or PE, and certainly any patient with unexplained DVT or PE should be evaluated for presence of APLAs.

Laboratory Diagnosis of Antiphospholipid Syndromes

Detection of Anticardiolipin Antibodies

The detection of ACLAs is straightforward, and there is general agreement that solid-phase ELISA is the method of choice (152–154). In the past, only IgG and IgA idiotypes have been assayed; however, with current recognition that IgM idiotypes, whether primary or secondary (especially drug-induced), also are associated with thrombosis, most laboratories are, or should be, assaying all three idiotypes. The idiotype distribution of ACLAs in patients with thrombosis is depicted in Table 14.5. Thus the appropriate assay for detecting ACLs is solid-phase ELISA, measuring all three (IgG, IgA, and IgM) idiotypes (28,31,155).

TABLE 14.5. IDIOTYPE DISTRIBUTION IN PATIENTS WITH THROMBOSIS AND ANTICARDIOLIPIN ANTIBODIES

36% have isolated IgG
17% have isolated IgM
14% have isolated IgA
33% have various mixtures

Ig, immunoglobulin.

Detection of Lupus Anticoagulants

In the presence of the LA, an abnormality exists in the phospholipid-dependent coagulation reactions including the PT, the aPTT, and the RVVT (7,11). The LA is directed not against a specific factor, but to phospholipids. The inhibitor does not exert an increasing effect with prolonged incubation with normal plasma, and thus this simple screen can be used to distinguish the lupus inhibitor from inhibitors that neutralize specific clotting factors. Incubation of the patient's plasma with normal plasma does not cause a sensitivity of the PTT to the inhibitor's effect, and one-stage assays for factors XII, XI, IX, and VII may yield low values when the standard dilutions of test plasma are used (11). Usually further dilution of the test plasma causes the measured level of these factors to approach the normal range; the exception occurs in rare patients with a decreased concentration of prothrombin, resulting from accelerated removal of prothrombin antigen–antibody complexes, sometimes seen in patients with SLE.

Multiple LA assays are currently in use. Sensitivity of the aPTT to the presence or absence of the LA is highly dependent on the reagents used. Many patients with thrombosis and the LA have normal aPTTs, even with the newer allegedly more "sensitive" reagents; thus the aPTT is *not* a reliable screening test for LAs and should not be used for this purpose (7,11,31,32,156–158). With suspicion of the presence of an LA, a more definitive test, preferably the dRVVT, should immediately be performed regardless of the aPTT. The lupus inhibitor is identified by the ability to bind phospholipid and inhibit phospholipid-dependent coagulant reactions. The assays available are based on the use of limiting amounts of phospholipid and therefore sensitized in platelet-poor plasma. Initially, a PT was performed with dilute tissue thromboplastin and a reduced number of platelets in the mixture; however, IgM inhibitors were missed. Subsequently, a "modified" RVVT was developed in which the venom is diluted to give a "normal" time of 23 to 27 seconds, and the phospholipid is then diluted to a minimal level that continues to support this range. A prolongation of this system will not correct with a mixture of patient and normal plasma; this system detects both IgG and IgM LAs (33). This assay is generally known as the dRVVT and appears the most sensitive of all assays for the LA (159). The KCT test also has been modified to assay for the LA inhibitor. In the KCT, platelet-poor plasma is mixed with varying proportions of test plasma and normal plasma. Kaolin is added, and time required for clotting is determined (11). The KCT is then plotted against proportions of patients' plasma with normal plasma; an inhibitor is assumed to be present when a small portion of test serum, in comparison with normal serum, prolongs the assay. A kaolin-activated PTT, with rabbit brain phospholipid in a standard and fourfold increased "high" lipid concentration to normalize or "out-inhibit" the abnormal "standard" aPTT, also has been used in diagnosis of the lupus inhibitor (11). This is known as the rabbit brain neutralization procedure, and although specific (because of rabbit brain neutralization), lacks sensitivity comparable to that of the dRVVT. The best test to detect the LA at present is the dRVVT; if this test is prolonged, the confirmation of a lupus inhibitor, by noting correction of the prolonged dRVVT by adding phospholipid in some form (unfortunately often platelet membrane derived) is required, especially if the patient is receiving warfarin or heparin therapy. Both heparin and warfarin also are capable of prolonging the dRVVT. Confirmation of an LA in these assays is by phospholipid neutralization (shortening) of the prolonged test (7,11,159). As a practical matter, most clinicians and laboratories are asked to evaluate patients for the LA after they have been given anticoagulant therapy. Both heparin and warfarin prolong most of these tests, including the most sensitive test, the dRVVT. If the patient is taking warfarin and the dRVVT is prolonged and then neutralized by appropriate phospholipid, an LA is confirmed (7,11). However, if the patient is taking heparin and the dRVVT is prolonged, the neutralization by platelet-derived phospholipid is not confirmatory, as large amounts of platelet-derived platelet factor 4 may inhibit the heparin effect to correct the test. For example, a commercially available platelet extract for the platelet neutralization procedure was found to contain about 100 IU per milliliter of platelet factor 4, and normal male freeze-thaw platelet extract, commonly prepared for "platelet or phospholipid neutralization procedures" in the clinical laboratory, contains about 95 IU per milliliter of platelet factor 4, enough to neutralize heparin and shorten a prolonged clotting test and render a false-positive result in the dRVVT or platelet neutralization procedure for an LA (7,11,160). As a practical matter, therefore, use of the dRVVT offers the most sensitive assay for detection of an LA. Neutralization of this test by a non–platelet-derived phospholipid, in particular cephalin (Bell–Alton extract) (161), which contains no platelet factor 4, makes this test the most specific as well.

Because of marked heterogeneity of APLAs, especially in the secondary APL syndromes, there is a correlation between elevated ACLAs and the LA in secondary APL-TSs. However, the LA and ACLAs are two separate entities, and most of the time, one occurs without the other being present, especially in the primary APL-TSs (6). The LA has a stronger association with binding phospholipids of a hexagonal composition such as phosphatidylcholine, or after membrane damage by infection, IL-1, or other mechanisms leading to change from the lamellar to hexagonal form, whereas ACLAs have an affinity to lamellar phospholipids in a bilayer (lamellar) composition (162).

Detection of "Subtypes"' of Antiphospholipid Antibodies

When suspecting thrombosis or RMS patients of having APLAs and noting negative assays for ACLAs or LAs, the clinician should suspect discordant subgroups and order assays for anti–β_2-GpI, and antibodies to phosphatidylserine, phosphatidylethanolamine, phosphatidylglycerol, phosphatidylinositol, annexin-V, and phosphatidylcholine. These are all available by enzyme immunoassay (EIA). It must be remembered that there is significant discordance between these subgroups and LAs or the three idiotypes of ACLAs; thus they must be recalled and tested for in the appropriate clinical situations discussed previously (163–168).

As mentioned earlier, discordance will be seen in a significant number of patients. In particular, many patients will have subgroups of APLA (β_2-GpI, antiphosphatidylserine, antiphosphatidylcholine, antiphosphatidylglycerol, antiphosphatidylinositol, and antiphosphatidylethanolamine in the absence of ACLAs (IgG, IgA, or IgM) or LA. Specifically, this will be seen in 7% of patients with APL-TS and DVT/PE (type I), 15% of those with coronary artery or peripheral arterial thrombosis (type II), 15% to 24% of those with cerebrovascular or retinal vascular thrombosis (type III), and in 22% of those with RMS (type V). All APLAs of importance, to date, are depicted in Table 14.6. The tests at the top are ordered first, and those at the bottom ordered if clinical suspicion of a subgroup is present. Figure 14.1 depicts an approach to the laboratory diagnosis of APL-TS.

TABLE 14.6. LABORATORY DIAGNOSIS OF ANTIPHOSPHOLIPID SYNDROMES

Suspicion of antiphospholipid syndrome (unexplained thrombosis, TIA, SSS; CAD, fetal loss, etc.)
Primary evaluation
Anticardiolipin antibodies (IgG, IgA, IgM)
Lupus anticoagulant (dRVVT)
Hexagonal phospholipid neutralization
β_2-glycoprotein-I (IgG, IgA, IgM)
Secondary evaluation
Antiphosphatidylserine (IgG, IgA, IgM)
Antiphosphatidylinositol (IgG, IgA, IgM)
Antiphosphatidylcholine (IgG, IgA, IgM)
Antiphosphatidylethanolamine (IgG, IgA, IgM)
Antiphosphatidylglycerol (IgG, IgA, IgM)
Antiannexin-V antibody

Ig, immunoglobulin; TIA, transient ischemic attack; SSS, small stroke syndrome; CAD, coronary artery disease; dRVVT, dilute Russell viper venom time.

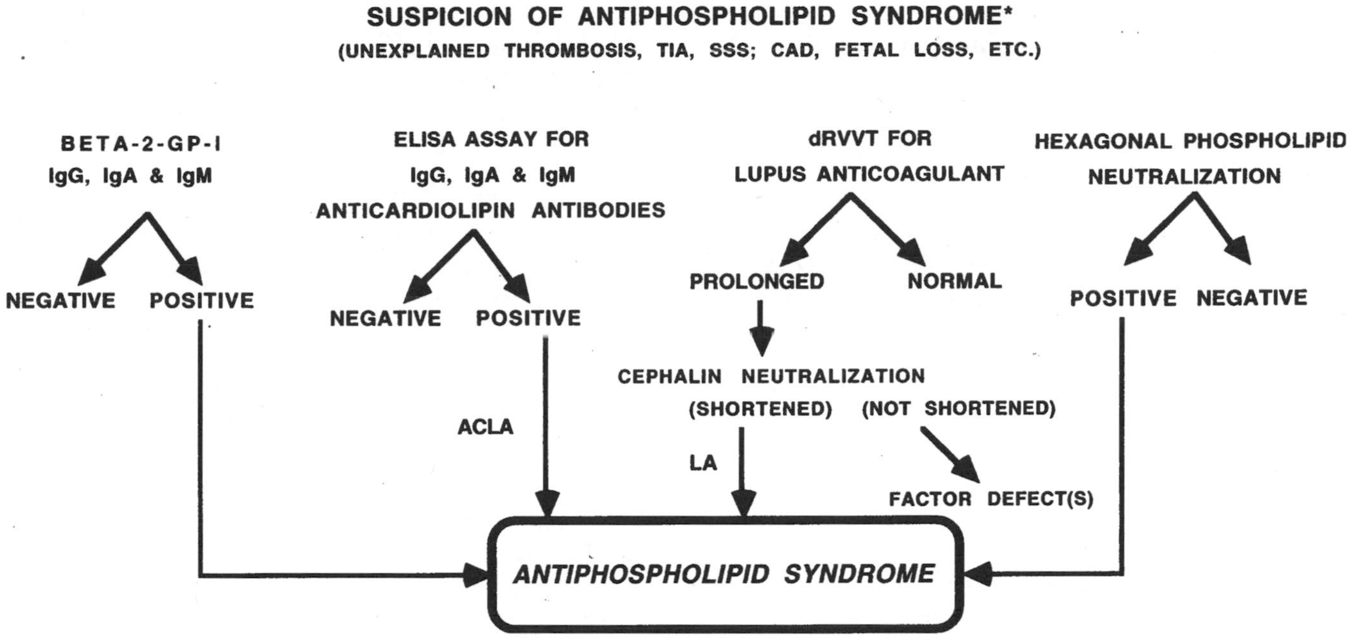

FIGURE 14.1. Laboratory diagnosis of antiphospholipid syndromes. *CAD,* coronary thrombosis; *SSS,* small stroke syndrome; *TIA,* transient ischemic attack. *If the laboratory diagnosis is negative and clinically indicated, do antiphosphatidylserine, antiphosphatidylcholine, antiphosphatidylinositol, antiphosphatidic acid, antiphosphatidylethanolamine, antiphosphatidylglycerol, and anti–annexin-V antibodies.

Summary

APLAs are strongly associated with thrombosis and are the most common of the acquired blood protein defects causing thrombosis. Although the precise mechanism(s) whereby APLAs alter hemostasis to induce a hypercoagulable state remain unclear, numerous theories, as previously discussed, have been advanced. The most common thrombotic events associated with ACLAs are DVT and PE (type I syndrome), coronary or peripheral artery thrombosis (type II syndrome), or cerebrovascular/retinal vessel thrombosis (type III syndrome), and occasionally patients have mixtures (type IV syndrome). Type V patients are those with APLAs and RMS. It is as yet unclear how many seemingly normal individuals who may never have manifestations of APL syndrome (type VI) have asymptomatic APLAs. The relative frequency of ACLAs in association with arterial and venous thrombosis strongly suggests that these should be looked for in any individual with unexplained thrombosis; all three idiotypes (IgG, IgA, and IgM) should be assessed. The type of syndrome (I through VI) should be defined if possible, as this may dictate both type and duration of both immediate and long-term anticoagulant therapy. Unlike those with ACLAs, patients with primary LA thrombosis syndrome usually have venous thrombosis. Because the aPTT is unreliable in patients with LA (prolonged in only about 40% to 50% of patients) and is not usually prolonged in patients with ACLAs, definitive tests including ELISA for ACLA, the dRVVT for LA, hexagonal phospholipid neutralization procedure and β_2-GpI (IgG, IgA, and IgM) should be immediately ordered with suspicion of APL syndrome or in individuals with otherwise unexplained thrombotic or thromboembolic events. If these are negative, in the appropriate clinical setting, subgroups also should be assessed. Finally, for most patients with APL-TS, warfarin therapy will fail and, except for retinal vascular thrombosis, and some types of antiplatelet therapy may fail; thus it is of major importance to make this diagnosis so patients can be treated with the most effective therapy for secondary prevention: LMWH or UFH in most instances, and clopidogrel in some instances.

Myeloproliferative Syndromes

Acute myocardial infarction, neurologic symptoms suggesting small vessel stroke; peripheral digital ischemia; DVT; PE; and cerebral, mesenteric, splenic, portal, and hepatic venous thrombosis have all been associated with myeloproliferative syndromes (169–171). Polycythemia vera may result in increased viscosity, leading to hypercoagulability. Treatment primarily consists of phlebotomy, with the goal to maintain the hematocrit at 40% to 45% (172). Patients with essential thrombocythemia also are at significantly increased risk of thrombosis. The risk of thrombosis appears to increase significantly above a platelet count of 650 × 10^9/L. Therapy may include hydroxyurea (173) or anagrelide (174). It has been well demonstrated that the longer the platelet count remains below 600×10^9/L, the lower the risk of thrombosis (175). Low-dose ASA also is recommended.

Trousseau Syndrome

Recurrent migratory polyphlebitis, including thrombosis of veins of the legs, neck, superficial veins of the thorax and abdomen, axillary and subclavian veins, cerebral veins, and mesenteric veins is a characteristic manifestation of Trousseau syndrome. Typically, the syndrome is associated with the presence of mucinous adenocarcinoma (see Chapter 12) (176,177). Effective long-term treatment requires full-dose anticoagulation with heparin or LMWH, as these patients are notoriously resistant to warfarin therapy. Dose-adjusted porcine UFH may be administered subcutaneously, or full-dose LMWH may be given. Warfarin is not efficacious.

Acquired Antithrombin Deficiency

Acquired deficiency of AT may occur in a variety of clinical settings. The most common of these conditions is DIC (178,179). In DIC, AT is complexed with circulating activated clotting factors (serine proteases) generated during the process of systemic activation of the procoagulant system (see Chapter 7). This considerably reduces functional AT levels. In addition, end-organ hepatic injury, accompanying the multiorgan system failure that frequently accompanies DIC, may reduce hepatic AT synthesis (180,181). In chronic liver disease (due to reduced synthesis), levels of AT decrease, but an increased risk of thrombosis usually does not follow because of other defects leading to a hemorrhagic tendency (182). Patients with nephrotic syndrome lose AT in the urine, and their blood become hypercoagulable (183). AT levels generally correlate with the severity of an acute thrombotic event. In the presence of active DVT or PE, functional levels typically decrease to 67% to 75% of normal human plasma, respectively (184). In DIC, AT levels may decrease much lower. Sepsis and other causes of cardiovascular collapse, as well as massive trauma, releasing large amounts of procoagulant into the systemic circulation (all variants of a DIC process), may rapidly reduce systemic AT functional levels. This abrupt decrease may contribute to the development of local and systemic thrombosis, and has significant therapeutic implications.

The management of patients with both inherited and acquired AT deficiency has advanced considerably with the wide availability of AT concentrates (185). Because patients with AT deficiency lack the available site of action for heparin, anticoagulation of patients with congenital deficiency with acute venous thrombosis or PE, with heparin alone, is ineffective. Administration of AT concentrates must accompany anticoagulation with heparin. AT concentrates also may be efficacious in patients with deficiency, even without heparin (186). Prophylaxis with AT for deficient patients in high-risk settings may be indicated; however, controlled studies are not available to confirm this. Pregnancy is a special risk for deficient patients. Subcutaneous heparin or LMWH is recommended throughout pregnancy. Warfarin is contraindicated because of teratogenicity. AT concentrates may be indicated at the time of greatest risk, during the puerperium and for obstetric emergencies (187).

Acquired AT deficiency must be categorized as to the cause of the abnormality before therapy is contemplated. In DIC, the clinical trigger for thrombosis must be treated for any therapy to be effective. Individuals with a decrease in AT due to primary liver disease require no treatment, as they may actually be at a greater risk of hemorrhage than of thrombosis, because of accompanying hematologic and coagulation abnormalities. Vinazzer et al. (188) demonstrated the efficacy of AT concentrates administration in patients with DIC, septic shock, and massive trauma. The formula for administration of therapeutic AT concentrates is as follows:

$$\text{Units required} = \frac{(\text{Desired} - \text{Baseline AT level}) \times \text{Weight (kg)}}{1.4}$$

Baseline AT level is expressed as percentage of normal level based on functional AT assay. Dosing frequency is generally every 6 to 12 hours, guided by repeated AT assays (189).

Generally, a dose of 50 U/kg is recommended for a patient with a baseline functional level of 50%. Repeated administration of 60% of the loading dose every 24 hours will usually maintain adequate levels in patients with deficiency (189). The dose requirement may be much higher in patients with DIC and with similar conditions that actively deplete AT.

Monitoring of patients with AT deficiency varies considerably between inherited and acquired states. Patients with the inherited disorder who experience recurrent thrombosis require life-long anticoagulation with warfarin and the determination of the PT at regular intervals [goal to maintain international normalized ratio (INR) of 2.0 to 3.0]. As the clinical circumstance changes, the intervals of follow-up and monitoring may change. For clinical purposes, the assay of choice is the functional AT assay, reported as percentage of normal human plasma. Immunologic assays of AT are of no clinical value. In the acutely ill patient receiving AT concentrates, repeated AT levels may be required at intervals of 6 to 12 hours.

Acquired Heparin Cofactor II Deficiency

Acquired deficiency of heparin cofactor II (HC-II) is well documented in DIC, as HC-II levels are markedly reduced (190). In contradistinction to the reduction noted in AT levels, HC-II is not decreased as the result of acute thrombosis (191) nor in nephrotic syndrome (192). Treatment is based on the clinical circumstances. Treatment with anticoagulation should proceed according to accepted guidelines for the clinical condition (193). Heparin will be effective in the presence of HC-II deficiency. Long-term anticoagulation and prophylaxis for high-risk situations should be considered for individuals with a history of recurrent thrombosis. Because the populations studied are small, firm recommendations are not available.

Acquired Protein C Deficiency

Acquired deficiency is detected in DIC, in the presence of acute thromboembolic disease, in severe liver disease (decreased hepatic synthesis), hemolytic uremic syndrome, and thrombotic thrombocytopenia purpura (194).

Treatment of acquired protein C deficiency requires a precise diagnosis and treatment of the underlying cause. Anticoagulation is the treatment of choice in patients with acquired protein C deficiency and thrombosis. Heparin or LMWH is used according to accepted guidelines for acute thrombotic events (195,196). Long-term anticoagulation with warfarin is indicated after an acute event and as subsequent secondary prophylaxis in those with acquired deficiency. Warfarin-induced skin necrosis is a major therapeutic problem (197–199). With the institution of warfarin, the reduction of protein C (half-life, 6 hours) occurs at a faster rate than the reduction in the other vitamin K–dependent factors II (half-life, 72 hours), VII, and X. This results in a transient hypercoagulable state, predisposing to thrombosis, including skin necrosis (175,200). Recent studies have demonstrated that this problem can be controlled by maintaining full anticoagulation with heparin until the PT is well into the therapeutic range (target INR, 3.0 to 3.5). Maintaining a therapeutic PT is, subsequently, essential to avoiding recurrent thrombosis. Despite therapeutic anticoagulation with warfarin, there are treatment failures. Long-term therapy with heparin/LMWH may be required. Protein C concentrates are now available for treatment failures (201).

Therapy is monitored with the appropriate laboratory test depending on the pharmacologic agent selected. The target INR for warfarin therapy is 3.0 to 3.5. Therapy with LMWH is weight adjusted and does not require monitoring, except for a platelet count every 2 days for the first 2 weeks of treatment. Although the measurement of the biologic and immunologic activity of protein C is required for diagnosis (202), follow-up analysis is not required. When evaluating a patient with unexplained thrombosis, however, it is essential to obtain the laboratory tests for protein C deficiency before therapy is initiated, because warfarin immediately reduces the vitamin K–dependent hepatic production of protein C. The levels of both protein C and S decrease to 40% to 60% of normal immediately and return to about 70% of normal after several weeks of therapy. Measurement of the protein C and S levels should wait for several weeks after initiation of warfarin therapy.

Acquired Protein S Deficiency

Acquired deficiency has been documented in a variety of conditions, including DIC (203), type I (204), and type II (205) diabetes mellitus, pregnancy (206), oral contraceptive use (207), nephrotic syndrome (208), liver disease (209), and essential thrombocythemia (210).

Management of patients with protein S deficiency is similar to that of those with protein C deficiency. Acute thrombosis is managed with heparin anticoagulation according to accepted guidelines, dependent on the site and severity of disease. Long-term anticoagulation with warfarin is indicated after heparin therapy for an acute event and for prophylaxis (195,196). Follow-up of patients involves repeated clinical evaluation in the acute setting, and monitoring is dependent on the form of anticoagulation selected. LMWH requires only periodic evaluation of the platelet count. Warfarin is monitored with the PT to maintain a target INR of 2.0 to 3.0. Repeated analysis of the protein S level is usually not required if evaluation is performed before initiation of warfarin therapy. Subsequent measurement should wait for several weeks, as discussed with protein C (201). In warfarin failures, long-term therapy with subcutaneous UFH or LMWH may be required. As with other thrombophilic disorders, the patient and family members should be counseled regarding the need to intervene in high-risk circumstances. These include but are not limited to the avoidance of oral contraceptives, control of obesity, prophylactic anticoagulation at the time of surgery, prolonged immobility, pregnancy, and the puerperium.

Acquired Fibrinolytic System Defects

A variety of clinical conditions are associated with elevated levels of fibrinolytic inhibitors leading to hypercoagulability, including diabetes mellitus (211), thrombotic thrombocytopenic purpura (212), myocardial infarction (213,214), malignancy, DVT and PE (215), scleroderma, pulmonary fibrosis, pregnancy, oral contraceptive use (216), serious infections, surgery, and other clinical conditions (217,218). Patients with generalized atherosclerosis may exhibit decreased plasminogen activity because of damage to the vascular intima.

Treatment of impaired fibrinolysis must include treatment of the underlying disease with the appropriate modalities, as well as anticoagulation. Caution must be exercised in the application of thrombolytic agents because, in the absence of adequate levels of plasminogen, t-PA, streptokinase, and urokinase may be less effective than expected.

Acquired deficiency of t-PA is identified in a variety of clinical conditions, including: coronary artery disease (especially in unstable angina, acute myocardial infarction, and after PTCA) (219–221), ulcerative colitis, and Crohn disease (222). Decreased levels of t-PA also are noted in patients with recurrent DVT, presumably due to vascular intimal injury (201). Increased t-PA is seen in histiocytosis X, cryptogenic fibrosing alveolitis (222,223), carcinoma of the breast (224), and female heavy smokers also taking oral contraceptives (225). t-PA inhibitor type I is decreased in non–insulin-dependent diabetes mellitus patients who are treated with insulin (226).

TABLE 14.7. RECOMMENDED LONG-TERM PHARMACOLOGIC THERAPY FOR SYMPTOMATIC THROMBOPHILIA

Disorder	Therapy
APC resistance	Warfarin (INR, 2.0–3.0); fixed, low-dose s.c. UFH or LMWH
FV Leiden	
FV Cambridge	
Prothrombin 20210A	
Factor XII deficiency (Hageman trait)	Fixed, low-dose s.c. UFH or LMWH
Dysfibrinogenemia	Fixed, low-dose s.c. UFH or LMWH, or warfarin (INR, 2.3–3.0)
Hyperhomocyst(e)inemia	Folic acid, 5 mg/day; consider additional vitamin B_6 (50 mg/day ASA prophylaxis for atherosclerosis)
Antithrombin deficiency	Warfarin (INR, 2.3–3.0); antithrombin concentrates for acute intervention or LMWH
Heparin cofactor II deficiency	Warfarin (INR, 2.0–3.0), fixed, low-dose s.c. UFH or LMWH
Protein C deficiency	Warfarin (INR, 2.0–3.0), fixed, low-dose s.c. UFH or LMWH
Protein S	Warfarin (INR, 2.0–3.0); fixed, low-dose s.c. UFH or LMWH
Plasminogen deficiency/inhibition	Warfarin (INR, 2.0–3.0); fixed, low-dose s.c. UFH or LMWH
Antiphospholipid antibodies	Dependent on syndrome type (see Table 3)
Platelet defects	
Wein–Penzing defect	ASA (81–325 mg/day)
Sticky platelet syndrome	
Myeloproliferative disorders	Phlebotomy, ASA (81–325 mg/day), anagrelide, hydroxyurea
Trousseau syndrome	PTT adjusted dose UFH i.v. or s.c. or LMWH (full dose)

ASA, acetylsalicylic acid; INR, international normalized ratio; s.c., subcutaneously; UFH, unfractionated heparin; LMWH, low-molecular-weight heparin; PTT, partial thromboplastin time; APC, activated protein C.

Treatment is based on therapy for the primary disease and antithrombotic therapy as needed. Awareness of the underlying decrease in fibrinolytic activity associated with decreased plasminogen activity should prompt greater attention to appropriate antithrombotic therapy, both with acute thrombosis and as prophylaxis in high-risk circumstances.

SUMMARY

In all patients with acquired thrombophilia, management is determined not solely by the presence of the laboratory abnormality but also by the clinical consequences. Prophylaxis in asymptomatic patients is reserved for those disorders with the highest risk of idiopathic thrombosis. The choice of pharmacologic agent will necessarily vary with the likelihood of life-threatening thrombosis. As with APA, intervention includes a spectrum from no treatment to full-dose anticoagulation. This summary notes that blinded, controlled studies to validate many of these recommendations are frequently lacking. Understanding of the pathophysiology of the disorder, review of the available studies and reports, and clinical experience must guide management decisions. Our recommendations for treatment of the hereditary and acquired thrombophilic disorders are presented in Table 14.7. Common drug regimens are presented in Table 14.8.

TABLE 14.8. RECOMMENDED MONITORING OF LONG-TERM PHARMACOLOGIC THERAPY

Drug	Monitoring
Heparin	CBC baseline and every 2 days for the first 15 days (UFH or LMWH) of therapy, and then weekly for the first month, and then monthly. Heparin levels (anti-Xa) weekly for the first month and then monthly. Bone density analysis baseline and every 6–12 mo. Liver function tests every 3 mo
Warfarin	CBC and PT/INR baseline then PT/INR monthly to every 2 mo in the most stable patients. Dose adjustments require repeated PT/INR weekly or more often. CBC every 1 to 3 months. Periodic UA and stool occult blood in selected patients
Aspirin	CBC baseline and then if any symptoms or signs of bleeding or GI side effects, do CBC. May take with liquid antacid. GI studies if indicated
Clopidogrel	CBC ADP aggregation and baseline; repeated CBC q week × 4 weeks and repeated ADP aggregation in 4 weeks to note blunted effect, and then CBC if any symptoms or signs of bleeding or GI side effects. GI studies if indicated

CBC, complete blood count; UFH, unfractionated heparin; LMWH, low-molecular-weight heparin; ADP, adenosine diphosphate; PT, prothrombin time; INR, international normalized ratio; UA, urinalysis; ADP, adenosine diphosphate; GI, gastrointestinal.

Finally, it must be emphasized that any patient with unexplained arterial or venous thrombosis should be evaluated for thrombophilia; only by defining the cause of thrombosis in this manner can rational primary and secondary preventive therapy be applied.

REFERENCES

1. Bick RL, Ancypa D. Blood protein defects associated with thrombosis: laboratory assessment. *Clin Lab Med* 1995;15:125–164.
2. Bick RL. Hypercoagulability and thrombosis. *Med Clin North Am* 1994;78:635–666.
3. Bick RL. Antiphospholipid thrombosis syndromes: etiology, pathophysiology, diagnosis and management. *Int J Hematol* 1997;65:193–213.
4. Oosting JD, Derksen RH, Bobbink IWG. Antiphospholipid antibodies directed against a combination of phospholipids with prothrombin, protein C or protein S: an explanation for their pathogenic mechanism? *Blood* 1993;81:2618–2625.
5. Bick RL. The antiphospholipid thrombosis syndromes: a common multidisciplinary medical problem. *J Clin Appl Thromb Hemost* 1997;3:270–283.
6. Bick RL, Baker WF. Anticardiolipin antibodies and thrombosis. *Hematol Oncol Clin North Am* 1992;6:1287–1300.
7. Bick RL, Baker WF. Antiphospholipid syndrome and thrombosis. *Semin Thromb Hemost* 1999;25:333.
8. Bick RL, Baker WF. The antiphospholipid and thrombosis syndromes. *Med Clin North Am* 1994;78:667–684.
9. Conley CL, Hartmann RC. A hemorrhagic disorder caused by circulating anticoagulant in patients with disseminated lupus erythematosus. *J Clin Invest* 1952;31:621–622.
10. Criel A, Collen D, Masson PL. A case of IgM antibodies which inhibit the contact activation of blood coagulation. *Thromb Res* 1978;12:833–836.
11. Kunkel L. Acquired circulating anticoagulants. *Hematol Oncol Clin North Am* 1992;6:1341–1358.
12. Coller BS, Hultin MB, Hoyer LW. Normal pregnancy in a patient with a prior postpartum factor VIII inhibitor: with observations on pathogenesis and prognosis. *Blood* 1981;58:619–624.
13. LeFrere JJ, Gozin D, Lerable J. Circulating anticoagulant in asymptomatic persons seropositive for human immunodeficiency virus [Letter]. *Ann Intern Med* 1988;108:771.
14. Taillan B, Roul C, Fuzibet JG. Circulating anticoagulant in patients seropositive for human immunodeficiency virus. *Ann Intern Med* 1989;87:405–407.
15. Davis S, Furie B, Griffin JH. Circulating inhibitors of blood coagulation associated with procainamide-induced lupus anticoagulants. *Am J Hematol* 1978;4:401–407.
16. Jeffrey RF. Transient lupus anticoagulant with Fansidar therapy. *Postgrad Med J* 1986;62:893–894.
17. Morgan M, Downs K, Chesterman CN, et al. Clinical analysis of 125 patients with the lupus anticoagulant. *Aust N Z J Med* 1993;23:151–156.
18. Bick RL, Ucar K. Hypercoagulability and thrombosis. *Hematol Oncol Clin North Am* 1992;6:1421–1431.
19. Schleider MA, Nachman RL, Jaffe EA. A clinical study of the lupus anticoagulant. *Blood* 1976;48:499–509.
20. Regan MG, Lackner H, Karpatkin S. Platelet function and coagulation profile in lupus erythematosus. *Ann Intern Med* 1974;81:462–468.
21. Mueh JR, Herbst KD, Rapaport SI. Thrombosis in patients with the "lupus"-type circulating anticoagulant. *Ann Intern Med* 1980;92:156–159.
22. Shapiro SS, Rajagopalon V. Hemorrhagic disorders associated with circulating inhibitors. In: Ratnoff OD, Forbes CD, eds. *Disorders of hemostasis.* Philadelphia: WB Saunders, 1996: 208–227.
23. Kampe CE. Clinical syndromes associated with lupus anticoagulants. *Semin Thromb Hemost* 1994;20:16–26.
24. Hinton RC. Neurological syndromes associated with antiphospholipid antibodies. *Semin Thromb Hemost* 1994;20:46–54.
25. Kleinknecht D, Bobrie G, Meyer O, et al. Recurrent thrombosis and renal vascular disease in a patient with lupus anticoagulant. *Nephrol Dial Transplant* 1989;4:051–050.
26. Pope JM, Canny CL, Bell DA. Cerebral ischemic events associated with endocarditis, retinal vascular disease and lupus anticoagulant. *Am J Med* 1991;90:299–309.
27. Baker WF, Bick RL. Antiphospholipid antibodies in coronary artery disease. *Semin Thromb Hemost* 1994;20:27–45.
28. Reyes H, Dearing L, Shoenfeld Y. Antiphospholipid antibodies: a critique of their heterogeneity and hegemony. *Semin Thromb Hemost* 1994;20:89–100.
29. Kaczor NA, Bickford NN, Triplett DA. Evaluation of different mixing study reagents and dilution effect in lupus anticoagulant testing. *J Clin Pathol* 1991;95:408–411.
30. Shapiro SS, Thagarajan P. Lupus anticoagulants. *Prog Hemost Thromb* 1982;6:263–285.
31. Ko J, Guaglianone P, Wolin M, et al. Variation in the sensitivity of an activated thromboplastin time reagent to the lupus anticoagulant. *Am J Clin Pathol* 1993;99:333(abst).
32. Bick RL. The antiphospholipid thrombosis syndromes: fact, fiction, confusion and controversy. *Am J Clin Pathol* 1993;100: 477–480.
33. Thiagarajan P, Pengo V, Shapiro SS. The use of the dilute Russell viper venom time for the diagnosis of lupus anticoagulants. *Blood* 1986;68:869–874.
34. McGehee WG, Patch MJ, Lingao JU. Detection of the lupus anticoagulant: a comparison of the kaolin clotting time with the tissue thromboplastin inhibition test. *Blood* 1983;(suppl)62: 276(abst).
35. Rosove MH, Ismail M, Koziol BJ. Lupus anticoagulants: improved diagnosis with a kaolin clotting time using rabbit brain phospholipid in standard and high concentrations. *Blood* 1986;68:472–478.
36. Bick RL. Hypercoagulability and thrombosis. In: *Disorders of thrombosis and hemostasis: clinical and laboratory practice.* Chicago: ASCP Press, 1992:261–290.
37. Harris EN. Immunology of antiphospholipid antibodies. In: Lahita R, ed. *Systemic lupus erythematosus.* 2nd ed. London: Churchill Livingstone, 1992:505–340.
38. Rauch J, Janoff AS. The nature of antiphospholipid antibodies. *J Rheumatol* 1992;19:1782–1785.
39. De Castellarnau C, Vila CL, Sancho MJ. Lupus anticoagulant, recurrent abortion, and prostacyclin production by cultured smooth muscle cells. *Lancet* 1983;2:1137–1138.
40. Sanfelippo MJ, Drayna CJ. Prekallikrein inhibition associated with the lupus anticoagulant: a mechanism for thrombosis. *Am J Clin Pathol* 1982;77:275–279.
41. Bick RL, Baker WF. Antiphospholipid and thrombosis syndromes. *Semin Thromb Hemost* 1994;20:3–15.
42. Roubey RAS. Autoantibodies to phospholipid-bonding plasma proteins: a new view of lupus anticoagulants and other "antiphospholipid" antibodies. *Blood* 1994;84:2854–2867.
43. Bick RL, Laughlin HR, Cohen B, et al. Fetal wastage syndrome due to blood protein/platelet defects: results of prevalence studies and treatment outcome with low-dose heparin and low-dose aspirin. *Clin Appl Thromb Hemost* 1995;1:286–292.

44. Bick RL. The antiphospholipid thrombosis (APL-T) syndromes: characteristics and recommendations for classification and treatment. *Am J Clin Pathol* 1991;96:424–425.
45. Rosove MH, Brewer PMC. Antiphospholipid thrombosis: clinical course after the first thrombotic event in 70 patients. *Ann Intern Med* 1992;117:303–308.
46. Bick RL, Baker WF. Deep vein thrombosis: prevalence of etiologic factors and results of management in 100 consecutive patients. *Semin Thromb Hemost* 1992;18:267–274.
47. Bick RL, Madden J, Heller KB, et al. Recurrent miscarriage: causes, evaluation, and treatment. *Medscape Womens Health* 1998;3:1–13.
48. Bick RL. Recurrent miscarriage syndrome and infertility caused by blood coagulation protein or platelet defects. *Hematol Oncol Clin North Am* 2000;14:1117–1131.
49. Bowie EJW, Thompson JH, Pascuzzi CA. Thrombosis in systemic lupus erythematosus despite circulating anticoagulant. *J Lab Clin Med* 1963;162:417–430.
50. Bell WR, Boss GR, Wolfson JS. Circulating anticoagulant in the procainamide-induced lupus syndrome. *Arch Intern Med* 1977;137:1471–1473.
51. Bick RL. The antiphospholipid thrombosis syndromes: lupus anticoagulants and anticardiolipin antibodies. *Adv Pathol Lab Med* 1995;8:391–423.
52. Espinoza LR, Hartmann RC. Significance of the lupus anticoagulant. *Am J Hematol* 1986;22:331–337.
53. Manoussakis MN, Tzioufas AG, Silis MP. High prevalence of anticardiolipin and other autoantibodies in a healthy elderly population. *Clin Exp Immunol* 1987;69:557–565.
54. Zarrabi MH, Zucker S, Miller F. Immunologic and coagulation disorders in chlorpromazine-treated patients. *Ann Intern Med* 1979;91:914–919.
55. Harris EN, Gharavi AE, Boey ML. Anticardiolipin antibodies: detection by radioimmunoassay and association with thrombosis in systemic lupus erythematosus. *Lancet* 1983;II:1211–1214.
56. Weidmann CE, Wallace D, Peter J. Studies of IgG, IgM and IgA antiphospholipid antibody isotypes in systemic lupus erythematosus. *J Rheumatol* 1988;15:74–79.
57. Asherson RA, Harris EN. Anticardiolipin antibodies: clinical associations. *Postgrad Med J* 1986;62:1081–1087.
58. Hughes GVR, Harris EN, Gharavi AE. The anticardiolipin syndrome. *J Rheumatol* 1986;13:486–489.
59. Triplett DA. Clinical significance of antiphospholipid antibodies. *Hemost Thromb* 1988;10:1–30.
60. Derue G, Englert H, Harris E. Fetal loss in systemic lupus: association with anticardiolipin antibodies. *Br J Obstet Gynecol* 1985;5:207–211.
61. Lubbe WF, Palmer SJ, Butler WS. Fetal survival after prednisolone suppression of maternal lupus anticoagulant. *Lancet* 1983;i:1361–1363.
62. Harris EN, Gharavi AE, Hedge U. Anticardiolipin antibodies in autoimmune thrombocytopenia purpura. *Br J Haematol* 1985;59:231.
63. Harris EN, Asherson RA, Gharavi AE. Thrombocytopenia in SLE and related autoimmune disorders: association with anticardiolipin antibodies. *Br J Haematol* 1985;59:227–230.
64. Bick RL, Kaplan H. Syndromes of thrombosis and hypercoagulability: congenital and acquired thrombophilias. *Med Clin North Am* 1998;82:409–458.
65. Rosove MH, Brewer P, Runge A. Simultaneous lupus anticoagulant and anticardiolipin assays and clinical detection of antiphospholipids. *Am J Hematol* 1989;32:148–149.
66. Tanne DT, Triplett DA, Levine SR. Antiphospholipid-protein antibodies and ischemic stroke: not just cardiolipin any more. *Stroke* 1998;29:1755–1758.
67. Bick RL. Antiphospholipid thrombosis syndromes. *J Clin Appl Thromb Hemost* 2001;7:241–258.
68. McNeil HP, Chesterman CN, Krilis SA. Anticardiolipin antibodies and lupus anticoagulants comprise separate antibody subgroups with different phospholipid binding characteristics. *Br J Haematol* 1989;73:506–513.
69. Shi BS, Chong BH, Chesterman CN. Beta-2-Glycoprotein I is a requirement for anticardiolipin antibodies binding to activated platelets: differences with lupus anticoagulants. *Blood* 1993;81:1255–1262.
70. Harris EN, Hughes GRV, Gharavi AE. Antiphospholipid antibodies: an elderly statesman dons new garments. *J Rheumatol* 1987;14:208–213.
71. Gharavi AE, Harris EN, Asherson RA. Anticardiolipin antibodies: isotype distribution and phospholipid specificity. *Ann Rheum Dis* 1987;46:1–6.
72. Carreras L, Defreyn G, Manchin S. Arterial thrombosis, intrauterine death and lupus anticoagulant: detection of immunoglobulin interfering with prostacyclin formation. *Lancet* 1981;1:244–246.
73. Cariou R, Tobelem G, Bellucci S. Effect of lupus anticoagulant on antithrombogenic properties of endothelial cells: inhibition of thrombomodulin-dependent protein C activation. *Thromb Haemost* 1988;60:54–58.
74. Cosgriff TM, Martin BA. Low functional and high antigenic antithrombin III level in a patient with the lupus anticoagulant. *Arthritis Rheum* 1981;24:94–96.
75. Khamashta MA, Harris EN, Gharavi AE. Immune mediated mechanism for thrombosis: antiphospholipid antibody binding to platelet membranes. *Ann Rheum Dis* 1988;47:849–853.
76. Sanfellipo MJ, Drayna CJ. Prekallikrein inhibition associated with the lupus anticoagulant. *Am J Clin Pathol* 1982;77:275–279.
77. Angeles-Cano E, Sultan Y, Clauvel JP. Predisposing factors to thrombosis in systemic lupus erythematosus: possible relationship to endothelial cell damage. *J Lab Clin Med* 1979;94:312–323.
78. Ruiz-Arguelles G. The activated protein C resistance phenotype of the antiphospholipid syndrome may follow a relapsing course. *Clin Appl Thromb Hemost* 1998;4:277–279.
79. Ginsburg KS, Liang MH, Newcomer L, et al. Anticardiolipin antibodies and the risk for ischemic stroke and venous thrombosis. *Ann Intern Med* 1992;117:997–1002.
80. Boey ML, Colaco CB, Gharavi AE. Thrombosis in SLE: striking association with the presence of circulating "lupus anticoagulant." *Br Med J* 1983;287:1021–1023.
81. Elias M, Eldor A. Thromboembolism in patients with the "lupus-like" circulating anticoagulant. *Arch Intern Med* 1984;144:510–515.
82. Hall S, Buettner H, Luthra HS. Occlusive retinal vascular disease in systemic lupus erythematosus. *J Rheumatol* 1984;11:96–98.
83. Asherson RA, Harris EN, Gharavi AE. Arterial occlusions associated with antibodies to anticardiolipin. *Arthritis Rheum* 1985;28:89(abst).
84. Hamilton ME. Superior mesenteric artery thrombosis associated with antiphospholipid syndrome. *West J Med* 1991;155:174–176.
85. Asherson RA, Harris EN, Gharavi AE. Aortic arch syndrome associated with anticardiolipin antibodies and the lupus anticoagulant. *Arthritis Rheum* 1985;28:594–595.
86. Asherson RA, Morgan SH, Harris EN. Arterial occlusion causing large bowel infarction: a reflection of clotting diathesis in SLE. *Clin Rheumatol* 1986;5:102–106.
87. Asherson RA, MacKay IR, Harris EN. Myocardial infarction in a young male with systemic lupus erythematosus, deep vein

thrombosis and antiphospholipid antibodies. *Br Heart J* 1986; 56:190–193.
88. Gavaghan TP, Krilis SA, Daggard GE. Anticardiolipin antibodies and occlusion of coronary artery bypass grafts. *Lancet* 1987; ii:977–978.
89. Morton KT, Gavaghan S, Krilis G. Coronary artery bypass graft failure: an autoimmune phenomenon? *Lancet* 1986;I: 1353–1354.
90. Hamsten A, Norberg R, Bjorkholm M. Antibodies to cardiolipin in young survivors of myocardial infarction: an association with recurrent cardiovascular events. *Lancet* 1986;I: 113–116.
91. Harpaz D, Sidi Y. Successful thrombolytic therapy for acute myocardial infarction in a patient with the antiphospholipid antibody syndrome. *Am Heart J* 1991;122:1492–1495.
92. Asherson RA, Khamashta MA, Ordi-Ros J. The "primary" antiphospholipid syndrome: major clinical and serological features. *Medicine* 1989;68:366–374.
93. Bick RL, Ismail Y, Baker WF. Coagulation abnormalities in patients with precocious coronary artery thrombosis and patients failing coronary artery bypass grafting and percutaneous transluminal coronary angioplasty. *Semin Thromb Hemost* 1993;19:411–417.
94. Galve E, Ordi J, Barquinero J. Valvular heart disease in the primary antiphospholipid syndrome. *Ann Intern Med* 1992;116: 293–298.
95. Chartash EK, Lans DM, Paget SA. Aortic insufficiency and mitral regurgitation in patients wirh systemic lupus erythematosus and the antiphospholipid syndrome. *Am J Med* 1989; 86:406–412.
96. Chartash EK, Paget SA, Lockshin MD. Lupus anticoagulant associated with aortic and mitral valve insufficiency. *Arthritis Rheum* 1986;29:95–96.
97. Leung WH, Wong KL, Wong CK. Association between antiphospholipid antibodies and cardiac abnormalities in patients with systemic lupus erythematosus. *Am J Med* 1990; 89:411–419.
98. Coppock MA, Safford RE, Danielson GK. Intracardiac thrombosis, phospholipid antibodies, and two-chambered right ventricle. *Br Heart J* 1988;60:455–458.
99. Reisner SA, Blumenfeld Z, Brenner B. Cardiac involvement in patients with primary antiphospholipid syndrome. *Circulation* 1990;(suppl III)82:398.
100. Weinstein C, Miller M, Axtens R. Livido reticularis associated with increased titers of anticardiolipin antibodies in systemic lupus erythematosus. *Arch Dermatol* 1987;123:596–600.
101. Eng AM. Cutaneous expressions of antiphospholipid syndromes. *Semin Thromb Hemost* 1994;20:71–78.
102. Englert H, Hawkes C, Boey M. Degos' disease: association with anticardiolipin antibodies and the lupus anticoagulant. *Br Med J* 1984;289:576–584.
103. Bird AG, Lendrum R, Asherson RA. Disseminated intravascular coagulation, antiphospholipid antibodies, and ischemic necrosis of extremities. *Ann Rheum Dis* 1987;46:251–255.
104. Wolf P, Peter-Soyer H, Auer-Grumbach P. Widespread cutaneous necrosis in a patient with rheumatoid arthritis associated with anticardiolipin antibodies. *Arch Dermatol* 1991;127: 1739–1740.
105. Ingram SB, Goodnight SH, Bennett RM. An unusual syndrome of a devastating noninflammatory vasculopathy associated with anticardiolipin antibodies: report of two cases. *Arthritis Rheum* 1987;30:1167–1172.
106. Levine SR, Langer SL, Albers JW. Sneddon's syndrome: an antiphospholipid antibody syndrome? *Neurology* 1988;38: 798–800.
107. Frampton G, Winer JB, Cameron JS. Severe Guillain-Barré syndrome: an association with IgA anti-cardiolipin antibody in a series of 92 patients. *J Neuroimmunol* 1988;19:133–139.
108. Levine S, Welch K. The spectrum of neurologic disease associated with anticardiolipin antibodies. *Arch Neurol* 1987;44: 876–490.
109. Oppenheimer S, Hoffbrand B. Optic neuritis and myelopathy in systemic lupus erythematosus. *Can J Neurol Sci* 1986;13: 129–132.
110. Harris EN, Gharavi AE, Asherson RA. Cerebral infarction in systemic lupus: association with anticardiolipin antibodies. *Clin Exp Rheumatol* 1984;2:47–51.
111. Williams RC. Cerebral infarction in systemic lupus: association with anticardiolipin antibodies. *Clin Exp Rheumatol* 1984;2:3.
112. Coull BM, Bourdette DN, Goodnight SH. Multiple cerebral infarctions and dementia associated with anticardiolipin antibodies. *Stroke* 1987;18:1107–1112.
113. Asherson RA, Khamashta MA, Hughes GRV. Sneddon's syndrome [Letter]. *Neurology* 1989;39:1138.
114. Moral A. Sneddon's syndrome with antiphospholipid antibodies and arteriopathy. *Stroke* 1991;22:1327–1328.
115. Sohngen D, Wehmeier A, Specker C. Antiphospholipid antibodies in systemic lupus erythematosus and Sneddon's syndrome. *Semin Thromb Hemost* 1994;20:55–63.
116. Levine SR, Brey RL, Joseph CLM. Risk of recurrent thromboembolic events in patients with focal cerebral ischemia and antiphospholipid antibodies. *Stroke* 1992;23(suppl I):29–32.
117. Levine SR, Diaczok IM, Deegan MJ. Recurrent stroke associated with thymoma and anticardiolipin antibodies. *Arch Neurol* 1987;44:678–679.
118. Brey RL, Hart RG, Sherman DG, et al. Antiphospholipid antibodies and cerebral ischemia in young people. *Neurology* 1990;40:1190–1196.
119. Toschi V, Motta A, Castelli C, et al. High prevalence of antiphosphatidylinositol antibodies in young patients with cerebral ischemia of undetermined cause. *Stroke* 1998;29: 1759–1764.
120. Nencini P, Baruffi MC, Abbate R, et al. Lupus anticoagulant and anticardiolipin antibodies in young adults with cerebral ischemia. *Stroke* 1992;23:189–193.
121. Carhaupoma JR, Mitsias P, Levine SR. Cerebral venous thrombosis and anticardiolipin antibodies. *Stroke* 1997;28 2363–2369.
122. Bick RL, Hinton RC. Prevalence of hereditary and acquired coagulation protein/platelet defects in patients with cerebral ischemia. *Blood* 1998;92:(suppl 1, pt 2):114(abstr).
123. Levine SR, Brey RL, Sawaya KL, et al. Recurrent stroke and thrombo-occlusive events in the antiphospholipid syndrome. *Ann. Neurol* 1995;38:119–124.
124. Brey R, for the APASS Group. Anticardiolipin antibodies are an independent risk factor for first ischemic stroke. *Neurology* 1993;43:2069–2073.
125. Hull RG, Harris N, Gharavi AE. Anticardiolipin antibodies: occurrence in Behçet's syndrome. *Ann Rheum Dis* 1984;43: 746–748.
126. Harris NE, Spinnato JA. Should anticardiolipin tests be performed in otherwise healthy pregnant women? *Am J Obstet Gynecol* 1991;165:1272–1275.
127. Buchanan NM, Khamashta MA, Morton KE, et al. A study of 100 high-risk lupus pregnancies. *Am J Reprod Immunol* 1992; 28:192–194.
128. Anticardiolipin antibodies: a risk factor for venous and arterial thrombosis [Editorial]. *Lancet* 1985;1:912.
129. Kwak JY, Gilman-Sachs A, Beaman KD, et al. Reproductive outcome in women with recurrent spontaneous abortions of alloimmune and autoimmune causes: preconception versus

postconception treatment. *Am J Obstet Gynecol* 1992;166: 1787–1795.

130. Bick RL. Recurrent miscarriage syndrome and infertility caused by blood coagulation protein or platelet defects. *Hematol Oncol Clin North Am* 2000;14:1117.
131. Lin QD. Investigation of the association between autoantibodies and recurrent abortions. *Chin J Obstet Gynecol* 1993;28:674–677.
132. Parazzini F, Acaia B, Faden D. Antiphospholipid antibodies and recurrent abortion. *Obstet Gynecol* 1991;77:854–858.
133. Grandone E, Margaglione M, Vecchione G. Antiphospholipid antibodies and risk of fetal loss: a pilot report of a cross-sectional study. *Thromb Haemost* 1993;69:597(abst).
134. Birdsall M, Pattison N, Chamley L. Antiphospholipid antibodies in pregnancy. *Aust N Z J Obstet Gynaecol* 1992;32:328–330.
135. Maclean MA, Cumming GP, McCall F. The prevalence of lupus anticoagulant and anticardiolipin antibodies in women with a history of first trimester miscarriages. *Br J Obstet Gynaecol* 1994; 101:103–106.
136. Howard MA, Firkin BG, Healy DL. Lupus anticoagulant in a woman with multiple spontaneous miscarriage. *Am J Hematol* 1987;26:175–178.
137. Taylor M, Cauchi MN, Buchanan RRC. The lupus anticoagulant, anticardiolipin antibodies, and recurrent miscarriage. *Am J Reprod Immunol* 1990;23:33–36.
138. Parke AL, Wilson D, Maier D. The prevalence of antiphospholipid antibodies in women with recurrent spontaneous abortion, women with successful pregnancies, and women who have never been pregnant. *Arthritis Rheum* 1991;34:1231–1235.
139. Kochenour NK, Branch DW, Rote NS. A new postpartum syndrome associated with antiphospholipid antibodies. *Obstet Gynecol* 1987;69:460–468.
140. Intrator L, Oksenhendler E, Desforges L. Anticardiolipin antibodies in HIV infected patients with or without immune thrombocytopenic purpura. *Br J Haematol* 1988;67:269–270.
141. Canoso RT, Zon LI, Groopman JE. Anticardiolipin antibodies associated with HTLV-III infection. *Br J Haematol* 1987;65: 495–498.
142. Panzer S, Stain C, Hartl H. Anticardiolipin antibodies are elevated in HIV-1 infected haemophiliacs but do not predict for disease progression. *Thromb Haemost* 1989;61:81–85.
143. Stimmler MM, Quismorio FP, McGehee WG. Anticardiolipin antibodies in acquired immunodeficiency syndrome. *Arch Intern Med* 1989;149:1833–1835.
144. Vaarala O, Palosuo T, Kleemola M. Anticardiolipin response in acute infections. *Clin Immunol Immunopathol* 1986;41:8–15.
145. Violi F, Ferro D, Quintarelli C. Dilute aPTT prolongation by antiphospholipid antibodies in patients with liver cirrhosis. *Thromb Haemost* 1990;63:183–186.
146. Harrison RL, Alperin JB, Kumar D. Concurrent lupus anticoagulants and prothrombin deficiency due to phenytoin use. *Arch. Pathol Lab Med* 1987;111:719–722.
147. Lillicrap DP, Pinto M, Benford K. Heterogeneity of laboratory test results for antiphospholipid antibodies in patients treated with chlorpromazine and other phenothiazines. *Am J Clin Pathol* 1990;93:771–775.
148. Walenga JM, Bick RL. Heparin-induced thrombocytopenia, paradoxical thromboembolism and other side effects of heparin therapy. *Cardiol Clin Annu Drug Ther* 1998;2:123–139.
149. Girolami B, Prandoni P, Rossi L, et al. Transaminase elevation in patients treated with unfractionated heparin or low molecular weight heparin for venous thromboembolism. *Clin Appl Thromb Hemost* 1998;4:126–128.
150. Schved JF, Dupuy-Fons C, Biron C. A prospective epidemiological study on the occurrence of antiphospholipid antibody: the Montpellier Antiphospholipid (MAP) Study. *Haemostasis* 1994;24:175–182.
151. Vila P, Hernandez MC, Lopez-Fernandez MF. Prevalence, follow-up and clinical significance of the anticardiolipin antibodies in normal subjects. *Thromb Haemost* 1994;72:209–213.
152. Bick RL, Ancypa D. The antiphospholipid and thrombosis syndromes: clinical and laboratory correlates. *Clin Lab Med* 1995; 15:63–84.
153. Falcon CR, Hoffer AM, Forastiero RR, et al. Clinical significance of various ELISA assays for detecting antiphospholipid antibodies. *Thromb Haemost* 1990;64:21–25.
154. Loizou S, McCrea JD, Rudge AC, et al. Measurement of anticardiolipin antibodies by an enzyme-linked immunosorbent assay (ELISA): standardization and quantitation of results. *Clin Exp Immunol* 1985;62:738–745.
155. Reyes H, Dearing L, Bick RL, et al. Laboratory diagnosis of antiphospholipid syndromes. *Clin Lab Med* 1995;15:85–108.
156. Triplett DA. Laboratory evaluation of circulating anticoagulants. In: Bick RL, Bennett RM, Brynes RK, eds. *Hematology: clinical and laboratory practice.* St. Louis: CV Mosby, 1993:1539–1548.
157. Mannucci PM, Canciani MT, Mari D, et al. The varied sensitivity of partial thromboplastin and prothrombin time reagents in the demonstration of the lupus-like inhibitor. *Scand J Haematol* 1979;22:423–432.
158. Bick RL, Pascoe HR, Laughlin WR. Efficacy of four common activated partial thromboplastin times in screening for the lupus anticoagulant. *Blood* 1994;84:82(abst).
159. Saxena R, Saraya AK, Kotte VK, et al. Evaluation of four coagulation tests to detect plasma lupus anticoagulants. *Am J Clin Pathol* 1991;96:755–758.
160. Exner T, Triplett DA, Taberner D, et al. Guidelines for testing and revised criteria for lupus anticoagulants. *Thromb Haemost* 1991;65:320–322.
161. Bell HG, Alton HG. A brain extract as a substitute for platelet suspensions in the thromboplastin generation test. *Nature* 1954;174:880–881.
162. Rauch J, Tannenbaum M, Janoff AS. Distinguishing plasma lupus anticoagulants from anti-factor antibodies using hexagonal (II) phase phospholipids. *Thromb Haemost* 1989;62: 892–896.
163. Cabral AR, Amigo MC, Cabiedes J, et al. The antiphospholipid/cofactor syndromes: a primary variant with antibodies to beta-2-glycoprotein-I but no antibodies detectable in standard antiphospholipid assays. *Am J Med* 1996;101:472–481.
164. Falcon CR, Hoffer AM, Carreras LO. Antiphosphatidylinositol antibodies as markers of the antiphospholipid syndrome. *Thromb Haemost* 1990;63:321–322.
165. Falcon CR, Hoffer AM, Carreras LO. Evaluation of the clinical and laboratory associations of antiphosphatidylethanolamine antibodies. *Thromb Res* 1990;59:383–388.
166. Sorice M, Circella A, Garofalo GT, et al. Anticardiolipin and anti-beta-2-GPI are two distinct populations of antibodies. *Thromb Haemost* 1996;75:303–308.
167. Martinuzzo ME, Forastiero RR, Carreras LO. Anti-beta-2-glycoprotein I antibodies: detection and association with thrombosis. *Br J Haematol* 1995;89:397–402.
168. Staub HL, Harris EN, Khamashta MA, et al. Antibody to phosphatidylethanolamine in a patient with lupus anticoagulant and thrombosis. *Ann Rheum Dis* 1989;8:166–169.
169. Wasserman LR, Gilbert HS. Complications of polycythemia vera. *Semin Hematol* 1966;3:199–208.
170. Jabaily J, Iland HJ, Laszlo J, et al. Neurologic manifestations of essential thrombocythemia. *Ann Intern Med* 1983;99:513–518.
171. Singh AK, Wetherly-Mein G. Microvascular occlusive lesions in primary thrombocythaemia. *Br J Haematol* 1977;36:553–564.
172. Conley CL. Polycythemia vera. *JAMA* 1990;263:2481–2483.
173. Cortelazzo S, Finazzi G, Ruggeri M, et al. Hydroxyurea for

patients with essential thrombocythemia and a high risk of thrombosis. *N Engl J Med* 1995;332:1132–1136.
174. Frenkel EP, Bick RL. Prothrombin G202010A gene mutation: heparin cofactor II defects, primary (essential) thrombocythemia and thrombohemorrhagic manifestations. *Semin Thromb Hemost* 1999;25:375–386.
175. Cortelazzo S, Viero P, Finazzi G, et al. Incidence and risk factors for thrombotic complications in a historical cohort of 100 patients with essential thrombocythemia. *J Clin Oncol* 1990;8: 556–562.
176. Sack GH Jr, Levin J, Bell WR. Trousseau's syndrome and other manifestations of chronic disseminated coagulopathy in patients with neoplasms: clinical, pathophysiologic and therapeutic features. *Medicine* 1977;56:1–37.
177. James WD. Trousseau's syndrome. *Int J Dermatol* 1984;23: 1–44, 205–206.
178. Bick RL, Kunkel L. Hypercoagulability and thrombosis. *Lab Med* 1992;23:233.
179. Hathaway W. Clinical aspects of antithrombin III deficiency. *Semin Hematol* 1991;28:19.
180. Bick RL. Disseminated intravascular coagulation. *Hematol Oncol Clin North Am* 1992;6:1259.
181. Bick RL, Baker WF. Disseminated intravascular coagulation syndromes. *Hematol Pathol* 1992;6:1.
182. Bick RL. *Disorders of thrombosis and hemostasis: clinical and laboratory practice.* Chicago: ASCP Press, 1992:175.
183. Kendall A, Lohmann R, Dosseter J. Nephrotic syndrome: a hypercoagulable state. *Arch Intern Med* 1971;127:1021.
184. Bick RL, McClain BJ. A comparison of the Protopath and DuPont ACA antithrombin III assays in 149 patients with DIC, deep vein thrombosis, and hereditary thrombophilia. *Am J Clin Pathol* 1984;82:371.
185. Menache D, O'Malley JP, Schorr JB, et al. Evaluation of the safety, recovery, half-life, and clinical efficacy of antithrombin III (human) in patients with hereditary antithrombin III deficiency. *Blood* 1990;75:33.
186. Vinazzer H. Hereditary and acquired antithrombin deficiency. *Semin Thromb Hemost* 1999;25:257.
187. Owen J. Antithrombin III replacement therapy in pregnancy. *Semin Hematol* 1991;28:46.
188. Vinnazer H. Antithrombin III in shock and disseminated intravascular coagulation. *Clin Appl Thromb Hemost* 1995; 257–263.
189. Schwartz RS, Bauer KA, Rosenberg RD, et al. Clinical experience with antithrombin III concentrate in treatment of congenital and acquired deficiency of antithrombin. *Am J Med* 1989; 87:53S.
190. Chaunsumrit A, Manco-Johnson MJ, Hathaway WE. Heparin cofactor II in adults and infants with thrombosis and DIC. *Am J Hematol* 1989;31:109.
191. Toulin P, Vitoux JF, Capron L. Heparin cofactor II in patients with deep venous thrombosis under heparin and oral anticoagulant therapy. *Thromb Res* 1988;49:479.
192. Grau E, Oliver A, Felez J. Plasma and urinary heparin cofactor II levels in patients with nephrotic syndrome. *Thromb Haemost* 1988;60:137.
193. Hirsh J, Hoak J. Management of deep vein thrombosis and pulmonary embolism: a statement for healthcare professionals. *Circulation* 1996;93:2212–2245.
194. Griffin JH. Clinical studies on protein C. *Semin Thromb Hemost* 1984;10:162.
195. Nicolaides AN. Prevention of venous thromboembolism: international consensus statement: guidelines complied in accordance with the scientific evidence. *Int Angiol* 2001;20:1.
196. Baker WF Jr, Bick RL. Deep vein thrombosis: diagnosis and management. *Med Clin North Am* 1994;82:685.
197. Broekmans AW, Bertina RM, Loeliger EA, et al. Protein C and the development of skin necrosis during anticoagulant therapy. *Thromb Haemost* 1983;49:251.
198. Zauber NP, Stark MW. Successful warfarin anticoagulation despite protein C deficiency and a history of warfarin necrosis. *Ann Intern Med* 1986;104:659–660.
199. Samama M, Horellou MH, Soria J, et al. Successful progressive anticoagulation in a severe protein C deficiency and previous skin necrosis at the initiation of oral anticoagulation treatment [Letter]. *Thromb Haemost* 1984;51:132–133.
200. Warkentin TE, Elavathil LJ, Hayward CP, et al. The pathogenesis of venous limb gangrene associated with heparin-induced thrombocytopenia. *Ann Intern Med* 1997;127:804–812.
201. Bick RL, Kaplan H. Syndromes of thrombosis and hypercoagulability: congenital and acquired thrombophilias. *Clin Appl Thromb Hemost* 1998;4:25–50.
202. Nizzi FA, Kaplan HS. Protein C and S deficiency. *Semin Thromb Hemost* 1999;25:265.
203. Heeb M, Mosher D, Griffin MH. Activation and complexation of protein C and cleavage and decrease of protein S in plasma of patients with intravascular coagulation. *Blood* 1989;73:455.
204. Schwarz HP, Schnernathaner G, Griffin JH. Decreased plasma levels of protein S in well-controlled type I diabetes mellitus. *Thromb Haemost* 1987;57:240.
205. Saito M, Kumabashiri I, Jokaji H. The levels of protein C and protein S in patients with type II diabetes mellitus. *Thromb Res* 1988;52:479.
206. Comp PC, Thurnau GR, Welsh J. Functional and immunological protein S levels are decreased during pregnancy. *Blood* 1986; 68:881.
207. Huisveld IA, Hospers JEH, Meijers JCM. Oral contraceptives reduce total protein S, but not free protein S. *Thromb Res* 1987; 45:109.
208. Vigano-D'Angelo S, D'Angelo A, Kaufman C. Protein S deficiency occurs in the nephrotic syndrome. *Ann Intern Med* 1987; 107:42.
209. D'Angelo A, Vigano-D'Angelo S, Esson CT, et al. Acquired deficiencies of protein S: protein S activity during oral anticoagulation, in liver disease, and in disseminated intravascular coagulation. *J Clin Invest* 1988;81:1445.
210. Conlan MG, Haire WD. Low protein S in essential thrombocythemia. *Am J Hematol* 1989;32:88.
211. Juhan-Vague I, Roul C, Alessi MC, et al. Increased plasminogen activator inhibitor activity in non-insulin dependent diabetic patients-relationship with plasma insulin. *Thromb Haemost* 1989;61:370.
212. Nalbandian RM, Henry RL, Bick RL. Thrombotic thrombocytopenic purpura: an extended editorial. *Semin Thromb Hemost* 1979;5:216.
213. Bick RL, Bishop RC, Shanbrom E. Fibrinolytic activity in acute myocardial infarction. *Am J Clin Pathol* 1972;57:359.
214. Collen D, Juhan-Vague I. Fibrinolysis and atherosclerosis. *Semin Thromb Hemost* 1988;14:180.
215. Mansfield MO. Alterations in fibrinolysis associated with surgery and venous thrombosis. *Br J Surg* 1972;59:754.
216. Bick RL, Thompson WB. Fibrinolytic activity: changes induced with oral contraceptives. *Obstet Gynecol* 1972;39:213.
217. Fareed J, Hoppensteadt DA, Jeske WP, et al. Acquired defects of fibrinolysis associated with thrombosis. *Semin Thromb Hemost* 1999;24:367.
218. Hedner U, Nilsson IM. Urokinase inhibitors in serum in a clinical series. *Acta Med Scand* 1971;1989:185–189.
219. Nilsson IM, Tehgborn LA. A family with thrombosis associated with high level of tissue plasminogen activator inhibitor. *Haemostasis* 1984;14:24.

220. Petaja M, Rasi V, Myllyla G. Familial hypofibrinolysis and venous thrombosis. *Br J Haematol* 1989;71:393.
221. Kirschstein W, Simianer S, Dempfle CE. Impaired fibrinolytic capacity and tissue plasminogen activator release in patients with restenosis after percutaneous transluminal coronary angioplasty (PTCA). *Thromb Haemost* 1989;62:772.
222. de Jong E, Porte RJ, Knot EA: Disturbed fibrinolysis in patients with inflammatory bowel disease. *Gut* 1989;30:188.
223. Robinson BW. Production of plasminogen activator by alveolar macrophages in normal subjects and patients with interstitial lung disease. *Thorax* 1988;43:508.
224. Duffy MJ, O'Grady P, Devaney D. Urokinase-plasminogen activator, a marker for aggressive breast carcinomas. *Cancer* 1988;62:531.
225. Kjaeldgaard A, Larsson B. Long-treatment with combined oral contraceptives and cigarette smoking associated with impaired activity of plasminogen activator. *Acta Obstet Gynecol Scand* 1986;65:219.

Disorders of Thrombosis and Hemostasis: Clinical and Laboratory Practice, Third Edition, edited by Rodger L. Bick.
Lippincott Williams & Wilkins, Philadelphia © 2002

15

THROMBOPROPHYLAXIS AND THROMBOSIS IN MEDICAL, SURGICAL, TRAUMA, AND OBSTETRIC/GYNECOLOGIC PATIENTS

RODGER L. BICK
SYLVIA K. HAAS

THROMBOSIS

Thrombosis is the most common single cause of death in the United States. More than two million individuals die each year from an arterial or venous thrombosis or the consequences thereof (1). About an equal number have nonfatal thrombosis [for example, deep vein thrombosis (DVT), nonfatal pulmonary embolus (PE), nonfatal cerebrovascular thrombosis (CVT), transient cerebral ischemic attacks (TIAs); 40% of these will have a fatal or nonfatal CVT within 1 year] (2), nonfatal coronary artery thrombosis, retinal vascular thrombosis (RVT), and other nonfatal thrombotic episodes. These numbers emphasize the scope of the problem; by contrast, about 560,000 will die this year in the United States from cancer; thus fatal thrombosis is about 4 times as prevalent as fatality from malignancy (1). Thrombosis therefore accounts for extraordinary morbidity, mortality, and cost of medical care (1). Many, if not most, episodes of thrombosis can be prevented by appropriate primary antithrombotic therapy; almost all instances of recurrence also can be prevented by appropriate choice of secondary therapy (3). About 80% to 90% of all unexplained episodes of venous thrombosis (nontraumatic and nonsurgical) and about 65% of arterial thromboses are associated with a blood-coagulation protein or platelet defect that can now be defined with respect to etiology (3,4). Of these, about 50% of all patients have a congenital and about 50% have an acquired blood-coagulation protein or platelet defect that caused or predisposed to the thrombotic event (1,3). To appreciate the scope of the problem, specific examples follow. The incidence of DVT in the United States is about 159 per 100,000 or about 450,000 per year. The overall incidence of PE in the United States is about 139 per 100,000 or about 355,000 cases per year (clinical data); the incidence of fatal PE in the United States is 94 per 100,000 or about 240,000 deaths (autopsy data) (5–8). The incidences of fatal and nonfatal thrombotic events are summarized in Table 15.1. The etiologies of hypercoagulability and overt thrombosis are becoming more clear and often definitive with enhanced knowledge of hemostasis and the development and extended use of testing systems for evaluating patients with thrombotic and thromboembolic disorders (9). With these test systems, in conjunction with careful clinical assessment of patients, about 80% to 90% of patients with thrombosis will have a defined etiology (1,3,4). Many of these will have an obvious clinical condition leading or contributing to thrombosis, and at least 50% to 80% will have an underlying hereditary or acquired blood-protein/platelet defect causing or predisposing to thrombosis. Many clinical conditions are associated with an increased risk of arterial or venous thrombosis and thromboembolism; the more common of these are summarized in Table 15.2 (1). It must be appreciated, however, that in many instances, clinical situations associated with thrombosis simply serve to unmask a congenital or acquired blood-coagulation protein/platelet defect in the patient. Cost-containing and effective management of thrombosis, reducing morbidity, mortality, and costs centers around three interrelated areas: (a) clear definition of the etiology or contributing factor(s) of thrombosis, (b) appropriate primary and then subsequent prophylactic therapy for acute events, and (c) appropriate secondary prevention (prevention of recurrence).

R. L. Bick: Department of Medicine and Pathology, University of Texas Southwestern Medical Center; Dallas Thrombosis/Hemostasis Clinical Center; ThromboCare Laboratories, Dallas, Texas.

S. K. Haas: Institut fur Experimentelle Onkologie und Therapieforschung, Technische Universität München, Munich, Germany.

TABLE 15.1. INCIDENCE OF THROMBOSIS IN UNITED STATES

Disease	U.S. Incidence/100,000	Total in United States/Year (Cases)	Definable Reason
Deep vein thrombosis (DVT)	159/100,000	450,000	≈80%
Pulmonary embolus (PE)	139/100,000	355,000	≈80%
Fatal pulmonary embolus	94/100,000	240,000	≈80%
Myocardial infarction (AMI)	600/100,000	1,500,000	≈67%
Fatal myocardial infarction	300/100,000	750,000	≈67%
Cerebrovascular thrombosis (CVT)	600/100,000	1,500,000	≈30%
Fatal cerebrovascular thrombosis	396/100,000	990,000	≈30%
Total serious thromboses in United States	1,498/100,000	5,785,000	≈50%
Total deaths from these thromboses	790/100,000	1,990,000	≈50%
All cancer in United States, 1996	544/100,000	1,359,150	
Cancer deaths in United States, 1996	222/100,000	554,740	

Definition of Etiology

Most instances of initial arterial and venous thrombosis are unexplained (unassociated with surgery, trauma, cardiac emboli, etc.). Most instances of first-event thrombosis are expensive with respect to cost of care; national average costs for DVT and PE, per episode (admission), are presented in Table 15.3 (10). An appreciation of these per-episode costs of care allows one to appreciate cost savings per patient for each primary or recurrent episode, which can often be prevented. Only by defining the etiology/predisposing factor(s) can appropriate primary and secondary therapy be provided to patients.

The common and rarer blood-coagulation protein/platelet defects leading to thrombosis are summarized in Table 15.4. In viewing this table, it must be remembered that most instances of thrombosis are without a clinical etiology, but often a clinical event associated with thrombosis is simply unmasking an underlying blood-coagulation protein/platelet defect already in the patient. The hereditary and acquired thrombophilias are discussed in Chapters 13 and 14.

TABLE 15.2. CLINICAL CAUSES OF THROMBOSIS

Clinical Conditions: Arterial	Clinical Conditions: Venous
Atherosclerosis	General surgery
Cigarette smoking	Orthopedic surgery
Hypertension	Arthroscopy
Diabetes mellitus	Trauma
LDL cholesterol	Malignancy
Hypertriglyceridemia	Immobility
Positive family history	Sepsis
Left ventricular failure	Congestive heart failure
Oral contraceptives	Nephrotic syndrome
Estrogens	Obesity
Lipoprotein (a)	Varicose veins
Polycythemia	Postphlebitic syndrome
Hyperviscosity syndromes	Oral contraceptives
Leukostasis syndromes	Estrogens
Thrombocythemia	Thrombocythemia

LDL, low-density lipoprotein.

Cost Containment

It is obviously of major importance to define individuals with these defects, as this allows (a) appropriate secondary antithrombotic therapy to decrease risks of recurrence, (b) determination of length of time the patient must remain on therapy for secondary prevention, and (c) testing of family members in those with a hereditary blood-coagulation protein or platelet defect (about 50% of all coagulation and platelet defects mentioned earlier), thus allowing primary prevention in appropriate relatives. The prevalence, as far as is known at present, of coagulation protein/platelet defects in common thrombotic disorders is shown in Table 15.5; this incidence will likely increase with additional prevalence/epidemiologic studies and certain subsequent discoveries of new defects (3,4,11).

Aside from mortality, significant additional morbidity occurs from both arterial or venous thrombotic events, including, but not limited to, paralysis (nonfatal thrombotic stroke), cardiac disability (repeated coronary events), loss or impairment of vision (retinal vascular thrombosis), recurrent miscarriage syndrome (placental vascular thrombosis), and stasis ulcers and other manifestations of postphlebitic syndrome (recurrent DVT), etc. It must be remembered and emphasized that a diagnosis of thrombosis is similar to and as generic as a diagnosis of "anemia"; one must, in all instances, as in anemia, ask next, *What is the etiology of the thrombosis?* (8). As in anemia, the specific and appropriate therapy is highly dependent on defining the etiology (8). Arterial and venous thrombosis can no longer be viewed as a generic diagnosis; approaching thrombosis in a generic manner probably accounts for not only

TABLE 15.3. COST AND LOS PER ADMISSION

Disease	Average Cost	Average Los
Deep vein thrombosis (DVT)	$9,337.00	6.3
Pulmonary embolus (PE)	$12,795.00	7.42

LOS, length of stay in days (United States).

TABLE 15.4. BLOOD PROTEIN/PLATELET DEFECTS LEADING TO THROMBOSIS

Antiphospholipid syndrome
APC resistance (factor V Leiden)
Sticky platelet syndrome
Prothrombin 20210A
MTHFR mutations
Protein S defects
Protein C defects
Antithrombin defects
Heparin cofactor II defects
Plasminogen defects
Factor XII defects
Dysfibrinogenemia
Homocystinemia
Lipoprotein A
Tissue plasminogen activator (t-PA) defects
Plasminogen activator inhibitor (PAI-1) defects
Tissue factor pathway inhibitor (TFPI) defects

APC, activated protein C; MTHFR, methylene tetrahydrofolate reductase.

many treatment failures, but also often confusing and conflicting results of clinical trials. Failure to make a specific diagnosis accounts for enhanced morbidity and mortality and exorbitant unnecessary medical costs for recurrent episodes. Most clinicians and investigators approaching thrombosis as a generic diagnosis fail to note that a very heterogeneous population is likely to be present, and outcomes will depend on designing therapy specific for a given etiology. For example, it is senseless to treat patients with thrombosis and sticky platelet syndrome with heparin or warfarin when they need only aspirin (12,13), nor would it make sense to treat a patient with antiphospholipid syndrome and thrombosis with aspirin (no response) or warfarin (65% failure rate) (4,14) when they respond most ideally to low molecular weight heparin (LMWH) or unfractionated heparin (UFH) and eventually potential long-term clopidogrel (4,14,15). Defining the defect and instituting appropriate therapy will save a minimum of $2,900,000.00 per 1,000 patients with DVT (3,8,16). The cost of defining the common blood-coagulation protein defects in these patients is $1,000.00 to $3,500.00 per patient (3,8,16). Thus an average cost of $1,100.00 × 1,000 DVT patients ($1,100,000) will save a minimum of $2,900,000.00 (1,3,8,16). A cost of $1,100.00 per 100 CVT patients ($110,000.00) will save a minimum of $350,000.00 (3,8,16–18). This does not account for additional savings such as rehabilitation, long-term care, long-term wound care for stasis ulcers/infection, etc., and thus the savings in morbidity is extraordinary and priceless.

Deep Vein Thrombosis

The incidence of DVT in the United States is about 159 per 100,000 or about 450,000 per year (5,6). A definable etiology can be found in 80% to 90% of these patients; this allows effective therapy to be delivered and allows the other advantages of defining the blood-coagulation protein or platelet defects, mentioned earlier, to be instituted. For example, about 28% of these patients will have antiphospholipid syndrome, and treatment with oral anticoagulants will fail in about 55% to 65% (recurrent thrombosis will develop while taking warfarin therapy) (4). Each of these failures will be readmitted at a cost of about $6,000.00 to $7,000.00, with an average length of stay (LOS) in the United States of about 6 to 7 days. About 30% to 50% of these patients also will have congenital coagulation protein or platelet defects; thus family members should be assessed

TABLE 15.5. PREVALENCE OF COAGULATION PROTEIN/PLATELET DEFECTS ASSOCIATED WITH THROMBOSIS IN COMMON DISORDERS

Defect	DVTPE (%)	CVT (%)	TIA (%)	CAT (%)	RVT (%)
Antiphospholipid syndrome	29	65	28.5	18	60
APC resistance (factor V Leiden)	18	3	14	?	7
Sticky platelet syndrome	14	19	30	18	13
Prothrombin 20210A	7	7	?	6	?
Protein S deficiency	6	?	?	7	?
Protein C deficiency	5.5	?	?	12	?
Antithrombin deficiency	4	3	?	5	?
t-PA deficiency	?	1	11	16	13
PAI-1 elevation	?	—	?	11	7
Plasminogen deficiency	2	?	?	?	?
Dysfibrinogenemia	?	?	?	?	?
Homocystinemia	?	?	?	?	?
Lipoprotein (a)	?	?	?	?	?
MTHFR mutations	?	?	?	?	?

DVT, deep vein thrombosis; PE, pulmonary embolus; CVT, cerebrovascular thrombosis; TIA, transient ischemic attacks; CAT, coronary artery thrombosis; RVT, retinal vascular thrombosis; APC, activated protein C; t-PA, tissue plasminogen activator; PAI, plasminogen activator inhibitor; MTHFR, methylene tetrahydrofolate reductase.

and spared a first event by instituting appropriate therapy at appropriate times, depending on clinical status [oral contraceptives, hormone-replacement therapy (HRT), impending surgery, trauma, etc.] (3). Obviously, antithrombotic therapy for the afflicted patient should generally be over the long term, not 6 weeks to 3 months (18). The cost of an evaluation for the common blood-coagulation protein/platelet defects is about $1,100.00 to $3,500.00; this is minimal when considering that if the patient has antiphospholipid syndrome (about 28% of patients with DVT/PE), warfarin or antiplatelet therapy will fail for 55% to 65% of patients, but low-dose subcutaneous porcine heparin every 12 hours or subcutaneous LMWH every 24 hours will fail for fewer than 1%. About 14% of DVT/PE patients will have sticky platelet syndrome (SPS), and warfarin or heparin/LMWH will fail for almost all, but aspirin (ASA) at 81 mg/day will fail for fewer than 1% (12,13). Activated protein C resistance defects (factor V Leiden, factor V Cambridge, factor V HR2 mutation, or factor V Hong Kong), protein C and S, and antithrombin deficiency, and prothrombin G20210A mutation are probably best treated with warfarins, unless recurrence occurs. Then LMWH is preferred. The rarer defects mentioned in Table 15.5 are probably best treated with warfarin or long-term heparin/LMWH, although more studies are needed to define ideal therapy for many. Thus the importance of effective therapy and the cost of effective therapy is negligible compared with the cost of recurrence, the morbidity of recurrence, and the impact on the quality of life. In addition, if simply offering "generic therapy," usually in the form of initial inpatient heparin for 5 to 7 days, followed by outpatient warfarin for 6 weeks to 6 months, those with blood-coagulation protein/platelet defects refractory to warfarin will have repeated thrombosis, and in 40% of these, chronic venous insufficiency (postphlebitic syndrome) will then develop; the sequelae of postphlebitic syndrome consist of a life-long experience of recurrent DVT/PE, often requiring multiple admissions, potential development of stasis ulcers requiring vigorous wound care and long-term expensive antibiotics, and other supportive therapy (19,20). The costs of allowing unnecessary recurrence and development of chronic venous insufficiency are exorbitant beyond calculations; the morbidity and potential mortality also are devastating. The cost containment for appropriately defining the precise etiology (blood-coagulation protein/platelet defect) in DVT/PE patients is summarized in Table 15.6. The approximate costs of heparin, LMWH, warfarin and ASA therapy are summarized in Table 15.7 (21,22).

TABLE 15.6. COST REDUCTION BY PREVENTION OF RECURRENCE (USE OF APPROPRIATE SECONDARY THERAPY)

Deep Vein Thrombosis	Cost of Acute Care
Deep vein thrombosis; 100 events/yr	$933,700.00
Assume 70% are candidates for evaluation	$636,690.00
Assume 80% have treatable findings	$522,872.00
Cost of evaluation	($75,950.00)
Savings per 100 DVT patients	$446,922.00

DVT, deep vein thrombosis.

TABLE 15.7. COSTS OF COMMON ANTITHROMBOTIC DRUGS: (FOR 5 DAYS OF THERAPY)

Drug	Cost
Unfractionated heparin[a]	$210.00
Low-molecular-weight heparin[b]	$209.60
Warfarin (coumadin @ 7.5 mg/day)[c]	$28.05
Aspirin (81 mg)	0.45

PTT, partial thromboplastin time; INR, international normalized ratio.
[a]Includes daily PTT at 1992 cost ($35.00) and intravenous or dose-adjusted.
[b]Assumes 70-kg patient (dalteparin).
[c]Assumes one prothrombin time (INR).

Prophylaxis

Numerous studies have provided evidence that patients who undergo surgery or trauma are at significant risk for developing venous thromboembolic complications, including PE, and that trauma, obstetric, gynecologic, and general medical patients also are at risk. Thus an important task for the clinician is to prevent DVT and its complications and morbid sequelae (PE, chronic venous insufficiency, compartmental compression syndromes, stasis ulcers, and other morbidity and mortality). It is important to define risk groups by quantifying risk(s) when possible, where prophylaxis must be considered. Unfortunately, the attitudes and opinions, and occasionally "myths" regarding prophylaxis show immense regional variability (23). Variations include the definition of risk groups, the numbers of patients receiving prophylaxis, and the prophylactic modalities used. Because of this, various "consensus conference" groups have been formed in attempts to alleviate these problems. Formerly there were at least three consensus conference groups, the American College of Chest Physicians (ACCP, begun in 1986) (24), the European Consensus Conference Groups (begun in 1991) (25), and the Scandinavian Consensus Conference Group (begun in 1995) (26). Since then, the International Consensus Conference group, derived from the European Group, has been formed and encompasses experts from the other groups (23,27). We tend to favor recommendations of the International Consensus Conference Group because of the wider base of expertise, the stronger emphasis on solid data, and the extensive experience of the European members in dealing with prophylaxis in surgery and trauma with low-dose UFH (LD-UFH) and LMWH, more than a decade longer experience than in

North America. The primary purpose of consensus guidelines is to provide optimal direction to the practicing physician/surgeon. If practice guidelines generated are successful, clinicians are assisted in decision making for individual patients and provided protection against unjustified malpractice actions (28). Guidelines should be considered "Standards of Care" if they meet five simple criteria: (a) they were developed for benefit of patient care and outcome, (b) they are supported by data from peer-reviewed medical literature, (c) they allow exceptions based on reasonable clinical judgment and clear medical (never financial) reasons for deviation, (d) there are no financial/cost-containment incentives/considerations in developing the guidelines, and (e) the guidelines are generally available to the majority of patients being considered (Table 15.8).

PE is responsible for approximately 150,000 to 240,000 deaths per year in the United States (29–31). The incidence of DVT in the United States is about 160/100,000 or 450,000 cases per year; about 30% to 50% of undetected, untreated DVT will progress to PE, and in about 40% with DVT, chronic venous insufficiency will develop, with the chances increasing about sixfold with each recurrent episode (1,20,32). Despite significant advances in prevention and treatment of venous thromboembolism (VTE; venous thrombosis with or without PE), PE remains the most common preventable cause of hospital death (33). VTE often occurs in the setting of surgery, trauma, and other medical conditions, but also may affect ambulant healthy individuals. Thus prevention is the key to reducing death and morbidity from VTE. Effective and safe prophylactic measures to prevent DVT, PE, and attendant sequelae are now available for most high-risk patients (34–36). Table 15.9 lists the ascending probability of DVT with surgical procedures and trauma (37). Recent studies revealed that despite innumerable consensus conference meetings and resultant publications, surgeons in the United States are apparently not yet offering appropriate prophylaxis to appropriate patients and appropriate numbers of patients (38,39). This chapter reviews and presents practical approaches to the prevention of VTE in surgical, trauma, obstetric, gynecologic, and general medical patients; the recommendations are based, largely but not totally, on recommendations of the International Consensus Groups and large clinical trials. For brevity, citations are limited to key studies, well-referenced reviews, and large analyses.

TABLE 15.8. GUIDELINES AND "STANDARDS OF CARE"

Guidelines may be considered standards of care if they meet the following criteria:
- They were developed for benefit of patient care and outcome
- They are supported by data from peer-reviewed medical literature
- They allow exceptions based on reasonable clinical judgment and clear medical (never financial) reasons for deviation
- There are no financial/cost-containment incentives/considerations in developing the guidelines
- The guidelines are generally available to the majority of patients being considered

TABLE 15.9. RISKS OF DVT IN SURGERY AND TRAUMA

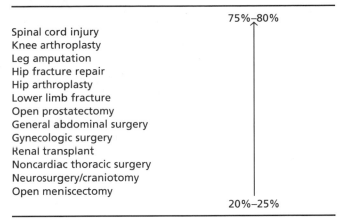

	75%–80% ↑
Spinal cord injury	
Knee arthroplasty	
Leg amputation	
Hip fracture repair	
Hip arthroplasty	
Lower limb fracture	
Open prostatectomy	
General abdominal surgery	
Gynecologic surgery	
Renal transplant	
Noncardiac thoracic surgery	
Neurosurgery/craniotomy	
Open meniscectomy	
	20%–25%

DVT, deep vein thrombosis.

VENOUS THROMBOEMBOLISM: THE PROBLEM AND THE NEED FOR PREVENTION

Numerous studies have provided evidence that surgical and medical patients are at risk of VTE, and therefore an important goal of clinical practice is to prevent DVT and its complications. Both epidemiologic and pathophysiologic data are important to allow accurate risk assessment and to define the patient groups that require prophylaxis.

When assessing risk, both the International Consensus Group (IC) and European Consensus Group (EC) classify patients according to exposing and predisposing risk factors for developing VTE. Patients are graded as low, medium, or high risk (Table 15.10). The Sixth ACCP Consensus Statement further refined these risk levels to highlight a group of patients at highest risk, including those with a history of VTE or malignant disease and major orthopedic surgery patients (Table 15.11) (40). In principle, introducing a fourth level of risk will refine the prophylactic regimen adopted and opti-

TABLE 15.10. LEVELS OF RISK

Risk of Thrombosis	Calf (%)	Proximal (%)	Fatal PE (%)
High risk (= 3)	40–80	10–30	>1
Moderate risk (= 2)	10–40	1–10	0.1–1.0
Low risk (= 1)	<10	<1	<0.1

PE, pulmonary embolism.

TABLE 15.11. CLASSIFICATION OF LEVEL OF RISK

	Risk			
	Calf Vein Thrombosis	Proximal Vein Thrombosis	Clinical PE	Fatal PE
Low	2%	0.4%	0.2%	0.002%
Uncomplicated minor surgery in patients 40 years old or younger with no clinical risk factors				
Moderate	10%–20%	2%–4%	1%–2%	0.1%–0.4%
Any surgery (major and minor) in patients 40–60 years old, but with no additional risk factors				
Major surgery in patients younger than 40 years but with no additional risk factors				
Minor surgery in patients with risk factors				
High	20%–40%	4%–8%	2%–4%	0.4%–1.0%
Major surgery in patients older than 60 years without additional risk factors				
Major surgery in patients 40 to 60 years old who have additional risk factors				
Patients with myocardial infarction and medical patients with risk factors				
Highest	40%–80%	10%–20%	4%–10%	1%–5%
Major surgery in patients older than 40 years plus prior VTE or malignant disease or hypercoagulable state				
Patients with elective major lower extremity orthopedic surgery, or hip fracture, or stroke, or multiple trauma, or spinal cord injury				

PE, pulmonary embolism; VTE, venous thromboembolism.

mize patient care, but it is unclear how this would be put into practice. Furthermore, the Sixth ACCP Consensus remains vague in some areas of risk classification (40).

Surgical Patients

During surgery, risk assessment is based on the exposing risk (type of surgery or trauma) and the predisposing risk (patient risk factors) (8,23,40). Major trauma, orthopedic surgery, and abdominal surgery procedures are the highest risk. Risk is further increased by predisposing factors such as increasing age, morbidity, malignancy, obesity, history of thromboembolism, varicose veins, inflammation, infection, HRT, oral contraceptives, venous stasis (such as "coach class syndrome") and thrombophilia, and modified by general care, including duration and type of anesthesia, pre- and postoperative immobilization, level of hydration, and the presence of sepsis.

Medical Patients

Although there are fewer available data compared with those for surgical patients, prospective studies have demonstrated that medical patients with acute myocardial infarction (AMI), stroke, and those treated in intensive care are also at increased risk of VTE (8). Recent studies provided firm evidence that certain acute medical illnesses are associated with an increased thromboembolic risk (8,42–45).

Recommendations for Thromboprophylaxis in Surgical and Medical Patients

Recommendations for VTE prophylaxis of surgical and medical patients include pharmacologic methods (including UFH, LMWH, aspirin, other antiplatelet agents, dextran, and warfarin) with or without mechanical methods [e.g., graduated compression stockings (GCSs) or intermittent pneumatic compression (IPC)]. Recommendations are graded A, B, or C according to the strength of clinical evidence (40).

There are no reported randomized trials of mechanical methods of prophylaxis such as GCSs or IPC in medical patients. Although there is no reason to believe that such methods would be less effective than in surgical patients, further studies are needed before clear recommendations can be made. All medical patients admitted to the hospital should be assessed for risk of VTE with predisposing and exposing risk factors (8,23), and prophylaxis considered for those at moderate or high risk.

Acute Myocardial Infarction

Low-dose and high-dose UFH can significantly reduce DVT in patients with AMI. According to the IC, antiplatelet therapy is recommended. In patients with AMI at high risk but in whom anticoagulants are contraindicated because of overt or high risk of bleeding, the addition of GCSs and/or IPC to aspirin may be considered. However, this is based on extrapolation of data from surgical patients (46). The Sixth ACCP Consensus recommended that subcutaneous LD-UFH or intravenous heparin be used in patients with AMI. These are grade 1A recommendations (40). Kher and Samama (43) recently addressed extended treatment with LMWHs in unstable coronary artery disease. These authors summarized as follows:

> In unstable angina, aspirin has been shown to reduce the incidence of death or acute myocardial infarction by more than 50%. Moreover, a meta-analysis of three randomized studies indicated that the risk of death or myocardial infarction was lower after 5 days of active treatment with both aspirin and unfractionated heparin than with aspirin alone.

LMWHs may be used as alternatives to unfractionated heparin. Several clinical trials strongly suggested that LMWHs are at least as effective as UFH in patients with unstable angina, with a number of advantages: subcutaneous administration, predictable and stable anticoagulant effect, and no need for laboratory monitoring. Evidence has been accumulated to support much longer periods of anticoagulant treatment than 5 to 6 days. Several studies have demonstrated a reactivation phenomenon of the underlying disease soon after discontinuation of heparin therapy, because of a persistent hypercoagulable state, which can last for several weeks after an acute episode of an unstable angina. In the FRISC trial, there was a further reduction in event rate with a prolonged once-daily treatment with dalteparin for 45 days, given only in patients with elevation of troponin T level on admission (high-risk patients). In the FRIC trial, no additional benefit was reported in using the same therapeutic regimen as in the FRISC trial. The reason was probably that this trial evaluated a lower risk population as compared with the previous one in the FRISC trial. Finally, in the TIMI IIB trial, no beneficial effect could be demonstrated with an extension of treatment with enoxaparin for 43 days. Several explanations were given to try to understand the lack of efficacy. For example, the dosage of enoxaparin was not adequate, and also patients at high risk were dropped from the prolonged-treatment phase because of early catheterization and revascularization. The remaining group of patients treated for 43 days was again at low risk. The FRISC II trial was a prospective, randomized, multicenter trial, comparing, according to a factorial design, invasive with noninvasive management and extended versus acute-phase dalteparin treatment in unstable coronary artery disease. On admission, all patients received aspirin, β blockers, calcium antagonists, and nitrates, according to clinical guidelines, and subcutaneous dalteparin, 120 IU/kg/12 hours, or UFH. At randomization, all patients were switched to the dalteparin regimen. In the selective noninvasive strategy, all continued the dalteparin regimen for 5 to 7 days and until an exercise test had been performed. In the early-intervention arm, the dalteparin was given for at least 5 days and always until the invasive procedure, which is usually performed within 7 days of admission. Thereafter, the randomized medication was given as twice-daily subcutaneous injections of either dalteparin or placebo. The randomized, twice-daily dose was 5,000 IU in women weighing less than 80 kg and men, less than 70 kg. Heavier patients received 7,500 IU twice daily. This treatment was given by self-injections for another 3 months. In this trial, 2,267 patients were included in the medical part of the study. The results at 3 months demonstrated a 19% relative and 12.3% absolute reduction in death or myocardial infarction in the dalteparin group, which was not statistically significant (p = 0.17). However, up to approximately 60 days during the prolonged treatment period, a clear difference in the incidence of death or MI was observed. At day 30, the results showed that the incidence of death or MI was 3.1% in the dalteparin group compared with 5.9% in the placebo group, a highly significant reduction of 47%, (p = 0.002). At 3 months there was a 13% reduction in death, MI, or revascularization, which was significant. The corresponding figure at day 30 was a 2% to 4% reduction in favor of dalteparin (p = 0.001). An increased risk of serious bleeding complications with extended dalteparin treatment compared with acute treatment (2.2% vs. 1.2%) was acceptable, given the clinical benefits. Importantly, as in the FRISC trial, the beneficial effect of extended treatment with dalteparin was confined to patients with elevated troponin T levels.

In the FRISC II trial, 2,457 patients were randomized to invasive compared with a noninvasive treatment. After 6 months, there was a decrease in the composite end point of death of MI of 9.4% in the invasive group (previously dalteparin-treated patients) compared with 12.1% in the noninvasive group (p = 0.031). After an invasive procedure, there was no benefit in continuing dalteparin in subsequent cardiac events. In the FRISC II trial, extended treatment with dalteparin, in addition to ASA and antiischemic medication, significantly reduced the risk of death and MI during the first 60 days of extended treatment. This benefit was still decreased at 90 days but was not significant. The authors concluded in their review,

> The dalteparin treatment can safely be used in patients who are candidates for percutaneous coronary intervention or coronary artery bypass surgery. The effects of long term dalteparin treatment are therefore useful for protection against further events while patients are waiting for invasive procedures. It is difficult to know if these excellent results are restricted to dalteparin or can be obtained by other LMWHs. A head-to-head comparison is required to answer this question.

Acute Stroke

Subcutaneous LD-UFH, LMWH, or heparinoid are effective in reducing the incidence of DVT in patients with ischemic stroke. However, it is essential to exclude intracranial hemorrhage before instituting thromboprophylaxis. In patients with hemorrhagic stroke, and in patients with ischemic stroke in whom the risks of prophylactic anticoagulant therapy are perceived to outweigh the benefits, GCSs and/or IPC are recommended, based on extrapolation of data from trials in neurosurgical patients and surgical patients (46). In patients with ischemic stroke and lower-extremity paralysis, LDUH and LMWH are effective. These are grade 1A recommendations. If anticoagulant prophylaxis is contraindicated, mechanical prophylaxis with elastic stockings (ESs) or IPC is recommended (grade 1C) (40). A recent venography-controlled study demonstrated that high-risk prophylactic doses of LMWH are more effective than LDUH in patients with lower-limb paresis due to acute ischemic stroke and are achieved without compromising patient safety (47,48).

Other Medical Patients

Patients with acute medical illnesses such as heart failure, chronic respiratory diseases, or severe chest infections, as well as critically ill patients, are at VTE risk. Prophylactic LDUH and high-dose LMWH prophylaxis are recommended in medical patients with disease-related risk factors and/or additional patient-related risk factors (46). This statement also is underlined by the latest ACCP Consensus, stating that in these patients, LDUH or LMWH is effective. These are grade A1 recommendations (40).

Two recent randomized, double-blind studies provided strong evidence that chronic respiratory disease and congestive heart failure patients are at significant risk of DVT. These trials suggested that once-daily high-dose LMWH provides effective prophylaxis (41,42). No trials described mechanical prophylaxis. Further studies are needed before clear recommendations can be made (46).

A recent meta-analysis confirmed the benefit of heparin prophylaxis in the prevention of VTE in internal medicine patients (excluding AMI or ischemic stroke). Seven randomized trials of UFH or LMWH in a total of 15,095 patients demonstrated a significant decrease in DVT and clinical PE as compared with controls. There was no significant difference in the incidence of major bleedings or deaths. Nine trials comparing LMWHs with UFH (4,559 patients) revealed that the efficacy of LMWHs assessed together was similar to that of UFH in terms of DVT, clinical PE, or mortality, but with reduced risk of major hemorrhage (45).

Efficacy of LMWH, low-dose subcutaneous UFH, or heparinoid in the prevention of DVT as documented by surveillance with objective methods (real-time color-flow Doppler, other ultrasound techniques, and/or phlebography) is established in acute medical patients (23,27,49).

Efficacy of LMWH or low-dose heparin (LDH), or moderate-dose UFH in reduction of total mortality in randomized studies of acute medical patients remains unclear. Most studies assessing the incidence of DVT in AMI were performed in the 1970s before the introduction of routine ASA and selective thrombolytic therapy. There is no evidence that earlier mobilization reduces the risk of DVT (50,51), but thrombolytic therapy and ASA have both been shown to reduce mortality. In addition, ASA reduces the rate of reinfarction and stroke. Some patients with AMI will receive full-dose anticoagulants (heparin and/or warfarin), either as prophylaxis to prevent rethrombosis in the coronary artery(s) after thrombolytic therapy or to prevent systemic embolism from a left ventricular mural thrombus (such as patients with anterior Q-wave infarction, severe left ventricular dysfunction, or mural thrombus at echocardiography) or from atrial fibrillation. In the absence of ASA, full-dose anticoagulants appear to be effective in preventing VTE, but there is no clear evidence that anticoagulants produce the additional benefit of PE reduction when given with ASA, which is now used routinely because of proven benefits. In patients with AMI who are at high risk for DVT but in whom anticoagulants are contraindicated because of overt or high risk of bleeding, the addition of GCSs and/or IPC to ASA may be considered (grade C recommendation based on extrapolation of data from trials in surgical patients) (23,27).

Risk-assessment guidelines for general medical patients are summarized in Fig. 15.1 (8,23).

In summary, it can be said that the European Consensus Statement, the ACCP Consensus 2001, the Scandinavian Consensus Statement 1995, and the International Consensus Statement 2001 had a great impact on the clinical acceptance of LMWHs by clinicians, physicians, and health authorities. In general, surgical and trauma patients with a risk score of 1.5 to 2.0 should be considered for prophylaxis, and if the score is greater than 2.0, prophylaxis is mandatory. The most effective prophylaxis, in descending order of efficacy, is LMWH [dalteparin (Fragmin), 2,500 to 5,000 anti-Xa units every 24 hours/enoxaparin (Lovenox) at 30 mg every 12 hours or 40 mg every 24 hours], followed by fixed LDUH at 2,500 to 5,000 units every 12 hours, followed by low-dose warfarin at a fixed dose of 1 mg every 24 hours or dose adjusted to prolong the prothrombin time by 1.5 to 3.0 seconds (29); GCS or IPC is less effective, but may be considered in those with contraindications to LMWH/LDUH [bleeding, history of heparin-induced thrombocytopenia (HIT), etc.].

Inferior vena cava filters have been used for almost 40 years for the potential prevention of PE and have been routinely inserted by the percutaneous route during the last decade, thus markedly increasing their use, with about 30,000 to 40,000 filters per year being placed in the United States (52–55). However, the widespread use of these filters for prevention of PE has been based on case reports, case studies, and uncontrolled, unblinded, and retrospective reviews. More recently, however, two randomized studies

EXPOSING RISK(S):

STROKE AGE > 70 CHF	*HIGH = 3*
IMMOBILITY HEART FAILURE OTHER THAN CONGESTIVE	*MODERATE = 2*
MINOR MEDICAL ILLNESSES	*LOW = 1*

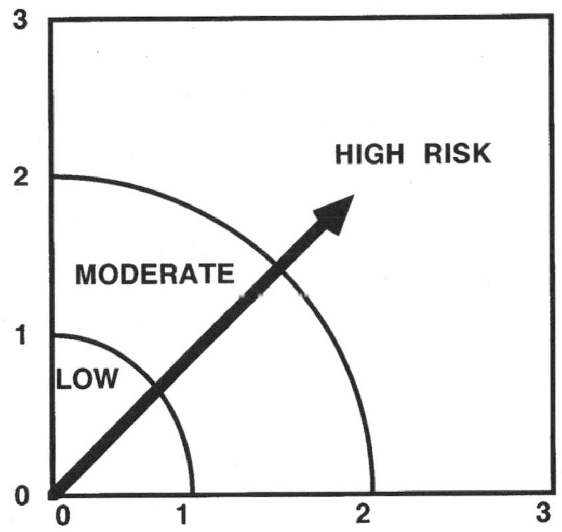

PREDISPOSING RISK(S):

HISTORY OF DVT / PE	1.5
AGE > 70 YEARS	1.5
THROMBOPHILIA*	1.5
MALIGNANCY	1.5
AGE > 60 YEARS	1.0
OBESITY	0.5
MAJOR VARICOSITIES	0.5
ESTROGENS / HRT	0.5
OC PILLS	0.5
INFLAMMATION / INFECTION	0.5

* = HEREDITARY OR ACQUIRED THROMBOPHILIA

FIGURE 15.1. Guidelines for risk assessment: general and orthopedic surgery.

were performed. The first demonstrated no difference in mortality between patients randomized to no filter versus filter, but did demonstrate a statistically significant increase in DVT at 2 years in those receiving filters (20.8% in filter group and 11.6% in no-filter group), suggesting that filters enhanced DVT but did not affect mortality from PE; another recent population-based analysis also demonstrated no benefit from filters with respect to mortality, but an enhanced risk of DVT (relative risk of DVT, 2.62 in the filter group and 1.14 in the no-filter group; this was also of statistical significance) (53,54). Thus it may be concluded that many filters (a) are placed unnecessarily, (b) do not reduce mortality from PE, and (c) increase significantly the chances of recurrent DVT. Perhaps the only true indication for a filter is in (a) the patient who has an absolute contraindication to any antithrombotic agent, or (b) a patient for whom the appropriate antithrombotic therapy fails, at the appropriate dose, for a specific thrombophilic disorder or risk factor(s). Clearly the indications for insertion of inferior vena cava filters must be much more clearly defined, as current use appears to do more damage (DVT) than good (any positive impact on mortality).

To assess risk in internal medicine patients, see guidelines in Fig. 15.1.

Treatment of Deep Vein Thrombosis

Cost-Effective Treatment of Deep Vein Thrombosis/Pulmonary Embolus

DVT is common, accounts for significant morbidity and moderate mortality through development of PE, and is associated with high costs of care, as previously delineated. Cost-effective and excellent care is possible by considering several important principles of therapy. This section is divided into cost-effective inpatient care for DVT with or without PE versus "early discharge"/outpatient care for DVT. There is not yet enough information to provide guidelines for outpatient management of PE. As a general principle, calf thrombosis should be treated the same as proximal vein thrombosis (50). Calf vein thrombosis, in the past, was treated by many with ASA, antiinflammatory, and local supportive measures; this is inappropriate treatment and not cost-effective. Although the majority of PE arise from proximal vein thrombosis, about 25% of PE arise from isolated calf vein thrombosis (51). Additional problems with calf vein thrombosis include propagation to proximal deep veins (30% of calf thrombi), destruction of or damage to venous valves, and subsequent late sequelae of chronic venous insufficiency (56). The goals of therapy for

DVT are arresting of thrombus growth; prevention of recurrence; limiting swelling, which may lead to compartmental compression syndrome with resultant interference with venous and arterial flow with gangrene/loss of limbs; and prevention of embolization, which may lead to significant morbidity (pulmonary hypertension, etc.) or mortality (50). The mainstay of initial treatment of DVT/PE is heparin/LMWH in some form (8,23). Thrombolytic therapy may be indicated for extensive or recurrent DVT/PE, as it clearly is associated with reduction in incidence of chronic venous insufficiency (56). However, costs and hemorrhagic complications limit indications for thrombolysis. Indications for thrombolysis have been reviewed (57,58) (see Chapter 19).

Inpatient Management of Acute Deep Venous Thrombosis/Pulmonary Embolus

In general, the initial therapy for inpatient care of DVT/PE is porcine mucosal unfractionated heparin (UFH) or fixed-dose LMWH. UFH may be given by the intravenous route or by a dose-adjusted subcutaneous (s.c.) route; the dose-adjusted s.c. route has clearly been shown to be equal to or better than the i.v. route (59–62). Intravenous UFH is given by i.v. bolus followed by infusion to maintain an activated partial thromboplastin time (aPTT) prolongation, which is equivalent to a therapeutic range of 0.30 to 0.70 anti-Xa units (50,59). Reliance on simple prolongation of the aPTT to 1.5 to 2.0 times baseline is no longer reliable with today's hypersensitive reagents and inconsistencies between collection in 3.2% and 3.8% citrate; thus all laboratories must calibrate the particular aPTT reagents used to a therapeutic anti-Xa range as defined earlier (23). Warfarin is started at the same time as i.v. UFH; UFH is continued for 5 days or longer and stopped when the international normalized ratio (INR) is approximately 2.0 for at least 48 hours (23). Dose-adjusted s.c. UFH is given as an s.c. injection every 12 hours, aiming for the same aPTT as mentioned earlier and initiating warfarin therapy as defined earlier. It should be noted that if using i.v. or dose-adjusted UFH for initial therapy for DVT/PE, it is imperative to reach a therapeutic range, as defined earlier, within 24 hours; if this is not achieved, the late recurrence is markedly increased (63). DVT/PE also may be treated with LMWH; in this instance, the dose is fixed and given every 12 hours or every 24 hours; the aPTT is not used to assess therapy, and the dose is not varied (50). Thus an aPTT is not needed. In general, heparin assays by anti-Xa assay also are unnecessary unless clinical changes suggest too much (hemorrhage) or too little (recurrence) LMWH or if the patient is unusually obese or small. See Table 15.12 for general indications for anti-Xa levels. With both modes of therapy (UFH or LMWH), frequent platelet counts are required to assure quick detection of heparin-induced thrombocytopenia, a rare complication of UFH or LMWH therapy and much less common with LMWH than with UFH (64).

TABLE 15.12. INDICATIONS FOR ANTI-XA LEVELS WITH LMW HEPARIN

Renal dysfunction
Hypotension/poor tissue perfusion
Obesity (>80 kg or BMI >30 kg/m^2)
Underweight (<50 kg or BMI <22 kg/m^2) or children
Change in clinical event(s) (bleeding/thrombosis/other)
Pregnancy

BMI, body mass index.

There have been more than 13 well-controlled double-blind randomized trials comparing UFH (i.v. or dose-adjusted s.c.) with LMWH for treatment of active DVT/PE (65–78). In all such trials, objective methods were used for initial diagnosis and confirmation of recurrence. These trials used a variety of LMWH preparations given once a day or twice a day, depending on brand. The results of these trials are summarized in Table 15.13. A meta-analysis of these trials demonstrated clear superiority of LMWH over UFH for treatment of active DVT (79). The recurrence rates are significantly reduced with LMWH, major hemorrhage (defined as intracranial bleed, retroperitoneal, required transfusion(s), caused disruption of therapy, necessitated surgery, or fatality) is significantly less, and mortality is significantly reduced. Because some of the studies included patients with PE, and others excluded PE, risk reduction of PE cannot be assessed in analysis of these trials. The magnitude of risk and cost reductions in the 4,354 patients assessed in these 13 trials is summarized in Table 15.13. The cost savings in risk reduction of recurrence in Table 15.13 is depicted as savings per 1,000 patients. The cost reduction in preventing major hemorrhage or development of chronic venous insufficiency is extraordinary and incalculable.

In summary, major cost containment and a major impact on quality of life through reduction of recurrence, reduction of bleeds, and reduction in development of

TABLE 15.13. SAVINGS USING LOW-MOLECULAR-WEIGHT HEPARIN VERSUS UNFRACTIONATED HEPARIN: RESULTS FROM 13 RANDOMIZED TRIALS

38.5% Reduction in recurrence	7.8% to 4.8%
45.1% Reduction in major bleeds	2% to 1.1%
24.7% Reduction in mortality	7% to 5.2%
Recurrent disease	
Cost/1,000 patients using UF heparin	$9,337,000.00
Cost/1,000 patients using LMW heparin	$6,535,900.00
Savings per 1,000 patients (recurrence reduction)	**$2,801,000.00**
Hemorrhage	
Cost/1,000 patients using UF heparin	$21,500.00
Cost/1,000 patients using LMW heparin	$11,825.00
Savings per 1,000 patients (bleeding reduction)	**$9,675.00**

LMW, low molecular weight; UF, unfractionated.

chronic venous insufficiency can be achieved by use of LMWH for inpatients with DVT with or without PE. Further cost containment is achieved by choosing appropriate long-term therapy for those patients with hereditary or acquired blood-coagulation protein/platelet defects causing DVT with or without PE, as discussed in the first section. It is unjustified and wasteful to give DVT/PE patients long-term warfarin after initial UFH or LMWH if they have a causative defect that is refractory to warfarin (e.g., antiphospholipid syndrome, SPS).

Outpatient/"Early Discharge" Management of Acute Deep Vein Thrombosis/Pulmonary Embolus

Recent studies have opened the door to another key question, perhaps the primary question of the next decade: What is the role of outpatient management for DVT? Particularly in North America, where cost containment, often driven by managed care, is of primary concern and clinicians are under increasing pressure to decrease costs through decreased hospital admissions, the recent publications presenting results of LMWHs in randomized trials demonstrating the clear safety and efficacy of home treatment or "early discharge" management of DVT have become of key interest (78,80–84). Suggested outpatient management guidelines for therapy are summarized in Table 15.14. There have been three well-designed randomized trials assessing inpatient treatment of DVT/PE with UFH versus outpatient management of DVT/PE with LMWH (82–84). These trials have included 1,104 patients, 550 treated in the outpatient LMWH group, and 554 in the inpatient group. There were 32 (5.8%) recurrences in the outpatient group and 37 (6.6%) recurrences in the inpatient group, representing a nonsignificant risk reduction of 12.2%. All bleeding was minor; there were 10 (1.8%) minor bleeds in the outpatient group and nine (1.6%) in the inpatient group. Unfortunately, two of the outpatient LMWH bleeds were accidental, consisting of a miscalculated 2.5× increased dose of LMWH and an intramuscular dose of LMWH. Assessing the trials and DVT patients in general, realistically only about 70% of DVT patients can be treated on an outpatient basis; the remaining 30% must be admitted because of comorbid conditions requiring hospitalization or must be admitted for 12 to 24 hours to initiate the items needed for successful outpatient management (discussed later); in this instance, those patients arriving late in the day at the physician office or hospital often require short-term admission to institute appropriate measures for successful outpatient therapy. Obviously if 70% of patients with DVT can be managed as outpatients, this represents a cost savings of about $4,900,000.00 per 1,000 patients with DVT. The following general principles of outpatient or "early discharge" management of DVT can be instituted, pending more results of randomized trials or, preferably, consensus-driven recommendations to provide additional information (Table 15.14).

TABLE 15.14. SUGGESTED GUIDELINES FOR OUTPATIENT MANAGEMENT OF DVT/PE

1. Admit for 24 h if no comorbid condition, or treat as outpatient if no comorbid condition and all below can be accomplished
2. CBC/platelet count on admission
3. Prothrombin time (PT/INR) and aPTT on admission
4. Teach patient applicable antiembolic exercises on admission (see below)
5. Start s.c. low-molecular-weight heparin (LMWH) as
   A. Dalteparin @ 200 U/kg q 24 h (available as 2,500 U/0.2 mL or 5,000 units/0.2 mL or multidose vials of 95,000 U/9.5 mL), Lindmarker regimen[a]
   OR
   B. Enoxaparin @ 1 mg/kg q 12 h (= 100 U/kg q 12 h) (30 mg or 40 mg amps): Levine regimen[b]
6. Instruct patient in self-injection of s.c. LMWH in anterior/lateral thighs or anterior abdominal wall (anterior or lateral thighs preferred, use rotating injection sites)
7. Measure for medium compression panty hose (LE) or upper extremity hose (UE) for use during waking hours only
8. Start warfarin @ 5 mg/day if <70 kg total body weight or 10 mg/day if >70 kg total body weight[c]
9. Discharge at 24 h if no comorbid conditions or discharge as soon as comorbid condition (not DVT) allows
10. Arrange home health care if patient/family cannot self-inject LMWH
11. Arrange outpatient prothrombin time/INR and CBC/platelet count at home or outpatient facility on days 3 and 5
12. Evaluate patient clinically (in office/clinic) on days 5 or 7; obtain prothrombin time/INR and CBC/platelet count days 5 and 7; stop LMWH when INR ≈2.0, and then adjust warfarin dose accordingly
13. See patient weekly until stable with long-term antithrombotic therapy
14. If young age patient (≤60) with unexplained DVT, consider evaluation for blood coagulation protein(s)/platelet defects (thrombophilia) leading to thrombosis
16. While hospitalized patient in bed, raise foot of bed, *straight,* with feet elevated 7 degrees to 10 degrees above hips; *never* put pillow(s) under popliteal fossae

[a]From Lindmarker P, Holmstrom KM, Granquist S, et al. Comparison of once-daily subcutaneous Fragmin with continuous intravenous unfractionated heparin in the treatment of deep vein thrombosis. *Thromb Haemost* 1994;72:186, with permission.
[b]From Levine M, Gent M, Hirsh J, et al. A comparison of low-molecular-weight heparin administered primarily at home with unfractionated heparin administered in the hospital for proximal deep-vein thrombosis. *N Engl J Med* 1996;334:677, with permission.
[c]Depending on clinical parameters (thrombophilia, platelet defects, etc., alternatives to oral anticoagulants may be indicated).
CBC, complete blood count; INR, international normalized ratio; aPTT, activated partial thromboplastin time; DVT, deep vein thrombosis.

Ancillary Measures for Management of Deep Venous Thrombosis

Several ancillary measures generally should be instituted for all patients with DVT of the extremities. These are use of medium compression pantyhose during waking hours for patients with lower extremity DVT, medium compression arm hose for those with upper extremity DVT, and the teaching of antiembolic exercises and correct body positioning as summarized later. These modalities, particularly appropriate exercises and body positioning, are of no or minimal cost and aid in preventing recurrence (16,23).

Antiembolic Leg Exercises

The patient should be instructed in antiembolic leg exercises consisting of dorsoplantar flexion of each foot at a time with the legs supported at the feet, legs straight and elevated above the hips approximately 7 to 10 degrees. These are to continue for 3 to 5 minutes, or until the calf-muscle group is fatigued, with initiation of muscle pain; then the opposite leg should be exercised in a similar manner. The patient should be told to do these exercises 4 to 6 times a day. The patient also should be instructed to not remain in a sitting position or indulge in other activities, such as car or airplane trips, with the thighs and knees bent, for more than 20 minutes at a time without straightening the legs through brief ambulation or leg stretching for a few minutes.

Antiembolic Arm Exercises

The patient should be instructed in antiembolic arm exercises consisting of palmar "squeezing" of each hand at a time with the arms elevated and straightened above the head. Holding a tennis ball in the hand, while squeezing, is excellent for this exercise. These should continue for 3 to 5 minutes, or until the arm muscles are fatigued, with initiation of muscle pain, and then the opposite arm should be exercised in a similar manner. The patient should be told to do these exercises 4 to 6 times a day. The patient also should be instructed to not remain in a position or indulge in other activities with the arms tightly bent at the elbow or shoulder for more than 20 minutes at a time, without stretching the arms straight for a few minutes.

Recent studies have demonstrated that home therapy can easily be accomplished by 70% to 80% of patients with both safety and efficacy and a high level of patient satisfaction is associated with home care of DVT (85,86).

Surgical Patients

General Surgery

Low Risk

The data are insufficient to make recommendations for low-risk general surgical patients. By extrapolation from studies in moderate-risk patients, some recommend use of GCSs in addition to early ambulation and adequate hydration (46). According to the Sixth ACCP Consensus, no specific prophylaxis other than early ambulation is recommended (grade 1C) (40).

Moderate Risk

Based on level I and level II data, low-dose heparin, LMWH, dextran, or ASA, with or without GCSs or continuous IPC, are recommended. Further studies should assess the relative benefit of GCSs or IPC in addition to pharmacologic methods and assess combined pharmacologic methods (heparin and ASA vs. heparin alone) (46). According to the Sixth ACCP Consensus, in moderate-risk general surgery patients who are undergoing minor procedures but have additional thrombosis risk factors, who have nonmajor surgery between the ages of 40 and 60 years, or who are undergoing major operations and are younger than 40 years with no additional clinical risk factors, it is recommended that LDUH, LMWH, IPC, or ESs be used. These are grade 1A recommendations (40). With regard to the recommendation of ESs, the European Working Group believes that the evidence on the efficacy of this modality in general surgery is meager and does not justify such a strong recommendation (87).

High Risk

Patients should receive prophylaxis as for moderate-risk patients (grade A, IC recommendation). In addition to single modalities, such as LDUH or LMWH, combined modalities of pharmacologic and mechanical methods should be considered (grade B, IC recommendation). In moderate-risk and high-risk patients, dextran and ASA are not the drugs of choice because of their limited efficacy for DVT prevention (46). According to the Sixth ACCP Consensus, in higher-risk general surgery patients who are older than 60 years or with additional risk factors or patients undergoing major surgery aged 40 to 60 years or with additional risk factors, it is recommended that LDUH, LMWH, or IPC be used. These are grade 1A recommendations. In higher-risk general surgery patients with a greater than usual risk of bleeding, the use of mechanical prophylaxis with ESs or IPC is recommended. This is a grade 1A recommendation (40).

In very-high-risk general surgery patients with multiple risk factors, it is recommended that effective pharmacologic methods (LDUH or LMWH) be combined with ESs or IPC. This is a grade 1C recommendation based on small studies and on extrapolation of data from other patient groups.

In selected very-high-risk general surgery patients, postdischarge LMWH or perioperative warfarin (INR, 2.0 to 3.0) therapy may be considered (grade 2C) (40).

Orthopedic Surgery

Clinical evidence concerning elective hip and knee surgery, hip fractures, major trauma, and arthroscopic surgery was recently reviewed (88).

Total Hip Replacement

The incidence of total DVT detected by venography after total hip replacement without prophylaxis is in the range of

51% [95% confidence interval (CI), 47 to 55]. A wide range of mechanical and pharmacologic prophylactic agents has been investigated (40). Of the mechanical methods, only IPC has been shown to be effective (40,46), although the incidence of proximal DVT is lower when pharmacologic prophylaxis is used (88). No increase in bleeding risk is associated with IPC use, but patient compliance after ambulation is problematic. GCSs alone are inadequate, but may be beneficial in combination with other approaches (88).

The Sixth ACCP Consensus recommended the use of LMWH (started 12 hours before surgery, 12 to 24 hours after surgery, or 4 to 6 hours after surgery at half the usual high-risk dose) or adjusted-dose warfarin, with a target INR of 2.0 to 3.0, started preoperatively or immediately after surgery. Adjusted-dose UFH started preoperatively may be used as an acceptable but more complex alternative (grade 2A). The use of ESs or IPC may provide additional efficacy (grade 2A). The use of LDUH, ASA, dextran, and IPC is not recommended because these options are less effective, although they may reduce the overall incidence of VTE (40). These recommendations are compatible with those of the International Consensus Panel (46).

The relative benefit of extending the duration of prophylaxis has been investigated, given the continuing trend toward early discharge. Four European studies demonstrated that venographically proven DVT was significantly reduced when patients received LMWH for up to 4 weeks after hospital discharge, compared with placebo (88). However, two recent cohort studies of patients receiving in-hospital prophylaxis for 9 to 14 days without extended outpatient prophylaxis confirmed a low incidence of clinical VTE after hip surgery. Although these cohort studies suggest that extended prophylaxis after total hip replacement surgery may not be necessary (88), the ACCP recommended additional trials in which objectively documented symptomatic VTE is the primary efficacy end point. For some Europeans, however, this seems like "going back to the future," because most of the recommendations of the ACCP Consensus are based on studies with surrogate end points. The question is not settled, and trying to reach a consensus may be premature (87).

Total Knee Replacement

Although it is performed more frequently than total hip replacement, there have been fewer randomized clinical trials of knee-replacement prophylaxis. IPC is effective, applied during or immediately after surgery, although compliance after early ambulation may be a problem. Five studies, comparing LMWH with either placebo or warfarin, all showed a decreased incidence of total DVT but no difference between the incidence of proximal DVT when using LMWH or warfarin. No studies have been published on the use of extended prophylaxis after discharge (88). The current ACCP recommendation is for LMWH, warfarin, or IPC. The use of LDUH is not recommended (40). The IC recommends IPC and LMWH, the latter being more effective than either warfarin or LDUH (46).

Hip Fracture

LDUH, LMWH, and adjusted-dose warfarin are effective. The incidence of VTE is higher in patients who have delayed fixation, so early intervention is important. Bleeding remains a concern (11). The current recommendations of the ACCP are for LMWH or adjusted-dose warfarin (grade 1B because the available data are limited). The use of LDUH may be an alternative option, but this is a grade 2B recommendation based on the very limited available data. The use of ASA alone is not recommended because it is less efficacious than other approaches (40). The IC recommends UFH, LMWH, a heparinoid, oral anticoagulants, dextran, and antiplatelet therapy. The limited effect of dextran and ASA on the incidence of DVT suggests these are not the drugs of choice (46).

Major Trauma

The current ACCP recommendation is for the use of LMWH if there is no contraindication (grade 1A). If LMWH prophylaxis will be delayed or is contraindicated because of concerns about bleeding, it is recommended that initial prophylaxis with a mechanical modality (ESs and/or IPC) be used (grade 1C) (40). The recommendations of the IC include UFH, LMWH, one heparinoid, and oral anticoagulants. Although dextran and ASA therapies were partially effective, they are not recommended (46).

Arthroscopic Surgery

Although case-finding studies have demonstrated that both proximal and distal DVT occur after arthroscopic surgery, and there are anecdotal reports of significant VTE, no clinical trials have determined the most appropriate form of prophylaxis (88).

Neurosurgery

VTE is a common complication of neurosurgery and is frequent with brain or spinal tumors. Recent trials and a meta-analysis indicated that LMWH and compression stockings in combination may be the method of choice in high-risk neurosurgery patients, a combination that balances bleeding risk with antithrombotic efficacy. The efficacy and safety of UFH, and the relative value compared with LMWH, have not been properly assessed (89). The Sixth ACCP consensus strongly recommended that IPC with or without ESs be used in patients undergoing intracranial neurosurgery (grade 1A). LMWH and LDUH may be acceptable alternatives. The combination of physical (IPC or ESs) and pharmacologic (LMWH or LDUH) prophylaxis modalities may be more effective than either modality alone in high-risk patients (40).

There are a number of unresolved issues regarding the prevention of VTE in neurosurgery, including the optimal duration of prophylaxis and the choice of the primary efficacy end point. Prophylaxis after hospital discharge may be of particular value, as a proportion of patients after surgery are left with a neurologic deficit such as hemiparesis or hemiparalysis (89). The clinical value of a venography-detected DVT remains unclear, and it is uncertain whether a reduction reflects a real advantage in term of clinical outcome. A large study to investigate the rate of clinical outcomes such as symptomatic VTE and major bleeding is required in patients undergoing elective neurosurgery (89).

Concerns about bleeding complications continue to limit the broad application of thromboprophylaxis after neurosurgery. Available LMWH clinical data seem to indicate that the risk of bleeding is positively balanced by the advantage in terms of prevention of VTE. However, although these trials were designed with sufficient statistical power to detect differences in efficacy, they were not of sufficient size to address differences in bleeding risk between LMWH and placebo. Moreover, patients with excessive surgery-related bleeding and potential risk factors for bleeding were excluded, as were patients undergoing neurosurgery for cerebral trauma or intracranial bleeding. Data concerning the safety of LMWH do not apply to these patients (89).

Generally, without prophylaxis, the frequency of fatal PE ranges from 0.1% to 0.8% in patients undergoing elective general surgery (29,90–94), 2% to 3% in patients undergoing elective hip replacement (95), and 4% to 7% in patients undergoing surgery for a fractured hip (96). Guidelines for risk assessment in general and orthopedic surgery are defined in Table 15.10 (23). The risk of postoperative DVT can be identified as low, moderate, or high, depending on the surgical procedure and the presence or absence of additional risk factors (23,91). See Figs. 15.2 and 15.3 for guidelines for assessing risk in general, orthopedic, and gynecologic surgery patients.

Surgery for major trauma or orthopedic surgery, followed by abdominal surgery, is associated with a risk of up to 30% (29). However, the degree of risk is increased by predisposing risk factors, including age, morbidity, malignancy, obesity, history of thromboembolism, immobility, varicose veins, recent operative procedures, and hereditary or acquired thrombophilia (8,23). These factors are further modified by general care including duration and type of anesthesia, pre- and postoperative immobilization, level of

EXPOSING RISK(S):

HIP / KNEE ARTHROPLASTY MAJOR SURGERY	*HIGH = 3*
SURGERY > 30 MIN. AGE > 40 FEMORAL FRACTURE IMMOBILIZING PLASTER CAST	*MODERATE = 2*
SURGERY < 30 MIN. TRAUMA / TIBIAL FRACTURES AMBULATORY PLASTER CAST ARTHROSCOPY	*LOW = 1*

PREDISPOSING RISK(S):

HISTORY OF DVT / PE	1.5
AGE > 70 YEARS	1.5
THROMBOPHILIA*	1.5
MALIGNANCY	1.5
AGE > 60 YEARS	1.0
OBESITY	0.5
MAJOR VARICOSITIES	0.5
ESTROGENS / HRT	0.5
OC PILLS	0.5
INFLAMMATION / INFECTION	0.5

* = HEREDITARY OR ACQUIRED THROMBOPHILIA

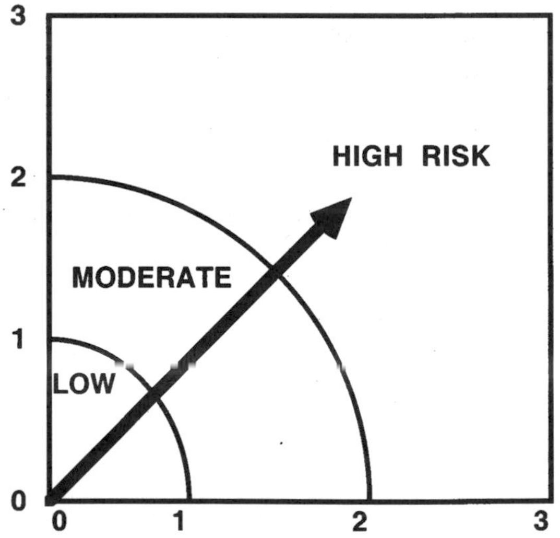

FIGURE 15.2. Guidelines for risk assessment: general and orthopedic surgery.

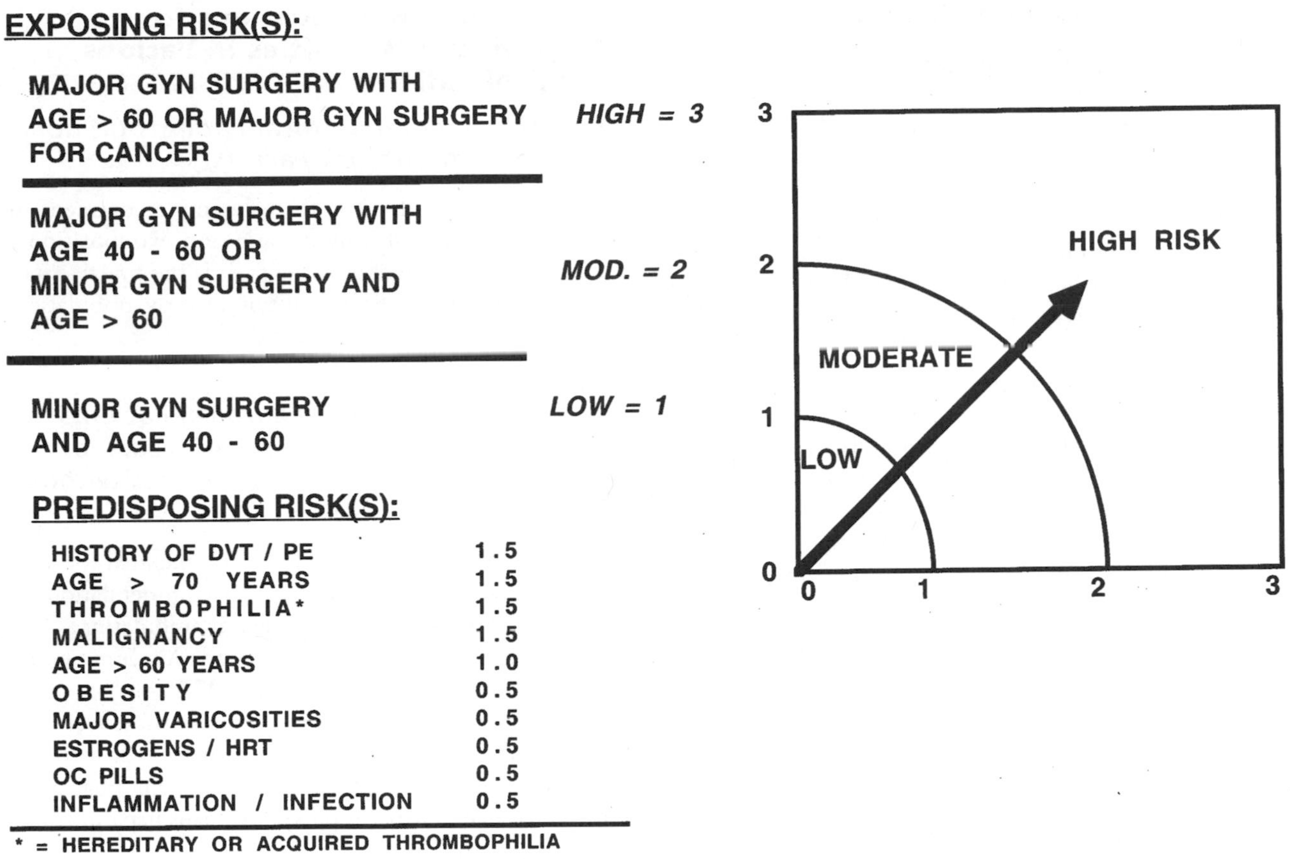

FIGURE 15.3. Guidelines for risk assessment: gynecologic surgery.

hydration, and the presence of sepsis (8,23). The assessment of risk in general and orthopedic surgery is given in Fig. 15.2. Thus the individual risk is determined by the type of surgery and an accumulation of predisposing factors [i.e., patients undergoing minor surgery but bearing several additional risk factors also may be at high risk for thromboembolic complications (23)].

APPROACHES TO THROMBOPROPHYLAXIS

The prophylactic measures most commonly used are LMWH, low-dose or adjusted-dose UFH, oral anticoagulants [(a) INR of 2 to 3, (b) fixed low-dose, or (c) dose-adjusted to prothrombin time, 1.3 to 1.5 seconds prolonged], IPC and GCSs, in probable descending order of efficacy depending on procedure and other clinical circumstances (23). Other less common measure include the use of ASA and i.v. dextran (23).

It has become standard practice to commence prophylaxis, for example, with low-dose heparin, before anesthesia in patients undergoing thoracic or abdominal surgery, and in Europe, prophylaxis is started the night before surgery in patients undergoing total hip or total knee replacement surgery (23). In North America, because of the concern related to postoperative bleeding, prophylaxis for patients having total knee or total hip replacement has often been started after surgery (97). This difference in the patterns of practice may account for the differences in the rates of postoperative venous thrombosis in Europe and North America (23). A recent randomized trial failed to note a significant difference in DVT or bleeding when LMWH was started preoperative or postoperatively (98).

Low-dose Heparin

The effectiveness of LDUH for preventing DVT has been established by multiple randomized clinical trials (34–36,92,99). Low-dose s.c. heparin is usually given in a dose of 5,000 units 2 hours before surgery, and then postoperatively every 8 or 12 hours. The incidence of major bleeding complications is not increased by low-dose heparin, but there is an increase in minor wound hematomas. The platelet count should be monitored every other day in all patients receiving low-dose heparin to detect heparin-induced thrombocytopenia (100). LDUH is relatively inexpensive, easily administered, and does not require monitoring, except mandatory platelet counts.

Low-molecular-weight Heparin

A number of LMWH fractions have been evaluated by randomized clinical trials in general surgical patients (101–109). In randomized clinical trials comparing LMWH with UFH, the LMWHs given once or twice daily are as effective or more effective in preventing thrombosis (101–109). The incidence of bleeding is significantly lower in patients receiving LMWH versus UFH as indicated by a reduction in wound hematomas, severe bleeding, and the number of patients requiring repeated surgery for bleeding (100).

Although the number of patients undergoing total knee replacement now equals those undergoing total hip replacements, there have been fewer trials in this patient population (110–113). The incidence of DVT with LMWH are significantly lower than those with warfarin (58–60,62). Recent studies have shown that LMWH is superior to LDUH in patients with multiple trauma (114,115).

Oral Anticoagulants

Warfarins can be started preoperatively, at the time of surgery, or in the early postoperative period; however, if started at the time of surgery or in the early postoperative period, warfarins may not prevent small venous thrombi from forming during surgery, or after surgery, as an antithrombotic effect is not achieved until the third or fourth postoperative day (23,29). However, oral anticoagulants may be effective in inhibiting the extension of thrombi and potentially prevent otherwise clinically significant VTE (23,29).

Low-dose warfarin, however, does not provide protection against DVT after hip or knee replacement (116).

Intermittent Leg Compression

Intermittent pneumatic leg compression is effective for preventing DVT in moderate-risk general surgical patients (117), in patients undergoing neurosurgery (118), and those undergoing cardiac surgery (119). In patients undergoing hip surgery, IPC of the calf is ineffective for proximal vein thrombosis (120).

Graduated Compression Stockings

GCSs are a simple, safe, and moderately effective form of thromboprophylaxis. GCSs are recommended in low-risk patients and only as an adjunct in those with medium and high risk (23). The only major contraindication is peripheral vascular disease. However, there is no conclusive evidence that GCSs are effective in reducing the incidence of fatal and nonfatal PE (23).

Specific Recommendations for Prophylactic Modalities in Various Surgical Patients

Low-risk General Surgical Patients (Minor Surgery without Risk Factors)

The data are insufficient to make any recommendations. On the basis of risk/benefit ratio and extrapolation from studies in moderate-risk patients, it is the practice in some countries to use GCSs in addition to early ambulation and adequate hydration (23,27,115).

Moderate-risk General Surgical Patients (Major Surgery, Older Than 40 Years, or Surgery for More Than 30 Minutes without Any Additional Risk Factors)

The use of LMWH or UFH is recommended for all moderate-risk patients. An alternative recommendation is IPC used continuously until the patient is ambulating, GCSs, or a combination of both. These are grade A recommendations based on level I or level II data (23,27,115).

Further studies are needed to assess the effect of using GCSs and/or IPC in addition to pharmacologic methods and to assess the combined effects of different pharmacologic methods such as heparin plus ASA versus heparin alone.

High-risk General Surgical Patients (Major Surgery, Older Than 60 Years, or Presence of Additional Risk Factors)

All should receive prophylaxis as for moderate-risk patients (grade A recommendation) (23,27,115). In addition to single modalities such as LMWH or UFH, combined modalities of pharmacologic (LMWH or UFH) and mechanical methods should be considered, as they may be more effective (grade B recommendation) (23,27,115).

In moderate- and high-risk patients, dextran and ASA are not the methods of choice because of their limited efficacy on DVT prevention, the anaphylactic reactions, and danger of cardiac overload associated with the former, the high dose of ASA (1,000 to 1,500) mg per day required, and the fact that oral medications are not possible for several days in patients having abdominal surgery (23,27,115).

Guidelines for scoring risk assessment in general and orthopedic surgical patients are summarized in Fig. 15.2.

Neurosurgery

Neurosurgery patients should be considered for mechanical methods of prophylaxis. In three randomized controlled studies involving a total of 422 patients, the incidence of DVT was reduced from 21.3% in controls to 6.0% in the prophylactic groups by using pneumatic compression (relative risk, 0.28; 95% CI, 0.16 to 0.51; grade A recommendation) (23,27,115).

Orthopedic Surgery and Trauma

Elective Hip Replacement

Fixed LDUH, 5,000 IU every 8 or 12 hours, is effective for reducing DVT (level I data) and PE (level II data) in patients having elective hip replacement. Increasing the dose leads to a greater risk of bleeding (23,27,115).

LMWH appears superior to UFH in reducing both DVT and PE for hip replacement surgery, but more studies are needed (23,27,115). Fixed "minidose" oral anticoagulant therapy is not effective (23,27,115).

Antiplatelet therapy (mainly ASA) in elective hip surgery is only moderately effective for protection against DVT (relative risk, 0.70; 95% CI, 0.61 to 0.82; level II evidence), but the observed reduction in the risk of PE is substantial (relative risk, 0.49; 95% CI, 0.26 to 0.92; level II evidence) (23,27,115). The effect of ASA on PE needs confirmation.

There are few data as to the efficacy of graduated elastic compression by itself after hip replacement, but its use in orthopedic surgery would be supported by data extrapolated from general surgery (grade C recommendation). IPC is effective (level I evidence) (23,27,115).

Elective Knee Replacement

Fewer studies are available on prophylaxis after knee replacement. Data from hip replacement should not be extrapolated to knee replacement (23).

IPC is effective (level I evidence). There is evidence that LMWH is more effective than warfarin and also more effective than UFH (level I evidence) (23,27,115). Some data support the combined use of regional anesthesia with graduated elastic compression. In most randomized controlled trials, after knee replacement, the absolute risk of DVT remains high despite prophylaxis (23).

Duration of Prophylaxis in Elective Orthopedic Surgery

The optimal duration of prophylaxis in elective orthopedic surgery has not been established. Because intraoperative risk factors are probably important, prophylaxis should ideally be started before surgery. A randomized comparison of preoperative and postoperative commencement of pharmacologic prophylaxis is necessary.

Most trials have studied prophylaxis for 7 to 10 days or until the patients are ambulatory; however, three recent randomized controlled studies in patients having hip arthroplasty indicated that more prolonged thromboprophylaxis with LMWH decreases the frequency of venographically detected DVT (23,27,115).

Emergency Orthopedic Surgery

The risks of DVT and PE, including fatal PE, are high in patients with hip fracture. Prophylaxis should be started as soon as possible after diagnosis and should be the same as recommended for elective hip surgery. The best results so far have been obtained from studies using LMWH (23,27,115). LDUH is effective in reduction of DVT, and although an overview of trials has not demonstrated a significant reduction in total PE, the observed effect was not different from that noted in general surgery, and there was a significant reduction in fatal PE (23,27,115).

Guidelines for risk assessment in orthopedic patients also are summarized in Fig. 15.2.

Multiple Trauma

Multiple trauma patients are at high risk for thrombosis, and LMWH represents the prophylaxis of choice (27,106, 121). IPC may be used when feasible, as this is unassociated with any bleeding risk. Other alternatives include LDUH or warfarin, based on extrapolation from other high-risk situations such as hip fracture and hip replacement surgery. Insertion of an inferior vena cava filter may be considered for very-high-risk situations in which anticoagulants may be contraindicated.

Acute Spinal Cord Injury Associated with Paralysis

LMWH is the most effective prophylaxis (115,122). Pneumatic compression is less effective. Combining IPC with LMWH or adjusted-dose heparin may provide additional benefit, but this is not yet supported by data.

Gynecologic Surgery

Low-risk Patients

These may receive prophylaxis. Turner et al. (123) reported a level I study that demonstrated a lower DVT rate with the use of graduated elastic compression (none vs. 4%; $p < 0.05$) (123). On the basis of this study, the risk/benefit ratio, and extrapolation from moderate-risk patients, GCSs may be used in addition to early ambulation and adequate hydration.

Moderate-risk Patients

LMWH and LDUH (5,000 units every 12 hours) are effective prophylaxis in medium-risk gynecologic surgery patients (grade A recommendation based on level I data) (23,27,115). By extrapolation from other types of surgery, IPC should also be considered because it is effective in higher risk patients (grade A recommendation). Adjusted-dose warfarin is not recommended for routine prophylaxis but may have a role when UFH/LMWH is contraindicated (a history of heparin-induced thrombocytopenia; grade A recommendation) (23,27,115).

High-risk Patients

LDUH (5,000 units every 8 hours) or IPC used continuously for at least 5 days provides effective prophylaxis (grade A recommendation). When these two modalities were compared in a randomized trial, their efficacy appeared to be equal, but more bleeding complications were associated with the use of low-dose heparin. Data evaluating LMWH and GCSs in high-risk gynecologic surgery patients are currently insufficient, but extrapolation from other high-risk surgical populations would suggest that LMWH is effective prophylaxis (23,27,115).

Guidelines for DVT/PE risk assessment for gynecologic surgical patients are summarized in Fig. 15.3.

Other Conditions

Pregnancy

Low-dose heparin prophylaxis is commonly used in pregnant patients at high risk for DVT and PE, such as those with previous DVT or PE and certain thrombophilias (see later), although data regarding efficacy from controlled trials are lacking (grade C recommendation). There are insufficient data on both the optimal timing and dosing schedule of low-dose heparin prophylaxis. There is substantial evidence for safety with low-dose ASA use in pregnancy. Although there is no direct evidence regarding ASA in preventing DVT or PE in pregnancy, its efficacy in other settings suggests that it may be worth considering (grade C recommendation) (22,26).

Oral anticoagulants are contraindicated for prophylaxis of VTE in the first trimester because of increased risk of embryopathies, and warfarin is associated with increased fetal and maternal–fetal bleeding in the second and particularly the third trimester. In the presence of contraindications to LMWH/UFH, oral anticoagulants may be considered, when justified, for prophylaxis in the second trimester because bleeding is uncommon at this stage (grade C recommendation).

The benefits of prophylaxis have not been demonstrated in patients undergoing cesarean section who do not have additional risk factors. Perioperative and postpartum prophylaxis should be considered if there are risk factors, par-

EXPOSING RISK(S):

HISTORY OF DVT OR PE	*HIGH = 3*
AGE > 40	*MODERATE = 2*
AGE < 40	*LOW = 1*

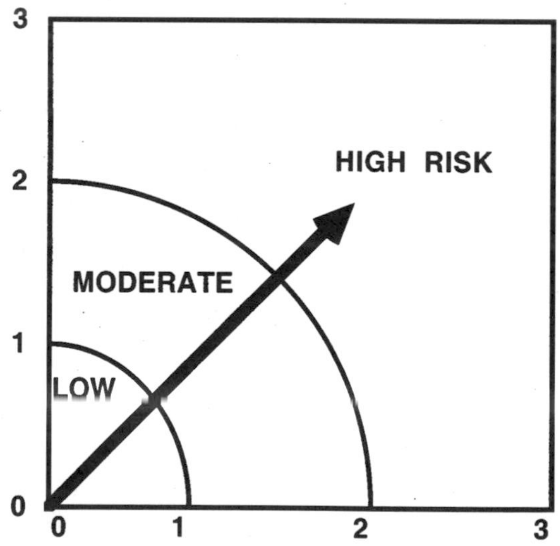

PREDISPOSING RISK(S):

HISTORY OF DVT / PE	1.5
AGE > 70 YEARS	1.5
THROMBOPHILIA*	1.5
MALIGNANCY	1.5
AGE > 60 YEARS	1.0
OBESITY	0.5
MAJOR VARICOSITIES	0.5
ESTROGENS / HRT	0.5
OC PILLS	0.5
INFLAMMATION / INFECTION	0.5

* = HEREDITARY OR ACQUIRED THROMBOPHILIA

FIGURE 15.4. Guidelines for risk assessment: obstetric surgery.

ticularly age older than 35 years, obesity, or previous DVT or PE or thrombophilia (grade C recommendation).

Dextran should be avoided in pregnancy, as an anaphylactic reaction may precipitate acute fetal distress. Dextran should be withheld during cesarean section until after delivery of the baby.

There are insufficient data on the use of LMWHs or mechanical methods in pregnancy. There is an urgent need for multicenter trials comparing standard heparin with LMWH in high-risk pregnant patients to assess efficacy, safety, and possible side effects, such as osteoporosis.

Women in whom thromboembolism develops during pregnancy should be treated with therapeutic levels of adjusted-dose s.c. heparin, which should be continued throughout pregnancy, labor, and delivery. Higher doses are required in late pregnancy, but the s.c. dose should be reduced in labor or before cesarean section to reduce the risk of hemorrhage at delivery. Anticoagulation is usually continued for at least 6 postpartum weeks, but the optimal duration of antithrombotic therapy has not been established in this setting (22,26).

Patients in whom thromboembolism develops during pregnancy or the puerperium should be referred for hematologic consultation. The management of thrombophilic conditions through pregnancy usually requires LMWH or adjusted-dose UFH with monitoring of the heparin effect and platelet counts (22,26). Pregnancy risk assessment is given in Fig. 15.4.

Combination Estrogen-containing Oral Contraceptives

These may be associated with increased risk of DVT in patients undergoing gynecologic surgery. Discontinuation of oral contraceptives 4 to 6 weeks before surgery should be considered, but this should be balanced against the risk of unwanted pregnancy. In the absence of other risk factors, there is insufficient evidence to support a policy of routinely stopping the combined pill before major surgery. LMWH/UFH prophylaxis is advisable if oral contraceptives have not been discontinued and additional risk factors are present. For emergency surgery, thromboprophylaxis should be provided in women taking the combined pill, as the risk of DVT is greater (grade C recommendation) (22,26).

Hormone-replacement Therapy

In the absence of other risk factors, there is currently insufficient evidence to support a policy of routinely stopping HRT before surgery. Although there are no data, LMWH/UFH prophylaxis is advisable where HRT has not been discontinued before surgery. In practice, most patients receiving HRT have additional risk factors (particularly age) that in themselves would be indications for thromboprophylaxis (grade C recommendation).

IMPACT OF CONSENSUS CONFERENCES ON THE CLINICAL ACCEPTANCE OF LOW-MOLECULAR-WEIGHT HEPARINS

The favorable assessment of LMWHs and the recommendation for use has encouraged numerous European clinicians to abandon dose-adjusted LDUH. The safety and efficacy of LMWHs coupled to a simple dosing regimen has facilitated home treatment and self-administration, significant factors in the acceptance of LMWHs. In the future, it is likely that regulatory authorities will require clinical trials to compare new compounds and formulations with fixed-dose LMWH or aPTT-adjusted UFH. In summary, the IC and the Sixth ACCP Consensus had a great impact on the clinical acceptance of LMWHs and helped in particular:

- to initiate various clinical trials to answer open key questions,
- to provide further evidence on the safety and efficacy profile of LMWHs,
- to consider LMWHs as individual compounds,
- to facilitate outpatient prophylaxis,
- to consider cost-effectiveness, and
- to set a new standard required by health authorities to use LMWH as a reference in future prophylaxis trials in high-risk patients.

THROMBOPROPHYLAXIS: CLINICAL PROGRESS IN 1999 AND 2000

During 1999 through 2001, a number of publications highlighted several issues that deserve further attention when deciding optimal prophylaxis regimens.

All Low-molecular-weight Heparins Are Not the Same

Preclinical studies have shown that the commercially available LMWHs differ in various biochemical, biophysical, and pharmacologic properties. They are prepared by different techniques have different molecular-weight distributions and pharmacodynamic characteristics, all of which may have significant clinical implications. In addition, differing dosing schedules have been used in various trials. Thus there are some substantial concerns that the efficacy and safety of LMWHs cannot be properly assessed by meta-analysis, a process that implies that the LMWHs are the same.

Consequently, a comparison of the therapeutic efficacy of LMWHs must be based on a wide variety of parameters (124). This is reflected in the modification of the Sixth ACCP Consensus, which excluded meta-analyses and now makes grade A recommendations based on single randomized trials alone (125). This approach has been very much appreciated by European and also some North American professionals. The issue of LMWH differentiation also has been extensively discussed by leading thrombosis experts at a Summit Conference in January 1999 (125).

Improved Risk Assessment for Venous Thromboembolism

Despite the publication of the ACCP and International Consensus Statements, many patients at risk of thrombosis will receive inadequate or no prophylaxis. One reason for failure to prescribe prophylaxis is underestimation of thromboembolic risk. Therefore the recent publication of a supplement volume to *Blood Coagulation and Fibrinolysis* discussing the development of risk-assessment models has been well received by practicing clinicians. These risk-assessment models take into account both the clinical setting and patient-related factors. A new category has been proposed to differentiate patients in need of very intensive prophylaxis (126).

Optimizing Surgical Prophylaxis: Prevention of Fatal Pulmonary Embolism

LMWHs have gradually replaced UFH as the standard of care in surgery thromboprophylaxis, but until recently, no prospective controlled study had investigated the efficacy of LMWH in preventing the most important efficacy end point: autopsy-proven fatal PE. A recent international trial compared the rates of fatal PE after surgery when patients received once-daily certoparin or UFH for a mean of 8 days, started before surgery (127). A total of 23,078 patients was randomized and underwent mainly general surgery (84%) or orthopedic and other surgical procedures (16%). Fatal PE was diagnosed in 17 (0.15%) patients receiving certoparin and 19 (0.17%) receiving UFH. This study demonstrates that single daily doses of the LMWH certoparin are at least as effective as UFH t.i.d. in the prevention of fatal PE.

Optimizing the Initiation of Surgical Prophylaxis

Although preoperative and postoperative initiation of prophylaxis for DVT with LMWH is effective, the relative efficacy and safety of these approaches is unknown. In the absence of a published level I trial, a meta-analysis of relevant trials in patients undergoing elective hip replacement was performed. Potential biases in the meta-analysis were minimized by analyzing randomized trials that met the criteria summarized in Table 15.15. LMWH initiated preoperatively was associated with a significant reduction in DVT compared with postoperative initiation (10.0% vs. 15.5%; $p = 0.02$), a benefit associated with a significant decrease in major bleeding (0.9% vs. 3.5%; $p = 0.01$). A randomized comparison of preoperative and postoperative initiation of pharmacologic prophylaxis of DVT would help resolve divergent practices for DVT prophylaxis between Europe and the North American countries, the United States and Canada, and would benefit thousands of patients on both continents (128).

TABLE 15.15. FACTORS INFLUENCING CLINICAL TRIAL RESULTS: SELECTED DIFFERENCES BETWEEN TRIAL DESIGNS THAT MAY INFLUENCE STUDY OUTCOME

Study location	Multicenter, national, international
Patient population	Size, risk profile
Comparator	Placebo, active treatment
Concomitant medications	Antiplatelet drugs
Surgical procedures	General, orthopedic, neurologic
Anesthesia type	Intubation, spinal, epidural
Dosing regimen	i.v., s.c.
Dosing duration	In-hospital, extended
Efficacy end point	Death, PE, DVT
Safety end point	Bleeding definition
Diagnosis of DVT	FUT, venography
Risk-stratification technique	

PE, pulmonary embolism; DVT, deep vein thrombosis; FUT, fibrinogen uptake test.

CONCLUSION

The International Consensus and the ACCP Sixth Consensus had a great impact on the clinical acceptance of LMWHs. These recommendations have been instrumental in initiating further clinical trials to answer key questions regarding thromboprophylaxis and in setting a new standard for patient care. The key to cost containment in management of DVT/PE is to (a) define the etiology (blood-coagulation protein/platelet defect) and institute appropriate long-term therapy as indicated and assess appropriate family members as indicated if a hereditary defect is found; and (b) use LMWH as inpatient management, saving a minimum of $210,000.00 per 1,000 patients simply from cost savings of recurrence, saving 17 lives per 1,000 patients, and saving exorbitant costs of care for patients with recurring and developing chronic venous insufficiency. The use of outpatient LMWH will save $4,900,000.00 per 1,000 patients if applied to the 70% of patients with DVT who fit criteria of no comorbid condition requiring hospitalization and arrive with a diagnosis early enough to be sent home or hospitalized for 24 hours or less. The simple defining of defects leading to unexplained thrombosis will add another $3,000,000.00 in savings per 1,000 patients with DVT and about $350,000.00 per 100 patients with thrombotic stroke. In those with TIAs, defining the defect and instituting appropriate antithrombotic therapy, thereby potentially saving about

30% from developing a thrombotic stroke, amounts to about $350,500.00 (30% of $1,168,500.00) in savings per 100 patients.

REFERENCES

1. Bick RL, Fareed J. Current status of thrombosis: a multidisciplinary medical issue and major American health problem: beyond the year 2000. *Clin Appl Thromb Hemost* 1997;3(suppl 1):1.
2. American Heart Association. *Heart and stroke: 1997.* Dallas, Tex: American Heart Association National Headquarters, 1996.
3. Bick RL, Kaplan H. Syndromes of thrombosis and hypercoagulability: congenital and acquired causes of thrombosis. *Med Clin North Am* 1998;82:409.
4. Bick RL, Jakway J, Baker WF. Deep vein thrombosis: prevalence of etiologic factors and results of management in 100 consecutive patients. *Semin Thromb Hemost* 1992;18:267.
5. Bergqvist D, Lundblad B. Incidence of venous thromboembolism in medical and surgical patients. In: Bergqvist D, Comerota A, Nicolaides A, et al., eds. *Prevention of venous thrombembolism.* London: Med-Orion Press, 1994:3.
6. Silverstein MD, Heit JA, Mohr DN, et al. Trends in the incidence of deep vein thrombosis and pulmonary embolism: a 25-year population-based study. *Arch Intern Med* 1998;158:585.
7. Ramaswami G, Nicolaides AN. The natural history of deep vein thrombosis. In: Bergqvist D, Comerota A, Nicolaides A, et al. *Prevention of venous thromboembolism.* London: Med-Orion Press, 1994:3.
8. Bick RL. Proficient and cost effective approaches for the prevention and treatment of venous thrombosis and thromboembolism. *Drugs* 2000;60:575.
9. Bick RL, Ancypa D. Blood protein defects associated with thrombosis: laboratory assessment. *Clin Lab Med* 1995;15:125.
10. *MedPar: the MedStat Group Outcomes analysis.* Nashville,Tenn: MedPar, Inforum, Medistat, 1998.
11. De Stefano V, Finazzi G, Mannucci PM. Inherited thrombophilia: pathogenesis, clinical syndromes and management. *Blood* 1996;87:3531.
12. Bick RL. Sticky platelet syndrome: a common cause of unexplained venous and arterial thrombosis: results of prevalence and treatment outcome. *Clin Appl Thromb Hemost* 1998;4:1.
13. Mammen EF. Sticky platelet syndrome. *Semin Thromb Hemost* 1999;24:361.
14. Bick RL, Baker WF. The antiphospholipid thrombosis syndrome and thrombosis. *Semin Thromb Hemost* 1999;25:333.
15. Bick RL. Antiphospholipid thrombosis syndromes: etiology, pathophysiology, diagnosis and management. *Int J Hematol* 1997;65:193.
16. Bick RL. Therapy for venous thrombosis: guidelines for a competent and cost-effective approach. *Clin Appl Thromb Hemost* 1999;5:2.
17. Bick RL, Hinton RC. Prevalence of hereditary and acquired coagulation protein/platelet defects in patients with cerebral ischemic events. *Blood* 1998;92(suppl 1):114.
18. Bick RL. Syndromes of thrombosis and hypercoagulability: congenital and acquired thrombophilias. *Clin Appl Thromb Hemost* 1998;4:25.
19. Beyth RJ, Cohen AM, Landefeld CS. Long-term outcomes of deep-vein thrombosis. *Arch Intern Med* 1995;155:1031.
20. Prandoni P, Lensing AWA, Cogo A, et al. The long-term clinical course of acute deep venous thrombosis. *Ann Intern Med* 1996;125:1.
21. Marshall J, Tu D. Dalteparin: a low molecular weight heparin. *PHD Pharm Lett* 1998;16:5.
22. Ardeparin and danaparoid for prevention of deep vein thrombosis. *Med Lett* 1997;39:94.
23. Bick RL, Haas SK. International consensus recommendations: summary statement and additional suggested guidelines. *Med Clin North Am* 1998;83:613.
24. American College of Chest Physicians. Conference on antithrombotic therapy. *Chest* 1986;89:1.
25. European Consensus Statement on the prevention of venous thromboembolism. *Int Angiol* 1992;11:151.
26. Waersted A, Westby O, Beerman B, eds. *Treatment of venous thrombosis and pulmonary embolism.* Oslo: Norwegian Medicines Control Authority, 1995. Medical Products Agency, 1995.
27. Prevention of venous thromboembolism: international consensus statement (guideline according to scientific evidence). *Int Angiol* 1997;16:3.
28. McIntyre K. Medicolegal implications of consensus statements. *Chest* 1995;108:502.
29. Hull RD, Pineo GF. Prophylaxis of deep venous thrombosis and pulmonary embolus: current recommendations. *Med Clin North Am* 1998;82:477.
30. Dismuke SE, Wagner EH. Pulmonary embolism as a cause of death: the changing mortality in hospitalized patients. *JAMA* 1986;255:2039.
31. Dalen JE, Alpert JS. Natural history of pulmonary embolism. *Prog Cardiovasc Dis* 1975;17:257.
32. Baker WF. Diagnosis of deep venous thrombosis and pulmonary embolism. *Med Clin North Am* 1998;82:459.
33. Anderson FA, Wheeler HB, Goldberg RJ, et al. A population-based perspective of the hospital incidence and case-fatality rates of deep vein thrombosis and pulmonary embolism. *Arch Intern Med* 1991;151:933.
34. Clagett GP, Reisch JS. Prevention of venous thromboembolism in general surgical patients: results of meta-analysis. *Ann Surg* 1988;208:227.
35. Collins R, Scrimgeour A, Yusef S, et al. Reduction in fatal pulmonary embolism and venous thrombosis by perioperative administration of subcutaneous heparin. *N Engl J Med* 1988; 318:1162.
36. Nicolaides AN (and committee). Prevention of venous thromboembolism: international consensus statement: guidelines compiled in accordance with scientific evidence. *Int Angiol* 2001;20:3.
37. Nicolaides AN. Prevention of thromboembolism: international consensus statement. In: Bergqvist D, Comerota AJ, Nicolaides AN, et al., eds. *Prevention of venous thromboembolism.* Los Angeles: Med-Orion Publishing, 1994:445.
38. Bratzler DW, Raskob GE, Murray CK, et al. Underuse of venous thromboembolism prophylaxis for general surgery patients. *Arch Intern Med* 1998;158:1909.
39. Gillies TE, Ruckley CV, Nixon SJ. Still missing the boat with fatal pulmonary embolism. *Br J Surg* 1996;83:1394.
40. Geerts WH, Heit JA, Clagett GP, et al. Prevention of venous thromboembolism. *Chest* 2001:119:132S–175S.
41. Samama MM, Cohen AT, Damron JY, et al. A comparison of enoxaparin with placebo for the prevention of venous thromboembolism in acutely ill medical patients. *N Engl J Med* 1999;341:793–800.
42. Kleber FX, Witt C, Flosbach CW, et al. Comparison of the low molecular weight heparin enoxaparin with unfractionated heparin in the prevention of venous thromboembolic events in medical patients with severe cardiopulmonary disease. *Thromb Haemost* 1999;82(suppl): 1552(abst).
43. Kher A, Samama MM. Low-molecular-weight heparins: weeks

or months instead of days of treatment. *J Clin Appl Thromb Hemost* 2001;314–320.
44. Goldhaber S. Venous thromboembolism prophylaxis in medical patients. *Thromb Haemost* 1999;82(suppl):899.
45. Mismetti P, Laporte-Simitsidis S, Tardy B, et al. Prevention of venous thromboembolism in internal medicine with unfractionated or low-molecular-weight heparins: a meta-analysis of randomised clinical trials. *Thromb Haemost* 2000;83:14.
46. Nicolaides AN, Bergqvist D, Hull R. Prevention of venous thromboembolism: international consensus statement (guideline according to scientific evidence). *Int Angiol* 1997;16:3.
47. Hillbom M, Erilä T, Flosbach CW, et al. Enoxaparin, a low molecular weight heparin, is superior to heparin in the prevention of deep vein thrombosis in patients with acute atherothrombotic stroke. *Thromb Haemost* 1999;(suppl:177 (abst).
48. Albers GW, Amarebhco P, Easton JD, et al. Antithrombotics and thrombolytic therapy for ischemic stroke. *Chest* 2001;119(suppl 1):300S.
49. Kakkar VV. Effectiveness and safety of low molecular weight heparins (LMWH) in the prevention of venous thromboembolism. *Thromb Haemost* 1995;74:364.
50. Haas SK. Treatment of deep venous thrombosis: current recommendations. *Med Clin North Am* 1998;82:495.
51. Philbrick JT, Becker DM. Calf deep vein thrombosis: a wolf in sheep's clothing? *Arch Intern Med* 1988;148:2131.
52. Greenfield LJ, Michna BA. Twelve-year clinical experience with the Greenfield vena cava filter. *Surgery* 1988;104:706.
53. Magnant JG, Walsh DB, Juravsky LI, et al. Current use of inferior vena cava filters. *J Vasc Surg* 1992;16:701.
54. Descousus H, Leizorocicz A, Parent F, et al. A clinical trial of vena caval filters in the prevention of pulmonary embolism in patients with proximal deep-vein thrombosis. *N Engl J Med* 1998;338:409.
55. White RH, Zhou H, Kim J, et al. A population-based study of the effectiveness of inferior vena cava filter use among patients with venous thromboembolism. *Arch Intern Med* 2000;1260: 2033.
56. Baker WF, Bick RL. Deep vein thrombosis: diagnosis and management. *Med Clin North Am* 1994;78:685.
57. Murano G, Bell WR. Thrombolytic therapy. In: Bick RL, Bennett JM, Byrnes RK, eds. *Hematology: clinical and laboratory practice.* St. Louis: Mosby, 1993:1633.
58. Bell WR. Thrombolytic therapy: agents, indications and laboratory monitoring. *Med Clin North Am* 1994;78:745.
59. Hoomes DW, Bura A, Mazzolai L, et al. Subcutaneous heparin compared with continuous intravenous heparin administration in the initial treatment of deep vein thrombosis: a meta-analysis. *Ann Intern Med* 1992;116:279.
60. Doyle DJ, Turpie AGG, Hirsh J, et al. Adjusted subcutaneous heparin or continuous intravenous heparin in patients with acute deep vein thrombosis. *Ann Intern Med* 1987;107:441.
61. Anderson G, Fagrell B, Holmgren K, et al. Subcutaneous administration of heparin: a randomized comparison with intravenous administration of heparin to patients with deep-vein thrombosis. *Thromb Res* 1982;27:631.
62. Hull RD, Raskob G, Hirsh J, et al. Continuous intravenous heparin compared with intermittent subcutaneous heparin in the initial treatment of proximal vein thrombosis. *N Engl J Med* 1986;315:1109.
63. Hull RD, Raskob GE, Brant RF, et al. The importance of initial treatment on long-term outcomes of antithrombotic therapy. *Arch Intern Med* 1997;157:2317.
64. Walenga JM, Bick RL. Heparin-induced thrombocytopenia, paradoxical thromboembolism, and other side effects of heparin therapy. *Med Clin North Am* 1998;82:635.
65. The Columbus Investigators. Low-molecular-weight heparin in the treatment of patients with venous thromboembolism. *N Engl J Med* 1997;337:657.
66. Duroux P. A Collaborative European Multicentre Study: a randomized trial of subcutaneous low molecular weight heparin (CY216) compared with intravenous unfractionated heparin in the treatment of deep vein thrombosis. *Thromb Haemost* 1991; 65:251.
67. Faivre R, Neuhart Y, Kieffer Y, et al. Un nouveau traitement des thromboses veineuses profondes: les fractions d'heparine de bas poids moleculaire: etude randomisee. *Presse Med* 1988;17:197.
68. Fiessinger JN, Lopez-Fernandez M, Gatterer E, et al. Once-daily subcutaneous dalteparin, a low molecular weight heparin, for the initial treatment of acute deep vein thrombosis. *Thromb Haemost* 1996;76:195.
69. Hull RD, Raskob GE, Pineo GF, et al. Subcutaneous low-molecular-weight heparin compared with continuous intravenous heparin in the treatment of proximal-vein thrombosis. *N Engl J Med* 1992;326:975.
70. Koopman MMW, et al. Treatment of venous thrombosis with intravenous unfractionated heparin administered in the hospital as compared with subcutaneous low-molecular- weight heparin administered at home. *N Engl J Med* 1996;334:682.
71. Levine M, Gent M, Hirsh J, et al. A comparison of low-molecular-weight heparin administered primarily at home with unfractionated heparin administered in the hospital for proximal deep-vein thrombosis. *N Engl J Med* 1996;334:677.
72. Lindmarker P, Holmstrom M, Granqvist S, et al. Comparison of once-daily subcutaneous Fragmin with continuous intravenous unfractionated heparin in the treatment of deep venous thrombosis. *Thromb Haemost* 1994;72:186.
73. Lopaciuk S, Meissner AJ, Filipecki S, et al. Subcutaneous low molecular weight heparin versus subcutaneous unfractionated heparin in the treatment of deep vein thrombosis: a Polish multicenter trial. *Thromb Haemost* 1992;68:14.
74. Luomanmaki K, and the Finnish Multicentre Group. Low molecular weight heparin (Fragmin) once daily vs continuous infusion of standard heparin in the treatment of DVT. *Haemostasis* 1994;24(suppl 1):248(abst).
75. Prandoni P, Lensing AWA, Buller HR, et al. Comparison of subcutaneous low-molecular-weight heparin with intravenous standard heparin in proximal deep-vein thrombosis. *Lancet* 1992;339:441.
76. Simonneau G, Charbonnier B, Decousus H, et al. Subcutaneous low molecular weight heparin compared with continuous intravenous unfractionated heparin in the initial treatment proximal vein thrombosis. *Arch Intern Med* 1993;153:1541.
77. Simonneau G, Sors H, Charbonnier B, et al. A comparison of low-molecular-weight heparin with unfractionated heparin for acute pulmonary embolism. *N Engl J Med* 1997;337:663.
78. Heissler FF, Bick RL. Dalteparin for the treatment of deep venous thrombosis and pulmonary embolism. *New Dev Vasc Dis* 2001;2:24–35.
79. van den Belt AGM, Prins MH, Lensing AWA, et al. Fixed dose subcutaneous low molecular weight heparins versus adjusted dose unfractionated heparin for venous thromboembolism (Cochrane review). In: *The Cochrane Library, issue 2.* Oxford: Update Software, 1998.
80. Hull RD, Raskob GE, Pineo GF, et al. The treatment of proximal vein thrombosis with subcutaneous low molecular weight heparin compared with continuous intravenous heparin: the Canadian-American Thrombosis Study Group. *Clin Appl Thromb Hemost* 1995;1:151.
81. Shafer AI. Low-molecular-weight heparin: an opportunity for home treatment of venous thrombosis [Editorial]. *N Engl J Med* 1996;334:724.

82. Koopman MMW, Prandoni P, Piovella F, et al. Treatment of venous thrombosis with intravenous unfractionated heparin administered in the hospital as compared with subcutaneous low-molecular-weight heparin administered at home. *N Engl J Med* 1996;334:682.
83. Levine M, Gent M, Hirsh J, et al. A comparison of low-molecular-weight heparin administered primarily at home with unfractionated heparin administered in the hospital for proximal deep-vein thrombosis. *N Engl J Med* 1996;334:677.
84. Lindmarker P, Holmstrom KM, Granquist S, et al. Comparison of once-daily subcutaneous Fragmin with continuous intravenous unfractionated heparin in the treatment of deep vein thrombosis. *Thromb Haemost* 1994;72:186.
85. Harrison L, McGinnis J, Crowther M, et al. Assessment of outpatient treatment of deep-vein thrombosis with low-molecular-weight heparin. *Arch Intern Med* 1998;158:2001.
86. Wells P, Kovacs M, Bormanis J, et al. Expanding eligibility for outpatient treatment of deep venous thrombosis and pulmonary embolus with low-molecular-weight heparin: a comparison of self-injection with home care injection. *Arch Intern Med* 1998;158:1809.
87. Verstraete M, Prentice CRM, Samama M, et al. A European view on the North American Sixth Consensus on antithrombotic therapy. *Chest* 2000;117:1755.
90. Kakkar VV, Adams PC. Preventive and therapeutic approach to venous thromboembolism: can death from pulmonary embolism be prevented? *J Am Coll Cardiol* 1986;8:146B.
91. Skinner DB, Salzman EW. Anticoagulant prophylaxis in surgical patients. *Surg Gynecol Obstet* 1967;125:741.
92. Shephard RM, White HA, Shirkey AL. Anticoagulant prophylaxis of thromboembolism in post-surgical patients. *Am J Surg* 1966;112:698.
93. International Multicentre Trial. Prevention of fatal postoperative pulmonary embolism by low doses of heparin. *Lancet* 1974;2:45–94.
94. Bergqvist D. Prevention in individual patient groups: general surgery. In: Bergqvist D, Comerota AJ, Nicolaides AN, et al., eds. *Prevention of venous thromboembolism.* Los Angeles: Med-Orion Publishing, 1994:243.
95. Coventry MB, Nolan DR, Beckenbaugh RD. "Delayed" prophylactic anticoagulation: a study of results and complications in 2,012 total hip arthroplasties. *J Bone Joint Surg* 1973;55:1487.
96. Eskeland G, Solheim K, Skhorten F. Anticoagulant prophylaxis, thromboembolism and mortality in elderly patients with hip fracture: a controlled clinical trial. *Acta Chir Scand* 1986;131:16.
97. Kearon C, Hirsh J. Starting prophylaxis for venous thromboembolism postoperatively. *Arch Intern Med* 1995;155:366.
98. Palareti G, Borghi B, Coccheri S, for the CITO Study Group. Postoperative versus preoperative initiation of deep-vein thrombosis prophylaxis with a low molecular weight heparin (Nadroparin) in elective hip replacement. *Clin Appl Thromb Hemost* 1996;2:18.
99. Hull RD, Hirsh J, Carter CJ, et al. Diagnostic efficacy of impedance plethysmography for clinically suspected deep-vein thrombosis: a randomized trial. *Ann Intern Med* 1985;102:21.
100. Walenga J, Bick RL. Heparin associated thrombocytopenia and other adverse effects of heparin therapy. *Cardiol Clin (Ann Drug Ther)* 1998;2:123.
101. Kakkar VV, Cohen AT, Edmonson RA, et al. Low molecular weight versus standard heparin for prevention of venous thromboembolism after major abdominal surgery. *Lancet* 1993;341:259.
102. Kakkar VV, Boeckl O, Boneau B, et al. Efficacy and safety of a low-molecular-weight heparin and standard unfractionated heparin for prophylaxis of postoperative venous thromboembolism: European multicenter trial. *World J Surg* 1997;21:2.
103. Bergqvist D, Matzsch T, Brumark U, et al. Low-molecular-weight heparin given the evening before surgery compared with conventional low-dose heparin in prevention of thrombosis. *Br J Surg* 1988;75:888.
104. Samama M, Bernard P, Bonnardot JP, et al. Low-molecular-weight heparin compared with unfractionated heparin in prevention of postoperative thrombosis. *Br J Surg* 1988;75:128.
105. The European Fraxiparin Study Group. Comparison of a low-molecular-weight heparin and unfractionated heparin for the prevention of deep vein thrombosis in patients undergoing abdominal surgery. *Br J Surg* 1988;75:1058.
106. Caen JP. A randomized double-blind study between a low-molecular-weight heparin Kabi 2165 and standard heparin in the prevention of deep-vein thrombosis in general surgery: a French multicentre trial. *Thromb Haemost* 1988;59:216.
107. Leizorovicz A, Picolet H, Peyrieux JC, et al. Prevention of perioperative deep vein thrombosis in general surgery: a multicentre double-blind study comparing two doses of logiparin and standard heparin. *Br J Surg* 1991;78:412.
108. Nurmohamed MT, Verhaeghe R, Haas S, et al. A comparative trial of a low molecular weight heparin (enoxaparin) versus standard heparin for the prophylaxis of postoperative deep vein thrombosis in general surgery. *Am J Surg* 1995;169:567.
109. Bergqvist D, Burmark US, Flordal PA, et al. Low molecular weight heparin started before surgery as prophylaxis against deep vein thrombosis: 2500 versus 500 XaI units in 2070 patients. *Br J Surg* 1995;82:496.
110. Leclerc JR, Geerts WH, Desjardins L, et al. Prevention of deep vein thrombosis after major knee surgery: a randomized, double-blind trial comparing a low-molecular-weight heparin fragment (enoxaparin) to placebo. *Thromb Haemost* 1992;67:417.
111. Leclerc JR, Geerts WH, Desjardins L, et al. Prevention of venous thromboembolism after knee arthroplasty: a randomized, double-blind trial comparing a low molecular weight heparin fragment (enoxparin) to warfarin. *Thromb Haemost* 1995;73:1103(abst).
112. Heit J, Berkowitz S, Bona R, et al. Efficacy and safety of Normiflow (a LMWH) compared to warfarin for prevention of venous thromboembolism following total knee replacement: a double-blind, dose-ranging study. *Thromb Haemost* 1995;73:A739(abst).
113. Nurmohamed MT, Rosendaal FR, Büller HR, et al. Low molecular weight heparin in the prophylaxis of venous thrombosis: a meta-analysis. *Lancet* 1992;340:152.
114. Geerts WH, Jay RM, Code KI, et al. A comparison of low-dose heparin with low-molecular-weight heparin as prophylaxis against venous thromboembolism after major trauma. *N Engl J Med* 1996;335:701.
115. Haas S. Recommendations for prophylaxis of venous thromboembolism: international consensus and the American College of Chest Physicians: Sixth Consensus Conference on antithrombotic therapy. *J Clin Appl Thromb Hemost* (in press).
116. Dale C, Gallus A, Wycherley A, et al. Prevention of venous thrombosis with minidose warfarin after joint replacement. *Br Med J* 1991;303:224.
117. Roberts VC, Sabri S, Beely AH, et al. The effect of intermittently applied external pressure on the hemodynamics of the lower limb in man. *Br J Surg* 1972;59:233.
118. Skillman JJ, Collins RR, Coe NP, et al. Prevention of deep vein thrombosis in neurosurgical patients: a controlled, randomized trial of external pneumatic compression boots. *Surgery* 1978;83:354.
119. Ramos R, Salem BI, Pawlikowski MP, et al. The efficacy of pneumatic compression stockings in the prevention of pulmonary embolism after cardiac surgery. *Chest* 1996;109:82.

120. Hull RD, Raskob G, Gent M, et al. Effectiveness of intermittent pneumatic leg compression for preventing deep vein thrombosis after total hip replacement. *JAMA* 1990;263:2313.
121. Geerts WH, Jay RM, Code KI. A comparison of low-dose heparin with low-molecular-weight heparin as prophylaxis against venous thromboembolism after major trauma. *N Engl J Med* 1996;335:701.
122. Clagett GP, Anderson FA, Heit J. Prevention of venous thromboembolism. *Chest* 1995;108:312s.
123. Turner GM, Cole SF, Brooks JH. The efficacy of graduated compression stockings in the prevention of deep vein thrombosis after major gynecological surgery. *Br J Obstet Gynecol* 1984;91:588.
124. Sarret M, Kher A, Toulemonde F. Prophylaxis of venous thromboembolism in general, oncological, gynecological and neurological surgery. In: Sarret M, Kher A, Toulemonde F, et al., eds. *Low molecular weight heparin.* New York: Marcel Dekker, 1999:296.
125. Haas SK, Wolf H, Encke A, et al. Prevention of fatal postoperative pulmonary embolism by low molecular weight heparin: a double blind comparison of certoparin and unfractionated heparin. *Thromb Haemost* 1999;82(suppl):1548(abst).
126. Fareed J, Haas S, Sasahara A, guest eds. Differentiation of low molecular weight heparins: applied and clinical considerations. *Semin Thromb Hemost* 1999;25(suppl):1.
127. Haas S, Turpie AGG, guest eds. From foundations to the future: building a new era in DVT management. *Blood Coagul Fibrinolysis* 1999;10(suppl):S1–S131.

Disorders of Thrombosis and Hemostasis: Clinical and Laboratory Practice, Third Edition, edited by Rodger L. Bick.
Lippincott Williams & Wilkins, Philadelphia © 2002

16

ORAL ANTITHROMBOTIC THERAPY: WARFARINS AND RELATED COMPOUNDS

GRAHAM F. PINEO
RUSSELL D. HULL

The oral anticoagulants are the most commonly used agents in the long-term prophylaxis and treatment of both arterial and venous thrombotic disorders. As new and expanded indications for their use are developed, such as the prevention of recurrent myocardial infarction or the treatment of systemic embolism in atrial fibrillation, the use of oral anticoagulants continues to increase. In North America, oral anticoagulants are commonly used for the prevention of venous thromboembolism after orthopedic surgery. In this chapter, we review the pharmacology of warfarin sodium, the most commonly used oral anticoagulant in North America, and discuss practical aspects of the use of this agent in the management of thrombotic disorders, with particular reference to the treatment of venous thromboembolism.

PHARMACOLOGY

The Vitamin K Cycle

Vitamin K is responsible for the posttranslational conversion of glutamate residues into Gla in a limited number of proteins, the best known of which are the blood-coagulation factors II, VII, IX, X, protein C, protein S, and protein Z, and bone matrix proteins. The best-known bone matrix proteins are osteocalcin and matrix Gla-protein (MGP) (1).

γ-Carboxyglutamic acid permits the binding of calcium by these proteins, and in the presence of calcium, the coagulation factors undergo a conformational change that is required for their binding to various active cofactors on cell surfaces (2). The reduced form of vitamin K (KH_2) acts as a coenzyme for carboxylase. The oxidation of vitamin (KH_2) by oxygen into vitamin K epoxide (KO) provides energy to fix carbon dioxide (CO_2) at the γ position of a glutamate residue (Fig. 16.1). The vitamin KO is then recycled, first by vitamin K epoxide reductase to vitamin K (quinone) and then by vitamin K reductase to vitamin KH_2 (hydroquinone). It is essential that each molecule of vitamin K be recycled several hundred times before being metabolized.

The oral anticoagulants inhibit vitamin KO reductase and possibly vitamin K reductase, thereby depleting vitamin KH_2 and causing the buildup of vitamin KO in the tissues such as the liver and plasma (Fig. 16.1).

The most important forms of vitamin K are phylloquinones (vitamin K_1) and menaquinones (vitamin K_2) (1).

Phylloquinones are found in green, leafy vegetables such as spinach, cabbage, and broccoli. Deficiencies of these vegetables in the diet can cause vitamin K deficiency, whereas excessive amounts can reverse the effects of oral anticoagulants. The menaquinones occur in various foods such as yogurt and organ meats. They also are produced by the bacterial flora of the colon and possibly the small intestine. Factors interfering with the production or absorption of these menaquinones (e.g., broad-spectrum antibiotics) may lead to vitamin K deficiency (3) and interference with anticoagulant control. Certain cephalosporins containing an *N*-methyl-thiotetrazole side chain may interfere directly with vitamin KO reductase in the liver (4), thereby leading to vitamin K deficiency. Most of the vitamin K stores in the liver are menaquinones, and it is thought that most of these originate from the diet rather than from intestinal flora (1).

Large doses of vitamin K can overcome the blockade of vitamin KH_2 by oral anticoagulants, presumably because vitamin K reductase is less sensitive to the coumarins than is vitamin KO reductase (Fig. 16.1) (1). This reversal of oral anticoagulants applies to the first-generation agents such as warfarin, but does not apply to the second-generation rodenticides known as the "superwarfarins," which have an extremely long half-life. Accidental consumption of these

G. F. Pineo and **R. D. Hull:** Department of Medicine, University of Calgary; Department of Medicine–Hematology, Foothills Hospital, Calgary, Alberta, Canada.

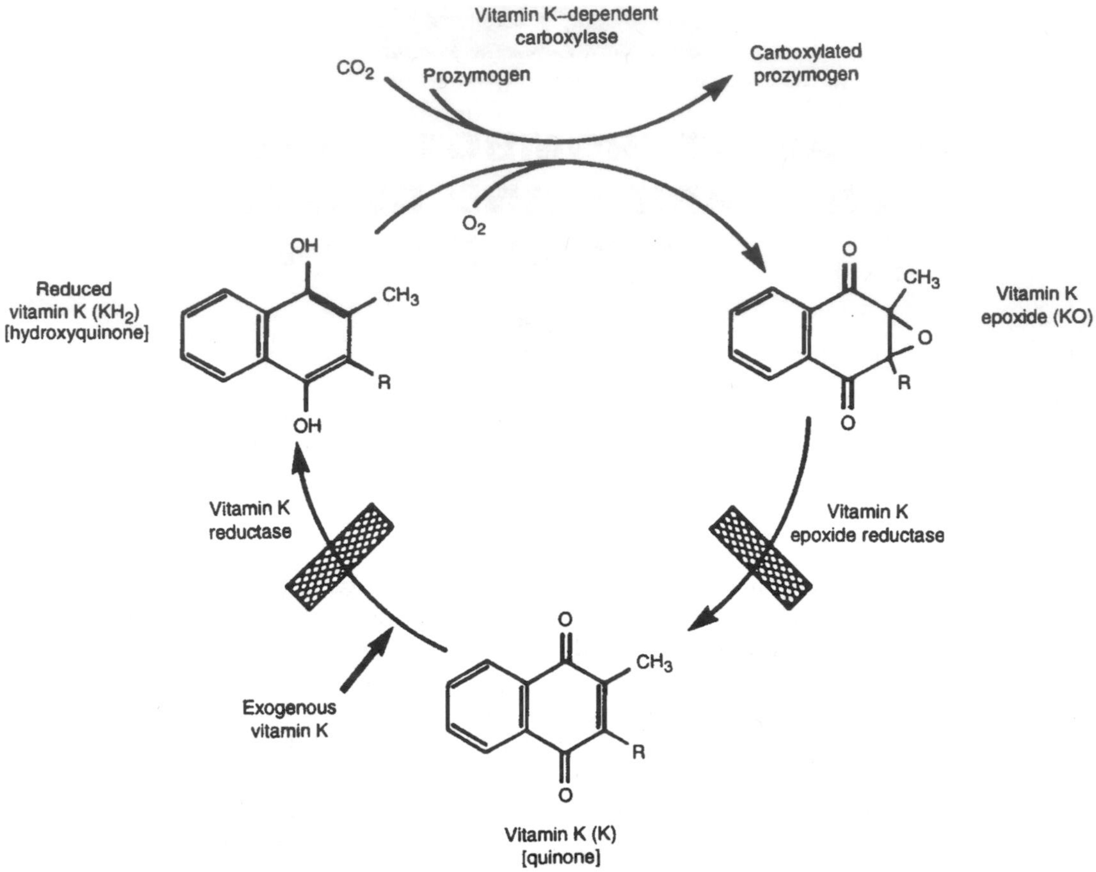

FIGURE 16.1. The vitamin K cycle: the effect of warfarin and exogenous vitamin K (phytomenadione). Vitamin K (quinone) is converted to reduced vitamin K (KH_2, hydroxyquinone) by vitamin K reductase. Vitamin KH_2 is the substrate for the carboxylation of prozymogens (e.g., factors II, VII, IX, X) to activate enzymes. Carbon dioxide and oxygen are required for this reaction, and vitamin KH_2 is converted to vitamin K epoxide (KO). Vitamin K is regenerated from vitamin KO by vitamin K epoxide reductase. Warfarin inhibits vitamin K epoxide reductase and, to some extent, vitamin K reductase (*hatched areas*). Exogenous vitamin K in large doses overcomes the blockage by warfarin, presumably because vitamin K reductase is less sensitive to warfarin than is vitamin K epoxide reductase (*arrow*). Reproduced from Furie B, Furie BC. Molecular basis of vitamin K-dependent gamma-carboxylation. *Blood* 1990;75:1753–1762, with permission.

agents requires repeated injections of vitamin K and fresh frozen plasma for up to 1 or 2 years to completely overcome their effects (5,6).

Pharmacokinetics and Pharmacodynamics of Warfarin

There are two distinct chemical groups of oral anticoagulants: the 4-hydroxy coumarin derivatives (e.g., warfarin sodium) and the indane-1,3-dione derivatives (e.g., phenindione) (7). The coumarin derivatives are the oral anticoagulants of choice because they are associated with fewer nonhemorrhagic side effects than are the indanedione derivatives. In North America, the most commonly used agent is coumarin (Coumadin–Bristol–Myers Squibb, Princeton, NJ, U.S.A.), but in recent years, various generic forms of warfarin sodium have been introduced.

Warfarin is a racemic mixture of stereoisomers (R and S forms). Warfarin is highly water soluble and is highly bioavailable (8). Peak absorption occurs at about 90 minutes, and the half-life is between 36 and 42 hours. Warfarin is highly protein bound (primarily albumin), and only the non–protein-bound material is biologically active. Any drug or chemical that also is bound to albumin may displace warfarin from its protein-binding sites and thereby increase the biologically active material (8). Warfarin is metabolized in the liver by the p450 system of enzymes. Interference with the p450 enzymes by various drugs or a mutation in the gene coding for one of the common p450 enzymes can markedly interfere with the metabolism of warfarin. Therefore the half-life of warfarin can vary markedly from one patient to another, and individual laboratory monitoring to determine drug dosing is mandatory.

The anticoagulant effect of warfarin is mediated by the inhibition of the vitamin K–dependent γ-carboxylation of coagulation factors II, VII, IX, and X (7,8). This results in the synthesis of immunologically detectable but biologically inactive forms of these coagulation proteins. Warfarin also inhibits the vitamin K–dependent γ-carboxylation of proteins C and S (9). Protein C circulates as a proenzyme that is activated on endothelial cells by the thrombin/thrombomodulin complex to form activated protein C. Activated protein C in the presence of protein S inhibits activated factor VIII and activated factor V activity (9). Therefore vitamin K antagonists such as warfarin create a biochemical paradox by producing an anticoagulant effect due to the inhibition of procoagulants (factors II, VII, IX, and X) and a potentially thrombogenic effect by impairing the synthesis of naturally occurring inhibitors of coagulation (proteins C and S) (9). Heparin or low-molecular-weight heparin and warfarin treatment should overlap by 4 to 5 days when warfarin treatment is initiated in patients with thrombotic disease.

The anticoagulant effect of warfarin is delayed until the normal clotting factors are cleared from the circulation, and the peak effect does not occur until 36 to 72 hours after drug administration (10). During the first few days of warfarin therapy, the prothrombin time (PT) reflects mainly the depression of factor VII, which has a half-life of 5 to 7 hours. Equilibrium levels of factors II, IX, and X are not reached until about 1 week after the initiation of therapy. The use of small initial daily doses (e.g., 5 mg) is the preferred approach for initiating warfarin treatment. The dose–response relation to warfarin therapy varies widely between individuals, and therefore, the dose must be carefully monitored to prevent overdosing or underdosing.

A number of factors influence the anticoagulant response of warfarin in individual patients; these include inaccuracies in laboratory testing and noncompliance of patients, but more importantly reflect the influence of dietary changes or the influence of drugs that interfere with the metabolism of warfarin. The availability of vitamin K can be influenced by dramatic changes in dietary intake or by drugs such as antibiotics, which interfere with the synthesis of vitamin K in the gastrointestinal tract. A wide variety of drugs may interact with warfarin. However, a critical appraisal of the literature reporting such interactions indicates that the evidence substantiating many of the claims is limited (11). The interactions of drugs and food with warfarin are reviewed in detail in a recent publication (8). Aspirin is particularly problematic because it interferes with platelet function, displaces warfarin from its protein binding, thus augmenting its biologic activities and, as with the nonsteroidal antiinflammatory drugs (NSAIDs), it may cause gastric erosions, thus creating a site for bleeding. Nonetheless, in certain patients, the use of aspirin and warfarin is indicated to improve efficacy, even though minor bleeding may be somewhat increased. It is important that patients be warned against taking any new drugs without the knowledge of their attending physician, and it is prudent to monitor the international normalized ratio (INR) more frequently when any drug (including natural compounds) is added or discontinued from the regimen of the patient being treated with an oral anticoagulant.

Laboratory Monitoring and Therapeutic Range

The laboratory test most commonly used to measure the effects of warfarin is the one-stage PT test. The PT is sensitive to reduced activity of factors II, VII, and X but is insensitive to reduced activity of factor IX. Confusion about the appropriate therapeutic range has occurred because the different tissue thromboplastins used for measuring the PT vary considerably in sensitivity to the vitamin K–dependent clotting factors and in response to warfarin (12). Rabbit brain thromboplastin, which has been widely used in North America, is less sensitive than is standardized human brain thromboplastin, which has been widely used in the United Kingdom and other parts of Europe. A PT ratio of 1.5 to 2.0 with rabbit brain thromboplastin (i.e., the traditional therapeutic range in North America) is equivalent to a ratio of 4.0 to 6.0 with human brain thromboplastin (12). Conversely, a two- to threefold increase in the PT with standardized human brain thromboplastin is equivalent to a 1.25- to 1.5-fold increase in the PT with a rabbit brain thromboplastin (12).

To promote standardization of the PT for monitoring oral anticoagulant therapy, the World Health Organization (WHO) developed an international reference thromboplastin from human brain tissue and recommended that the PT ratio be expressed as the INR (8). The INR is the PT ratio obtained by testing a given sample by using the WHO reference thromboplastin. For practical clinical purposes, the INR for a given plasma sample is equivalent to the PT ratio obtained by using a standardized human brain thromboplastin known as the Manchester Comparative Reagent, which has been widely used in the United Kingdom (8). In recent years, thromboplastins with a high sensitivity have been commonly used. Many centers have been using the recombinant tissue factor, which has an Institute for Scientific Information (ISI) value 0.9 to 1.0, giving an INR equivalent to the PT ratio.

Warfarin is administered in an initial dose of 5 to 7.5 mg per day for the first 2 days, and the daily dose is then adjusted according to the INR. Heparin or low-molecular-weight heparin therapy is discontinued on the fourth or fifth day after initiation of warfarin therapy, provided the INR is prolonged into the recommended therapeutic range (INR, 2.0 to 3.0) for at least two consecutive days (8). Because some individuals are either fast or slow metabolizers of the drug, the selection of the correct dosage of warfarin must be individualized. Therefore, frequent INR determinations are required initially to establish therapeutic anticoagulation.

Once the anticoagulant effect and patient's warfarin dose requirements are stable, the INR should be monitored every 1 to 3 weeks throughout the course of warfarin therapy. However, if there are factors that may produce an unpredictable response to warfarin (e.g., concomitant drug therapy) (11), the INR should be monitored more frequently to minimize the risk of complications due to poor anticoagulant control.

LONG-TERM TREATMENT OF VENOUS THROMBOEMBOLISM

Patients with established venous thrombosis or pulmonary embolism require long-term anticoagulant therapy to prevent recurrent disease (8,12). Warfarin therapy is highly effective and is preferred in most patients. Adjusted-dose subcutaneous heparin is the treatment of choice if long-term oral anticoagulants are contraindicated, such as in pregnancy. Adjusted-dose, subcutaneous heparin, or unmonitored low-molecular-weight heparin have been used for the long-term treatment of patients in whom oral anticoagulant therapy proves to be very difficult to control. In patients with proximal vein thrombosis, long-term therapy with warfarin reduces the frequency of objectively documented recurrent venous thromboembolism from 47% to 2% (13). The use of a less intense warfarin regimen (INR, 2 to 3) markedly reduces the risk of bleeding from 20% to 4%, without loss of effectiveness, in comparison with more intense warfarin (12). With the improved safety of oral anticoagulant therapy with a less intense warfarin regimen, there has been renewed interest in evaluating the long-term treatment of thrombotic disorders. In clinical trials in patients with atrial fibrillation, it has been shown that oral anticoagulant treatment can be given safely with a low risk of major bleeding complications (1% to 2% per year) (14). In trials such as these, the safety of oral anticoagulant treatment depends heavily on the maintenance of a narrow therapeutic INR range. When the INR falls below the therapeutic range, the incidence of thrombotic stroke increases, whereas when the INR exceeds a level of 3.5 to 5.0, the incidence of major hemorrhage markedly increases. These and other studies have emphasized the importance of maintaining careful control of oral anticoagulant therapy, particularly with the use of anticoagulant management clinics if oral anticoagulants are going to be used for extended periods.

Data from clinical trials indicating an unacceptably high incidence of recurrent venous thromboembolism, in patients with proximal deep vein thrombosis who are treated according to the current practice with intravenous heparin for several days, followed by oral anticoagulant treatment for 3 to 6 months, have been further reasons for renewed interest in longer-term treatment of venous thromboembolism (13,15–19). These studies indicate that patients with deep vein thrombosis who are treated according to current clinical practice face an unfavorable long-term prognosis. Three groups of patients who have a guarded prognosis have been identified: patients with idiopathic, recurrent venous thromboembolism; patients who are carriers of genetic mutations that predispose to venous thromboembolism, such as the factor V Leiden mutation; and patients with cancer (20,21).

OPTIMAL DURATION OF ORAL ANTICOAGULANTS AFTER A FIRST EPISODE OF DEEP VEIN THROMBOSIS

It has been recommended that all patients with a first episode of venous thromboembolism receive warfarin therapy for at least 12 weeks. Attempts to decrease the treatment to 4 weeks (22,23) or 6 weeks (18) resulted in higher rates of recurrent thromboembolism in comparison with either 12 or 26 weeks of treatment (11% to 18% recurrent thromboembolism in the following 1 to 2 years). Most of the recurrent thromboembolic events occurred in the 6 to 8 weeks immediately after anticoagulant treatment was stopped, and the incidence was higher in patients with continuing risk factors, such as cancer and immobilization (18, 23). Treatment with oral anticoagulants for 6 months reduced the incidence of recurrent thromboembolic events, but there was a cumulative incidence of recurrent events at 2 years (11%) and an ongoing risk of recurrent thromboembolism of approximately 5% to 6% per year (18). In patients with a first episode of idiopathic venous thromboembolism treated with intravenous heparin followed by warfarin for 3 months, continuation of warfarin for 24 months led to a significant reduction in the incidence of recurrent venous thromboembolism when compared with placebo (24). This continued risk of recurrent thromboembolism even with 6 months' treatment after a first episode of deep vein thrombosis has encouraged the development of clinical trials evaluating the effectiveness of long-term anticoagulant treatment beyond 6 months. Clinical trials are currently under way to determine if long treatment of anticoagulation with a targeted of INR of 1.5 to 2.0 can decrease the incidence of recurrent thromboembolism without an increase in major bleeding when compared with a targeted INR of 2.0 to 3.0 or with placebo treatment. It will be a few years before the results of these clinical trials are available.

Optimal Duration of Oral Anticoagulant Treatment in Patients with Recurrent Deep Vein Thrombosis

In a multicenter clinical trial, Schulman et al. (19) randomized patients with a first recurrent episode of venous thromboembolism to receive either 6 months or continued oral anticoagulants indefinitely, with a targeted INR of 2.0 to

2.85 (19). The analysis was reported at 4 years. In the patients receiving anticoagulants for 6 months, recurrent thromboembolism occurred in 20.7%, compared with 2.6% of patients on the indefinite treatment ($p < 0.001$). However, the rates of major bleeding were 2.7% in the 6-month group, compared with 8.6% in the indefinite group. In the indefinite group, two of the major hemorrhages were fatal, whereas there were no fatal hemorrhages in the 6-month group. This study showed that extending the duration of oral anticoagulants for approximately 4 years resulted in a significant decrease in the incidence of recurrent venous thromboembolism, but with a higher incidence of major bleeding. Without a mortality difference, the risk of hemorrhage versus the benefit of decreased recurrent thromboembolism with the use of extended warfarin treatment remains uncertain and will require further clinical trials.

From the sixth American College of Chest Physicians Consensus Conference on Antithrombotic Therapy, the following recommendations were made (25). Oral anticoagulant therapy should be continued for at least 3 months to prolong the prothrombin time to a targeted INR of 2.5 (range, 2.0 to 3.0). Patients with reversible or time-limited risk factors can be treated for 3 to 6 months. Patients with a first episode of idiopathic venous thromboembolism should be treated for at least 6 months. Patients with recurrent venous thromboembolism or a continuing risk factor such as cancer, antithrombin deficiency states, or antiphospholipid syndrome should be treated indefinitely. Patients with activated protein C resistance (factor V Leiden) should probably receive indefinite treatment if they have recurrent disease, are homozygous for the gene, or have multiple thrombophilic conditions. Accumulated evidence indicates that symptomatic isolated calf vein thrombosis should be treated with anticoagulants for at least 3 months (25).

PREVENTION OF VENOUS THROMBOEMBOLISM

The use of oral anticoagulant treatment with a targeted INR of 2 to 3 is effective in the prevention of venous thrombosis after hip fracture or total hip or total knee replacement (26,27). However, recent studies have demonstrated that the use of low-molecular-weight heparin in close proximity to surgery is more effective than oral anticoagulants after total hip replacement (28). Oral anticoagulants with an INR of 2 to 3 also are effective in preventing venous thrombosis after gynecologic surgery (29).

PREVENTION OF ISCHEMIC STROKE IN PATIENTS WITH ATRIAL FIBRILLATION

In five randomized clinical trials in patients with atrial fibrillation, the efficacy and safety of warfarin was compared with aspirin treatment (30–34). In all studies, warfarin was superior to aspirin in the prevention of ischemic stroke, and there was little difference in the rate of major or intracranial bleeding (30–34). Minor bleeding was seen more frequently with warfarin treatment.

The EAFT trial compared the anticoagulant treatment, aspirin, and placebo in the prevention of ischemic stroke in patients with atrial fibrillation (35). Compared with placebo, there was a significant decrease in the incidence of stroke with warfarin but an insignificant difference in risk reduction with aspirin. In the SPAF III trial, adjusted-dose warfarin with a targeted INR of 2 to 3 was more effective than a fixed dose of warfarin (1 to 3 mg/day) plus aspirin (325 mg/day) in patients with atrial fibrillation at high risk of embolism (36). Aspirin alone was sufficient in patients with atrial fibrillation at low risk of thromboembolism.

LONG-TERM ANTICOAGULATION IN PATIENTS WITH CARDIOVASCULAR DISORDERS

Oral anticoagulants have been used in the primary or secondary prevention of myocardial infarction and in patients with a variety of prosthetic heart valves. Low-intensity warfarin plus aspirin has been compared with aspirin alone in the primary prevention of acute ischemic coronary events (i.e., death or nonfatal myocardial infarction). In the CARS study (Coumadin Aspirin Reinfarction Study), fixed low-dose-intensity warfarin was similar to aspirin in the prevention of death or myocardial infarction (37). In the Thrombosis Prevention Trial, adjusted-dose warfarin with a targeted INR of 1.3 to 1.8 plus aspirin was compared with aspirin alone in the prevention of death or myocardial infarction (38). The combination of warfarin and aspirin was effective in reducing these outcomes, whereas either warfarin or aspirin given alone did not produce a significant reduction in these end points. In these low-intensity warfarin studies, it is apparent that the dose of warfarin must be adjusted to an INR of at least 1.5 when combined with aspirin to achieve a therapeutic benefit.

The multitude of clinical trials comparing warfarin of varying intensity with either placebo or aspirin has recently been reviewed in a meta-analysis (39). From this analysis, it was shown that moderate to high-intensity warfarin was more effective than either aspirin or placebo but with an increased incidence of major bleeding. Although low-fixed-dose unmonitored warfarin plus aspirin was more effective than aspirin, it did produce an increase in major bleeding. Moderately intense warfarin plus aspirin was superior to aspirin alone, with only a marginal and nonsignificant increase in major bleeding.

Warfarin has been used for the prevention of thromboembolic events in patients with a variety of prosthetic heart valves (40,41). The data are reviewed in the recent

Consensus Conference of the American College of Chest Physicians (42). In general, warfarin with a targeted INR of 2.5 to 3.5 is recommended for most patients with mechanical prosthetic valves. An INR of 2.0 to 3.0 is recommended with bioprosthetic valves and low-risk patients with bileaflet mechanical valves in the aortic position.

Adverse Effects

The major side effect of oral anticoagulant therapy is bleeding (43). Bleeding during well-controlled oral anticoagulant therapy is usually due to surgery or other forms of trauma, or to local lesions, such as peptic ulcer or carcinoma (43). Spontaneous bleeding may occur if warfarin is given in an excessive dose, resulting in marked prolongation of the INR; this bleeding may be severe and even life threatening. The risk of bleeding can be substantially reduced by adjustment of the warfarin dose to achieve a less intense anticoagulant effect than was traditionally used in North America (INR, 2.0 to 3.0; prothrombin time, 1.25 to 1.5 times control value obtained by using a rabbit brain thromboplastin, such as Simplastin or Dade-C) (12).

Nonhemorrhagic side effects of oral anticoagulant differ according to whether coumarin derivatives (e.g., warfarin sodium) or indanediones are administered. Such side effects are uncommon with coumarin anticoagulants, and the coumarins are therefore the oral anticoagulants of choice.

Coumarin-induced skin necrosis is a rare but serious complication that requires immediate cessation of oral anticoagulant therapy (44,45). It usually occurs between 3 and 10 days after therapy has commenced, is more common in women, and most often involves areas of abundant subcutaneous tissues, such as the abdomen, buttocks, thighs, and breast. The mechanism of coumarin-induced skin necrosis, which is associated with microvascular thrombosis, is uncertain but appears to be related, at least in some patients, to depression of protein C level. Patients with congenital deficiencies of protein C may be particularly prone to the development of coumarin skin necrosis.

Oral anticoagulants cross the placenta and may cause fetal malformations when used during pregnancy (46–48). Two specific fetopathic syndromes are associated with oral anticoagulant administration during pregnancy. Treatment with oral anticoagulants during weeks 12 to 16 of gestation may induce the syndrome of warfarin embryopathy in the fetus. This syndrome consists of skeletal abnormalities ranging from stippled epiphyses to frank skeletal hypoplasia. Although most of the reported cases have occurred in infants of mothers receiving warfarin, this syndrome also has been reported to result from phenindanedione or acenocoumarin administration. Oral anticoagulant administration during the second or third trimester of pregnancy may result in central nervous system abnormalities in the fetus, including abnormalities of the ventricular system (Dandy–Walker malformation), dorsal midline dysplasia, and optic atrophy. Therefore the use of oral anticoagulants is contraindicated at any time during pregnancy, and they should not be used in women planning a pregnancy. Adjusted-dose heparin or low-molecular-weight heparin can safely be given throughout pregnancy in patients with venous thromboembolism, and from that observation, indications have been extrapolated to include patients requiring anticoagulation to prevent systemic embolism from prosthetic heart valves (47).

Management of Patients Receiving Long-term Oral Anticoagulants Requiring Surgical Intervention

Physicians are commonly confronted with the problem of managing oral anticoagulants in individuals who require temporary interruption of treatment for surgery or other invasive procedures (49–54). In the absence of data from randomized clinical trials, recommendations can be made based only on cohort studies, retrospective reviews, and expert opinions. The most common conditions requiring long-term anticoagulant therapy are atrial fibrillation, mechanical or prosthetic heart valve replacement, and venous thromboembolism (55). For each of these conditions, the risk of arterial or venous thromboembolism, when anticoagulants have been discontinued, must be weighed against the risk of bleeding if intravenous heparin is applied before or after the surgical procedure, or if oral anticoagulant therapy is continued at the therapeutic level. The possible choices based on the risk/benefit assessment in the individual patient include (40):

1. discontinuing warfarin for 3 to 5 days before the procedure to allow the INR to return to normal and then restarting therapy shortly after surgery,
2. reducing the warfarin dose to maintain an INR in the lower or subtherapeutic range during the surgical procedure, or
3. discontinuing warfarin and treating the patient in the hospital with intravenous heparin before and after the surgical procedure, until warfarin therapy can be reinstituted. Low-molecular-weight heparin is now being used in some of the circumstances.

In a recent review that attempted to estimate the risk/benefit for the temporary discontinuation of oral anticoagulants and the temporary use of heparin in patients with different conditions requiring oral anticoagulation, further revised recommendations were made (55).

Low-molecular-weight heparin, which can be given by once- or twice-daily subcutaneous injection, offers a convenient alternative to intravenous unfractionated heparin for patients requiring temporary interruption of warfarin therapy for invasive procedures. Although no randomized clinical trials have been carried out, in a large cohort study, patients with mechanical heart valves, atrial fibrillation, or venous thromboembolism who required an interruption of anticoagulant therapy for various surgical procedures were given low-molecular-weight heparin in therapeutic doses after warfarin had been discontinued for 4 to 5 days before the procedure (56). The low-molecular-weight heparin was discontinued 12 hours before the procedure and recommenced within 8 to 12 hours after surgery, at which time warfarin was restarted. With this protocol, patients were off warfarin for an average of 5.4 days, and they received low-molecular-weight heparin an average of 9.3 days. Only one patient experienced major bleeding. Two other small studies have shown that low-molecular-weight heparin in either therapeutic or prophylactic doses was effective and safe in a similar setting and indicated that low-molecular-weight heparin provides a convenient and less costly alternative to intravenous unfractionated heparin for the temporary interruption of anticoagulant therapy (57,58).

ANTIDOTE TO ORAL ANTICOAGULANT AGENTS

The antidote to the vitamin K antagonists is vitamin K_1. If an excessive increase of the INR occurs, the treatment depends on the degree of the increase and whether the patient is bleeding (59). If the increase is mild and the patient is not bleeding, no specific treatment is necessary, other than reduction in the warfarin dose. The INR can be expected to decrease during the next 24 hours with this approach. With more marked increase of the INR in patients who are not bleeding, treatment with small doses of vitamin K_1, given either orally or by subcutaneous injection (1 to 2 mg) could be considered. With very marked increase of the INR, particularly in a patient who is either actively bleeding or at risk for bleeding, the coagulation defect should be corrected.

Reported side effects of vitamin K include flushing, dizziness, tachycardia, hypotension, dyspnea, and sweating (59). Intravenous administration of vitamin K_1 should be performed with caution to avoid inducing an anaphylactoid reaction. The risk of anaphylactoid reaction can be reduced by slow intravenous (i.v.) administration of vitamin K_1, at a rate no faster than 1 mg/min, i.v. In most patients, i.v. administration of vitamin K_1 produces a demonstrable effect on the INR within 6 to 8 hours and corrects the increased INR within 12 to 24 hours. Because the half-life of vitamin K_1 is less than that of warfarin sodium, a repeated course of vitamin K_1 may be necessary. If bleeding is very severe and life threatening, vitamin K therapy can be supplemented with concentrates of factors II, VII, IX, and X.

ALTERNATIVE APPROACHES TO THE MANAGEMENT OF ORAL ANTICOAGULANT THERAPY

Anticoagulant Management Clinics

In recent years, a large number of anticoagulation management clinics have been developed, initially in Europe and more recently in North America. As described by Ansell et al. (60–62), these anticoagulation management clinics provide coordinated services for patients requiring long-term anticoagulation therapy. Although there have been no randomized clinical trials comparing routine medical care with care given in anticoagulant management clinics, there is evidence that patients managed in these clinics are within the targeted INR a larger percentage of the time and therefore there would be expected to have a decrease in the incidence of thromboembolism as well as of major bleeding (62). Cost analysis based on the data from a number of reports comparing routine medical care with anticoagulation management clinics indicates that anticoagulant management clinics are capable of achieving cost saving that should be equal to the cost of running the clinics themselves.

Computer programs are now available for the data management for anticoagulant management clinics, and one system has been developed for the ongoing prescribing of warfarin once patients have a stable INR on at least two occasions. In an interesting report, it was shown that the computer was superior to experienced hematologists in the ordering of warfarin, with a higher percentage of patients achieving their targeted INR a greater amount of time with the use of the computer program (63).

Point-of-care International Normalized Ratio Testing

A number of instruments are now available for the measurement of capillary INRs on finger sampling of whole blood. INRs performed with these instruments compare well with venous samples, and numerous studies have indicated that many patients are capable of both self-testing and self-management of their warfarin dosing (64–66). Some studies have indicated that self-management of warfarin therapy using point-of-care INR testing has resulted in higher INR compliance with fewer tests when compared with physician-managed patients (66).

REFERENCES

1. Vermeer C. Gamma-carboxylglutamate-containing proteins and the vitamin K-dependent carboxylase. *Biochem J* 1990;266: 625–636.
2. Furie B, Furie BC. Molecular basis of vitamin K-dependent gamma-carboxylation. *Blood* 1990;75:1753–1762.
3. Pineo GF, Gallus AS, Hirsh J. Unexpected vitamin K deficiency in hospitalized patients. *Can Med Assoc J* 1973;109:880–883.

4. Lipsky JJ. Antibiotic-associated hypoprothrombinaemia. *J Antimicrob Chemother* 1998;21:281–300.
5. Exner DV, Brien WF, Murphy MJ. Superwarfarin ingestion. *Can Med Assoc J* 1992;146:34–35.
6. Lipton RA, Klass EM. Human ingestion of a "superwarfarin" rodenticide resulting in a prolonged anticoagulant effect. *JAMA* 1984;252:3004–3005.
7. Freedman MD. Oral anticoagulants: pharmacodynamics, clinical indication and adverse effects. *J Clin Pharmacol* 1992;32: 196–209.
8. Hirsh J, Dalen JE, Deykin D, et al. Oral anticoagulants; mechanism of action, clinical effectiveness, and optimal therapeutic range. *Chest* 2001;119:8S–21S.
9. Clouse LH, Comp PC. The regulation of hemostasis: the protein C system. *N Engl J Med* 1986;314:1298–1304.
10. O'Reilly RA, Aggeler PM. Studies on coumarin anticoagulant drugs: initiation of warfarin therapy without a loading dose. *Circulation* 1968;368:169–177.
11. Wells PS, Holbrook AM, Crowther R, et al. Warfarin and its drug/food interactions; a critical appraisal of the literature. *Ann Intern Med* 1994;121:676–683.
12. Hull R, Hirsh J, Jay R, et al. Different intensities of oral anticoagulant therapy in the treatment of proximal-vein thrombosis. *N Engl J Med* 1982;307:1676–1681.
13. Hull R, Carter C, Jay R, et al. The diagnosis of acute recurrent deep-vein thrombosis: a diagnostic challenge. *Circulation* 1983; 67:901–906.
14. Laupacis A, Albers G, Dalen J, et al. Antithrombotic therapy in atrial fibrillation. *Chest* 1995;108:352S–359S.
15. Prandoni P, Lensing AWA, Cogo A, et al. The long-term clinical course of acute deep venous thrombosis. *Ann Intern Med* 1996; 125:1–7.
16. Beyth RJ, Cohen AM, Landefeld CS. Long-term outcomes of deep vein thrombosis. *Arch Intern Med* 1995;155:1031–1037.
17. Franzeck UK, Schaich I, Jager KA, et al. Prospective 12 year follow-up study of clinical and hemodynamic sequelae after deep vein thrombosis in low-risk patients (Zurich study). *Circulation* 1996;93:74–79.
18. Schulman S, Rhedin AS, Lindmarker P, et al. A comparison of six week with six months of oral anticoagulation therapy after a first episode of venous thromboembolism. *N Engl J Med* 1995; 332:1661–1665.
19. Schulman S, Granqvist S, Holmstrom M, et al. The duration of oral anticoagulant therapy after a second episode of venous thromboembolism. *N Engl J Med* 1997;336:393–398.
20. Prandoni P, Lensing A, Buller H, et al. Deep vein thrombosis and the incidence of subsequent symptomatic cancer. *N Engl J Med* 1992;327:1128–1133.
21. Simioni P, Prandoni P, Lensing AWA, et al. The risk of recurrent venous thromboembolism in patients with an Arg^{506}Gln mutation in the gene for factor V (factor V Leiden). *N Engl J Med* 1997;336:339–403.
22. Research Committee of the British Thoracic Society. Optimum duration of anticoagulation for deep vein thrombosis and pulmonary embolism. *Lancet* 1992;340:873–876.
23. Levine MN, Hirsh J, Gent M, et al. Optimal duration of oral anticoagulation therapy: a randomized trial comparing four weeks with three months of warfarin in patients with proximal deep vein thrombosis. *Thromb Haemost* 1995;74:606–611.
24. Kearon C, Gent M, Hirsh J, et al. Extended anticoagulation prevented recurrence after a first episode of idiopathic venous thromboembolism. *N Engl J Med* 1999;340:901–907.
25. Hyers T, Agnelli G, Hull R, et al. Antithrombotic therapy for venous thromboembolic disease. *Chest* 119;S176–S193.
26. Powers PJ, Gent M, Jay RM, et al. A randomized trial of less intense postoperative warfarin or aspirin therapy in the prevention of venous thromboembolism after surgery for fractured hip. *Arch Intern Med* 1989;149:771–774.
27. Geerts WH, Heit JA, Clagett P, et al. Prevention of venous thromboembolism. *Chest* 119;S132–S175.
28. Hull RD, Pineo GF, Francis C, et al. Low-molecular-weight heparin prophylaxis using dalteparin close to surgery versus warfarin in hip arthroplasty patients. *Arch Intern Med* 2000;160:2199–2207.
29. Taberner DA, Poller L, Burslem RW, et al. Oral anticoagulants controlled by the British comparative thromboplastin versus low-dose heparin in prophylaxis of deep vein thrombosis. *Br Med J* 1978;1:272–274.
30. The Stroke Prevention in Atrial Fibrillation Investigators. The Stroke Prevention in Atrial Fibrillation study: final results. *Circulation* 1991;84:527–539.
31. The Boston Area Anticoagulation Trial for Atrial Fibrillation Investigators. The effect of low-dose warfarin on the risk of stroke in patients with nonrheumatic atrial fibrillation. *N Engl J Med* 1990;323:1505–1511.
32. Ezekowitz MD, Bridgers SL, James KE, et al. Warfarin in the prevention of stroke associated with nonrheumatic atrial fibrillation: Veterans Affairs stroke prevention in nonrheumatic atrial fibrillation investigators [published erratum appears in *N Engl J Med* 1993;328:148. *N Engl J Med* 1992;20:1406–1412.
33. Petersen P, Boysan G, Godtfredsen J, et al. Placebo-controlled, randomized trial of warfarin and aspirin for prevention of thromboembolic complication in chronic atrial fibrillation: the Copenhagen AFASAK Study. *Lancet* 1989;1:175–179.
34. Connoly SJ, Laupacis A, Gent M, et al. Canadian Atrial Fibrillation Anticoagulation (CAFA) Study. *J Am Coll Cardiol* 1991; 18:349–355.
35. European Atrial Fibrillation Trial Study Group. Secondary prevention in non-rheumatic atrial fibrillation after transient ischaemic attack or minor stroke. *Lancet* 1993;342:1255–1262.
36. Stroke Prevention in Atrial Fibrillation Investigators (SPAF III). Adjusted dose warfarin versus low-intensity, fixed dose warfarin plus aspirin for high-risk patients with atrial fibrillation: Stroke Prevention in Atrial Fibrillation III randomized clinical trial. *Lancet* 1996;348:633–638.
37. CARS Study Investigators. Randomised double-blind trial of fixed low-dose warfarin with aspirin after myocardial infarction. (Coumadin Aspirin Reinfarction Study). *Lancet* 1997;348: 389–396.
38. The Medical Research Council's General Practice Research Framework. Thrombosis Prevention Trial: randomized trial of low-intensity oral anticoagulation with warfarin and low-dose aspirin in the primary prevention of ischaemic heart disease in men at increased risk. *Lancet* 1998;351:233–241.
39. Anand SS, Yusuf S. Oral anticoagulant therapy in patients with coronary artery disease: a meta-analysis. *JAMA* 1999;1:2058–2067.
40. Stein PD, Alpert JS, Copeland JG, et al. Antithrombotic therapy in patients with mechanical and biological prosthetic heart valves. *Chest* 1995;108:3715–3795.
41. Cannegieter SC, Rosendaal FR, Wintzen AR, et al. The optimal intensity of oral anticoagulant therapy in patients with mechanical heart valve prostheses: the Leiden artificial valve and anticoagulation study. *N Engl J Med* 1995;333:11–17.
42. Stein PD, Alpert JS, Bussey HI, et al. Antithrombotic therapy in patients with mechanical and biological prosthetic heart valves. *Chest* 119:S220–S227.
43. Levine MN, Raskob GE, Hirsh J. Hemorrhagic complication of long term anticoagulant therapy. *Chest* 1989;95(suppl 2):26S.
44. Grimaudo V, Gueissaz F, Hauert J, et al. Necrosis of skin induced by coumarin in a patient deficient in protein. *Br Med J* 1989; 298:233.
45. Becker CG. Oral anticoagulant therapy of skin necrosis: speculation on pathogenesis. *Adv Exp Med Biol* 1987;214:217.

46. Hall JG, Pauli RM, Wilson KM. Maternal and fetal sequelae of anticoagulation during pregnancy. *Am J Med* 1980;68:122.
47. Ginsberg JS, Hirsh J. Use of antithrombotic agents during pregnancy. *Chest* 1995;100:305S–311S.
48. Iturbe-Alessio I, del Carmen Fonseca M, Mutchinik O, et al. Risks of anticoagulant therapy in pregnant women with artificial heart valves. *N Engl J Med* 1986;315:1390.
49. Rustad H, Myhre E. Surgery during anticoagulant treatment. *Acta Med Scand* 1963;173:115–119.
50. McIntyre H. Management during dental surgery of patients on anticoagulants. *Lancet* 1966;2:99–100.
51. Tinker JH, Tarhan S. Discontinuing anticoagulant therapy in surgical patients with cardiac valve prostheses. *JAMA* 1978; 239:730–739.
52. Katholi RE, Nolan SP, McGuire LB. The management of anticoagulation during noncardiac operations in patients with prosthetic heart valves. *Am Heart J* 1978;96:163–165.
53. Bodnar AG, Hutter AM. Anticoagulation in valvular heart disease preoperatively and postoperatively. *Cardiovasc Clin* 1984; 14:247–264.
54. Eckman MH, Beshansky JR, Duranad-Zaleski I, et al. Anticoagulation for noncardiac procedures in patients with prosthetic heart valves. *JAMA* 1990;263:1513–1521.
55. Kearon C, Hirsh J. Management of anticoagulation before and after elective surgery. *N Engl J Med* 1997;336:1506–1511.
56. Johnson J, Turpie AGG. Temporary discontinuation of oral anticoagulants: role of low molecular weight heparin. *Thromb Haemost* 1999;suppl:62–63.
57. Tinmouth A, Kovacs MJ, Cruikshank M, et al. Out-patient perioperative and peri-procedure treatment with dalteparin for chronically anticoagulated patients at high risk for thromboembolic complications. *Thromb Haemost* 1999;suppl:662.
58. Spanderfer JM, Lynch S, Weitz HH, et al. Use of enoxaparin for the chronically anticoagulated patient before and after procedures. *Am J Cardiol* 1999;84:478–480.
59. Ansell J, Hirsh J, Dalen J, et al. Managing oral anticoagulant therapy. *Chest* 119;S22–S38.
60. Ansell JE, Hughes R. Evolving models of warfarin management: anticoagulation clinics, patient self-monitoring and patient self-management. *Am Heart J* 1996;132:1095–1100.
61. Ansell J. Anticoagulation management as a risk factor for adverse events: grounds for improvement. *J Thromb Thrombolysis* 1998; 5:S13–S18.
62. Ansell JE, Buttaro ML, Voltis-Thomas O, et al. Consensus guidelines for co-ordinated outpatient oral anticoagulation therapy management. *Ann Pharmocther* 1997;31:604–615.
63. Poller L, Shiach CR, MacCallum PK, et al. Multicentre randomized study of computerized anticoagulant dosage: European concerted action on anticoagulation. *Lancet* 1998:352:1505–1509.
64. Leaning KE, Ansell JE. Advances in the monitoring of oral anticoagulation. *J Thromb Thrombolysis* 1996;3:377–383.
65. White RH, McCurdy SA, von Marensdorff H, et al. Home prothrombin time monitoring after initiation of warfarin therapy. *Ann Intern Med* 1989;111:730–737.
66. Bernardo A. Experience with patient self-management of oral anticoagulation. *J Thromb Thrombolysis* 1996;2:321–325.

Disorders of Thrombosis and Hemostasis: Clinical and Laboratory Practice, Third Edition, edited by Rodger L. Bick.
Lippincott Williams & Wilkins, Philadelphia © 2002

17

HEPARIN AND LOW-MOLECULAR-WEIGHT HEPARINS

RODGER L. BICK

Unfractionated heparin (UFH) has been in use for more than five decades. Initially UFH was used for the treatment of active thrombosis, initially by intravenous (i.v.) pushes, and then in the past 20 years by bolus followed by infusion; this was typically followed by outpatient warfarin therapy for secondary prevention. About three decades ago, in the early 1970s, it was found that subcutaneous (s.c.) low-dose UFH also was an excellent thromboprophylactic agent for a variety of high-risk medical and surgical conditions (1). About the same time, low-molecular-weight heparins (LMWHs) were developed and subjected to clinical trials to assess thromboprophylaxis in high-risk surgery and medical conditions and were generally found equal or superior to UFH (2). The first LMWH to receive approval for clinical use, approved in Europe in 1986, was dalteparin (Fragmin). During the 1990s, many studies compared the efficacy of LMWH with that of UFH for the treatment of active thrombotic events (2). Some of these trials encompassed outpatient/home therapy with a variety of different LMWHs, which were given s.c. by the patient or, when necessary, by home health visits (3).

The past decade has been associated with marked changes in concepts and recommendations for antithrombotic therapy. These changes have accelerated during the past several years and are expected to continue to change rapidly, contingent on the availability of new information from randomized clinical trials. Much of what physicians have done in the past, from both the therapeutic and the laboratory-monitoring standpoints, are founded on tradition rather than solid data. Finally, one must carefully distinguish between antithrombotic therapy (prevention of thrombosis, extension of existing thrombosis, or development of embolus) and anticoagulant therapy (the prolongation of a clotting or hemostasis test). We are often guilty of focusing on the anticoagulant aspects of a drug or treatment regimen rather than on the antithrombotic aspects. New knowledge and sound clinical trial data should now shift our focus from the prolongation of laboratory tests to the patient. Controversy, confusion, and misuse continue regarding short- and long-term management of venous thrombosis and thromboembolism.

R. L. Bick: Department of Medicine and Pathology, University of Texas Southwestern Medical Center; Dallas Thrombosis/Hemostasis Clinical Center; ThromboCare Laboratories, Dallas, Texas.

HISTORY

Heparin was first discovered by McLean (4,5) in 1916 while he was a second-year medical student. At that time, he was studying procoagulant effects of phospholipids and "thromboplastin" and noted a strong inhibitory activity, extracted from dog liver, which he referred to as "heparphosphatid" (4,5). He shared his discovery with his mentor, Howell, who used the term "heparin" for this new potent anticoagulant (6). Although Howell and his collaborator, Holt, are often credited with "discovering" heparin, it was in fact McLean's discovery. Subsequently, it was noted this "heparin" could be extracted from a number of tissues, including lung, intestine, mast cells, and other tissues. By the early 1930s, heparin, particularly from porcine intestine, had entered clinical use as an antithrombotic (7).

CHARACTERISTICS

Unfractionated Heparin

Sodium heparin may be derived from porcine intestinal mucosa (standardized for use as an anticoagulant), or from beef lung for commercial use. Many preparations use benzyl alcohol as a preservative; some brands are available without preservative.

The pharmacologic potency is determined by biologic assay, using a United States Pharmacopeia (USP) reference standard based on units of heparin activity per milligram. For clinical use, potency is measured by the activated partial thromboplastin time (aPTT), which must be calibrated to anti-Xa activity, discussed subsequently. The pH range is 5.0 to 7.5.

Heparin is a heterogeneous group of straight-chain anionic mucopolysaccharides, called glycosaminoglycans, having anticoagulant properties. The molecular mass is variable, being between 5,000 to 30,000, with a mean of about 15,000 (50 monosaccharide units) daltons. Although others may be present, the main sugars occurring in heparin are (a) (α)-L-iduronic acid-2-sulfate, (b) 2-deoxy-2-sulfamino-(α)-D-glucose-6-sulfate, (c) (β)-D-glucuronic acid, (d) 2-acetamido-2-deoxy-(α)-D-glucose, and (e) (α)-L-iduronic acid. These sugars are present in decreasing amounts, usually in the order (b) > (a) > (d) > (c) > (e), and are joined by glycosidic linkages, forming polymers of varying sizes. Heparin is strongly acidic because of its content of covalently linked sulfate and carboxylic acid groups. In heparin sodium, the acidic protons of the sulfate units are partially replaced by sodium ions. Heparin acts at multiple sites in the normal coagulation system. The multiple actions of heparin are given in Table 17.1 (8). Small amounts of heparin in combination with antithrombin III (heparin cofactor) can inhibit thrombosis by inactivating activated factor X and inhibiting the conversion of prothrombin to thrombin. Once active thrombosis has developed, larger amounts of heparin can inhibit further coagulation by inactivating thrombin and preventing the conversion of fibrinogen to fibrin. Heparin also prevents the formation of a stable fibrin clot by inhibiting the activation of the fibrin-stabilizing factor.

The template bleeding time (TBT) is usually unaffected by heparin. The aPTT and clotting time are prolonged by full therapeutic doses of heparin; in most cases, it is not measurably affected by low doses of heparin or prophylactic doses of s.c. heparin. Peak plasma levels of heparin are achieved 2 to 4 hours after s.c. administration, although there are considerable individual variations. Log linear plots of heparin plasma concentrations with time, for a wide range of dose levels, are linear, which suggests the absence of zero-order processes. Liver and the reticuloendothelial system are the sites of biotransformation. The biphasic elimination curve, a rapidly declining α phase ($t_{1/2}$ = 10 minutes), and after age 40 years, a slower β phase, indicates uptake in organs. The absence of a relation between anticoagulant half-life and concentration half-life may reflect factors such as protein binding of heparin. Heparin does not have fibrinolytic activity; therefore it will not lyse existing clots. Intravenous heparin has a very short plasma half-life without a bolus; a plasma half-life of about 30 minutes occurs if preceded by a bolus of 25 U/kg (1,750 units for a 70-kg patient), and to 60 minutes if preceded by a bolus of 100 U/kg (7,000 U for a 70-kg patient), and up to 150 minutes if preceded by a bolus of 400 U/kg (28,000 U for a 70-kg patient) (9). Given by the i.v. or s.c. route, UFH binds to endothelium, macrophages, histidine-rich glycoprotein, platelet factor 4 (PF-4), vitronectin, fibrinogen, lipoproteins, and von Willebrand factor. These binding characteristics account for instances of heparin "resistance," as discussed later in this chapter. UFH is cleared primarily by the liver.

TABLE 17.1. ACTIVITIES OF HEPARIN/LMW HEPARIN

Acceleration of antithrombin activity
Release of TFPI
Acceleration of HC-II activity
Release of t-PA
Binding to IIa (ionic)
Binding to IXa (ionic)
Binding to XIa (ionic)
Inhibition of plasmin
Inhibition of trypsin
Inhibition of vascular SMCs
Inhibition of renal mesangial cells
Enhancement of vascular angiogenesis
Activation of lipoprotein lipase
Activation of hepatic lipase
Inhibition of complement C1s
Inhibition of complement C1q
Inhibition of complement C3a
Inhibition of acetylcholine esterase

These activities of heparins are not inhibited by low-density lipoprotein (LDL) or platelet factor 4 (PF-4), two compounds that may bind with heparin.
TFPI, tissue factor pathway inhibitor; SMCs, smooth-muscle cells; HC, heparin cofactor; t-PA, tissue plasminogen activator.

UFH may be reversed by protamine sulfate. Protamines are simple proteins of low molecular weight that are rich in arginine and strongly basic. They occur in the sperm of salmon and certain other species of fish. Protamine sulfate occurs as fine white or off-white amorphous or crystalline powder. It is sparingly soluble in water. The pH is between 6 and 7. The cationic hydrogenated protamine at a pH of 6.8 to 7.1 reacts with anionic heparin at a pH of 5.0 to 7.5 to form an inactive complex. Protamine sulfate injection, USP, is a sterile, isotonic solution of protamine sulfate. It acts as a heparin antagonist and is itself also a weak anticoagulant. Protamine sulfate is administered i.v. When administered alone, protamine has an anticoagulant effect. However, when it is given in the presence of heparin (which is strongly acidic), a stable salt is formed, and the anticoagulant activity of both drugs is lost. Protamine sulfate has a rapid onset of action. Neutralization of UFH occurs within 5 minutes after i.v. administration of an appropriate dose of protamine sulfate. Although the metabolic fate of the heparin–protamine complex has not been elucidated, it has been postulated that protamine sulfate in the heparin–protamine complex may be partially metabolized or may be lysed by fibrinolysis, thus freeing heparin. Protamine sulfate is indicated primarily in the treatment of heparin overdosage.

Hyperheparinemia or bleeding has been reported in experimental animals and in some patients 30 minutes to

18 hours after cardiac surgery (under cardiopulmonary bypass) in spite of complete neutralization of heparin by adequate doses of protamine sulfate at the end of the operation. It is important to keep the patient under close observation after cardiac surgery. Additional doses of protamine sulfate should be administered if indicated by coagulation studies, such as the heparin titration test with protamine and the determination of plasma thrombin time.

A rapid administration of protamine sulfate can cause severe hypotensive and anaphylactoid reactions. Because of the anticoagulant effect of protamine, it is unwise to give more than 50 mg over a short period unless a larger dose is clearly needed. Patients with a history of allergy to fish may develop hypersensitivity reactions to protamine, although to date no relation has been established between allergic reactions to protamine and fish allergy. Previous exposure to protamine can induce a humoral immune response and predispose susceptible individuals to the development of untoward reactions from the subsequent use of this drug. Patients exposed to protamine through the use of protamine-containing insulin or during heparin neutralization may experience life-threatening reactions and fatal anaphylaxis on receiving large doses of protamine i.v. Severe reactions to i.v. protamine can occur in the absence of local or systemic allergic reactions to s.c. injection of protamine-containing insulin. Reports of the presence of antiprotamine antibodies in the sera of infertile or vasectomized men suggest that some of these individuals may react to use of protamine sulfate. Fatal anaphylaxis has been reported in one patient with no history of allergies (10). Protamine sulfate has been shown to be incompatible with certain antibiotics, including several of the cephalosporins and penicillins. It is not known whether protamine sulfate can cause fetal harm when administered to a pregnant woman or can affect reproduction capacity. Protamine sulfate should be given to a pregnant woman only if clearly needed. It also is not known whether this drug is excreted in human milk. Because many drugs are excreted in human milk, caution should be exercised when protamine sulfate is administered to a nursing woman. Other serious adverse reactions may occur with protamine sulfate: the i.v. administration of protamine sulfate may cause a sudden decrease in blood pressure and bradycardia. Other reactions include transitory flushing and feeling of warmth, dyspnea, nausea, vomiting, and lassitude. Back pain has been reported in conscious patients undergoing such procedures as cardiac catheterization. Severe adverse reactions have been reported including (a) anaphylaxis that resulted in severe respiratory distress, circulatory collapse, and capillary leak syndrome; and (b) anaphylactoid reactions with circulatory collapse, capillary leak, and noncardiogenic pulmonary edema; acute pulmonary hypertension has been reported. Complement activation by the heparin–protamine complexes, release of lysosomal enzymes from neutrophils, and prostaglandin and thromboxane generation have been associated with the development of anaphylactoid reactions. Severe and potentially irreversible circulatory collapse associated with myocardial failure and reduced cardiac output also may occur. The mechanism(s) of this reaction and the role played by concurrent factors are unclear. High-protein, noncardiogenic pulmonary edema associated with the use of protamine has been reported in patients on cardiopulmonary bypass who are undergoing cardiovascular surgery. Rapid administration of protamine is more likely to result in bradycardia, dyspnea, a sensation of warmth, flushing, and severe hypotension; hypertension also has occurred. Thus the drug should be given by slow i.v. infusion. Protamine sulfate injection should be given by very slow i.v. injection over a 10-minute period in doses not to exceed 50 mg. Because fatal anaphylactic and anaphylactoid reactions have been reported after the administration of protamine sulfate, the drug should be given only when resuscitation techniques and treatment of anaphylactic and anaphylactoid shock are readily available. An overdose of protamine sulfate may cause bleeding. Protamine has a weak anticoagulant effect due to an interaction with platelets and with many proteins including fibrinogen. This effect should be distinguished from the rebound anticoagulation that may occur 30 minutes to 18 hours after the reversal of heparin with protamine.

Each milligram of protamine sulfate neutralizes approximately 90 USP units of heparin activity derived from lung tissue or about 115 USP units of heparin activity derived from intestinal mucosa. The dosage of protamine sulfate should be guided by blood-coagulation studies (calibrated aPTT). Protamine sulfate has been shown to be incompatible with certain antibiotics, including several of the cephalosporins and penicillins. Because heparin disappears rapidly from the circulation, the dose of protamine sulfate required also decreases rapidly with the time elapsed after i.v. injection of heparin. For example, if the protamine sulfate is administered 30 minutes after the heparin, one half the usual dose may be sufficient.

UFH is derived from pork (porcine) or beef. The salt may be sodium or calcium. One difficulty with UFH is that varying sources and preparations can give differing clinical and laboratory results. Differing heparin preparations can give different aPTT results with similar reagents. Therefore, comparative results of clinical trials are difficult to interpret (8). Likewise, different PTT reagents can render different results with the same UFH, again making results of comparative clinical trials difficult to compare. Comparative differences among UFHs are summarized in Table 17.2. UFH can be given by i.v. infusion or by s.c. intermittent dose, usually twice daily. There is, however, a paucity of clinical trials that provide information regarding fixed-dose s.c. heparin versus dose-adjusted s.c. heparin. Most trials for acute events have compared i.v. heparin with fixed-dose UFH or i.v. heparin with dose-adjusted s.c. UFH. Trials are now needed to compare s.c. fixed-dose with s.c. dose-

TABLE 17.2. CHARACTERISTICS OF DIFFERENT HEPARIN PREPARATIONS

Source	
Beef lung	Porcine mucosal
Lower anti-Xa activity	Higher anti-Xa activity
Higher anti-IIa activity	Lower anti-IIa activity
Lower % LMW fractions	Higher % LMW fractions
Higher incidence of bleeding	Lower incidence of bleeding
Higher incidence of HIT/HITT	Lower incidence of HIT/HITT
Less antithrombotic efficacy	More antithrombotic efficacy
Salt	
Sodium	Calcium
Higher incidence of bleeding	Lower incidence of bleeding
Lower anti-Xa activity	Higher anti-Xa activity
Equal anti-IIa activity	Equal anti-IIa activity
Lower plasma levels by s.c. route	Higher plasma levels by s.c. route
Molecular weight	
Higher molecular weight	Lower molecular weight
Higher incidence of bleeding	Lower incidence of bleeding
Lower anti-Xa activity	Higher anti-Xa activity
Higher anti-IIa activity	Lower anti-IIa activity
Shorter s.c. half-life	Longer s.c. half-life
Lower efficacy	Higher efficacy

s.c., subcutaneous; HIT/HITT, heparin-induced thrombocytopenia/thrombosis; LMW, low molecular weight.

adjusted UFH for acute events. In using dose-adjusted s.c. UFH or i.v. UFH, laboratory monitoring is usually recommended but remains controversial, as discussed later. Fixed-dose UFH and LMWH usually require no laboratory monitoring other than platelet counts (8). UFH is cleared primarily by the liver, and LMWH is cleared primarily by the kidneys. This must be considered in patients with end-organ failure.

Low-Molecular-Weight Heparins

More than two decades ago, it was noted that fragments of heparin also had potent antithrombotic activity, primarily against factor Xa. Therefore the concept of fractionated LMWH was developed. There are several ways in which heparin is fractionated to derive LMWH, including use of heparinase, nitrous acid depolymerization, and other depolymerization techniques. Most LMWHs have a mean molecular mass of 3,000 to 7,000 daltons. Many different LMWHs are available world-wide. Each has differing characteristics, which are summarized in Table 17.3 (11–13). LMWH acts by enhancing the inhibition of factor Xa and thrombin by antithrombin. In humans, LMWH potentiates preferentially the inhibition of coagulation factor Xa, while only slightly affecting clotting times, such as the aPTT.

LMWH generally does not produce a significant change in platelet aggregation, fibrinolysis, or global clotting tests such as prothrombin time (PT), thrombin time (TT). or aPTT. Subcutaneous administration of LMWH for 7 consecutive days to patients undergoing abdominal surgery did not markedly affect the aPTT, PF-4, or lipoprotein lipase. Mean peak levels of plasma anti–factor Xa activity after single s.c. doses of 2,500, 5,000, and 10,000 IU of one LMWH (dalteparin) were 0.19 ± 0.04, 0.41 ± 0.07, and

TABLE 17.3. DIFFERENCES IN U.S. FDA-APPROVED LMW HEPARINS

Characteristics	Dalteparin	Enoxiparin (Lovenox)	Ardeparin	Tinzaparin
Percentage molecular weight <2,500	4%	15%	6%	7.90%
Percentage molecular weight >7,500	25%	37%	35%	31%
Anti-Xa activity (1 U/mg)	148	98	60	89
USP potency (U/mg)	75	53	70	60
Antithrombotic activity (intravenous)	14	9	5	14
Bleeding index (intravenous)	0.3	0.5	0.9	0.76
Bleeding index (subcutaneous)	0.45	0.68	0.35	0.71
TFPI release	110	120	130	168
Anti-Xa/Anti-IIa ratio	2.7	3.6	2.1	1.9

TFPI, tissue factor pathway inhibitor; FDA, Food and Drug Administration; LMW, low molecular weight.

0.82 ± 0.10 IU/mL, respectively, and were attained in about 4 hours in most subjects. Absolute bioavailability in healthy volunteers, measured as the anti–factor Xa activity, was 87% ± 6%. Increasing the dose from 2,500 to 10,000 IU resulted in an overall increase in anti–factor Xa activity that was greater than proportional by about one third. With LMWHs, peak anti–factor Xa activity increased more or less linearly with dose over the same dose range.

The volume of distribution for LMWH anti–factor Xa activity is 40 to 60 mL/kg. The mean plasma clearances of LMWH anti–factor Xa activity in normal volunteers after single i.v. bolus doses of 30 and 120 anti–factor Xa IU/kg is 24.6 ± 5.4 and 15.6 ± 2.4 mL/h/kg, respectively. The corresponding mean disposition half-lives are 1.47 ± 0.3 and 2.5 ± 0.3 hours. After i.v. doses of 40 and 60 IU/kg, mean terminal half-lives are 2.1 ± 0.3 and 2.3 ± 0.4 hours, respectively. Longer apparent terminal half-lives (3 to 5 hours) are observed after such dosing, possibly because of delayed absorption. In patients with chronic renal insufficiency requiring hemodialysis, the mean terminal half-life of anti–factor Xa activity after a single i.v. dose of 5,000 IU of LMWH is 5.7 ± 2.0 hours, considerably longer than values observed in healthy volunteers; therefore greater accumulation can be expected in patients with renal compromise, as LMWH is primarily cleared by the renal route. Unlike UFH, LMWH lacks binding to histidine-rich glycoprotein, PF-4, vitronectin, fibrinogen, lipoproteins, von Willebrand factor, and other acute-phase reactants, thus accounting for less "resistance" to LMWH than is seen with UFH. Table 17.4 lists reasons for heparin "resistance." As with UFH, LMWH does not cross the placental barrier and can therefore be used during pregnancy.

TABLE 17.4. HEPARIN "RESISTANCE"

1. Unfractionated heparin only binding to[a]
   A. Fibrinogen
   B. von Willebrand factor
   C. Fibronectin
   D. Vitronectin
   E. Lipoproteins
   F. Platelet factor 4
   G. Histadine-rich glycoprotein
2. LMW heparin and unfractionated heparin "resistance"[b]
   Fibrin-bound thrombin maintains enzymatic ability to
   A. Convert fibrinogen to fibrin
   B. Activate factor V to Va and factor VIII to VIIIa
   C. Activate platelets

[a]All these hemostasis components also are acute-phase reactants and may be elevated during disease, including arterial/venous thrombosis; all bind unfractionated heparin. LMW heparin does not bind to these "acute phase" hemostasis components, and thus LMW heparin resistance does not develop.
[b]These problems apply to both unfractionated heparin and LMW heparin and may lead to "resistance" or less than ideal response. These activities also most likely account for both "resistance" and rethrombosis ("rebound thrombosis") when heparin/LMW heparin is stopped, particularly in cardiovascular disorders.

Mechanisms of Action

UFH has traditionally been believed to exert its antithrombotic/anticoagulant effects by inhibition of factors Xa and IIa. The activity of UFH is primarily against factor IIa (thrombin). Hence, it prolongs the aPTT, the TT, and the activated clotting time (ACT). In addition, only 30% of UPS heparin binds to antithrombin, and therefore, as discussed later, only 30% is available to accelerate the serine protease–inhibitory activity of antithrombin (1,3,14). It has been generally accepted that coagulation occurs in a cybernetic manner, with fibrin deposition and lysis occurring as a continuous process (15–18). The manifestations of normal hemostasis versus increased fibrin deposition (thrombosis) or increased fibrinolysis (hemorrhage) depend on a delicate balance between the procoagulant system and associated inhibitors and between the fibrinolytic system and its associated inhibitors (17,19–22). The primary inhibitor of the procoagulant system is antithrombin, although significant inhibition also comes about through tissue factor pathway inhibitor (TFPI), plasminogen activator inhibitor (PAI-1), protein C, and protein S. The comparative roles of heparin cofactor II and TFPI remain to be defined, but TFPI is probably much more important than previously recognized. Antithrombins were first described in 1939 by Brinkhous et al. (23), and the first large survey of antithrombins was reported by Seegers et al. in 1952 (24). Antithrombin has activity not only against thrombin but also against other serine proteases generated during coagulation, including factors Xa, IXa, XIa, plasmin, kallikrein, and factor XIIa (25–29). Inhibition of factor Xa most closely correlates with clinical inhibition of thrombus formation, and inhibition of factor Xa appears to be much more important than inhibition of factor IIa with respect to the efficacy of heparin (3,30,31). Inhibition of IIa (thrombin) best correlates with prolongation of in vitro coagulation tests (aPTT, TT, and ACT). In most instances, especially with respect to antithrombin-III activity against thrombin and factor Xa, this activity is markedly accelerated by addition of heparin. The kinetics of this heparin–antithrombin–serine protease reaction have been elegantly described by Yin et al. (25,33,34). When the hemostasis system is driven in the procoagulant direction with the attendant generation of serine proteases and eventual fibrin formation, antithrombin consumption occurs, because antithrombin-III combines irreversibly with activated clotting factors, and this complex is then removed from the circulation. In the absence of heparin, antithrombin appears to inactivate thrombin in a progressive, irreversible manner that follows second-order kinetics (35,36). In addition, antithrombin inactivates other serine proteases, as previously discussed, although with slower reactivity in the absence of heparin than its inhibition of thrombin (27–29,37–39). In the presence of heparin, inactivation of thrombin and factor Xa is markedly accelerated and is almost instantaneous. However, there are differences depending on the differing molecular weights and other characteristics of the particular heparin used (30–33). Heparin interacts with antithrombin by binding to lysine residues of the antithrombin molecule and that this markedly accelerates the inhibitory activity of antithrombin with respect to serine proteases (34,35). However, heparin also combines directly with thrombin and factor Xa, and therefore it is still a matter of controversy as to whether the neutralization of thrombin and factor Xa by antithrombin is due to the interaction of heparin with antithrombin or to the interaction of heparin with the particular serine protease (40–43). Alternatively, another proposed mechanism is that a molecule of heparin may act to bind antithrombin and thrombin or Xa (44). However, these mechanisms appear to differ with differing heparin preparations and also appear to be different with respect to the antithrombin inhibition of thrombin versus the antithrombin inhibition of factor Xa (31–33,45,46). Differing molecular weight fractions of heparin have markedly different activities with respect to the interaction of antithrombin and thrombin, antithrombin and factor Xa, or interaction with the vasculature (31–33,45,46). During these processes, heparin appears not to be consumed. After formation of the heparin–antithrombin–serine protease complex, heparin dissociates from the complex, thus acting as a catalyst, and then becomes available to interact with more antithrombin or serine protease (47).

Endogenous heparin is rarely detected in the blood in significant amounts. However, it has been suggested that very low doses of heparin or of semisynthetic heparin analogues may release endogenous glycosaminoglycans, which then activate antithrombin to inhibit serine proteases (25,46,48–51). When exogenous heparin is delivered to the blood compartment, it is rapidly absorbed by the surface of endothelial cells. This endothelium-bound heparin may be far more important than heparin circulating in the bloodstream with respect to thrombus prevention in humans (1,52). In addition, it appears that the subspecies of heparin preparation used and the differing routes of delivery may preferentially lead to more or less heparin bound to the endothelium. In theory, therefore, those preparations or modes of delivery that lead to more endothelial-bound heparin and less heparin in the bloodstream may be the most efficacious for clinical use (1,52). In this regard, it should be recognized that some of the vascular proteoglycans other than heparin also are able to interact with antithrombin and enhance the rate of inhibition of thrombin and factor Xa. This activity appears to be limited to dermatan sulfate and heparan sulfate (50,53,54). The obvious major physiologic significance of this is implied but not yet conclusively proven. In addition, some evidence exists that the use of ultra-low-dose heparin or semisynthetic heparin analogues may accelerate endogenous vascular glycosaminoglycan-induced, antithrombin-mediated inhibition of serine proteases (48,49,55). Of particular significance is recent evidence that up to 40% to 50% of the antithrombotic activity of heparin is due to heparin-induced endothelial release of TFPI (56–58).

Most studies have shown that the physiologic range of antithrombin in normal human blood is quite narrow, and in addition, decreases in antithrombin levels may be of major clinical relevance when heparin (particularly unfractionated) anticoagulation is chosen (25,46,59,60). Most patients respond to heparin if the biologic antithrombin level is greater than 60%. However, many will not respond ideally if biologic antithrombin levels are less than 40% activity (25). Formerly, increased "anticoagulant activity" of heparin has been defined by noting of prolonged global tests of coagulation, primarily the aPTT, the ACT, the TT, and other similar tests. However, it has long been known that simple prolongation of these tests does not correlate well with efficacy, nor do the tests correlate with clinical bleeding (61–63). Now that the properties of different heparin preparations are becoming more clear, it is easy to explain this lack of correlation between global clotting tests and the clinical efficacy of heparin. No assay yet exists to ideally measure the clinical efficacy of heparin. However, as discussed later, the anti-Xa assay using the synthetic substrate S-2222 is probably the most reasonable assay to use at present (46,64). Heparin/LMWHs have many more advantageous activities, including modulation of cytokines, inhibition of complement components, and lipoprotein lipase–like activity. Many of the potentially antithrombotic activities of heparins/LMWHs are not measurable in any clinically applicable or available tests. The many activities of heparin/LMWH are summarized in Table 17.1.

Dosing of Heparin and Low-molecular-weight Heparin

The doses used are dependent on treating an active event (primary therapy) or offering heparin/LMWH for prophylaxis (secondary therapy).

Acute thrombotic events are treated with UFH by either the dose-adjusted i.v. or dose-adjusted s.c. route with a *calibrated/standardized* aPTT or anti-Xa assay. The calibrated aPTT is discussed in the subsequent section on laboratory monitoring. When using the i.v. route, UFH is preceded by a bolus of 5,000 to 10,000 units, followed by a constant infusion to maintain a therapeutic heparin level, as determined by the calibrated/standardized aPTT or anti-Xa assay. It has been demonstrated in multiple randomized trials that therapeutic levels must be achieved by 24 hours or the recurrence rate is increased fourfold to sixfold for several months (65–67). In addition, it has been demonstrated that although warfarin is traditionally started on day 1 of UFH therapy, the heparin therapy must continue for at least 5 days or, again, the recurrence rate is fourfold to sixfold increased for several months. Thus even though the international normalized ratio

(INR) may reach a therapeutic range (usually INR of 2.0 to 3.0) before day 5, the UFH must be continued through day 5. Several standardized nomograms exist for using UFH and are designed to help achieve a therapeutic range within 24 hours. Some are weight adjusted, and some are aPTT-adjusted. The most popular protocols used are depicted in Table 17.5. When starting UFH, a baseline PT, calibrated/standardized aPTT, complete blood count (CBC), and platelet count must be obtained. The aPTT should be repeated every 4 hours until a therapeutic range is achieved (calibrated/standardized aPTT greater than 1.5 × mean control) and to assure that a therapeutic range is achieved within the 24-hour window for maximal efficacy. If need be, the aPTT should be done more often if difficulty is encountered in achieving adequate prolongation (calibrated/standardized aPTT greater than 1.5 × mean control).

UFH also may be given by the s.c. route for acute events. Ten Cate et al. and others first demonstrated this through a large meta-analysis in 1992 and before (68,69). Indeed, use of s.c. heparin for acute thrombosis has been shown to be at least as effective and appears to be associated with less bleeding than when given by the i.v. route. When using s.c. UFH for acute thrombosis, the same principles as for i.v. heparin apply. Appropriate laboratory evaluation must be done before commencing heparin therapy. Most clinicians use an i.v. bolus of 5,000 to 10,000 units, and then start s.c. heparin at an every-12-hour dose schedule. As with i.v. heparin, the dose is adjusted, by calibrated/standardized aPTT, done every 4 hours, until a therapeutic effect is achieved. As with i.v. heparin use, a therapeutic range must be achieved within 24 hours, and the patient must remain in a therapeutic range through day 5; failure to achieve either will increase the recurrence rate fourfold to sixfold in the future. Thus even though the warfarin, typically started on day 1 of therapy, has reached a therapeutic range (INR, 2.0 to 3.0), the s.c. heparin must continue through day 5 (70,71).

Low-molecular-weight Heparin

LMWH has been shown to be equally effective, if not more effective, than UFH in numerous clinical trials and meta-analyses. The significant decrease in recurrence and the possibility of outpatient use in about 70% of patients with deep vein thrombosis (DVT) with or without asymptomatic pulmonary embolus (PE) has made use of LMWH desirable. Several trials have demonstrated the safety and efficacy of treating PE with the use of LMWH in the outpatient setting. In addition, LMWH appears to be associated with less bleeding, less frequent recurrence, and increased survival; these characteristics and outpatient treatment have a major impact on both quality of life and cost of care. As with use of UFH, baseline laboratory studies, most important, a CBC and platelet count must be obtained. The aPTT and PT should be obtained. Doses of LMWH vary according to the manufacturer. The two most popular regimens are the use of dalteparin (Fragmin) at 200 units/kg/24 hours ("Lindmarker regimen") or enoxaparin (Lovenox) at 1.0 mg/kg/12 hours ("Levine regimen"). Both regimens are given as a fixed dose, unless a particular clini-

TABLE 17.5. HEPARIN PROTOCOLS FOR TREATMENT OF THROMBOSIS/THROMBOEMBOLISM

Protocol 1:[a]

1. Intravenous bolus of 5,000 units
2. Continue intravenous infusion at 1,860 units/h
3. Adjust dose per nomogram to maintain calibrated aPTT at >1.5 s
4. Calibrated aPTT every 4 h for first 24 h to assure therapeutic level reached by first 24 h
5. If calibrated aPTT is therapeutic and remains so, change calibrated aPTT to every 24 h, unless it becomes subtherapeutic; then repeat steps 1–4. To achieve therapeutic calibrateed aPTT (>1.5) s after dose-adjustment nomogram

Calibrated aPTT	Dose change/h	Dose Change/24 h
<45 s	Add 242 U/h	Add 5,800 units
46–64 s	Add 120 U/h	Add 2,900 units
65–85 s	None	Stop 1 h, repeat aPTT 4 h after restarting same dose heparin
86–110	Deduct 242 U/h	Stop heparin 1 h; delete 2,900 units/24 h; repeat aPTT 4 h after restart
>110 s	Deduct 120 U/h	Stop 1 h; delete 5,800 units/24 h; repeat aPTT 4 h after restart

Protocol 2: (weight adjusted)[b]

Initial dose:	80 U/kg bolus, then 80 U/kg/h
aPTT <35 s	80 U/kg bolus, then 4 U/kg/h
aPTT 35–45 s	40 U/kg bolus, then 2 U/kg/h
aPTT 46–70 s	No change in dose
aPTT 71–90 s	Decrease dose/infusion by 2 U/kg/h
aPTT >90 s	Hold heparin 1 h, then decrease dose by 3 U/kg/h

aPTT, activated partial thromboplastin time.
[a]From Hull RD, Raskob G, Rosenbloom D. Optimal therapeutic level of heparin in patients with venous thrombosis. *Arch Intern Med* 1992;152:1589, with permission.

TABLE 17.6. INDICATIONS FOR ANTI-XA LEVELS

1. Renal compromise/dysfunction
2. Hypotension/poor tissue perfusion
3. Obesity (>80 kg or BMI >30 kg/m^2)
4. Underweight/emaciated (<50 kg or BMI <22 kg/m^2)
5. Children
6. Change in clinical events (recurrent thrombosis or hemorrhage)
7. Pregnancy
8. Compliance issues (are injections being given)
9. Unresolved issues (may change in future)

BMI, body mass index.

cal change occurs, and there is good reason to change the dose. Monitoring of therapy with the aPTT is generally not necessary, but certain circumstances, although uncommon, mandate anti-Xa levels. These circumstances are summarized in Table 17.6. Other laboratory monitoring is discussed in the subsequent section on laboratory monitoring of heparin therapy. Several modalities must be instituted for outpatient therapy of acute events with LMWH. As mentioned, about 70% of patients with DVT are candidates for outpatient therapy. Those with comorbid conditions mandating hospitalization and those patients arriving at a hospital or clinic "after hours" are admitted. The after-hours patients can usually be discharged to home care in 12 to 24 hours for continuation of home therapy. The patients, before being sent home, must be taught how to administer the s.c. LMWH, they must be instructed in appropriate antiembolic exercises (discussed later), and baseline laboratory values must be obtained. As with UFH, LMWH therapy must be continued for at least 5 days, or the recurrence rate is unacceptably increased (70,71). A protocol for outpatient management of DVT with or without asymptomatic or minor PE is summarized in Table 17.7.

Laboratory Monitoring

Despite more than a decade of reliable data from published studies, there remains confusion regarding monitoring of i.v. UFH therapy and dose-adjusted s.c. heparin therapy in acute events. Many well-controlled studies have clearly demonstrated very poor or no correlation between prolongation of the aPTT and therapeutic heparin levels, safety (hemorrhage), or efficacy (rethrombosis, extension, or embolus) of therapeutic UFH (summarized in refs. 72–74). As early as 1989, the American College of Chest Physicians (ACCP) consensus conference recommendations on antithrombotic therapy recognized this and recommended that all aPTT reagents be correlated to a therapeutic anti-Xa level or protamine titration level. The therapeutic range of the anti-Xa assay is 0.35 to 0.8/1.0 U/mL, and a therapeutic level using the protamine titration is 0.2 to 0.4 U/mL. This recommendation has been repeated at each subsequent ACCP North American Consensus Conference recommendation meeting and the publications thereof in 1989, 1992, 1995, 1998, and 2001 (75–79). Finally, a decade after the National Institutes of Health (NIH)/ACCP North American Committee recommendations, this also became a recommendation of the College of American Pathologists (CAP) XXXI Consensus Conference on moni-

TABLE 17.7. SUGGESTED GUIDELINES FOR THE OUTPATIENT OR "EARLY DISCHARGE" MANAGEMENT OF DVT

1. If necessary, admit for 12–24 h if no comorbid condition, or treat as outpatient if no comorbid condition and all below can be accomplished
2. CBC/platelet count and prothrombin time (PT) and aPTT on admission
3. Teach patient applicable antiembolic exercises (see text)
4. Start subcutaneous (s.c.) LMW heparin as
   A. Fragmin (dalteparin) @ 200 units/kg/24 h (available as 2,500 units/0.2 mL or 5,000 units/0.2-mL ampules, or 95,000 U/9.5 mL multidose vial) "Lindmarker regimen"
   OR
   B. Lovenox (Enoxaparin) @ 1 mg/kg/12 h (≈100 units/kg/12 h) (30 mg or 40-mg ampules): "Levine regimen"
5. Instruct patient in self-injection of s.c. LMW heparin in anterior or lateral thighs or anterior abdominal wall (anterior or lateral thighs preferred; use rotating injection sites)
6. Measure for medium-compression panty hose (LE) or upper-extremity hose (UE) for use during waking hours only; use 24–48 h after starting therapy
7. Start warfarin @ 5 mg/day on day 1 and monitor INR (see no. 15)
8. Discharge at 12–24 h if no comorbid conditions or discharge as soon as comorbid condition (not DVT) allows
9. Arrange home health if patient/family cannot self-inject LMW heparin
10. Arrange outpatient prothrombin time/INR and CBC/platelet count at home on day 3
11. Evaluate patient clinically (in office/clinic) on day 5 or 7; obtain prothrombin time and CBC/platelet count days 5 and 7. Stop LMWH when INR ≈ 2.0, and then adjust warfarin dose accordingly, assuming patient has had ≥5 days of LMWH
12. See patient weekly until stable with long-term antithrombotic therapy
13. If young age or a patient with unexplained DVT, consider evaluation for blood coagulation protein(s)/platelet defects leading to thrombosis: (hereditary or acquired thrombophilias). Always consider occult malignancy in appropriate clinical situation
14. While hospitalized patient in bed, raise foot of bed *straight,* with lower extremities elevated 7 degrees to 10 degrees above hips; *never* put pillow(s) under popliteal fossae
15. Depending on clinical parameters/thrombophilia (platelet defects, etc., alternatives to oral anticoagulants may be indicated; for example, antiphospholipid syndrome, sticky platelet syndrome)

INR, International normalized ratio; LMWH, low-molecular-weight heparin; CBC, complete blood count; aPTT, activated partial thromboplastin time; DVT, deep vein thrombosis.

toring of antithrombotic therapy (80). Because the aPTT can vary with (a) reagents, (b) equipment, and (c) type of heparin used, it is imperative that all hospitals calibrate/standardize their aPTT to a therapeutic anti-Xa level of 0.35 to 0.8/1.0 or protamine titration of 0.2 to 0.4. This must be done for every given aPTT reagent, including lot number changes, and/or equipment system, and for each heparin used (including lot number changes). Thus it is important to correlate this activity with the pharmacy so a single lot of aPTT reagents and a single lot of a particular heparin is ordered for at least a year. Any changes in reagents, equipment, or heparin mandate that the calibration be repeated. Thus the therapeutic range for the aPTT must be established for each reagent and type of UFH; to use a fixed noncalibrated ratio of 1.5 to 2.5 is no longer acceptable and must be abandoned.

When using LMWH for an active event (treatment), the dose is fixed, depending on manufacturer or clinical trials results; the aPTT is generally not prolonged, and the standardized/calibrated aPTT is not needed. Anti-Xa levels also are not generally needed when using LMWH; the exceptions to this and indications for performing anti-Xa levels when using LMWH for active events or for prophylaxis are given in Table 17.6. The anti-Xa level for prophylaxis, using UFH or LMWH, is lower than that for treatment and is 0.1 to 0.35 anti-Xa U/mL (8). As previously stated, for therapeutic use, treatment of an active event, the heparin or LMWH must be delivered for a minimum of 5 days; this applies to both i.v. and s.c. UFH (70,71). This also applies to s.c. LMWH used for an active event (70,71). A CBC and platelet count are mandatory before commencing heparin/LMWH therapy for either an active event or for prophylaxis. The platelet count should be repeated at least every 2 days while the patient is receiving heparin/LMWH and continued for 14 days to avoid heparin-induced thrombocytopenia (HIT/HITT). The original ACCP recommendations were "daily platelet counts for all heparin, all routes and all doses (77); however, this is impractical, and every other day should suffice for detecting HIT/HITT (8). The package inserts for UFH, and others, recommend "frequent" platelet counts during and after heparin/LMWH therapy; this is impractical without a clear definition of "frequent."

Side Effects/Adverse Reactions to Heparin and Low-molecular-weight Heparin

Heparin has been the most important anticoagulant in clinical use for the past half century. It is effective, relatively inexpensive, and readily available. Even today, it represents the most common agent for the treatment of acute thrombosis. Its extensive clinical use has commonly led to complacency and even disregard of the potential complications that relate to its use in the therapeutic setting. Although bleeding is the most obvious potential complication of heparin therapy, a very common sequel is HIT, which further can be complicated by the advent of thrombosis. Less common complications include osteoporosis, skin reactions, eosinophilia, alopecia, liver dysfunction, anaphylaxis, and hyperkalemia. This section characterizes these potential, sometimes quite serious, sequelae (Table 17.8).

TABLE 17.8. SIDE EFFECTS OF HEPARIN THERAPY

Potentially Severe	(Generally) Mild
Bleeding	Heparin-associated osteoporosis
Acute heparin "anaphylaxis"	Skin reactions
	Urticaria
	Erythematous papules
	Skin necrosis
Heparin-induced thrombocytopenia	Abnormal liver-function tests
	Eosinophilia
	Hyperkalemia
	Hypoaldosteronism
	Priapism
	Alopecia

HEPARIN-INDUCED THROMBOCYTOPENIA

Although heparin-induced, immune-mediated, thrombocytopenia (HIT-II) was first described by Fidlar and Jacques in 1948 (81), the characterization of clinical manifestations associated with this finding, definition of the potential sequelae, delineation of laboratory features, and recognition of the related therapeutic concepts have largely evolved only during the past decade (82–97).

Two clinical forms of HIT are now recognized. The first, now commonly termed HIT type I (HIT-I) is a nonidiosyncratic, nonimmunologic form (Table 17.9). The thrombocytopenia occurs early in the exposure, within the first few days of therapy in the heparin naïve, and within hours

TABLE 17.9. HEPARIN-INDUCED THROMBOCYTOPENIA TYPE 1: NONIMMUNE; NONIDIOSYNCRATIC

Episode of thrombocytopenia occurs early in exposure: generally in first few days in naive and in first hours in previously exposed
Mild thrombocytopenia: ≈10%–20% decrease in platelet numbers
Clinical manifestations: None
Mechanism: Heparin-induced platelet aggregation
True incidence: uncertain, but common
Biologic issues: Episode transient, counts normalize even with continued therapy
Therapy: None
Relation to HIT II: Unclear, but probably none

HIT, heparin-induced thrombocytopenia.

in the patient previously exposed to heparin. The decline in platelet numbers is usually modest (about 10% to 20%), and is not associated with any clinical manifestations. The decline in platelet numbers is the result of platelet aggregation by mechanism(s) that are currently uncertain; nevertheless, the aggregation is associated with platelet sequestration and increased consumption. High(er)-molecular-weight heparins have the greatest likelihood of producing this change. Of particular interest is that the episodes are transient, and platelet counts normalize by unknown mechanisms, in spite of continued exposure to heparin. Presently there is no evidence that this clinical–laboratory event is related to the more serious immune form of HIT-II.

By contrast, HIT-II is an immune-mediated lesion with serious clinical sequelae and significant morbidity and mortality (87,89,93,95,97). Some have considered this lesion to have two subtypes, HIT-II and HITT-II, the latter serving to recognize the presence of thrombosis, which is often the important clinical result of immune HIT. Table 17.10 lists the common clinical characteristics of this lesion. Although the usual recognition of the decreased number of platelets is generally after several days of therapy (3 to 14 days), with the median day being day 10, prior exposure to heparin can result in precipitate declines in circulating platelet numbers within hours. Most instances of HIT/HITT-II also involve antibodies to the multimolecular heparin/PF-4 complex [immunoglobulin G (IgG), IgA, or IgM idiotypes]; however, rarer antibodies appear to be against platelet membrane interleukin 8 (IL-8) or platelet membrane neutrophil activating peptide-2 (protein) receptors; these rarer forms may not behave typically with respect to temporal relations with heparin delivery or degree of decrease in platelet count.

Historically, and no longer appropriate, the parameter of diagnostic recognition was a decrease in platelets to less than 100×10^9/L. However, it has now become quite clear that clinical sequelae can occur when a significant decline in platelet numbers occurs, even when the usual parameter of true thrombocytopenia (less than 100×10^9/L) is not present (97). Therefore no specific platelet number should trigger suspicion of the presence of HIT-II. Currently, the best working rule is that the diagnosis must be strongly suspected if the platelet count decreases by 30% from the baseline and should be strongly considered diagnostic, unless ruled out, when the platelet count has declined to 50% of baseline levels (8,97,98). This implies that the thrombocytopenia may be relative rather than absolute, because the patients' baseline values may be in the 250 to 400×10^9/L range, a circumstance that is particularly true in surgical patients. Postoperative patients who have undergone cardiac surgery (particularly bypass procedures) have special criteria, because most such patients have platelet counts in the 100 to 150×10^9/L range during the first postoperative day. In such circumstances, the diagnosis of HIT-II should be based on a platelet count that is reduced 30% to 50% from the day 1 postoperative platelet count (97). An appropriate postoperative clinical parameter is that for any patient whose platelet count declines 20% to 30% from a day 1 postoperative value, the physician should suspect HIT-II and monitor such individuals with daily platelet counts.

When suspecting HIT in any medical or surgical patient, it is extremely important to graph out the platelet count, noting the rate of decline and temporal relations to heparin administration. Typically the rate of decline, as with other immune-mediated thrombocytopenias, is quite rapid and generally even more rapid than that of other immune thrombocytopenias and typically much more rapid than that in nonimmune causes of thrombocytopenia [disseminated intravascular coagulation (DIC), other mechanisms of consumption, hypersplenism, and marrow-suppressive mechanisms, including medications, sepsis, and other causes].

A very important clinical rule is that HIT-II can occur with any amount of heparin, any type of heparin, administered by any route. Although it is most common with the continuous infusion of UFH, it has occurred with heparin flushes as low as 500 U/day, and even with heparin-coated catheters with which the delivery can be as low as 3 U/hour (99,100).

An important component of HIT-II is the development of thrombotic lesions. This is ominous and is associated with significant morbidity and mortality. Its threat, therapeutic urgency, and treatment complexities are such that the term

TABLE 17.10. CLINICAL FEATURES OF HEPARIN-INDUCED THROMBOCYTOPENIA TYPE II: IMMUNOLOGICAL

- Usual onset at day 3–14 (median, day 10)
- Nadir platelet count: usually 30–60,000, but may be as low as 5,000. The most appropriate definition is a 50% decrease in platelet numbers from the baseline values
- Risk factors
  - Occurs with all methods of administration
    - Most common: continuous infusion of unfractionated heparin
    - Seen: heparin flushes: 500 U/day heparin-coated catheters: 3 U/h
    - Higher with i.v. than s.c. administration
    - Greater: bovine > porcine > LMWH
  - Can occur within hours in previously treated patients
  - Increased incidence with recent surgery (primarily venous problems)
  - Increased incidence with preexisting cardiovascular disease (primarily arterial)
- Absent risks
  - Equal in men and women:
  - Age not a factor
  - No relation to inherited deficiency or founder defects of clotting factors

LMWH, low-molecular-weight heparin.

HITT has been applied to highlight this sequence, and considerable effort has been expended to attempt to define risk factors for this occurrence (101,102). It should be noted that even with very severe thrombocytopenia (counts less than 10 $\times 10^9$/L), thrombosis is a more common sequel than bleeding. It merits stress that in earlier literature regarding HIT-II, the event of vascular thrombosis was almost entirely correlated with large-vessel arterial occlusions. Indeed the term "white clot syndrome" had been used to highlight the event of a massive, arterial occlusion of the lower extremity (101,103,104). Clinical experience has now identified thrombotic sequelae in both the arterial and venous circulation (99,104,105). Unfortunately, in a given patient in whom HIT-II has developed, the clinician cannot predict the subsequent advent of thrombosis. It is, however, now evident that in patients in whom HIT-II develops in juxtaposition to recent surgery, the thrombosis occurs most commonly in the venous circulation, including microcirculation. By contrast, the occurrence of HIT-II in patients with preexisting cardiovascular disease commonly results in arterial occlusions (99,102,106). PE also are quite common in both medical and surgical patients developing HITT. Attempts to characterize the risks better have noted that the incidence of HIT-II is similar in men and women, and age is not a factor. Therefore, with strong suspicion of HITT, not only must the heparin be immediately discontinued, but also a careful search for evidence of thrombosis initiated. The presence of inherited deficiencies of clotting factors (i.e., antithrombin, protein C, or protein S) or founder mutations (i.e., factor V Leiden, prothrombin G20210A) also do not correlate with either the occurrence of HIT-II or the thrombotic sequelae (i.e., HITT).

The diagnostic criteria for HIT-II are shown in Table 17.11. Although past definitions have included a definable platelet number to denote the degree of thrombocytopenia, these parameters no longer apply, as discussed earlier. Classically one would expect that another cause of the thrombocytopenia has been excluded. Unfortunately, the temporal events in HIT-II are often so abrupt that a long, agonizing clinical evaluation of other potential mechanisms to explain the thrombocytopenia often can contribute to severe clinical sequelae (97,98). Therefore this criterion is interpreted to mean that clinical judgment has eliminated other causes (including noting the rate of platelet count decrease, temporal relations with heparin, and evaluation of comorbid conditions and medications) and that HIT-II is the most likely responsible diagnosis. A delay in diagnosis and therapy while awaiting a serologic confirmation or other "diagnostic HIT/HITT test" also is no longer acceptable. From the studies of Walenga et al. (97,98), the multiplicity of tests and lack of an absolute "gold standard" further emphasize the importance of clinical judgment. An important basis for such a conclusion is related to some of the complex temporal relations in the clinical features of HIT-II. Thus as many as 45% of the thrombotic episodes of HIT-II occur in the first 48 hours after identification of the thrombocytopenia. A delay in diagnosis to await laboratory confirmation can, therefore, result in serious clinical risk to the patient. It must also, as discussed previously, not be assumed that other comorbid conditions or medications are automatically responsible for the thrombocytopenia.

TABLE 17.11. HEPARIN-INDUCED THROMBOCYTOPENIA TYPE II: IMMUNE–IDIOSYNCRATIC

Common diagnostic criteria
- Thrombocytopenia: decrease of 30% from baseline, strongly suggestive; decrease of ≥50% from baseline platelet count is diagnostic if no. 2
- Absence of other cause
- Confirmation by a heparin-associated antibody assay
- Return to normal platelet numbers when heparin stopped

A second issue relates to comorbid diseases. Thus concurrent illness can alter the pattern and severity of onset of HIT-II. An even more difficult aspect of HIT-II is the circumstance of "delayed onset of HIT-II." Clinical features and thrombocytopenia have been seen to develop 7 to 14 days *after* discontinuing the heparin therapy, and thrombosis has been described up to 1 month after heparin discontinuation (95). Although it is uncommon, the clinician must be aware of such potential; this further complicates the role of confirmatory testing. A related caveat is of clinical concern. The comorbid condition of the patient can have a significant effect on this pattern of development and similarly can affect the expected temporal pattern of repair of circulating platelet numbers after cessation of the heparin.

Several clinical laboratory features are characteristic. Thus although thrombocytopenia is the cardinal laboratory feature, bleeding is uncommon. Thrombosis, by contrast, is the clinical event that primarily results in morbidity and mortality in HIT-II. As mentioned, the classic descriptions defined the white-clot syndrome with an associated abrupt occlusion of a major artery. Although this does represent a dramatic event of acute emergency care requirement, it is now clear that more common are thrombi in small arterial and arteriolar beds as well as venous occlusive lesions; the latter are estimated to occur with threefold frequency over larger arterial lesions (87,89,92,93,96–98,101,103). PEs also are common. Important clinical clues to the potential occurrence of HIT-II include the recognition of "relative" heparin resistance during induction of heparin therapy or the presence of unexplained chills, fever, and constitutional symptoms. Four other rare clinical events can occur as part of the evolution of HIT-II, and these should alert the physician to the development of the syndrome. These are (a) skin necrosis, (b) transient global amnesia, (c) thrombosis on a present prosthetic value, or (d) bleeding into the adrenal glands with the abrupt development of adrenal insufficiency.

The true incidence of HIT-II is not certain, although an occurrence in 3% to 5% of all heparin-treated individuals is a reasonable figure. The diagnostic parameters are not absolute. In the past, significant or severe thrombocytopenia was the initial and frequently only identifying marker. The recent clinical observations have now more clearly defined a 50% decrease from baseline platelet levels (97,98). It also has been common to demand a "confirmatory" laboratory test. As has been well defined, no single laboratory test recognizes all clinical cases of HIT-II, and many medical centers actually lack the ability even to perform such assays (97,98). Therefore, if the incidence data required absolute confirmatory testing, the number of cases identified would be greatly reduced. In addition, the absolute incidence is affected by comorbid conditions, so that patients seen with a thrombosis for heparin therapy or who are given heparin for thrombosis prophylaxis during an orthopedic surgical procedure have a higher incidence than that in general hospital populations (107–111). Incidence figures also relate to the mode of heparin therapy, as it is well established that continuous infusion is more commonly associated with HIT-II than is intermittent UFH; each is more common than therapy with LMWHs.

Even more difficult is the delineation of the incidence of the most important clinical sequelae of HIT-II, thrombosis. Estimates of such a thrombosis in a patient with HIT-II are as high as 35% or more, and in those patients with such a thrombosis, amputation rates of 25% and mortality of 25% to 30% have been reported (87,89,94,95,97,105). The incidence of HITT-II appears to be about 1% (one per 100 patients) of patients receiving UFH for 5 days (112,113). All such data must be considered tentative until firm diagnostic criteria are more widely accepted and prospective studies are done in which the comorbid conditions are well documented. Although our current incidence data may be "soft," it is clear that morbidity and mortality in HIT-II are significant; therefore, the clinical recognition of the syndrome and proper therapy are critical. Finally, data from a variety of centers have suggested that the occurrence of HIT-II predicts future significant thrombotic events, further emphasizing the importance of clinical awareness.

Several controversies still exist in the emerging clinical understanding of HIT-II. First, the level of platelet numbers or change of platelet numbers from the baseline level to serve as the clinical parameter of diagnosis and thereby provide the parameter to perform other laboratory studies and alter therapy is not yet absolutely established. Second, the issue of whether incidence can be defined only by a specific serologic assay continues to be controversial and will probably always be so, as long as no single absolute assay defines all cases. We believe that the clinical evidence that up to 45% of the thrombotic episodes occur in the first 48 hours of the recognition of HIT-II strongly interdicts "waiting for laboratory confirmation" before therapeutic action, particularly in the current era when excellent alternatives to heparin are available. Third, the exact incidence of thrombosis is not well defined in HIT-II, but is thought to be 1% of those receiving UFH for 5 days. Fourth, whether the clinical sense that an HIT-II thrombosis is clinically more dangerous in circumstances in which the patient is being treated with heparin for a present thrombosis, and the true role of comorbid conditions are not settled issues. Fifth, the relation of an uncommonly described event, that of the paradoxic thrombotic complication of venous limb gangrene in patients receiving heparin during their transition to oral anticoagulant therapy with coumadin, is not fully clarified. However, many of these patients are now known to have an acquired protein C or S deficiency, which may accentuate or precipitate this problem (114).

Treatment of Heparin-induced Thrombocytopenia/Heparin-induced Thrombocytopenia and Thrombosis

Several immediate measures must be undertaken as soon as a clinical diagnosis of HIT/HITT is made. The first imperative measure is to stop heparin immediately; like any immune-mediated adverse reaction, the "antigen" (heparin) must be promptly removed. Next, the clinician must make a decision regarding need for rapid institution of alternative antithrombotic therapy. In many patients, the underlying thrombosis or hypercoagulable condition for which the patient was initially given heparin will still be present; in this case, rapid institution of alternate antithrombotic therapy is needed. When making a diagnosis of HIT, the clinician also must immediately suspect the possibility of thrombosis/thromboembolism (HITT-II) and institute a diligent search for thrombosis, such as color-flow Doppler of the lower extremity deep veins, ventilation/perfusion scan (V/P lung scan), magnetic resonance angiography (MRA) of abdominal vasculature, and other studies to search for thrombosis. Obviously if this search is positive for clinical or occult thrombosis, rapid institution of antithrombotic therapy also is indicated. The only agents currently FDA approved for this purpose are recombinant hirudin (lepirudin) and argatroban for rapid institution of antithrombotic therapy in HIT/HITT-II. If no thrombosis is present and the clinical condition for which the patient was initially administered heparin has abated, rapid or routine administration of warfarin may be considered. However, before embarking on this approach, it is mandatory that functional protein C and protein S levels be measured. For those patients needing rapid warfarin, a protocol for quick warfarin administration, within 24 hours, has been recently published (115). If the patient requires only prophylactic therapy with heparin and has a prior or current record of HIT/HITT-II, then lepirudin, at 10 to 20 mg s.c. every 12 hours, has been advocated (116). Table 17.12 provides a practical summary of treatment for HIT/HITT-II.

TABLE 17.12. MANAGEMENT OF HEPARIN-INDUCED THROMBOCYTOPENIA TYPE II

Stop all heparin immediately. Alternate rapid-onset antithrombotic therapy if original condition persists
- Lepirudin at 0.4-mg/kg bolus followed by 0.15-mg/kg infusion and adjust to maintain the aPTT at 1.5–3.0 times median of normal aPTT
- Argatroban: 2 units/kg/min, then adjust to maintain aPTT at 1.5–3.0 times median of normal aPTT

Assess immediately for evidence of occult thrombosis; rapid-onset antithrombotic if suspected or found

If heparin/LMW heparin needed for prophylaxis, may use lepirudin at 20–30 mg subcutaneously every 12 h

aPTT, activated partial thromboplastin time; LMW, low molecular weight.

Bleeding

The most common and more regularly anticipated complication of heparin therapy is bleeding (111,117–122). The true incidence of major bleeding has been sought, but is only an estimate, commonly ranging between 6% and 14% (119,120). Hirsh et al. (99,119,120) emphasized important variables relative to heparin-related bleeding. These are (a) the dose of heparin administered, (b) the method of administration (i.e., continuous vs. intermittent), and (c) the comorbid and concomitant therapy administered. Thus heparin therapy is more commonly associated with bleeding when given to chronic alcoholics (117). More complex and not completely resolved is the consideration that bleeding is more commonly seen in patients taking aspirin (117,120–122). Because this is not an uncommon treatment combination in patients with arterial vascular disease, clinical vigilance for bleeding is the only intelligent approach. Both bleeding and major hemorrhage appear to be much less frequent with use of LMWH as compared with UFH (8).

Acute Heparin Reaction (? Anaphylaxis)

A rare, but potentially lethal acute reaction to heparin can occur. The event is abrupt and clinically dramatic (123). It has been most commonly seen in patients previously treated with heparin. It again merits emphasis that the heparin exposure need not be a quantitative one, because it has occurred with heparin exposure as minimal as heparin flush or use of a heparin-coated catheter. Symptoms occur dramatically within 5 to 10 minutes of institution of the heparin bolus and include abrupt onset of chills and fever, tachycardia, diaphoresis, and nausea. Hypotension may be noted, although some patients have become abruptly and transiently hypertensive. Retrosternal chest pain with the pattern of an acute myocardial infarction is common. Finally, a global amnesia syndrome has been linked to the crisis event. This anaphylaxis-like reaction has all of the features of an Ig E–stimulated response. Immediate cessation of the heparin is critical. Other nonheparin antithrombotic agents should be used to treat the patient. This author has seen three cases of anaphylaxis to enoxaparin (Lovenox); none had a prior heparin exposure.

Heparin-associated Osteoporosis

Prolonged heparin exposure has been correlated with the development of osteoporosis (124,125). The clinical features that led to the evaluation of this finding were the unexpected development of bone pain or the identification of vertebral body or rib fractures. The clinical correlate was that the patient had been receiving long-term heparin (in excess of 6 months) and usually at daily doses in excess of 15,000 anti-Xa units (99). Limited epidemiologic and controlled studies are available to define the incidence of heparin-associated osteoporosis. In addition, many of the studies have focused on pregnant patients, because such patients are a group likely to have a long duration of therapy. However, because pregnancy itself is commonly associated with osteoporosis, such data must be cautiously interpreted. Howell et al. (126), in randomized trials, identified a 5% incidence of vertebral fractures in women treated during their pregnancy with UFH. Monreal et al. (127), in a randomized study of 40 men and 40 women (mean age, 68 years) receiving long-term heparin therapy, identified a 10% incidence of vertebral fractures. Six of the seven occurred with UFH, and the seventh with LMWH (Fragmin). A very interesting finding in this study was that there was no difference in bone density between the group with fractures compared with those without fractures. They could not show a correlation between the lumbar bone density and the dose or duration of therapy (127).

Barbour et al. (128) evaluated the subclinical occurrence of heparin-associated osteoporosis in pregnancy by means of bone densitometry in a prospective, consecutive cohort of 14 pregnant women requiring heparin therapy and 14 pregnant controls matched for age, race, and smoking status. Proximal femur bone-density measurements were taken at baseline, immediately postpartum, and 6 months postpartum in the cases and controls. Vertebral measurements also were obtained on both groups immediately postpartum and 6 months postpartum. Bone density relative to heparin dose and duration was examined. Five (36%) of 14 cases had a 10% decrease from their baseline proximal femur measurements to their immediate postpartum values, whereas none occurred in the 14 matched controls (p = 0.04). Mean proximal femur bone-density measurements also decreased, and this difference was still statistically significant 6 months postpartum (p = 0.03). This study concluded that no clear dose–response relation could be demonstrated, and that UFH adversely affected bone density in about 33% of exposed patients (128).

Dahlman (129) studied the effect of long-term heparin treatment during pregnancy and the incidence of osteoporotic fractures and thromboembolic recurrence. Long-term s.c. prophylaxis with heparin twice daily in pregnancy was used in 184 individuals. The dose of heparin was adjusted to anti–factor Xa activity or aPTT; different regimens were given depending on risk stratification. Symptomatic osteoporotic fractures of the spine occurred postpartum in four (2.2%) women. Their mean dosage of heparin ranged from 15,000 to 30,000 IU/24 hours (mean, 24,500 IU/24 hours), and their duration of treatment was from 7 to 27 weeks (mean, 17 weeks). It is of interest that in spite of prophylaxis with heparin, thromboembolic complications occurred in five women. Thus osteoporotic vertebral fractures were found in 2.2%, and these did correlate with the amount of heparin administered. There were no thromboembolic events, thrombocytopenias, or excessive hemorrhage. Hunt et al. (130), during a study of LMWH (Fragmin) for thromboprophylaxis in 34 high-risk pregnancies, identified one woman in whom a postpartum osteoporotic vertebral collapse developed. This woman had no other risk factors for osteoporosis. Parenthetically, this study did support the efficacy of LMWH in preventing recurrent thromboembolic disease in pregnant women at high risk. In this study, the incidence of osteoporotic fracture was 3%; however, bone-density studies to assess asymptomatic osteoporosis were not reported.

Douketis et al. (131), in a prospective matched cohort, studied the effects of long-term (more than 1 month) UFH therapy on lumbar spine bone density. Twenty-five women who received heparin during pregnancy and 25 matched controls underwent dual-photon absorptiometry of the lumbar spine in the postpartum period. None of 25 heparin-treated patients developed fractures. Heparin-treated patients had a 0.082 g/cm (2) lower bone density compared with untreated controls, which was statistically significant ($p = 0.0077$). There were six matched pairs in which only the heparin-treated patient had a bone density less than 1.0 g/cm (2), compared with only one pair in which only the control patient had a bone density below this level ($p = 0.089$). The duration of heparin therapy, the mean daily dose, and the total dose of heparin were not at levels of independent significance. They concluded that long-term heparin therapy was associated with a significant reduction in bone density, although fractures are uncommon. They could not show a correlation between the lumbar bone density and the dose or duration of heparin therapy. This is in contradistinction to the generally held views that heparin-induced osteoporosis is related to the dose and duration of therapy (97,98).

A variety of studies have focused on the mechanism whereby heparin affects bone metabolism and structure. Muir et al. (132) treated rats with once-daily s.c. injections of UFH or saline for 8 to 32 days, monitored the effects on bone histomorphometrically, and measured urinary type 1 collagen cross-linked pyrridinoline (PYD) and serum alkaline phosphatase as surrogate markers of bone resorption and formation. Biochemical markers of bone turnover showed that heparin produced a dose-dependent decrease in serum alkaline phosphatase and a transient increase in urinary PYD, thus confirming the histomorphometric data. They concluded that heparin decreases trabecular bone volume both by decreasing the rate of bone formation and by increasing the rate of bone resorption. In a subsequent study (133), this group evaluated the effect of LMWH in a similar model system. It was found that both UFH and LMWH decreased cancellous bone volume in a dose-dependent fashion, but UFH caused significantly more bone loss than did the LMWH. The biochemical markers of bone turnover demonstrated that both heparins produced a dose-dependent decrease in serum alkaline phosphatase, consistent with reduced bone formation, whereas only the UFH caused an increase in urinary PYD, consistent with increased bone resorption. They concluded that UFH decreases cancerous bone volume both by decreasing the rate of bone formation and by increasing the rate of bone resorption; in contrast, LMWH causes less osteopenia because it decreases only the rate of bone formation (133).

Panagakos et al. (134) demonstrated that heparin induces osteoporosis by enhancing the effects of other bone-resorbing factors, particularly parathyroid hormone. Shaughnessy et al. (135) further examined the issue of calcium loss by an in vitro calcium-release assay and demonstrated that size and sulfation of the heparins were the major determinants of the promotion of bone resorption. Their extrapolation was that LMWH preparations would, therefore, reduce the risk of the expected heparin-associated osteoporosis.

Murray et al. (136) examined bone density in a rabbit model. A reduction in cortical and trabecular bone density was seen with UFH ($p < 0.05$) and HMWH ($p < 0.01$), but not with LMWH.

Thus heparin-associated osteoporosis is a clinically uncommon event occurring in fewer than 5% of long-term heparin-treated patients. The evidence supports a lesser risk with LMWH than with UFH. The mechanisms appear related to impaired bone deposition and formation plus enhanced bone resorption with UFH. A change in new-bone deposition appears to be the major mechanism with LMWH. Most clinical evidence supports the view that a long duration of therapy (i.e., greater than 6 months) and a higher dose of heparin increases the risk of bone changes. From these observations, we currently recommend that bone-density studies be done in patients whose duration of therapy will be greater than 6 months at an equivalent of 20,000 anti-Xa U/day, or at 3 months if the dose will exceed 20,000 anti-X U/day. In addition, we encourage calcium supplements. If the patient is going to be receiving low-dose s.c. UFH or LMWH for 1 year or more, baseline bone-density studies are recommended, and repeated comparative studies should be done yearly; if a significant change occurs and continued heparin is required, alendronate should be started (137).

Heparin-related Skin Reactions

Three general types of skin reactions can occur with heparin therapy (97,98,138). The most common are those seen in patients being treated with s.c. heparin. These are small ecchymotic or erythematous papular or nodular lesions that are slightly tender and generally less than 1 cm in size. These occur at the sites of injection. Although at times these are the result of violated sterile technique and therefore represent infections, most are sterile and require no change in therapy except the selection of an alternate site. The exact mechanism is not certain, but local cytokine release is the current working concept.

A second skin reaction is that of urticarial, often pruritic, lesions; again largely at the sites of s.c. injection. These allergic reactions have commonly been associated with the vehicle for the heparin and can often be avoided by either a change in the brand of heparin or the use of an antihistamine at the time of the injections.

Heparin-induced skin necrosis is the most serious form of dermal reaction and fortunately the least common (138–143). These lesions have many features similar to coumadin necrosis, but the pathophysiology is distinctly different. The route and form of heparin is unrelated to this occurrence. Commonly these begin 5 to 10 days into the heparin therapy and are manifest on the extremities, abdominal wall, or nose; several of the case reports highlight their occurrence on the dorsum of the hand (61–63). The onset is abrupt with a dusky or erythematous plaque-like lesion that can rapidly evolve into hemorrhagic bullae with necrosis. The exact pathophysiologic basis for these necrotic lesions is not clear. The antibodies found in HIT have been seen in many of the patients in whom it has been sought, yet only about 25% of them will actually develop HIT-II. These lesions signal an immediate need to discontinue the heparin therapy and select an appropriate alternative agent.

Altered Liver-function Tests

Abnormal liver-function studies, primarily a transaminasemia of minimal degree, have been correlated with long-term heparin administration. The finding is uncommon, and the pathophysiologic mechanisms have never been defined. These changes revert to normal when the heparin is discontinued.

Heparin and Eosinophilia

Eosinophilia occurs in 5% to 10% of patients receiving either UFH or LMWH therapy (97,98,144). The eosinophilia is asymptomatic. In almost all of the patients, it is unrelated to systemic allergic reactions, dermal allergic reactions, skin necrosis, or any other evident symptom complex. It is not associated with any physiologic changes or sequelae. The eosinophilia abates 4 to 8 weeks after cessation of the heparin therapy. The current hypothesis relative to this occurrence is the activation of CD4 cells, with the subsequent release of granulocyte–macrophage colony-stimulating factor (GM-CSF), IL-3, and IL-5, which can induce eosinophilia (145).

Hyperkalemia, Hypoaldosteronism, and Related Metabolic Abnormalities

Prolonged heparin therapy has been recognized to be associated with functional hypoaldosteronism, hyperkalemia, and correlated metabolic abnormalities (99,146,147). Although it is rare, the evidence supports heparin suppression of synthesis of aldosterone (147). Cessation of the heparin results in resolution of the metabolic abnormalities and return to normal.

Priapism

Priapism has been considered to be a possible complication of heparin therapy (99). In the few reports available, it is not clear whether specificity of a vascular occlusive event is present or whether this simply represents thrombosis as part of an HIT-II event. We favor the latter pathophysiologic explanation.

Alopecia

Alopecia has been related to long-term heparin therapy (97–99). Neither its occurrence nor potential pathophysiologic mechanisms have been well defined, but it appears to be rare.

Epidural Bleeding, Hematomas, and Paralysis with Low-molecular-weight Heparins

In December of 1997, the FDA released a public health advisory warning of more than 30 cases of patients developing epidural or spinal hematomas, some with permanent paralysis. All cases reported in the United States were with the concomitant use of enoxaparin. In May of 1998, the FDA again released a report with 50 cases of epidural/spinal hematoma, some with permanent paralysis. Of all four LMWHs, including dalteparin (Fragmin), ardeparin (Normiflo), and danaparoid (Orgaron), only enoxaparin

(Lovenox) was the concurrent LMWH involved. It is unclear why this particular LMWH appears to be the only one associated with this catastrophic event.

REFERENCES

1. Jaques LB, McDuffie HM. The chemical and anticoagulant nature of heparin. *Semin Thromb Hemost* 1978;4:277.
2. Hirsh J. Mechanisms of action and monitoring of anticoagulants. *Semin Thromb Hemost* 1986;12:1.
3. Thomas DP. Heparin. *Clin Haematol* 1981;10:443.
4. McLean J. The thromboplastic action of cephalin. *Am J Physiol* 1916;41:250.
5. McLean J. The discovery of heparin. *Circulation* 1959;19:75.
6. Howell WH, Holt E. Two new factors in blood and physiological reactions. *Am J Physiol* 1918;47:328.
7. Coyne E. Heparin: past, present and future. In: Lundblad RL, Brown WV, Mann KG, et al., eds. *Chemistry and biology of heparin.* North Holland, NY: Elsevier, 1981:9.
8. Bick RL. Heparin therapy and monitoring: guidelines and practice parameters for clinical and laboratory approaches. *Clin Appl Thromb Hemost* 1996;2:12.
9. Hirsh J, Raschke R, Warkentin TE, et al. Heparin: mechanisms of action, pharmacokinetics, dosing considerations, monitoring, efficacy and safety. *Chest* 1995;108(suppl):258.
10. Protamine sulfate. In: *Physicians Desk Reference.* Montvale, NJ: Medical Economics Company, Inc., 2001:1768.
11. Bick RL, Fareed J. Low molecular weight heparins: differences and similarities in approved preparations in the United States. *Clin Appl Thromb Hemost* 1999;5:63–66.
12. Bick RL. Low molecular weight heparins in the outpatient management of venous thromboembolism. *Semin Thromb Hemost* 1999;25(suppl 3):97.
13. Fareed J, Hoppensteadt DA, Jeske WP. The available low molecular weight heparin preparations are not the same. *J Clin Appl Thromb Hemost* 1997;(suppl 1)3:38.
14. Thomas DP. Heparin: low molecular weight heparin, and heparin analogues. *Br J Haematol* 1984;58:385.
15. Alkjaersig N, Roy L, Fletcher A. Analysis of gel exclusion chromatographic data by chromatographic plate theory analysis: application to plasma fibrinogen chromatography. *Thromb Res* 1973;3:525.
16. Irwin JF, Seegers WH, Andary TJ, et al. Blood coagulation as a cybernetic system: control of autoprothrombin-C (Xa) formation. *Thromb Res* 1975; 6;431.
17. Muller-Berghaus G. Pathophysiology of generalized intravascular coagulation. *Semin Thromb Hemost* 1977;3:209.
18. Seegers WH, Irwin JF, Hivegas AB. Blood coagulation: a cybernetic system modified in hemophilia. *Proc IX Congr World Fed Hemophilia* 1974; 3(abst).
19. Harpel PC, Rosenberg RD. Alpha-2-macroglobulin and antithrombin-heparin cofactor: modulators of hemostasis and inflammatory reactions. *Prog Hemost Thromb* 1976;3:145.
20. Mammen EF. Physiology and biochemistry of blood coagulation. In: Bang NU, Belier FK, Deutsch E, et al., eds. *Thrombosis and bleeding disorders: theory and methods.* New York: Academic Press, 1971:1.
21. Murano G. "The Hageman connection": interrelationships between complement, kinins, and coagulation. *Am J Hematol* 1978;4:409.
22. Seegers WH. Use and regulation of blood clotting mechanisms. In: Seegers WH, ed. *Blood clotting enzymology.* New York: Academic Press, 1971:1.
23. Brinkhous KM, Smith HP, Warner ED, et al. Inhibition of blood clotting and unidentified substances which act in conjunction with heparin to prevent the conversion of prothrombin to thrombin. *Am J Physiol* 1939;125:683.
24. Seegers WH, Miller KD, Andrews EB, et al. Fundamental interaction and effect of storage, other adsorbents, and blood clotting in plasma antithrombin activity. *Am J Physiol* 1952; 169:700.
25. Bick RL. Clinical relevance of antithrombin III. *Semin Thromb Hemost* 1982;8:276.
26. Abildgaard U, Graven K, Godal HC. Assay of progressive antithrombin in plasma. *Thromb Diath Haemorrh* 1970;34:224.
27. Seegers WH, Cole ER, Harmison CR, et al. Neutralization of autoprothrombin-C activity with antithrombin. *Can J Biochem* 1964;42:359.
28. Seegers WH, Schroer H, Kagami M. Interaction of purified autoprothrombin I with antithrombin. *Can J Biochem* 1964;42: 425.
29. Vennerod AM, Laake K, Soleberg AK, et al. Inactivation and binding of human plasma kallikrein by antithrombin III and heparin. *Thromb Res* 1976;9:457.
31. Anderson LO, Barrowcliffe TW, Holmer E, et al. Molecular weight dependency of the heparin potentiated inhibition of thrombin and activated factor X: effect of heparin neutralization in plasma. *Thromb Res* 1979;15:521.
32. Johnson EA, Kirkwood TBL, Sterling Y, et al. Four heparin preparations: anti-Xa potentiating effect of heparin after subcutaneous injection. *Thromb Haemost* 1976;35:586.
33. Holmer E, Lindahl U, Backstrom G, et al. Anticoagulant activities and effects on platelets of a heparin fragment with high affinity for antithrombin. *Thromb Res* 1980;18:861.
34. Yin ET. Effect of heparin on the neutralization of factor Xa and thrombin by the plasma alpha-2-globulin inhibitor. *Thromb Diath Haemorrh* 1975;33:43.
35. Abildgaard U. Binding of thrombin to antithrombin III. *Scand J Clin Lab Invest* 1969;24:23.
36. Bentley PG, Kakkar VV, Scully MF, et al. An objective study of alternative methods of heparin administration. *Thromb Res* 1980;18:177.
37. Kurachi K, Schmer G, Hermodson M, et al. Inhibition of bovine factor IXa by antithrombin-III. *Biochemistry* 1976;15: 368.
38. Lahiri B, Rosenberg RD, Talamo RC, et al. Antithrombin-III: an inhibitor of human plasma kallikrein. *Fed Proc* 1974;33: 642(abst).
39. Stead N, Kaplan AP, Rosenberg RD. Inhibition of activated factor XII by antithrombin-heparin cofactor. *J Biol Chem* 1976; 251:6481
40. Hook M, Bjork 1, Hopwood J, et al. Anticoagulant action of heparin: separation of high-activity and low-activity heparin species by affinity chromatography on immobilized antithrombin. *FEBS Lett* 1976;66:90.
41. Li E, Orton H, Feinman R. The interaction of thrombin and heparin: proflavine dye binding studies. *Biochemistry* 1974;13: 5012.
42. Walker F, Esmon C. The molecular mechanism of heparin action, II: separation of functionally different heparins by affinity chromatography. *Thromb Res* 1979;14:219.
43. Yin E, Eisenkramer L, Butler J. Heparin interaction with activated factor X and its inhibitor. *Adv Exp Med Biol* 1974;52:239.
44. Pomerantz M, Owen W. A catalytic role for heparin: evidence of a ternary complex of heparin cofactor, thrombin, and heparin. *Biochim Biophys Acta* 1978;535:66.
45. Nordeman B, Nordling K, Bjork I. A differential effect of low-affinity heparin on the inhibition of thrombin and factor Xa by antithrombin. *Thromb Res* 1980;17:595.

46. Thomas D, Merton R, Lewis W, et al. Studies in man and experimental animals of a low molecular weight heparin fraction. *Thromb Haemost* 1981;45:214.
47. Carlstrom A, Lieden K, Bjork I. Decreased binding of heparin to antithrombins following the interaction between antithrombin and thrombin. *Thromb Res* 1977;11:785.
48. Negus D, Friedgood A, Cox JJ, et al. Ultra-low dose intravenous heparin in the prevention of postoperative deep-vein thrombosis. *Lancet* 1980;1:891.
49. Thomas DP, Barrowcliffe TW, Merton RE, et al. In vivo release of anti-Xa clotting activity by a heparin analogue. *Thromb Res* 1980;17:831.
50. Thomas DP, Merton RE, Barrowcliffe TW, et al. Anti-factor Xa activity of heparan sulfate. *Thromb Res* 1979;14:501.
51. Marcum JA, Rosenberg RD. Role of endothelial cell surface heparin-like polysaccharides. *Ann N Y Acad Sci* 1989;556:81.
52. Jaques L, Mahadoo J. Pharmacodynamics and clinical effectiveness of heparin. *Semin Thromb Hemost* 1978;4:298.
53. Hatton M, Berry L, Regoeczi E. Inhibition of thrombin by anti-thrombin III in the presence of certain glycosaminoglycans found in the mammalian aorta. *Thromb Res* 1978;13:655.
54. Wight T. Vessel proteoglycans and thrombogenesis. *Prog Hemost Thromb* 1980;5:1.
55. Kakkar VV, Lawrence D, Bentley PG, et al. A comparative study of low doses of heparin and a heparin analogue in the prevention of postoperative deep vein thrombosis. *Thromb Res* 1978;13:111.
56. Bick RL, Fareed J, Walenga J, et al. Heparin releasable tissue factor pathway inhibitor during interventional cardiovascular procedures. *Blood* 1994; 84:81.
57. Fareed J, Callas D, Hoppensteadt D, et al. Tissue factor antigen levels in various biological fluids. *Blood Coagul Fibrinolysis* 1995;6:1.
58. Fareed J, Pifarre R, Leya F, et al. Platelet factor 4 and antithrombin III are not the sole determinants of the heparinization response. *Circulation* 1994;90:180.
59. Bick RL, Kovacs I, Fekete L. A new two-stage functional assay for antithrombin III (heparin co-factor): clinical and laboratory evaluation. *Thromb Res* 1976;8:745.
60. Odegard O, Lie M, Abildgaard U. Heparin cofactor activity measured with an amidolytic method. *Thromb Res* 1975;6:287.
61. Teiem AN, Abildgaard R. On the value of the activated partial thromboplastin time in monitoring heparin therapy. *Thromb Haemost* 1976;35:592.
62. Shapiro GA, Huntzinger SW, Wilson JE. Variation among commercial activated partial thromboplastin time reagents in response to heparin therapy. *Am J Clin Pathol* 1977;67:477.
63. Bick RL, McClain BJ. A comparison of five activated partial thromboplastin times and the activated clotting time during heparin therapy. *Thromb Haemost* 1983;50:236.
64. Denson KWE, Bonnar J. The measurement of heparin: a method based on the potentiation of anti-factor Xa. *Thromb Diath Haemorrh* 1973;30:471.
65. Hull RD, Raskob GE, Hirsh J. Continuous intravenous heparin compared with intermittent subcutaneous heparin in the initial treatment of proximal-vein thrombosis. *N Engl J. Med* 1986; 315:1109.
66. Haas S. Treatment of deep venous thrombosis and pulmonary embolism: current recommendations. *Cardiol Clin Annu Drug Ther* 1998;2:99.
67. Hull RD, Raskob G, Rosenbloom D. Optimal therapeutic level of heparin in patients with venous thrombosis. *Arch Intern Med* 1992;152:1589.
68. Hoomes DW, Bura A, Mazzolai L, et al. Subcutaneous heparin compared with continuous intravenous heparin administered in the initial treatment of deep vein thrombosis. *Ann Intern Med* 1992;116:279.
69. Anderson G, Fagrell B, Holmgren K, et al. Subcutaneous administration of heparin: a randomized trial comparison with intravenous administration of heparin to patients with deep-vein thrombosis. *Thromb Res* 1982;27:631.
70. Hull RD, Raskob G, Rosenbloom D. Heparin for 5 days compared to 10 days in the initial treatment of proximal venous thrombosis. *N Engl J Med* 1990;322:1260.
71. Haas S. Treatment of deep venous thrombosis and pulmonary embolism: current recommendations. *Med Clin North Am* 1998;82:495.
72. Stevenson KJ, Easton AC, Curry A, et al. The reliability of the activated partial time methods and the relationship to lipid composition and ultrastructure. *Thromb Haemost* 1986;55:250.
73. Shofjania AM, Tetreault J, Turnbull G. The variat6ions between heparin sensitivity of different lots of activated partial thromboplastin time reagent produced by the same manufacturer. *Am J Clin Pehtol* 1988;89:19.
74. Baker BA, Adelman MD, Smith PA, et al. Inability of the activated partial thromboplastin time to predict heparin levels. *Arch Intern Med* 1997;157:2475.
75. Dalen J, Hirsh J, eds. Second ACCP Consensus Conference on Antithrombotic Therapy. *Chest* 1989;95(suppl):1.
76. Dalen J, Hirsh J, eds. Third ACCP Consensus Conference on Antithrombotic Therapy. *Chest* 1992;102(suppl):303.
77. Dalen J, Hirsh J, eds. Fourth ACCP Consensus Conference on Antithrombotic Therapy. *Chest* 1995;108(suppl):225.
78. Dalen J, Hirsh J, eds. Fifth ACCP Consensus Conference on Antithrombotic Therapy. *Chest* 1998;114(suppl):439.
79. Dalen J, Hirsh J, eds. Sixth ACCP Consensus Conference on Antithrombotic Therapy. *Chest* 2001;119(suppl):1.
80. Laposata M, Green D, Van Cott EM, et al. College of American Pathologists Conference XXXI on laboratory monitoring of anticoagulant therapy. *Arch Pathol Lab Med* 1998;122:799.
81. Fidlar E, Jaques LB. The effect of commercial heparin on the platelet count. *J Lab Clin Med* 1948;33:1410.
82. Nelson JC, Lerner RG, Goldstein R, et al. Heparin-induced thrombocytopenia. *Arch Intern Med* 1978;138:548.
83. Ansell J, Slepchuk N Jr, Kumar R, et al. Heparin induced thrombocytopenia: a prospective study. *Thromb Haemost* 1980; 43:61.
84. King DJ, Kelton JG. Heparin associated thrombocytopenia. *Ann Intern Med* 1984;100:535.
85. Chong BH, Ismail F. The mechanism of heparin-induced platelet aggregation. *Eur J Haematol* 1989;43:245.
86. Warkentin TE, Kelton JG. Heparin and platelets. *Hematol Oncol Clin North Am* 1990;4:243.
87. Boshkov LK, Warkentin TE, Hayward CPM, et al. Heparin induced thrombocytopenia and thrombosis: clinical and laboratory studies. *Br J Hemost* 1993;84:322.
88. Chong BH. Heparin induced thrombocytopenia. *Br J Haemost* 1995;89:431.
89. Aster RH. Heparin-induced thrombocytopenia and thrombosis. *N Engl J Med* 1995;332:1374.
90. Kelton JG, Warkentin TE. Diagnosis of heparin-induced thrombocytopenia: still a journey, not yet a destination [Editorial]. *Am J Clin Pathol* 1995;104:611.
91. Schmitt BP, Adelman B. Heparin associated thrombocytopenia: a critical review and pooled analysis. *Am J Med Sci* 1993;305: 208.
92. Mumer R, Schulman IC, Wolf DJ, et al. Heparin induced thrombocytopenia thrombosis after cardiopulmonary bypass. *Ann Thorac Surg* 1994;14:1764.
93. Shorten GD, Comunale ME. Heparin induced thrombocytopenia. *J Cardiother Vasc Anesth* 1996;10:521.

94. Kibbe MR, Rhee RY. Heparin induced thrombocytopenia: pathophysiology. *Semin Vasc Surg* 1996;9:284.
95. Warkentin TE, Kelton JG. A 14 year study of heparin induced thrombocytopenia. *Am J Med* 1996;101:502.
96. Jackson MR, Krishnamurti C, Aylesworth CA. Diagnosis of heparin induced thrombocytopenia in the vascular surgery patient. *Surgery* 1997;121:419.
97. Walenga JM, Bick RL. Heparin-induced thrombocytopenia, paradoxical thromboembolism, and other side effects of heparin therapy. *Cardiol Clin Annu Drug Ther* 1998;2:123.
98. Walenga JM, Bick RL. Heparin-induced thrombocytopenia, paradoxical thromboembolism, and other side effects of heparin therapy. *Med Clin North Am* 1998;82:635.
99. Hirsh J, Raschke R, Warkentin TE, et al. Heparin: mechanism of action, pharmacokinetics, dosing considerations, monitoring, efficacy, and safety. *Chest* 1995;108:259S.
100. Moberg P, Geary V, Sheikh M. Heparin-induced thrombocytopenia: a possible complication of heparin-coated pulmonary artery catheters. *J Cardiothorac Anesth* 1990;4:266.
101. Weismann RE, Tobin RW. Arterial embolism occurring during systemic heparin therapy. *Arch Surg* 1958;76:219.
102. Abhyankar V, Kouides P, Phatak P. Heparin-induced thrombocytopenia is a cause of thromboembolism following coronary by-pass surgery. *Blood* 1995;86:846(abst).
103. Towne JB, Bernhard VM, Hussey C, et al. White clot syndrome: peripheral vascular complications of heparin therapy. *Arch Surg* 1979;114:372.
104. Stanton PE Jr, Evans JR, Lefemine AA, et al. White clot syndrome. *South Med J* 1988;81:616.
105. Battey PM, Salam AA. Venous gangrene associated with heparin-induced thrombocytopenia. *Surgery* 1985;97:618.
106. Kappa JR, Risher CA, Todd B. Intraoperative management of patients with heparin-induced thrombocytopenia. *Ann Thorac Surg* 1990;49:714.
107. Green D, Martin GJ, Shoichet SH, et al. Thrombocytopenia in a prospective, randomized, double blind trial of bovine and porcine heparin. *Am J Med Sci* 1984;288:60.
108. Powers PJ, Kelton JG, Carter CJ. Studies on the frequency of heparin-associated thrombocytopenia. *Thromb Res* 1984;33:439.
109. Ansell JE, Price JM, Beckner RR. Heparin induced thrombocytopenia: what is its real frequency? *Chest* 1985;88:878.
110. Warkentin TE, Levine MN, Hirsch, J, et al. Heparin-induced thrombocytopenia in patients treated with low-molecular-weight heparin or unfractionated heparin. *N Engl J Med* 1995;332:1330.
111. Thomas DP. Heparin prophylaxis and treatment of venous thromboembolism. *Semin Hematol* 1978;15:1.
112. Hirsh J, Warkentin TE, Raschke R, et al. Heparin and low molecular weight heparin: mechanisms of action, pharmacokinetics, dosing considerations, monitoring, efficacy and safety. *Chest* 1998;114(suppl):489.
113. Warkentin TE. Clinical presentation of heparin-induced thrombocytopenia. *Semin Hematol* 1998;35(suppl):9.
114. Warkentin TE. Limitations of conventional treatment options for heparin-induced thrombocytopenia. *Semin Hematol* 1998;35(suppl):17.
115. Neverre DR, Digiovanni A. Hypercoagulability and the management of anticoagulant therapy in surgical patients: review and recommendations. *J Endovasc Surg* 1998;5:282.
116. Eriksson BI, Ekman S, Kalebo P. Prevention of deep-vein thrombosis after total hip replacement: direct thrombin inhibition with recombinant hirudin CGP 39393. *Lancet* 1996;347:635.
117. Walker AM, Jick H. Prediction of bleeding during heparin therapy. *JAMA* 1980;244:1209.
118. Salzman EW, Deykin D, Shapiro RM, et al. Management of heparin therapy. *N Engl J Med* 1975;292;1046.
119. Levine M, Hirsh J. Hemorrhagic complications of anticoagulant therapy. *Semin Thromb Hemost* 1986;12:39.
120. Hirsh J. Heparin. *N Engl J Med* 1991;327:1565.
121. Morabia A. Heparin doses and major bleedings. *Lancet* 1986;1:1278.
122. Yett HS, Skillman JJ, Salzman EW. The hazards of aspirin plus heparin. *N Engl J Med* 1978;298:1092.
123. Warkentin TE, Soutar RL, Panju A. Acute systemic reactions to intravenous bolus heparin therapy: characterization and relationship to heparin induced thrombocytopenia. *Blood* 1992;80:160(abst).
124. Jaffe MD, Willis PW. Multiple fractures associated with long-term sodium heparin therapy. *JAMA* 1965;193:152.
125. Levine M. Non-hemorrhagic complications of anticoagulant therapy. *Semin Thromb Hemost* 1986;12:63.
126. Howell R, Fidler J, Letsky E, et al. The risks of antenatal subcutaneous heparin prophylaxis: a controlled trial. *Br J Obstet Gynaecol* 1983;90:1124.
127. Monreal M, Lafoz E, Olive A, et al. Comparison of subcutaneous unfractionated heparin with low molecular weight heparin (Fragmin) in patients with venous thromboembolism and contraindications to coumarin. *Thromb Haemost* 1994;71:7.
128. Barbour LA, Kick SD, Steiner JF, et al. A prospective study of heparin-induced osteoporosis in pregnancy using bone densitometry. *Am J Obstet Gynecol* 1994;170:862.
129. Dahlman TC. Osteoporotic fractures and the recurrence of thromboembolism during pregnancy and the puerperium in 184 women undergoing thromboprophylaxis with heparin. *Am J Obstet Gynecol* 1993;168:1265.
130. Hunt BJ, Doughy H, Majumdar G, et al. Thromboprophylaxis with low molecular weight heparin (Fragmin) in high risk pregnancies. *Thromb Haemost* 1997;77:39.
131. Douketis J, Ginsberg JS, Burrows RF, et al. The effects of long-term therapy during pregnancy on bone density: a prospective matched cohort study: a prospective matched cohort study. *Thromb Haemost* 1996;75:254.
132. Muir JM, Andrew M, Hirsh J, et al. Histomorphometric analysis of the effects of standard heparin on trabecular bone in vivo. *Blood* 1996;88:1314.
133. Muir JM, Hirsh J, Weitz JI, et al. A histomorphometric comparison of the effects of heparin and low-molecular-weight heparin on cancellous bone in rats. *Blood* 1997;89:3236.
134. Panagakos FS, Jandinski JJ, Feder L, et al. Heparin fails to potentiate the effects of IL-1 beta-mediated bone resorption of fetal rat long bones in vitro. *Biochimie* 1995;77:915.
135. Shaughnesy SG, Young E, Deschamps P, et al. The effects of low molecular weight and standard heparin on calcium loss from fetal rat calvaria. *Blood* 1995;86:1368.
136. Murray WJ, Lindo VS, Kakkar VV, et al. Long term administration of heparin and heparin fractions and osteoporosis in experimental animals. *Blood Coagul Fibrinolysis* 1995;6:113.
137. Bick RL. Heparin therapy and monitoring: guidelines and practice parameters for clinical and laboratory approaches. *J Clin Appl Thromb Hemost* 1996;2(suppl):12.
138. Warkentin TE. Heparin-induced skin lesions. *Br J Haematol* 1996;92:494.
139. Hill J, Caprini JA, Robbins JL. An unusual complication of minidose heparin therapy. *Clin Orthop* 1976;118:130.
140. White PW, Sadd JR, Wensel RE. Thrombotic complications of heparin therapy. *Ann Surg* 1979;190:595.
141. Kelly RA, Gelfand JA, Pincus SH. Cutaneous necrosis caused by systemically administered heparin. *JAMA* 1981;246:1582.
142. Hall JC, McConahay D, Gibson D, et al. Heparin necrosis: an anticoagulation syndrome. *JAMA* 1980;244:1831.

143. Levine LE, Bernstein JE, Soltani K. Heparin-induced cutaneous necrosis unrelated to injection sites. *Arch Dermatol* 1983;119: 400.
144. Bircher AJ, Itin PH, Buchner SA. Skin lesions, hypereosinophilia and subcutaneous heparin. *N Engl J Med* 1994;343:861.
145. Giustolisi R, Guglielmo P, di Raimondo F, et al. Hypereosinophilia and subcutaneous heparin. *N Engl J Med* 1993;342: 1371.
146. Lechy D, Gantt C, Linn V. Heparin-induced hypoaldosteronism. *JAMA* 1981;246:2189.
147. Aull L, Chao H, Coy K. Heparin-induced hyperkalemia. *Ann Pharmacother* 1990;24:244.
148. Food and Drug Administration. *Reports of epidural or spinal hematomas with the concurrent use of low molecular weight heparin and spinalepidural anesthesia or spinal puncture.* Washington, DC: FDA Public Health Advisory, USDHHS, December 15, 1997.
149. Food and Drug Administration. *Low molecular weight heparinsheparinoids and spinalepidural anesthesia.* Washington, DC: US FDA MedWatch, May 6, 1998.

Disorders of Thrombosis and Hemostasis: Clinical and Laboratory Practice, Third Edition, edited by Rodger L. Bick.
Lippincott Williams & Wilkins, Philadelphia © 2002

18

ANTIPLATELET THERAPY

HANS KLAUS BREDDIN

Platelets have receptors for agonist molecules such as adenosine diphosphate (ADP), collagen, or proteases as thrombin. Platelets as adhesive cells also bind to many subendothelial and plasma molecules. During platelet activation, changes occur in the cytoskeleton and outside–in signaling.

After blood sampling, platelets change their shape by forming pseudopods, followed by swelling. The velocity of this process is temperature dependent. Whereas it takes an hour at 37°C for 80% of the platelets in platelet-rich plasma (PRP) to change their shape, the same degree of shape change is observed after 20 minutes at room temperature. In parallel to the shape change, the aggregation response of PRP increases. Platelets have to be fixed at blood sampling to retain their disk shape (Fig. 18.1A and B and Fig. 18.2A). In freshly prepared PRP, agonists like ADP or collagen induce the formation of reversible aggregates (Fig. 18.1C and 18.2B), a rapid shape change (Fig. 18.1D), and the release of constituents (Fig. 18.2C), followed by irreversible aggregation (Fig. 18.2D).

The presently used aggregation inhibitors do not interfere with shape change. Aggregation studies in vitro cannot be directly translated into the in vivo situation because platelet populations as they develop ex vivo during the preparation of PRP do not exist in vivo.

The originally disk-shaped platelets swell and membrane glycoproteins such as GpIIb/IIIa and GpIb, as well as other activation proteins, surface.

Low-affinity platelet glycoprotein receptors for adhesive molecules on the platelet membrane such as GpIIb/IIIa are activated, leading to high affinity (e.g., for fibrin) and to subsequent aggregation. GpIIb/IIIa changes its conformation during this activation process, so that it can bind fibrinogen, von Willebrand factor (vWF), or fibronectin. Fibrinogen bound to GpIIb/IIIa also binds to resting platelets, thereby leading to their activation. Platelet adhesion and aggregation at high shear stress is mediated by GpIb but also by GpIIb/IIIa. Another activation antigen is P-selectin (CD62). This and other molecules can be detected by the combination of monoclonal antibodies and immunohistologic staining or by flow cytometry. The GpIb–V–IX complex is involved in platelet interactions with exposed subendothelium and with vWF. GpIb is the vWF receptor.

PHARMACOLOGY OF PLATELET-FUNCTION INHIBITORS

Aspirin

Aspirin has antithrombotic effects by inhibiting platelet function. It mildly prolongs the bleeding time and blocks thromboxane A_2 (TXA_2) formation by inhibiting cyclooxygenase in platelets but also the vascular synthesis of prostaglandin I_2 (PGI_2).

Cyclooxygenase exists in two isoforms, COX-1 and COX-2. Acetylsalicylic acid (ASA) at antithrombotic (low) doses inhibits COX-1; it blocks the enzymatic function of COX after acetylation of the amino acid Tyr385 and binds to Ser530, thereby preventing arachidonic acid to reach the enzyme (1).

After single ASA doses of 100 mg, thromboxane synthesis in platelets is almost totally suppressed. ASA also has a slight inhibiting effect on thrombin generation (2), which is not observed with ticlopidine.

Aspirin Resistance

The response to aspirin varies in healthy volunteers and in patients. There are hypo- and hyperresponders. ASA resistance has been described in single patients but also under certain clinical conditions. It is discussed whether, in cerebrovascular disease, higher ASA doses are needed in comparison to those in coronary disease or whether some diabetics are more ASA resistant (3,4).

The COX-2 gene is probably expressed in atherosclerotic vessels, leading to a 100-fold expression of prostaglandin

H. K. Breddin: International Institute of Thrombosis and Vascular Diseases, Frankfurt/Main, Germany.

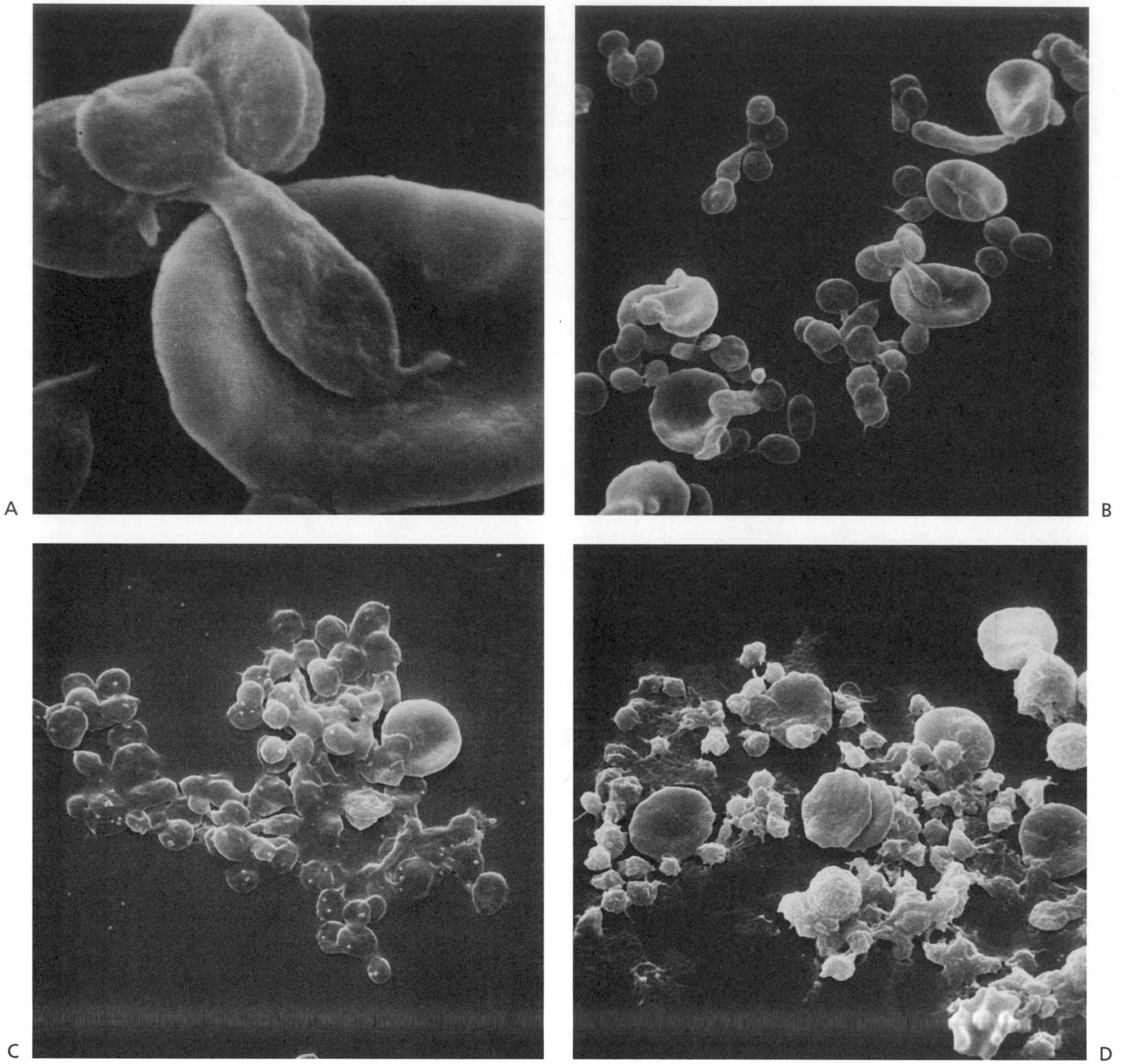

FIGURE 18.1. Raster electron microscopy. **A:** Platelets fixed at blood sampling. A handle-shaped platelet on an erythrocyte with a small pseudopod and several disk-like platelets. Original magnification, ×10,000. **B:** Platelets fixed at blood sampling. The majority of platelets retained the disk-like form; only a few platelets have pseudopods. Original magnification, ×2,000. **C:** Reversible aggregate, several platelets are swollen; some granule-like material is visible on the surface of some platelets. Original magnification, ×2,000. **D:** Aggregate, most platelets have pseudopods and are swollen; some platelets seem fused. Original magnification, ×2,000.

synthesis in the vessel wall (5). Under these conditions, a retrograde transfer of precursors from the vessel wall to adhering platelets may increase their thromboxane synthesis. This mechanism could explain the generally increased thromboxane synthesis in cardiovascular diseases (6).

High doses of ASA (500 mg) inhibit thrombin formation in whole blood (2). Lower doses (300 mg/day) inhibit thrombin formation in PRP, with a marked intraindividual variation (1). How this mechanism is correlated with the inhibition of thromboxane synthesis in platelets and to

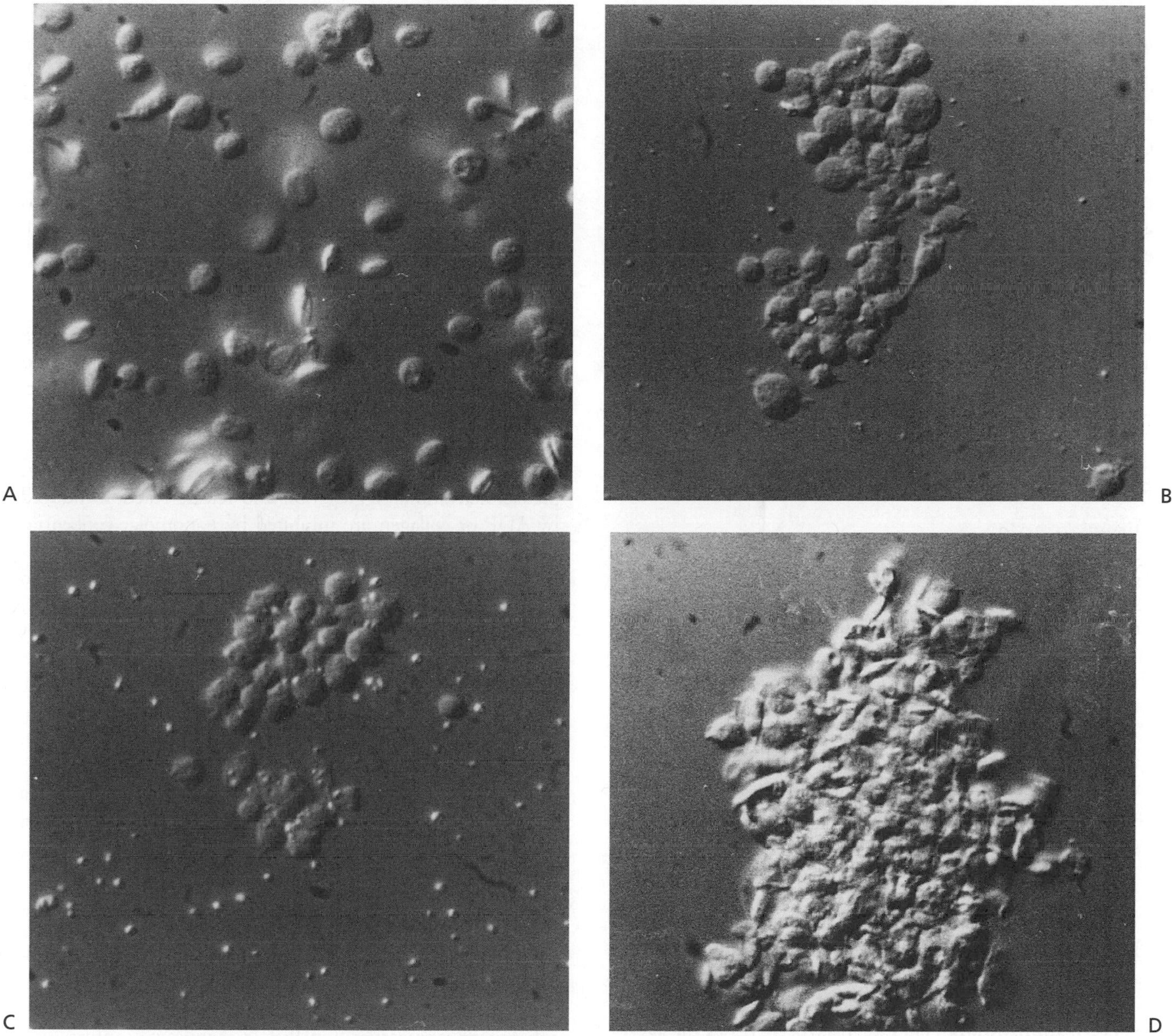

FIGURE 18.2. Interference contrast microscopy (Nomarski optics); original magnification, ×2,000. **A:** Platelets fixed at blood sampling display their disk-like form. **B:** Reversible aggregate; most platelets are partly swollen; many have pseudopods. **C:** Reversible aggregate after partial release. In the center, some platelets are fused. Many small released particles are visible. **D:** Irreversible aggregate. Most platelets are fused, but some on the surface of the aggregate still look intact.

what extent it may explain ASA resistance in a clinical setting requires further evaluation.

Ticlopidine/Clopidogrel

The thienopyridines ticlopidine and clopidogrel are inactive in vitro. Their in vivo inhibiting effect on platelet aggregation is probably due to the formation of an active metabolite in the liver (7). Both drugs inhibit ADP-induced aggregation. This effect is retarded and reaches its maximum after several (4 to 5) days of treatment. It is caused by the interference with a glycoprotein receptor for ADP on the platelet membrane (8,9). The binding of fibrinogen to the GpIIb/IIIa complex triggered by ADP is dramatically inhibited. Thienopyridines inhibit irreversibly and noncompetitively the binding of ADP to the platelet $P2Y_{(AC)}$ receptor (7). This inhibition is not due to a direct modification of the glycoprotein complex. Clopidogrel is 6 times more active than ticlopidine in inhibiting ADP-induced platelet aggregation in humans. Ticlopidine and clopidogrel both mildly prolong the bleeding time. ASA and ticlopidine inhibit only amplification pathways of platelet activation.

Both ASA and ticlopidine have a long-lasting effect because they irreversibly inhibit circulating platelets in contrast to dipyridamole, prostacyclin, or its analogues or GpIIb/IIIa-receptor antagonists. There is a gradual reduction of platelet inhibition when new platelets enter the circulation. The risk of bleeding is reduced about 3 or 4 days after the last intake. The maximal aggregation-inhibiting effect of the standard dose of ticlopidine, 250 mg twice daily, or of clopidogrel, 75 mg once daily, is reached after 3 to 5 days of oral administration. The sensitivity to ASA and ticlopidine/clopidogrel has a marked individual variation, as far as the time to reach an inhibition of aggregation and its intensity, as well as the effects on platelet activation and bleeding time are concerned.

Phosphodiesterase Inhibitors

Dipyridamole

Dipyridamole stimulates platelet membrane adenylate cyclase. It inhibits phosphodiesterase, thus preventing the degradation of cyclic adenosine monophosphate (cAMP) to AMP. In addition, it decreases adenosine uptake and degradation and increases plasma adenosine levels (10). The platelet function-inhibiting effects of dipyridamole are relatively brief. After single oral doses of 75 mg, the antiaggregating effect lasts for about 3 hours. This short duration of the platelet-inhibiting effect may be mainly responsible for the lack of increased bleeding in patients receiving dipyridamole, but also for the negative results in clinical trials.

Cilostazol

Cilostazol, a selective phosphodiesterase 3 inhibitor, has vasodilatory and antiplatelet activities. It inhibits ADP- and collagen-induced aggregation and has antithrombotic effects in animal studies (11). Cilostazol increases the aggregation-inhibiting effect of ASA in human volunteers (12).

Thromboxane-receptor Antagonists

Several drugs have been developed to inhibit or interfere with thromboxane formation (e.g., thromboxane synthase inhibitors) (13–15) or thromboxane-receptor antagonists (6–18).

Thromboxane synthase inhibitors selectively block TXA_2 formation but may increase the level of PGG_2/H_2, which are potent aggregating agents and vasoconstrictors stimulating the same platelet receptor as TXA_2, resulting in an inconsistent platelet inhibition (19,20). Complete and selective inhibition of the effects of TXA_2 as well as PGG_2/H_2 on platelets may be achieved with TXA_2-receptor antagonists (21).

Schenk et al. (22) studied the effects of HN-11500 ($C_{14}H_{15}NO_5S_2$;5-[2(phenyl-sulfonyl)amino-ethyl]-2-thienyloxyacetic acid), a new thromboxane-receptor antagonist (22). Platelet aggregation induced by the thromboxane mimetic U 46 619 and platelet adhesion to siliconized glass were significantly and dose-dependently inhibited. The effect lasted between 3 and 4 hours (10 mg) and 8 hours (400 mg), and correlated well with pharmacokinetic data. HN-11500 also is a strong antithrombotic agent in a rat thrombosis model (23).

Prostaglandins

Prostaglandin E_1 (PGE_1) and prostacyclin (PGI_2) are strong vasodilators. Higher doses reduce vascular resistance and mean blood pressure. The observed favorable effect in patients with progressive vascular disease and microcirculatory disorder probably is caused by the vasodilatory effects and microcirculatory improvement. PGE_1 and PGI_2 (Iloprost) inhibit platelet activation. Aggregation and release reaction induced by ADP or collagen are inhibited by nanomolar concentrations in vitro but also ex vivo, probably by a platelet receptor–dependent activation of adenylate cyclase, which leads to an intracellular increase of cAMP. After an infusion of PGE_1 or PGI_2, the platelet-inhibiting effect lasts only for minutes (24). PGI_2 also inhibits leukocyte adhesion.

High doses of prostacyclin have strong antithrombotic effects in different animal models. The adhesion of platelets to the damaged endothelial wall is mainly inhibited (25). Because prostaglandins are not primary platelet-function inhibitors and because in patients treated with these drugs, a platelet-function inhibition cannot be measured, the clinical trials with PGE_1 or prostacyclin are not discussed in detail.

Glycoprotein IIb/IIIa–receptor Antagonists

Low-affinity platelet glycoprotein receptors for adhesive molecules on the platelet membrane such as GpIIb/IIIa are activated, leading to high affinity (e.g., for fibrinogen) and to subsequent aggregation. GpIIb/IIIa changes its confirmation during this activation process, so that it can bind fibrinogen, vWF, or fibronectin. The heterodimer GpIIb/IIIa complex is a member of the integrin family of receptors, which mediates platelet aggregation and adhesion to collagen (26). Expression of the GpIIb/IIIa complex and its binding to fibrinogen is believed to be the final common pathway for all platelet agonists. The amino acid sequence Arg-Gly-Asp (RGD) or RGDS of fibrinogen, vWF, and fibronectin bind to the activated GpIIb/IIIa receptor. GpIIb/IIIa-receptor antagonists can be divided into three classes: RGD or Lysin-Gly-Asp (KGD) peptides, RGD-mimicking nonpeptides, and monoclonal antibodies (mAbs) like the modified human–mouse chimeric mAb c7E3Fab (abciximab). They dose-dependently inhibit platelet aggregation induced by ADP, collagen, and other agonists, fibrinogen binding, and in vitro platelet adhesion. They also strongly prolong the bleeding time (26,27).

Platelet-induced thrombin generation also is markedly reduced (27,28). The mAb abciximab or the peptides/peptidomimetics eptifibatide and tirofiban are currently used for intravenous (i.v.) short-term treatment (up to 72 hours). So far, all clinical data on the efficacy of these drugs were generated with underlying comedication with ASA. Inhibitory effects of GpIIb/IIIa-receptor antagonists on platelet granular secretion have rarely been investigated. Tsao et al. (29) reported that at concentrations of the antagonists abciximab and the peptide DMP728 that inhibited platelet aggregation by 80% to 90%, neither had any effect on CD62 expression. Furthermore, a lack of significant effect was demonstrated on platelet granular secretion induced by either thrombin or ADP. Formation of TXA_2, which acts as a vascular smooth muscle mitogen, was not compromised under the peptidomimetic agent fradafiban, despite complete inhibition of fibrinogen binding. Klinckhardt et al. (30) observed only a small inhibitory effect of abciximab and a new compound designed for oral use, SR121566A, on CD62 or CD63 expression.

Platelet membrane GpIIb/IIIa inhibitors such as abciximab, tirofiban, or eptifibatide have much stronger effects than ASA or ticlopidine/clopidogrel. After cessation of the i.v. infusion of the presently available drugs, a partial normalization of platelet function is achieved within a relatively short time of usually a few hours. This is in contrast to the long-lasting effects of either ASA or the thienopyridines ticlopidine and clopidogrel, with which the platelet-function inhibition lasts for several days after treatment discontinuation.

CLINICAL TRIAL RESULTS

General Remarks

Antithrombotic drugs may inhibit new vascular occlusions. The detection of new vascular occlusions during long-term treatment is a suitable end point in coronary or peripheral arterial occlusive disease. An antithrombotic agent also may improve the walking distance if it is administered for long periods, because in the treated patient group, fewer thrombotic occlusions may be expected than in the control group. In several clinical trials of platelet-function inhibitors (e.g., ticlopidine or cilostazol) in patients with peripheral arterial occlusive disease (PAOD), the improvement of the pain-free or maximal walking distance has been used as the clinical end point. This parameter also has been propagated with the assumption that it can be objectively measured. In reality this is, however, very difficult. Obviously the walking distance is not a useful end point for such trials.

Aspirin

Aspirin in Peripheral Arterial Disease

Acetylsalicylic acid (ASA, aspirin) has been used in patients with peripheral arterial occlusive disease (PAOD) in daily doses ranging between 50 and 1,500 mg. Most earlier studies were performed with 1,000 to 1,500 mg/day.

We observed in 1968 and 1969 an inhibition of spontaneously enhanced platelet aggregation and clinical improvement in patients with PAOD during treatment with 3 × 500 mg of ASA (31,32).

In a patient with Raynaud syndrome and fingertip necroses, Fitzgerald and Butterfield (33) saw a marked clinical improvement with 300 mg ASA/day. Similar effects were described by Vreeken and van Aken (34) in patients with spontaneously enhanced platelet aggregation. Biermer et al. (35) and Preston et al. (36) observed a marked clinical improvement in ASA-treated patients with multiple thromboses with thrombocytosis.

Aspirin after Vascular Surgery

ASA was effective in several clinical studies in patients who had undergone vascular surgery (Table 18.1) (37–41). Some of these studies also made it likely that after suboptimal reconstruction, ASA medication is advantageous. In patients with endarterectomy in the femoropopliteal region receiving ASA or ASA in combination with dipyridamole, reocclusions were significantly reduced compared with those in a group receiving a vitamin K antagonist (39). The same authors observed a nonsignificantly lower reocclusion rate in patients with venous bypass operations treated with a vitamin K antagonist compared with combined treatment with ASA and dipyridamole after an observation period of 2 years (40). Green et al. (41) found a significantly higher patency rate in patients with polytetrafluoroethylene (PTFE) prostheses above the knee, if they were treated with ASA or with ASA and dipyridamole, compared with placebo.

Edmonson et al. (44) demonstrated that a 3-month treatment period with a low-molecular-weight heparin (LMWH) in patients after bypass operations after 1 year significantly reduced reocclusions compared with treatment with ASA and dipyridamole. The difference was more pronounced in patients with a preoperatively reduced outflow.

ASA in doses of 1.5 g/day reduced reocclusions in patients after vascular surgery. ASA had no effect on vascular mortality. There was no evidence that ASA reduced the progression of atherosclerotic lesions.

There is no conclusive evidence on the best dose of ASA for the prevention of reocclusions after reconstructive vascular surgery. Most surgeons in Europe use 100 to 300 mg/day. Prophylaxis should probably begin as early as possible after the operation.

Prevention of Reocclusions after Percutaneous Transluminal Angioplasty

In several trials, the effect of ASA on reocclusions after angioplasty was compared with that of placebo or oral anticoagulants (Table 18.2). These studies were relatively small

TABLE 18.1. CLINICAL STUDIES ON THE EFFICACY OF ASA AFTER VASCULAR SURGERY

End Authors	Year	Medic.	Patients (No.)	Dose (mgday)	Patency Rate (%)	End Point	Controls	Controls (No.)	Patency Rate (%)	Duration	P
Zekert et al.	1976	ASA	149	1,500	88	Reoccl. after vasc. surgery	Placebo	150	81	14 days	NS
Ehresmann et al.	1977	ASA	215	1,500	53	Reoccl. after vasc. surgery	Placebo	213	47	1 yr	<0.03
Brunner et al.	1979	ASA + Dip.	61	1,000 225	73	Reoccl. after bypass	Vit K antag.	30	66	3 mo–2 yr	NS
Bollinger et al.	1981	ASA + Dip.	81	1,000 225	80	Reoccl. after TEA	Vit K antag.	39	58	3 mo–2 yr	<0.02
Broomè et al.	1982	ASA	83	1,000	85	Reoccl. after TEA	Placebo	64	65	2 yr	<0.001
Albert et al.	1982	ASA	37	1,500	86	Reoccl. after TEA	Vit K antag.	28	93	2 yr	NS
		ASA	11	1,500	55	Reoccl. after bypass	Vit K antag.	10	90	2 yr	NS
Kohler et al.	1984	ASA + Dip.	44	975 225	43	Reoccl. after vasc. surgery	Placebo	44	33	2 yr	NS
Raithel et al.	1986	ASA	59	1,500	82	Reoccl. after bypass	Pentox.	59	67	1 yr	<0.05
Clyne et al.	1987	ASA + Dip.	49	300 400	83	Reoccl. after bypass	Placebo	44	72	1 yr	NS
		ASA + Dip.	29	300 400	85	Reoccl. after bypass	Placebo	26	53	1 yr	0.005
Edmonson et al.	1994	LMWH	103	2,500 U	[a]	Reoccl. after bypass	ASA 300, dip	103	(a)	1 yr	<0.01

[a]Patency rate in the LMWH-group 20% higher than in the ASA + dipyridamole group.
ASA, acetylsalicylic acid; Dip, dipyridamole; TEA, thromboendauterectomy; LMWH, low-molecular-weight heparin.

TABLE 18.2. CLINICAL STUDIES ON THE EFFECT OF ASA ON THE PATENCY RATE AFTER SUCCESSFUL PERIPHERAL TRANSLUMINAL ANGIOPLASTY (PTA)

Authors	Year	Medic.	Dose (mgday)	Control Group	Patient n.	Reocclusion Rate (%)	Controls n.	Reocclusion Rate (%)	Duration	p
Zeitler et al.	1973	ASA	1,500	vit.K-anta.	87	4.6	19	21	10 days	<0.05
				ASA + vt.K-anta.	90	6.7			10 days	NS
Hess et al.	1978	ASA	990	ASA + 225 mg dip.	50		60	16	14 days	NS
Staiger	1980	ASA	1,500		33	21	39	36	5 mo	?
		ASA	1,500		28	25				
		Dipyrid.	225							
Heiss et al.	1990	ASA + Dipyrid.	990 225	Placebo	47	38	47	60	6 mo	<0.05
		ASA + Dipyrid.	300 225		47	53			6 mo	NS
Ranke et al.	1992	ASA	990	ASA 50	175	15.1	112	16	1 yr	NS
Weichert et al.	1993	ASA	1,000	ASA 300	111	18	112	16	1 yr	NS
Minar et al.	1995	ASA	1,000	ASA 100	102	45	105	43	2 yr	NS

ASA, acetylsalicylic acid; dip, dipyridamole; anta, antagonist.

(45–48) and showed no significant differences between the ASA-treated and the control groups.

In three newer studies, different doses of ASA have been compared in patients after percutaneous transluminal angioplasty (PTA). In a double-blind study of 359 patients, Ranke et al. (49) detected no difference in the reocclusion rate between daily doses of ASA of 50 and 900 mg. But in the 50 mg/day ASA group, gastrointestinal side effects (peptic ulcers and erosive gastritis), needing transfusions were significantly less frequent compared with those in the 900 mg/day group (1.1% and 5.1%; $p = 0.03$). In a similar randomized double-blind study in patients after successful PTA receiving either 2 × 150 mg ASA/day (n = 112) or 2 × 500 mg ASA/day (n = 111), the reocclusion rate after 1 year was almost identical. Gastrointestinal side effects leading to cessation of the medication were slightly but not significantly more frequent in the high-dose group (n = 21) compared with the lower-dose group (n = 16) (50). In a third double-blind prospective study in 207 patients receiving either 1,000 mg or 100 mg ASA/day, after 2 years, 36 reocclusions had occurred in both the high- and the low-dose treatment groups (51).

These studies demonstrated that in this indication, a daily dose of 50 to 300 mg ASA is as effective as 1 g/day. However, it still remains uncertain whether ASA really prevents reocclusions after PTA. Further studies with newer antithrombotic agents may lead to better prevention of reocclusions.

Prevention of New Vascular Occlusions in Patients with Peripheral Artery Occlusive Disease

The few small studies in this area are listed in Table 18.3 (52–55). In four of five studies, a significant difference in favor of ASA was reported. The ASA dose in these studies was relatively high, varying between 900 mg and 1.5 g/day.

New studies in comparison with vitamin K antagonists but also with combinations of low-dose ASA with low-dose vitamin K antagonists are promising. An LMWH was more

TABLE 18.3. CLINICAL STUDIES ON THE EFFECT OF ASPIRIN IN PATIENTS WITH PERIPHERAL ARTERIAL OCCLUSIVE DISEASE

Authors	Year	Medic.	Dose (mgday)	Control Group	End Point	Patient No.	Patency Rate (%)	Control No.	Patency Rate (%)	Durat.	P Value
Linke	1975	ASA	1,500	Placebo	Reocclusions	50	68	50	44	3 yr	NS
Hess et al.	1978	ASA	1,500	Placebo	Reocclusions	134	94	124	86.3	2 yr	<0.05
Schoop et al.	1963	ASA	990	Placebo	Reocclusions	100	80	100	40	2 yr	<0.05
		ASA + dip.	990	Placebo	Reocclusions	100	63			<0.05	
Hess et al.	1985	ASA	990	Placebo	Angiographic score system	67	(a)	69	[a]	2 yr	<0.01
		ASA + dip.	990			63	(a)				

ASA, acetylsalicylic acid; dip, dipyridamole.

effective than ASA in one recent study (44). In the near future, new antithrombotic drugs (thrombin inhibitors, thromboxane-receptor antagonists, platelet membrane GpIIb/IIIa inhibitors, and others) will probably be compared with ASA.

In the American Physician's Health Study, 22,071 male physicians aged 40 to 84 years received every second day 325 mg ASA or placebo for a mean of 60 months. In 20 participants in the ASA group and in 36 physicians in the placebo group, peripheral vascular surgery had to be performed ($p = 0.03$). The authors concluded that continuous treatment with low-dose ASA reduced the need for peripheral vascular reconstructions (56).

Peripheral Arterial Occlusive Disease and Vascular Risk

Patients with PAOD frequently also have coronary heart disease. There is an inverse correlation between ankle/brachial pressure index and manifest coronary heart disease (57). In PAOD patients, the risk of early death is clearly increased (58). The data of the "antiplatelet trialist's group" (59) impressively showed that total mortality is reduced in PAOD patients treated with ASA.

Aspirin in Cerebrovascular Disease

ASA in doses of 50 and 1,300 mg/day was effective in the secondary prevention after transitory ischemic attacks or incomplete stroke in several placebo-controlled trials (60,61). A large meta-analysis of all ASA studies reported no difference between the risk reduction of low and medium ASA doses (75 to 325 mg/day) and high doses (more than 900 mg/day) (59). Two very large studies on about 20,000 patients each recently demonstrated that 160 or 300 mg ASA/day significantly reduced new strokes and death in patients with recent strokes (62,63). It is not yet clear which is the optimal ASA dose in the secondary prevention of cerebrovascular diseases. In the ESPS-2 studies (64), a low ASA dose of 75 mg/day was marginally effective. If the increasing number of nonresponders with low ASA doses is considered, the minimal daily dose in these patients should be 300 mg/day.

Aspirin in Coronary Heart Disease

After Craven's observation in 1950 (65) that patients receiving high doses of ASA for rheumatic disease had fewer myocardial infarctions (MIs), ASA has become one of the most effective drugs in the treatment of coronary heart disease.

Primary Prophylaxis

The American Physicians' Health Study (66), a double-blind, placebo-controlled investigation included 22,071 male physicians aged 40 to 84 years. Half of them received ASA (325 mg) every second day, and the other half, placebo. The study was stopped after 5 years because of a highly significant reduction of 47% ($p < 0.0001$) of the incidence of MIs in the ASA-treated group. In the placebo group, 239 MIs had occurred (26 fatal), but in the ASA group, only 139 MIs (10 fatal). However, the total incidence of cardiovascular death in both groups was not significant. The positive effect of ASA in this study was not confirmed in a British study with 5,139 male physicians (67).

With the presently available data, a primary prophylaxis with ASA, especially concerning the side effects of this drug, cannot be recommended.

Myocardial Infarction

Cardiff I 1974 was the first study on the incidence of reinfarction in patients with recent MI (68) followed by a German/Austrian study (69). Both studies showed a reduction of reinfarctions in the ASA-treated groups. Further studies were published in the following years. In none of these trials was the reinfarction reduction significant with ASA. The daily ASA dose varied between 300 and 1,500 mg.

The first clinical trial that convincingly demonstrated the effect of ASA in patients with acute MI was the ISIS-2 trial (70). ASA in this large study was as effective as thrombolytic treatment with streptokinase and reduced mortality within the first 35 days after the acute MI. The protective effects of ASA and streptokinase were additive, so mortality in the combined group was 8% compared with 13.2% in the placebo group. Since the ISIS-2 study on 17,000 patients, ASA has become a standard treatment in acute MI. The protective effect also has been shown in later studies after 15 months and 4 years (71).

The largest meta-analysis on the effect of ASA was published by the Antiplatelet Trialists' Collaboration Group (72), in which the results of 174 studies in 70,000 high-risk patients (atherosclerotic vascular disease) were included (Fig. 18.3). ASA has been used in doses between 75 and 1,500 mg/day. The analysis showed no dose dependency of the protective effects. The incidence of vascular end points was 17.1% in the control group and 13.6% in the ASA group. This corresponds to the relative risk reduction of 20.5% ($p < 0.00001$).

Because of the low side-effect rate, ASA has become the treatment of choice in patients with acute MI if no additional factors as ventricular thrombi, ventricular fibrillation, or valvular defects require treatment with oral anticoagulants. The daily ASA dose lies between 100 and 300 mg. However, if the increasing number of nonresponders with low ASA doses is considered, 300 mg/day should be generally used.

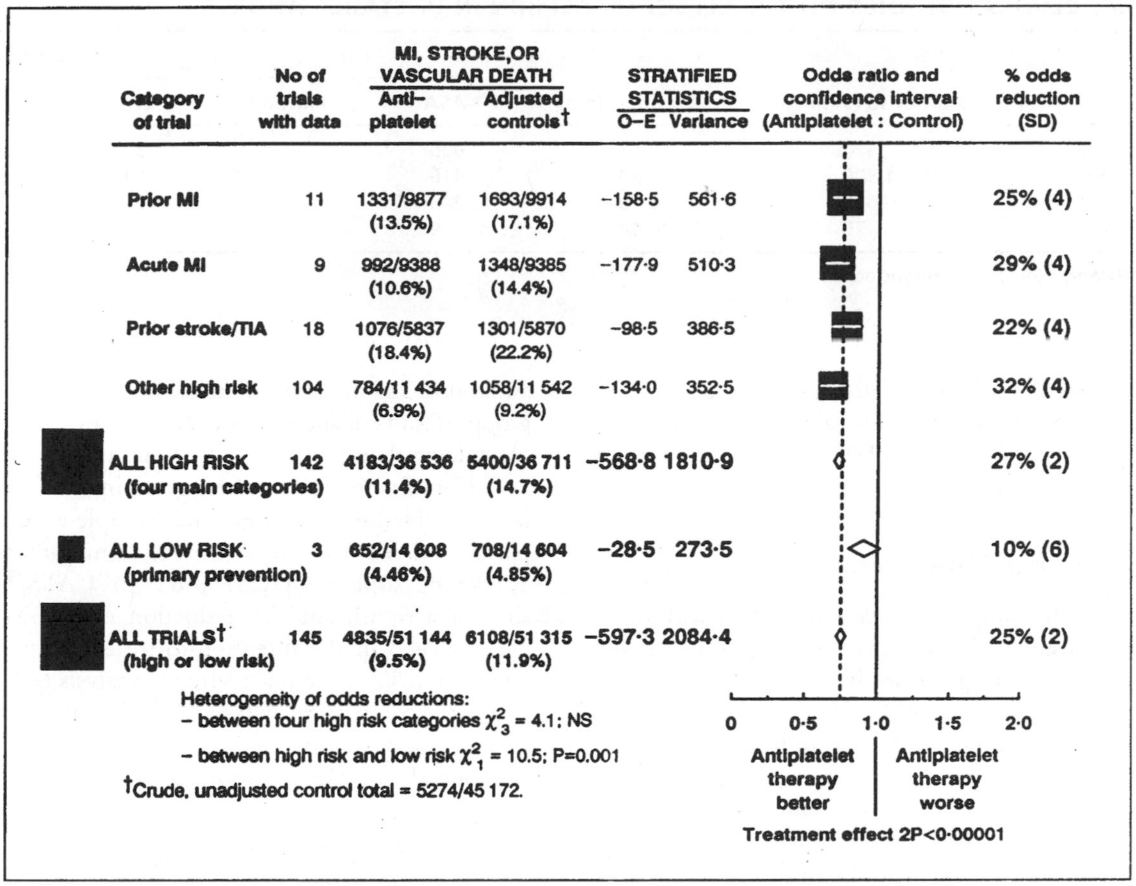

FIGURE 18.3. Proportional effects of antiplatelet therapy: 145 trials on vascular events (myocardial infarction, stroke, or vascular death) in four main high-risk categories of trial and in low risk (primary prevention). *TIA,* transient ischemic attack. Stratified ratio of odds of an event in treatment groups to that in control groups is plotted for each group of trials (*black square*) along with its 99% confidence interval (*horizontal line*). Overview of results for certain subtotals (and 95% confidence intervals) are represented by *diamonds*. Odds reductions observed in particular groups of trials are given to right of vertical line. (From Antiplatelet Trialists' Collaboration. Collaborative overview of randomized trials of antiplatelet therapy, I: prevention of death, myocardial infarction and stroke by prolonged antiplatelet therapy in various categories of patients. *BMJ* 1994;308:81–106, with permission.)

Aspirin in Unstable Angina

Since a study of Lewis et al. (73), unstable angina is one of the classic indications for ASA in coronary heart disease. In this study, 1,266 patients with unstable angina received either 324 mg/day ASA or placebo and were observed for 3 months. In the ASA group, the rate of nonfatal MIs was reduced from 6.9% to 3.4%, and total mortality, from 3.3% to 1.6%. The incidence of a cumulative end point, cardiovascular events, was significantly reduced from 10.1% to 5.0%.

Several other randomized, placebo-controlled trials on the effect of ASA in unstable angina have been performed (74–76). ASA was used in doses between 75 and 1,300 mg/day and led to an about 50% reduction of events in comparison with placebo (Table 18.4).

Stable Angina Pectoris

Since the positive results of the ASA trials in unstable angina, ASA has frequently been used in stable angina without scientific evidence. Only the subgroup analysis of the Physicians' Health Study by Manson et al. (77) showed that in patients who had angina pectoris at entry, the MI incidence was reduced by 87%. The Swedish Angina Pectoris Trial (78) demonstrated that 75 mg ASA daily in patients with stable angina reduced MIs by 39%.

TABLE 18.4. CLINICAL STUDIES ON THE EFFECT OF ASPIRIN IN UNSTABLE ANGINA

Study	ASA dose (1 mg/d)	Duration (mo)	No.		Reduction of	
			ASA	Placebo	Events	Mortality
Lewis et al. 1983	324	3	625	641	51%	51%
Cairns et al. 1985	1,300	20	416	139	51%	71%
Theroux et al. 1988	650	6 days	243	236	72%	—[a]
RISC trial 1990	75	14	399	397	50%	NS

NS, not significant; ASA, acetylsalicylic acid.
[a]No mortality.

The Antiplatelet Trialists' Collaboration Group (72), in a meta-analysis of seven trials, also calculated a significant reduction of all vascular events of 33% in patients treated with ASA in stable angina.

Ticlopidine and Clopidogrel

Stiegler et al. (79) compared a 1-year treatment with ticlopidine with placebo in 43 patients with PAOD. Patients had angiography entering the study and after 1 year (79). An angiographic score was used and showed a significant decrease in the ticlopidine group as an indicator of a reduction of new vascular lesions. The authors assumed that ticlopidine reduces thrombotic progression of atherosclerotic lesions.

Several later studies showed a significant increase in walking distance in patients with PAOD (80–84). An increased walking distance is, however, not a suitable end point to detect effects of antithrombotic agents in PAOD.

The Swedish Ticlopidine Multicenter Study (STIMS) was published in 1990 (85). The investigators assumed that intermittent claudication is an indicator of a generalized atherosclerosis with increased morbidity and mortality by cardio- and cerebrovascular events. It was the aim of the study to test whether the occurrence of fatal and nonfatal MIs, ischemic stroke, or transient ischemic attacks (TIAs) in patients with PAOD can be reduced by long-term treatment with ticlopidine.

In six Swedish clinical centers, 687 patients received either 2 × 250 mg ticlopidine/day or placebo. The mean observation period was 5 to 6 years. The sum of all primary end points in the placebo group was 113 (33.1%) compared with 96 (27.7%) in the ticlopidine group. If only patients receiving treatment until the end of the observation period were evaluated, the difference of the sum of all primary end points between the two groups was statistically significant, with a p value of 0.007. Total mortality in the ticlopidine group (18.5%) was by 29.1% lower than that in the placebo group (26.1%). Cause of death was ischemic heart disease in 54 patients of the placebo group compared with 31 in the ticlopidine group.

In a retrospective analysis, Bergqvist et al. (86) evaluated the need for vascular surgery in patients of the STIMS trial and found a significant difference in favor of the ticlopidine group. Results of such secondary analyses are, however, less convincing than the results of prospective trials.

Ticlopidine has been investigated in two large randomized, double-blind studies after complete stroke against placebo (CATS) (87) or after TIA and minor stroke against 1,300 mg aspirin (TASS) (88). In CATS, ticlopidine showed a significant risk reduction of 23.3% compared with placebo in the intention-to-treat analysis (p = 0.02) and of 30.2% in the on-treatment analysis (p = 0.006). In the direct comparison with ASA, ticlopidine was superior, with a risk reduction of 12% (p = 0.048). Studies with clopidogrel have not yet been performed.

Results of the CAPRIE Study

Clopidogrel is a successor of ticlopidine. In the large CAPRIE study (CAPRIE Steering Committee, 1996) (89), more than 19,000 patients were treated with either 325 mg ASA or once-daily 75 mg clopidogrel and were observed for a mean of 1.9 years. Included were 6,491 patients with a stroke within the preceding 6 months, 6,302 patients with an MI within the preceding 35 days, and 6,452 patients with a PAOD. Primary end points were new strokes, recurrent or new MIs, intracranial bleeding, and leg amputations.

Strokes, MI, and vascular death were significantly less frequent in the clopidogrel group compared with the ASA-treated group (relative risk reduction, 8.7%). For the three very large subgroups, the results were divergent. In the group with recent MIs, the effect of ASA was slightly better than that of clopidogrel (relative risk reduction for ASA, 3.7%). In the group with recent stroke, the risk reduction was in favor of clopidogrel, with 7.3%. The best results for clopidogrel were observed in the PAOD group, with a risk reduction compared with ASA of 23.8%. In this group, however, the main difference was due to a reduction of new MIs in the clopidogrel-treated patients. The number of amputations in the total group was 52 with clopidogrel and 47 with ASA.

No direct conclusions on the effect of clopidogrel on peripheral arterial disease can be drawn from the CAPRIE study. Why new MIs were reduced so clearly in the patients with PAOD receiving clopidogrel remains an interesting question.

Combined Use of Aspirin and Ticlopidine/Clopidogrel in Stenting

Recent reports by cardiologists (90–92) have led to a wide acceptance of the combination of ASA and ticlopidine in patients receiving coronary stents. These studies made it likely that the combined use of ticlopidine and ASA after stenting reduced the bleeding incidence in comparison with the former use of vitamin K antagonists and that the reocclusion rate after stenting is markedly less than that seen with oral anticoagulation. Thebauldt et al. (93) reported in 1977 that ASA does not increase the effect of ticlopidine on ADP induced aggregation, but that it increased the effect of ASA on collagen-induced aggregation. ASA and ticlopidine prolonged the bleeding time slightly in comparison with ASA alone. The combination of high-dose ASA with ticlopidine led to a marked prolongation of the bleeding time in all volunteers except one. Beyond any doubt, patients using both drugs will come to emergency coronary artery bypass graft (CABG) more frequently in the future, as the combined use of these two platelet-function inhibitors is increasing.

Side Effects of Ticlopidine and Clopidogrel

The most frequent side effects with ticlopidine treatment are neutropenia, thrombocytopenia, and aplastic anemia in about 1% to 2%, diarrhea in 20% to 25%, and skin changes (rash) in about 5%. In contrast, in the CAPRIE study with clopidogrel, side effects were not more frequent than in the ASA group.

Phosphodiesterase Inhibitors

Dipyridamole

Several studies in patients with MI in which ASA and dipyridamole were combined led to inconclusive results. The effect of dipyridamole with ASA did not exceed that of ASA alone. Dipyridamole has been used at doses of 2×75 mg/day. At this dose, dipyridamole inhibits platelet aggregation only for a few hours. The effect of dipyridamole can probably be increased by using it in a sustained release form. The European Stroke Study (ESPS) (64) was the first to show a positive effect of a combination of such a retarded dipyridamole form (2×200 mg/day) in comparison with ASA alone in patients with recent stroke. Further studies are necessary before dipyridamole will have a verified place in combined treatments.

Cilostazol

Cilostazol was more effective than pentoxifylline in patients with moderate to severe intermittent claudication (94). However, the end point that was influenced in this study was the walking distance after a treatment period of 24 weeks. Cilostazol may be a potent platelet-function inhibitor, but it certainly has other, mainly vasodilatory effects. Further studies are necessary to establish its clinical role as an antiplatelet agent.

Glycoprotein IIb/IIIa–receptor Antagonists

Studies with Intravenous Glycoprotein IIb/IIIa Inhibitors

The first drug effectively used in clinical trials was the chimeric monoclonal 7E3 Fab (abciximab), created through genetic recombination. This new hybrid molecule consists of mouse-derived variable antibody regions linked to the constant region derived from human immunoglobulin. Abciximab was successfully used in large trials in high-risk patients undergoing percutaneous transluminal coronary angioplasty (PTCA) [EPIC (95), EPILOG (96)] and in unstable angina [CAPTURE (97)]. There were, however, increased procedural bleeding complications 2 to 3 times more frequently than with placebo in the EPIC trial. The reduction of heparin apparently reduced the excess bleeding in the EPILOG and CAPTURE trials.

Tirofiban is an i.v. nonpeptide GpIIb/IIIa-receptor antagonist that specifically inhibits fibrinogen-dependent platelet aggregation and prolongs the bleeding time. Three large clinical trials [RESTORE (98), PRISM (99), and PRISM PLUS (100)] showed that, when administered with a standard heparin and ASA regimen, tirofiban reduces the risk of ischemic complications in patients with unstable angina/non–q-wave MI and in patients undergoing PTCA.

Eptifibatide also has been studied in large clinical trials [IMPACT II (101), PURSUIT (102)] and effectively reduced death and MI in patients with acute coronary syndromes. Similarly, lamifiban was effective in 3- to 5-day infusion in the PARAGON (103) trial. The i.v. drugs have shown marked efficacy in comparison with heparin plus ASA alone. It is possible that underdosing occurred in some patients and that close monitoring would improve the results of the i.v. agents. In the studies with i.v. GpIIb/IIIa inhibitors, an optimal amount of platelet-function inhibition, which could be correlated with efficacy or bleeding complications, has not yet been established.

Studies with Oral Glycoprotein IIb/IIIa–receptor Antagonists

GpIIb/IIIa inhibitors such as orbofiban, sibrafiban, and xemilofiban have been developed for oral use. They are prodrugs that after absorption are split in the liver to generate the active compound.

Three large clinical trials with orbofiban [OPUS (104)], sibrafiban [SYMPHONY (105)], and xemilofiban [EXCITE (106)] have been performed in patients who had experienced acute coronary syndromes. Almost 27,000 patients were included, but the trials led to disappointing results (Table 18.5). These new drugs are very effective in

TABLE 18.5. CLINICAL TRIALS WITH ORAL GP IIB/IIIA INHIBITORS; DEATH / MYOCARDIAL INFARCTION

Study	No.	Placebo (%)	Fiban (%)	Odds Ratio	χ p Value
EXCITE	7,232	9.10	8.74	0.95	0.60
OPUS	10,302	4.50	5.25	1.17	0.10
SYMPHONY	9,169	7.00	7.65	1.10	0.26
All	26,703	6.60	7.00	1.07	0.29

GP, glycoprotein.

human volunteers, and they all strongly inhibit platelet function. Probably multiple factors have been responsible for the failure of the new drugs.

- In contrast to the i.v. short-term trials, patients did not receive ASA and heparin.
- The effect of all agents studied was relatively brief. The omission of even one single dose probably led to insufficient platelet-function inhibition at least for some time.
- A large variation of platelet inhibition in the study population is very likely, because there was no close monitoring of drug effects in individual patients. In contrast to ASA in the control population, a relevant number of patients did not receive adequate protection.
- The wide variation of platelet-function inhibition depending on bioavailability, differences in platelet counts, fibrinogen content, and receptor density on the platelet surface may have further influenced the treatment effects.
- In addition, it has been suggested that a rebound phenomenon may occur in some underdosed patients, leading to increased platelet activation, thereby fully counteracting the desired drug effects.

Some of these problems will have to be solved in the near future. A therapeutic platelet-function inhibition probably has to be established throughout the dosing interval.

Monitoring of the Effects of Glycoprotein IIb/IIIa Inhibitors

The extent of platelet-function inhibition necessary for a therapeutic effect of these agents has never been clearly defined. Future new clinical trials with i.v., subcutaneous, or oral agents or with drug combinations may lead to better efficacy and improve safety if patients are monitored. There is no agreement on the methods to be used and on the intensity of platelet-function inhibition. None of the available methods is sufficiently standardized.

A bedside test should be able to measure platelet function and possibly also coagulation. A therapeutic window must be defined between no response and overdosing. The standard dose of GpIIb/IIIa antagonist may not be ideal for the individual patient. More valid data on the effect of monitoring on clinical results and its clinical relevance can be expected from future clinical trials.

The only test that seems to be relatively robust at the moment is the rapid platelet-function analyzer (RPFA) from Accumetrics (Ultegra Systems, Accumetrics, San Diego, CA, U.S.A.) (107–109). RPFA is perhaps too sensitive, and inhibition greater than 95% might be a dangerous range. The test probably is specific for GpIIb/IIIa inhibitors, but whether it is influenced by interactions with thienopyridines has not yet been shown. Clinical data on the efficacy and safety should provide further information. Other functional platelet parameters show a high variability, which in part is due to preanalytic factors (platelet activation) and technical variations of the procedure. An important factor is the anticoagulant used for blood sampling (110). Conventional methods like (turbidimetric) light-transmittance aggregometry depend on agonist, agonist concentration, and anticoagulation, all of which significantly influence the results. It has been suggested and widely adopted to use ADP as inducer at a 20 μ*M* concentration and to assume that more than 80% inhibition compared with normal or baseline values should be the therapeutic target. However, this has never been validated. Quality assurance, reliability, and standardization of conventional platelet function tests in principle are possible and urgently needed. New clinical trials with oral inhibitors will not do without close monitoring. Among the available tests, conventional aggregation will still be a useful parameter. Collagen-induced aggregation may be more suitable than ADP-induced aggregation if the method can be standardized and if a well-standardized collagen is used. New simple tests have been proposed, but they need further evaluation.

Interactions with Anticoagulants and Other Antiplatelet Agents

Klinckhardt et al. (111) showed that additive enhancement of inhibitory effects of GpIIb/IIIa inhibitors to underlying monotherapy with ASA and clopidogrel was selective for ASA- or clopidogrel-specific effects. However, although clopidogrel alone has no effect on collagen-induced aggregation, the inhibitory effects of a new compound, SR121566A, on collagen-induced aggregation were augmented with clopidogrel. The combination of ASA and clopidogrel clearly enhanced the inhibitory effects on both inducers, and in collagen-induced aggregation with SR121566A, a supraadditive effect was observed. The body of data characterizing the pharmacodynamic interaction between GpIIb/IIIa antagonists and either ASA or ticlopidine is small, and no data have been published for clopidogrel or a combination of clopidogrel and ASA. Umemura et al. (112) determined the inhibitory effects of tirofiban and ticlopidine on platelet aggregation and bleeding time in five healthy male volunteers. Inhibition of ADP-induced platelet aggregation (5 μM final concentration) with tirofiban was enhanced by ticlopidine in an additive manner. However, although ticlopidine had no independent effect on collagen-induced aggregation in that study, tirofiban-induced inhibition also was significantly enhanced by approximately 30%, coinciding with Klinckhardt's observations. No data on platelet secretory parameters have been reported from this study.

ASA and clopidogrel reinforced inhibitory effects of GpIIb/IIIa antagonists on collagen- and ADP-induced aggregation. It might be speculated to what extent comedication with one or both platelet-aggregation inhibitors might contribute to the clinical efficacy of GpIIb/IIIa inhibitors. However, more clinical data would be needed to substantiate the perspectives of a combination of long-term GpIIb/IIIa inhibition by oral agents with clopidogrel.

Although heparin seems to be a pivotal component of the antithrombotic regimen with GpIIb/IIIa inhibitors, it also contributes to the risk profile of this therapy [i.e., bleeding and thrombocytopenia (113)]. Klinkhardt et al. (111) demonstrated that UFH seems to attenuate platelet aggregation and fibrinogen binding, whereas application of the LMWH reviparin did not affect the pharmacodynamic profile of the GpIIb/IIIa antagonists abciximab and tirofiban. A possible (seen from a pharmacodynamic viewpoint) advantage of the LMWH is reflected by a comparable or even better outcome in clinical studies, as suggested by first reports.

Platelet-function Inhibitors in the Prevention of Venous Thromboses and Pulmonary Embolism

ASA has been used for the prophylaxis of postoperative deep vein thrombosis and pulmonary embolism even before low-dose heparin prophylaxis was generally used. Several small studies were published between 1974 and 1980 (114–119). In many of these early trials, high ASA doses between 1,000 and 1,500 mg/day were used.

A meta-analysis of the Antiplatelet Trialists' Collaboration Group (120) included 53 trials and came to the conclusion that platelet-function inhibitors should be considered alone or combined with heparin for the prophylaxis of deep vein thrombosis or pulmonary embolism. This conclusion has been frequently repeated. It was hypothesized that ASA could replace heparins as a cheap and effective form of thrombosis prophylaxis. This, however, is not acceptable. The high ASA doses used in the early trials may have led to better results than the presently advocated 100 to 300 mg/day. Many of the early trials did not fulfill present criteria for clinical trials, and larger well-planned studies such as those of the British Medical Research Council (121) did not show an effect of ASA on postoperative thrombosis.

A very large study on 13,356 patients with hip fracture and on 4,088 patients with elective arthroplasty (PEP Study) (122) was recently published. Patients received 160 mg ASA daily or placebo. Treatment started preoperatively and lasted for 35 days. Any other thromboprophylaxis was allowed. There was a significant reduction of pulmonary embolism of 43% and of symptomatic deep vein thrombosis of 29%. The observed incidence of pulmonary embolism or deep vein thrombosis was extraordinary low, with 1.6% in the ASA group and 2.5% in the placebo group. Because symptomatic pulmonary embolus or thrombosis was the end point in this study, it seems doubtful that the data of this large study are representative.

The therapeutic effect of unfractionated heparins seems to be much greater than that found in the Antiplatelet Trialists' meta-analysis. However, ASA probably has a mild antithrombotic effect in the prevention of postoperative thrombosis and could be used if no heparin is available. In this indication, ASA is less effective than present day LMWH prophylaxis and therefore cannot be regarded as a method of choice.

REFERENCES

1. Otto JC, Smith WL. Prostaglandin endoperoxide synthases 1 and 2. *J Lipid Med* 1995;12:139–156.
2. Kessels H, Beguin S, Nandree H, et al. Measurement of thrombin generation in whole blood: the effect of heparin and aspirin. *Thromb Haemost* 1994;72:78–83.
3. Barnett HJM, Kaste M, Meldrum H, et al. Aspirin dose in stroke prevention: beautiful hypotheses slain by ugly facts. *Stroke* 1996;27:588–592.
4. Mori TA, Vandongen T, Douglas AJ, et al. Differential effect of aspirin on platelet aggregation in IDDM. *Diabetes* 1992;41: 261–266.
5. Rimarachin JA, Jacobson JA, Szabo P, et al. Regulation of cyclooxygenase-2 expression in aortic smooth muscle cells. *Arterioscler Thromb* 1994;14:1021–1031.
6. FitzGerald GA, Healy C, Daugherty J. Thromboxane A_2 biosynthesis in human disease. *Fed Proc* 1987;46:154–158.
7. Savi P, Nurden P, Nurden AT, et al. Clopidogrel: a review of its mechanism of action. *Platelets* 1998;9:251–255.
8. Schrör K. Clinical pharmacology of the adenosine diphosphate (ADP) receptor antagonist, clopidogrel. *Vasc Med* 1998;3: 247–251.
9. Weber A-A, Schrör K. Thienopyridine (ticlopidine, clopidogrel). *Hämostaseologie* 1998;18:180–191.
10. Best LC, McGuire MB, Jones PBB, et al. Mode of action of

dipyridamole on human platelets. *Thromb Res* 1979;16: 367–379.
11. Hirose H, Mashiko S, Kimura T, et al. Antithrombotic activity of NSP-513, a novel selective phosphodiesterase 3 inhibitor, on femoral arterial thrombosis induced by physical stenosis and electrical current: comparison of antithrombotic and hemodynamic effects. *J Cardiovasc Pharmacol* 2000;35:586–594.
12. Mallikaarjun S, Forbes WP, Bramer SL. Interaction potential and tolerability of the coadministration of cilostazol and aspirin. *Clin Pharmacokinet* 1999;37(suppl.2):87–93.
13. Burke S, Lefer AM, Smith GM, et al. Prevention of extension of ischemic damage following acute myocardial ischemia by dazoxiben, a new thromboxane synthetase inhibitor. *Br J Clin Pharmacol* 1983;15(suppl 1):97–101.
14. Fitzgerald GA, Reilly IA, Pedersen AK. The biochemical pharmacology of thromboxane synthase inhibition in man. *Circulation* 1985;72:1194–1201.
15. Verstraete M. Thromboxane synthase inhibition, thromboxane/endoperoxide receptor blockade and molecules with the dual property. *Drugs Today* 1993;29:221–232.
16. French SB, Prasad R, Leese P, et al. Pharmacodynamics substituted 1,3-dioxane (ICI 192,605), a novel thromboxane A_2 receptor antagonist. *Clin Pharmacol Ther* 1991;49:141.
17. Lardy C, Rousselot C, Chavernac G, et al. Antiaggregant and antivasospastic properties of the new thromboxane A_2 antagonist sodium 4-[[1-[[[(4-chlorophenyl)sulfonyl]amino]methyl]-cyclopentyl]methyl]benzene acetate. *Arzneimittelforshung Drug Res* 1994;44:1196–1202.
18. Patscheke H, Staiger C, Neugebauer G, et al. Inhibition of platelet activation in man by the selective thromboxane receptor antagonist "BM 13 177" (sulotroban). In: Schrör K, ed. *Prostaglandins and other eicosanoids in the cardiovascular system. Proc 2nd Int Symp Nörnberg, Fürth,* Basal: Karger, 1995:504–508.
19. Vargaftig BB, Chignard M, Lecouedic JP, et al. One, two, three or more pathways for platelet aggregation. *Acta Med Scand* 1980;642:23–29.
20. Bertele V, Cerletti G, Schieppati A, et al. Inhibition of thromboxane synthetase does not necessarily prevent platelet aggregation. *Lancet* 1981;1:1057–1058.
21. Fellier H, Kühberger E, Stimmeder D, et al. HN-11 500, a novel antithrombotic agent: effects in various in vitro models. *8th international conference on prostaglandins and related compounds,* Montreal. Abstract Book 1992:18, abstr. no. 62.
22. Schenk JF, Radziwon P, Fellier H, et al. Antiplatelet and anticoagulant effects of HN-11 500, a selective thromboxane receptor antagonist. *Thromb Res* 2001;103:79–91.
23. Giedrojc J, Fellier H, Breddin HK. Individual and combined effects of a thromboxane receptor antagonist and different antithrombotic agents in a rat microcirculatory thrombosis model. *Haemostasis* 1992;22:322–329.
24. Schenk J, Breddin HK. PGE_1 bei perkutaner transluminaler Angioplastie: Pathophysiologische und klinische Aspekte. *Perfusion* 1994;12:442–448.
25. Giedrojc J, Breddin HK. Effects of combination of a prostacyclin analogue (cicaprost) with different antithrombotic agents in a rat microcirculatory thrombosis model. *Int J Microcirc Clin Exp* 1992;11:277–286.
26. Coller BS. Platelet GPIIb/IIIa antagonists: the first anti-integrin receptor therapeutics. *J Clin Invest* 1997;100(suppl 11): S57–S60.
27. Harder S, Kirchmaier CM, Krzywanek HJ, et al. Pharmacokinetics and pharmacodynamic effects of a new antibody glycoprotein IIb/IIIa inhibitor (YM337) in healthy subjects. *Circulation* 1999;100:1175–1181.
28. Klinkhardt U, Kirchmaier CM, Westrup D, et al. Ex vivo/In vivo interaction between ASA, clopidogrel and GP IIb/IIIa inhibitors. *Hämostaseologie* 1999;19:112–114.
29. Tsao PW, Forsythe MS, Mousa SA. Dissociation between the antiaggregatory and antisecretory effects of platelet integrin alpha IIb beta 3 (GPIIb/IIIa) antagonist, c7E3 and DMP 728. *Thromb Res* 1997;88:137–146.
30. Klinckhardt U, Kirchmaier CM, Westrup D, et al. Differential in vitro effects of the platelet glycoprotein IIb/IIIa inhibitors abciximab or SR121566 on platelet aggregation, fibrinogen binding and platelet secretory parameters. *Thromb Res* 2000; 97:201–207.
31. Breddin HK. *Die Thrombozytenfunktion bei hämorrhagischen Diathesen, Thrombosen und Gefässkrankheiten.* Stuttgart: Schattauer, 1968.
32. Scharrer I, Schepping M, Breddin K. Thromboseprophylaxe mit Aspirin? *Klin Wochenschr* 1969;47:1318–1324.
33. Fitzgerald DE, Butterfield WJH. A case of increased platelet anti-heparin factor in a patient with Raynaud's phenomena and gangrene treated by aspirin. *Angiology* 1969;20:317–324.
34. Vreeken J, van Aken WG. Spontaneous aggregation of blood platelets as a cause of idiopathic thrombosis and recurrent painful toes and fingers. *Lancet* 1971;2:1394–1397.
35. Biermer R, Boneu B, Guiraud B, et al. Aspirin and recurrent painful toes and fingers in thrombocythemia. *Lancet* 1972;1: 432.
36. Preston FE, Emmanuel IG, Winfield DA, et al. Essential thrombocythaemia and peripheral gangrene. *BMJ* 1974;3: 548–552.
37. Ehresmann U, Alemany D, Loew D. Prophylaxe von Rezidivverschlüssen nach Revaskularisationseingriffen mit Acetylsalizylsäure. *Med Welt* 1977;28:1157–1162.
38. Zekert F, Kohn P, Vormittag E. Eine randomisierte Studie über die postoperative Thromboseprophylaxe mit Acetylsalizylsäure. *Med Welt* 1976;30:1372–1373.
39. Bollinger A, Schneider E, Pouliadis G, et al. Thrombozytenfunktionshemmer und Antikoagulantien nach gefässrekonstruktiven Eingriffen im femoro-poplitealen Bereich: resultate einer prospektiven Studie. In: Breddin HK, ed. *Thrombose und Atherogenese, Risikofaktoren bei gefässchirurgischen Eingriffen Beckenthrombose.* Baden-Baden: Witstrock, 1981:276–279.
40. Brunner U, Bollinger A, Schneider E, et al. Endarteriektomie und autologer Venenbypass: Rezidivprophylaxe mit Aggregationshemmern und Antikoagulantien. In: Wagener O, Kubina VK, eds. *Der Rezidivverschluss nach Gefässrekonstruktionen an der unteren Extremität.* Wien: Egermann, 1979:99–107.
41. Green RM, Roedersheimer RL, de Weese JA. Effects of aspirin and dipyridamole on expanded polytetrafluorethylene graft patency *Surgery* 1982;92:1016–1026.
42. Raithel D, Kaprzak P, Noppeney T. Rezidivprophylaxe nach femoropoplitealer Rekonstruktion mit PTFE-Prothesen. *Med Welt* 1986;37:644–650.
43. Clyne GAC, Archer TJ, Atuhaire LK, et al. Randomized controlled trial of a short course of aspirin and dipyridamole (Persantin) for femoral grafts. *Br J Surg* 1987;74:246–248.
44. Edmonson RA, Cohen AT, Das SK, et al. Low molecular weight heparin versus aspirin and dipyridamole after femoropopliteal bypass grafting. *Lancet* 1994;344:914–918.
45. Zeitler E, Reichold J, Schoop W, et al. Acetylsalizylsäure auf das Frühergebnis nach perkutaner Rekanalisation arterieller Obliterationen nach Dotter. *Dtsch Med Wochenschr* 1973;98: 1285–1288.
46. Hess H, Müller-Fassbender H, Ingrisch H, et al. Wiederverschlüssen nach Rekanalisation obliterierter Arterien mit der Kathetermethode. *Dtsch Med Wochenschr* 1978;103: 1994–1997.

47. Staiger J, Mathias K, Friederich M, et al. Perkutane Katheterkanalisation (Dotter-Technik) bei peripherer arterieller Verschlusskrankheit. *HerzKreisl* 1980;9:383–386.
48. Heiss HW, Just H, Middleton D, et al. Reocclusion prophylaxis with dipyridamole combined with acetylsalicylic acid following PTA. *Angiology* 1990;41:263–269.
49. Ranke C, Creutzig A, Luska G, et al. Controlled trial of high versus low dose aspirin treatment after percutaneous transluminal angioplasty in patients with peripheral vascular disease. *Clin Invest* 1994;72:673–680.
50. Weichert W, Meentz H, Abt K, et al. Acetylsalicylic acid reocclusion prophylaxis after angioplasty (ARPA Study). *Vasa* 1994; 23:57–65.
51. Minar E, Ahmadi A, Koppensteiner R, et al. Comparison of effects of high dose and low dose aspirin on restenosis after femoropopliteal percutaneous transluminal angioplasty. *Circulation* 1995;91:2167–2173.
52. Linke H. Langzeitprophylaxe mit ASS (Colfarit) bei arteriellen Angiopathien, insbesondere bei der Angiopathia diabetica. In: Marx R, Breddin HK, eds. *Colfarit Symposium III.* Köln: Bayer, 1975:88–103.
53. Hess H, Keil-Kuri E. Theoretische Grundlagen der Prophylaxe obliterierender Arteriopathien mit Aggregationshemmern und Ergebnisse einer Langzeitstudie mit ASS (Colfarit). In: Marx R, Breddin HK, eds. *Colfarit Symposium III.* Köln: Bayer, 1975: 80–87.
54. Schoop W. Prognose und Prophylaxe der peripheren arteriellen Verschlusskrankheit. In: Trübestein C, ed. *Arterielle Verschlusskrankheit und tiefe Bein-Beckenvenenthrombose.* Stuttgart: Thieme, 1984:172–176.
55. Hess H, Mietaschk A, Deichsel G. Drug induced inhibition of platelet function delays progression of peripheral occlusive arterial disease. *Lancet* 1985;1:415–419.
56. Goldhaber SZ, Manson JE, Stampfer MJ, et al. Low dose aspirin and subsequent peripheral arterial surgery in the Physicians Health Study. *Lancet* 1992;340:143–145.
57. Newman AB, Siscovick DS, Manolio TA, et al. Ankle-arm index as a marker of atherosclerosis in the cardiovascular health study. *Circulation* 1993;88:837–845.
58. Ogren M, Jungquist G, Hedblad B, et al. Non-invasively detected carotid stenosis and ischemic heart disease in men with leg arteriosclerosis. *Lancet* 1993;342:1138–1141.
59. Antiplatelet Trialists' Collaboration. Collaborative overview of randomised trials of antiplatelet therapy, II: maintenance of vascular graft or arterial patency by antiplatelet therapy. *BMJ* 1994; 308:159–168.
60. Dyken ML, Barnett JHM, Easton D, et al. Low-dose aspirin and stroke: "it ain't necessarily so." *Stroke* 1992;23:1395–1399.
61. Fields WS, Lemak NA, Frankowski RF, et al. Controlled trial of aspirin in cerebral ischemia. *Stroke* 1977;8:301–316.
62. CAST (Chinese Acute Stroke Trial) Collaborative Group. Randomised placebo-controlled trial of early aspirin use in 20,000 patients with acute ischaemic stroke. *Lancet* 1997;349: 1641–1649.
63. International Stroke Trial Collaborative Group. The International Stroke Trial (IST): a randomised trial of aspirin, subcutaneous heparin, both, or neither among 19435 patients with acute ischaemic stroke. *Lancet* 1997;349:1569–1581.
64. Diener HC, Cunha L, Forbes C, et al. European Stroke Prevention Study 2: dipyridamole and acetylsalicylic acid in the secondary prevention of stroke. *J Neuol Sci* 1996;143:1–13.
65. Craven LL. Acetylsalicylic acid, possible prevention of coronary thrombosis. *Ann West Med Surg* 1950;4:95–96.
66. Steering Committee of the Physicians' Health Study Research Group. Final report on the aspirin component of the ongoing Physicians' Health Study. *N Engl J Med* 1989;321:129–135.
67. Peto R, Gray R, Collings R, et al. Randomized trial of prophylactic daily aspirin in British male doctors. *BMJ* 1988;296: 313–316.
68. Elwood PC, Cochrane AL, Burr ML, et al. A randomized controlled trial of acetylsalicylic acid in the secondary prevention of mortality from myocardial infarction. *BMJ* 1974;268:436–440.
69. Breddin HK, Loew D, Lechner K, et al. The German-Austrian Aspirin Trial: a comparison of acetylsalicylic acid, placebo and phenprocoumon in secondary prevention of myocardial infarction. *Circulation* 1980;62(suppl V):V63–V72.
70. ISIS-2 (Second International Study of Infarct Survival) Collaborative Study Group. Randomized trial of intravenous streptokinase, oral aspirin, both, or neither among 17,187 cases of suspected acute myocardial infarction: ISIS-2. *Lancet* 1988;II: 349–360.
71. Baignent C, Collins F (for the ISIS Collaborative Group, Oxford). ISIS-2: 4-year mortality follow-up of 17,187 patients after fibrinolytic and antiplatelet therapy in suspected acute myocardial infarction. *Circulation* 1993;88:I291.
72. Antiplatelet Trialists' Collaboration. Collaborative overview of randomized trials of antiplatelet therapy, I: prevention of death, myocardial infarction and stroke by prolonged antiplatelet therapy in various categories of patients. *BMJ* 1994;308:81–106.
73. Lewis HD, Davis JW, Archibald DG, et al. Protective effects of aspirin against acute myocardial infarction and death in men with unstable angina: results of a Veterans Administration Cooperative Study. *N Engl J Med* 1983;309:396–403.
74. Cairns JA, Gent M, Singer J, et al. Aspirin, sulfinpyrazone, or both in unstable angina: results of a Canadian multicenter trial. *N Engl J Med* 1985;313:1369–1375.
75. Théroux P, Quimet H, McCans J, et al. Aspirin heparin or both to treat acute unstable angina. *N Engl J Med* 1988;319: 1105–1111.
76. The RISC Group. Risk of myocardial infarction and death during treatment with low dose aspirin and intravenous heparin in men with unstable coronary artery disease. *Lancet* 1990;336: 827–830.
77. Manson JE, Grobbee DE, Stampfer MJ, et al. Aspirin in the primary prevention of angina pectoris in a randomized trails of United States physicians. *Am J Med* 1990;89:772–776.
78. Juul-Möller S, Edvardsson N, Jahnmatz B, et al. [Swedish Angina Pectoris Aspirin Trial Group (SAPAT) group]. Double-blind trial of aspirin in primary prevention of myocardial infarction in patients with stable chronic angina pectoris. *Lancet* 1992;340:1421–1425.
79. Stiegler H, Hess H, Mietaschk A, et al. Von Ticlopidin auf die periphere obliterierende Arteriopathie. *Dtsch Med Wochenschr* 1984;109:1240–1243.
80. Ellis DJ. Treatment of intermittent claudication with ticlopidine. Abstr. 32nd, Meeting of the International Committee on Thrombosis and Haemostasis and the 9th Congress of the Mediterranean League against Thromboembolic Diseases, Jerusalem, June 1–6, 1986.
81. Arcan JC, Blanchard J, Boissel JP, et al. Multicenter double blind study of ticlopidine in the treatment of intermittent claudication and the prevention of its complications. *Angiology* 1988;39:802–811.
82. Balsano F, Coccheri S, Libretti A, et al. Ticlopidine in the treatment of intermittent claudication, a 21 month double blind trial. *J Lab Clin Med* 1989;114:84–91.
83. Cloarec M, Arcan JC, Caillard PH, et al. Double blind clinical trial of ticlopidine versus placebo in peripheral atherosclerotic disease of the legs. *Angiologie* 1988;5(suppl 77):14–20.

84. Boissel JP, Peyrieux JC, Destors JM. Is it possible to reduce the risk of cardiovascular events in subjects suffering from intermittent claudication of the lower limbs? *Thromb Haemost* 1989;62: 681–685.
85. Janzon L, Bergqvist D, Boberg J, et al. Prevention of myocardial infarction and stroke in patients with intermittent claudication; effects of ticlopidine: results from STIMS, Swedish Ticlopidine Multicentre Study. *J Intern Med* 1990;227:301–308.
86. Bergqvist D, Almgren B, Dickinson JP. Reduction of requirement for leg vascular surgery during long term treatment of claudicant patients with ticlopidine: results of Swedish Ticlopidine Multicenter Study (STIMS). *Eur J Vasc Endovasc Surg* 1995;10:69–76.
87. Gent M, Blakely JA, Easton JD, et al. The Canadian American Ticlopidine Study (CATS) in thromboembolic stroke. *Lancet* 1989;I:1215–1220.
88. Hass WK, Easton JD, Adams HP Jr, et al. A randomized trial comparing ticlopidine hydrochloride with aspirin for the prevention of stroke in high-risk patients. *N Engl J Med* 1989;321: 501–507.
89. CAPRIE Steering Committee. A randomised, blinded, trial of clopidogrel versus aspirin in patients at risk of ichaemic events (CAPRIE). *Lancet* 1996;348:1329–1339.
90. Colombo A, Hall P, Nakamura S, et al. Intracoronary stenting without anticoagulation accomplished with intravascular ultrasound guidance. *Circulation* 1995;91:1677–1688.
91. Garcia-Cantu E, Spaulding C, Corcos T, et al. Stent implantation in acute myocardial infarction. *Am J Cardiol* 1996;77: 451–454.
92. Serruys PW, Emanuelsson H, van der Giessen W, et al. Heparin coated Palmaz-Schatz stents in human coronary arteries: early outcome of the Benestent II pilot study. *Circulation* 1996;93: 412–422.
93. Thebault JJ, Blatrix CE, Blanchard JF, et al. The interactions of ticlopidine and aspirin in normal subjects. *J Intern Med Res* 1977;5:405–411.
94. Dawson DL, Cutler BS, Hiatt WR, et al. A comparison of cilostazol and pentoxifylline for treating intermittent claudication. *Am J Med* 2000;109:523–530.
95. EPIC investigators. Use of a monoclonal antibody directed against the platelet glycoprotein IIb/IIIa receptor in high risk coronary angioplasty. *N Engl J Med* 1994;330:956–961.
96. EPILOG investigators. Platelet glycoprotein IIb/IIIa receptor blockade and low dose heparin during percutaneous coronary revascularization. *N Engl J Med* 1997;36:1689–1696.
97. CAPTURE investigators. Randomised placebo-controlled trial of abciximab before and during coronary intervention in refractory unstable angina: the CAPTURE study. *Lancet* 1997;349: 1429–1435.
98. RESTORE investigators. Effects of platelet glycoprotein IIb/IIIa blockade with tirofiban on adverse cardiac events in patients with unstable angina or acute myocardial infarction undergoing coronary angioplasty. *Circulation* 1997;96: 1445–1453.
99. Platelet Receptor Inhibition in Ischemic Syndrome Management (PRISM) study investigators. A comparison of aspirin plus tirofiban with aspirin plus heparin for unstable angina. *N Engl J Med* 1998;338:498–505.
100. Platelet Receptor Inhibition in Ischemic Syndrome Management in Patients Limited by Unstable Signs and Symptoms (PRISM+PLUS) investigators. Inhibition of the platelet glycoprotein IIb/IIIa receptor with tirofiban in unstable angina and non-Q-wave myocardial infarction. *N Engl J Med* 1998;338: 1488–1497.
101. IMPACT II investigators. Randomized placebo-controlled trial of effect of eptifibatide on complications of percutaneous coronary intervention IMPACT II. *Lancet* 1997;349:1422–1428.
102. PURSUIT trial investigators. Inhibition of platelet glycoprotein IIb/IIIa with eptifibatide in patients with acute coronary syndromes. *N Engl J Med* 1998;339:436–443.
103. PARAGON investigators. International, randomized, controlled trial of lamifiban (a platelet glycoprotein IIb/IIIa inhibitor), heparin, or both in unstable angina: Platelet IIb/IIIa Antagonism for Reduction of Acute coronary syndrome events in a Global Organization Network. *Circulation* 1998;97:2386–2395.
104. Holmes MB, Sebel BE, Cannon CP, et al. Increased platelet reactivity in patients given orbofiban after acute coronary syndrome: an OPUS-TIMI 16 substudy: orbofiban in patients with unstable coronary syndromes: thrombolysis myocardial infarction. *Am J Cardiol* 2000;85:491–493.
105. SYMPHONY investigators. Comparison of sibrafiban with aspirin for prevention of cardiovascular events after acute coronary syndromes: a randomized trial: the SYMPHONY investigators: Sibrafiban versus aspirin to Yield Maximum Protection from ischemic events post-acute coronary syndromes. *Lancet* 2000;355:337–345.
106. O'Neill WW, Serruys P, Knudtson M, et al. Long term treatment with glycoprotein-receptor antagonist after percutaneous coronary revascularization: EXCITE trial investigators: evaluation of oral xemilofiban in controlling thrombotic events. *N Engl J Med* 2000;342:1316–1324.
107. Smith JW, Steinhubl SR, Lincoff AM, et al. Rapid platelet function assay: an automated and quantitative cartridge-based method. *Circulation* 1999;99:620–625.
108. Storey RF, May JA, Wilcox RG, et al. Whole blood assay of inhibition of platelet aggregation by glycoprotein IIb/IIIa antagonists: comparison with other aggregation methodologies. *Thromb Haemost* 1999;82:1307–1311.
109. Steinhubl SR, Kottke-Marchant K, Moliterno DJ, et al. Attainment and maintenance of platelet inhibition through standard dosing of abciximab in diabetic and nondiabetic patients undergoing percutaneous coronary intervention. *Circulation* 1999; 100:1977–1982.
110. Storey RF, Wilcox RG, Heptinstall S. Differential effects of glycoprotein IIb/IIIa antagonists on platelet microaggregate and macroaggregate formation and effect of anticoagulant on antagonist potency. *Circulation* 1998;98:1616–1621.
111. Klinckhardt U, Breddin HK, Esslinger et al. Interaction between the LMWH reviparin and aspirin in healthy volunteers. *Clin Pharmacol* 2000;49:337–341.
112. Umemura K, Kondo K, Nakashima N. Enhancement by ticlopidine of the inhibitory effect on in vitro platelet aggregation of the glycoprotein IIb/IIIa inhibitor tirofiban. *Thromb Haemost* 1997;76:1381–1384.
113. Aguirre FV, Topol EJ, Ferguson JJ, et al. Bleeding complications with the chimeric antibody to platelet glycoprotein IIb/IIIa integrin in patients undergoing percutaneous coronary intervention. *Circulation* 1995;91:2882–2890.
114. Zekert F. Prophylaxe von Phlebothrombosen und Lungenembolien mit Aggregationshemmern. In: Zekert F, ed. *Thrombosen, Embolien Aggregationshemmer Chirurgie.* Stuttgart: Schattauer, 1975:75–88.
115. Clagett GP, Schneider P, Rosoff CB, et al. The influence of aspirin on postoperative platelet kinetics and venous thrombosis. *Surgery* 1975;77:61–74.
116. Zekert F. Prophylaxis of postoperative thromboembolism with acetylsalicylic acid and dihydroergotamine. In: Balas P, ed. *Angiology: new developments.* New York: Plenum, 1980:1173–1176.
117. Harjola P, Meurala H, Frick MH. Prevention of deep venous thrombosis and thrombo-embolism by dipyridamole and

acetylsalicylic acid after reconstructive arterial surgery. *J Cardiovasc Surg* 1980;21:451–454.
118. Morris GK, Mitchell JR. Preventing venous thromboembolism in elderly patients with hip fractures: studies of low-dose heparin, dipyridamole, aspirin and flurbiprofen. *BMJ* 1977;I:535–537.
119. Harris WH, Salzman EW, Athanasoulis CA, et al. Aspirin prophylaxis of venous thromboembolism after total hip replacement. *N Engl J Med* 1977;297:1246–1249.
120. Antiplatelet Trialists' Collaboration. Collaborative overview of randomised trials of antiplatelet therapy, III: reduction in venous thrombosis and pulmonary embolism by antiplatelet prophylaxis among surgical and medical patients. *BMJ* 1994; 308:235–246.
121. Medical Research Council. Effect of aspirin on postoperative venous thrombosis. *Lancet* 1972;II:441–444.
122. Anonymous. Prevention of pulmonary embolism and deep vein thrombosis with low dose aspirin: pulmonary embolism prevention (PEP) trial. *Lancet* 2000;355:1295–1302.

Disorders of Thrombosis and Hemostasis: Clinical and Laboratory Practice, Third Edition, edited by Rodger L. Bick.
Lippincott Williams & Wilkins, Philadelphia © 2002

19

THROMBOLYTIC THERAPY

WILLIAM F. BAKER, JR.

Since the first trial was published in 1959 (1), thrombolytic therapy has evolved to become an important therapeutic option for patients with arterial and venous thrombosis. A variety of thrombolytic agents are available; however, all are plasminogen activators. The primary mechanism of action is to convert plasminogen to plasmin. Plasmin then cleaves fibrinogen and fibrin into fibrin degradation products. The ideal thrombolytic agent would cause complete clot dissolution without triggering systemic fibrinogenolysis.

Thrombolytic agents play a very specific role in the treatment of thrombosis and are used in conjunction with other agents to enhance and sustain clinical efficacy in achieving and sustaining vascular patency (2). The majority of acute myocardial infarctions (AMIs) result from acute coronary artery thrombosis at the site of an atherosclerotic plaque. Thrombolytic therapy is among the first-line strategies for patients with AMI. Acute cerebrovascular thrombosis has become another important application of thrombolysis. Clinical studies are further defining the role of these agents and their proper use. The indications for thrombolysis for venous thromboembolic (VTE) disease are less clear. Both systemic and catheter-directed approaches have been used with variable success.

This chapter provides an overview of the role of thrombolytic agents in treatment of thrombosed vessels and clearly separates these agents as a class from the antithrombotic agents and antiplatelet agents. Following this is a discussion of the specific mechanism of action and pharmacology of each of the currently available agents. In view of the large number of clinical trials seeking to define the optimal strategy for use of thrombolysis in arterial and venous thrombosis, the final section focuses on specific disease entities and the application of thrombolytic therapy to each, with reference to the recent literature.

W. F. Baker, Jr.: Department of Medicine, Center for Health Sciences, University of California at Los Angeles, Los Angeles, California; Department of Medicine, Kern Medical Center, Bakersfield, California; and California Clinical Thrombosis Center, Bakersfield, California.

OVERVIEW OF THE ROLE OF THROMBOLYTIC AGENTS

The primary goal of thrombolytic therapy is the rapid recanalization of the thrombosed artery or vein. All thrombolytic agents activate plasminogen to plasmin, which then acts to degrade fibrin clots, fibrinogen, and other plasma proteins including factors V, VIII, IX, XI, and XII, components of complement, growth hormone, adrenocorticotropic hormone, and insulin (3,4). Plasmin is inactivated by a number of plasmin inhibitors, including the rapidly acting and potent α_2-antiplasmin, and the slow acting α_2-macroglobulin (5,6). The commonly used thrombolytic agents have included urokinase (UK), streptokinase (SK), alteplase [recombinant tissue plasminogen activator (rt-PA)] and anistreplase [anisoylated streptokinase activator complex (APSAC)]. Newer agents include reteplase (r-PA), tenecteplase (TNKt-PA), saruplase (scu-PA), lanoteplase (n-PA), and staphylokinase (STAR) (7–9). The mechanism of action of fibrinolytic agents in relation to the intrinsic pathways of thrombosis and fibrinolysis is depicted in Fig. 19.1. The goal is to induce local pathologic clot dissolution without inducing systemic fibrinogenolysis or disrupting physiologic thrombi necessary for normal hemostatic balance. Laboratory abnormalities induced by the infusion of the plasminogen activators are markers for thrombosis and for the extent of systemic fibrinogenolysis (Table 19.1).

Thrombolytic agents act uniquely to activate the intrinsic fibrinolytic system. This is in clear contrast to the indirect-acting (heparin) and direct-acting (hirudin) antithrombin agents, which inhibit the action of thrombin to activate fibrinogen to fibrin. Antiplatelet agents act by a variety of mechanisms to inhibit platelet adhesion, aggregation, activation, or binding to thrombin [glycoprotein (Gp)IIb/IIIa agents] but have no direct activity on the fibrinolytic system. Both antithrombin agents and antiplatelet agents, however, are used in conjunction with thrombolytic agents to sustain vascular patency.

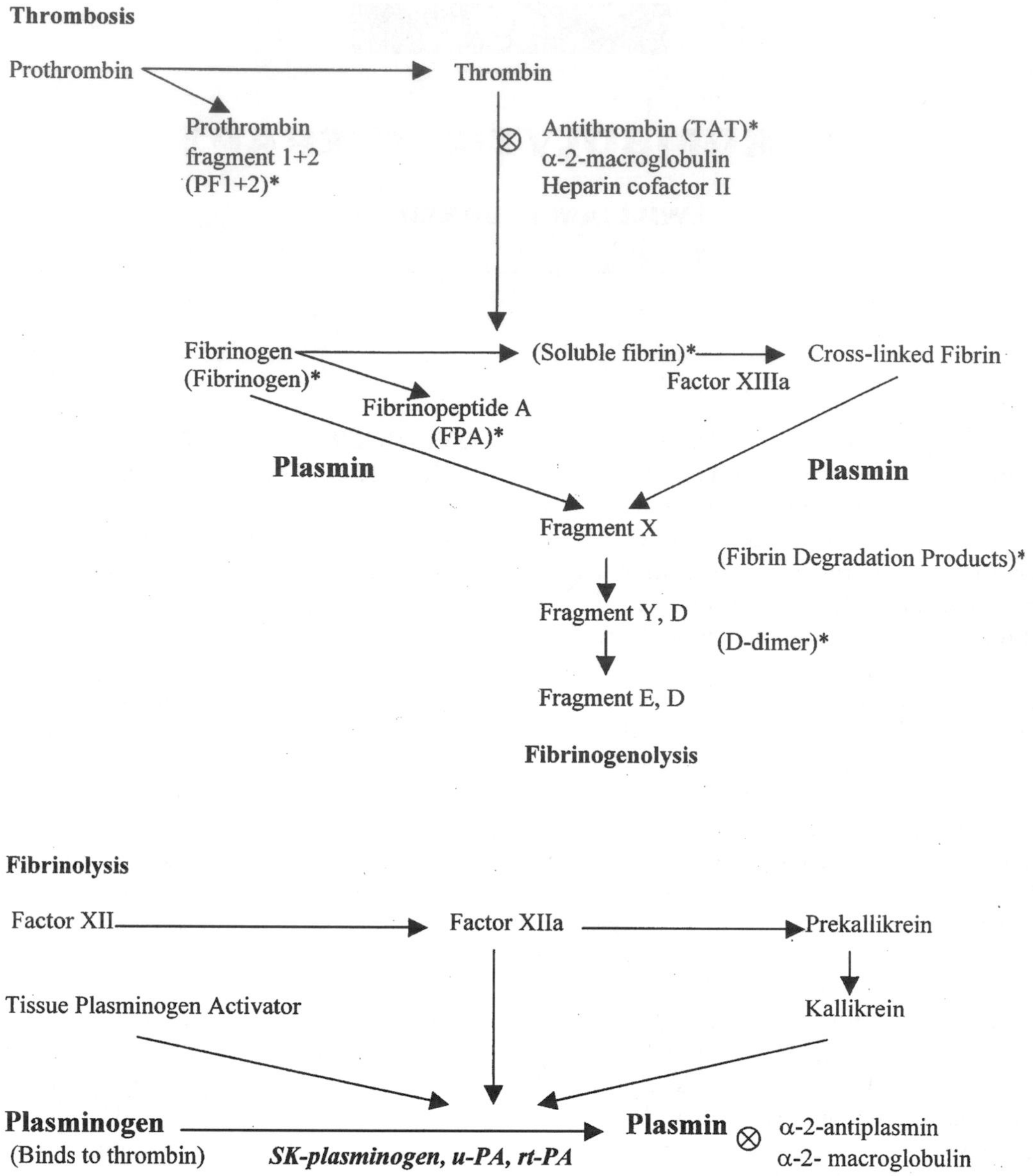

FIGURE 19.1. Pathways of thrombosis and fibrinolysis. The *circled X* represents inhibitors. Therapeutic thrombolytic agents include streptokinase (*SK*), *u-PA*, and recombinant tissue-type plasminogen activator (*rt-PA*). *Asterisks* represent laboratory markers. (Adapted from Bick RL. Physiology of hemostasis. In: *Disorders of thrombosis and hemostasis*. Chicago: ASCP Press, 1992:1–26.)

TABLE 19.1. LABORATORY MARKERS OF THROMBOSIS, THROMBOLYSIS, AND FIBRINOGENOLYSIS

Marker	Level	Etiology	Manifestations
Fibrinogen	Decreased	Circulating plasmin	Thrombolysis/hemorrhage
D-dimer	Elevated	Plasmin cleavage of fibrin	Thrombolysis
Fibrin degradation products (FDPs)	Elevated	Plasmin cleavage of fibrinogen and fibrin	Thrombolysis
Template bleeding time	Prolonged	Platelet dysfunction due to FDPs	Hemorrhage
Thrombin–antithrombin	Elevated	Circulating thrombin inactivated by antithrombin	Thrombosis
Prothrombin F 1 + 2	Elevated	Prothrombin conversion to thrombin	Thrombosis
Soluble fibrin	Elevated	Formation of fibrin aggregates	Thrombosis
Fibrinopeptide A	Elevated	Cleaved from fibrinogen by thrombin	Thrombosis

Thrombus Characteristics

Thrombus characteristics are an important determinant of the effectiveness of thrombolytic therapy (10). The susceptibility of the thrombus to thrombolysis is influenced by a number of factors: (a) thrombus size, (b) the surface area of thrombus exposed to the surrounding blood, (c) the extent of fibrin cross-linking, (d) thrombus age and extent of invasion with collagen and fibroblasts, (e) thrombus location, and (f) local blood-flow rates (10). Pulmonary vascular thrombi present for longer than 7 days have been demonstrated to be relatively resistant to thrombolysis (11). Areas of slow blood flow are more resistant to thrombolysis, as may be thrombi in side-branch arteries adjacent to larger widely patent arteries because of the Bernoulli effect (10). Thrombi with a surface area at least 50% in contact with flowing blood are more likely to respond to thrombolytic agents than are thrombi in areas with little surface contact to flowing blood. Only a single end of an obstructive thrombus is exposed to flowing blood and thus available to the direct action of circulating plasmin. Once surface lysis is initiated, the improvement of intraluminal blood flow exposes an increasing surface area of the thrombus to the thrombolytic agent, and lysis is accelerated and may be sustained (10).

STRUCTURE, FUNCTION, AND PHARMACOLOGY OF THROMBOLYTIC AGENTS

Streptokinase

SK is a bacterial enzyme first discovered in 1933, isolated from the broth of Lancefield group C β-hemolytic streptococci. In vivo fibrinolytic activity in humans was first reported in 1959 (12). The single-chain protein contains 414 amino acid residues and has a molecular size of 47.0 to 50.2 kDa (13). There are three structurally autonomous folded domains (14) and a fourth less structured carboxy-terminal tail (15). The active regions are linked by a flexible protein chain and may be found in partially folded states (16,17). The region Ser60–Asn90 is responsible for human plasminogen activation, and the sequence Val58–Arg219, together with Tyr252–Ala316 is required for the conversion of plasminogen to plasmin in the plasminogen–SK complex (18).

The equimolar complex of SK and plasminogen forms a complex that induces a conformational change in the plasminogen moiety exposing an active site (19). The active site of the SK–plasminogen complex catalyzes the conversion of plasminogen to plasmin (20) and of the SK–plasminogen complex to the SK–plasmin complex through an intramolecular peptide bond cleavage (21). Progressive degradation into smaller fragments culminates in the loss of activity. SK activity increases in the presence of fibrinogen, fibrin, and the fibrin degradation products, fragments D and E (22). Fibrinogen increases the rate of formation of the SK–plasminogen complex active sites (23) and stimulates plasminogen activity (24).

SK activates both circulating and fibrin-bound plasminogen. Fibrin binding of the SK–plasmin complex occurs through the five kringle regions of the plasmin moiety and localizes to areas of fibrin deposition (20). The SK–plasmin complex is not inhibited by α_2-antiplasmin, as is the SK–plasminogen complex, thus facilitating the activation of clot-bound plasminogen (25). With the degradation of fibrin, locally bound SK plasmin and SK plasminogen are stimulated, accelerating the process of clot lysis. The degradation of both SK complexes reduces plasminogen-activator activity. Circulating SK complexes convert plasminogen to plasmin, resulting in systemic plasminemia, fibrinogen degradation, and prothrombinase-mediated activation of thrombin (26). In addition to direct effects on fibrinolytic pathways, SK indirectly induces a defect in platelet aggregation. Newly generated fibrin degradation products compete with already depleted levels of fibrinogen for the platelet GpIIb/IIIa receptor (27).

Although the initial half-life of SK is a mere 10 to 20 minutes (28), prolonged effects due to slow hepatic clearance, the persistence of fibrin(ogen) degradation products, depletion of fibrinogen and other procoagulant factors, and prolonged SK plasminogen-activator activity result in a terminal SK half-life of 83 minutes (1) and a biologic half-life as long as 3 hours (29). Measurable laboratory changes with both SK and urokinase therapy include decreased fibrinogen, plasminogen, α_2-antiplasmin, clotting factors V, VIII:c, IX, XI, XII, prolonged activated partial thromboplastin time (aPTT), prolonged prothrombin time (PT), elevated plasmin levels, elevated fibrin(ogen) degradation products, and elevated B-β 15-42–related peptides (30,31).

Because SK is a bacterial product, it is antigenic and may induce an allergic reaction accompanied by hypotension, rash, and fever in as many as 13% of patients (32). The administration of diphenhydramine hydrochloride and intravenous glucocorticoid is effective for allergic reactions; they are usually administered prophylactically. Anti-SK antibodies [immunoglobulin G (IgG)] are generated after administration of SK and may persist for up to 54 months. The result is decreased SK activity if it is readministered. Other consequences of SK immunogenicity may include a serum sickness–type syndrome (33) and bronchospasm (34).

Anistreplase

Anisoylated, lys-plasminogen-streptokinase activator complex (APSAC, or anistreplase) is a complex of human plasminogen and SK, in which the active site of plasminogen has been acylated, rendering the plasminogen inert to activation or inhibition by circulating plasma proteins (35). The result is a longer half-life (92 minutes) but basically the same plasminogen-activating effect as SK (36,37). After administration, deacylation occurs, resulting in activation of plasminogen for several hours.

The noncovalently bound SK and lys-plasminogen complex has a molecular mass of 131 kDa. The catalytically active center is protected by the *p*-anisoyl group, covalently bound to Ser740. Production of the compound is facilitated by the inverse acylating agent *p*-amidinophenyl-*p*′-anisate-HCL (APAN). APAN is reacted with the SK–plasminogen complex (38). In contrast, the SK–plasmin complex does not undergo multiacylation (37). Because the chemical alteration of the SK–plasminogen complex does not affect the kringle region, the fibrin-binding properties are maintained (36). The active center is protected from the inactivating action of α_2-antiplasmin and α_2-macroglobulin (39).

The net effect of anisoylation is rapid, effective, and sustained thrombolytic effect, while avoiding the acute hypotension seen with SK (40). APSAC has powerful fibrin-binding activity (41), is more potent as a lytic agent than SK, but has greater plasma stability (37) and longer circulation time (39). APSAC is not, however, fibrin specific, may induce systemic proteolysis, and is equally as antigenic as SK. APSAC does result in less depletion of fibrinogen (characteristic of systemic fibrinogenolysis) than SK–plasmin or urokinase but more than alteplase (41).

The rate of deacylation is rapid, following first-order kinetics. Slower hepatic clearance and less inactivation by plasma inhibitors underlie the prolonged half-life compared with SK (39). The antigenicity of APSAC, generating anti-SK antibodies, explains the decrease in effectiveness observed with repeated doses for up to 54 months (42). The rate of allergic reactions is lower than that with SK. These include rash, bronchospasm, and erythema (43).

Urokinase

In contradistinction to tissue-type plasminogen activators (t-PA), derived from tissue and vascular cells, urokinase is derived from kidney cells and urine (urokinase-type plasminogen activators, u-PA) (44). Urokinase is a serine protease consisting of two polypeptide chains of 20 and 34 kDa, respectively, linked by a single disulfide bond. The process of synthesis involves isolation of a single-chain precursor from urine (45), plasma (46), and cell culture (47). The 411 amino acid single-chain urokinase-type PA (scu-PA) with a molecular mass of 54 kDa is converted to the high-molecular-weight (HMW) two-chain u-PA (tcu-PA). This conversion results from limited hydrolysis of the Lys158–Ile159 peptide bond by plasmin and kallikrein (47). The peptide contains an amino-terminal and a carboxy-terminal end with a catalytically active center of Asp255, His204, and Ser356 (48). The chains are linked by a Cys279 disulfide bond, and scu-PA includes an additional 12 disulfide bonds dispersed throughout the protein. Hydrolysis of the Glu143–Leu144 bond cleaves the amino-terminal 143 amino acids and results in a low-molecular-weight (LMW) scu-PA. This product is up to 5 times less active than scu-PA in a fibrin clot assay and is less sensitive to activation by plasmin. The additional cleavage of HMW tcu-PA at Lys135-Lys136 results in a 33-kDa peptide, which is the commercially available urokinase in the United States (19). Distinct regions of urokinase include the amino-terminal receptor binding; epidermal growth factor–like domain; the central, kringle region; and the carboxy-terminal, catalytic, serine protease domain (48). The kringle domain consists of two helices, one of which is unique, and the other resembles the t-PA kringle 2. Other features include a binding site for anionic polysaccharides like heparin and structural characteristics similar to those of other serine proteases such as t-PA, factor XII, and complement factor (19,49).

Activation of plasminogen by several forms of u-PA has been studied, and the kinetic parameters of the enzymatic reactions have been determined (50). When scu-PA and plasminogen are combined, plasmin and HMW tcu-PA are generated. Aprotinin and other plasmin inhibitors block the production of HMW tcu-PA. Plasmin is, however, generated from plasminogen. Study of the enzymatic properties of scu-PA indicates that it functions primarily as a proenzyme (19). When scu-PA is exposed to thrombus, plasminogen and clot lysis occurs with the additional result of generation of HMW tcu-PA. Such plasminogen activation requires the presence of fibrin, despite the lack of direct fibrin–scu-PA binding (51). It appears that fibrin mediates the plasminogen activation by scu-PA, as limited plasmin digestion of fibrin results in exposure of the carboxy-terminal binding site of fibrin. Glu-plasminogen binds to the exposed carboxy-terminal sites, inducing a conformational change, which provides a favorable substrate for scu-PA. The process of plasminogen activation to plasmin proceeds and is amplified by the generation of HMW tcu-PA and additional carboxy-terminal lysine residues (52). Cell-surface localization of scu-PA appears to play an important role in the mechanism of action. Several cell types, including endothelial cells, possess a urokinase-type plasminogen activator receptor (u-PAR) (53). The presence of receptor-bound scu-PA and cell-bound plasminogen is required for enhanced generation of plasmin (54). The surface of the endothelial cell serves as a template for assembly of scu-PA/tcu-PA and plasminogen–plasmin. This proximation of all necessary components promotes plasmin generation and fibrinolysis (19).

The serine protease inhibitors, plasminogen activator inhibitor type-1 (PAI-1), plasminogen activator inhibitor type-2 (PAI-2), and protease nexin-1 (PN) modulate both circulating and receptor-bound urokinase. Bound complexes are internalized and degraded through α_2-macroglobulin/low-density lipoprotein receptor–associated protein (α_2-MR/LRP) (55,56). Fibrin, fibrinogen, fibrin degradation products, as well as long-chain fatty acids and lysine analogues such as ω-aminocarboxylic acids accelerate the plasminogen activation by HMW tcu-PA from twofold to 10-fold (19,52,57). Heparin stimulates the enzymatic activity of both scu-PA and tcu-PA, but to a greater degree for scu-PA (58). The inhibitory effect of PAI-1 toward tcu-PA also is accentuated by heparin and heparan sulfate (59). Primary clearance of urokinase is through hepatic metabolism, and the half-life is a feature of the protein itself rather than dependent on inactivation by inhibitors (60).

Clinical application of u-PA has included the use of HMW tcu-PA, LMW tcu-PA, and a recombinant, full-length, nonglycosylated scu-PA, saruplase (61). Urokinase is no longer available in the United States because of manufacturer production problems.

Saruplase

The scu-PA demonstrates little intrinsic enzymatic activity. Specificity for fibrin is high, as the amino acid sequence is very similar to that of t-PA. The half-life is short, as the scu-PA circulates bound to a specific inhibitor. Fibrinolytic activity appears when the scu-PA inhibitor complex dissociates in the presence of fibrin.

Tissue-type Plasminogen Activator

The t-PA was first purified from uterine tissue and subsequently determined to be found in the same form in other tissues, including the vascular endothelium (62,63). Recombinant t-PA (rt-PA) was first produced from a melanoma cell extract (64) and subsequently from *Escherichia coli* (65).

t-PA is a single-chain serine protease consisting of 527 amino acids at a molecular mass of 68 kDa (65). A free cysteine residue is present at position 83, and there are 17 other disulfide bonds (66). Hydrolysis of the Arg275–Ile276 bond, catalyzed by plasmin, kallikrein factor, Xa, and other serine proteases, produces a two-chain t-PA consisting of a heavy chain of amino acids 1–275 and a light chain of 275–527 (19). The kringle regions are included in the heavy chain, and the serine protease activity, in the light chain. Five domains are designated based on homology with other functional proteins including fibronectin (finger domain), epidermal growth factor (residues 50–87), plasminogen kringle regions (K1 and K2 kringle regions, residues 87–176 and 176–262, respectively), serine protease trypsin (residues 276–527), and the catalytic center of the serine protease domain (His322, Asp371, and Ser478) (19). Further study of the structure and functional characteristics of the various domains indicate that the insertion loop Lys296–Arg304 plays an important role in specificity for fibrin and binding of PAI-1 (19). Of additional importance is the formation of a bridge between Lys429 and Asp477, which appears to play a role in the high catalytic activity of single-chain t-PA, providing stability to the catalytically active protease domain without unmasking the Ile276 amino terminus (67).

The enzymatic activity of t-PA has been found to follow Michaelis–Menten kinetics. A range of kinetic values has been reported, apparently due to differences in the activity of single-chain versus double-chain t-PA. In the presence of fibrin, however, these differences are minimal (68). t-PA binds specifically and with high affinity to intact fibrin. Although t-PA binds to the carboxy terminal lysine residues of degraded fibrin, it does so less efficiently than endogenous plasminogen, which competes for these binding sites.

On binding to fibrin, the catalytic efficiency of plasminogen activation by fibrin is promptly increased. Exclusive to single-chain t-PA, a ternary complex is formed involving fibrin, t-PA, and plasminogen. Structural and kinetic studies further demonstrate that in spite of the homology between the protease domain and trypsin, t-PA specifically recognizes one or more structural features of native plasminogen (69). As described by Bauer et al. (70), t-PA–mediated fibrinolysis involves a three-step process. On the addition of t-PA, protofibrils are formed, with an average length about 10 times that of fibrinogen. The length of this phase increases as the concentration of t-PA increases. A second phase follows, in which there is sudden elongation and lateral aggregation of the fibrin fibers. This phase is especially pronounced with low concentrations of t-PA and is accompanied by the formation of fragment X. Disorganization of the fibers follows in the third phase, and fragments Y and D are formed. Plasmin then internally degrades the fibers, resulting in the formation of long, loose bundles subsequently disintegrated into thin filaments. At high t-PA concentrations, the maximal rate of plasmin generation occurs before the onset of the second phase, whereas at low concentrations, the peak plasmin generation follows. Overall, the rate of plasmin formation is equivalent across all concentrations of t-PA.

Other clinically relevant observations regarding the activity of t-PA include lipid-induced modification of plasminogen activation and PAI-1 modulation of t-PA amidolytic activity. As with platelets (71,72), monocytes (73), and endothelial cells (74), cell-associated t-PA appears to be more efficacious than free t-PA. It also has been noted that apo(a), which is homologous with plasminogen, binds with lysine many sites available for plasminogen on the surface of fibrin, interfering with thrombolysis (75). PAI-1 recognizes two binding sites on fibrin and, as it accumulates in the thrombus, inhibits t-PA–mediated plasmin generation (76). PAI-1 also binds directly to t-PA, inhibiting the F and K2 domains from binding fibrin (77).

When administered by intravenous injection to humans, single-chain t-PA has a plasma volume distribution of 3.5 to 5.4 L, and the double-chain form, a distribution of 3.8 to 6.6 L. The single-chain form has an initial half-life of 3.6 to 4.6 minutes and a terminal half-life of 39 to 53 minutes. Double-chain t-PA has an initial half-life of 4.1 to 6.3 minutes and a terminal half-life of 41 to 50 minutes (78). Intravenous bolus administration of single-chain t-PA may achieve as much as a 45% higher steady-state plasma concentration than slower methods of infusion, without affecting the plasma half-life (79). In the hope of increasing the terminal half-life without reducing efficacy, a variety of methods of infusion have been evaluated, and novel forms of t-PA have been produced.

Hepatic clearance of single-chain t-PA occurs at a rate of 520 to 1,000 mL/min, and of double-chain t-PA, 450 to 640 mL/min (80). Clearance may be delayed, based on levels of PAI-1 present, as the formation of t-PA/PAI-1 complexes is cleared at a slower rate than active t-PA (81). Recombinant t-PA (alteplase) is not antigenic; thus the reactions seen with SK and UK are generally absent. Anaphylaxis has been observed, characterized by the presence of IgE antibodies to alteplase (82).

Variants Of Tissue Plasminogen Activator

In addition to the original, commercially available compound single-chain alteplase (rt-PA), other variants of t-PA have been produced in an attempt to prolong the half-life and/or to increase efficacy, while reducing the degree of systemic fibrinogenolysis. These include the two-chain t-PA duteplase (83); the deletion mutant reteplase (84); the deletion mutant n-PA, lanoteplase (85); and TNKt-PA, tenectoplase (86,87) with several amino acid substitutions. All of these variants of t-PA exhibit the same mode of action as t-PA, converting plasminogen to plasmin.

Duteplase

Duteplase is a double-chain form of t-PA. Although it appears to possess biologic effects similar to those of single-chain t-PA, large studies did not demonstrate superiority over SK, and production of the compound was halted (88).

Reteplase

Reteplase (r-PA) is a single-chain t-PA mutant in which the finger, epidermal growth factor, and kringle-1 domains have been deleted, leaving the kringle-2 and serine protease domains (84). The half-life is doubled compared with that of t-PA, permitting effective double-bolus therapy of 10 U, 30 minutes apart. Systemic depletion of fibrinogen is less than that of SK but greater than that of t-PA. The absence of the finger domain decreases the affinity of r-PA for fibrin, compared with t-PA (89,90). Whereas t-PA and other mutants exhibit hepatic clearance, r-PA is cleared primarily by the kidney (88).

Tenectoplase

TNKt-PA (tenectoplase) differs from wild-type t-PA only in amino acid substitutions of threonine 103 with asparagine, asparagine 117 with glutamine in the kringle-1 domain, and a tetra-alanine substitution at positions 296 to 299 in the protease domain (91). Compared with t-PA, TNKt-PA demonstrates greater fibrin specificity, a prolonged half-life, and relative resistance to PAI-1 (87,92). The TIMI 10A trial demonstrated a plasma half-life from 11 to 20 minutes, compared with 3.5 minutes for t-PA (93). Systemic fibrinogenolysis was less, as measured by less decrease in fibrinogen and plasminogen levels (5% to 15% with TNKt-Pa compared with 40% to 50% with t-PA) (94). There also was 4 to 5 times less consumption of α_2-antiplasmin and lower levels of plasmin–α_2-antiplasmin complexes than seen with t-PA. The enhanced fibrin specificity of TNKt-PA, compared with alteplase, underlies the efficacy when given as a single bolus (9).

Lanoteplase

Lanoteplase, the deletion mutant n-PA, substitutes glycine for asparagine at position 117, removing the glycosylation site in the first kringle domain (85). The finger domain and epidermal growth factor domains are deleted. The result is a very long half-life (30 to 45 minutes), permitting single-bolus administration. Lacking the finger domain, it has less affinity for fibrin than does t-PA. The InTIME trial demonstrated comparable efficacy and superior combined TIMI grade 2 and 3 flow at 90 minutes with n-PA compared with t-PA (85). The structural characteristics of thrombolytic agents are outlined in Table 19.2.

Staphylokinase

Staphylokinase is isolated from *Staphylococcus* sp. as a 15.5-kDa protein consisting of two folded domains of similar size with a dumbbell shape (95,96). Staphylokinase forms a 1:1 stoichiometric complex with plasminogen, is converted to plasmin, and then activates other plasminogen molecules to plasmin as well. A Met26 residue is involved, the loss of which eliminates fibrinolytic activity (97). In experimental systems, staphylokinase is highly effective at clot lysis, without significantly reducing fibrinogen, plasminogen, or α_2-antiplasmin levels. By comparison, SK yields much less clot lysis with substantial decreases in fibrinogen, plasminogen, and α_2-antiplasmin levels, and t-PA yields effective clot lysis at low doses, but at higher doses, significantly depletes plasminogen, which results in diminution of local fibrinolysis (98). Recombinant staphylokinase (STAR) has been compared with rt-PA in patients with AMI. At doses of 10 or 20 mg intravenously over 30 minutes for STAR and weight-based dose for rt-PA, TIMI grade 3 flow (normal antegrade flow) at 90 minutes was achieved in 62% of STAR patients and in 58% of rt-PA patients. Fibrinogen levels

TABLE 19.2. STRUCTURAL CHARACTERISTICS OF THROMBOLYTIC AGENTS

Agent	Molecular Mass (kDa)	Structure	Mutation
Streptokinase	47–50.2	414 amino acids 4 folded domains	Native
Urokinase	54	411 amino acids 3 domains: EGF, K, P	Native
Anistreplase	131 (SK-PGN)	SK-PGN + *p*-anisoyl	Native SK
rt-PA	68	527 amino acids 5 domains: F, EGF, K1 + K2, P, C	Native
r-PA	39.6	355 amino acids Absent F, EGF, K1; K2, P preserved	Single-chain deletion
TNKt PA	65	527 amino acids T103N, N117Q, KHRR 296-299AAAA	Point substitutions
n-PA	—	N117G substitution; absent F, EGF, domains; K1 + K2, P preserved	Point substitutions, domain deletions

EGF, epidermal growth-factor domain; F, finger domain; K, kringle domain; P, serine protease domain; C, catalytic center; PGN, plasminogen.
Data from Leopold J, Keaney J, Loscalzo, J. Pharmacology of thrombolytic agents. In: Schafer JL, ed. *Thrombosis hemorrhage.* Vol 1. Baltimore: Williams & Wilkins, 1998:1215–1258; and Ohman EM, Harrington RACPC, Agnelli G, et al. Intravenous thrombolysis in acute myocardial infarction. *Chest* 2001;119:253s–277s.

decreased significantly by rt-PA but not by STAR. In spite of the known antigenicity of staphylokinase, no allergic reactions were observed in this study. There also were no cases of STAR-related hemorrhage (99). STAR also has been used intraarterially for acute peripheral arterial occlusion (100). A mutant form of staphylokinase has been produced in attempt to reduce the immunogenic potential. Fibrin specificity and potency are retained with less antigenicity (101).

Chimeric Agents

A variety of chimeric agents have been produced in an attempt to enhance efficacy as therapeutic thrombolytic agents. The objective has been to increase potency, increase fibrin specificity, and reduce systemic fibrinogenolysis. These have included products of u-PA (102); splicing of fragments of u-PA to t-PA (t-PA/u-PA) (103); t-PA–based proteins combining the amino terminal portion of t-PA and serine protease region of scu-PA (104); and a variety of other proteins using component domains of t-PA and u-PA. As the result of experiments with a variety of chimeric derivatives, it has become clear that there is not a correlation between specific thrombolytic activity (percentage of clot lysis per unit concentration of circulating plasminogen activator) and thrombolytic potency (percentage of lysis per unit dose per kilogram of body weight). Thus it is not possible to extrapolate molecular properties to clinical effect. Even though the functional domains mediating plasminogen activation are present, the difficulty in producing three-dimensional compounds with the correct primary sequence has been repeatedly demonstrated (19).

CLINICAL THERAPEUTICS

Procoagulant Effect

Although it is clear that thrombolytic agents promote thrombolysis through the activation of the plasminogen–plasmin system, it also has been observed that a procoagulant effect may result (105–107). This is of particular importance in patients with acute myocardial infarction (AMI), in whom reocclusion remains a major challenge. Analysis of molecular markers of coagulation indicates that patients with AMI present in a hypercoagulable state with elevations of PAI-1, t-PA mass concentration, fibrinogen, factor XII, thrombin–antithrombin complexes (TATs), kallikrein, plasmin, and D-dimer (105). In a comparison of SK, rt-PA, and untreated AMI patients, SK was found to exert a greater procoagulant effect, as measured by relative increases in thrombin activation (increase in TAT complexes), a more prolonged increase in kallikrein activity, higher levels of D-dimer, and greater reductions in fibrinogen, with persistent elevations after 48 hours (105).

In addition to activation of the contact phase of coagulation, the intrinsic coagulation pathways, and the intrinsic fibrinolytic system, platelet activation plays a major role in coronary arterial thrombosis (108–113). Coronary thrombi are platelet rich, and both platelet activation and aggregation are accentuated after therapeutic thrombolysis (114–116). Antiplatelet therapy with aspirin and GpIIb/IIIa–receptor blocking agents has proven to be of substantial value in sustaining patency and now plays an important adjunctive role to thrombolytic agents (109–113,116–119). Evaluation of platelet aggregation and receptor expression by flow cytometry in AMI patients after therapy with reteplase and alteplase reveals potentially

TABLE 19.3. THE "IDEAL" THROMBOLYTIC AGENT

Characteristics	Clinical Advantages
Rapid thrombolysis	Prompt restoration of arterial or venous blood flow
Fibrin specificity	Targets areas of acute thrombus with reduced systemic fibrinolysis
Sustained duration of action	Maintains patency; no early reocclusion
Thrombus specific	Avoids effects on fibrinogen, other coagulation proteins, yet does not impair primary hemostasis
Low risk of hemorrhage	Reduced risk of cerebral and other sites of occult hemorrhage; compatible with immediate acute interventional procedures
Absence of systemic side effects	Nonantigenic, avoids systemic fibrinolysis
Low cost	Availability across a wide economic spectrum

important differences between the two agents (120). At 24 hours, aggregation was enhanced more after reteplase than after alteplase (120). In a similar pattern, platelet-receptor expression (GpIIb/IIIa, very late antigen-2, platelet/endothelial cell adhesion molecule-1) also was increased (120). Both reteplase and alteplase exhibited decreased receptor expression at 3 to 6 hours, followed by progressive increase at 12 and 24 hours (120). Comparison of platelet aggregation with measures of thrombin generation (TAT complexes) and endogenous fibrinolysis (PAI-1) indicated that platelet aggregation is the primary determinant of risk for both early and late reocclusion (121). Clearly, antiplatelet therapy plays an important adjunctive role during thrombolytic therapy, and this may be even more important at 24 hours than early on. Some differences may exist between thrombolytic agents in the time course and degree of enhancement of platelet activity, but all exhibit measurable increases in platelet aggregation (119–121).

The "Ideal" Thrombolytic Agent

Advances in experimental evaluation, pharmaceutical development, and clinical application have made it abundantly clear that the "ideal" thrombolytic agent has yet to be developed. The properties of the ideal agent are outlined in Table 19.3. These properties include (a) rapid and effective thrombolysis without rethrombosis; (b) lack of activation or depletion of coagulation proteins, of platelets, or activation of the intrinsic fibrinolytic system; (c) absence of systemic toxicity; and (d) specificity for pathologically thrombosed vessels, sparing physiologic hemostatic plugs. Utility must be demonstrated across a range of therapeutic indications from acute coronary and cerebral thrombosis to venous thrombosis and pulmonary embolism (PE) in patients with significant comorbidities and at low cost. A comparison of the commercially available agents is presented in Table 19.4. The "ideal" has yet to emerge. Ongoing laboratory evaluation and clinical trials will more clearly delineate the superiority of the available newer agents compared with others and point to superior agents and approaches to management. It now appears that a variety of adjunctive therapies are required to achieve all of the goals of an ideal thrombolytic. Adjunctive therapies to the presently available thrombolytics are summarized in Table 19.5. Sustaining patency in the face of incomplete thrombolysis and/or postthrombolytic hypercoagulability is the major role for adjunctive agents.

Myocardial Infarction

Since Herrick's description of AMI in 1912 (122), it has become recognized that nearly 90% of patients with AMI have acute coronary thrombosis (123). Numerous studies demonstrated the clinical efficacy of thrombolytic agents in opening the thrombosed coronary artery (124–133). Reperfusion success is measured primarily against the standard set by the Thrombolytics in Myocardial Infarction trial, which designated occlusion as TIMI grade 0 to 1 flow, and patency as TIMI grade 2 to 3 flow (grade 3 as normal

TABLE 19.4. COMPARISON OF THROMBOLYTIC AGENTS IN ACUTE MYOCARDIAL INFARCTION

Agent	Clot Lysis	Fibrin Specific	Half-life	IC Bleed	Cost
Streptokinase	44%–85%	No	~23 min	.5%	Low
Anistreplase	60%–72%	>SK < rt-PA	~2 h	.6%	Low
Alteplase	60%–88%	>Urokinase	~4 min	.9%	High
Reteplase	63%–85%	=Alteplase	~58 min	.8%	High
Tenectoplase	54%–88%	>Alteplase	~20 min	.9%	High

Clot lysis reflects TIMI grade 2 or 3 flow. Percentages from half-life and intracranial bleed are approximations from a number of studies.
IC, intracranial; rt-PA, recombinant tissue plasminogen activator; SK, streptokinase; TIMI, thrombolysis in myocardial infarction.
References: Streptokinase (131,151,274); Anistreplase (146,148,275); Alteplase (86,148,151); Reteplase (86,90,276); Tenectoplase (8,9,94).

TABLE 19.5. ADJUNCTIVE THERAPY TO THROMBOLYTIC AGENTS

Agent	Mechanism of Action
Antithrombin agents	
Heparin	Antithrombin activation to inhibit anti-Xa and factor II
Low-molecular-weight heparin	Antithrombin activation to inhibit anti-Xa
Hirudin (log)	Direct antithrombin inhibition
Argatroban	Direct antithrombin inhibition
PPACK	Direct antithrombin inhibition
Antiplatelet agents	
Aspirin	Cyclooxygenase inhibitor
Dipyridamole	Phosphodiesterase inhibition
Ticlopidine	Blocks exposure of platelet GPIIb/IIIa
Clopidogrel	Inhibits ADP-mediated activation of platelet GPIIb/IIIa
Abciximab	Antagonist to platelet GPIIb/IIIa
Tirofiban	Antagonist to platelet GPIIb/IIIa
Eptifibatide	Antagonist to platelet GPIIb/IIIa

GP, glycoprotein; ADP, adenosine diphosphate.

antegrade flow) (125). Consistent reductions in mortality have been demonstrated; however, failure to restore normal antegrade flow occurs in 45%, and the mortality rate with thrombolytic therapy remains at 7% to 10% (119). The earlier therapy is instituted after symptom onset, the greater the potential for a reduction in time-dependent myocardial injury (134). Early intervention also correlates with an increase in survival benefit. The avoidance of ischemic injury preserves myocardial function and improves electrical stability (135).

The major factors in distinguishing the various thrombolytic agents have been the early (90 minute) and late success at achieving reperfusion, the rate of reocclusion, mortality, and the risk of hemorrhage. Studies have varied primarily in the choice of thrombolytic agent, the dose regimen, and the use of adjunctive agents to sustain patency.

Clinical Trials in Acute Myocardial Infarction

Streptokinase

Although published studies of SK use in the setting of AMI appeared as early as 1959 (1), dose-ranging trials were not carried out until the 1980s (136). Angiographic trials that assessed patency and recanalization demonstrated an overall patency rate of 44% at 60 minutes and 48% at 90 minutes. Pooled meta-analyses indicated a patency rate of 72% at approximately 2 to 3 hours after therapy onset and 75% to 85% at 24 to 21 days (137). These rates were substantially higher than those of control patients, similar to the rates with anistreplase, but less than the patency rates achieved with alteplase. Mortality with SK was evaluated in the Gruppo Italiano per lo Studio Steptokinasi nell'Infarto Miocardico (GISSI-1) trial (138), the Intravenous Streptokinase in Acute Myocardial Infarction study (ISAM) (139), and the International Study of Infarct Survival (ISIS)-2 trial (140). Although only 14% of patients received aspirin and 62% received heparin (now well-accepted adjunctive therapies), in-hospital mortality was reduced by 18% compared with standard therapy. Mortality reduction was greatest in those patients treated within 1 hour (47%), and less for those treated within 3 hours (23%) and within 6 hours (17%). Similar to findings of GISSI-2 (138), an 11% reduction in 21-day mortality was found in the ISAM trial (139). The ISIS-2 trial, a large double-blind placebo-controlled trial of SK in AMI, determined a 25% reduction in 35-day mortality for patients randomized to SK, compared with placebo. The synergistic effects of aspirin with SK were clearly demonstrated, producing a 42% reduction in mortality compared with placebo with combination therapy. Confirming the data from other studies, patients who were treated within 6 hours, and even up to 12 hours, experienced the greatest reduction in mortality risk (140). A meta-analysis of SK trials confirmed this consistent in-hospital and late mortality benefit (maintained up to 1 year). Benefit can be expected for patients with symptoms of AMI treated within 12 hours of symptom onset. The attendant risk of cerebral hemorrhage is approximately four per 1,000 patients treated (141).

Alteplase

The first comparative trial between alteplase and SK, Thrombolysis in Myocardial Infarction-1 (TIMI-1), demonstrated a 90-minute reperfusion rate of 62% with alteplase compared with 31% with SK (142). Independent of baseline angiographic findings, the patency rate was 70% for alteplase and 43% for SK (142). Subsequent angiographic trials demonstrated similar superior TIMI grade 3 flow rates (normal antegrade flow) with the 3-hour infusion of alteplase compared with SK and anistreplase (143). Higher rates of reperfusion were subsequently demonstrated with an "accelerated" dosing regimen of alteplase (144). Although it appeared that early reperfusion correlated with lowered mortality, the GISSI-2 (145) and ISIS-3 (146) trials raised doubts concerning this concept. The strong evidence provided by the Global Utilization of Streptokinase and t-PA for Occluded Coronary Arteries-1 (GUSTO-1) trial (124,147) of a relation between early reperfusion and survival suggests that the heparin protocol used in the GISSI-2 and International Study of Infarct Survival-3 (ISIS-3) trials (subcutaneous heparin rather than intravenous heparin) was the primary cause for the disparate results of these studies. In the GUSTO trial, all patients received aspirin but were otherwise randomized to receive either SK (with subcutaneous or intravenous heparin), "accelerated" dose regimen alteplase with intravenous heparin, or combination fibrinolytic therapy. Mortality was significantly reduced in the "accelerated" alteplase arm compared with the other regimens (124). The relative mortality improvement with alteplase over SK (absolute reduction of 1%) was questioned as to its significance. It has been pointed out that this represents one life saved of the seven expected deaths in 100 treated patients (88). Subgroup analysis consistently confirmed the superiority of alteplase. Higher 90-minute patency rates corresponding to increased rates of TIMI grade 3 flow were present in the alteplase patients (124,147). The TIMI 4 trial (148) compared alteplase, anistreplase, and their combination. Aspirin and intravenous heparin were administered to all patients. A 78% 60-minute patency rate was demonstrated with alteplase compared with only 60% with anistreplase or the combination. Similarly higher 90-minute TIMI grade 3 flow was demonstrated with alteplase. Composite end points and 1-year mortality also were better with alteplase.

The alteplase comparative trials have clearly demonstrated not only the superiority of alteplase as a fibrinolytic agent but also the importance of intravenous heparin and aspirin. As the mortality in patients with early reocclusion of an infarct-related artery is at least 3 times higher than if the vessel remains patent, adjunctive agents to maintain patency are clearly critical to early and late mortality. With this understanding, it is not surprising that the GISSI-2 and ISIS-3 trials, lacking effective regimens of aspirin and intravenous heparin, failed to demonstrate the improvement in mortality observed with GUSTO-1 and TIMI-4. Furthermore, the most effective dose regimen for alteplase is the front-loaded or "accelerated" regimen. A trial of a double-bolus regimen was less effective and associated with an increased rate of hemorrhagic stroke (1.12% vs. 0.8%) (149). Cost-effectiveness analysis determined that thrombolysis with alteplase may save the lives of 11 patients for every 1,000 treated at a cost of $32,678 per year of life saved (150).

In the GUSTO-1 trial, intracranial hemorrhage was observed in only 0.5% of SK patients, 0.7% of alteplase patients, and 0.9% of the combination patients (124,147). Subsequent review of studies including a total of 71,073 patients demonstrated an intracranial hemorrhage risk with rt-PA of 0.88% [confirmed by brain computed tomography (CT) or magnetic resonance imaging]. Increased risk for intracranial hemorrhage was associated with older age, female sex, black ethnicity, systolic blood pressure of 140 mm Hg or more, diastolic blood pressure of 100 mm Hg or more, history of stroke, rt-PA dose greater than 1.5 mg/kg, and lower body weight (151).

Reteplase

The initial trial of reteplase (r-PA) examined three dosing regimens and demonstrated a 90-minute TIMI grade 3 flow rate of 63% with reteplase and 49% with alteplase (152,153). Subsequently, the larger Reteplase Angiographic Phase II International Dose-finding (RAPID-2) trial (89) again demonstrated superior patency rates for r-PA compared with alteplase. Combining the two RAPID trials, the 90-minute TIMI grade 3 flow was 61% for r-PA (10 U, followed by a second 10 U, 28 minutes later) and 45% for alteplase. The result was a clear mortality advantage for the r-PA patients (3.1% for r-PA vs. 8.4% for alteplase). Reteplase and SK were compared in the International Joint Efficacy Comparison of Thrombolytics (INJECT) study, and r-PA was found to be at least as effective as SK at reducing mortality (9% for r-PA vs. 9.5% for SK). In the GUSTO-3 study (90), r-PA and rt-PA were compared in an attempt to confirm the apparent mortality benefit with r-PA seen in other studies. In this trial, the superior 90-minute TIMI grade 3 flow of r-PA was not found to correlate with improved mortality over rt-PA. Similarly, the complications of stroke, bleeding, and intracranial hemorrhage also were not significantly different (90). The results of the GUSTO-3 trial support the concept that at least an absolute increase in TIMI grade 3 flow of 20% is required to reduce mortality significantly (88).

Tenectoplase

Tenectoplase (TNKt-PA) was tested in the TIMI-10A (94) and TIMI-10B (9) trials. Use of the 50-mg dose of TNKt-PA was discontinued because of excess bleeding. The 90-minute TIMI grade 3 flow with the 40-mg dose was similar to that with alteplase. The Assessment of the Safety and Efficacy of a New Thrombolytic Agent-1 (ASSENT-1) trial examined weight-based dosing and noted that the TIMI grade 3 flow was 62% to 63% for TNKt-PA doses of 0.5 mg/kg compared with 51% to 54% with lower doses (7).

Evaluation of various subsets, however, indicated that patients who were treated more than 4 hours after symptom onset experienced improved outcomes with TNKt-PA. In considering data from the GUSTO-3 trial comparing r-PA with alteplase, it appears that a more fibrin-specific agent (TNKt-PA > rt-PA > r-PA) may be more efficacious in patients who are seen at greater than 4 hours after the onset of symptoms (90).

Evaluation of the intracranial hemorrhage rate in the ASSENT-1 (7) (no hemorrhages) and TIMI-10B (9) (three hemorrhages in 78 patients) trials indicated that the dose of heparin played a significant role in hemorrhagic risk. Reduction of the heparin dose (body weight more than 67 kg) from a 5,000-U bolus followed by an infusion of 1,000 U/h to a 4,000-U bolus followed by an infusion of 800 U/h reduced the rate of major bleeding and intracranial hemorrhage in patients receiving either alteplase or tenectoplase. As a result, the ASSENT-2 trial used the lower-dose regimen of heparin. In this trial, the mortality rate was essentially the same, and TNKt-PA and alteplase appeared statistically equivalent.

The rate of serious bleeding in the TIMI-10B trials and the ASSENT-1 trials was significantly less with TNKt-PA compared with alteplase (154). In the ASSENT-2 trial, the rate of intracranial hemorrhage was 0.93% for TNKt-PA and 0.94% for alteplase. For the highest-risk subset for intracranial hemorrhage (women older than 75 years and 67 kg or less), the risk was 1.1% for TNKt-PA and 3.0% for alteplase (86,155). It appears that the more fibrin-specific agent TNKt-PA may be associated with a lower risk of hemorrhage.

Saruplase

Saruplase (scu-PA) has been compared in clinical trials to SK and alteplase. An angiographic trial demonstrated equivalency with SK. A higher rate of intracranial hemorrhage was found with scu-PA (0.9%) compared with SK (0.3%) (156,157).

Lanoteplase

Lanoteplase (n-PA) has been compared with alteplase in an angiographic trial, which demonstrated a 90-minute TIMI grade 3 flow of 83% for n-PA and 71% for alteplase (158). Thirty-day mortality was similar, but the rate of intracranial hemorrhage was significantly higher in the patients receiving n-PA (1.13% for n-PA vs. 0.62% for rt-PA) (159).

Staphylokinase

Recombinant staphylokinase (STAR) has been evaluated in two randomized trials. In the first, TIMI grade 3 flow was achieved in 62% compared with 58% of patients with alteplase (99). In the second, the Collaborative Angiographic Patency Trial of Recombinant Staphylokinase (CAPTORS) study (160), a range of doses was tested from 15 to 45 mg. Similar 62% flow rates were achieved with no relation to dose.

Adjunctive Agents

A variety of adjunctive strategies are used in conjunction with thrombolytic agents in the setting of AMI (Table 19.5). The objective is to sustain vascular patency achieved with effective thrombolysis. Characteristic of coronary thrombi is the presence of thrombin, which actively converts fibrinogen to fibrin, induces platelet aggregation, and activates factor XIII, which cross-links and stabilizes the fibrin clot. With the activation of plasminogen and release of plasmin, effective local and systemic fibrinolysis, and fibrinogenolysis, the clot may be lysed; however, activated and aggregated platelets as well as thrombin remain. The residual presence of these key components of obstructive clot underlies the need for adjunctive pharmacologic agents. Those used have included aspirin and the GpIIb/IIIa inhibitors as antiplatelet agents and the indirect antithrombin agent heparin and the direct antithrombin inhibitors hirudin (161), bivalrudin (162), argatroban (163), efegatran (164), and inogatran (165).

Antiplatelet Therapy

The benefit of adding aspirin to thrombolytic therapy has been clearly established since the ISIS-2 trial (166) and is standard therapy for all patients with AMI. The addition of GpIIb/IIIa agents to fibrinolytic agents has been evaluated in a number of trials (117,119,167). Improvement has been demonstrated in electrocardiographic (ECG) evidence of infarction and in angiographic patency. Trials of the full doses used for patients treated with percutaneous coronary angioplasty have suggested an increased bleeding risk (111,117,168,169). Reduced-dose protocols using full-dose abciximab with half-dose reteplase demonstrate improved rates of perfusion compared with thrombolytic therapy without abciximab (167,170).

Antithrombin Therapy

Heparin

Heparin has been the primary antithrombin agent for all indications since it was first discovered by McLean in 1912 (171). The primary action of heparin is indirect, through induction of a conformational change in antithrombin, enhancing its avidity for thrombin. As the primary inhibitor of thrombin, antithrombin effectively modulates the coagulation cascade, preventing thrombin from acting on fibrinogen to produce fibrin. Clot-bound thrombin is, however, not accessible to heparin (172). Heparin is effective, as clot lysis proceeds, in preventing rethrombosis by inhibiting circulating thrombin. Heparin has been demonstrated to be essential to maintain patency in vessels opened by rt-PA, r-PA, TNKt-PA, n-PA, and other similar agents (173,174). The TIMI and Intravenous n-PA for Treatment of Infarcting Myocardium Early (InTIME) trials confirm that lower doses of heparin also correlate with a reduction in the risk for intracranial hemorrhage (175). Current American College of Cardiology/American Heart Association (ACC/AHA) guidelines advise a dose of heparin of 60 U/kg (up to 4,000 U) bolus followed by an infusion of 12 U/kg/h (up to 1,000 U/h) (176). The current recommendations of the American College of Chest Physicians Consensus Conference on Antithrombotic Therapy include either the weight-adjusted protocol as recommended by the ACC/AHA or the standard-dose regimen of 5,000-U bolus followed by an infusion of 1,000 U/h, adjusted to maintain an aPTT of 50 to 70 seconds (88).

Low-molecular-weight heparin (LMWH), clearly demonstrated to be efficacious in unstable angina and non–Q-wave MI, has been evaluated in conjunction with SK thrombolytic therapy in two trials (177). The results demonstrate a reduced risk of left ventricular mural thrombosis formation and possible decreased risk of recurrent MI within 30 days (178).

Direct Antithrombin Agents

The direct-acting antithrombin agents bind to thrombin selectively and, essentially, irreversibly (161). Hirudin binds to thrombin at two sites. The carboxy terminus binds to the thrombin substrate-recognition site responsible for binding to platelets (179) and to fibrinogen (180). The amino terminus binds to the thrombin catalytic site responsible for cleaving fibrinogen to fibrin and fibrinopeptide A (180). Desirudin (recombinant hirudin) in conjunction with thrombolysis was tested in the TIMI-5 (148), TIMI-6 (181), TIMI-9 (182), and GUSTO-2 (183) trials. With hirudin, a more stable aPTT was achieved, and there was no thrombocytopenia. In the TIMI-5 (148) and GUSTO-2B (183) trials, there was a lower rate of reinfarction. The TIMI-9B trial (182) demonstrated a nonsignificant reduction in rate of reinfarction but no difference in the 30-day composite end point of death, MI, severe congestive heart failure, or shock. Lepirudin was evaluated in the Hirudin for the Improvement of Thrombolysis (HIT-3) (184) and HIT-4 (185) trials. In the HIT-3 trial, an excess risk of intracranial hemorrhage was observed. With a reduction in the dose of lepirudin, this risk was not different from that with heparin in the HIT-4 trial. Lepirudin, in conjunction with SK, was not, however, superior to heparin in the rate of TIMI grade 3 flow. Hirulog versus heparin with SK demonstrated a trend to improved TIMI grade 3 flow (162,186). Although they are an intriguing adjunct to thrombolytic agents, it is not yet clear that there are significant advantages with the use of the direct-acting antithrombin agents over heparin.

Cerebrovascular Thrombosis

The application of thrombolytic therapy to patients with acute ischemic stroke is based on the understanding that, as in AMI, the majority of these events (approximately 80%) result from intravascular thrombosis (187,188). The progression from acute cerebral ischemia to irreversible infarction was recognized to be time dependent (189). Early studies were limited by the lack of availability of CT imaging and were abandoned as the result of concern regarding intracranial hemorrhage (190,191). Meta-analysis of the available trials indicated, however, the potential benefit of thrombolysis (192). In 1995, the National Institute of Neurologic Disorders and Stroke Study Group (NINDS) published the first major clinical trial clearly demonstrating the benefit of thrombolytic therapy (rt-PA) in acute ischemic stroke (193). Clinical-outcome measures were standardized by using the National Institutes of Health Stroke Scale (NIHSS) in Part I of the trial and in Part II, the Barthel Index (BI), modified Rankin Scale (mRS), and Glasgow Outcome Scale (GOS) were added. The study protocol included only patients within 3 hours of symptom onset and without evidence of intracerebral hemorrhage on the pretreatment CT brain scan. Initial results indicated efficacy and safety in patients who were seen within 3 hours of symptom onset and without evidence of major acute abnormalities on CT brain scan. In view of the recognized association between uncontrolled hypertension and intracerebral hemorrhage, the blood pressure of all patients was carefully controlled within the range of less than 185 mm Hg systolic and 110 mm Hg diastolic. The dose of rt-PA was 0.9 mg/kg administered 10% as a bolus and the remainder as an infusion over a 1-hour period. Part I results demonstrated no significant difference between patients receiving rt-PA and those with placebo, at 24 hours. Subsequent analysis and 3-month follow-up data indicated benefit from rt-PA in all measurements of outcome. The patients treated with rt-PA were 30% less likely to be disabled than were the placebo-treated patients. The 3-month mortality rate was 17% in the rt-PA group and 21% in the placebo group. All stroke subtypes fared similarly, and the risk of symptomatic cerebral hemorrhage was 6.4% for rt-PA patients and 0.6% for placebo patients. Whereas the risk of hemorrhage was greatest among the patients with cerebral edema, mass effect, and the greatest degree of clinical deficit, the potential for benefit also was greatest. At the 12-month follow-up mark, benefit once again was demonstrated in the treated patients, with a 30% reduction in disability compared with placebo patients.

The European and Australian trials, European Cooperative Acute Stroke Study (ECASS-I) (194), and ECASS-II (195) were of significantly different design and yielded quite different results. In ECASS-I (194), treatment consisted of rt-PA at a dose of 1.1 mg/kg (maximum of 100 mg) versus placebo. The window for treatment was within 6 hours of symptom onset. At 3 months, 41% of the rt-PA–treated patients experienced minimal or no disability, compared with 29% of the placebo patients. Intracerebral hemorrhage was a major problem, seen in 19.8% of treated patients and 6.8% of controls. The ECASS-II trial used dosing of rt-PA similar to that in the NINDS trial (0.9 mg/kg, up to 90 kg), during a 6-hour window. Benefit in 90-day mRS scores could be demonstrated from rt-PA (54.3%) versus placebo (46%). No difference could be demonstrated between rt-PA patients and controls in death rate, but there was a significantly increased rate of intracerebral hemorrhage (8.8% vs. 3.4%). This further pointed to the importance of the 3-hour window between symptom onset and intervention with thrombolysis.

The Alteplase Thrombolysis for Acute Noninterventional Therapy in Ischemic Stroke (ATLANTIS) trial (196,197), originally begun in 1991 and modified several times, was eventually terminated in 1998 because of lack of demonstrable benefit between rt-PA and placebo patients (excellent recovery in 32% of placebo and 34% of rt-PA patients) and an excess of intracerebral hemorrhage (7.0% in rt-PA patients and 1.1% in placebo). All three SK trials (198–200) also were terminated early because of an increase in early mortality and intracranial hemorrhage.

Intraarterial administration of recombinant pro-urokinase (rpro-UK) has been evaluated in the Pro-urokinase for Acute Cerebral Thrombosis (PROACT) (201) and PROACT-II (202) trials. The original PROACT trial (201) used rpro-UK infusion directly into the thrombosed artery via supraselective catheter. Intravenous heparin infusion was concomitantly administered in all patients. Outcomes and mortality at 90 days favored the rpro-UK–treated patients but did not reach statistical significance. Hemorrhagic transformation occurred in 15.4% of treated rpro-UK and 7.1% of placebo patients. The PROACT-II trial compared intraarterial rpro-UK (9 mg) with heparin versus heparin alone (heparin, 2,000-U bolus, and 500 U/h for 4 hours in both). Favorable outcomes were demonstrated to an mRS of 2 or less in 40% of rpro-UK patients and 25% of controls. Mortality was 25% and 27% in the rpro-UK and placebo arms, respectively, and the rate of symptomatic intracerebral hemorrhage was 10% for rpro-UK and 2% for controls. TIMI grade 3 flow was achieved in 66% of rpro-UK patients and 10% of controls. Currently, intraarterial thrombolytic therapy for ischemic stroke remains experimental and is not approved by the Food and Drug Administration (FDA).

Meta-analysis of thrombolytic therapy in acute ischemic stroke currently indicates that significant benefit may result from the administration of intravenous rt-PA in patients treated within 6 hours of symptom onset. The greatest benefit and lowest risk of hemorrhagic transformation, however, is measured in patients treated within 3 hours of symptom onset (203,204). Adherence to the NINDS (193) protocol offers the greatest potential for successful outcome at the lowest risk. The report of acute hemopericardium in patients with recent myocardial ischemia who are treated with intravenous rt-PA for acute stroke within a few days of a cardiac event suggests caution in this subset of patients (205).

Venous Thromboembolism

The indications for thrombolytic therapy in VTE are less clear than in other clinical settings. Whereas acute PE may cause hemodynamic instability and sudden death, the presentation of deep vein thrombosis (DVT) is usually less acute, and time-dependent tissue injury does not occur in the same manner as acute arterial occlusion. Complete clot lysis is not critical or likely in the low-flow venous circulation (206–209). Compared with arterial thrombi, venous thrombi are usually present for a much longer period and are in a greater state of cross-linked maturation when clinically diagnosed. The objective of thrombolysis is immediately to relieve hemodynamic instability due to massive PE, more quickly to restore venous flow in hopes of immediately reducing the pain and swelling of iliofemoral DVT, and to reduce the risk of postphlebitic syndrome (approximately 25% among patients with proximal DVT) (210,211–217). The major question has been whether such immediate intervention with thrombolytic agents is superior to standard anticoagulation therapy with unfractionated heparin or LMWH. A number of clinical trials have attempted to answer this question.

Pulmonary Embolism

In the treatment of acute PE, SK, UK, and rt-PA have all been well studied (218). Large clinical trials performed in the 1970s demonstrated that infusion of SK for 24 hours and UK for 12 hours were similarly efficacious and superior to heparin in the rate of early recanalization (206–208). Alteplase has been demonstrated to be of similar efficacy (209,219–222). At 24 hours, reduction in pulmonary vascular resistance by 25% was demonstrated with thrombolysis compared with 4% with intravenous unfractionated heparin alone. Ventilation/perfusion lung scans were improved at 24 and 72 hours with thrombolysis but were comparable to heparin later (206,207,223). The risk of intracranial hemorrhage in patients treated with thrombolytic agents for VTE has consistently been in the range of 1% to 2% (224). Double-bolus reteplase also has been compared with alteplase with similar efficacy and safety (225). Therapy consists of SK as a 250,000-U loading dose followed by infusion of 100,000 U/h for 24 hours. UK is dosed as 4,400 IU/kg loading dose followed by infusion of 2,200 IU/kg/h for 12 hours (226). Laboratory monitoring with SK and UK is directed primarily to document systemic fibrinolysis. Prolongation of the aPTT or thrombin time (TT) allows documentation of fibrinolysis. Heparin may be initiated when the aPTT or TT returns to less than 2 times normal (226). Alteplase is administered as a 100-mg infusion over a 2-hour period. Reteplase is not currently approved for use in PE but has been studied at a dose of two intravenous boluses of 10 U, 28 minutes apart (225). Heparin should not be infused concurrent with SK or UK but is optional with rt-PA and r-PA. There is no evidence that catheter-directed therapy is superior to systemic therapy with rt-PA (227). After any thrombolytic therapy, full-dose anticoagulation with intravenous unfractionated heparin or LMWH is required to prevent rethrombosis. Current clinical use of thrombolytic agents in patients with PE is most often confined to those with hemodynamic instability (228) or echocardiographic evidence of right ventricular dysfunction (226,229). The recommendation of the AHA has been to consider rt-PA therapy in patients with the potential for greatest benefit, such as those with syncope, hypotension, or submassive PE in the presence of premorbid cardiac or pulmonary disease (230). As a life-saving measure, rt-PA has also been used in patients for whom thrombolytic therapy is ordinarily considered contraindicated, including those with recent general surgery (231) or neurosurgery (232), pregnancy (233), and those with cardiac arrest requiring cardiopulmonary resuscitation (234,235). In patients with massive PE, thrombolysis has been combined with embolus fragmentation by a rotating pigtail catheter (236).

Deep Vein Thrombosis

Thrombolytic therapy for DVT has produced evidence of early benefit with relatively low risk. Although the incidence of symptomatic postphlebitic syndrome may be reduced from 40% in heparin patients to 10% in patients treated with thrombolysis (237), there is controversy regarding the long-term clinical impact of early thrombolytic therapy (212–215, 238). Recommendations have been to consider thrombolysis in young patients with acute iliofemoral thrombosis at high risk for postphlebitic syndrome and at low risk for hemorrhage. FDA approval is for 48 hours of UK and for 72 hours of SK (226). Dosing for DVT is the same as that for PE; however, the infusion dose of SK or UK may be required for a longer time to achieve satisfactory clinical improvement. Catheter-directed therapy has emerged as an option for the delivery of thrombolytic agents. Recanalization rates as high as 90% are achieved, and the procedure may be combined with the placement of an intravascular stent (239–242). Clots as old as 4 weeks may be amenable to treatment. Unfortunately, the rate of intracerebral hemorrhage has been reported as high as 11% (243); death may still result from PE, and the long-term clinical benefit of early clot lysis remains unclear (226).

Peripheral Arterial Thrombosis

Acute thrombosis of peripheral arteries presents a similar problem as acute coronary thrombosis, that of acute, time-dependent tissue ischemia proceeding to infarction. The application of thrombolytic therapy to acute peripheral arterial thrombosis has been met with considerable success in opening the occluded artery (244–251). The clinical outcome with thrombolysis is contrasted with the recognized benefit of early surgical intervention. The apparent benefit of thrombolysis is balanced against the risk of intracranial hemorrhage.

The majority of patients with peripheral arterial occlusion have atherosclerosis and other risk factors associated with an increased risk of hemorrhage. Thrombolysis may especially be efficacious for small peripheral artery occlusion not amenable to surgical therapy. In addition to thrombolysis for acute thrombosis, angioplasty or surgery may still be required for definitive treatment to sustain vascular patency (244–251).

Clinical trials have demonstrated the benefit of thrombolysis in peripheral arterial thrombosis. The earliest reported randomized trial in 1994 used catheter-directed UK and achieved successful reperfusion in 70% and facilitated angioplasty in another 30%. Hospital limb salvage was equal to that achieved with surgery; however, the 1-year mortality was 16% in the thrombolytic patients and 42% in the surgery patients (252). Recombinant UK has been used in the same study design, with similar results at reperfusion. Major hemorrhage occurred in 13% of thrombolytic patients (1.5% intracranial hemorrhage) and 6% of surgery patients (253). Alteplase was studied in a similar manner and demonstrated no clear advantage over surgical management (254). Experience has demonstrated effective thrombolysis in both native vessels and thrombosed arterial grafts (255,256). Alteplase and UK have emerged as superior to SK for reperfusion (80% vs. 64%) and risk of hemorrhage (5% vs. 25%) (257,258). Staphylokinase also is effective at achieving reperfusion but is associated with a risk of fatal intracranial hemorrhage (2.1%) (259). No comparative trials clearly demonstrate superiority of one agent over the other or definitively confirm a higher rate of limb salvage with thrombolysis versus surgery (260). Patients who do not achieve recanalization with immediate thrombolysis (rt-PA, 2 to 10 mg over a 3-hour period) have been treated with an intraarterial infusion of prostaglandin E_1 (2.1 mL/h for 3 hours) alternating with rt-PA, 3 mg every 3 hours, and concomitant intravenous unfractionated heparin (15,000 U/24 hours to slightly prolong the aPTT), over as long as 13 days (mean, 2.8 ± 2.2). This regimen achieved a successful recanalization rate of 61% in patients for whom initial thrombolysis failed. Subsequent angioplasty, where appropriate, has yielded 1-year patency rates as high as 90%. At 3 years, the rate of patency was not statistically different in patients treated with short-term versus extended-course rt-PA (261).

Miscellaneous Disorders

A number of clinical applications of thrombolytic therapy have evolved from experience in the treatment of arterial and venous thrombosis. Cerebral venous sinus thrombosis and intraventricular hemorrhage (262) have been treated effectively with thrombolysis. Unusual foci of arterial thrombosis amenable to treatment with catheter-directed thrombolysis include the axillary/subclavian vein (263, 264), the mesenteric artery and venous system, the superior and inferior vena cava (particularly when compressed by tumor), portal vein thrombosis (265,266), and peripheral arterial occlusion due to heparin-induced thrombocytopenia with thrombosis. Thrombolytic therapy is recommended as first-line strategy in patients with mechanical valves who experience valve thrombosis. Patients responding to thrombolytic therapy generally do not subsequently require surgery (267,268). Thrombosis of other devices for which thrombolytic agents are used include vena caval filters, peripheral and central access catheters, arteriovenous cannulae, and dialysis catheters. In all instances, the potential benefit must be weighed against the potential for life-threatening hemorrhage (260).

COMPLICATIONS OF THROMBOLYTIC THERAPY

The primary risk of thrombolytic therapy is hemorrhage. Of greatest concern is life-threatening major hemorrhage and intracranial hemorrhage. Clinical trials clearly indicate that the risk of hemorrhage is greater with thrombolytic

TABLE 19.6. CLINICAL APPLICATIONS OF THROMBOLYTIC AGENTS

Agent	Clinical Use	Dose
Streptokinase	AMI	1.5 mU i.v. over 1 h or 20 kU intracoronary, then 2 kU per min for 60 min
	PE	250 kU i.v. over 0.5 h, then 100 kU/h for 24 h (72 h if concurrent DVT)
	DVT	250 kU i.v. over 0.5 h, then 100 kU/h for 72 h
	PAO	250 kU i.v. over 0.5 h, then 100 kU/h for 24–72 h
	AV	250 kU intracannula, then clamp for 2 h
Anistreplase	AMI	30 U i.v. over 2 to 5 min
Urokinase	AMI	6 kU/kg per min for ≤2 h i.c.
	PE	4.4-kU/kg bolus, then 4.4 kU/h for 12 h i.v.
	PAO	4 kU per min for 4 h, then 4 kU per min for ≤48 h
	CC	5 kU intracatheter
Alteplase	AMI	15-mg bolus i.v., then 50-mg infusion over 30 min, then 35 mg over next 60 min (>67 kg), if ≤67 kg, use weight-based (maximal dose of 100 mg)
	PE	100 mg by i.v. infusion over 2 h
	AIS	0.9 mg/kg i.v. over 60 min with 10% of dose as initial bolus (maximal 90 mg total dose)
	DVT	10 mg intracatheter, then 1 to 2 mg/h for 12 h (not FDA approved)
Reteplase	AMI	10 U i.v. over 2 min, wait 28 min, then repeat
	PE	10 U i.v. over 2 min, wait 28 min, then repeat (not FDA approved)
Tenecteplase	AMI	30 to 50 mg i.v. bolus (weight based)
Lanoteplase	AMI	15 to 120 kU/kg over 2 to 4 min (not FDA approved)

mu, million units; kU, thousand units; i.v., intravenous; AMI, acute myocardial infarction; AIS, acute ischemic stroke; PAO, peripheral arterial occlusion; AV, arteriovenous cannulae occlusion; CC, catheter clearance; PE, pulmonary embolus; DVT, deep vein thrombosis; FDA, Food and Drug Administration.

therapy than with placebo or with anticoagulation alone, in all clinical settings. Careful case selection and strict adherence to established protocols will help to mitigate the risk of hemorrhage. The clinical applications of the available thrombolytic agents are summarized in Table 19.6, and the contraindications, in Table 19.7.

Management of hemorrhage will depend on the severity of bleeding, the clinical manifestations, and the overall setting. Massive hemorrhage with hemodynamic instability requires immediate reversal of systemic fibrinogenolysis. If hemorrhage occurs, the thrombolytic agent should immediately be discontinued, and emergency laboratory testing performed, including a fibrinogen level and TBT. The nadir of fibrinogen levels may remain low for as long as 24 hours after rt-PA (269). Normal hepatic production may take 24 to 36 hours to replenish fibrinogen. Therapeutic repletion of fibrinogen can be achieved with fresh frozen plasma or cryoprecipitate. Platelet dysfunction may result from circulating fibrin(ogen) degradation products, and an abnormal TBT should be followed by platelet transfusions.

If hemorrhage occurs during the duration of action of the thrombolytic agent, reversal may be achieved with ε-aminocaproic acid or aprotinin (260). Emergency interventional procedures or surgery such as coronary artery bypass are not unusual in AMI. In such circumstances, an excess of bleeding can be expected and should be anticipated (270,271). Reversal of systemic fibrinogenolysis, repletion of fibrinogen with fresh frozen plasma or cryoprecipitate, and platelet transfusion can allow surgery to proceed. The period of hemorrhagic risk at sites of vascular trauma may

TABLE 19.7. CONTRAINDICATIONS TO THROMBOLYTIC THERAPY

Recent (within 10 days) major surgery
Recent (within 10 days) puncture of noncompressible organ or vessel
Recent (within 10 days) gastrointestinal or genitourinary bleeding
Recent (within 10 days) trauma
Recent (within 3 months) intracranial or intraspinal surgery, serious head trauma, or stroke
Uncontrolled hypertension with systolic ≥180 mm Hg or diastolic ≥110 mm Hg
Intracranial neoplasm, arteriovenous malformation, or aneurysm
Strong probability of intracardiac thrombus
Subacute bacterial endocarditis
Acute pericarditis
Hemorrhagic diathesis
Major hepatic dysfunction (reteplase may be safer because of renal metabolism)
Pregnancy
Hemorrhagic ophthalmopathy (e.g., diabetic retinopathy)
Current use of anticoagulants (especially warfarin)
Septic thrombophlebitis or thrombosed and infected AV fistula
Demonstrated allergy to thrombolytic agent (especially streptokinase, anistreplase)
Administration of streptokinase or anistreplase within the preceding 2 years or more (antibodies may persist as long as 54 months)
Age >75 years (relative contraindication)

Contraindications are relative and not absolute. Benefit versus risk should be weighed on a patient-by-patient basis.
AV, arteriovenous.

TABLE 19.8. COMPLICATIONS OF THROMBOLYTIC THERAPY

Complication	Etiology	Management
Hemorrhage	Fibrinogenolysis (fibrinogen low)	ε-Aminocaproic acid or aprotonin (particularly during thrombolysis); FFP, cryoprecipitate (may be required ≤36)
	Platelet dysfunction (TBT prolonged)	Platelet transfusion (requirement determined by TBT)
Embolization	Partial thrombolysis	Continue thrombolytic infusion, add adjunctive agents
Hypotension, rash, fever	Anaphylaxis	Intravenous fluids, vasopressors glucocorticoids, antihistamines

TBT, template bleeding time; FFP, fresh frozen plasma.

extend for up to 10 days. Precautions should be taken to avoid soft-tissue or invasive trauma in all patients who receive thrombolytic agents, and careful attention should be given to mechanical measures to assist hemostasis at sites of venous and arterial puncture.

Other potential complications of thrombolytic therapy include allergic reactions and distal embolization. Immunogenic reactions to SK are well described and can occasionally be observed with rt-PA (82,209,272). Management includes the prophylactic administration of glucocorticoid and diphenhydramine to SK patients and similar therapy as needed with other agents. Hypotension may occur in up to 12% of patients receiving SK or APSAC and in about 7% of patients treated with rt-PA (273). Management requires infusions of intravenous fluid and occasionally vasopressors.

Patients treated for peripheral arterial thrombosis may exhibit peripheral embolization to digits up to 20% of the time (247). Patients with DVT and PE rarely exhibit clinical manifestations of thromboembolism as a direct result of thrombolysis (260). Continued infusion of the thrombolytic agent is usually effective at lysis of peripheral emboli. Table 19.8 summarizes the management of complications.

SUMMARY

The therapeutic use of thrombolytic agents is the natural result of the increasing understanding of the pathophysiologic mechanisms underlying normal and deranged thrombosis and fibrinolysis. Plasminogen activators capable of increasing the production of plasmin are demonstrated to exhibit considerable efficacy in the treatment of a variety of arterial and venous thrombotic disorders. The ideal thrombolytic agent has yet to be developed, but the desired clinical result of rapid opening of the thrombosed vessel without reocclusion, without activation of systemic fibrinogenolysis, and without a risk of hemorrhage are well defined. Clinical studies clearly demonstrate that the addition of a variety of adjunctive agents to the available thrombolytics enhances benefit without inordinate risk. Newer agents and new protocols for use of existing therapies offer the promise of saving many who would otherwise die of coronary or cerebral arterial thrombosis or VTE.

REFERENCES

1. Fletcher A, Sherry S, Alkjaersig N, et al. The maintenance of a sustained thrombolytic state in man, II: clinical observations on patients with myocardial infarction and other thromboembolic disorders. *J Clin Invest* 1959;38:11–19.
2. (GISSI-1) Gruppo Italiano per lo Studio Steptokinasi nell'Infarto Miocardico. Effectiveness of intravenous thrombolytic treatment in acute myocardial infarction. *Lancet* 1986;1: 397–401.
3. McNicol G. The fibrinolytic system. *Postgrad Med J* 1973;49 (suppl):10–17.
4. Bick R. Physiology of hemostasis. In: *Disorders of thrombosis and hemostasis: clinical and laboratory practice* Chicago: ASCP Press, 1992:1–27.
5. Bick R. Physiology of hemostasis and thrombosis. In: *Disorders of hemostasis and thrombosis: principles of clinical practice.* New York: Thieme, 1985:1–30.
6. Aoki N, Moroi M, Matsuda M. The behavior of alpha-2-plasmin inhibitor in fibrinolytic states. *J Clin Invest* 1977;60:361.
7. Van de Werf FCC, Luyten A, Houbracken K, et al. Safety assessment of a single bolus administration of TNK tissue-plasminogen activator in acute myocardial infarction: the ASSENT-1 trial. *Am Heart J* 1999;137:786–791.
8. ASSENT Investigators. Single-bolus tenecteplase compared with front-loaded alteplase in acute myocardial infarction: the ASSENT-2 double-blind randomised trial. *Lancet* 1999;354: 716–722.
9. Cannon CP, McCabe GC, Adgey CH, et al. TNK-tissue plasminogen activator compared with front-loaded alteplase in acute myocardial infarction: results of the TIMI 10B trial. *Circulation* 1998;98:2805–2814.
10. Bell W. Thrombolytic therapy: agents, indications, and laboratory monitoring. *Med Clin North Am* 1994;78:745–764.
11. Bell W, Black E, DeMets D, et al. Urokinase-streptokinase embolism trial, phase 2 results. *JAMA* 1974;229:1606–1613.
12. Johnson A, McCarty W. The lysis of artificially induced intravascular clots in man by intravenous infusion of streptokinase. *J Clin Invest* 1959;38:1627–1643.
13. Jackson KWTJ. Complete amino acid sequence of streptokinase and its homology with serine proteases. *Biochemistry* 1982;21: 6620–6625.
14. Medved LVSD, Ingham KC. Domain structure, stability and interactions in streptokinase. *Eur J Biochem* 1996;239: 333–339.
15. Parrado JC-LF, Smith RA, et al. The domain organization of streptokinase: nuclear magnetic resonance, circular dichroism, and functional characterization of proteolytic fragments. *Protein Sci* 1996;5:693–704.
16. Damaschun GDH, Gast K, et al. Streptokinase is a flexible multi-domain protein. *Eur Biophys J* 1992;20:355–361.

17. Malke HSK, Gase K, et al. The streptokinase gene: allelic variation, genomic environment and expression control. *Dev Biol Stand* 1995;85:183–193.
18. Young KCSG, Chang YF, et al. Interaction of streptokinase and plasminogen: studies with truncated streptokinase peptides. *J Biol Chem* 1995;270:29601–29606.
19. Leopold J, Keaney J, Loscalzo J. Pharmacology of thrombolytic agents. In: Schafer JL, ed. *Thrombosis hemorrhage.* Vol 1. Baltimore: Williams & Wilkins, 1998:1215–1258.
20. Reddy KNMG. Mechanism of activation of human plasminogen by streptokinase: presence of an active center in streptokinase-plasminogen complex. *J Biol Chem* 1972;247: 1683–1691.
21. Summaria LWR, Boreisha IG, et al. A virgin enzyme derived from human plasminogen: specific cleavage of the arginyl-560-valyl peptide bond in the diisopropoxyphosphinyl virgin enzyme by plasminogen activators. *Biochemistry* 1982;21: 2056–2059.
22. Takada YTA. Kinetic analyses of potentiation of plasminogen activation by streptokinase in the presence of fibrin or its degradation products. *Haemostasis* 1987;16:1–7.
23. Chibber BAMJ, Castellino FJ. Effects of human fibrinogen and its cleavage products on activation of human plasminogen by streptokinase. *Biochemistry* 1985;24:3429–3434.
24. Camiolo SMMG, Evers JL, et al. Augmentation of streptokinase activator activity by fibrinogen or fibrin. *Thromb Res* 1980; 17:697–706.
25. Wiman B. On the reaction of plasmin or plasmin-streptokinase complex with aprotinin or α-2-antiplasmin. *Thromb Res* 1980; 17:143–152.
26. Brommer EJMP. Thrombin generation induced by the intrinsic or extrinsic pathway is accelerated by streptokinase, independent of plasminogen. *Thromb Haemost* 1993;70:995–997.
27. Gouin ILT, Morel MC, et al. In vitro effects of plasmin on human platelet function in plasma: inhibition of aggregation caused by fibrinogenolysis. *Circulation* 1992;85:935–941.
28. Bick R. Thrombolytic therapy. In: *Disorders of thrombosis and hemostasis: clinical and laboratory practice.* Chicago: ASCP Press, 1992:313–317.
29. Col J, Col-De Beys C, Renkin J, et al. Pharmacokinetics, thrombolytic efficacy and hemorrhagic risk of different streptokinase regimens in heparin-treated acute myocardial infarction. *Am J Cardiol* 1989;63:1185–1192.
30. Bell W. Thrombolytic therapy: a comparison between urokinase and streptokinase. *Semin Thromb Hemost* 1975;2:1–11.
31. Bick R. Clinical implications of molecular markers on hemostasis and thrombosis. *Semin Thromb Hemost* 1984;10: 290–304.
32. Figueredo V, Amidon T, Wolfe C. Thrombolysis after acute myocardial infarction: who should be added to inclusion criteria? *Postgrad Med J* 1994;96:30–40.
33. Lee H, Yule S, McKenzie A, et al. Hypersensitivity reactions to streptokinase in patients in patients with high pre-treatment antistreptokinase antibody and neutralization titers. *Eur Heart J* 1993;14:1640–1643.
34. Anonymous. Long-term effects of intravenous thrombolysis in acute myocardial infarction: final report of the GISSI Study: Gruppo Italiano per lo Studio della Streptokinasi nell'Infarto Miocardico (GISSI). *Lancet* 1987;ii:871–874.
35. Fears R. Development of anisoylated plasminogen-streptokinase activator complex from the acyl enzyme complex. *Semin Thromb Hemost* 1989;15:129.
36. Smith R, Dyse R, English P. Acyl-enzymes as thrombolytic agents in a rabbit model of venous thrombosis. *Thromb Haemost* 1982;47:269.
37. Smith R, Dupe R, English P, et al. Fibrinolysis with acyl-enzymes: a new approach to thrombolytic therapy. *Nature* 1981;290:505–508.
38. Anderson J. Development and evaluation of anisoylated plasminogen streptokinase activator complex (APSAC) as a second generation thrombolytic agent [Review]. *J Am Coll Cardiol* 1987;10:22B–27B.
39. Fears R, Ferres H, Standring R. The protective effect of acylation on the stability of anisoylated plasminogen streptokinase activator complex in human plasma. *Drugs* 1987;33(suppl): 57–63.
40. Green J, Dupe R, Smith R, et al. Comparison of the hypotensive effects of streptokinase-(human) plasmin activator complex and BRL 26921 (p-anisoylated streptokinase-plasminogen activator complex) in the dog after high dose bolus administration. *Thromb Res* 1984;36:29–36.
41. Ferres H. Preclinical pharmacological evaluation of anisoylated plasminogen streptokinase activator complex [Review]. *Drugs* 1987;33(suppl):33–50.
42. Lee H, Cross S, Davidson R, et al. Raised levels of antistreptokinase antibody and neutralization titres from 4 days to 54 months after administration of streptokinase or anistreplase. *Eur Heart J* 1993;14:84–89.
43. Johnson E, Gregeen R. An interim report of the efficacy and safety of anisoylated plasminogen activator complex (APSAC). *Drugs* 1987;33(suppl 3):298–311.
44. Collen D. Report of the Subcommittee on Fibrinolysis; San Diego, CA, July 13, 1985. *Thromb Haemost* 1985;54:893.
45. Husain S, Gurewich W, Lipinski B. Purification and partial characterization of a single-chain high-molecular-weight form of urokinase from human urine. *Arch Biochem Biophys* 1983; 220:31–38.
46. Wun T, Schleuning W, Reich E. Isolation and characterization of urokinase from human plasma. *J Biol Chem* 1982;257: 3276–3283.
47. Wun T, Ossowski L, Reich E. A proenzyme form of human urokinase. *J Biol Chem* 1982;257:7262–7268.
48. Riccio A, Grimaldi G, Verde P, et al. The human urokinase-plasminogen activator gene and its promotor. *Nucleic Acids Res* 1985;13:2759–2771.
49. Spraggon G, Phillips C, Nowak U, et al. The crystal structure of the catalytic domain of human urokinase-type plasminogen activator. *Structure* 1995;3:681–691.
50. Collen D, Zamarron C, Lijnen H, et al. Activation of plasminogen by pro-urokinase II: kinetics. *J Biol Chem* 1986;621: 1259–1266.
51. Pannell R, Gurewich V. Pro-urokinase: a study of its stability in plasma and of a mechanism for its selective fibrinolytic effect. *Blood* 1986;67:1215–1223.
52. Pannell R, Black J, Gurewich V. Complementary modes of action of tissue-type plasminogen activator and pro-urokinase by which their synergistic effect on clot lysis may be explained. *J Clin Invest* 1988;81:853–859.
53. Pepper M, Sappino A, Stocklin R, et al. Up-regulation of urokinase receptor expression on migrating endothelial cells. *J Cell Biol* 1993;122:673–684.
54. Ellis V, Scully M, Kakkar V. Plasminogen activation initiated by single-chain urokinase-type plasminogen activator: potentiation by U937 monocytes. *J Biol Chem* 1989;264:2185–2188.
55. Heegard C, Simonsen A, Oka K, et al. Very low density lipoprotein receptor binds and mediates endocytosis of urokinase-type plasminogen activator-type-1 plasminogen activator inhibitor complex. *J Biol Chem* 1995;270:20855–20861.
56. Nykjaer A, Petersen C, Moller B, et al. Purified alpha 2-macroglobulin receptor/LDL receptor-related protein binds urokinase plasminogen activator inhibitor type-1 complex: evidence that the alpha 2-macroglobulin receptor mediates cellular

degradation of urokinase receptor-bound complexes. *J Biol Chem* 1992;267:14543–14546.
57. Higazi A, Mazar A, Wang J, et al. Single-chain urokinase-type plasminogen activator bound to its receptor is relatively resistant to plasminogen activator inhibitor type 1. *Blood* 1996; 87:3545–3549.
58. Linjen H, Collen D. Stimulation by heparin of the plasmin-mediated conversion of single-chain and two-chain urokinase-type plasminogen activator. *Thromb Res* 1986;43:687–690.
59. Urano T, Serizawa K, Takada Y, et al. Heparin and heparan sulfate enhancement of the inhibitory activity of plasminogen activator inhibitor type-1 toward urokinase type plasminogen activator. *Biochim Biophys Acta* 1994;1201:217–222.
60. Stump D, Kieckens L, De Cock F, et al. Pharmacokinetics of single-chain forms of urokinase-type plasminogen activator. *J Pharmacol Exp Ther* 1987;242:245–250.
61. Diefenbach C, Erbel R, Pop T, et al. Recombinant single-chain urokinase-type plasminogen activator during acute myocardial infarction. *Am J Cardiol* 1988;61:966–970.
62. Rijken D, Wijngaards G, Zaal-De Jong M, et al. Purification and partial characterization of plasminogen activator from human uterine tissue. *Biochim Biophys Acta* 1979;580:140–153.
63. Rijken D, Wijngaards G, Welbergen J. Relationship between tissue plasminogen activator and the activities in blood and vascular wall. *Thromb Res* 1980;18:815–830.
64. Collen D, Rijken D, Van Damme J, et al. Purification of human tissue-type plasminogen activator in centigram quantities from human melanoma cell culture fluid and its conditioning for use in vivo. *Thromb Haemost* 1982;48:294–296.
65. Pennica D, Holmes W, Kohr W, et al. Cloning and expression of human tissue-type plasminogen activator cDNA in *E. coli. Nature* 1983;301:214–221.
66. Linjen H, Collen D. Mechanism of plasminogen activation by mammalian plasminogen activators. *Enzyme* 1988;40:90–96.
67. Lamba D, Bauer M, Huber R, et al. The 2.3 A crystal structure of the catalytic domain of recombinant two-chain human tissue-type plasminogen activator. *J Mol Biol* 1996;258:117–135.
68. Loscalzo J. Structural and kinetic comparison of recombinant human single- and two-chain tissue plasminogen activator. *J Clin Invest* 1988;82:1391–1397.
69. Madison E, Coombs G, Corey D. Substrate specificity of tissue type plasminogen activator: characterization of the fibrin specificity of t-PA for plasminogen. *J Biol Chem* 1996;270:7558–7562.
70. Bauer R, Hansen S, Jones G, et al. Fibrin structures during tissue-type plasminogen activator-mediated fibrinolysis studied by laser light scattering: relation to fibrin enhancement of plasminogen activation. *Eur Biophys J* 1994;23:239–252.
71. Stricker R, Wong D, Shiu D, et al. Activation of plasminogen by tissue plasminogen activator on normal and thromboasthenic platelets: effects on surface proteins and platelet aggregation. *Blood* 1986;68:275–280.
72. Gao S, Morser J, McLean K, et al. Differential effect of platelets on plasminogen activation by tissue plasminogen activator, urokinase, and streptokinase. *Thromb Res* 1990;58:421–433.
73. Felez J, Chanquia C, Levin E, et al. Binding of tissue plasminogen activator to human monocytes and monocytoid cells. *Blood* 1991;78:2318–2327.
74. Hajjar K, Hamel N, Harpel P, et al. Binding of tissue plasminogen activator to cultured human endothelial cells. *J Clin Invest* 1987;80:1712–1719.
75. Angles-Cano E, Hervio L, Rouy D, et al. Effects of lipoprotein(a) on the binding of plasminogen to fibrin and its activation by fibrin-bound tissue-type plasminogen activator. *Chem Phys Lipids* 1994;67–68:369–380.
76. Reilly C, Hutzelmann J. Plasminogen activator inhibitor-1 binds to fibrin and inhibits tissue-type plasminogen activator-mediated fibrin dissolution. *J Biol Chem* 1992;267: 17128–17135.
77. Kaneko M, Sakata Y, Matsuda M, et al. Interactions between the finger and kringle-2 domains of tissue-type plasminogen activator inhibitor-1. *J Biochem* 1992;111:244–248.
78. Verstraete M, Su C, Tanswell P, et al. Pharmacokinetics and effects on fibrinolytic and coagulant parameters of two doses of recombinant tissue-type plasminogen activator in healthy volunteers. *Thromb Haemost* 1986;56:1–5.
79. Tanswell P, Tebbe U, Neuhaus K, et al. Pharmacokinetics and fibrin specificity of alteplase during accelerated infusions in acute myocardial infarction. *J Am Coll Cardiol* 1992;19: 1071–1075.
80. Garabedian H, Gold H, Leinbach R, et al. Comparative properties of two clinical preparations of recombinant human tissue-type plasminogen activator in patients with acute myocardial infarction. *J Am Coll Cardiol* 1987;9:599–607.
81. Chandler W, Alessi M, Aillaud M, et al. Clearance of tissue plasminogen activator (TPA) and TPA/plasminogen activator type 1(PAI-1) complex. *Circulation* 1997;96:761–768.
82. Rudolf J, Grond M, Prince W, et al. Evidence of anaphylaxy after alteplase infusion. *Stroke* 1999;30:1142–1143.
83. Berger HJ, Pizzo S. Preparation of polyethylene glycol-tissue plasminogen activator adducts that retain functional activity: characteristics and behavior in three animal species. *Blood* 1988; 71:1641–1647.
84. Burck P, Berg D, Warrick M, et al. Characterized of a modified human tissue plasminogen activator comprising a kringle-2 and a protease domain. *J Biol Chem* 1990;265:5170–5177.
85. Cody R. Results from late breaking trials sessions ACC '97. *J Am Coll Cardiol* 1997;30:1–7.
86. ASSENT Investigators. Single-bolus tenecteplase compared with front-loaded alteplase in acute myocardial infarction: the ASSENT-2 double-blind randomised trial. *Lancet* 1999;354: 716–722.
87. Keyt B, Paoni P, Refino C, et al. A faster-acting and more potent form of tissue plasminogen activator. *Proc Natl Acad Sci U S A* 1994;91:3670–3674.
88. Ohman EM, Harrington RACPC, Agnelli G, et al. Intravenous thrombolysis in acute myocardial infarction. *Chest* 2001;119: 253S–277S.
89. Bode C, Smalling RW, Berg G, et al. Randomized comparison of coronary thrombolysis achieved with double-bolus reteplase (recombinant plasminogen activator) and front-loaded accelerated alteplase (recombinant tissue plasminogen activator) in patients with acute myocardial infarction. *Circulation* 1996;94:891–898.
90. GUSTO Investigators. The global use of strategies to open occluded coronary arteries (GUSTO III): a comparison of reteplase with alteplase for acute myocardial infarction. *N Engl J Med* 1997;337:1118–1123.
91. Keyt B, Paoni N, Refino C, et al. A faster-acting and more potent form of tissue plasminogen activator. *Proc Natl Acad Sci U S A* 1994;91:3670–3674.
92. Paoni N, Keyt B, Refino C, et al. A slow clearing, fibrin specific, PAI-1 resistant variant of t-PA (T103N, KHRR 296-299). *Thromb Haemost* 1993;70:307–312.
93. Tanswell P, Tebbe U, Neuhaus KL, et al. Pharmacokinetics and fibrin specificity of alteplase during accelerated infusion in acute myocardial infarction. *J Am Coll Cardiol* 1992;19:1071–1075.
94. Cannon C, McCabe C, Gibson C, et al. TNK-tissue plasminogen activator in acute myocardial infraction: results of the Thrombolysis in Myocardial Infarction (TIMI) 10A dose-ranging trial. *Circulation* 1997;95:351–356.
95. Sako T, Tsuchida N. Nucleotide sequence of the staphylokinase gene from *Staphylococcus aureus. Nucleic Acids Res* 1983;11: 7679–7693.

96. Damaschun GDH, Gast K, et al. Biophysical and conformational properties of staphylokinase in solution. *Biochim Biophys Acta* 1993;1161:244–248.
97. Schlott B, Hartmann M, Guhrs K, et al. Functional properties of recombinant staphylokinase variants obtained by site-specific mutagenesis of methionine-26. *Biochim Biophys Acta* 1994; 1204:235–242.
98. Hauptmann KE, Glusa E. Differential effects of staphylokinase, streptokinase and tissue-type plasminogen activator on the lysis of retracted human plasma clots and fibrinolytic parameters in vitro. *Blood Coagul Fibrinolysis* 1995;6:579–583.
99. Vanderschueren S, Barrios L, Kerdsinchai P, et al. A randomized trial of recombinant staphylokinase versus alteplase for coronary artery patency in acute myocardial infarction: the STAR Trial Group. *Circulation* 1995;92:2044–2049.
100. Vanderschueren S, Stockx L, Wilms G, et al. Thrombolytic therapy of peripheral arterial occlusion with recombinant staphylokinase. *Circulation* 1995;92:2050–2057.
101. Collen D, Bernaerts R, Declerck P, et al. Recombinant staphylokinase variants with altered immunoreactivity, I: construction and characterization. *Circulation* 1996;94:197–206.
102. Robbins K, Tanaka Y, Gulba D, et al. Covalent molecular weight approximately 92,000 hybrid plasminogen activator derived from human plasmin amino terminal and urokinase carboxy terminal domains. *Biochemistry* 1986;25:3603–3611.
103. Pennica D, Holmes W, Kohr W, et al. Cloning and expression of human tissue-type plasminogen activator cDNA in *E. coli*. *Nature* 1983;301:214–221.
104. Gheysen D, Lijnen HR, Pierard L, et al. Characterization of a recombinant fusion protein of the finger domain of tissue-type plasminogen activator with a truncated single chain urokinase-type plasminogen activator. *J Biol Chem* 1987;262: 11779–11784.
105. Hoffmeister HM, Szabo S, Kastner C, et al. Thrombolytic therapy in acute myocardial infarction: comparison of procoagulant effects of streptokinase and alteplase regimens with focus on kallikrein system and plasmin. *Circulation* 1998;98:2527–2533.
106. Rapold H. Promotion of thrombin activity by thrombolytic therapy without simultaneous anticoagulation. *Lancet* 1990;1: 481–482.
107. Eisenberg P, Miletich J, Sobel B, et al. Factors responsible for the differential procoagulant effects of diverse plasminogen activators in plasma. *Fibrinolysis* 1991;5:217–224.
108. Davies M, Thomas A, Knapman P. Intra-myocardial platelet aggregation in patients with unstable angina suffering sudden ischemic cardiac death. *Circulation* 1986;73:418–427.
109. Nicolini FA, Lee P, Rios G, et al. Combination of platelet fibrinogen receptor antagonist and direct thrombin inhibitor at low doses markedly improves thrombolysis. *Circulation* 1994; 89:1802–1809.
110. Roux S, Tschoff T, Kuhn H, et al. Effects of heparin, aspirin, and synthetic glycoprotein IIb/IIIa receptor antagonist on coronary reperfusion and reocclusion after thrombolysis with tissue-type plasminogen activator in the dog. *J Pharmacol Exp Ther* 1993;264:501–508.
111. Ohman EM, Kleiman N, Gacioch G, et al. Combined accelerated tissue-plasminogen activator and glycoprotein IIb/IIIa integrin receptor blockade with Integrilin in acute myocardial infarction: results of a randomized, placebo-controlled dose-ranging trial. *Circulation* 1997;95:846–854.
112. Moliterno DJ, Harrington RA, Krucoff MW, et al. More complete and stable reperfusion with platelet IIb/IIIa antagonism plus thrombolysis for AMI: the PARADIGM trial. *Circulation* 1996;94(suppl I):I553(abst).
113. Rote W, Mu D, Bates E, et al. Prevention of rethrombosis after coronary thrombolysis in chronic canine model: adjunctive therapy with monoclonal antibody 7E3 F(ab′) 2 fragment. *J Cardiovasc Pharmacol* 1994;23:194–202.
114. Cronberg S. Effect of fibrinolysis on adhesion and aggregation of human platelets. *Thromb Diath Haemorrhage* 1968;19: 474–482.
115. Terres W, Unmus S, Mathey DG, et al. Effect of streptokinase, urokinase and tissue plasminogen activator on platelet aggregability and stability of platelet aggregates. *Cardiovasc Res* 1990; 67:1175–1181.
116. Fitzgerald D, Catella F, Roy L, et al. Marked platelet activation in vivo after intravenous streptokinase in patients with acute myocardial infarction. *Circulation* 1988;77:142–150.
117. Kleiman N, Ohman M, Califf R, et al. Profound inhibition of platelet aggregation with monoclonal antibody 7E3 fab following thrombolytic therapy: results of the TAMI 8 pilot study. *J Am Coll Cardiol* 1993;22:381–389.
118. White H, Van De Werf F. Thrombolysis for acute myocardial infarction. *Circulation* 1998;97:1632–1646.
119. Coulter S, Cannon C, Ault K, et al. High levels of platelet inhibition with abciximab despite heightened platelet activation and aggregation during thrombolysis for acute myocardial infarction: results from TIMI (Thrombolysis in Myocardial Infarction) 14. *Circulation* 2000;101:2690–2695.
120. Gurbel PA, Serebruany VL, Shustov AR, et al. Effects of reteplase and alteplase on platelet aggregation and major receptor expression during the first 24 hours of acute myocardial infarction treatment. *J Am Coll Cardiol* 1997;31:1466–1473.
121. Nordt TK, Moser M, Kohler B, et al. Augmented platelet aggregation as predictor of reocclusion after thrombolysis in acute myocardial infarction. *Thromb Haemost* 1998;80:881–886.
122. Herrick J. Clinical features of sudden obstruction of the coronary arteries. *JAMA* 1912;59:2015–2020.
123. DeWood M, Spores J, Notshe R, et al. Prevalence of total coronary occlusion during the early hours of transmural myocardial infarction. *N Engl J Med* 1980;303:897–902.
124. The GUSTO Trial Investigators. An international randomized trial comparing four thrombolytic strategies for acute myocardial infarction. *N Engl J Med* 1993;329:673–682.
125. Chesebro JH, Knaterud G, Roberts R, et al. Thrombolysis in acute myocardial infarction (TIMI) trial, phase 1: a comparison between intravenous plasminogen activator and intravenous streptokinase. *Circulation* 1987;76:142–154.
126. Verstraete M, Bleifeld W, Bory M, et al. Randomized trial of intravenous recombinant tissue-type plasminogen activator versus intravenous streptokinase in acute myocardial infarction. *Lancet* 1985;1:842–847.
127. Verstraete M, Bleifeld W, Brower R, et al. Double blind randomized trial of intravenous tissue-type plasminogen activator versus placebo in acute myocardial infarction. *Lancet* 1985; 2:956–969.
128. Sheehan FH, Braunwald E, Canner P, et al. The effect of intravenous thrombolytic therapy on left ventricular function: a report on tissue-type plasminogen activator and streptokinase from the thrombolysis in myocardial infarction (TIMI phase I) trial. *Circulation* 1987;75:817–829.
129. PTSG Group. Randomized double-blind trial of recombinant pro-urokinase against streptokinase in acute myocardial infarction. *Lancet* 1989;1:863–868.
130. (GISSI) Gruppo Italiano per lo Studio Steptokinasi nell'Infarto Miocardico. Effectiveness of intravenous thrombolytic treatment in acute myocardial infarction. *Lancet* 1986;1:397–402.
131. ISIS-2 (Second International Study of Infarct Survival) Group. Collaborative randomized trial of intravenous streptokinase, oral aspirin, both or neither among 17,187 cases of suspected acute myocardial infarction. *Lancet* 1988;2:349–360.
132. AIMS Trial Study Group. Effect of intravenous APSAC on mor-

tality after acute myocardial infarction: preliminary report of a placebo-controlled clinical trial. *Lancet* 1988;1:545–549.
133. Wilcox R, VanderLippe G, Olsson C, et al. Trial of tissue plasminogen activator for mortality reduction in acute myocardial infarction: Anglo-Scandinavia study of early thrombolysis (ASSET). *Lancet* 1988;2:525–530.
134. Morrison LJ, Verbeek PR, McDonald AC, et al. Mortality and prehospital thrombolysis for acute myocardial infarction: a meta-analysis. *JAMA* 2000;283:2686–2692.
135. Carnendran L, Steinberg J. Does an open infarct-related artery after myocardial infarction improve electrical stability. *Prog Cardiovasc Dis* 2000;42:439–454.
136. Six A, Louwerenburg H, Braams R, et al. A double-blind randomized multicenter dose-ranging trial of streptokinase in acute myocardial infarction. *Am J Cardiol* 1990;65:119–123.
137. Granger CB, White HD, Bates ER, et al. A pooled analysis of coronary arterial patency and left ventricular function after intravenous thrombolysis for acute myocardial infarction. *Am J Cardiol* 1994;74:1220–1228.
138. (GISSI) Gruppo Italiano per lo Studio Steptokinasi nell'Infarto Miocardico. Effectiveness of intravenous thrombolytic treatment in acute myocardial infarction. *Lancet* 1986;1:397–402.
139. The ISAM Study Group. A prospective trial of intravenous streptokinase in acute myocardial infarction (ISAM): mortality, morbidity, and infarct size at 21 days. *N Engl J Med* 1986;314: 1465–1471.
140. ISIS-2 (Second International Study of Infarct Survival) Collaborative Group. Randomised trial of intravenous streptokinase, oral aspirin, both or neither among 17,187 cases of suspected acute myocardial infarction: ISIS-2. *Lancet* 1988;2:349–360.
141. FTFCG Group. Indications for fibrinolytic therapy in suspected acute myocardial infarction: collaborative overview of early mortality and major morbidity results from all randomised trials of more than 1000 patients. *Lancet* 1994;343:311–322.
142. The TIMI Study Group. Thrombolysis in Myocardial Infarction (TIMI) trial phase I findings. *N Engl J Med* 1985;312: 932–936.
143. Granger C, Califf R, Topol EJ. Thrombolytic therapy for acute myocardial infarction. *Drugs* 1992;44:293–325.
144. Neuhaus R, VonEssen R, Tebbe U, et al. Improved thrombolysis in acute myocardial infarction with front-loaded administration of alteplase: results of the rt-PA-APSAC patency study (TAPS). *J Am Coll Cardiol* 1992;19:885–891.
145. GISSI-2, and International Study Group. Six-month survival in 20,891 patients with acute myocardial infarction randomized between alteplase and streptokinase with or without heparin. *Eur Heart J* 1992;13:1692–1697.
146. Third International Study of Infarct Survival (ISIS-3) Collaborative Group. ISIS-3: a randomized comparison of streptokinase versus tissue plasminogen activator versus anistreplase and of aspirin plus heparin versus aspirin alone among 41,299 cases of suspected acute myocardial infarction. *Lancet* 1992;339:753–770.
147. The GUSTO Angiographic Investigators. The effects of tissue plasminogen activator, streptokinase, or both on coronary-artery patency, ventricular function, and survival after acute myocardial infarction. *N Engl J Med* 1993;329:1615–1622.
148. Cannon CP, McCabe CH, Diver DJ, et al. Comparison of front-loaded recombinant tissue-type plasminogen activator, anistreplase and combination thrombolytic therapy for acute myocardial infarction: results of the Thrombolysis in Myocardial Infarction (TIMI) 4 trial. *J Am Coll Cardiol* 1994;24:1604–1610.
149. The COBALT Investigators. The continuous infusion versus double-bolus administration of alteplase (COBALT): a comparison of continuous infusion of alteplase with double-bolus administration for acute myocardial infarction. *N Engl J Med* 1997;337:1124–1130.
150. Mark DB, Hlatky M, Califf RM, et al. Cost effectiveness of thrombolytic therapy with tissue plasminogen activator as compared to streptokinase for acute myocardial infarction. *N Engl J Med* 1995;332:1418–1424.
151. Gurwitz JH, Gore JM, Goldberg RJ, et al. Risk for intracranial hemorrhage after tissue plasminogen activator treatment of acute myocardial infarction. *Ann Intern Med* 1998;129:597–604.
152. Bode C, Nordt TK, Peter K, et al. Patency trials with reteplase (r-PA): what do they tell us? *Am J Cardiol* 1996;78:16–19.
153. Smalling R, Bode C, Kalbfleisch J, et al. More rapid, complete, and stable coronary thrombolysis with bolus administration of reteplase compared with alteplase infusion in acute myocardial infarction. *Circulation* 1995;91:2725–2732.
154. Fox N, Cannon C, Berioli S, et al. Rates of serious bleeding events requiring transfusion in AMI patients treated with TNK-tPA. *J Am Coll Cardiol* 1999;33:279.
155. Barron HV, Fox N, Berioli S, et al. Comparison of intracranial hemorrhage rates in patients treated with rt-PA and TNKt-PA: impact of gender, age and low body weight. *Circulation* 1999; 100:I1.
156. Bar F, Meyer J, Vermeer F, et al. Comparison of saruplase and alteplase in acute myocardial infarction: SESAM Study Group; the study in Europe with saruplase and alteplase in myocardial infarction. *Am J Cardiol* 1997;79:727–732.
157. Tebbe U, Michels R, Adgey J, et al. Randomized, double-blind study comparing saruplase with streptokinase therapy in acute myocardial infarction: the COMPASS equivalence trial. *J Am Coll Cardiol* 1998;31:487–493.
158. den Heijer P, Vermeer F, Ambrosioni E, et al. Evaluation of a weight-adjusted single-bolus plasminogen activator in patients with myocardial infarction: a double-blind, randomized angiographic trial of lanoteplase versus reteplase. *Circulation* 1998; 98:2117–2125.
159. The In TIME-II Investigators. Intravenous NPA for the treatment of single-bolus lanoteplase vs accelerated alteplase for the treatment of patients with acute myocardial infarction. *Eur Heart J* 2000;21:2005–2013.
160. Armstrong P, Burton J, Palisaitis D, et al. Collaborative angiographic patency trial of recombinant staphylokinase (CAPTORS). *Am Heart J* 2000;139:820–823.
161. Markwardt F. Hirudin and its derivatives ad anticoagulant agents. *Thromb Haemost* 1991;66:141–152.
162. White H, Aylward P, Frey M, et al. Randomized, double-blind comparison of hirulog versus heparin in patients receiving streptokinase and aspirin for acute myocardial infarction (HERO). *Circulation* 1997;96:2155–2161.
163. Jang IK, Giugliano RP, Massey T, et al. A randomized, blinded study of two doses of Novastin (brand of argatroban) versus heparin as adjunctive therapy to recombinant tissue-plasminogen activator (accelerated administration) in acute myocardial infarction: rationale and design of the myocardial infarction using Novastin and T-PA (MINT) study. *J Thromb Thrombolysis* 1998;5:49–52.
164. Fung A, Lorch G, Cambier P, et al. Efegetran sulfate as an adjunct to streptokinase versus heparin as an adjunct to tissue plasminogen activator in patients with acute myocardial infarction. *Am Heart J* 1999;138:696–704.
165. Thrombin Inhibition in Myocardial Ischemia (TRIM) Group. A low molecular weight, selective thrombin inhibitor, inogatran, vs heparin, in unstable coronary artery disease in 1209 patients: a randomized, dose-finding study. *Eur Heart J* 1997; 18:1416–1425.
166. ISIS-2 (Second International Study of Infarct Survival) Collaborative Group. Randomised trial of intravenous streptokinase, oral aspirin, both, or neither among 17,187 cases of suspected acute myocardial infarction: ISIS-2. *Lancet* 1988;2:349–360.

167. Antman EM, Giugliano RP, Gibson CM, et al. Abciximab facilitates the rate and extent of thrombolysis: results of the thrombolysis in myocardial infarction (TIMI 4) trial. *Circulation* 1999;99:2720–2732.
168. The PARADIGM Investigators. Combining thrombolysis with the platelet glycoprotein IIa/IIIb inhibitor lamifiban: results of the Platelet Aggregation Receptor Antagonist Dose Investigation and reperfusion gain in myocardial infarction (PARADIGM). *J Am Coll Cardiol.* 1998;32:2003–2010.
169. Topol EJ. Toward a new frontier in myocardial perfusion therapy: emerging platelet preeminence. *Circulation* 1998;97: 211–218.
170. Strategies for Patency Enhancement in the Emergency Department (SPEED) Group. Trial of abciximab with and without low-dose reteplase for acute myocardial infarction: strategies for patency enhancement in the emergency department (SPEED). *Circulation* 2000;101:2788–2794.
171. McLean J. The thromboplastic action of cephalin. *Am J Physiol* 1912;41:250–257.
172. Weitz J, Hudoba M, Massel D, et al. Clot-bound thrombin is protected from inhibition by heparin-antithrombin III but susceptible to inactivation by antithrombin III-independent inhibitors. *J Clin Invest* 1990;86:385–391.
173. Bleich S, Nichols T, Schumacher R, et al. Effect of heparin on coronary arterial patency after thrombolysis with tissue plasminogen activator in acute myocardial infarction. *Am J Cardiol* 1990;66:1412–1417.
174. Hsia J, Hamilton W, Kleiman N, et al. A comparison between heparin and low-dose aspirin as adjunctive therapy with tissue plasminogen activator for acute myocardial infarction. *N Engl J Med* 1990;323:1433–1437.
175. Giugliano RP, Cutler S, Llevadot J. Risk of intracranial hemorrhage with accelerated tPA: importance of heparin dose. *Circulation* 1999;100:I650.
176. Ryan T, EM. A, Brooks N, et al. Update: ACC/AHA guidelines for the management of patients with acute myocardial infarction: a report of the American College of Cardiology/American Heart Association Task Force on Practice Guidelines (Committee on Management of Acute Myocardial Infarction). *J Am Coll Cardiol* 1999;34:890–911.
177. Kontny F, Dale J, Abildgaard U, et al. Randomized trial of low molecular weight heparin (dalteparin) in prevention of left ventricular mural thrombus formation and arterial embolism after acute myocardial infarction: the Fragmin in Acute Myocardial Infarction (FRAMI) Study. *J Am Coll Cardiol* 1997;39: 962–969.
178. Glick A, Kornowski R, Michowich Y, et al. Reduction of reinfarction and angina with the use of low-molecular-weight heparin therapy after streptokinase (and heparin) in acute myocardial infarction. *Am J Cardiol* 1996;77:1145–1148.
179. Vu T, Hung D, Wheaton V, et al. Molecular cloning of a functional thrombin receptor reveals a novel proteolytic mechanism of receptor activation. *Cell* 1991;64:1057–1068.
180. Rydel T, Ravichandran K, Tulinsky A, et al. The structure of a complex of recombinant hirudin and human-thrombin. *Science* 1990;249:277–280.
181. Lee L. Initial experience with hirudin and streptokinase in acute myocardial infarction: results of the Thrombolysis in Myocardial Infarction (TIMI) 6 trial. *Am J Cardiol* 1995;75:7–13.
182. Antman EM. Hirudin in acute myocardial infarction: thrombolysis and thrombin in Myocardial Infarction (TIMI) 9b trial. *Circulation* 1996;94:911–921.
183. Investigators in the Global Use of Strategies to Open Occluded Coronary Arteries (GUSTO), IIb. A comparison of recombinant hirudin with heparin for the treatment of acute coronary syndromes. *N Engl J Med* 1996;335:775–782.
184. Neuhaus K, von Essen R, Tebbe U, et al. Safety observations from the pilot phase of the randomized r-Hirudin for Improvement of Thrombolysis (HITT-III) study: a study of the Arbeirsgemeinschaft Leitender Kardiologischer Krankenhausarzte (ALKK). *Circulation* 1994;90:1638–1642.
185. Neuhaus KL, Molhoek GP, Zeymer U, et al. Recombinant hirudin (lepirudin) for the improvement of thrombolysis with streptokinase in acute myocardial infarction: results of the HIT-4 trial. *J Am Coll Cardiol* 1999;34:966–973.
186. Theroux P, Perez-Villa F, Waters D, et al. Randomized double-blind comparison of two doses of Hirulog with heparin as adjunctive therapy to streptokinase to promote early patency of the infarct related artery in acute myocardial infarction. *Circulation* 1995;91:2132–2139.
187. Fieschi C, Argentino C, Weschler L, et al. Clinical and instrumental evaluation of patients with ischemic stroke within the first six hours. *J Neurol Sci* 1989;91:311–322.
188. del Zoppo G, Poeck P, Pessin M. Recombinant tissue plasminogen activator in acute thrombotic and embolic stroke. *Ann Neurol* 1992;32:78–86.
189. Siesjo B. Pathophysiology and treatment of focal cerebral ischemia, I: pathophysiology. *J Neurosurg* 1992;77:169–184.
190. Levine S, Brott T. Thrombolytic therapy in cerebrovascular disorders. *Prog Cardiovasc Dis* 1992;34:235–262.
191. Brott T, Broderick J, Kothari R. Thrombolytic therapy for stroke. *Curr Opin Neurol* 1994;7:25–35.
192. Wardlaw JM, Warlow C. Thrombolysis in acute ischemic stroke: does it work? *Stroke* 1992;23:1826–1839.
193. The National Institute of Neurological Disorders and Stroke rt-PA Study Group. Tissue plasminogen activator for acute ischemic stroke. *N Engl J Med* 1995;333:1581–1587.
194. Hacke W, Kaste M, Fieschi C, et al. Intravenous thrombolysis with recombinant tissue plasminogen activator for acute hemispheric stroke: the European Cooperative Stroke Study (ECASS). *JAMA* 1995;274:1017–1025.
195. Hacke W, Kaste M, Fieschi C, et al. Randomized double-blind placebo controlled trial of thrombolytic therapy with intravenous alteplase in acute ischemic stroke (ECASS II): second European-Australian Acute Stroke Study Investigators. *Lancet* 1998;352:1245–1251.
196. Clark W, Wissman S, Albers G, et al. Recombinant tissue-type plasminogen activator (alteplase) for ischemic stroke 3-5 hours after symptom onset. *JAMA* 1999;282:2019–2026.
197. Clark W, Albers G, Madden K, et al. The rt-PA (alteplase) 0 to 6-hour acute stroke trial, Pt. A: results of a double-blind, placebo-controlled multicenter study: thrombolytic therapy in acute ischemic stroke study investigators. *Stroke* 2000; 31:811–816.
198. The Multicenter Acute Stroke Trial-Europe Study Group. Thrombolytic therapy with streptokinase in acute ischemic stroke. *N Engl J Med* 1996;335:145–150.
199. The Australian Streptokinase (ASK) Trial Study Group. Streptokinase for acute ischemic stroke with relationship to time of admission. *JAMA* 1996;276:961–966.
200. Multicenter Acute Stroke Trial-Italy (MAST-I) Group. Randomized controlled trial of streptokinase, aspirin and combination of both in treatment of acute ischemic stroke. *Lancet* 1995; 346:1509–1514.
201. del Zoppo G, Higashida R, Furlan R, et al. PROACT: a phase II randomized trial of recombinant pro-urokinase by direct delivery in acute middle cerebral artery stroke. *Stroke* 1998;29: 4–11.
202. Furlan A, Higashida F, Wechsler L, et al. A randomized trial of intra-arterial prourokinase for acute ischemic stroke due to middle cerebral artery occlusion. *JAMA* 1999;282:2003–2011.
203. Wardlaw J, Warlow C, Counsell C. Systematic review of evi-

dence of thrombolytic therapy for acute ischemic stroke. *Lancet* 1997;350:607.

204. Hacke W, Brott T, Caplan L, et al. Thrombolysis in acute ischemic stroke: controlled trials and clinical experience. *Neurology* 1999;53(suppl 4):S3–S14.
205. Albers G, Amarenco P, Easton D, et al. Antithrombotic and thrombolytic therapy for ischemic stroke. *Chest* 2001;119S: 300S–3320S.
206. Urokinase Pulmonary Embolism Trial. Urokinase pulmonary embolism: phase I results. *JAMA* 1970;214:2163–2172.
207. UPE: Urokinase Pulmonary Embolism Trial. Phase II results. *JAMA* 1974;229:1606–1613.
208. Marder V. The use of thrombolytic agents: choice of patient, drug administration, laboratory monitoring. *Ann Intern Med* 1979;90:802–808.
209. Goldhaber SZ, Kessler C, Heit J, et al. Randomised controlled trial of recombinant tissue plasminogen activator versus urokinase in the treatment of acute pulmonary embolism. *Lancet* 1988;2:293–298.
210. Immelman E, Jeffrey P. The post-phlebitic syndrome: pathophysiology prevention and management. *Clin Chest Med* 1984; 5:537.
211. Arnesen H, Hoiseth A, Ly B. Streptokinase or heparin in the treatment of deep vein thrombosis: results of a prospective trial. *Acta Med Scand* 1982;211:65.
212. Elliott M, Imelman E, Jeffrey P, et al. A comparative randomized trial of heparin versus streptokinase in the treatment of acute proximal venous thrombosis: an interim report of a prospective trial. *Br J Surg* 1979;66:383–843.
213. Watz R, Savidge G. Rapid thrombolysis and preservation of valvular venous function in high deep vein thrombosis. *Acta Med Scand* 1979;205:293–298.
214. Common H, Seaman A, Rosch J, et al. Deep vein thrombosis treated with streptokinase or heparin: follow-up of a randomized study. *Angiology* 1976;27:645–654.
215. Johanson L, Nylander G, Hedner U, et al. comparison of streptokinase with heparin: late results in the treatment of deep vein thrombosis. *Acta Med Scand* 1979;296:93–98.
216. Kakkar V, Lawrence DA. Hemodynamic and clinical assessment after therapy of acute deep vein thrombosis. *Am J Surg* 1985; 10:54–63.
217. Prandoni P, Lensing AW, Cogo A, et al. The long-term clinical course of acute deep venous thrombosis. *Ann Intern Med* 1996; 125:1–7.
218. Marder V, Sherry S. Thrombolytic therapy: current status. *N Engl J Med* 1988;318:1512–1520; 1585–1594.
219. Goldhaber SZ, Meyerovitz M, Green D, et al. Randomized controlled trial of tissue plasminogen activator in proximal deep venous thrombosis. *Am J Med* 1990;88:235–240.
220. Goldhaber SZ, Haire W, Feldstein M. Alteplase versus heparin in acute pulmonary embolism: randomized trial assessing right-ventricular function and pulmonary perfusion. *Lancet* 1993; 341:507–511.
221. Goldhaber SZ, Agnelli G, Levine MN. Reduced dose alteplase versus conventional alteplase for pulmonary thrombolysis: an international multicenter randomized trial: Bolus Alteplase Pulmonary Embolism Group. *Chest* 1994;106:718–724.
222. Meneveau N, Schiele F, Metz D, et al. Comparative efficacy of a two-hour regimen of streptokinase versus alteplase in acute massive pulmonary embolism: immediate clinical and hemodynamic outcome and one-year follow-up. *J Am Coll Cardiol* 1998;31:1057–1063.
223. Kostantinides S, Tiede N, Geibel A, et al. Comparison of alteplase versus heparin for resolution of major embolism. *Am J Cardiol* 1998;82:966–970.
224. Sharma G, Burleson V, Sasahara A, et al. Effect of thrombolytic therapy on pulmonary blood capillary blood volume in patients with pulmonary embolism. *N Engl J Med* 1980;303:842–845.
225. Tebbe U, Graf A, Kamke W, et al. Hemodynamic effects of double bolus reteplase versus alteplase infusion in massive pulmonary embolism. *Am Heart J* 1999;138:39–44.
226. Hyers T, Agnelli G, Hull RD, et al. Antithrombotic therapy for venous thromboembolic disease. *Chest* 2001;119S:176S–193S.
227. Verstraete M, Miller G, Bounameaux H, et al. Intravenous and intrapulmonary recombinant tissue-type plasminogen activator in the treatment of acute massive pulmonary embolism. *Circulation* 1988;77:353.
228. Dalen JE, Alpert JS. Thrombolytic therapy for pulmonary embolism: is it effective? is it safe? when is it indicated? *Arch Intern Med* 1997;157:2550–2556.
229. McConnell M, Solomon S, Rayan M, et al. Regional right ventricular dysfunction detected by echocardiography in acute pulmonary embolism. *Am J Cardiol* 1996;78:469–473.
230. Hirsh J, Hoak J. Management of deep vein thrombosis and pulmonary embolism: a statement for healthcare professionals. *Circulation* 1996;93:2212–2245.
231. Nasraway S, Kabani N, Lawrence K. Thrombolytic therapy for pulmonary embolism: reversal of shock in the early postoperative period. *Pharmacotherapy* 1994;14:616.
232. Severi P, LoPinto G, Poggio R, et al. Urokinase thrombolytic therapy of pulmonary embolism in neurosurgically treated patients. *Surg Neurol* 1994;42:469.
233. Mazeka P, Oakley C. Massive pulmonary embolism in pregnancy treated with streptokinase and percutaneous catheter fragmentation. *Eur Heart J* 1994;15:1281.
234. Kurkciyan I, Meron G, Sterz F, et al. Pulmonary embolism as a cause of cardiac arrest. *Arch Intern Med* 2000;160:1529–1535.
235. Bottinger B, Reim S, Diezel G, et al. High-dose bolus injection of urokinase: use during cardiopulmonary resuscitation for massive pulmonary embolism. *Chest* 1994;106:1281.
236. Schmitz-Rode T, Janssens U, Duda SH, et al. Massive pulmonary embolism: percutaneous emergency treatment by pigtail rotation catheter. *J Am Coll Cardiol* 2000;36:375–380.
237. Turpie AG, Levine M, Hirsh J, et al. Tissue plasminogen activator vs heparin in DVT: results of a randomized trial. *Chest* 1990;97:172S.
238. Arnesen H, Hoiseth A, Ly B. Streptokinase or heparin in the treatment of deep vein thrombosis: follow-up results of a prospective trial. *Acad Med Scand* 1982;211:65.
239. Camerota A, Aldridge S, Cohen G, et al. A strategy of aggressive regional therapy for acute iliofemoral venous thrombosis with contemporary venous thrombectomy or catheter-directed thrombolysis. *J Vasc Surg* 1994;20:244.
240. Semba C, Dake M. Iliofemoral deep venous thrombosis: aggressive therapy with catheter-directed thrombolysis. *Radiology* 1994;191:487.
241. Vehaeghe R, Stockx L, Lacroix H, et al. Catheter-directed lysis of iliofemoral vein thrombosis with the use of rt-PA. *Eur Radiol* 1997;7:996.
242. Bjarnason H, Kruse J, Azinger D, et al. Iliofemoral deep vein thrombosis: safety and efficacy outcome during 5 years of catheter-directed thrombolytic therapy. *J Vasc Intervent Radiol* 1997;8:405.
243. Mewissen M, Seabrook G, Meissner M, et al. Catheter-directed thrombolysis for lower extremity deep venous thrombosis: report of a national multicenter registry. *Radiology* 1999;211: 39.
244. Verstraete M, Vermylen J, Donati M. The effect of streptokinase infusion of chronic arterial occlusions and stenosis. *Ann Intern Med* 1971;74:377.
245. Cotton L, Flute P, Tsapogas M. Popliteal artery thrombosis treated with streptokinase. *Lancet* 1962;2:1081.

246. Amery A, Deloof W, Vermylen J, et al. Outcome of recent thromboembolic occlusion of limb arteries treated with streptokinase. *Br J Med* 1970;4:639.
247. Sicard G, Schier J, Totty W, et al. Thrombolytic therapy for acute arterial occlusion. *J Vasc Surg* 1985;2:65.
248. Hallet J, Greenwood L, Yrizzary J, et al. Statistical determinants of success and complications of thrombolytic therapy for arterial occlusion of lower extremity. *Surg Gynecol Obstet* 1985;161: 431.
249. Chaise L, Camerota A, Soulen R, et al. Selective intra-arterial streptokinase therapy in the immediate postoperative period. *JAMA* 1982;247:2397.
250. Hess H, Ingrisch H, Mietaschk A, et al. Local low-dose thrombolytic therapy of peripheral arterial occlusions. *N Engl J Med* 1982;307:1627.
251. Berni G, Bandyk D, Zierler R, et al. Streptokinase treatment of acute arterial occlusion. *Ann Surg* 1983;198:185.
252. Ouriel K, Shortell C, de Weese J, et al. A comparison of thrombolytic therapy with operative revascularization in the initial treatment of acute peripheral arterial ischemia. *J Vasc Surg* 1994; 19:1021.
253. Ouriel K, Veith F, Sasahara A, et al. A comparison of recombinant urokinase with vascular surgery as initial treatment for acute arterial occlusion of the legs. *N Engl J Med* 1998;338: 1105.
254. The STILE Investigators. Results of a prospective randomized trial evaluating surgery versus thrombolysis for ischemia of the lower extremity: the STILE Trial. *Ann Surg* 1994;220:251.
255. van Breda A, Robison J, Feldman L, et al. Local thrombolysis in the treatment of arterial graft occlusions. *J Vasc Surg* 1984;1: 103.
256. Gardiner GA Jr, Koltun W, Kandarpa K, et al. Thrombolysis of occluded femoropopliteal grafts. *AJR Am J Roentgenol* 1986; 147:621.
257. Belkin M, Belkin B, Bucknam C, et al. Intra-arterial fibrinolytic therapy: efficacy of streptokinase vs. urokinase. *Arch Surg* 1986; 121:769.
258. McNamara T, Fischer J. Thrombolysis of peripheral arterial and graft occlusions: improved results using high-dose urokinase. *AJR Am J Roentgenol* 1985;144:769.
259. Heymans S, Vanderschueren S, Verhaege R, et al. Outcome and one year follow-up of intra-arterial staphylokinase in 191 patients with peripheral arterial occlusions. *Thromb Haemost* 2000;83:666.
260. Marder VJ. Thrombolytic therapy: foundations and results. In: Colman R, Hirsh J, Marder VJ, et al., eds. *Hemostasis and thrombosis: basic principles and clinical practice.* 4th ed. Philadelphia: Lippincott Williams & Wilkins, 2001:1475–1495.
261. Kroger K, Buss D, Rudofsky G. Retrospective analysis of rt-PA thrombolysis combined with PGE1 in patients with peripheral arterial occlusions. *Angiology* 2000;52:377–383.
262. Murr K, Rhoney D, Coplin W. Urokinase in the treatment of intraventricular hemorrhage. *Ann Pharmacother* 1998;32: 256–258.
263. Lee W, Hill B, Harris EJ, et al. Surgical intervention is not required for all patients with subclavian vein thrombosis. *J Vasc Surg* 2000;32:57–67.
264. Urschel HC Jr, Razzuk MA. Paget-Schroetter syndrome: what is the best management? *Ann Thorac Surg* 2000;69:1663–1668; discussion 1668–1669.
265. Leebeek F, Lameris J, van Buren H, et al. Budd-Chiari syndrome, portal vein and mesenteric vein thrombosis in a patient homozygous for factor V Leiden mutation treated by TIPS and thrombolysis. *Br J Haematol* 1998;102:929–931.
266. Bhattacharjya T, Olliff S, Bhattacharlya S, et al. Percutaneous portal vein thrombolysis and endovascular stent for management of posttransplant portal venous conduit thrombosis. *Transplantation* 2000;69:2195–2198.
267. Silber H, Khan S, Matloff J, et al. The St. Jude valve: thrombolysis as the first line of therapy for cardiac valve thrombosis. *Circulation* 1993;87:30–37.
268. Shapira Y, Herz I, Vaturi M, et al. Thrombolysis is an effective and safe therapy in stuck mitral valves in the absence of high-risk thrombi. *J Am Coll Cardiol* 2000;35:1874–1880.
269. Stump D, Califf R, Topol EJ, et al. Pharmacodynamics of thrombolysis with tissue-type plasminogen activator: correlation with characteristics of and clinical outcomes in patients with acute myocardial infarction. *Circulation* 1989;80:1222.
270. Lee K, Mandell J, Rankin J, et al. Immediate versus delayed coronary grafting after streptokinase treatment. *J Thorac Cardiovasc Surg* 1988;95:216.
271. TIMI Research Group. Immediate versus delayed catheterization and angioplasty following thrombolytic therapy for acute MI: TIMI II A results. *JAMA* 1988;260:2849.
272. Francis G, Brenner B, Leddy J, et al. Angioedema during therapy with recombinant tissue plasminogen activator. *Br J Haematol* 1991;77:562.
273. Third International Study of Infarct Survival (ISIS-3) Collaborative Group. ISIS-3: a randomized comparison of streptokinase vs tissue plasminogen activator vs anistreplase and of aspirin plus heparin vs aspirin alone among 41,299 cases of suspected acute myocardial infarction. *Lancet* 1992;339:753–770.
274. Gore JM, Granger C, Simoons ML, et al. Stroke after thrombolysis: mortality and functional outcomes in the GUSTO-1 trial: global use of strategies to open occluded coronary artery. *Circulation* 1995;92:2811–2818.
275. Anderson J, Sorensen S, Moreno F, et al. Multicenter patency trial of intravenous anistreplase in acute myocardial infarction: theTEAM-2 Study Investigators. *Circulation* 1991;83:126–140.
276. International Joint Efficacy Comparison of Thrombolytics. Randomized, double-blind comparison of reteplase double-bolus administration with streptokinase in acute myocardial infarction (INJECT): trial to investigate equivalence. *Lancet* 1995;346:329–336.

Disorders of Thrombosis and Hemostasis: Clinical and Laboratory Practice, Third Edition, edited by Rodger L. Bick.
Lippincott Williams & Wilkins, Philadelphia © 2002

20

HEMOSTATIC FACTORS IN ATHEROTHROMBOTIC DISEASE

YALE S. ARKEL
DE-HUI W. KU

Arterial occlusive disease is intimately associated with the hemostatic system. The management of atherothrombotic disease includes the use of anticoagulants, antiplatelet agents, and fibrinolytic agents. One of the central pathways for the progression of arterial occlusive disease is the generation of tissue factor and the activation of the coagulation pathway. Although very defined hemostatic abnormalities have been associated with an increased risk for venous thrombosis, the associations in the arterial events are less clear.

Several studies looked at arterial occlusive events and the hemostatic system. We review some of the representative studies over the last few years, particularly those that have shown evidence for the association and give us some insight into the mechanism for the hemostatic role in the atherothrombotic process.

An epidemiologic survey, to assess the risk profiles of early and advanced atherosclerosis, was reported by Willeit et al. (1). In this study, approximately 1,000 subjects were recruited at ages 40 to 79; half were men; the subjects were followed up for 5 years (1990 through 1995). During this time, 62 died [26 of myocardial infarction (MI) and stroke]. Follow-up was completed in 826 subjects with a 96.5% completion rate. Among the risk factors related to the hemostatic system noted to be significant for early atherogenesis was lipoprotein a [Lp(a)] greater than 30 g/L, and, for advanced stenotic atherosclerosis, Lp(a), factor V gene mutation, high fibrinogen level, low antithrombin, and a high platelet count. One of the conclusions that can be drawn from the study is that some hemostatic factors, such as increased fibrinogen, factor V Leiden (FVL), increased platelet count, and Lp(a), may be related to progression of atherosclerotic disease and may predispose to the atherosclerotic process.

Hemostatic factors and the prediction of ischemic heart disease and stroke in patients with claudication were reported by Smith et al. (2). In a cohort study with a 6-year follow-up, the hemostatic and rheologic factors were correlated with incident ischemic heart disease (IHD), stroke, and peripheral arterial disease. Patients, 607, with intermittent claudication were evaluated. The median levels of fibrinogen, von Willebrand factor (vWF), tissue plasminogen activator (t-PA), D-dimer (DD), and whole blood viscosity were statistically higher in those who experienced a vascular event. After adjusting for age and sex, DD was associated with risk for nonfatal MI ($p < 0.01$). Fibrinogen and DD were associated with total coronary events ($p < 0.05$). The risk for stroke was related to t-PA and blood viscosity ($p < 0.05$ and 0.01). All the relations became weaker and nonsignificant when adjusted for cigarette smoking, systolic blood pressure (BP), glucose, and baseline IHD. This study revealed data that seem to be fairly consistent in other studies. Increased fibrinogen is an adverse finding with MI and peripheral arterial disease and is a persistent finding with arterial disease. The increased blood viscosity may be related to a degree to the fibrinogen level. Abnormalities in the fibrinolytic system have been noted in patients with progressive arterial disease. Although increased t-PA has been noted in this study, most other studies noted that the increase in plasminogen activator inhibitor 1 (PAI-1) levels correlated most with atherothrombotic disease.

Tracy et al. (The Cardiovascular Health Study) (3) assessed the relation of fibrinogen and factors VII and VIII to incident cardiovascular disease and death in the elderly. They recruited 5,201 patients, all 65 years or older. Their findings showed a definite relation to the development of cardiovascular disease with elevated factor VIII (FVIII) and fibrinogen. The FVII levels were less convincing. They found that fibrinogen was significantly associated with

Y. S. Arkel and D-H. W. Ku: Departments of Obstetrics/Gynecology and Maternal/Fetal Medicine, Thrombophilia Research Program, New York University School of Medicine, New York, New York.

coronary artery disease (CAD) events and stroke in men, with an increased mortality within 2.5 years. FVIII was significantly associated with CAD and mortality in men, and with women, there was an association with transient ischemic attack (TIA)/stroke. For both these factors, there was a higher percentage of patients who died. FVII was associated significantly with angina in men and with death in women. In general, the FVII was not consistently associated with cerebrovascular disease (CVD).

The authors concluded that the use of fibrinogen and FVIII assays might be of benefit in assessing risk for CVD and mortality. Araujo et al. (4), in a study of 100 random blood donors, 70 men and 30 women, median age of 41, and 52 consecutive and unrelated patients, 41 men and 11 women, median age 60, from North Portugal, and determined the genetic risk factors in acute coronary disease. The patients had a diagnosis of MI or unstable angina. They looked at FVL, PLA2, prothrombin gene mutation G20210A (PGM), and the polymorphism for the gene for methylenetetrahydrofolate reductase, MTHFR. There was a statistically significant finding of the PLA2 polymorphism in the patients. This was amplified in the patients younger than 60 years ($p < 0.05$ overall, and for the younger than 60 year group, $p < 0.025$).

These studies indicate that aspects of the hemostasis system and coagulation factors play a role in atherothrombotic disease. There is evidence that Lp(a) (which can affect the fibrinolytic process on the vessel surface), fibrinogen (which can enhance platelet reactivity, increase thrombin production and blood rheology), factor VIII (which can affect thrombin production), and PAI-1 (which can delay fibrinolysis), when increased, are risk factors for atherothrombotic disease.

Several investigators have assessed the occurrence of arterial occlusive events in the younger age group. Childhood stroke patients were studied for hypercoagulable markers (5). Infants and children aged 6 months to 16 years, with first onset of spontaneous ischemic stroke over a 3-year period, were compared with 148 consecutive white patients, median age, 4.5 years (6 months to 16 years) with a male-to-female ratio of 1:1.1. A control population of 296 age- and sex-matched white controls [potential bone marrow donors and those undergoing elective surgery; median age, 5 years (6 months to16 years)] were studied. There was a statistically significant occurrence of increased levels of Lp(a) and an increased incidence of FVL, PGM 20210A, and the mutation for MTHFR mutation in affected children. The findings are summarized in Table 20.1. There have been previous reports of little influence of FVL, protein C deficiency (PCD), and PGM20210A in arterial thrombosis, such as with MI and stroke (6–9), whereas other studies have suggested that a relation does exist in young patients with stroke (10–16). These studies reveal the importance of elevated Lp(a) as a risk factor for spontaneous stroke in childhood. Lp(a) previously was identified as an independent risk factor for both MI and atherothrombotic stroke in young adults.

TABLE 20.1. CHILDHOOD STROKE

Childhood Stroke	Patients	Controls	Significance
Single risk factor			
Lp(a) >30 mg/dL	26.4%	4.7%	<0.0001
FVL	20.2%	4%	<0.0001
PCD	6%	0.67%	0.001
PGM	6%	1.3%	0.01
MTHFR (TT677)	23.6%	10.4%	<0.0001
Combined risk factors			
FVL + Lp(a) >30 mg/dL	7.4%	0.3%	<0.0001
FVL + MTHFR (TT677)	3.3%	—	0.004

Data from refs. 5 and 13.
FVL, factor V Leiden; PCD, protein C deficiency; PGM, prothrombin gene mutation 20210A; MTHFR, gene mutation (TT677) for methylenetetrahydrofolate reductase; Lp(a), lipoprotein (a).

Lp(a) is a risk factor for venous thrombosis in childhood as well as for peripartum stroke in neonates. It has homology to plasminogen and has been shown to be associated with a decreased fibrinolytic activity. It is an independent risk factor for both MI and atherothrombotic stroke in young adults.

In this study, both the TT677 genotype of the MTHFR polymorphism and slightly elevated homocysteine (HCYT) were risk factors for stroke in childhood. The HCYT levels did not reach the level noted in adults with stroke. The data indicate that FVL, PGM, and PCD play a role in children and young adults with stroke.

In a separate study from Brazil, no significant relation to thrombophilic factors was noted in young whites with ischemic stroke. However, there was a trend to a relation with homozygous MTHFR-T in the patients of African origin (17).

In the adult population, the study of the FVL mutation and acute stroke is less convincing. Catto et al. (18) studied 386 patients with acute stroke for the FVL gene mutation and thrombin generation. FVL was not a factor in elderly adults with stroke. The marker of thrombin generation (PF1.2) is increased in acute stroke and at 3 months after the episode. This suggests that a prothrombotic state with increased thrombin generation is ongoing in stroke patients.

THE PROTEIN C SYSTEM (PROTEIN C, PROTEIN S, THROMBOMODULIN, AND ACTIVATED PROTEIN C)

Abnormalities in the protein C (PC) system have been noted in venous thrombosis and venous thromboembolism. The correlation with arterial disease is not as well established.

Esmon et al. (19) in a discussion of the PC system pointed out that the PC response is dependent on the generation of thrombin, and activated PC (APC) is initiated when thrombin binds to thrombomodulin (TM). The activation process takes place on the endothelial surface. The thrombin/TM complex is the activator of PC and has no ability to activate platelets or to clot fibrinogen. PC activation is enhanced when PC binds to the endothelial cell PC receptor (EPCR). This is accomplished by the increase in the affinity of the thrombin/TM complex for PC. The PC inhibitor and antithrombin rapidly inactivate the thrombin/TM complex. Once APC is formed, it proteolytically inactivates factors Va and VIIIa and limits thrombin production. Abnormalities in PS with FVL will increase the risk for thrombosis due to the decreased cleavage of factor V at Arg306 (20). Deficiencies in the TM or polymorphisms in the TM gene may result in an increased thrombotic risk. Alterations in the 5′ regulatory region of the TM gene have been reported with MI. As noted earlier, the APC system is involved in the control of the inflammatory response. The PC pathway is critical to preventing thrombosis in the microcirculation. EPCR is noted on the endothelial cell, with the greatest level of expression on the large vessels, with the arteries having higher levels. EPCR functions by providing the negatively charged phospholipid for PC to be activated. The involvement of the APC system in other aspects of the hemostatic process has been described. The profibrinolytic properties of APC have been suggested to be a direct function of APC. However, Bajzar et al. (21) demonstrated that the profibrinolytic effect of APC is due to the decrease in thrombin generation secondary to the effect of APC on factor Va and VIIIa. This results in less thrombin and subsequently less in thrombin-activated fibrinolysis inhibitor (TAFI) production. The decrease TAFI produces a fibrin molecule that is less resistant to lysis. This is thought to be the reason that factor XI–deficient patients have bleeding at sites that are richer in fibrinolytic enzymes, such as oral mucosa. Factor XI has a major effect on the generation of TAFI. Mizutani et al. (22) demonstrated the effect that APC has on the activation of leukocytes. In a rat renal perfusion model, they demonstrated that APC infusion prevented the ischemia/reperfusion (I/R) damage to the kidney in a manner independent of the anticoagulant effect but dependent on serine protease activity. The APC significantly inhibited the increase in tumor necrosis factor (TNF), interleukin-8, and myeloperoxidase. Their findings indicated that APC protects against I/R-induced renal injury by inhibiting the activation of leukocytes. APC therefore can affect the hemostatic process through mechanisms other than purely its anticoagulant properties in the degradation of factor Va and factor VIIIa. It affects the leukocyte inflammatory response and by downregulating thrombin generation and TAFI, it modulates the lysis of fibrin. The inflammatory process has been shown to be a major factor in the risk for coronary artery disease (94,97).

As has been noted, FVL is an inherited cause of resistance to activated protein C (APCR). However, other causes of APCR have been described. These may be due to other factor V gene polymorphisms, the R2 group, or acquired disorders such as the anticardiolipin syndrome.

The incidence of APCR in arterial disorders has been studied. Kiechl et al. (23), by using the standard commercial activated partial thromboplastin time (aPTT)-based Coatest (Chromogenix) looked at APCR as a predictor of advanced atherosclerosis and arterial disease in 826 subjects. In the patients being treated with warfarin, factor V–depleted plasma was used in the test. Their data revealed a strong independent association between APCR and risk for stenosis greater than 40% in carotid and/or femoral arteries ($p < 0.0001$). APCR also was a significant risk predictor of prevalent nonfatal CVD. Those with fatal CVD had significantly lower ratios for APCR than those with other causes of death or those alive with no CVD. This would indicate that APCR is a significant risk factor, when using the original aPTT test system, of arterial disease and should be included in the evaluation of arterial risk factors. The cause of the APCR in the non-FVL patients is unclear. They raised the possibility of an elevated FVIIII as an explanation for the APCR.

Nowak-Gottl et al. (13) found that the FVL mutation plays a role in childhood stroke. They looked at 14 infants over a 2-year period, neonates to age 18 years, who were treated for ischemic stroke. They noted that most of the strokes involved the left middle cerebral artery (eight of 14; three right middle cerebral, one vertebral, one cerebellar, and one posterior communicating). Three children had underlying cardiac disorders with major congenital defects; others had DM (one), mitochondrial disease (MELAS; one), and thrombotic thrombocytopenia purpura (one). Inherited thrombophilia was found in 10 of 14, with FVL in five, PC deficiency in three, and increased Lp(a) in two.

The authors concluded from their data that deficiencies in the PC system play an important role in the etiology of childhood stroke. The hemostatic factors require other triggering factors such as underlying diseases, central lines, or vascular damage after cardiac catheterization that may promote thromboembolism in infants and children who have inherited disorders of the clotting system.

It should be noted that, in this study, PGM 20210A was not assessed; neither was HCYT measured. We reported a young male with stroke who had been noted to have a mild PC deficiency. When evaluated in our laboratory, PGM 20210A was diagnosed. It was our thought that many of the previously reported strokes in youngsters with PC deficiency may have had other thrombophilic abnormalities, such as PGM 20210A, not as yet detected. We suggested that a combination of PC deficiency and PGM 20210A might be a stroke risk factor in younger patients (24).

Prothrombotic disorders in infants and children, newborns to 18-year-olds, with arterial ischemic stroke or sinovenous thrombosis and cerebral thromboembolism were studied by deVeber et al. (25). They found one or more abnormal results in 38% of the 92 patients and 21 of 35 had multiple abnormal tests: anticardiolipin antibodies in 33%, lupus inhibitor in 8%, an unusually high incidence of plasminogen deficiency was noted in 9.5%; APCR in 9%, PC deficiency in 7%, free PS deficiency in 11.5%, and antithrombin III (AT-III) deficiency in 12.5%. They did not separate the data of sinovenous versus arterial thrombosis. The number of patients with plasminogen abnormalities seems a bit high, as does the number of patients with low ATIII.

Simioni (26) reported a tendency to abnormal APCR and stroke in young patients using original aPTT-based assay for APCR. All the patients had FVL performed. They described three children with stroke from three different families who had FVL and APCR. They recommended case–control studies.

De Stefano et al. (27) looked at the PGM 202110A as a risk factor for cerebrovascular ischemic disease in patients younger than 50 years. They found a significantly higher incidence of PGM 20210A in the patients versus controls. The odds ratio (OR) for stroke with PGM was 5.1. A total of 72 patients was studied. Austrian children with stroke had a higher incidence of FVL, whereas the PGM 20210A did not seem to present a risk (28). Longstreth et al. (29) found that neither FVL nor PGM 20210A added to the risk of stroke in young women aged 18 to 44 years. Margaglione et al. (30) studied 202 patients younger than 50 years, 105 men and 97 women, with ischemic stroke. The median age was 39 years, and the range, 3 to 50 years. Patients with FVL and to a lesser extent MTHFR had an independently higher estimated risk of having a history of ischemic stroke. The FVL mutation is independently associated with the occurrence of ischemic stroke. The greater association in women suggests the possibility of an interaction of this genotype with female hormones. In addition to fibrinogen, hypertension, and smoking, the authors found an independent positive impact on stroke with FVL and to a smaller degree with MTHFR. When the gender of the patients was included, the FVL took on a more significant value for a risk factor. This report supports the findings in other studies, which indicated that thrombophilic factors such as FVL are important risk factors for stroke in younger patients, particularly in women, and more particularly in those who smoke. In this study, the PGM did not reach statistically significant values.

The impact of the altered ability to respond to thrombin with the activation of the APC system has been addressed in atherosclerotic animals. The impaired anticoagulant response to the infusion of thrombin in atherosclerotic monkeys was demonstrated to be associated with an acquired defect in the ability to stimulate the APC system (31). Monkeys fed an atherosclerosis-producing diet compared with controls had statistically less response to the thrombin infusion as compared with the control group. It was also noted that the atherosclerotic diet–fed monkeys had increased HCYT, and the use of B vitamins did not alter their response to thrombin. The authors concluded that in atherogenesis, there is altered ability to activate the natural APC anticoagulant system.

Contrary to some of these studies, Renner et al. (32) did not find an association of FVL or the PGM with peripheral arterial occlusive disease (PAOD). They studied 336 patients with documented PAOD. The patients' mean age was 68.7 years ± 9.7 years, which was significantly older than controls. The study found that PGM 20210A and FVL were not significantly different in the patients compared with the controls. In this study, the patient and control populations were not well matched.

Mansourati et al. (33) addressed the occurrence of coronary occlusive disease with normal-appearing vessels on angiography. They looked at the prevalence of FVL in a selected group of patients with MI and normal coronary angiograms and compared this group with normal controls and other patients with MI and significant coronary stenosis. All the groups were ethnically matched, with 244 MI and CAD patients screened. A total of 107 patients was included in the group with MI without CAD. Their results revealed that of the 400 controls, 5% had FVL, 244 patients with a premature MI and CAD, FVL was noted in 4.5%; and in 107 with MI and no CAD, 12.1% had FVL. The difference is statistically significant. The only other significant difference between both groups was a higher proportion of hypercholesterolemic patients in the CAD group. Normal coronary angiography with MI was found in 1% to 3% of the cases. It is most usually noted in younger patients with risk factors for CAD. Therapeutic implications are unclear, but further studies are indicated to assess whether anticoagulation treatment would be beneficial. Testing for FVL may well be in order for the younger patients with coronary occlusive disease, particularly in those without evidence of coronary vessel disease.

Lipoprotein (a) [Lp(a)] has been related to the onset of atherogenic disease. The level of Lp(a) is determined by apo(a) polymorphisms and is marginally affected by environmental factors. Increased levels of Lp(a) have been reported in CAD and ischemic stroke. The Lp(a) is thought to interfere with fibrinolysis and to promote thrombosis. Lp(a) accelerates atherogenesis.

Willeit et al. (34) evaluated the impact of Lp(a) in the development of carotid artery disease in asymptomatic patients. The patients studied were participants in the Bruneck Ischemic Heart disease and Stroke Prevention Study and were 1,000 men and women, aged 40 to 79 years, randomly selected. Logistic regression analysis revealed a significant ($p < 0.001$) binary association between Lp(a) and carotid artery disease. The threshold value is at 32 mg/dL. The OR with elevated Lp(a) was 4.7 for carotid stenosis. This was significantly greater than for nonstenosis, with a value of $p < 0.05$. High Lp(a) levels were more prevalent in CAD and PAOD. A synergistic effect of fibrinogen and Lp(a) on the occurrence of carotid atherosclerosis across the lower to medium fibrinogen levels was noted.

Tissue Factor Activity and Arterial Disease

Tissue factor activity (TFa) is one of the most important activators of the coagulation cascade and in particular is related to the events that occur in diseased arterial vessels. It is thought to play a central role in atheroma-induced thrombosis (35–39). Monocytes–macrophages (MO-MP) can generate TFa when stimulated by several agonists or inducers. Mulhfelder et al. (40) demonstrated that the contents of an atheromatous plaque could induce monocytes to generate TFa (40). Tissue factor is a lipidated integral membrane-bound glycoprotein with potent promoter activity of blood coagulation. TFa complexes with factor VII/VIIa to hydrolytically activate factor X and factor IX, which leads to increased formation of thrombin and the subsequent fibrin clot (41,42). TF messenger RNA (mRNA) and TF antigen have been detected in the adventitia of arteries. The adventitia is usually shielded from the blood elements. TFa has been induced in vitro in endothelial cells, and TF mRNA has been induced in the muscularis after balloon injury of the vessel. Two elements of the circulating blood cells that are implicated in plaque-induced thrombogenesis are the blood platelets and monocytes (MO). MO-MP may be induced to generate TFa and have a well-established thrombogenic activity. Bacterial endotoxin (lipopolysaccharide, LPS), antigen–antibody complexes, complement fragments, and lipoproteins can induce MO-TFa (43–48). MO-TFa occurs in vivo, as demonstrated in peripheral blood MOs in humans, and it was recently reported that MOs from patients with coronary ischemia bear TF antigen, in MP removed from atheromatous plaques have TFa. TFa has been obtained from coronary arteries at the time of surgery (49–53). TF is found in human atherosclerotic plaques within the extracellular lipid-rich core, macrophages, smooth muscle cells, adventitia, and endothelium. Blood TF antigen and activity increase progressively with unstable angina and MI. Khajuria and Houston (54) demonstrated the induction of MO-TF expression by homocysteine (54). They demonstrated that homocysteine at physiologic levels induces MO-TF and concluded that homocysteine is a cause for increased TF production and increases the risk for thrombosis. Muhfelder et al. (40) demonstrated that atheromatous plaque extracts may contain substantial amounts of TFa and that the plaques may induce MO-TFa. They further theorized that specific inhibition of TFa and MO-TF generation may be an appropriate form of anticoagulation during angioplasty.

MO-TF expression is enhanced in women who smoke and use oral contraceptives (OCs). Smoking compounds the risk of thromboembolism in women taking OCs. TF expression was measured by using mRNA and protein levels in unstimulated cells and LPS-stimulated cells. A clotting activity for TFa was used. The data indicated that the use of OCs and smoking are associated with an increase in MO-TF expression in premenopausal women. Further enhancement of TF in women who smoke and use OCs may explain the synergistic effect of smoking on the risk of thromboembolic events with OCs (55). The impact of TF activity in circulating MOs in thrombosis was studied in younger stroke patients (56). In this study, patients younger than 50 years were assessed. TF antigen was significantly increased in the patients with acute and chronic disease versus controls with $p < 0.01$ and $p < 0.05$, respectively. The TFa revealed increased values in the acute and chronic patients with $p < 0.05$ only for the acute-phase patients. The PF-1.2 and TAT were increased with statistical significance in the acute and chronic patients, with the DD showing a significant increase in the chronic group. The authors suggested that platelet activation contributes to MO-TF expression and would imply that antiplatelet drugs such as aspirin (ASA) might decrease the stroke risk. They suggested that the use of anti-TF antibodies may be of benefit in the acute stroke patient. The polymorphisms of the TF-promoter genes were assessed by Arnaud et al. (57). They found that the 1208-D haplotype is not associated with coronary thrombosis but is associated with reduced plasma TF levels and a lower risk of venous thrombosis.

The transfer of TF from leukocytes to platelets is mediated by CD15 and TF, as reported by Rauch et al. (58). They described thrombogenic TF on leukocyte-derived microparticles and their incorporation into human thrombi. The transfer of TF leukocyte-derived particles is dependent on the interaction of CD15 and TF with platelets. The antagonism of the interaction of CD15 with P-selectin and therefore the direct interaction of TF with platelets suggest a possible novel therapeutic approach to prevent thrombosis.

Marcucci et al. (59) studied the presence of TF and homocysteine levels in IHD with recurrence after angioplasty (59). In this study, they showed that TF, TFPI, and TAT levels are correlated with HCYT plasma levels in IHD, which provides evidence of an in vivo pathophysiologic mechanism of hyperhomocystinemia. The clinical recurrences and TF and HCYT values must be evaluated in larger numbers of patients.

Factor VII is the target of TF, and the TFa/FVIIa complex is the vehicle for the extrinsic pathway of coagulation activation. Factor VII has been extensively studied in relation to arterial thrombotic disease. FVIIa is positively correlated to serum triglycerides and less consistently to serum cholesterol and has been found in some studies to predict coronary heart disease. FVIIa has been found to be increased in acute coronary syndromes (60,61). Patients with combined hyperlipidemia commonly show changes in hemostatic variables associated with increased risk for developing thrombotic events.

These have been associated with increased procoagulant activity and with inhibition of the fibrinolytic potential. There is evidence that factor VII is activated to FVIIa during alimentary lipemia (62). However, a consistent correlation of FVII with arterial disease is not present.

Hyperhomocystinemia in Atherosclerosis

In the last two decades, a growing amount of interest has focused on mild-to-moderate hyperhomocystinemia as a risk factor of thromboembolic diseases. Two important features distinguish hyperhomocystinemia from other known risk factors for thrombosis: (a) it is associated with increased risk for both arterial and venous thrombosis; and (b) it may be corrected with safe and relatively inexpensive therapeutic approaches by dietary supplementation of folic acid and vitamin B complexes.

High homocysteine in the blood can arise from three primary causes. The first is a genetic defect that impairs homocysteine metabolism. Several different genetic defects have been identified, such as mutations in the MTHFR and cystathionine β-synthase (CBS) activities. Consuming too much methionine-rich food also can elevate homocysteine levels. Probably the most important contribution to an elevated homocysteine level is inadequate intake of folic acid, vitamins B complexes, and betaine.

The mechanisms by which hyperhomocystinemia might predispose to thrombosis are not fully understood. In vivo studies showed that homocysteine can cause desquamation of endothelial cells in baboons (63). In vitro studies showed that copper and oxygen were required in homocysteine-induced endothelial injury, which suggests that production of hydrogen peroxide is responsible for the toxic effect. Other studies showed that homocysteine can interfere with PC activation and TM expression (64 65), increase endothelial cell TF activity (66), inhibit t-PA binding (67), increase DNA synthesis in aortic smooth muscle cells (68), and impair generation of and decrease bioavailability of endothelium-derived relaxing factor/nitric oxide (69–71).

In 1969, McCully (72) first reported the presence of severe atherosclerotic lesions in patients with homocystinuria and hypothesized the pathogenic link between hyperhomocystinemia and atherogenesis (72). Several epidemiologic studies have confirmed his initial hypothesis by showing that mild to moderate hyperhomocystinemia also is associated with increased risk of cardiovascular disease (73,74). Since then, case–control and cross-sectional studies clearly indicated that mild to moderate hyperhomocystinemia is associated with increased risk of arterial thrombosis. However, the prospective studies of the association of hyperhomocystinemia and the risk of arterial disease in initial healthy subjects have given contrasting results. Therefore, additional studies are needed to clarify the relation between hyperhomocystinemia and arterial disease. Most important, randomized, placebo-controlled, double-blind trials of the effects of nutritional supplements on thrombotic risk reduction are needed.

Tissue Factor Pathway Inhibitor

TFPI plays an important role in the antithrombotic properties of vessel walls by inhibiting extrinsic pathway coagulation processes (75,76).

- Intravascular TFPI consists of free and Lp-bound forms.
- There is a circulating free form without carrier in preheparin and a heparin-releasable TFPI from endothelial cells.
- In animal studies, recombinant TFPI has prevented thrombosis.
- Increased TFPI has been observed in patients with MI (77).

TFPI has been demonstrated to be inversely correlated with high-density lipoprotein (HDL) cholesterol and postheparin lipoprotein lipase but proportional to apolipoprotein (a-II) (78).

The partial depletion of TFPI during subcutaneous (s.c.) administration of unfractionated heparin (UFH), but not with low-molecular-weight heparin (LMWH) was reported by Bendz et al. (79). TFPI is released to circulating blood after intravenous and s.c. injections of heparin. This may contribute to the antithrombotic effect of heparin. TFPI activity and antigen have been shown to be depleted after continuous infusion of heparin but not with s.c. administration of LMWH. In this study, a crossover experiment included the s.c. administration of UH and LMWH to 12 healthy normal subjects. The free TFPI antigen decreased 44% from baseline with UH twice daily on day 1 and to preinjection level on day 5. Free TFPI antigen decreased to 50%, 56%, and 27% on days 2, 3, and 5, respectively, compared with day 1. Minimal depletion was noted with the LMWHs. This may explain the differences noted between the UFH and LMWH in their antithrombotic effects.

Hemostatic risk factors for IHD were correlated with lifestyle in the Caerphilly Study (80). As has been previously shown, DD, t-PA antigen, vWF antigen, fibrinogen, and plasma viscosity were associated with subsequent IHD in men aged 49 to 65 years in the Caerphilly Study from South Wales. In this report, the contribution of lifestyle factors to the plasma levels of these factors for IHD was studied in 2,188 men. Most of the hemostatic variables increased with age and smoking. Increasing use of alcohol was associated with increases in t-PA and PAI-1, with decreases in fibrinogen and WBC. t-PA, PAI-1 fibrinogen, and viscosity were positively associated with body mass. This would be in line with the reported relation of fat cells with PAI-1, particularly in diabetics. Increased leisure-time activity associated inversely with DD, vWF, fibrinogen, and viscosity. t-PA, PAI-1 plasma viscosity were associated with blood pressure (BP), cholesterol, and triglycerides, but not with Lp(a) or HCYT. This study suggests that the hemostatic markers, which are associated with poor risk for IHD, can be affected by modifications in lifestyles. Folsom et al. (81) and the ARIC investigators examined the association of hemostatic variables with prevalent CVD and asymptomatic carotid artery atherosclerosis (81). Patients with CVD had 10 to 19 mg/dL higher fibrinogen concentrations compared with those without CVD. Factor VII was higher in the female patients with CVD. FVIII and vWF were higher in participants with CVD in all race- and sex-specific groups, although not always at $p < 0.05$. There was no association with PC, AT-III, or aPTT.

- In patients free of previous CVD, when an age-adjusted relation of carotid artery intimal medial wall thickness with hemostatic factors were assessed, the only consistent association was for fibrinogen.
- This was significantly greater in men versus women.
- Therefore fibrinogen is related to development of CVD by being

1. An important determinant of the amount of fibrin formed during thrombosis
2. A determinant of blood viscosity
3. A mediator of platelet aggregation.

- Many studies have shown that increased fibrinogen levels are associated with a greater occurrence of CAD, PAOD, TIA, stroke, and cardiovascular events in stroke survivors.
- This study of the positive correlation of fibrinogen and carotid disease in asymptomatic patients implies that fibrinogen is important in atherogenesis.
- The most important lifestyle determinant of fibrinogen is smoking, but the fibrinogen relation with carotid atherosclerosis is present in nonsmokers as well as smokers.

Factor VIII and von Willebrand Factor

The previously described study revealed that FVIII correlated with prevalent CVD but not with asymptomatic carotid artery disease. The findings were most notable for men with intermittent claudication. Other prospective studies reported factor VIII to be positively but nonsignificantly associated with coronary disease incidence and significantly associated with prevalent cerebrovascular disease. Other prospective data revealed an association of FVIII with ischemic events among vascular disease patients. vWF has been associated with clinical CVD but not with asymptomatic carotid atherosclerosis and may be involved more with the acute thrombotic component of CVD than with atherogenesis.

O'Donnell et al. (82) demonstrated that the elevation of FVIII:c in VTE is persistent and independent of the acute-phase response. There was no correlation between FVIII and either C-reactive protein (CRP) or fibrinogen. Increased FVIII levels after VTE are persistent, independent of the acute-phase reaction and may represent a constitutional risk factor for VTE. This raises the possible relation of the association of increased FVIII with thrombotic arterial disease.

Factor XI and Thrombosis

Meijers et al. (83) reported the increased levels of factor XI as a risk factor for venous thrombosis. The authors postulated that the elevated FXI leads to increased thrombin production on a long-term basis. The role of factor XI in coagulation is twofold: by generating thrombin, it contributes to the formation of fibrin and helps to protect fibrin from rapid proteolysis. They then postulated that high levels of factor XI with the secondary generation of thrombin leads to a prolonged downregulation of fibrinolysis by the effect of TAFI and therefore increases the risk of thrombosis. The enhanced risk when an elevated factor XI is combined with FVL, and increases in the levels of FVIII, prothrombin, and fibrinogen are compatible with data indicating an increased risk with multiple abnormalities. The elevated FVIII and prothrombin may increase the prothrombotic tendency by increasing thrombin generation.

Factor IX and Thrombosis

The relation of high levels of factor IX and the risk for venous thrombosis was reported by van Hylckama Vlieg et al. (84). They found a twofold to threefold increased risk for individuals with factor IX levels greater than 129%. The risk was higher in women. Overall the findings show that increased factor IX is a common risk factor for DVT. At present the relation to possible arterial disease has not been determined.

FIBRINOLYSIS AND ARTERIAL DISEASE

Significant data indicate a strong correlation of abnormalities in the components of the fibrinolytic system with arterial disease and atherothrombosis. Circadian fluctuations in the fibrinolytic factors may have relevance to the time of onset of MI, sudden death, and stroke (85).

Thrombin-activatable Fibrinolysis Inhibitor (Carboxypeptidase U)

Broze and Higuchi (86) described coagulation-dependent inhibition of fibrinolysis and the role of carboxypeptidase-U (CPU) in the premature lysis of clots in hemophilia plasma.

- Resistance to clot lysis by t-PA related to the amount of thrombin that is generated.

- Thrombin → activates carboxypeptidase → CPU (TAFI).
- The previously described increase in fibrinolysis by APC is probably due to the decrease in the thrombin generation with increased APC activity.
- TM enhances the thrombin activation of CPU more than 1,000-fold.
- In the study of Broze and Higuchi (86), the activity of CPU, due to thrombin, may in part explain the requirement of factors VIII, IX, and XI for sustained hemostasis.
- CPU-dependent inhibition of fibrinolysis is associated with a decrease in the generation of plasmin activity within the fibrin clot.
- CPU removes the lysine from the carboxy-terminal basic residues from fibrin polypeptides produced by plasmin.

TAFI levels and their influence in the clot-lysis time in healthy individuals was described by Mosnier et al. (87). TAFI is activated by relatively high concentrations of thrombin that exceed the thrombin concentration required for fibrin formation. The authors showed that the concentration of TAFI affects the rate of clot lysis. The data indicate that increased levels of TAFI might result in an increased risk for thrombosis, and decreased levels of TAFI might result in bleeding disorder. The variations of TAFI antigen in healthy subjects were assessed by Chetaille et al. (88). The broad range of antigen in normal subjects was 41% to 259%. Gender and pregnancy did not affect values. Data from our laboratory indicate that TAFI tends to increase during the trimesters of pregnancy. (unpublished data). There was a positive correlation of TAFI and age in female subjects. The TAFI levels were lower in African male patients compared with age-matched whites. In a study of patients undergoing coronary bypass surgery, increased levels of TAFI were noted in symptomatic men with coronary artery disease (89). In a rabbit arterial thrombolysis model, the effect of an inhibitor to TAFI activity (TAFI*a*), isolated from the potato tuber, was assessed in conjunction with t-PA. The results indicated that inhibitors of TAFI*a* might comprise novel and very effective adjuncts to t-PA and improve thrombolytic therapy to achieve clot lysis and vessel patency. The use of both agents did not adversely affect blood pressure, aPTT, TT, fibrinogen, or α_2-antiplasmin concentrations. More data are necessary to understand the degree of importance of TAFI in arterial thrombosis and atherothrombosis. However, we may consider the contribution of TAFI to delayed fibrinolysis, and in combination with other components of the lytic system, such as PAI-1, as being integral to the thrombotic process.

Plasminogen Activator Inhibitor-1

Kohler and Grant (90) reviewed the subject of PAI-1 and coronary artery disease. We summarize some of their comments.

The association of high levels of PAI-1 with the suppression of fibrinolysis has been associated with the development of MI. Further evidence of the involvement of the lytic pathway in MI is the finding of elevated t-PA and DD as risk factors for MI (90). PAI-1 is a fast-acting inhibitor of the plasminogen activation process. It is produced by the vascular endothelium, is present in platelets, and is an important regulatory component of fibrinolysis. The other antifibrinolytic is α_2-antiplasmin, which is a specific plasmin inhibitor bound to polymerizing fibrin by activated FXIII. Thrombin stimulates platelet release of PAI-1 to the platelet surface. Thrombin stimulates the synthesis of PAI-1 in endothelial cells. PAI-1 binds to fibrin and so retains its inhibitory activity to t-PA and u-PA. t-PA increases fibrinolysis during the early stages of fibrin formation on ruptured atherosclerotic plaques, whereas fully formed fibrin, with highly polymerized and cross-linked fibrin, is resistant to lysis by t-PA.

The association of PAI-1 with CAD is supported by the finding of high plasma levels of PAI-1 associated with thrombotic disorders. PAI-1 is noted to be an independent risk factor for reinfarction for those younger than 45 years. There is an association of CAD with low fibrinolytic activity. The European Concerted Action on Thrombosis and disabilities study revealed high plasma levels of PAI-1 activity and antigen associated with angina pectoris. The association decreased after adjustment for insulin resistance, body mass, and serum triglycerides and cholesterol. A Swedish study revealed a high prevalence of CAD with high PAI-1 and with predictive value for the first occurrence of an MI. High PAI-1 predicts subsequent MI with stable angina and is associated with angiographic evidence of progressive CAD in young men with a history of MI. Patients with diabetes mellitus type 2 (DM-2) have increased amounts of PAI-1 in their atheromatous plaques. Increased mRNA for PAI-1 is noted in severely atherosclerotic arteries compared with normal arteries. Interventions that reduce insulin resistance and cause weight loss are accompanied by a reduction in PAI-1. Control of hyperglycemia decreases plasma PAI-1 activity in DM-2. Postmenopausal women receiving estrogen have lower PAI-1 levels than those not receiving hormone-replacement therapy (HRT). Premenopausal women have lower PAI-1 levels than do postmenopausal women. Angiotensin II stimulates production of PAI-1 in cultured endothelial cells and vascular smooth muscle cells. Inhibition of the angiotensin-converting enzyme may limit progression of cardiovascular disease by reducing PAI-1 concentrations.

These findings suggest that PAI-1 could play a direct role in the development of advanced atherosclerotic plaque.

The effect of local PAI-1 overexpression in rat carotid arteries was shown to enhance endothelial regeneration while inhibiting intimal thickening. Hasenstab et al. (92) reported that the laboratory model, in which the denuded luminal surface of rat carotid artery smooth muscle cells transduced with replication-defective retrovirus encoding rat PAI-1, resulted in localized gene overexpression of PAI-1. This was associated with increased mural thrombus accumulation at 4 days but decreased neointimal area by 30% and 25% at 1 and 2 weeks, respectively. PAI-1 overexpression does not alter matrix accumulation at 1 week. Increased PAI-1 expression in the rat artery enhances thrombosis and endothelial regeneration while inhibiting intimal thickening. These results suggest that PAI-1 could play a direct role in the development of advanced atherosclerotic plaque and in the repair of the diseased vessel after fibrous cap disruption.

Factor XIII and Thrombolysis

Factor XIIIa bonds are covalently introduced into the fibrin structure that causes an irreversible end-to-end fusion of fibrin particles (93).

A therapeutic aim for thrombotic tendencies would be to block the factor XIIIa–mediated reactions in a controlled manner without interfering with the primary clotting time. Cross-linking inhibitors can reduce clot stiffness and resistance to lysis. This can enhance greatly the susceptibilities of thrombi for digestion by lytic agents. A protein isolated from a giant Amazon leech has been described to possess similar properties. Positive results have been obtained with a monoclonal antibody directed against the thrombin cleavage site of factor XIII, which blocked the activation of the zymogen.

SUMMARY

This survey lists but a few of the studies that have addressed the issues related to the hemostatic system and arterial thrombosis (Fig. 20.1). Obviously the voluminous literature related to the use of the antithrombotic agents would require a much more extensive discussion, beyond the scope of this chapter.

The existing data indicate that hemostatic factors play a major role in the pathophysiology of arterial atherothrombotic disease. There is strong evidence that increased fibrinogen, PAI-1, and factor VIII have predictive value. The

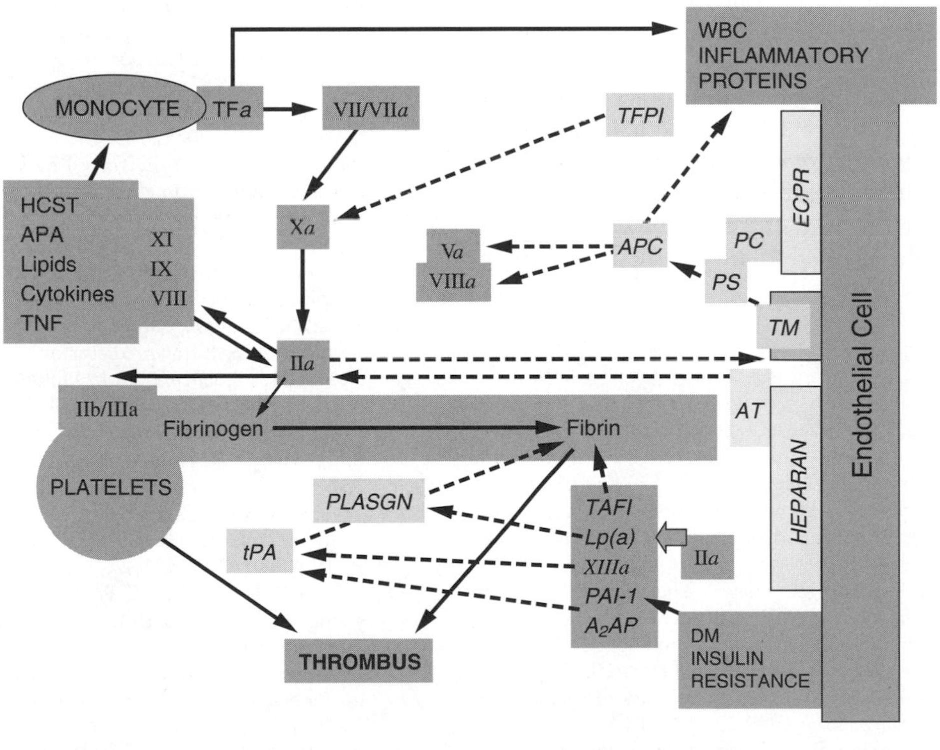

FIGURE 20.1. Major hemostatic factors demonstrated to be involved in the atherothrombotic process. *VII*, factor VII; *TFPI*, tissue factor pathway inhibitor; *APC*, activated protein C; *V*, factor V; *VIII*, factor VIII; *XI*, factor XI; *IX*, factor IX; *X*, factor X; *HCYT*, homocysteine; *APA*, antiphospholipid antibody; *TNF*, tumor necrosis factor; *PC*, protein C; *PS*, protein S; *TM*, thrombomodulin; *EPCR*, endothelial protein C receptor; *AT*, antithrombin; *IIa*, thrombin; *XIIIa*, activated factor XIII; *TAFI*, thrombin activatable fibrinolysis inhibitor; *PAI-1*, plasminogen activator inhibitor-1; α_2AP, α_2-antiplasmin; *IIbIIIa*, platelet glycoprotein IIb/IIIa; (*a*), activated factor; *Lp(a)*, lipoprotein (a); *PLASGN*, plasminogen; *DM*, diabetes mellitus.

thrombophilia abnormalities such as factor V Leiden and PGM 20210A most likely are factors in selected patient groups in which there are other risk factors at play. There are convincing data that younger women who smoke are at greater risk for arterial thrombosis, particularly coronary, when there is a thrombophilia abnormality. The data suggesting that resistance to APC is associated with progression of arterial disease and arterial occlusive events require further exploration. There are sufficient findings to suggest that the APC system is involved in the atherothrombotic process. The recent data related to TAFI increase the speculation that fibrin that is resistant to lysis may be an important contributor to the arterial lesion. One can speculate that a combination of increased TAFI, PAI-1, and a down-regulated APC system could be involved in some patients with atherothrombotic disease. The expanding number of abnormalities in the hemostatic system may make it more appropriate to study the patient thought to be at risk for arterial disease with an expanded array of tests that monitor the prothrombotic and fibrinolytic systems. The relation of the inflammatory process and CVD has been noted in several studies (94–98). The impacts of the inflammatory proteins and activated white cells on the hemostatic and thrombotic pathways are now being studied, but data already clearly indicate a strong interrelation, as we indicated in the section on TF. Obviously the justification for testing will depend on further studies and the development of standardized and reliably informative assays. Several gene polymorphisms for platelet antigens and other coagulation-related proteins have been reported in some of the arterial diseases. To date their impact is marginal. We need functional assays that reflect the imbalance of the hemostatic system and possibly its interaction with the inflammatory proteins and leukocytes.

REFERENCES

1. Willeit J, Kiechl S, Oberhollenzer F, et al. Distinct risk profiles of early and advanced atherosclerosis: prospective results from the Bruneck Study. *Arterioscler Thromb Vasc Biol* 2000;20:529–537.
2. Smith FB, Rumley A, Lee AJ, et al. Haemostatic factors and the prediction of ischaemic heart disease and stroke in claudicants. *Br J Haematol* 1998;100:758–763.
3. Tracy R, Arnold AM, Etinger W, et al. The relationship of fibrinogen and factors VII and VIII to incident cardiovascular disease and death in the elderly: results from the Cardiovascular Health Study. *Arterioscler Thromb Vasc Biol* 1999;19:1776–1783.
4. Araujo F, Santos A, Araujo V, et al. Genetic risk factors in acute coronary disease. *Haemostasis* 1999;29:212–218.
5. Nowack-Gottl U, Strater R, Heinecke A, et al. Lipoprotein (a) and genetic polymorphisms of clotting factor V, prothrombin, MTHFR are risk factors of spontaneous ischemic stroke in childhood. *Blood* 1999;94:3678–3682.
6. Catto A, Carter A, Ireland H, et al. FV Leiden and thrombin generation in relation to the development of acute stroke. *Arterioscler Thromb Vasc Biol* 1995;15:783.
7. Press RD, Liu XY, Beamer N, et al. Ischemic stroke in the elderly. *Stroke* 1996;27:44.
8. Martinelli I, Franchi F, Akwan S, et al. The PGM is not associated with cerebral ischemia [Letter]. *Blood* 1997;90:3806.
9. Longstreth WT, Rosendaal FR, Siscovick DS, et al. Risk of stroke in young women and FVL and PGM. *Stroke* 1998;29:577.
10. DeVeber G, Monagle P, Chan A, et al. Prothrombotic disorders in infants and children with cerebral thromboembolism. *Arch Neurol* 1998;55:1539.
11. Gansean V, Kelsey H, Cookson J, et al. Activated protein C resistance in childhood stroke [Letter]. *Lancet* 1996;347:260.
12. Simioni P, DeRonde H, Prandoni P, et al. Ischemic stroke in young patients with activated protein C resistance: a report of three cases belonging to three different kindreds. *Stroke* 1995; 26:885.
13. Nowak-Gottl U, Strater R, Dubbers A, et al. Ischemic stroke in infancy and childhood: role of FV Leiden. *Blood Coagul Fibrinolysis* 1996;7:684.
14. Zenz W, Bodo Z, Plotho J, et al. Factor V Leiden and PGM in children with stroke. *Thromb Haemost* 1998;80:763.
15. Halbmayer WM, Haushofer A, Herman KM, et al. PGM: a risk factor for juvenile stroke? Result of a pilot study. *Blood Coagul Fibrinolysis* 1998;9:209.
16. De Stefano V, Chiusolo P, Paciaroni K, et al. PGM is a risk factor for cerebrovascular ischemic disease in young patients. *Blood* 1998;91:3562.
17. Voetsch B, Damasceno BP, Camargo ECS, et al. Inherited thrombophilia as a risk factor for the development of ischemic stroke in young adults. *Thromb Haemost* 2000;83:229–233.
18. Catto A, Carter A, Ireland H, et al. *Arterioscler Thromb Vasc Biol* 1995;15:783.
19. Esmon CT, Xu J, Gu JM, et al. Endothelial protein C receptor. *Thromb Haemost* 1999;82:251–258.
20. Giri TK, Yamazaki T, Sala N, et al. Deficient APC-cofactor activity of protein S Heerlen in degradation of factor Va Leiden: a possible mechanism of synergism between thrombophilic risk factors. *Blood* 2000;96:523–531.
21. Bajzar L, Nesheim ME, Tracy PB. The profibrinolytic effect of activated protein C in clots formed from plasma is TAFI-dependent. *Blood* 1996;88:2093–2100.
22. Mizutani A, Okajima K, Uchiba M, et al. Activated protein C reduces ischemic/reperfusion-induced renal injury in rats by inhibiting leukocyte activation. *Blood* 2000;95:3781–3787.
23. Kiechl S, Muigg A, Santer P, et al. Poor response to APC as a prominent risk factor predictor of advanced atherosclerosis and arterial disease. *Circulation* 1999;99:614–619.
24. Arkel Y, Ku D, Gibson D, et al. Ischemic stroke in a young patient with protein C deficiency and prothrombin gene mutation G20210A. *Blood Coagul Fibrinolysis* 1998;9: 757–760.
25. deVeber G, Monagle P, Chan A, et al. Prothrombotic disorders in infants and children with cerebral thromboembolism. *Arch Neurol* 1998;55:1539–1543.
26. Simino P, de Rhonde H, Prandoni P, et al. Ischemic stroke in young patients with activated protein C resistance. *Stroke* 1995; 26:885–890.
27. De Stefano V, Chiusolo P, Pascorini K, et al. PGM is a risk factor for cerebrovascular ischemic disease in young patients. *Blood* 1998;91:3562–3565.
28. Zenz W, Bodo Z, Plotho J, et al. FVL and PGM in children with ischemic stroke. *Thromb Haemost* 1998;80:763–766.
29. Longstreth WT, Rosendaal FR, Siscovick DS, et al. Risk of stroke in young women and FVL and PGM. *Stroke* 1998;29:577–580.
30. Margaglione M, D'Andrea G, Giuliani N, et al. Inherited prothrombotic conditions and premature ischemic stroke. *Arterioscler Thromb Vasc Biol* 1999;19:1751–1756.
31. Lentz SR, Fernandez JA, Griffen J, et al. Impaired anticoagulant response to infusion of thrombin in atherosclerotic monkeys

associated with acquired defects in the protein C system. *Arterioscler Thromb Vasc Biol* 1999;19:1744–1750.
32. Renner W, Koppel H, Brodmann M, et al. PGM and FVL and peripheral arterial occlusive disease. *Thromb Haemost* 2000;83: 20–22.
33. Mansourati J, DaCosta A, Munier S, et al. Prevalence of factor V Leiden in patients with MI and normal coronary angiography. *Thromb Haemost* 2000;83:822–825.
34. Willeit J, Kiechl S, Santer P, et al. Lipoprotein(a) and asymptomatic carotid artery disease: evidence of a prominent role in the evolution of advanced carotid plaques: the Bruneck Study. *Stroke* 1995;26:1582–1587.
35. Constantinides P. Plaque fissures in human coronary thrombosis. *J Atheroscler Res* 1966;6:1–17.
36. Davies MJ, Thomas AC. Plaque fissuring: the cause of acute MI, sudden ischemic death, and crescendo angina. *Br Heart J* 1985; 53:363–373.
37. Fuster V, Badimon L, Badimon JJ, et al. The pathogenesis of coronary artery disease and the acute coronary syndromes: parts 1 and 2. *N Engl J Med* 1992;326:242–250, 310–318.
38. Levin DC, Fallon JT. Significance of the angiographic morphology of localized coronary stenosis: histopathologic correlations. *Circulation* 1982;66:316–320.
39. Ross R. Atherosclerosis: a defense mechanism gone awry. *Am J Pathol* 1993;143:987–1002.
40. Muhfelder T, Teodorescu V, Rand J, et al. Human atheromatous plaque extracts induce tissue factor activity in monocytes and also express constitutive TFa. *Thromb Haemost* 1999;81:146–150.
41. Nemerson Y. Tissue factor and hemostasis. *Blood* 1988;71:1–8.
42. Osterud B, Rapaport SI. Activation of factor IX by the reaction product of TF and factor VII: additional pathway for initiating blood coagulation. *Proc Natl Acad Sci U S A* 1977;74:5260–5264.
43. Niemetz J, Fani K. Role of leukocytes in blood coagulation and the generalized Schwartzman reaction. *Nat New Biol* 1971;232: 247–248.
44. Niemetz J. The coagulant activity of leukocytes: tissue factor activity. *J Clin Invest* 1972;51:307–313.
45. Rothberger H, Zimmerman TS, Spielgelberg HL, et al. Leukocytes procoagulant activity: enhancement of production in vitro by IgG and antigen-antibody complexes. *J Clin Invest* 1977;59: 549–557.
46. Muhlfelder T, Niemetz J, Kreutzer Beebe D, et al. C5 chemotactic fragment induces leukocyte production of tissue factor activity-link between complement and coagulation. *J Clin Invest* 1981;67:1614–1622.
47. Levy GA, Schwartz BS, Curtiss LK, et al. Plasma lipoprotein induction and suppression of the generation of cellular procoagulant activity in vitro: requirements for cellular collaboration. *J Clin Invest* 1981;67:1614–1622.
48. Schwartz BS, Levy GA, Curtiss LK, et al. Plasma lipoprotein induction and suppression of the generation of cellular procoagulant activity in vitro: two procoagulant activities are produced by peripheral blood mononuclear cells. *J Clin Invest* 1981;67: 1650–1658.
49. Thiagarajan P, Niemetz J. Procoagulant-tissue factor activity of circulating peripheral blood leukocytes: results of in vivo studies. *Thromb Res* 1980;17:891–896.
50. Osterud B, Glaegstad T. Increased tissue thromboplastin activity in monocytes of patients with meningococcal infection. *Thromb Haemost* 1983;49:5–7.
51. Leatham PM, Tooze JA, Camm AJ. Increased monocyte factor expression in coronary disease. *Br Heart J* 1995;73:10–13.
52. Tipping PA, Malliarros J, Holdworth SR. Procoagulant activity expression by macrophages from atheromatous vascular plaques. *Atherosclerosis* 1989;79:237–243.
53. Marmur JD, Thiruviikraman SV, Fyfe BS, et al. Identification of active tissue factor in human coronary atheroma. *Circulation* 1996;94:1226–1232.
54. Khajuria A, Houston DS. Induction of monocyte tissue factor expression by homocysteine: a possible mechanism for thrombosis. *Blood* 2000;96:966–972.
55. Kapplemayer J, Berecki D, Misz M, et al. Monocytes express tissue factor in young women who smoke and use oral contraceptives. *Thromb Haemost* 1999;82:1614–1620.
56. Kapplemayer J, Berecki D, Misz M, et al. Monocytes express tissue factor in young patients with cerebral ischemia. *Cerebrovasc Dis* 1998;8:235–239.
57. Arnaud E, Barbalat V, Nicaud V, et al. Polymorphisms in the 5′-regulatory region of the TF gene and the risk of MI and venous thromboembolism: the ECTIM and PATHROS Studies. *Arterioscler Thromb Vasc Biol* 2000;20:892–898.
58. Rauch U, Bonderman D, Bohrmann B, et al. Transfer of tissue factor from leukocytes to platelets is mediated by CD15 and tissue factor. *Blood* 2000;96:170–175.
59. Marcuci R, Prisco D, Brunelli T, et al. Tissue factor and HCYT levels in ischemic heart disease are associated with angiographically documented clinical recurrences after angioplasty. *Thromb Haemost* 2000;83:826–832.
60. Ruddock V, Meade TW. FVII activity and ischemic heart disease. *Am J Med* 1994;87:403–406.
61. Hamsten A, Wiman B, deFaire B, et al. Increased plasma levels of rapid inhibitory tissue plasminogen activator in young survivors of MI. *N Engl J Med* 1985;313:1557–1563.
62. Silveira A, Karpe F, Blomback M, et al. Activation of coagulation factor VII during alimentary lipemia. *Arterioscler Thromb* 1994; 14:60–90.
63. Harker LA, Ross R, Slichter SJ, et al. Homocystine-induced arteriosclerosis: the role of endothelial cell injury and platelet response in its genesis. *J Clin Invest* 1976;58:731–741.
64. Rodgers GM, Conn MT. Homocysteine, an atherogenic stimulus, reduces protein C activation by arterial and venous endothelial cells. *Blood* 1990;75:895–901.
65. Lentz SR, Sadler JE. Inhibition of thrombomodulin surface expression and protein C activation by the thrombogenic agent homocysteine. *J Clin Invest* 1991;88:1906–1914.
66. Fryer RH, Wilson BD, Gubler DB, et al. Homocysteine, a risk factor for premature vascular disease and thrombosis, induces tissue factor activity in endothelial cells. *Arterioscler Thromb* 1993; 13:1327–1332.
67. Hajjar KA. Homocysteine-induced modulation of tissue plasminogen activator binding to its endothelial cell membrane receptor. *J Clin Invest* 1993;91:2873–2879.
68. Tsai J-C, Perrella MA, Yoshizumi M, et al. Promotion of vascular smooth muscle cell growth by homocysteine: a link to atherosclerosis. *Proc Natl Acad Sci U S A* 1994;91:6369–6373.
69. Stamler JS, Osborne JA, Jaraki O, et al. Adverse vascular effects of homocysteine are modulated by endothelium-derived relaxing factor and related oxides of nitrogen. *J Clin Invest* 1993;91: 308–318.
70. Welch GN, Upchurch GR Jr, Loscalzo J. Hyperhomocysteinemia and atherothrombosis. *Ann N Y Acad Sci* 1997;811:48–58.
71. Upchurch GR Jr, Welch GN, Fabian AJ, et al. Homocysteine decreases bioavailable nitric oxide by a mechanism involving glutathione peroxidase. *J Biol Chem* 1997;272:17012–17017.
72. McCully KS. Vascular pathology of homocysteinemia: implications for the pathogenesis of atherosclerosis. *Am J Pathol* 1969; 56:111–128.
73. D'Angelo A, Selhub J. Homocysteine and thrombotic disease. *Blood* 1997;90:1–11.
74. Refsum H, Ueland PM, Nygard O, et al. Homocysteine and cardiovascular disease. *Annu Rev Med* 1998;49:31–62.
75. Novotny WF. TFPI. *Semin Thromb Hemost* 1994;20:101–108.

76. Broze GJ. TFPI. *Thromb Haemost* 1995;74:90–93.
77. Sandset PM, Sirnes PA, Abildgaard U. Factor VII and extrinsic pathway inhibitor in acute coronary disease. *Br J Haematol* 1989; 72:391–396.
78. Kawaguchi A, Miyao Y, Noguchi T, et al. Intravascular free TFPI is inversely correlated with HDL cholesterol and postheparin lipoprotein lipase but proportional to apolipoprotein A-II. *Arterioscler Thromb Vasc Biol* 2000;20:251–258.
79. Bendz B, Hansen JB, Andersen TO, et al. Partial depletion of TFPI during administration of subcutaneous unfractionated heparin and not with LMWH. *Br J Haematol* 1999;107: 756–762.
80. Yarnell JWG, Sweetnam PM, Rumley A, et al. Lifestyle and hemostatic risk factors for IHD: the Caerphilly Study. *Arterioscler Thromb Vasc Biol* 2000;20:271–279.
81. Folsom AR, Wu Kenneth K, Shahar E, et al. Association of hemostatic variables with prevalent cardiovascular disease and asymptomatic carotid artery atherosclerosis. *Arterioscler Thromb* 1993;13:1829–1836.
82. O'Donnell J, Mumford AD, Manning RA, et al. Elevation of FVIII:C in VTE is persistent and independent of acute phase response. *Thromb Haemost* 2000;83:10–13.
83. Meijers JCM, Tekelenburg WLH, Bouma BN, et al. High levels of coagulation factor XI as a risk factor for venous thrombosis. *N Engl J Med* 2000;342:696–701.
84. van Hylckama Vlieg A, van der Linden IK, Bertina RM, et al. High levels of factor IX increase the risk of venous thrombosis. *Blood* 2000;95:3678–3682.
85. Andreotti F, Davies GJ, Hackett DR, et al. Major circadian fluctuations in fibrinolytic factors and possible relevance to time of onset of MI, sudden death and stroke. *Am J Cardiol* 1988;62: 635–637.
86. Broze GJ, Higuchi DA. Coagulation-dependent inhibition of fibrinolysis: role of carboxypeptidase-U and the premature lysis of clots from hemophilia plasma. *Blood* 1996;88:3815–3823.
87. Mosnier LO, von dem Borne PA, Meijers JCM, et al. Plasma TAFI levels influence the clot lysis time in healthy individuals in the presence of an intact intrinsic pathway of coagulation. *Thromb Haemost* 1998;80:829–835.
88. Chetaille P, Alessi MC, Kouassi D, et al. Plasma TAFI antigen variations in healthy subjects. *Thromb Haemost* 2000;83: 902–905.
89. Silveira A, Schatteman K, Goosens F, et al. Plasma procarboxypeptidase U in men with symptomatic coronary artery disease. *Thromb Haemost* 2000;84:364–368.
90. Kohler HP, Grant PJ. Plasminogen-activator inhibitor type 1 and coronary artery disease. *N Engl J Med* 2000;342:1792–1801.
91. Deleted.
92. Hasenstab D, Lea H, Clowes AW. Local PAI-1 over expression in the rat carotid artery enhances thrombosis and endothelial regeneration while inhibiting intimal thickening. *Arterioscler Thromb Vasc Biol* 2000;20:853–859.
93. Laszlo L. Research on clot stabilization provides clues for improving thrombolytic therapies: Sol Sherry lecture in thrombosis. *Arterioscler Thromb Vasc Biol* 2000;20:2–9.
94. Ridker PM, Hennekens CH, Buring JE, et al. C-reactive protein and other markers of inflammation in the prediction of cardiovascular disease in women. *N Engl J Med* 2000;342:836–843.
95. Gussekloo J, Schaap MCL, Frohlich M, et al. CRP is a strong but nonspecific risk factor of fatal stroke in elderly persons. *Arterioscler Thromb Vasc Biol* 2000;20:1047–1051.
96. Ford ES, Giles WH. Serum CRP and self-reported stroke. *Arterioscler Thromb Vasc Biol* 2000;20:1052–1056.
97. Strandberg TE, Tilvis RS. CRP, cardiovascular risk factors, and mortality in a prospective study in the elderly. *Arterioscler Thromb Vasc Biol* 2000;20:1057–1060.
98. Mosorin M, Surcel HM, Laurila A, et al. Detection of *Chlamydia pneumoniae*-reactive T lymphocytes in human atherosclerotic plaques of carotid artery. *Arterioscler Thromb Vasc Biol* 2000;20: 1061–1067.

Disorders of Thrombosis and Hemostasis: Clinical and Laboratory Practice, Third Edition, edited by Rodger L. Bick.
Lippincott Williams & Wilkins, Philadelphia © 2002

SUBJECT INDEX

Note: Page numbers followed by f indicate figures; page numbers followed by t indicate tables.

A

Abciximab, for hereditary thrombophilic disorders, 287, 287t
ABG analysis. *See* Arterial blood gas (ABG) analysis
Acidosis, in DIC, 147
ACLAs. *See* Anticardiolipin antibodies (ACLAs)
Actinomycin D, hemostasis effects of, 275
Activated partial thromboplastin time (aPTT)
  in factor V defects, 120
  in factor X defects, 125
  in factor XI defects, 125–126
  in fibrinogen defects, 118
  in hemophilia A, 122
  in prothrombin defects, 119
Activated protein C (APCR), in atherosclerosis, 423
Activation, intrinsic, 11, 11f
Acute myocardial infarction (AMI), 283–284
  clinical trials in, 405–407
  thrombolytic therapy for, 397, 404, 404t
  thromboprophylaxis in, 330–331
Acute spinal cord injury, paralysis associated with, deep venous thrombosis after, prevention of, 341
Adenylate cyclase
  inhibition of, thromboxane A_2 in, 8
  stimulation of, prostacyclin in, 8
Adhesion molecules, in hemostasis, 23–24, 24t
Afibrinogenemia, congenital, 117t, 118–119, 118t
Age
  as factor in hemolytic–uremic syndrome, 98
  as factor in primary thrombocythemia, 109
Aggregation defects, secondary, 61, 62t
Aggregation pattern, platelet, normal, 82–83, 83f
Aggregometer(s), described, 82
Alopecia, heparin and, 373
Alport syndrome, 93
Alteplase
  in acute myocardial infarction, 404t
    clinical trials of, 405–406
  clinical applications of, 411t
Amniotic fluid embolism (AFE), syndrome of, 139–140
  causes of, 140–141, 141t
  characteristics of, 141, 141t
  diagnosis of, 143–144
  incidence of, 140
  management of, 144–148, 144t, 145t, 148f
  maternal deaths due to, 140
  pathophysiology of, 141–143, 142f, 143f
    hemostasis, 142–143, 142f
    pulmonary, 142
  risk factors associated with, 140–141, 141t
  signs and symptoms of, 141
Amyloidosis, 40t, 46t, 47–48
Anagrelide, for primary thrombocythemia, 110
Anaphylaxis, heparin and, 371
Anemia
  aplastic, 94, 94t
  correction of, 172
Anesthesia/anesthetics, platelet dysfunction due to, 71t
Angina pectoris
  stable, aspirin in, clinical trials of, results of, 387–388
  unstable, aspirin in, clinical trials of, results of, 387, 388t
Angiography
  CT, in pulmonary embolus evaluation, 258
  pulmonary, in pulmonary embolus evaluation, 258
Anistreplase
  in acute myocardial infarction, 404t
  clinical applications of, 411t
  structure, function, and pharmacology of, 399–400, 403t
Antibiotic(s), platelet dysfunction due to, 70, 70t
Antibody(ies)
  to activated protein C, 238
  anticardiolipin, and thrombosis. *See* Anticardiolipin antibodies (ACLAs)
  anti–factor IX, acquired, 228
  antiphospholipid, 303–304, 303t
    subtypes of, detection of, 314, 314t, 315f
  anti–von Willebrand factor, detection of, 232–233
  to prothrombin, 237–238
  "subgroup," and thrombosis, 307–310
Anticardiolipin(s)
  and autoimmune collagen disease, 309
  and cardiac disease, 308
  and cutaneous manifestations, 308
  and neurologic syndromes, 309
  and obstetric syndromes, 309–310
  and venous–arterial thrombosis, 308
Anticardiolipin antibodies (ACLAs)
  detection of, 313, 313t
  syndromes of thrombosis associated with, 310–311, 311t, 312t
  and thrombosis, 307–310
Anticardiolipin thrombosis syndrome, miscellaneous disorders and, 310
Anticoagulant(s)
  circulating. *See* Blood coagulation inhibitors
  heparan sulfate, 237
  heparin-like, 237
  for hereditary thrombophilic disorders, 286–288, 286t, 288t
  lupus
    detection of, 313–314
    and thrombosis, 304–307. *See also* Lupus anticoagulant (LA)–thrombosis syndrome
  oral, 349–357. *See also* Warfarin
    adverse effects of, 354
    after first episode of deep venous thrombosis, optimal duration of, 352–353
    alternative approaches to, 355
    antidote to, 355
    for cardiovascular disorders, 353–355
    long-term, in patients requiring surgery, 354–355
    for recurrent deep venous thrombosis, optimal duration of, 352–353
    in thromboprophylaxis, 340
    for venous thromboembolism, 352
    in venous thromboembolism prevention, 353
Anticoagulant management clinics, 355
Antiembolic arm exercises, for deep venous thrombosis, 336
Antiembolic leg exercises, for deep venous thrombosis, 336
Anti–factor IX antibodies, acquired, 228
Antigen(s), von Willebrand, 1
Anti-inflammatory drugs, platelet dysfunction owing to, 71t
Antineoplastic therapy
  for thrombocytopenia, intensity of, 95, 95t
  for thrombosis in malignancy, 266
Antiphospholipid antibodies, subtypes of, detection of, 314, 314t, 315f
Antiphospholipid syndromes, 303–304
  classification of, 310–311, 311t, 312t
  clinical presentations of, 312, 312t
  drugs associated with, 312, 312t
  laboratory diagnosis of, 313–314, 313t, 314t, 315f
  prevalence of, 313
Antiphospholipid thrombosis syndromes (APL-TS), 303–304, 303t
α_2-Antiplasmin, in plasmin activity inhibition, 17–18, 18f
α_2-Antiplasmin defects, 128, 128t
Antiplatelet activity, evaluation of, 81–82
Antiplatelet therapy, 379–395. *See also specific drug, e.g.,* Aspirin
  in acute myocardial infarction, clinical trials of, 407
  clinical trials of, results of, 383–391, 384t, 385t, 387f, 388t, 390t
  for hereditary thrombophilic disorders, 287, 287t
  pharmacology of, 379–383, 380f, 381f
Antithrombin deficiency, 291–292
  acquired, 316
Antithrombin therapy, in acute myocardial infarction, clinical trials of, 407–408
Antithrombin–heparin inhibitor activity, 21, 21f
Antithrombotic drugs, costs of, 328, 328t
Antithrombotic therapy, oral, 349–357. *See also* Anticoagulant(s), oral; Warfarin
Anti–von Willebrand factor antibody, detection of, 232–233
Aplastic anemia, 94, 94t
aPTT. *See* Activated partial thromboplastin time (aPTT)
Ardeparin, characteristics of, 362t

Arm exercises, antiembolic, for deep venous thrombosis, 336
Arterial blood gas (ABG) analysis, in pulmonary embolus evaluation, 257
Arterial catheters, thrombohemorrhagic complications of, 201
Arterial occlusive disease, hemostatic factors in, 421–432. *See also* Atherothrombotic disease, hemostatic factors in
Arterial thrombosis, risk factors for, 262t
Arthroscopic surgery, deep venous thrombosis after, treatment of, 337
L-Asparaginase therapy, hemostasis effects of, 274–275
Aspirin
  for acquired thrombophilia, 318t
  in acute myocardial infarction, clinical trials in, 407
  after vascular surgery, clinical trials of, results of, 383, 384t
  brand names of common drugs containing, 71t
  in cerebrovascular disease, clinical trials of, results of, 386
  clinical trials of, results of, 383–388, 384t, 385t, 387f, 388t
  in coronary heart disease, clinical trials of, results of, 386
  costs of, 328, 328t
  for hereditary thrombophilic disorders, 287, 287t, 288t
  in myocardial infarction, clinical trials of, results of, 386, 387f
  in PAOD, clinical trials of, results of, 383, 386
  platelet dysfunction due to, 71t
  platelet function inhibition by, 379–381
  as platelet-function inhibitor, 46–47
  in prevention of new vascular occlusions in patients with PAOD, clinical trials of, results of, 385–386, 385t
  in prevention of reocclusions after percutaneous transluminal angioplasty, clinical trials of, results of, 383, 385, 385t
  in stable angina pectoris, clinical trials of, results of, 387–388
  in unstable angina, clinical trials of, results of, 387, 388t
Aspirin-like effect, hereditary, 60t, 63–64, 63f, 63t
Atherosclerosis
  hyperhomocystinemia in, 426
  risk factors for, 421
Atherothrombotic disease
  hemostatic factors in, 421–432
    clinical studies of, 421–422
    factor VIII, 427
    fibrinolysis, 427–429, 429f
    historical background of, 421–422
    PAI-1, 428–429, 429f
    protein C system, 422–425
    tissue factor activity, 425–426
    tissue factor pathway inhibitor, 426–427
    von Willebrand factor, 427
Athrombia, essential, 60t, 61, 61t
Atrial fibrillation, ischemic stroke in patients with, prevention of, oral anticoagulants in, 353
Autoimmune collagen disease, anticardiolipins and, 309
Autoimmune disorders, 40t, 46t, 48, 49t
Autoplex, 221
Azathioprine, for acquired coagulation factor VIII inhibitors, 223, 223t

B

Behçet syndrome, 49–50
Bernard–Soulier syndrome, 60t, 61, 61t, 93
  platelet defects in, 84
Bleeding
  epidural, heparin and, 373–374
  heparin and, 360–361, 371, 373–374
Blood coagulation inhibitors
  acquired, 213–249. *See also specific inhibitor, e.g.,* Coagulation factor VIII inhibitors
    antibodies and inhibitors for prothrombin, 237–238
    antibodies and inhibitors of activated protein C, 238
    circulating heparan–heparin-like anticoagulants, 237
    factor IX inhibitors, in hemophilia B, 228
    factor V inhibitors, 234–237
    factor VIII inhibitors, 214–225
    factor XI inhibitors, 225–227
    factor XIII inhibitors, 238–239
    von Willebrand disease, 228–234
  defined, 213
  diagnosis of, 213–214
  presence of, indicators of, 213
Blood coagulation system, inhibitors affecting. *See* Blood coagulation inhibitors
Blood protein/platelet defects, thrombosis due to, 326, 327t
Blue sclerae syndrome, 40t, 42, 42t
Bone marrow transplantation, hemostasis and, 275
Brittle bones syndrome, 40t, 42, 42t
Burn victims, DIC in, 147

C

C3a, in hemostasis, 23
C5a, in hemostasis, 23
Caffeine, in phosphodiesterase inhibition, 6, 8
Cancer
  mortality due to, 325
  prostate, thrombosis in, 266
CAPRIE study, results of, 388
γ-Carboxyglutamic acid (calcium-binding group), 14, 15f
Carboxypeptidase, in atherosclerosis, 428
Cardiac disease, anticardiolipins and, 308
Cardiac surgery
  bleeding due to, prevention of, 190–191, 191t
  defects in, 197–198
  DIC in, 195–196
  isolated coagulation factor defects in, 195, 196f
  platelet dysfunction in, 64t, 66–67, 66f, 67f, 193–195, 194f
  primary fibrinolysis, 196–197
  thrombocytopenia during, 191–193, 192f
Cardiopulmonary bypass (CPB) surgery
  hemorrhage in
    diagnosis of, 198–199, 198t, 199t
    management of, 200
  hemostasis in, pathophysiology of, 198, 198t
  platelet counts during, 192, 192f
  platelet dysfunction in, 64t, 66–67, 66f, 67f
  vascular defects associated with, 50
Cardiovascular bypass surgery, thrombotic and hemorrhagic problems during, 177–211
Cardiovascular diseases
  DIC and, 147–148
  increased platelet consumption or destruction effects on, thrombocytopenia due to, 101
  treatment of, oral anticoagulants in, 353–355
Cardiovascular procedures, thrombotic and hemorrhagic problems during, 177–211
Catheter(s)
  arterial, thrombohemorrhagic complications of, 201
  thrombosis related to, malignancy-related, 275–276, 276f, 277t
  venous, thrombohemorrhagic complications of, 201
Cerebrovascular disease, aspirin in, clinical trials of, results of, 386
Cerebrovascular thrombosis, 284
  incidence of, 284
  thrombolytic therapy for, clinical trials in, 408–409
Chédiak–Higashi syndrome, 61
Chemotherapy
  cytoreductive agents in, for primary thrombocythemia, 109–110
  hemostasis effects of, 274–275
Chest radiography, in pulmonary embolus evaluation, 255–256, 257
Children, stroke in, 422, 422t
Chimeric agents, 403
Christmas disease, 123–124, 124t
Chromosome location, coagulation factor information by, 10, 10t
Chronic renal failure
  bleeding manifestations in, 170
  pathogenesis of, 170–171, 170t
  in uremic patients, 171, 171t
Cilostazol
  clinical trials of, results of, 389
  platelet function inhibition by, 382
Cirrhosis
  Laënnec-type, in Osler–Weber–Rendu disease, 45

liver, 165–168, 165t, 167t. *See also* Liver cirrhosis
Clopidogrel
for acquired thrombophilia, 318t
clinical trials of, results of, 388–389
for hereditary thrombophilic disorders, 287, 287t, 288t
side effects of, 389
Coagulation, kinins and, 20, 20f, 21f
Coagulation factor(s)
chromosomal location containing, information related to, 10, 10t
information related to, chromosomal location containing, 183t
synonyms for, 9–10, 10t, 182, 183t
Coagulation factor disorders
hereditary, 117–137. *See also specific disorder*
α_2-antiplasmin defects, 128, 128t
causes of, 117
clinical manifestations of, 117
detection of, 117
factor IX defects, 123–124, 124t
factor V defects, 117t, 119–120, 120t
factor VII defects, 120–121, 120t, 121t
factor VIII:c defects, 121–123, 121t–123t. *See also* Hemophilia A
factor X defects, 124–125, 125t
factor XI defects, 125–126, 126t
factor XII (Hageman factor) defects, 126, 126t
factor XIII defects, 128–129, 129t
fibrinogen defects, 117–119, 117t, 118t
kininogen defects, 127, 127t
Passovoy deficiency, 133
plasminogen activator inhibitor defects, 128, 128t
prekallikrein defects, 127, 127t
prothrombin defects, 119, 119t
pseudo–von Willebrand disease, 133
rare defects, 133
types of, 117t
von Willebrand disease, 129–133, 130t, 131t
isolated, in cardiac surgery, 195, 196f
Coagulation factor IX, and thrombosis, 427
Coagulation factor IX inhibitors, in hemophilia B, 228
Coagulation factor IXa
formation of, 182–183
generation of, 10, 10f
Coagulation factor V, defined, 234
Coagulation factor V Cambridge, 289
Coagulation factor V Hong Kong, 289
Coagulation factor V HR2 haplotype, 289
Coagulation factor V inhibitors, 234–237
bovine thrombin and, 235–236
conditions associated with, 236
defined, 234
features of, 235
historical background of, 234
postoperative, 235–236
treatment of, 236–237
Coagulation factor V Leiden, 288–289
Coagulation factor VII, 11–12
Coagulation factor VIII, and von Willebrand factor, in atherosclerosis, 427
Coagulation Factor VIII Inhibitor Bypassing Activity (FEIBA)–VH, 221
Coagulation factor VIII inhibitors, 214–225
acquired, 215–219, 217t
management of, 223–225, 223t
immunosuppressive therapy in, 223–224, 223t
initial approach to, 223
detection of, general approach to, 214–215
disorders associated with, 217t
hemophilia A patients with, acute bleeding in, management of, 222t, 224
pregnancy-related, 219–220
treatment of, 220–223, 222t
Coagulation factor Xa
formation of, 183–184
generation of, 11–12, 11f, 12f
Coagulation factor XI
defined, 225
and thrombosis, 427
Coagulation factor XI inhibitors, 225–227
Coagulation factor XII (Hageman factor), 290
activation of, 10, 10f
Coagulation factor XII (Hageman factor)–dependent activation of fibrinolysis, 15, 17, 17f
Coagulation factor XIII, and thrombolysis, 429, 429f
Coagulation factor XIII inhibitors, 238–239
Coagulation factors, 9–10, 10t
Coagulation protein system, 9–15, 9t, 10f, 10t, 11f–16f, 14t
factor IXa generation, 10, 10f
factor Xa generation, 11–12, 11f, 12f
fibrin generation, 14–15, 15f, 16f
in hemostasis, 182–184, 183t, 184f, 185f
thrombin generation, 12–14, 12f–14f, 14t
Coagulation reactions, stoichiometry in, 13–14, 13f
Coagulopathy(ies), consumptive. *See* Disseminated intravascular coagulation (DIC)
Cocaine, in antiphospholipid thrombosis syndrome, 312t
Complement activation, and hemostasis, 18–19, 19f, 186–187, 187t
Complement system, 19f, 186, 187f
Compression stockings, graduated, in thromboprophylaxis, 340
Compression ultrasonography, real-time B-mode, in deep venous thrombosis evaluation, 256
Computed tomographic angiography (CTA), spiral, in pulmonary embolus evaluation, 258
Congenital dysfibrinogenemia, 290
Congenital marrow infiltrative disorders, 93
Congenital platelet-production defects, thrombocytopenia due to, 92–93, 92t
Congestive splenomegaly. *See* Hypersplenism
Consumptive coagulopathy. *See* Disseminated intravascular coagulation (DIC)
Contraceptive(s), oral, estrogen-containing, deep venous thrombosis after, prevention of, 343
Contrast venography, ascending, in deep venous thrombosis evaluation, 257
Coronary artery thrombosis, 283–284
incidence of, 283
mortality rates in, 283
Coronary heart disease, aspirin in, clinical trials of, results of, 386
Cyclooxygenase, in platelet function, 182
Cyclophosphamide, for acquired coagulation factor VIII inhibitors, 224, 223t
Cytokine(s), in hemostasis, 23
Cytoreductive chemotherapeutic agents, for primary thrombocythemia, 109–110
Cytosine arabinoside, hemostasis effects of, 275

D

Dalteparin, characteristics of, 362t
Deep vein thrombosis. *See* Deep venous thrombosis (DVT)
Deep venous thrombosis (DVT), 251–264, 327–329, 328t, 329t. *See also* Pulmonary embolus (PE)
causes of, 251–252, 283
defects associated with, 283
diagnosis of, 251
ascending contrast venography in, 257
laboratory studies in, 258–259
MRI in, 257
patient history in, 252–253, 259f, 260f
physical examination in, 253–256, 259f, 260f
real-time B-mode compression ultrasound in, 256
real-time B-mode ultrasound with color Doppler in, 256–257
strategies in, 259–262, 259f–262f, 262t
first episode of, oral anticoagulants after, optimal duration of, 352–353
incidence of, 283, 325, 326t, 327
lower extremity, diagnosis of, 251, 252t
presentation of, 252
prevention of, 328–329, 329t
clinical progress in 1999 and 2000, 343–344, 344t
estrogen-containing oral contraceptives and, 343
low-dose heparin in, 339
low-molecular-weight heparin in, 340
oral anticoagulants in, 340

Deep venous thrombosis (DVT) (*contd.*)
in surgical patients, 340–343, 342f
acute spinal cord injury associated with paralysis, 341
approaches to, 339–343, 342f
general surgery, 340
graduated compression stockings for, 340
gynecologic surgery, 341–343, 342f
HRT and, 343
intermittent pneumatic leg compression and, 340
neurosurgery, 340–341
optimization of, 344
orthopedic surgery, 341
pregnancy-related, 342–343, 342t
trauma-related, 341
pulmonary embolism in. *See* Pulmonary embolus (PE)
recurrence of
prevention of, cost reduction by, 328, 328t
treatment of, oral anticoagulants in, 352–353
risk factors for, 262t
in surgery and trauma, 329, 329t
"standards of care" for, 329, 329t
thrombolytic therapy for, clinical trials in, 409–410
treatment of, 333–339
ancillary measures in, 335–336
antiembolic arm exercises in, 336
antiembolic leg exercises in, 336
cost-effective, 333–334
costs of common antithrombotic drugs, 328, 328t
"early discharge," guidelines for, 366, 366t
inpatient, 334–335, 334t
low-molecular-weight heparin in, 334–335, 334t
outpatient/"early discharge," 335, 335t
in surgical patients, 336–339, 338f, 339f
after arthroscopic surgery, 337
after general surgery, 336
after hip fracture, 337
after neurosurgery, 337–339, 338f, 339f
after orthopedic surgery, 336–337
after total hip replacement, 336–337
after total knee replacement, 337
after trauma, 337
Degos disease, skin lesions of, 308
Desirudin, in acute myocardial infarction, clinical trials in, 408
Diabetes mellitus, 46t, 48–49
DIC. *See* Disseminated intravascular coagulation (DIC)
Dipyridamole
clinical trials of, results of, 389
for hereditary thrombophilic disorders, 287, 287t
in phosphodiesterase inhibition, 6, 8
platelet function inhibition by, 382
Disseminated intravascular coagulation (DIC), 139–164. *See also* Amniotic fluid embolism (AFE), syndrome of
acidosis in, 147
in burn victims, 147
in cardiac surgery, 195–196
cardiovascular diseases associated with, 147–148
causes of, 139–143, 140t, 141t, 142f, 143f, 146–147
clinical findings in, 149–150, 150t
defined, 140
described, 139
disorders associated with, 140t, 147–148
eclampsia in, 145, 145t
fibrinolysis in, 166
fulminant, 154–157, 155t
in gynecologic patients, 145–148, 148f
HELLP syndrome in, 145
hematologic disorders and, 147
HIV in, 146
kinin system in, activation of, 149
laboratory diagnosis of, 151–154, 154t
global coagulation tests in, 151–152
molecular markers in, 152–154, 154t
in leukemia, 268–270, 269t, 270t
in liver cirrhosis, 166
"low-grade," 157
malignancy-related, 146
diagnosis of, 270–271
treatment of, 271, 271t
morphologic findings in, 150–151
in obstetrics, 139–143, 140t, 141t, 142f, 143f
pathophysiology of, 139, 148–149
in placental abruption, 144
plasmin in, 149
platelet count in, 153
preeclampsia in, 145, 145t
in retained-fetus syndrome, 144
septicemia in, 146
signs and symptoms of, 149–150, 150t
in syndrome of amniotic fluid embolism, 139–143, 140t, 141t, 142f, 143f. *See also* Amniotic fluid embolism (AFE), syndrome of
management of, 144–148, 144t, 145t, 148f
systemic thrombin activity in, consequences of, 148–149
thrombocytopenia due to, 98–99, 99t
treatment of, 154–157, 155t
triggering mechanisms for, 148, 148f
vascular disorders associated with, 147
viremias associated with, 146
Diuretic(s), platelet dysfunction due to, 71t
Doppler ultrasonography
color, real-time B-mode with, in deep venous thrombosis evaluation, 256–257
in pulmonary embolus evaluation, 256
Drug(s)
effects on platelets, 100–101
marrow suppression with, 94–95, 93t, 94t
platelet dysfunction owing to, 69–70, 70t–79t, 75
with unknown mechanisms of action on platelet function, 69
vasculitis caused by, 40t, 46t, 50, 50t–52t
Duteplase, structure, function, and pharmacology of, 402
Dysfibrinogenemia, 118, 118t, 166
congenital, 290
Dysprothrombinemia, 119

E

ECG. *See* Electrocardiography (ECG)
Eclampsia, 48–49
DIC and, 145, 145t
Ehlers–Danlos syndrome, 40–41, 40t, 41t
Electrocardiography (ECG), in pulmonary embolus evaluation, 257
Endothelial sloughing, 2, 2f, 3f
and atheroma formation, 3f
Endothelium
with "gaps," 6, 6f
in hemostasis, 23
properties of, 1–2, 2t
Enoxiparin, characteristics of, 362t
Eosinophilia, heparin and, 373
Essential athrombia, 60t, 61, 61t
Estrogen(s), in oral contraceptives, deep venous thrombosis after, prevention of, 343
Exercise(s)
arm, antiembolic, for deep venous thrombosis, 336
leg, antiembolic, for deep venous thrombosis, 336
Extremity(ies), lower, deep venous thrombosis of, diagnosis of, 251, 252t

F

Factor(s). *See under* Coagulation factor
Fanconi syndrome, 92–93, 92t
Fibrin
conversion from fibrinogen, 184f
conversion of fibrinogen to, 14–15, 15f
formation of, 184, 184f, 185f
key reactions in, 185f
generation of, 14–15, 15f, 16f
Fibrin clot, formation of, reactions in, 10, 10t
Fibrin(ogen) degradation products, formation of, 17–18, 18f, 186, 186f
Fibrinogen, 290
conversion to fibrin, 14–15, 15f, 184f
defects of. *See* Fibrinogen defects
structure of, 16f
synthesis of, 117–118
Fibrinogen defects, 117–119, 117t, 118t
afibrinogenemia, 117t, 118–119, 118t
classification of, 118
hypofibrinogenemia, 117t, 118–119, 118t
qualitative, 118, 118t
quantitative, 118, 118t
Fibrinogen molecule, described, 117

Fibrinogenolysis, laboratory markers of, 397, 398t
Fibrinolysis
  and arterial disease, 428–429, 429f
  Hageman factor–dependent activation of, 15, 17, 17f
  impaired, acquired, 317–318
  in liver cirrhosis, 166
  pathways of, 398f
  primary, in cardiac surgery, 196–197
Fibrino(geno)lysis, primary, in solid tumors, 272
Fibrinolytic defects, thrombosis due to, 293–294
Fibrinolytic system, 15, 17–18, 17f, 18f
  defects of, acquired, 317–318
  in hemostasis, 184–186, 185f, 186f
  modulation of, 17
  physiologic activation pathways for, 15
  physiology of, 185f
Fibronectin, in hemostasis, 22–23, 189–190
Fletcher factor, 20
Fracture(s), hip, deep venous thrombosis after, treatment of, 337
Fragility, in hemostasis, 178

G

Giant cavernous hemangiomata, 40t, 44
Glanzmann thrombasthenia, 60t, 61, 61t
Global coagulation tests, in DIC, 151–152
Glomerulonephritis, 172
Glycoprotein(s), platelet membrane, 8, 9t, 182, 182t
Glycoprotein IIb/IIIa inhibitors
  effects of, monitoring of, clinical trials of, results of, 390
  interactions with anticoagulants and other antiplatelet agents, 390–391
  intravenous, clinical trials of, results of, 389
Glycoprotein IIb/IIIa–receptor antagonists
  clinical trials of, results of, 389–391, 390t
  oral, clinical trials of, results of, 389–390, 390t
  platelet function inhibition by, 382–383
Glycosaminoglycan(s), 360
Gray platelet syndrome, 93
Gynecologic surgery, deep venous thrombosis after, prevention of, 341–343, 342f
Gynecology, DIC syndromes unique to, 145–148, 148f

H

Hageman factor (factor XII), activation of, 10, 10f
Hageman factor (factor XII)–dependent activation of fibrinolysis, 15, 17, 17f
Hageman trait, 290
Heart valves, prosthetic, thrombohemorrhagic complications of, 203–204
HELLP (hemolysis, elevated liver enzymes, and low platelet) syndrome, DIC and, 145
Hematologic disorders, DIC and, 147
Hematoma(s), heparin and, 373–374
Hemolytic–uremic syndrome, 98–99, 99t
  age of onset of, 98
  clinical findings in, 98–99, 99t
  described, 98
  laboratory findings in, 99, 99t
  treatment of, 99
Hemophilia A, 121–123, 121t–123t
  acquired, 215–219, 217t
    bleeding episodes in, management of, 224–225
  alloantibodies against, 122
  aPTT in, 122
  assessment of, 122
  carrier status of, 123
  clinical manifestations of, 121–122, 121t, 122t
  coagulation factor VIII inhibitors in, acute bleeding in patients with, management of, 222t, 224
  described, 121
  diagnosis of, 122
  hallmark of, 122, 122t
  incidence of, 121
  severity of, 121–122, 121t
  treatment of, 122–123, 123t
  whole blood clotting time in, 122
Hemophilia B, 123–124, 124t
  clinical features of, 123–124, 124t
  factor IX inhibitors in, 228
  synonyms for, 123
  variants of, 124, 124t
Hemorrhage
  cardiopulmonary bypass
    diagnosis of, 198–199, 198t, 199t
    management of, 200
  clinical assessment of, 31–37
    family history in, 32–33
    laboratory testing in, 34–35
    patient history in, 31–33
    physical examination in, 33–34
  disorders related to, classification of, 36, 36t
  in leukemias, 267–268, 267t
  platelets and, 272–273
  in solid tumors, 269–270, 269t
Hemostasis
  anatomic compartments involved in, 177
  and bone marrow transplantation, 275
  during cardiac surgery, pathology of, 190–200
  cardiopulmonary bypass, pathophysiology of, 198, 198t
  chemotherapy effects on, 274–275
  coagulation protein system in, 182–184, 183t, 184f, 185f
  cohesion, 8
  complement activation and, 18–19, 19f, 186–187, 187t
  defects of
    in liver diseases, 165
    liver transplantation in, 168–169
    in renal diseases, 170–172, 170t, 171t
    screening tests for, 36–37, 37t
    vitamin K deficiency and, 169–170, 170t
  defined, 177
  disorders of, bleeding-associated, hereditary vs. acquired, 31
  fibrinolytic system in, 15, 17–18, 17f, 18f, 184–186, 185f, 186f
  inhibitor mechanisms in, 20–22, 21f, 21t, 22f, 22t
  inhibitor systems in, 187–189, 188t, 189f
  interactive components in, 22–24, 24t
  kinin(s) in, generation of, 187, 188f
  kinins and, 20, 20f, 21f
  in malignant paraprotein disorders, 273–274
  physiology of, 1–29, 177–190. *See also specific component, e.g.,* Platelet(s)
    understanding of, importance of, 1
  plasma protein functions in, 9–22, 182–190, 183t, 184f–189f, 188t
  platelet function in, 4–9, 4f–8f, 4t, 5t, 179–182, 179t, 180f, 181f, 182t
  screening tests for, 36, 36t
  vascular function in, 1–3, 2f, 2t, 3f, 177–178, 178f
Hemostasis system, compartments of, 1, 2f
Heparan sulfate anticoagulant, 237
Heparin, 359–377
  for acquired thrombophilia, 318t
  activities of, 360, 360t
  in acute myocardial infarction, clinical trials in, 407
  acute reaction to, 371
  alopecia due to, 373
  altered liver-function tests due to, 373
  anaphylaxis due to, 371
  bleeding due to, 371
  characteristics of, 359–367
  complications of, 371–374
  for DIC, 144
  dosing of, 364–365, 365t
  eosinophilia due to, 373
  for hereditary thrombophilic disorders, 286–288, 286t, 288t
  historical background of, 359
  hyperkalemia due to, 373
  hypoaldosteronism due to, 373
  low-dose, in thromboprophylaxis, 339
  low-molecular-weight, 359–377
    characteristics of, 362–363, 362t, 363t
    clinical acceptance of, impact of consensus conferences on, 343
    costs of, 328, 328t
    for deep venous thrombosis, 334–335, 334t
    differences among, 343–344
    dosing of, 365–366, 365t, 366t
    epidural bleeding due to, 373–374
    hematomas due to, 373–374
    laboratory monitoring of, 366–367
    mechanisms of action of, 363–364
    paralysis due to, 373–374
    side effects of, 367, 367t
    in thromboprophylaxis, 340

Heparin (*contd.*)
mechanisms of action of, 363–364
osteoporosis due to, 371–373
priapism due to, 373
"resistance" of, 363, 363t
side effects of, 367, 367t
skin reactions due to, 373
thrombocytopenia due to, 104–106, 104t, 105t, 367–371, 367t–369t, 371t. *See also* Thrombocytopenia, heparin-induced
for thrombosis/thromboembolism, 365, 365t
unfractionated
activities of, 360, 360t
bleeding due to, 360–361
characteristics of, 359–362, 360t, 362t
costs of, 328, 328t
described, 359
effects on template bleeding time, 360
laboratory monitoring of, 366–367
pharmacologic potency of, 359–360
reversal of, 360–361
Heparin cofactor II (HC–II), 292
deficiency of, acquired, 316–317
Heparin-like anticoagulant, 237
Hepatic venoocclusive disease, 275
Hereditary aspirin-like defects, 60t, 63–64, 63f, 63t
Hereditary coagulation protein defects, 117–137. *See also specific defect and* Coagulation factor disorders, hereditary
Hereditary hemorrhagic telangiectasia (HHT). *See* Osler–Weber–Rendu disease
Hereditary storage pool defect, 60t, 61–63, 62f, 62t
Hereditary thrombophilic disorders, 283–302. *See also* Thrombophilic disorders, hereditary
Hermansky–Pudlak syndrome, 61
High responders, defined, 215
Hip fracture, deep venous thrombosis after, treatment of, 337
Hip replacement
deep venous thrombosis after, prevention of, 341
total, deep venous thrombosis after, treatment of, 336–337
Hirudin, in acute myocardial infarction, clinical trials in, 407–408
HIV. *See* Human immunodeficiency virus (HIV)
Homocyst(e)inemia, 290–291
Homocystinurea, 40t, 43–44
Hormone-replacement therapy (HRT), deep venous thrombosis after, prevention of, 343
HRT. *See* Hormone-replacement therapy (HRT)
Human immunodeficiency virus (HIV), in DIC, 146
Hydralazine, in antiphospholipid thrombosis syndrome, 312t
Hydroxyurea, for primary thrombocythemia, 109–110
Hypercoagulability
causes of, 325
malignancy-related, 265–266, 266t
Hyperheparinemia, heparin and, 360–361
Hyperhomocystinemia, 43–44
in atherosclerosis, 426
Hyperkalemia, heparin and, 373
Hypersplenism
causes of, 97, 97t
thrombocytopenia in, 97, 97t
clinical features of, 97
laboratory features of, 97
Hypertension, malignant, 48–49
Hypoaldosteronism, heparin and, 373
Hypofibrinogenemia, 117t, 118–119, 118t
Hypoprothrombinemia, 119, 119t
Hypothermia, thrombocytopenia in, 97

I

Immune system, platelet destruction due to, thrombocytopenia resulting from, 101–106, 104t, 105t
Immune thrombocytopenic purpura (ITP), 101–106, 104t, 105t
acute, 101–102
chronic, 102–103
clinical findings in, 102
described, 102
presentation of, 102
treatment of, 102–103
platelet dysfunction in, 64t, 68, 68f
during pregnancy, 103
Immunoglobulin(s), 213. *See also* Blood coagulation inhibitors
for acquired coagulation factor VIII inhibitors, 224, 223t
Immunoglobulin-like proteins, in hemostasis, 23
Immunosuppressive therapy, for acquired coagulation factor VIII inhibitors, 223–224, 223t
Infection(s)
decreased platelet production and, 94t, 95–96, 95t
effects on platelets, 100–101
Inhibitor systems, 20–22, 21f, 21t, 22f, 22t
in hemostasis, 187–189, 188t, 189f
Integrin(s), in hemostasis, 23
Interferon-α
in antiphospholipid thrombosis syndrome, 312t
for primary thrombocythemia, 110
Intermittent leg compression, in thromboprophylaxis, 340
International normalized ratio testing, point-of-care, 355
Intraaortic balloon pump (IABP), thrombohemorrhagic complications of, 201–202
Intraplatelet biochemistry, 6, 7f, 180, 181f
Intrinsic activation, 11, 11f
Ischemic stroke, prevention of, in patients with atrial fibrillation, oral anticoagulants in, 353

K

Kaolin clotting time (KCT) test, in LA-thrombosis syndrome, 305
Kasabach–Merritt syndrome, 44, 147
Kinin(s), and coagulation, 20, 20f, 21f
Kinin generation, in hemostasis, 187, 188f
Kinin system, activation of, in DIC, 149
Kininogen defects, 127, 127t
Knee replacement, deep venous thrombosis after, prevention of, 341

L

Laënnec-type cirrhosis, in Osler–Weber–Rendu disease, 45
Lanoteplase
in acute myocardial infarction, clinical trials in, 407
clinical applications of, 411t
structure, function, and pharmacology of, 402, 403t
Leg compression, intermittent, in thromboprophylaxis, 340
Leg exercises, antiembolic, for deep venous thrombosis, 336
Lepirudin, in acute myocardial infarction, clinical trials in, 408
Leukemia(s)
acute, 267
acute granulocytic, 267
acute monocytic, 267
acute myelogenous, 267
acute myelomonocytic, 267
acute promyelocytic, 267
chronic myelogenous, 267–268
chronic myeloid, 267
defective hemostasis associated with, 269t
DIC in, 268–270, 269t, 270t
hemorrhage in, 267–268, 267t
thrombocytopenia in, mechanisms of, 267, 267t
Liver cirrhosis, 165–168, 165t, 167t
abnormal factor production in, 166
bleeding manifestations of, 165
fibrinolysis in, 166
impaired synthesis in, 166
increased factor consumption in, 166
laboratory tests in, 167, 167t
management of, 167–168
pathogenesis of, 165–166, 165t
portal vein thrombosis due to, 169
shunt placement in, 169
thrombocytopathy in, 167
thrombocytopenia in, 166–167
Liver diseases
hemostasis defects with, 165
mild to moderate, 168, 168t
platelet dysfunction in, 64t, 67–68
thrombohemorrhagic defects in, 165–170, 165t, 167t, 168t
Liver transplantation, hemostasis defects with, 168–169

Liver-function tests, altered, heparin and, 373
Low responders, defined, 215
Lower extremities, deep venous thrombosis of, diagnosis of, 251, 252t
Low-molecular-weight heparins (LMWHs). *See* Heparin, low-molecular-weight
Lupus anticoagulant(s)
detection of, 313–314
and thrombosis, 304–307. *See also* Lupus anticoagulant (LA)–thrombosis syndrome
Lupus anticoagulant (LA)–thrombosis syndrome, 304–307
clinical subclassification in, 306
described, 304
elevated ACLAs in, 305–306
kaolin clotting time test in, 305
prevalence of, 305
treatment of, 306–307
venous systems involved in, 305

M

Magnetic resonance imaging (MRI), in deep venous thrombosis evaluation, 257
Malignancy
acquired, von Willebrand disease–related, 268, 268t
issues related to, 231, 232t
catheter-related thrombosis in, 275–276, 276f, 277t
DIC in
diagnosis of, 270–271
leukemias, 268–270, 269t, 270t
treatment of, 271, 271t
hemorrhage in, thrombocytopenia and, 272–273
platelet-function defects related to, 273
solid tumors
hemorrhage associated with, 269–270, 269t
primary fibrino(geno)lysis in, 272
thrombohemorrhagic defects associated with, 265–282
thrombosis in, 265–266, 266t. *See also* Thrombosis, malignancy-related
underlying, in *de novo* thrombotic disease, 277–278, 278t
Malignant hypertension, 48–49
Malignant paraprotein disorders, 46t, 47–48
hemostasis in, 273–274
Marfan syndrome, 40t, 41–42, 42t
Marrow infiltrative disorders, 94, 94t
Maturation/metabolic defects, 94t, 96
May–Hegglin anomaly, 93
Megakaryocytic marrow aplasia, 94, 94t
Melphalan, hemostasis effects of, 275
Menaquinone(s), 349, 350f
Mitomycin, hemostasis effects of, 275
Molecular markers, in DIC, 152–154, 154t
Monocyte(s), in hemostasis, 23
MRI. *See* Magnetic resonance imaging (MRI)
Multiple myeloma, hemostasis in, 274
Mutation(s), prothrombin G20210A, 289–290
Myelodysplastic syndromes, platelet dysfunction in, 64t, 66
Myeloma, multiple, hemostasis in, 274
Myeloproliferative syndromes, 64t, 66, 315–318
acquired antithrombin deficiency, 316
acquired fibrinolytic system defects, 317–318
acquired heparin cofactor II deficiency, 316–317
acquired protein C deficiency, 317
acquired protein S deficiency, 317
Trousseau syndrome, 316
Myocardial infarction
acute, 283–284. *See also* Acute myocardial infarction (AMI)
aspirin in, clinical trials of, results of, 386, 387f
thrombolytic therapy for, 404–408, 404t, 405t

N

Neonate(s)
increased platelet destruction or consumption in, thrombocytopenia due to, 98
platelet-production defects in, thrombocytopenia due to, 92–93, 92t
Nephrotic syndrome, 172
Neurologic syndromes, anticardiolipins and, 309
Neurosurgery, deep venous thrombosis after
prevention of, 340–341
treatment of, 337–339, 338f, 339f
Neutrophil(s), in hemostasis, 23

O

Obstetric syndromes, anticardiolipins and, 309–310
Obstetrical accidents, DIC in, 139–143, 140t, 141t, 142f, 143f
Oral contraceptives, estrogen-containing, deep venous thrombosis after, prevention of, 343
Orthopedic surgery, deep venous thrombosis after, prevention of, 341
Osler–Weber–Rendu disease, 39–40, 40t, 44–46, 46t
characteristics of, 45, 46t
described, 44–45
family history of, 44
incidence of, 44
laboratory findings in, 45
Laënnec-type cirrhosis in, 45
telangiectatic lesions of, 45
treatment of, 45–46
Osteogenesis imperfecta, 40t, 42, 42t
Osteoporosis, heparin and, 371–373

P

PAI-1. *See* Plasminogen activator inhibitor-1 (PAI-1)
PAOD. *See* Peripheral arterial occlusive disease (PAOD)
Papaverine, in phosphodiesterase inhibition, 6
Paralysis
acute spinal cord injury associated with, deep venous thrombosis after, prevention of, 341
heparin and, 373–374
Paraprotein disorders
malignant, 46t, 47–48
hemostasis in, 273–274
platelet dysfunction in, 64, 64t, 65f
Paroxysmal nocturnal hemoglobinemia (PNH), thrombocytopenia and, 96
Passovoy deficiency, 133
Percutaneous transluminal angioplasty (PTA), reocclusions after, prevention of, aspirin in, 383, 385, 385t
Peripheral arterial occlusive disease (PAOD)
aspirin in, clinical trials of, results of, 383
occlusions in, prevention of, aspirin in, 385–386, 385t
vascular risk associated with, 386
Peripheral arterial thrombosis, thrombolytic therapy for, clinical trials in, 410
Permeability, in hemostasis, 178
Phenothiazines, in antiphospholipid thrombosis syndrome, 312t
Phenytoin, in antiphospholipid thrombosis syndrome, 312t
Phosphodiesterase
inhibition of, 6, 8
in platelet function, 180
Phosphodiesterase inhibitors
clinical trials of, results of, 389
platelet function inhibition by, 382
Phospholipase A_2, in platelet function, 180–181
Phylloquinone(s), 349, 350f
Placental abruption, DIC in, 144
Plasma protein, functions of, 9–22, 9t
coagulation protein system in, 9–15, 9t, 10f, 10t, 11f–16f, 14t
in hemostasis, 182–190, 183t, 184f–189f, 188t
Plasma thromboplastin antecedent (PTA). *See* Coagulation factor XI
Plasma thromboplastin component (PTC), 123–124, 124t
Plasmin, in DIC, 149
Plasminogen activator(s), mechanism of action of, 397
Plasminogen activator inhibitor defects, 128, 128t
Plasminogen activator inhibitor-1 (PAI-1), in atherosclerosis, 428–429, 429f
Platelet(s)
activation of, 379
assessment of, methods in, 9
adhesion, 8
bleeding associated with, 272–273
compounds released from, 5, 5t
consumption of. *See* Platelet consumption

Platelet(s) (*contd.*)
  decreased production of, thrombocytopenia due to, 92–97
  drugs toxic to, 100–101
  endothelial gaps filled by, 177, 178f
  filling endothelial gaps, 3f
  functions of, 4–9, 4f–8f, 4t, 5t
    in hemostasis, 179–182, 179t, 180f, 181f, 182t
    normal, factors necessary for, 4, 4t
    prostaglandins in, 8, 8f
    summary of, 6, 7f
  in hemostasis, 23
  hyperactive "prethrombotic," 70–71, 80–82, 80t, 81t
  infections toxic to, 100–101
  moderately activated, 5–6, 5f
  morphology of, 4, 4t
Platelet consumption, increased
  acquired, thrombocytopenia due to, 98–101, 99t, 100t
  cardiovascular diseases and, thrombocytopenia due to, 101
  neonatal, thrombocytopenia due to, 98
Platelet count
  during cardiopulmonary bypass surgery, 192, 192f
  in DIC, 153
Platelet defects. *See also* Platelet-function defects
  clinical findings of, 59, 59t
  quantitative, 91–92
  types of, 59–60, 59t, 60t
Platelet destruction
  immune-induced, thrombocytopenia due to, 101–106, 104t, 105t
  increased
    cardiovascular diseases and, thrombocytopenia due to, 101
    neonatal, thrombocytopenia due to, 98
    thrombocytopenia due to, 98–101, 99t, 100t
Platelet distribution, altered, thrombocytopenia secondary to, 97–98, 97t
Platelet factors, 5, 5t
  named, 179, 179t
Platelet function
  drugs with unknown mechanisms of action on, 69
  laboratory evaluation of, 59, 60t, 82–84, 82t, 83f
Platelet hyperactivity, evaluation of, 81–82
Platelet lumi-aggregation patterns, normal, 82–83, 83f
Platelet membrane glycoproteins (PMGPs), 8, 9t, 182, 182t
Platelet membrane phospholipid (platelet factor 3) selectivity, in procoagulant activity, 14, 14t
Platelet membrane receptors, drugs interfering with, 69
Platelet open canalicular system, transmission electron micrograph of, 4, 4f
Platelet phosphodiesterase activity, drugs inhibiting, 69
Platelet proteins, 4–5, 5t
  in hemostasis, 179, 179t
Platelet-aggregation patterns, normal, 82–83, 83f
Platelet-function defects, 59–90. *See also* Platelet defects
  acquired, 64–68, 64t, 65f–67f
    cardiopulmonary bypass–related, 64t, 66–67, 66f, 67f
    liver disease–related, 64t, 67–68
    myelodysplastic syndromes, 64t, 66
    myeloproliferative syndromes, 64t, 66
    paraprotein disorders, 64, 64t, 65f
    uremia, 64, 64t, 65f
  in cardiac surgery, 193–195, 194f
  drug-induced, 69–70, 70t–79t, 75
    classification of drugs, 69–70, 70t–79t
  hereditary, 60–64, 60t–63t, 62f, 63f
    Bernard–Soulier syndrome, 60t, 61, 61t, 84
    Glanzmann thrombasthenia, 60t, 61, 61t
    hereditary aspirin-like defects, 60t, 63–64, 63f, 63t
    hereditary storage pool defect, 60t, 61–63, 62f, 62t
  hyperactive platelets, 70–71, 80–82, 80t, 81t
  laboratory evaluation of, 82–84, 82t, 83f
  malignancy-related, 273
  miscellaneous disorders and, 64t, 68–82, 68f, 70t–81t
Platelet-function inhibitors
  pharmacology of, 379–383, 380f, 381f
    aspirin, 379–381
    cilostazol, 382
    dipyridamole, 382
    glycoprotein IIb/IIIa–receptor antagonists, 382–383
    phosphodiesterase inhibitors, 382
    prostaglandins, 382
    thromboxane-receptor antagonists, 382
    ticlopidine/clopidogrel, 381–382
  in prevention of venous thromboses and pulmonary embolism, 391
Platelet-production defects
  acquired, 93–97, 94t, 95t
    thrombocytopenia due to, 93–97, 94t, 95t
  congenital, thrombocytopenia due to, 92–93, 92t
  infections associated with, 94t, 95–96, 95t
  neonatal, thrombocytopenia due to, 92–93, 92t
  renal failure due to, 96
PMGPs. *See* Platelet membrane glycoproteins (PMGPs)
Polymerization I, 15, 16f
Polymerization II, 15, 16f
Portal vein thrombosis, liver cirrhosis and, 169
Posttransfusion purpura, 106
Prednisolone, for acquired coagulation factor VIII inhibitors, 223, 223t
Preeclampsia, DIC and, 145, 145t
Pregnancy
  deep venous thrombosis after, prevention of, 342–343, 342t
  DIC in, 139–143, 140t, 141t, 142f, 143f
  factor VIII inhibitors associated with, 219–220
  immune thrombocytopenic purpura during, 103
Prekallikrein, 20
Prekallikrein defects, 127, 127t
Priapism, heparin and, 373
Primary fibrino(geno)lysis, in solid tumors, 272
Primary phospholipid syndrome, anticardiolipins and, 309
Procainamide, in antiphospholipid thrombosis syndrome, 312t
Procoagulant reactions, 10, 10t
Proconvertin deficiency, 120–121, 120t, 121t
Prostacyclin, in adenylate cyclase stimulation, 8
Prostaglandin(s)
  in platelet function, 180–181, 181f
  platelet function inhibition by, 382
  in platelet/endothelial function, 8, 8f
Prostaglandin pathways, drug inhibition of, 69
Prostate cancer, thrombosis in, 266
Prosthetic devices, thrombohemorrhagic complications of, 200–204
Prosthetic heart valves, thrombohemorrhagic complications of, 203–204
Protamine sulfate, in heparin reversal, 360–361
Protein(s)
  hereditary defects of, 117–137. *See also specific defect and* Coagulation factor disorders, hereditary
  immunoglobulin-like, in hemostasis, 23
  plasma, functions of
    coagulation protein system in, 9–15, 9t, 10f, 10t, 11f–16f, 14t
    in hemostasis, 182–190, 183t, 184f–189f, 188t
  platelet, 4–5, 5t
    in hemostasis, 179, 179t
Protein C
  activity of, 188, 189f
  antibodies of, 238
  functions of, 22, 22f, 22t
  inhibitors of, 238
Protein C deficiency, 292
  acquired, 317
Protein C system, in atherosclerosis, 422–425
Protein S
  activity of, 188, 189f
  functions of, 22, 22f, 22t
Protein S deficiency, 293
  acquired, 317

Proteoglycan(s), in hemostasis, 23
Prothrombin
antibodies to, 237–238
defects of, 119, 119t
inhibitors for, 237–238
Prothrombin complex concentrates, in factor VIII inhibitor management, 220–223, 222t
Prothrombin G20210A mutation, 289–290
Pseudothrombocytopenia, 92
Pseudothrombocytosis, 107
Pseudo–von Willebrand disease, 133
Pseudoxanthoma elasticum, 40t, 42–43, 43t
Psychiatric drugs, platelet dysfunction owing to, 71t
Pulmonary angiography, in pulmonary embolus evaluation, 258
Pulmonary embolism. *See* Pulmonary embolus (PE)
Pulmonary embolus (PE), 251–264, 283. *See also* Deep venous thrombosis (DVT)
causes of, 251–252
diagnosis of, 251
ABG analysis in, 257
chest radiography in, 255–256, 257
Doppler ultrasonography in, 256
ECG in, 257
laboratory studies in, 258–259
patient history in, 252–253, 259f, 260f
physical examination in, 253–256, 259f, 260f
pulmonary angiography in, 258
SCTA in, 258
V/Q match in, 257–258
fatal, prevention of, 344
incidence of, 283, 325, 326t
mortality rates in, 251
presentation of, 252
prevention of, platelet-function inhibitors in, 391
risk factors for, 262t
symptoms of, 251
thrombolytic therapy for, clinical trials in, 409
treatment of, 333–339
cost-effective, 333–334
inpatient, 334–335, 334t
outpatient/"early discharge," 335, 335t
Purpura, posttransfusion, 106

Q
Quinidine, in antiphospholipid thrombosis syndrome, 312t
Quinine, in antiphospholipid thrombosis syndrome, 312t

R
Radiography, chest, in pulmonary embolus evaluation, 255–256, 257
"Reactive" thrombocytosis, 108–109
Real-time B-mode compression ultrasound (CUS), in deep venous thrombosis evaluation, 256
Real-time B-mode ultrasound with color Doppler, in deep venous thrombosis evaluation, 256–257
Recurrent miscarriage syndrome, 284
Renal diseases
hemostasis defects with, 170–172, 170t, 171t
thrombohemorrhagic defects in, 170–172, 170t, 171t
chronic renal failure, 170–171, 170t, 171t
uremia, 170–171, 170t, 171t
Renal failure
chronic. *See* Chronic renal failure
platelet-production defects and, 96
Responder(s)
high, defined, 215
low, defined, 215
Retained-fetus syndrome, DIC in, 144
Reteplase
in acute myocardial infarction, 404t
clinical trials in, 406
clinical applications of, 411t
structure, function, and pharmacology of, 402, 403t
RMS
APLAs in, incidence of, 310
characteristics of, 309
treatment of, 309–310

S
Saruplase
in acute myocardial infarction, clinical trials in, 407
structure, function, and pharmacology of, 401
SCTA. *See* Spiral computed tomographic angiography (SCTA)
Selectin(s), in hemostasis, 23
Septicemia, in DIC, 146
Skin reactions, heparin-related, 373
SLE. *See* Systemic lupus erythematosus (SLE)
Sloughing, endothelial, and atheroma formation, 3f
Sneddon syndrome, 308
Spinal cord injury, acute, paralysis associated with, deep venous thrombosis after, prevention of, 341
Spiral computed tomographic angiography (SCTA), in pulmonary embolus evaluation, 258
Splenectomy, for chronic immune thrombocytopenic purpura, 103
Splenomegaly, congestive. *See* Hypersplenism
Staphylokinase
in acute myocardial infarction, clinical trials in, 407
structure, function, and pharmacology of, 402–403
Sticky platelet syndrome (SPS), 70, 75, 80, 80t, 294–295
described, 70
diagnostic criteria for, 80, 80t
normal ranges for, 75, 80, 80t
prevalence of, 70, 75
in thrombosis, incidence of, 80, 80t
Stoichiometry, in coagulation reactions, 13–14, 13f
Streptokinase
in acute myocardial infarction, 404t
clinical trials in, 405
clinical applications of, 411t
structure, function, and pharmacology of, 399, 403t
Stroke
acute, thromboprophylaxis in, 331–332
childhood, 422, 422t
ischemic, prevention of, in patients with atrial fibrillation, oral anticoagulants in, 353
Subendothelium, properties of, 1, 2t
Sulfadoxine and pyrimethamine, in antiphospholipid thrombosis syndrome, 312t
Swedish Ticlopidine Multicenter Study (STIMS), 388
Systemic lupus erythematosus (SLE), thromboembolism in, 304
Systemic thrombin activity, in DIC, consequences of, 148–149

T
TAR syndrome, 61
TAR-baby syndrome, 92–93
Template bleeding time (TBT)
in hemorrhage assessment, 34–35
heparin effects on, 360
prolongation of, in vascular disorder assessment, 39
Tenectoplase
in acute myocardial infarction, 404t
clinical trials in, 406–407
clinical applications of, 411t
structure, function, and pharmacology of, 402, 403t
Thrombasthenia, Glanzmann, 60t, 61, 61t
Thrombin
bovine, factor V inhibitors related to, 235–236
formation of, 184
generation of, 12–14, 12f–14f, 14t
Thrombin-activated fibrinolysis inhibitor (TAFI), in atherosclerosis, 427–428
Thrombin-activated fibrinolysis inhibitor (TAFI) production, in atherosclerosis, 423
Thrombocythemia, 106–110, 108t
clinical features of, 91
defined, 106–107
essential. *See* Thrombocythemia, primary (essential)
laboratory assessment of, 91–92
primary (essential), 107–110, 108t
age as factor in, 109
described, 107
diagnostic criteria for, 108, 108t
differential diagnosis of, 108
endovascular changes in, 109

Platelet(s) (*contd.*)
laboratory features of, 108
obstetric complications in, 109
pathophysiology of, 109
presentation of, 107–108
treatment of, 109
Thrombocythemia vera. *See* Thrombocythemia, primary (essential)
Thrombocytopathy, in liver cirrhosis, 167
Thrombocytopenia
altered platelet distribution and, 97–98, 97t
with antineoplastic therapy, intensity of, 95, 95t
in cardiac surgery, 191–193, 192f
clinical features of, 91
congenital, maternal disorders and, 93
cyclic, 94t, 95
decreased platelet production and, 92–97, 92t, 94t, 95t
acquired, 93–97, 94t, 95t
congenital, 92–93, 92t
neonatal, 92–93, 92t
DIC and, 98–99, 99t
dilutional, 92
drug-induced, 103–106, 104t, 105t
hemorrhage associated with, malignancy-related, 272–273
hemorrhage in leukemias due to, 267, 267t
heparin-induced, 104–106, 104t, 105t, 367–371, 367t–369t, 371t. *See also* Heparin, thrombocytopenia due to
causes of, 104
clinical features of, 368–369, 369t
clinical forms of, 367–368, 367t
comorbid diseases associated with, 106
historical background of, 367
incidence of, 106
treatment of, 106, 370, 371t
type I, 367–368, 367t
type II, 369–370, 369t
immune-mediated, 103–106, 104t, 105t
increased platelet consumption or destruction and, 98–110
laboratory assessment of, 91–92
in liver cirrhosis, 166–167
marrow suppression with drugs and, 94–95, 93t, 94t
in paroxysmal nocturnal hemoglobinemia, 96
treatment of, general issues in, 96–97
Thrombocytopenia absent radii syndrome (TAR syndrome), 61
Thrombocytosis, 106–110, 107t
clinical features of, 91
defined, 106
described, 107, 107t
laboratory assessment of, 91–92
"reactive," 108–109
Thromboembolism
in SLE, 304
treatment of, heparin in, 365, 365t
venous, 329–333. *See also* Venous thromboembolism
Thromboembolus, clinical approach to, 251–264. *See also* Deep venous thrombosis (DVT)
Thrombohemorrhagic defects
in liver and renal diseases, 165–175. *See also* Renal diseases, thrombohemorrhagic defects in
malignancy-related, 265–282
Thrombolysis
factor XIII and, 429, 429f
laboratory markers of, 397, 398t
Thrombolytic therapy, 397–419. *See also specific agents, e.g.*, Streptokinase
for acute myocardial infarction, 397, 404, 404t
adjunctive agents in, clinical trials in, 407
adjunctive therapy to, 404, 405t
agents in, 399–403, 403t
alteplase in
in acute myocardial infarction, 404t, 405–406
clinical applications of, 411t
anistreplase in, 399–400, 403t, 404t
clinical applications of, 411t
antiplatelet therapy in. *See* Antiplatelet therapy
antithrombin therapy in, clinical trials in, 407–408
for cerebrovascular thrombosis, clinical trials in, 408–409
chimeric agents in, 403
clinical applications of, 411t
clinical uses of, 403–410, 404t, 405t
complications of, 410–412, 411t, 412t
contraindications to, 411t
for deep venous thrombosis, clinical trials in, 409–410
desirudin in, clinical trials in, 408
duteplase in, 402
effectiveness of, thrombus characteristics in, 399
goal of, 397
heparin in. *See* Heparin
hirudin in, clinical trials in, 407–408
"ideal" agent, 404t
indications for, 397
lanetoplase in, 402, 403t
lanoteplase in
in acute myocardial infarction, 407
clinical applications of, 411t
lepirudin in, clinical trials in, 408
in myocardial infarction, 404–408, 404t, 405t
for peripheral arterial thrombosis, clinical trials in, 410
procoagulant effect of, 403–404
for pulmonary embolism, clinical trials in, 409
reteplase in, 402, 403t
in acute myocardial infarction, 404t, 406
clinical applications of, 411t
role of, overview of, 397–399, 398f, 398t
saruplase in, 401
in acute myocardial infarction, 407
staphylokinase in, 402–403
in acute myocardial infarction, 407
streptokinase in, 399, 403t
in acute myocardial infarction, 404t, 405
clinical applications of, 411t
structural characteristics of, 403t
tenectoplase in
in acute myocardial infarction, 404t, 406–407
clinical applications of, 411t
t-PA in. *See* Tissue plasminogen activator (t-PA)
urokinase in, 400–401, 403t
clinical applications of, 411t
for venous thromboembolism, clinical trials in, 409
Thrombomodulin, 2
Thrombophilia
acquired, 303–324. *See also* Antiphospholipid syndromes
treatment of, 318, 318t
vs. hereditary thrombophilia, 303, 303t
defined, 303
hereditary, *vs.* acquired thrombophilia, 303, 303t
hereditary platelet defects and, 294–295, 295t
Thrombophilic disorders, hereditary, 283–302. *See also specific disorder*
antithrombin deficiency, 291–292
cerebrovascular thrombosis, 284
coronary artery thrombosis, 283–284
deep venous thrombosis, 283
dysfibrinogenemia, 290
factor V Cambridge, 289
factor V Hong Kong, 289
factor V HR2 haplotype, 289
factor V Leiden, 288–289
factor XII, 290
fibrinolytic defects, 293–294
heparin cofactor II, 292
homocyst(e)inemia, 290–291
platelet defects, 294–295, 295t
protein C deficiency, 292
protein S deficiency, 293
prothrombin G20210A mutation, 289–290
pulmonary embolus, 283
recurrent miscarriage syndrome, 284
sticky platelet syndrome, 294–295
treatment of
anticoagulants in, 286–288, 286t, 288t
antiplatelet agents in, 287, 287t
pharmacologic, 286–288, 286t–288t
types of, 285, 285t
Wein–Penzing defect, 294
Thrombopoietin (TPO), for chronic immune thrombocytopenic purpura, 103
Thrombopoietin (TPO) serum levels, in thrombocytopenia assessment, 91
Thromboprophylaxis, approaches to, 339–343, 342f. *See also* Deep venous thrombosis (DVT), prevention of
Thrombosis, 325–348. *See also* Deep venous thrombosis (DVT)

ACLA-related, 310–311, 311t, 312t
anticardiolipin antibodies and, 307–310
arterial, risk factors for, 262t
blood protein/platelet defects and, 326, 327t
catheter-related, in malignancy, 275–276, 276f, 277t
causes of, 283, 284–286, 284t, 325, 326, 326t, 327t
cerebrovascular
incidence of, 284
thrombolytic therapy for, clinical trials in, 408–409
clinical approach to, 251–264. *See also* Deep venous thrombosis (DVT)
coronary artery, 283–284
incidence of, 283
mortality rates in, 283
costs related to, 326, 326t
containment of, 326–327, 327t
factor IX and, 428
factor XI and, 427
fibrinolytic defects and, 293–294
hypercoagulability and, 265–266, 266t
incidence of, 284, 285t, 325, 326t
laboratory markers of, 397, 398t
lupus anticoagulants and, 304–307. *See also* Lupus anticoagulant (LA)–thrombosis syndrome
malignancy-related, 265–266, 266t
hemorrhage, 267–268, 267t
leukemias, 267–268, 267t
management of, 266–267
pathophysiology of, 265–266, 266t
morbidity associated with, 325
mortality due to, 283, 325
pathways of, 398f
peripheral arterial, thrombolytic therapy for, clinical trials in, 410
of portal circulation, 169
portal vein, liver cirrhosis and, 169
prevention of, platelet-function inhibitors in, 391
sticky platelet syndrome in, incidence of, 80, 80t
"subgroup" antibodies and, 307–310
treatment of, heparin in, 365, 365t
venous–arterial, anticardiolipins and, 308
Thrombotic thrombocytopenia purpura (TTP), 99–100, 100t
Thrombotic–thromboembolic disease, underlying malignancy in, 277–278, 278t
Thromboxane A_2
in adenylate cyclase inhibition, 8
in platelet function, 181
Thromboxane-receptor antagonists, platelet function inhibition by, 382
Thrombus, characteristics of, in determination of effectiveness of thrombolytic therapy, 399
Ticlopidine
clinical trials of, results of, 388–389
for hereditary thrombophilic disorders, 287, 287t
side effects of, 389
Ticlopidine/clopidogrel, platelet function inhibition by, 381–382
Tinzaparin, characteristics of, 362t
Tissue factor, 11
and tissue factor pathway inhibitor, 11–12, 12f
Tissue factor activity (TFa), and arterial disease, 425–426
Tissue factor pathway inhibitor (TFPI), 11–12, 12f
in atherosclerosis, 426–427
Tissue plasminogen, variants of, 402–403, 403t
Tissue plasminogen activator (t-PA)
for partial thrombotic occlusion of central venous catheter, 276, 276f
for total thrombotic occlusion of central venous catheter, 276, 277f
Tissue-type plasminogen activator (t-PA), structure, function, and pharmacology of, 401–402, 403t
TNKt-PA. *See* Tenectoplase
Total hip replacement, deep venous thrombosis after, treatment of, 336–337
Total knee replacement, deep venous thrombosis after, treatment of, 337
t-PA. *See* Tissue-type plasminogen activator (t-PA)
Transient ischemic attacks (TIAs), drug-induced, 80–81, 80t
Transplantation
bone marrow, hemostasis and, 275
liver, hemostasis defects with, 168–169
Trauma, deep venous thrombosis after
prevention of, 341
treatment of, 337
Trousseau syndrome, 316
Tumor(s), solid
hemorrhage associated with, 269–270, 269t
primary fibrino(geno)lysis in, 272

U

Ultrasonography
compression, real-time B-mode, in deep venous thrombosis evaluation, 256
Doppler
color, real-time B-mode with, in deep venous thrombosis evaluation, 256–257
in pulmonary embolus evaluation, 256
Uremia
chronic renal failure and, 171, 171t
hemostasis defects with, 170–171, 170t, 171t
management of, 171–172
platelet dysfunction in, 64, 64t, 65f
Urokinase
clinical applications of, 411t
structure, function, and pharmacology of, 400–401, 403t

V

Vascular damage, consequences of, 3f
Vascular disorders
acquired, 40t, 46–50, 46t, 49t–52t
amyloidosis, 40t, 46t, 47–48
autoimmune disorders, 40t, 46t, 48, 49t
Behçet syndrome, 49–50
cardiopulmonary bypass–related, 50
described, 40
diabetes mellitus, 46t, 48–49
drug-induced vasculitis, 40t, 46t, 50, 50t–52t
eclampsia, 48–49
immune-associated, 40t, 46t, 48–49
malignant hypertension, 48–49
malignant paraprotein disorders, 46t, 47–48
mechanisms of, 46, 46t
types of, 40t, 46, 46t
causes of, 40, 40t
classification of, 39, 40t
clinical findings in, 39, 39t
determinants of, 40, 40t
DIC associated with, 147
hereditary, 40–46, 40t–43t, 46t
Ehlers–Danlos syndrome, 40–41, 40t, 41t
giant cavernous hemangiomata, 40t, 44
homocystinurea, 40t, 43–44
hyperhomocystinemia, 43–44
Kasabach–Merritt syndrome, 44
Marfan syndrome, 40t, 41–42, 42t
Osler–Weber–Rendu disease, 40t, 44–46, 46t
osteogenesis imperfecta, 40t, 42, 42t
pseudoxanthoma elasticum, 40t, 42–43, 43t
types of, 40t
immune-associated, 48, 49t
immune-mediated disorders associated with, 48, 49t
laboratory findings in, 50, 53, 53t
presentation of, 39
thrombohemorrhagic, 39–58
Vascular function, in hemostasis, 177–178, 178f
Vascular permeability, 1
Vascular shunts, thrombohemorrhagic complications of, 202–203
Vascular surgery, aspirin after, clinical trials of, results of, 383, 384t
Vascular system, function of, 1–3, 2f, 2t, 3f
Vasculature
disorders of. *See* Vascular disorders
properties of, 1, 2t
Vasculitis, infectious agents associated with, 48, 49t
Vasoconstriction, 1, 2t
in hemostasis, 178
Venography, contrast, ascending, in deep venous thrombosis evaluation, 257
Venoocclusive disease, hepatic, 275
Venous catheters, thrombohemorrhagic complications of, 201

Venous thromboembolism, 329–333, 329t, 330t, 333f. *See also* Deep venous thrombosis (DVT)
  in medical patients
    prevention of, 330–333, 333f
    risk factors for, 330–333, 333f
  prevention of, oral anticoagulants in, 353
  risk assessment for, improvements in, 344
  risk factors for, 329–330, 329t, 330t
    assessment guidelines for, 333f
  in surgical patients
    prevention of, 330–332, 333f
    risk factors for, 329t, 330, 330t
  thrombolytic therapy for, clinical trials in, 409
  treatment of, long-term, oral anticoagulants in, 352
Venous–arterial thrombosis, anticardiolipins and, 308
Ventilation/perfusion lung scan, in pulmonary embolus evaluation, 257–258
Vinblastine, hemostasis effects of, 275
Vincristine, hemostasis effects of, 275
Viremia(s), in DIC, 146
Vitamin K
  absence of, proteins induced by, 14, 14f
  forms of, 349–350, 350f
  function of, 349
Vitamin K cycle, 349–350, 350f
Vitamin K deficiency, hemostasis defects with, 169–170, 170t
Vitamin K1, as antidote to vitamin K antagonists, 355
Vitamin K–dependent coagulation factors, 14, 14f
von Willebrand antigen, 1
von Willebrand disease, 129–133, 130t, 131t, 228–234
  acquired
    antibody-induced, 230
    causes of, 229–230
    diagnosis of, 231–233
    disorders associated with, 231, 232t
    malignancies associated with, 268, 268t
      issues related to, 231, 232t
    management of, 233–234
    non–antibody-induced, 230–231
  assessment of, 130–131
  clinical presentation of, 130, 131t
  defined, 228
  described, 129, 130, 228–229
  diagnosis of, 129
  forms of, 130–133, 131t
  incidence of, 129
  type 1, 131–132, 131t
  type 2, 131t, 132
  type 3, 131t, 133
von Willebrand factor (vWF), 1
  in thrombotic thrombocytopenia purpura, 99–100
von Willebrand factor (vWF) replacement therapy, 233
V/Q. *See* Ventilation/perfusion lung scan

W

Warfarin
  for acquired thrombophilia, 318t
  anticoagulant effect of, 351
  for cardiovascular disorders, 353–355
  costs of, 328, 328t
  for hereditary thrombophilic disorders, 286–288, 286t, 288t
  laboratory monitoring with, 351–352
  pharmacodynamics of, 350–351
  pharmacokinetics of, 350–351
  pharmacology of, 349–352
  therapeutic range of, 351–352
  for thrombosis in malignancy, 266–267
Weibel–Palade bodies, 1–2
Wein–Penzing defect, 70, 294
Westermark sign, 255
Win Rho SDF, for chronic immune thrombocytopenic purpura, 103
Wiskott–Aldrich syndrome, 61, 93